Refractive Eye Surgery, Second Edition

List of Contributors

LASIK section:
Howard N. Straub, DO
Director, Colorado Eye Institute
Past president American Academy of Osteopathic Ophthalmology.
Author's first refractive surgery fellow and co-instructor for a series of courses on radial keratotomy and keratomileusis.

ICRS (Intacs):
Daniel S. Durrie, MD
Assistant Clinical Professor of Ophthalmology
Kansas University Medical Center
Kansas City, KS
&
Director of Refractive Services
Hunkeler Eye Centers
Kansas City, MO and Overland Park, KS

Scleral reinforcement:
Frank B. Thompson, MD
[retired]

Scleral expansion hyperopia:
Ronald Schachar, PhD, MD
Spencer Thornton, MD

Topography:
Terry E. Burris, M.D.
&
Debby Holmes-Higgin, M.S., M.P.H.
Corneal Topography Research Center
Northwest Corneal Services
Portland, OR 97225

Thomas A. Silvestrini, MS
Kera Vision, Inc.
Fremont, CA

Phillip C. Baker, MS
Baker Consulting
Walnut Grove, CA

Complications of refractive eye surgery:
Eric J. Linebarger, MD
Assistant Clinical Professor of Ophthalmology
University of California San Diego
Shiley Eye Center
La Jolla, CA; Director of Cornea and Refractive Surgery
Sharp Rees-Stealy Medical Group
San Diego, CA

Alexander Hatsis, MD, FACS
Director of Refractive Surgery
Nassau County Medical Center
East Meadow, NY

Stephen D. McLeod, M.D.
Assistant Clinical Professor of Ophthalmology
Co-Director, Refractive Surgery Service
University of California San Francisco
Department of Ophthalmology
San Francisco, CA 94143-0730

Others delineated within the text

Refractive Eye Surgery, Second Edition

Leo D. Bores MD
MEDICAL RESEARCH DIRECTOR
OPHTHALMIC INTERNATIONAL, INC.
FOUNTAIN HILLS, ARIZONA

WITH A CONTRIBUTION BY
Richard D. Smith MD

FOREWORD BY
José I. Barraquer

b

Editorial Offices:
Commerce Place, 350 Main Street, Malden, Massachusetts 02148, USA
Osney Mead, Oxford OX2 0EL, England
25 John Street, London WC1N 2BL, England
23 Ainslie Place, Edinburgh EH3 6AJ, Scotland
54 University Street, Carlton, Victoria 3053, Australia
Other Editorial Offices:
Blackwell Wissenschafts-Verlag GmbH, Kurfürstendamm 57, 10707 Berlin, Germany
Blackwell Science KK, MG Kodenmacho Building, 7-10 Kodenmacho Nihombashi, Chuo-ku, Tokyo 104, Japan

Distributors:
USA
Blackwell Science, Inc.
Commerce Place
350 Main Street
Malden, Massachusetts 02148
(Telephone orders: 800-215-1000 or 781-388-8250; fax orders: 781-388-8270)

Canada
Login Brothers Book Company
324 Saulteaux Crescent
Winnipeg, Manitoba R3J 3T2
(Telephone orders: 204-837-2987)

Australia
Blackwell Science Pty, Ltd.
54 University Street
Carlton, Victoria 3053
(Telephone orders: 03-9347-0300;
fax orders: 03-9349-3016)

Outside North America and Australia
Blackwell Science, Ltd.
c/o Marston Book Services, Ltd.
P.O. Box 269
Abingdon
Oxon OX14 4YN
England
(Telephone orders: 44-01235-465500;
fax orders: 44-01235-465555)

Acquisitions: Chris Davis
Development: Julia Casson
Production: Textbook Writers Associates
Manufacturing: Lisa Flanagan
Marketing Manager: Anne Stone
Cover design by ColourMark
Typeset by Circle Graphics
Printed and bound by Walsworth Publishing Company

Printed in the United States of America
00 01 02 03 5 4 3 2 1

Library of Congress Cataloging-in-Publication Data

Bores, Leo D.
Refractive eye surgery / by Leo D. Bores.—2nd ed.
p. ; cm.
Includes bibliographical references and index.
ISBN 0-632-04364-4
1. Refractive keratoplasty. I. Title.
[DNLM: 1. Refractive Errors–surgery. 2. Cornea–surgery. 3. Keratotomy, Radial.
WW 300 B731r2001]
RE336 .B67 2001
617.7'1—dc21

00-056420

This textbook is respectfully dedicated to a dear friend and colleague –
Svatyslav Nicholœvich Fyodorov, M.D.
1927–2000

Contents

Foreword

The author of this magnificent book, Dr Leo Bores, was the one to introduce radial keratotomy to the western world for the correction of myopic ametropia, a technique originally developed by Sato in 1951 and later perfected by Fyodorov in 1977, using incisions only in the anterior face of the cornea and reducing the size of the optical zone.

Dr Bores has developed instruments and technical features to improve refractive interventions on the cornea, among them the design of diamond and sapphire blades, a corneal topographer model, an adjustable progressive increment cut turbine engine microkeratotome, keratotomy instruments, the use of centrifugal incisions, etc., instruments and techniques widely publicized in multiple journals and lectures, and which now have been gathered in this book where his experience is presented in full detail.

He puts special emphasis on the specific aspects that, if overlooked, lead to adverse results. His entire book is a paradigm of Lister's statement: "Success depends on the attention paid to details," details that the attentive reader will find in every chapter and sometimes in each paragraph.

Refractive corneal surgery has been in the past decades and is still one of the new frontiers of ophthalmology. Its basis has been well established both for lamellar and relaxation techniques. For the latter since the end of the nineteenth century and for the former since 1964, where we demonstrated that, to correct myopia, thickness must be subtracted from the center of the cornea or increased in its periphery, and that to correct hyperopia, thickness must be added to the center of the cornea or subtracted from its periphery. Procedures involving subtraction were called keratomileusis and those involving addition received the name of keratophakia.

Procedures without freezing and laser exeresis are some recent examples of surface and intrastromal keratomileusis, without requiring a change in the procedure's name. This has been done in some cases giving the impression that the procedure in question is somehow new.

Keratotomies remain keratotomies be they straight, centrifugal or centripetal, curved, transversal, etc.; be they performed with steel, diamond, sapphire, or ruby blades; and keratomileusis remains keratomileusis, be it performed with a lathe, a microkeratome, a laser, or other exeresis procedures.

Perhaps, in the near future, and in order to avoid surgery altogether, it will be possible to soften the cornea, modify its shape, and harden it again so as to maintain its new form, thus correcting the refractive, spherical, and meridional errors in a non-surgical way.

My warmest congratulations to Dr Bores, promoter of these techniques and author of this book.

José I. Barraquer

Preface

This book had its beginning in the first moments of a meeting that took place almost fourteen years ago on a cold, bleak, February morning between two men—one Russian and one American. The decision that led to that meeting had been taken approximately six months previously and seemingly by accident. Yet that decision and what came out of that meeting seem almost to have been fated.

During the spring of 1975, I had reached a crisis in my life that necessitated a change in direction. Many choices presented themselves, but the one path I chose was to completely narrow my focus to two things—my family and my profession. I began to cast about for interesting things with which to get involved. I was quite facile in the anterior segment, and I liked the idea and potential of intraocular lens implants. So I arranged to borrow two Copeland lenses from Henry Hirschman, a fellow Kresge Eye alumnus, with some vague promises about "paying him back." He parted with them quite easily, which, on reflection, should have made me nervous. These I implanted without much difficulty but not without some reservations about their design. These lenses were the first ever implanted in Detroit and occasioned some comment—a lot of which was negative. Additionally, I had had no formal instruction in implantation techniques, having "learned" by attending a few presentations elsewhere (not a process generally to be recommended), so I decided to seek out an education, preferably abroad.

Since the pioneering work in intraocular lenses (IOLs) had been done mostly in England and Holland, it was there that I intended to go. Having already made plans to visit Jan Worst in Gronigen in February, I chanced to mention my proposed excursion to Jo Isaacson, a colleague and former mentor. He considered what I had said and then uttered the fateful words: "Why not visit Fyodorov? No one's seen him for about 5 years—might be interesting." (I've often wondered whether Jo has ever reflected on what his casual comment unleashed.) I was somewhat aghast—a trip to a place Winston Churchill had so aptly described as a "riddle wrapped in a mystery inside an enigma" was not quite what I had originally planned. Yet the thought piqued me. I did, after all, need to get away from everything as much as I wanted to learn new things, and where better to "get away," to get shut of the world, than in Russia? "But," said I, "how do I find this Fyodorov?" half hoping that there would be no answer. "Call Miles Galin," said Jo, writing down the number, "He should know."

Miles Galin, as I subsequently learned, is not all that easy to reach, but through some "miracle," he happened to be in his "snuggery" that day and less acerbic than usual. He took my call. "Why do you want to see Fyodorov?" he demanded in that slightly nasal and imperious tone that is so Miles. "To learn how to implant lenses," said I, unabashed. "Here's his phone number," said he. "Tell him that I recommended you. Goodbye." So I called immediately, not thinking about the time difference, but

I got Fyodorov himself on the phone—he'd been working late. At that time, his English was what can only be described as scanty, whereas my Russian was worse, consisting of *da* and *nyet*. "Yes!" he exclaimed, "You are friend of Miles! You will come visit me for two weeks. We will show you all. I will send you invitation for visa. Christmoose merry!" and he hung up.

There were still some minor details to settle before going, however. First, I had no passport, but luckily, the U.S. Passport Office had just streamlined its operation, and I got one in 10 days. I submitted a photocopy of it and my completed visa application along with Fyodorov's cable to the Soviet embassy in Washington. Now, never let it be said that naiveté is all bad. Had I been more worldly or sophisticated or knowledgeable, I would have *known* that there was no way that the visa would be ready in time. After all, it was only six weeks before I was due to leave, and we're talking the Soviet Union here. The travel agent, whose trepidations were echoed by my friends, was not hopeful, and even the Soviet embassy suggested that I might reconsider my travel timetable. But again, some "miracle" intervened, and the visa arrived, again in 10 days. Three miracles in a row—I was beginning to get a little nervous. However, I had said that I was going, so armed with my *Berlitz Guide to Russian for Travelers* and some Kaopectate, I went off to visit Fyodorov at No. 10 Lobninskaya Ulitza, Moscow, U.S.S.R.—in February 1976.

I landed at Sherymetevo Airport Number 2 on a Sunday afternoon. It was snowing, and the sky was gray. But of course it was snowing, of course the sky was gray! It was February! This was Russia! Didn't the song say something about ". . . more skies of gray than any Russian play," etc.? I disembarked from the plane under brooding clouds into an odorous yellow bus that took me to the old terminal, a dark concrete building of indeterminate age. "Bleaker and bleaker," said Alice. I unloaded and passed within, traversing some invisible threshold from bleakness into chaos. Therein I had my first taste of the real Soviet Union—I got into a line. The border guards (passport control) were very solemn and very young. The way they stared at the arrivees, I half expected to be arrested and carted away to Lubyanka at any second. So far, Russia was living up to its advance billing.

Suitcase inspection was next, but I had been primed by my travel agent—I had placed a pack of cigarettes on top of my clothes. The pack vanished instantly, and I was waved through—another miracle—everyone else was being "sifted." I passed on through the gate into still more chaos—shades of Dante. Now what was I supposed to do? Fortunately, the professor had sent someone to meet me—Dr. Topolovna. Somehow she had found me among the throng, but it turned out that she had even less English than the professor, and my Russian had not improved in the interim. So we stared helplessly at each other for a time until I heard my name called. I looked toward the sound, which was coming from a row of tables at which a woman was looking in my direction expectantly. When I looked back to my new acquaintance, she had vanished!

The woman who had called out to me was with Intourist and spoke passable English. She handed me a fistful of vouchers and rattled off some instructions before passing me off to a rather disreputable looking specimen who turned out to be my driver to the hotel. Between him and me and a *nisilchik* (porter), we managed to get my baggage into his black Volga (for a time, I thought Volga meant "black," because I didn't see one in any other color until years later). After a mildly harrowing ride into the city, I was deposited at the *Gastanyeetza Nationale*—National Hotel—right across from the Kremlin. I turned over my passport and vouchers to the reception desk and was taken upstairs, where I was introduced to the floor lady—the Cerberus of the room keys. She unlocked the 9-foot-tall, etched-glass door and ushered me into a baroque room right out of *Doctor Zhivago*. I set my bag down, and closed the door—I had arrived in Moscow.

The next morning, Dima, the professor's personal driver, collected me at the hotel and rocketed me to the clinic. Dima was a Tartar, and his car had two speeds—stop and go-like-blazes. The clinic was a rather decrepit looking building set among an apartment complex and surrounded by a drunkenly leaning concrete fence. I found out later that the building was actually an annex to a gynecologic hospital nearby and that Fyodorov had it "on loan." I walked up the brick steps, through the double-doored entry, and into a time warp.

My first impression was that I had been somehow transported back to the past into a hospital existing in the United States some 50 or 60 years earlier. All the equipment and furnishings, the rooms, everything seemed like photos of some bygone age come suddenly alive. I followed my driver up the stairs to the second floor, down the hall to a solitary door on the left, opened it, and stepped into an adventure that changed my life and the lives of countless thousands—forever.

I wasn't sure what I expected, but what I got was the greeting "Aha! Louva Boris!" and a bear hug. I gasped "Professor Fyodorov?" in that wheezy, throaty style that comes either from nervousness or from having one's breath squeezed out, or both. He looked a little like Khrushchev but with hair cut to a flat-topped brush. He had an enormous chest and wide shoulders with large hands and fingers (I was to find out a little later just how skilled those hands and fingers were). His eyes were bright, and he had an engaging smile that lighted his entire face as well as most of the room. He offered me tea, which I accepted. He was gruff. He was direct. I liked him instantly.

He also was very gracious and open and true to his word. In the next few days he "showed me all," as he had said he would. I had been there but two days when he announced that he wanted to show me something else. He then introduced me to a procedure involving making radiating incisions in the corneal stroma that he said was "against *blizarukist* [nearsightedness]." My initial reaction was one of disbelief, a reaction that I'm sure everyone experiences when first exposed to this procedure. After all—it seemed rather a bizarre solution to the "spectacle problem." In addition, I knew something of Sato's work. It hadn't worked for Sato, why should it work for Fyodorov? Could this perhaps be another Russian "reinvention" of previous technology? He sensed my hesitation because he said, "No, it is not Sato procedure. We do incisions only from outside." Still, I would have left it at that had it not been for one thing: Slava and I had become fast friends in those past two days.

Everyone who meets Svyataslav Nicholævich Fyodorov is struck by the charisma of the man—I was no exception. However, there seemed to be something deeper between us, almost as though we had known each other for a thousand years. It was a mutual connection that had manifested itself the very first instant we met. We soon began to communicate *dusha-a-dusha,* or soul to soul. We quickly found that we thought very much alike, and there was understanding and absolute candor between us. In some instances we would finish each others sentences; at other times no sentences at all were necessary. Somehow, despite the barrier of language, we understood and trusted one another—completely. Therefore, when he explained this procedure to me, I was disposed to believe him, despite my initial reservations.

I was allowed to examine, without interference, all the available patients who had had the surgery to that point—there were 135 in all, and it took several days to round them up. Each had unaided visual acuity ranging from 6/5 to 6/9 (20/15 to 20/30) with a follow-up period ranging from 2 weeks to 2 years. An examination of their records showed that preoperatively they all had unaided vision of 0.04 (20/100) or less (Cyrillic numerals are the same as ours). If the records were correct, and there was no reason to believe that they were not, then there was no question that the corneas of these patients had become flatter as a consequence of this bizarre surgery "against *blizarukist.*"

I suggested that I would like to check the next group of preoperative patients personally. I carefully recorded the examinations and matched them with the names both on the chart and on their wristbands. I also followed them into the operating room and observed their surgery. Postoperatively, I found that their corneas had become flatter and that the myopia had disappeared. In some cases the refractions were on the plus side. It being Friday, and since I was going by train to Leningrad that evening, I would have the weekend to ponder this phenomenon and to offer comment. On my return to Moscow early Monday morning, I found Slava there to greet me at the train station. He asked if I felt like doing a "little surgery." When I replied positively, he said "Good!" because he had eight patients cases lined up for me, four of whom were to undergo keratotomy. I broke out in a sweat despite the temperature being –20°F.

We were whisked to the hospital, where we exchanged mufti for hospital attire. After scrubbing up, I was led into the operating theater, where I was gowned and then seated, gloveless, at the operating microscope—an Opton (which is a Zeiss in disguise). My assistant was Boris Feldman, M.D., the "interpreter" who had been with me most of the previous week. His English was terrible, and I didn't know a *britva* from a *nosh.* I looked around for Slava, but he had unaccountably vanished! Then I looked through the scope at the case before me. "Ye merciful Gods!" I thought (this is not what I actually thought, but it's close). It was a hypermature membranous cataract! The eye was already open, and Boris handed me—two hooks! "Jehosophat!" thought I (which is not what I thought, but . . . well, you get the picture). Here I was, a stranger in a strange land trying to perform eye surgery with strange tools and not a familiar face in sight! The feeling was right up there with the sensation of falling off a building.

So I did what I always do in situations like this—put myself on automatic pilot. On closing the eye after having lost only a small bit of vitreous and implanting my very first "Sputnik" IOL, a disembodied voice said: "Very nice, Louva! You may operate in my clinic anytime you want." I looked around, and then it hit me—Slava had been watching the whole thing via television! But I wasn't thinking about the joke he had just played on me (he 'fessed up later) but about what he had just said. I have never told him just how much that simple statement meant to me at that time or since, but I would not trade that moment for any other in the world.

Within a few minutes, Slava rejoined me in the OR, and we began my first "dosaged dissection of the circumferential ligament of Kokott" (which was what Fyodorov called the surgery, a somewhat droll name that I subsequently changed to—*radial keratotomy*—at my wife Leara's suggestion). At that time, the surgery was done "free hand" with an unguarded razor blade held in a blade breaker. Slava assisted and guided me step-by-step through each case. It was a peak experience for me, needless to say. The incisions were all made beginning outside the limbus and moving in toward the optic center—a nerve-wracking proposition I can assure you. After each stroke of the knife, a "dipstick" gauge was used to check the depth of the incision. Thirty-two incisions were each made in this manner. One week later we did the other eye of each patient. In each case, corneal flattening occurred, and the myopia vanished. Furthermore, the fellow corneas were still flat.

Needless to say, I was thrilled—I also was apprehensive because if this operation really worked, and it certainly seemed that it did, it should be introduced into the United States. The potential of this procedure for doing great good was enormous. Considering the temperament of my colleagues, however, there also was an enormous potential for personal disaster. After all—who the devil was this upstart Leo Bores? Supposing that it did not work after all? *Chort voz me*—the devil take me!

When I returned to the United States, I tested the waters. I conferred with some of the other physicians who had visited Fyodorov but had not known about this operation. They all gave me the same answer: "Too risky," "Too variable," "Too unpredictable," "Won't last," etc. Others mentioned Sato. So I decided to lay low. In addition, the follow-up in the Russian series had only been 2 years, hardly enough time to decide if the method really effected a permanent corneal change.

Nevertheless, I mentioned it, almost in jest, to a couple of problem patients of mine. They weren't very happy with their glasses and were having difficulties with their contact lenses as well. I must confess that I was not prepared for their reaction. They practically exploded. They demanded the procedure on the spot. "Never mind the follow–up; just get me out of these damned glasses!" was one of the milder retorts. This was my initiation into the world of myopes. I had not realized until that moment just how trapped and helpless many of these people felt—how dependent they were on a simple visual aid. I began to realize that myopia was a very real problem—a congenital anomaly that we were "treating" with crutches.

In the fall of 1976, Slava came to the United States as my guest and stayed at my home in Detroit, Michigan. I arranged for him to give a lecture at the Kresge Eye Institute on the topic of "dosaged dissection"—the response was polite but indifferent.

In May of 1977, I returned to Moscow, bringing with me a retinue of well-known eye surgeons from the United States, including the late Bill Valloton, then director of the Storm Eye Institute at the University of South Carolina, in Charleston. My chief resident, Steve Gianarelli, accompanied us as well. The others were shown the procedure—and again, the response was one of indifference. Steve and I examined the patients that I had operated on the year before. Very little change had taken place in the shape of their corneas, and they were still seeing well. I also examined the records of some of the earlier patients, as well as more of the previous patients themselves. They were all doing well. There were no regressions (beyond that expected in the first 3 months), no infections, and no decompensatory changes in the cornea. "Now," said Slava, "you will do in the United States!"

However, the possibility of being "burned at the stake" still loomed before me. If I did do it, while I may be thought of as some sort of god by my patients, I felt that I was bound to be "God something else" to my colleagues. Steve opined that that sort of possibility had never stopped me before this and suggested that I purchase a pair of asbestos BVDs and a flak jacket and get on with it.

Considerable dialogue followed between Slava and myself vis-à-vis this procedure in the ensuing months. Finally, in the early spring of 1978, he showed me the records of the patients that I had operated on 2 years previously. That, coupled with the good results and 4 years of follow-up on almost 200 other Soviet patients, was sufficient—I had to get off dead center. Therefore, in November of 1978, when Bob Jampel (my department chief) was out of town, I "sneaked" a patient into the hospital and did the operation under general anesthesia (the Russians at that time were doing the surgery under topical anesthesia, consisting of 1% tetracaine). That first patient was a young black woman in her thirties who had bilateral myopia of −3.25 D and a long history of contact lens intolerance with skin irritation from her spectacles. She had been a patient of mine for years and had begun nursing school with my wife.

I must tell you that doing the first eye—all alone—was the most trying and difficult experience in my entire life. It was worse than doing that first patient in Russia. Unless you have been there, it is impossible to appreciate the degree of stress such a situation can engender. Your whole life passes in front of your eyes like an old-time movie. I was "assisted" by an ignorant first-year eye resident who, mercifully, shall remain nameless and who bombarded me with incessant and inane questions and who, I'm sure, ran off bleating to the chief as soon as he was able. Sweat poured from my body in torrents. I wanted to be elsewhere. A voice within me kept crying out—"What the h--- are you doing here Bores?" "Everything is cool," thought I. After all—4 years of experience were in the can. This procedure worked! "Oh yeah?" said the voice, "Suppose you blow it?" Meanwhile, I was filming it, and as I worked away, the room began to fill up with spectators. Through the whispering, I caught words like—"What is it *this* time?" ". . . crazy bastard!" "Fantastic!" "He's gone bonkers!" ". . . never a dull moment with Bores around!" etc. But I didn't "blow it"—it was fantastic, and 2 weeks later I operated on her other eye. Her uncorrected visual acuity was 20/25 (where it has remained to this day). The operation worked—as it was supposed to and as I really knew it would deep down.

In January, I proudly presented my patient at Grand Rounds and showed the film that I had made. I also presented some of the Russian data—zero response! Correction, there was one question: "Isn't this the Sato procedure?" and that from one of the most learned of the group. Apparently no one had been listening. By that time, however, I was totally convinced that any attempt by me to communicate this idea to my esteemed local colleagues was an exercise in futility. It was obvious that I was hearing different music than they were and marching to a different drummer altogether.

I therefore decided that the best course of action was to proceed according to my convictions. The chief—bless him—looked the other way while I did two more patients before he "asked" that I submit a proper research protocol to the university human research committee, which I did. It was a carefully constructed protocol that met all the requirements of the National Institutes of Health (NIH), the Hague Convention, and the University Safety in Human Research Guidelines. It passed with flying colors and was pronounced by the chairman of the Human Research Committee, Dr. Prasad, as the best example of such a protocol he had ever seen—and well it should be, having been modeled on the one devised for IOLs written by Miles Galin. It later became the basis of other such protocols throughout the world, including the PERK study.

I also decided that this procedure was too big for just one man. Accordingly, I set up the framework for the National Radial Keratotomy Study Group and went about selecting individuals whom I felt were "team players" and not afraid to stick with a program. Thus the stage was set for what followed—the start of a new era in the annals of eye surgery and the birth of a new subspecialty—refractive eye surgery. The stage also was set for a fire storm of criticism and rebuke hardly to be imagined. I did expect some controversy based on the response to the surgery by my local colleagues. It was still a shock and trial, though, when it really "hit the fan."

The mildest criticism offered was that radial keratotomy was not new, that it had been done before, and that it didn't work (referring to the Sato operation). Of course, the wheel is not new either; it had been done before as well—lo these many years ago. However, no one confuses the earlier product with our new and modern wheel, and I doubt that anyone would care to return to that older design.

Worse was the accusation that we were irresponsibly endangering vision by incising normal corneal tissue in an effort to cure something that was not even a disease. We were branded as "buccaneers" capitalizing on people's fears and misinformation (a sword, as later shown, that cuts both ways—see *Lasers*). But we knew that we were not the monsters we had been painted to be. We also knew that the critics were wrong. Myopia *is* a congenital "disease." It is every bit as disabling, as disheartening a handicap as a withered arm or leg or a cleft palate. It meets the conventional definition of a handicap in that it requires an external or artificial appliance for the afflicted to function normally. It interferes with normal functions as much as deformed limbs. It can be life-threatening as well. Furthermore, visual appliances are a hoax and a cruel joke on the patient. Their presence engenders false hope and breeds dependence. Patients are fooled into thinking that they can see, but when the appliances are lost, the patient is lost.

This disease causes discrimination both consciously and subconsciously. "Men don't make passes at girls who wear glasses" is not just a clever jingle—it is an insight into a strong social prejudice. Manufacturers recognize this and "fancy up" spectacles to make the wearer "more attractive." But in truth, the wearer is isolated—behind a window—peering out at the world—as if from a prison cell.

Contact lenses are also an attempt to remove the stigma. There is no denying that, for some, contact lenses provide the only hope of usable vision. But there is also no question that this type of wearer is in the minority. Most people wear contacts because "they look terrible in glasses." They may not admit this. Their usual explanation is that they "see better." Anyone who has fitted more than two pairs of contact lenses will recognize the contact lens "failures" who insist that they won't give up the lenses because they "see better" (even when the patient's best corrected vision with contacts may be 20/30 as opposed to 20/15 with spectacles).

Yet who is to say that they don't see better? What do we mean by "see better" anyway? There is ample evidence to show that vision is more than reading the small print on an eye chart—witness the small success of the Bates method. Yet, for lack of the ability to read that chart without a visual aid, doors are closed to the afflicted. How many potential Neil Armstrongs or Amelia Earharts are sitting out their lives on the side lines—not even getting a chance to participate?

Anyone can visualize a small child with a leg brace—a victim of a congenital defect. Everyone can see that her progress is impaired. Who would deny her the right to discard that brace—that crutch—that dependence? It would take an insensitive person indeed not to picture her joy at running and climbing unencumbered. It would take a granite heart to state, "She gets along well enough with her braces—she can survive and function well enough." However, only a champion of mediocrity and the status quo would opt for that kind of choice. Why should a visual handicap not entitle an individual to relief? Why should he or she be doomed to the status quo? Why cannot such people partake of the "forbidden fruit"? Who gave us the mandate to make that judgment anyway?

Still, someone invariably will say: "Surely this argument is all nonsense. What has the patient's sense of well-being got to do with it? What does 'quality of life' have to do with the 'sacred' art and science of medicine? The patient has no choice. He or she is incapable of choice. How could anyone be so irresponsible as to propose to actually cut into a normal cornea—just to do away with glasses? That's utter foolishness! Why, any fool can see that it's dangerous. It exposes the eye to infection! The whole idea is utter nonsense!" However, like the measurement of time and space, the concept of nonsense is relative, and we can always be sure when we use it that from some frame of reference it applies to us. Reality is never as we suppose it to be or wish it to be. Experience is the only reality. What is—is. There is no "supposed to be." The only "truth" is what is there. Perishing few of the frightful things that were "supposed" to happen with this surgery have ever happened!

I had hoped that recognition of this Zen-like concept of reality on the part of detractors, well meaning and otherwise, would have ended the discussion and let us get back to the task at hand, namely, refining the "wheel." Unfortunately, this hope was not to be realized for some years. It seems that there is a tendency for those of the species *Homo sapiens* to look with suspicion on anything not personally created. While in the past this had great survival value, its usefulness has diminished in a cooperative society. Some have developed this tendency to a fine art and have carried it to the extreme of telling others how to order their lives (witness the "Carrie Nations" of the world). This propensity is defended under the guise of *teaching* the "great unwashed" the *error* of their ways. The common denominator here is the belief that *others* are incapable of thought and that only the *professor* possesses the qualities of honesty, knowledge, and forthrightness. Do I hear an "Amen," brothers and sisters?

This phenomenon was not confined to just my situation. Trokel and Munnerlyn encountered the same problem early in the history of excimer laser surgery of the eye. Which prompts me to cry: "Ye merciful gods—will there be no respite?" Where, pray, do these "seers" and keepers of ultimate "wisdom," who have, unfortunately, elbowed their way into controlling positions, come from? "History does not repeat itself—only human beings do." So goes the saying, and how true it is. After having been thrashed completely over their opposition to penetrating keratoplasty, vitrectomy, alpha-chymotrypsin, intraocular lenses, and radial keratotomy—the "nay-sayers" persist in saying nay. How quaint. How old. How utterly boring—perhaps they're betting on being "right" one of these times. Considering their dismal track record, my advice would be to stay away from Las Vegas—the disease of chronic recurring wrongness is obviously incurable. Many of these down-putters are, no doubt, puffing up about their eventual acceptance of radial keratotomy, and many have wriggled their way into the forefront of the excimer laser arena with LASIK. It has been said that the essence of human beings is their intelligence and that the essence of intelligence is learning from one's mistakes. This does not speak well of the nay-sayers. In scientific and medical endeavors there will always be disagreement—this is healthy. Discourse and open-mindedness are the key to medical progress—suppression and censorship are its death. Oliver Wendell Holmes, Jr., said it quite well:

> When men have realized that time has upset many fighting faiths, they may come to believe even more than they believe the very foundations of their own conduct that the ultimate good desired is better reached by free trade in ideas—that the best test of truth is the power of the thought to get itself accepted in the competition of the market, and that truth is the only ground upon which their wishes safely can be carried out.

I address this additional thought to the young reader who is both new on this scene and who is experiencing his or her greening within the profession: Study and heed the lessons of medical history—recent and remote—so that you will not be included among those mean spirited of your colleagues to whom nothing is sacred but their own petrified opinion. Admit to yourself the possibility, nay, the probability, that you will often be mistaken in your views. And have a care to husband your opinion and remember that "It is better to keep silent and be thought a fool than to speak and remove all doubt" (Abraham Lincoln).

It hardly seems possible that almost twenty-five years have passed since that first visit to Hospital No. 81, 10 Lobninskaya Street. When it all began, much of what has transpired since was then only a dream. When the contents of my first radial keratotomy syllabus were transcribed, a battle was raging over what had begun as a simple and earnest desire to improve the lives of an unrecognized group of sufferers—myopes. Since then, the storm of that war has passed by, leaving only sporadic "guerrilla" action. Energy has been turned to the more important task of furthering the art of refractive surgery. During these past sixteen-plus years there has been born a new subspecialty—refractive eye surgery. To be sure, such surgery had been done before (*ca.*1713?) but quietly and by very few. Not until I performed that first radial keratotomy in 1978 did that interest change from a tiny spark into a raging fire. The knowledge that I have been instrumental in igniting and fanning those flames has sustained me through some very dark times. All in all, I think that I acted wisely.

I must confess, though, that during the early part of this adventure, I became quite empathetic to the frontiersmen's penchant for lynching rustlers and claim jumpers. That, however, is a story best left for another time and another place. Suffice to say that it has been said, and a wise saying it is, that "defeat is an orphan, while success has many fathers."

I've often been asked whether it was all worth it; the ostracizing, the bashing, the name-calling? In the final analysis, did I succeed in what I set out to do? Perhaps Ralph Waldo Emerson said it for me:

> To laugh often and much; to win the respect of intelligent people and affection of children; to earn the appreciation of honest critics and endure the betrayal of false friends; to appreciate beauty, to find the best in others; to leave the world a little better, whether by a healthy child, a garden patch,

or a redeemed social condition; to know even one
life has breathed easier because you have lived.
This is to have succeeded.

Notice: The indications and dosages of all drugs in this book have been recommended in the medical literature and conform to the practices of the general community. The medications described and treatment prescriptions suggested do not necessarily have specific approval by the Food and Drug Administration (FDA) for use in the diseases and dosages for which they are recommended. The package insert for each drug should be consulted for use and dosage as approved by the FDA. Because standards for usage change, it is advisable to keep abreast of revised recommendations, particularly those concerning new drugs.

Leo D. Bores, MD
Scottsdale, Arizona

Acknowledgments

No one can be the sole author of a work of this magnitude—no matter how fervently he may wish it or how hard he may try to accomplish it. The ghosts of authors past are forever peering over the writer's shoulder—whispering criticism and advice. At times, the murmuring can become so insistent and strident as to cause the writer to temporarily lose his identity. Sometimes the "conversation" takes on the flavor of a fireside chat with friends:

> Whate'er I feel I cannot feel alone.
> When I am happiest or most forlorn,
> Uncounted friends, whom I have never known
> Rejoicing stand or grieving by my side,
> These nameless, faceless friends of mine who died
> A thousand years or more e'er I was born.
>
> Rosalind Murray

In fact, the very process of such an undertaking triggers a metamorphosis in thought and being. It is not possible to come away from such an experience with a whole skin. Had I realized this potential hazard at the outset, perhaps I would have declined the challenge. Perhaps—but not likely. Such an opportunity is not proffered to all who seek it—thus one must grasp the nettle. *Carpe diem. Kismet.*

Fortunately, I had help. First, of course, from Richard Smith, my coauthor, who initially had to be bludgeoned into acquiescence. To him was assigned the task of writing the chapter on corneal anatomy and the pathology of corneal wound healing. Heavy stuff, that. To his credit, he did admirably. Frank Thompson was next on my "hit list." My man Vito convinced Frank to supply materials for the chapter on scleral reinforcement. This contribution is, in fact, fitting. It is not possible to do justice to that subject without incorporating the important work of this distinguished pioneer. Howard Straub, my first refractive surgery fellow and a person I've always been able to count on through thick and thin, obliged me with the material on laser in situ keratomileusis (LASIK)—a subject on which he is an expert.

To my good friend and fellow adventurer, Akira Momose, go the laurels for shedding light on the early days of refractive surgery in Japan—ala Sato. His own work on posterior scleral support is not without merit. It would have been difficult, to say the least, to write the ametropia chapter without the help and encouragement of "Doctor Myopia"—Brian Curtin. His monumental work, *The Myopias,* is recommended reading for all refractive surgeons—aspiring or other. And if the text of the current treatise sometimes transcends the usual pedantic style expected of a work of this type, thank Guido Majno. His wonderful book, *The Healing Hand: Man and Wound in the Ancient World,* proved to me that it is possible to be scholarly without being stuffy. I am indebted as well to Professor Gabriel van Rij of the Academisch Ziekenhuis, Gronigen, The Netherlands, for the history of Lans and other Dutch investigators. The "Learned Man"—Houdijn Beekhuis, M.D.—kept me in stitches with his droll perspectives on certain aspects of medicine; it was enlightening to say the least.

To all the ghosts—Imhotep, Hippocrates, Aristotle, Galen, Al-Hazen, Keppler, Tadini, Boerhaave, Young—to name but a few—my profound and humble thanks. Take a break.

My earnest and heartfelt good wishes go out to those others of my colleagues (cited throughout the text and in the List of Contributors) without whose support much of this treatise would be figureless. Absent the able assistance of Dick Wolf, curator of Harvard's Countway Library, and Reva Hurtes, librarian and rare book guru at the Bascom Palmer Eye Institute, we would be without many of our historic illustrations. My profound thanks to Karla VanderSypen, head of the Rare Book Room at the library of the University of Michigan, and especially to Mary Lou Goldstein, chief librarian at Scottsdale Memorial Hospital North and her able assistant Deborah LaBarbera, who provided assistance above and beyond their requirement to do so. Kudos as well to the charming May Cheney, whose beautiful artwork graces these pages throughout.

I am particularly indebted to my professional critics, who continually provided me with stimulation and helped me to remember exactly what it was that I was trying to accomplish with refractive surgery. This kept me from becoming lazy and complacent and forced me to weigh everything that I said carefully and to be prepared to back it up—it still does.

I have enjoyed the support and encouragement of my many friends as well as my family from the very beginning of this medical adventure. Much of what lies within these pages was stimulated both by experience and by intimate discussions with these friends, but of course, none of this was accomplished without episodes of depression and self-doubt. The example of Slava Fyodorov, as he struggled to build his dream, was a constant inspiration to me. The numerous "skull sessions" with him were always sure to strike sparks of inspiration in us both. I am grateful to my long-suffering wife Leara, who gave back as good as she got and then some. She has provided insight into areas of which I was untutored and used her "sharp stick" when I got down and feeling sorry for myself, as well as suggesting the name—radial keratotomy—for the procedure. To her and to Molly, my secretary at the Kresge Eye Institute; to Ella, Karen, Kathy, and Laura, my tough assistants; and to Bob and Jane and Carlo and Mahmud and all the other patients too numerous to name who played a part—my undying gratitude. I hope that I have not let you down. To Mother Nature—I got the message, and thanks.

Finally, to the late Professor A. D. Ruedeman, Sr., my first *sensei,* whose gruff model of bulldog determination and no-nonsense approach to medicine has served me well; to my gentlemanly chief—the late Windsor S. Davies—who inherited the rough beginnings and put the final polish on a brash young eye resident; to my mentor and friend—the late José Ignacio Barraquer—whose paradigm of diligence and rectitude is always before me; and of course, to my dear friend Slava, I dedicate this text.

Leo D. Bores, MD
Scottsdale, Arizona

Refractive Eye Surgery

1
Introduction to the Second Edition

Caveats for the prudent and thoughtful

This section might better be entitled "The Dutch Uncle Speaks and About Time Too!" because there is an unfortunate tendency among our ophthalmic brethren to credit science over art and to ignore clinical experience. This is to say that $x + y$ must always equal z because science says so—anything else is looked down on and with a sneer as anecdotal. *Anecdotal,* however, is defined in the *Oxford English Dictionary* as "things unpublished" or "hitherto private or unpublished narrative or details of history." The word is often used disparagingly by a certain group of individuals (who obviously do not know what it really means) to discredit careful clinical observations by "outsiders" and is part and parcel of the NIH ("Not Invented Here") syndrome. As a foot-slogger of long experience, I have been sufficiently pummeled by the realities of medicine to tell you flatly that "it ain't necessarily so." The natterings of rear-echelon commandos do not signify.

When I first began to teach radial keratotomy, I felt that it was incumbent on me to explain that the response to the surgery may not be what the surgeon expects. I had to remind erstwhile refractive surgeons of the old cliché: "Man proposes and God [nature] disposes." In short—what happens to the eye happens, and we must live with that—all that we've been taught to the contrary. Basically, this meant that the budding refractive surgeon must be of Zen to be successful and that one had to accept the fact that there is no *should* or *ought to be*—there is only what is. This is not to say that there is no cause and effect—that there surely is. It is merely to say that the cause portion of the equation may not be as you suppose.

Experiments in modern Gestalt psychology demonstrate a universal need to discover familiar patterns in apparently random occurrences, to bring order out of chaos, to explain the unexplainable. But this quest for comfort and security sometimes leads to bizarre conclusions: *The cock crows at daybreak, and the sun also rises. Hence the sun rises in response to the crowing of the cock.* Ridiculous to be sure, but it was once also earnestly believed, supported by sublime and elegant proofs that adequately explained most observed phenomena, that the sun rotated around the Earth. We have subsequently discovered another reality.

In the early days of radial keratotomy, there were encounters that caused me great consternation. Frequently, I would find myself approached by some shiny-faced youth (occasionally not so shiny-faced nor youthful) who would introduce himself or herself and then immediately set to explaining how radial keratotomy worked, and of course, he or she had it all figured out because he or she held a degree in engineering. I once witnessed an electrical engineer damn near electrocute himself because he had overlooked the fact that a sweaty sock inside a rubber-soled shoe with a hole in it provides an excellent electrical pathway to a wet floor—but I digress. Most of the theories put forth by my shiny-faced protagonists were amusing, but some were downright terrifying. Fortunately, reality has a way of burning away fancy if you let it. Still, the tendency to credit vapid musings over nitty-gritty reality persists, especially when garnished with numbers—preferably arranged into complex equations.

We seem to have forgotten—if we indeed ever knew it—that mathematics is an artificial construct and that an inch—isn't. Mathematical expressions may be useful in explaining some of the phenomena we experience in this singularity, but they are not real. They have been bent, twisted, and bludgeoned until they concur with real-life experiences—sometimes. If we are lucky, this happens most of the time. However, sometimes it doesn't. Sometimes the product of mathematical manipulation is a phantasm. And all too often the prestidigitators who deal with such obscurities accept and preach these results as holy writ.

We humans also have a tendency to bestow a certain cachet on those who seem in mastery of a discipline with which we have little experience. Hence the awe accorded to physicians, the clergy, and rich folks. It must be remembered, though, that all these people put their pantaloons on—one leg at a time.

Then, too, it is said that *there are none so self-righteous as the converted sinner*. This would certainly apply to those among us who have recently acquired wealth in the form of new technology (read "toys"). Such a thing causes a burning desire to proselytize—to spread the word—often before the true situation becomes completely understood and often ending in causing great harm. Case in point—sphere-based topography of the cornea (see Chapter 6).

We have today the singular phenomenon of seemingly intelligent men rushing about and proclaiming that "this and that" are happening on the cornea and that therefore you must do "this and that" to surgically correct them. In the meantime, the reality that the refractive power of the eye is a reflection of an entire system—is completely ignored.

Well then, if all this science is mucking up the picture, why should we give our attention and time to this business of corneal topography, wavefront technology (interferometric and adaptive optics), and biomechanics? The answer is: Because the wise person will consider all things and file away those which do not fit. How does one know which things to keep and which to file? We can do what paleontologists do to reconstruct a dinosaur—a creature never seen by human beings. They simply gather together all the parts, set aside those which do not look like a "Thingamasaurus," and assemble the rest.

It may be thought that I am merely being droll, but this is exactly what paleontologists do. Of course, like all magicians—they cheat. They have prepared themselves to perform this feat of legerdemain in advance by studying the bones of modern creatures and the way the muscles and tendons attach to those bones and the effect on bone growth of different stimuli. Hence they have provided themselves with the tools necessary to sort out that which is important and that which is not, and they never throw anything away. Note that earlier I said *file away*, not throw away.

Can we do less? Certainly not. The study of biomechanics and the other things is vital to carrying forward our surgical techniques. It is just that we must apply what we discover with great caution. More importantly we needs must seek out those relationships and properties which best describe the true situation. In constructing our description, the best language to use may be that of mathematics. But we must be prepared to coin new terms and expressions to use when it is evident that the old ones will not do and lay in a goodly supply of salt as well.

What's contained herein

Some things have changed since the premier edition of this book first saw the light of day. For example, photoablative refractive keratectomy (PRK)—the darling of the laser crowd—has pretty much gone away, except for "touching up" post-radial keratotomy cases and perhaps in myopia under 4 D. During this same period, thermokeratoplasty (TK) and hexagonal keratotomy (HK) also have gone the way of the dodo—and a good thing too. HK destabilized the cornea to a fare-thee-well, and changes in corneal shape through denaturization of the stroma by heat continue to be both unpredictable and short-lived into the bargain. Sunrises' laser TK technique was sent back by the Food and Drug Administration "for repair" on the grounds that the results do not last. Hyperopic lamellar keratotomy (HLK) also went down for the count, as did automated lamellar keratectomy (ALK).

The king is dead

I have mixed emotions about PRK because it turns out that the Food and Drug Administration was right. Why do I say the Food and Drug Administration was right? Because it delayed approval of widespread use of of excimer laser PRK in this country—and a good thing too! It didn't work that well, you see. The darling of the laser cult turned out to have feet of clay.

LASIK

Laser in situ keratomileusis (LASIK) is the new darling of the laser crowd, and it has caught on well around the world. It is a good procedure, but it requires thinking. Greater care needs be taken with lamellar surgery—the principles of which are laid out in the chapter on lamellar refractive surgery (see Chapter 10). Unfortunately, too many practitioners treat this procedure as a "no-brainer." Not good, especially since it can introduce corneal aberrations that reduce visual efficiency big time, and then there's this interesting phenomenon of the increasing incidence of dry eye following LASIK (see Chapter 15).

Corneal topography

I had thought that by now everyone would have seen the error of their ways. But alas, it was not to be. Practitioners still have not got the message that meridional slope values (provided by sphere-based Placido's disk systems) do not provide enough information to describe the true shape of the cornea. All the mathematical gymnastics in the world will not provide the missing data, and the fact remains that such devices are nowhere to be found in laboratories dealing with precision optics. Huxley said that this was the terrible tragedy of science: "When a beautiful theory is destroyed by an ugly fact." Is it any wonder that current topographic maps still have only entertainment value, using as they do Placido's disk and slit-scan interpolation of corneal curvature? Fortunately, some laser manufacturers are beginning to catch on that wavefront and interferometric technology is the proper way to reshape the corneal surface (see Chapters 6 and 11). We can but hope.

Telescopic implants for macular degeneration

Alas, this saga is pretty much in suspended animation. The AMO lens did not work as well as first thought and the study was suspended. There is still hope, however, in a multi-objective Israeli implant being tested by Dr. Issac Lipshitz.

Long live the king

Radial keratotomy (RK)—which was to have been done to death by PRK—is still being performed in considerable and increasing numbers by the "unenlightened" around the world for the simple reason that it works well for the degrees of myopia for which it was designed. Though some lasers have been approved to treat corneal astigmatism, nothing works better nor is more predictable than RK so far.

Taken all together, it is still an exciting time to be a refractive eye surgeon.

Introduction to the First Edition

It has long been an axiom of mine that the little things are infinitely the most important. [Sir Arthur Conan Doyle]

This work is about a new type of eye surgery—refractive eye surgery—designed primarily to remove the visual handicap of ametropia, chiefly myopia. To be sure, hyperopia and astigmatism take their toll in diminished vision. However, it is myopia that is, by far, the greatest scourge and toward which the majority of our energies have been focused. This treatise is designed to prepare the beginning refractive surgeon for this adventure by providing a firm grounding in basic fundamentals and techniques and to assist the general ophthalmologist in understanding these methodologies. The experienced refractive surgeon will find much that is of value within these pages as well. All aspects of the problem including hyperopia and astigmatism are included, and practical tips and methods of surgical treatment are detailed.

This work is not, however, encyclopedic, nor does it attempt to be. The author has found through experience that eclecticism has no place in refractive surgery. If ever the old saw—*too many cooks spoil the broth*—were true, it is surely here. All too often instruction courses are given whose many guest speakers present so many differing points of view, undoubtedly in the spirit of nonbias, that the erstwhile refractive surgeon goes away more confused and bewildered than before. It is just not possible, however, to "mix-and-match" with this surgery. The beginning refractive surgeon cannot be eclectic in his or her surgical approach and expect it to be effective. Nor are they in any position to decide what to choose and what to discard. They must first adopt the surgical method of a particular, experienced surgeon and follow his or her method assiduously until such time that they have become absolutely confident in their understanding of all the nuances of the surgery. Then and only then will it be possible for the surgeon to "vary the theme" and strike off on his or her own. Thus this present work emerges as the point of view of one individual—with a little help from friends—admixed with a tincture of philosophy to give it some spice.

Refractive eye surgery is defined as that surgery on the eye which acts to change the light-bending characteristics of that eye. This definition would include such things as cataract surgery—with or without the implantation of an intraocular lens. This discussion will, however, confine itself to surgery performed on the cornea, sclera, or lens of the eye specifically for modifying its refractive characteristics.

In 1708, Hermann Boerhaave suggested that high myopia could perhaps be treated by couching the clear lens in such patients. Von Haller, in 1746, may well have tried it, but it was not until 1894 that Fukala published his first reports on the technique of clear lens extraction for myopia. In 1869, Snellen, in an article published in the German literature, discussed the possibilities of correcting corneal astigmatism, possibly drawing on the attempts of Von Galezowski to achieve the same purpose through resection of a crescentric piece from the cornea. Bates, in 1894, described a surgical technique for such modification and reported a number of patients, as did Lans in 1898. Thus the search for effective surgical means to modify ametropia began.

The evolution of such surgical techniques resembles, in many ways, the development of manned flight. As experience and technical skills improve, early and more primitive efforts give way to more advanced ideas and methods. Sometimes, ideas that were discarded previously or not implemented because of technical deficiencies are revived at a later time when they are capable of being used or their worth fully recognized.

Parallel with these and other technological advances have come changes in the psychosocial makeup of human society. In the early days, the battle against disease was black and white. Disease was once thought of as God's punishment to the ungodly and meddling with its progress sinful. As medicine advanced, the subject of preventative medicine began to play a more important role. Today there is more emphasis on the quality of life and the human condition than ever before, and procedures designed to modify human existence, such as genetic engineering, plastic and reconstructive surgery, and refractive surgery of the eye are being employed.

Throughout such evolution, however, the innovator not only must battle those specific problems which accompany the treatment itself but also must confront and surmount those generated by the actions and attitudes of his or her contemporaries and colleagues. Such circumstances are, of course, not new, and given the nature of human beings, they are very likely to continue.

There are currently five methods of surgically modifying the corneal curvature in general usage. These are

1 Mechanical modulation of corneal shape—keratomileusis
2 Relaxing incisions—radial keratotomy
3 Corneal onlays—epikeratophakia
4 Corneal inlays—keratophakia
5 Tissue replacement—keratoplasty

Of these five, the latter—keratoplasty—does not always have as its primary goal (except in cases of keratoconus) the modification of the corneal curvature and so will be discussed only incidentally. Additionally, clear lens extraction or intraocular lens implantation can be employed to reduce high myopia, and scleral reinforcement can shorten axial length and prevent further elongation of the globe. Such approaches to the problem, once considered bizarre and risky, are now being entertained more seriously as primary or alternative treatments of ametropia.

To be successful as a refractive surgeon, the ophthalmologist must develop a special mind-set. He or she must come to terms with the fact that refractive surgery is truly microsurgery and that microns count. He or she must not be swayed by the argument that because biologic systems are variable in nature, precision is unnecessary in the performance of this surgery. It is vital that the surgeon make precise those things which he or she can control and minimize the imprecision of those things which he or she cannot. He or she also must avoid the tendency to "simplify" the surgical decision-making process *ad absurdum*.

There is a strong tendency by the neophyte to take shortcuts and because of inexperience to overlook data deemed insignificant. However, as in no other aspect of ophthalmology, the careful gathering and integration of numerous parameters to affect a desirable end result is paramount. As never before, the beginning surgeons cannot rely on their common sense to guide them through their learning experience. They cannot "wing it." They must instead rely on the hard-won experience of their brother and sister surgeons who have gone before. As John Dickinson said: "Experience must be our only guide. Reason may mislead us." Because of this fact, this surgery finds no place for instant experts and their incisional configuration of the month. Good ideas will still be good ideas six months or a year from now. Sudden flashes of inspiration are too often found to be mere glints of the egoist's eye that pale when exposed to the harsh light of time and reality. Small changes in technique often made for no other reason than that "it seemed right" can produce a domino effect not apparent for some time, perhaps years.

Radial keratotomy is a case in point. This surgery is said to be simple and that it is not necessary to do "all those measurements." If it were possible to perform this surgery optimally through the consideration of only a few parameters or by consultation of rigid tables—then those who have labored long and hard to bring this surgery about would be doing it the simple way.

Such simplifications have led, for example, to overcorrections and progression of effect after radial keratotomy. It was such "innovation" that produced circular radial keratotomy in some 30 patients with resulting increased myopia, nonhealing, and marsupialization of the wounds. This was done by an "expert" some seven days after taking his first course in radial keratotomy. It was another "expert" who kept his patients on topical steroids four times daily for more than six months to "enhance the effect" of his ineffective surgical technique and induced cataracts. It was another "expert" who overextended his blade in the presence of a flat chamber and incised the anterior capsule of the lens. It was still another "expert" who neglected to cover his patient with antibiotics after a microperforation and the eye then went on to develop endophthalmitis.

This surgery is simple to watch being done by an expert, who often makes it look so easy. After all, how could it be hard to make a cut on the eye? It is done all the time. But the incision made for a cataract extraction is not expected to produce a precisely modulated change in corneal curvature—it is expected only to provide access to the anterior chamber. This surgery is only simple to "screw up." There are too many factors involved, all supported by clinical results over time, to take the casual approach. It is possible to guide an aircraft to a landing or simply to "arrive." One also can "arrive" on the first floor by leaping from the tenth, but the results would not be as satisfactory as taking the elevator. Some surgeons find the elevator too slow for their tastes and insist on leaping—taking their patients with them.

All these surgeries continue to evoke controversy despite successful application of the basic principles and techniques. Some of the cautious statements that were made in the beginning were valid then but not today. Moreover, some problems previously trumpeted have resulted from inappropriate application or execution of these procedures and are not inherent—as once believed.

These cases have served to emphasize a point often overlooked: This surgery is microsurgery in its strictest sense. It requires of the surgeon a particular mind-set. He or she must convert from "macro" to "micro" thinking. He or she must think in terms of microns instead of millimeters. He or she must pay attention to preoperative testing as never before. He or she must consider and weigh as significant parameters that heretofore seemed "not to matter." It should not be surprising that some surgeons fail in this conversion. A gifted cataract surgeon may not make a gifted microrefractive surgeon. If it happens to you, don't blame the surgery—some of us can't ride skate boards very well either. *Kismet.*

This is no place for the casual or occasional surgeon. This is no province for the surgical dilettante. None of these techniques are simple despite their appearance, and some are on a par with open-heart surgery in their complexity. No general surgeon would dream of performing open-heart surgery, leaving that to specialists. So too refractive surgery. There are a myriad of small details that must be considered constantly, and concentration on the patient at hand is essential to success. Such necessity does not fit in well with the general practice of ophthalmology. The proper performance of this surgery is best left to specialists who have dedicated themselves to it and are prepared to continue to dedicate themselves to it. Teaching of these techniques should not be done as a matter of course in a residency program, but afterwards in a program devoted to refractive surgery alone. This represents a shift in my previous position on this subject. However, continued misapplication of these techniques by general ophthalmic surgeons has made this shift in opinion necessary.

This is not a definitive text—no text on this subject could ever be—rather, consider it a primer on refractive eye surgery. The type of surgery I am describing is undergoing an evolution of impressive dimension. Still the basics have not changed. The rationale behind each technique remains. It is hoped that the refractive surgeon, beginner and shellback, will find within these pages those tools necessary to take the next step, whenever or where ever that might be. Thus the thrust of this text is as a foundation, a sheet-anchor from whence one can cast off on the great adventure that is refractive surgery.

2
The Nature of Ametropia

The newly invented optick glasses are immoral since they pervert the natural sight, and make things appear in an unnatural and false light. [Mr Cross, Vicar of Chew Magna, Somersetshire, England (13th century)]

Introduction and historical background

Nearsighted people have sought ways to get rid of their glasses for centuries. Tradition says the ancient (presumably myopic) Chinese slept with sandbags on their eyes to flatten their corneas. It is certain Purkinje tried the same thing in the 1820s with only temporary improvement of his 5 D of myopia. In the mid 1800s, a Dr. J Ball advertised a small mallet mounted on a spring in an eye cup that struck the cornea through the closed eyelid, pounding it flat. "It restores your eyesight and renders spectacles useless," he claimed. "Professor" Charles Tyrell claimed a similar effect from the use of his Ideal Sight Restorer at the turn of the century (Figures 2.1 and 2.2) [1]. Ridiculous perhaps, ineffectual certainly, but not all such notions were either ridiculous or ineffectual—they may have just been untimely. Timing, as someone once said, is everything. This is especially true in medicine. Methods considered bizarre, far-fetched, impractical, or fantastical in some yesteryear, are not so seen today. That being true, who can say what the verdict of tomorrow will be?

It is not possible to say with assurance just who it was that first conceived of treating ametropia or altering the refractive power of the eye surgically. Perhaps some long-forgotten troglodyte had his myopic vision restored after an injury—before his visual handicap led to his demise—and may have wondered over it. It is not clear that the ancients (before Aristotle) even recognized ametropia as such. Nevertheless, many of these early physicians were astute observers, and many of their medical techniques made sense even if they seemed to have ascribed the cure to supernatural intervention. Certainly visual problems other than that due to disease were observed and treated from the earliest of times, but we lack direct and pertinent documentation of such treatments.

The Egyptians had a long and apparently deserved reputation as physicians *swnw* (sounou). Homer speaks of Egypt in Book IV of the *Odyssey*:

> In that country the fertile soil produces all kinds of juices which may have a good or bad effect. There everybody is a physician and surpasses in experience all other men; because verily they are from the family of Paeon.

That Egyptian medicine was apparently sacerdotal does not mean that superstition held sway over common sense, despite some modern views to the contrary. Their knowledge of treatment of trauma was quite advanced and thorough, as evidenced by the Edwin Smith surgical and Ebers papyri [2–4]. Figure 2.3 shows the Stele of Iry (2400 BC), the earliest known ophthalmologist, while Figure 2.4 shows a physician treating an eye.

However, except for some references to weak vision and remedies for this and other problems which could have been cataract, there is no indication that the Egyptians (or for that matter, the Sumerians) knew anything about myopia, hyperopia, or presbyopia. Likewise, while there is

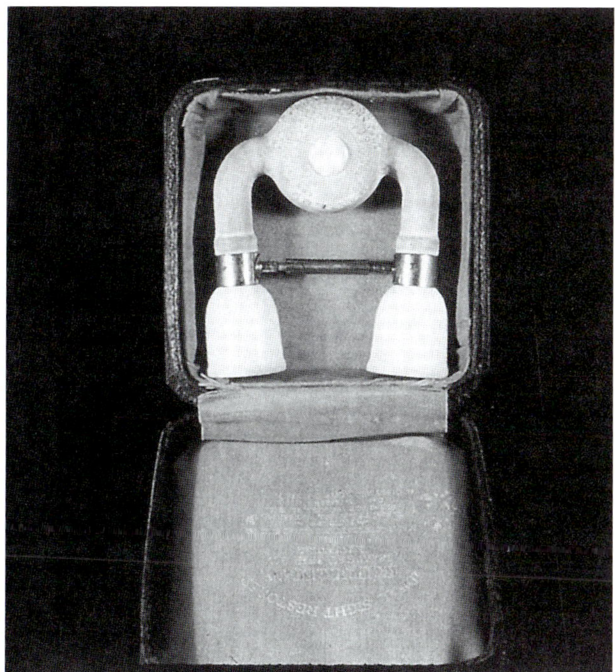

Fig. 2.1 The Ideal Sight Restorer of "Professor" Tyrell, circa 1909 (Andrew Ferry, MD).

evidence of the use of magnifying lenses by lapidaries in Nineveh, such usage is not described in extant Egyptian writings but may have been known and kept as a guild secret (Figure 2.5). Nothing resembling spectacles has been found either in inscriptions or with any mummies. While early Greeks borrowed much from the Egyptians and were familiar both with the magnifying as well as the heating potential of a water-filled glass globe, it is not clear whether such knowledge came from other cultures or originated with the Greeks themselves.

Aristotle and myopia

The first real discussion or mention of refractive errors came later in the works of Aristotle who lived about

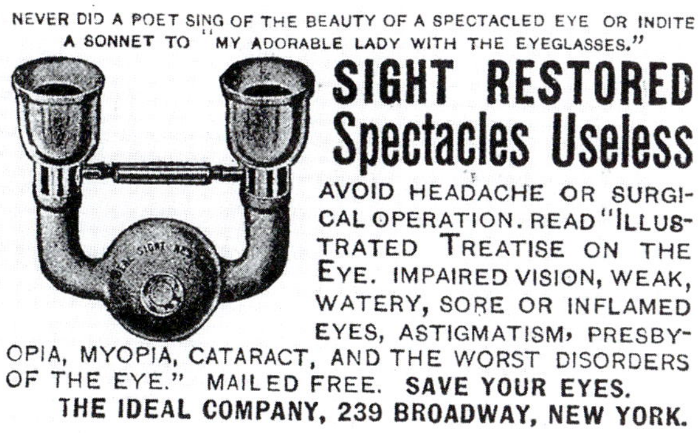

NEVER DID A POET SING OF THE BEAUTY OF A SPECTACLED EYE OR INDITE A SONNET TO "MY ADORABLE LADY WITH THE EYEGLASSES."

SIGHT RESTORED
Spectacles Useless

AVOID HEADACHE OR SURGICAL OPERATION. READ "ILLUSTRATED TREATISE ON THE EYE. IMPAIRED VISION, WEAK, WATERY, SORE OR INFLAMED EYES, ASTIGMATISM, PRESBYOPIA, MYOPIA, CATARACT, AND THE WORST DISORDERS OF THE EYE." MAILED FREE. **SAVE YOUR EYES.**

THE IDEAL COMPANY, 239 BROADWAY, NEW YORK.

Fig. 2.2 Advertisement extolling the virtues of the Sight Restorer (Andrew Ferry, MD).

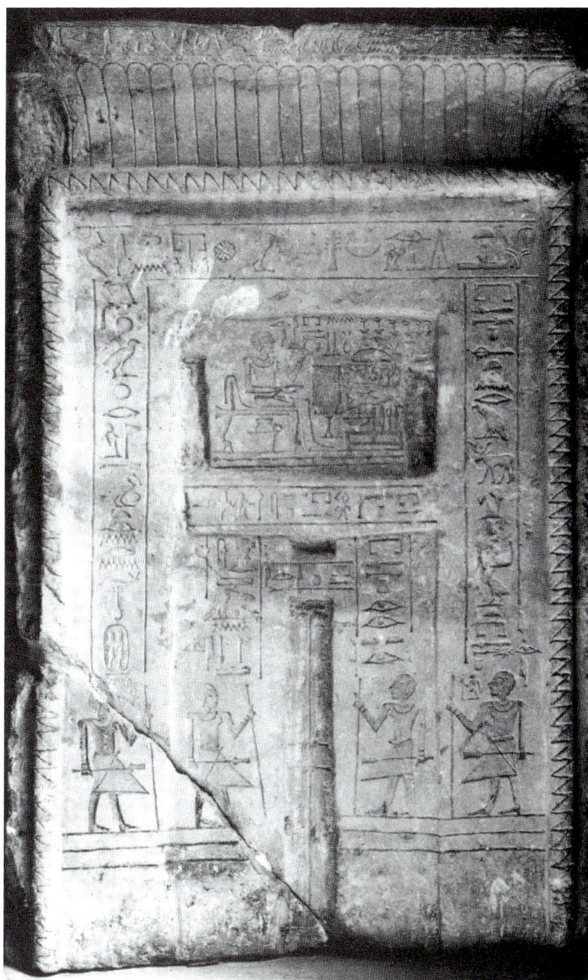

Fig. 2.3 The Stele of Iry (2400 BC)—the first ophthalmologist (Kunsthistorisches Museum, Vienna).

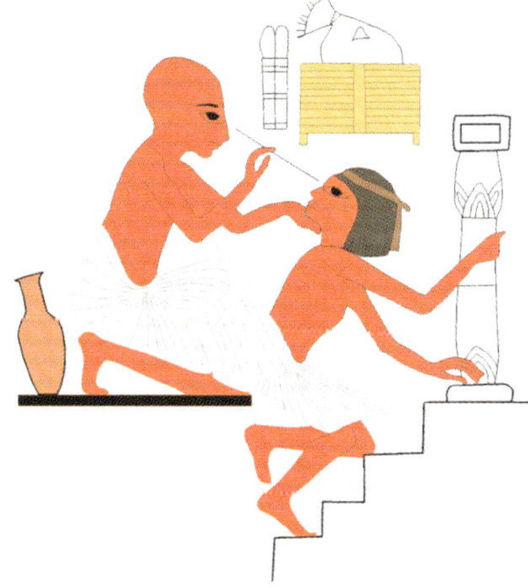

Fig. 2.4 An inscription from the temple of Ipuy showing a physician or his assistant probably removing an ocular foreign body at a construction site.

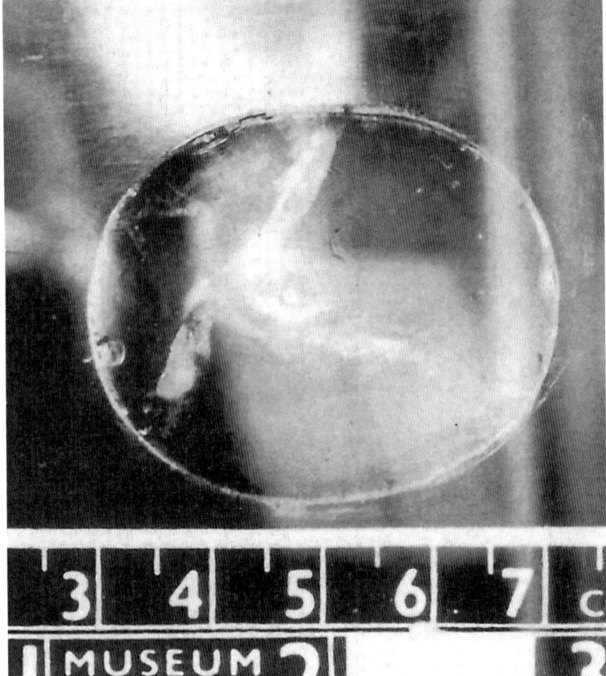

Fig. 2.5 A polished crystal excavated at Nineveh that might have been used as a magnifying lens (British Museum, London).

100 years after Hippocrates and therefore before the collection of Hippocratic books was completed. These books by Aristotle should be able to show us what the Greeks of the classical period and shortly after it knew about this topic. Unfortunately, those works which would primarily be concerned with this field, the so-called *Problems* of Aristotle, do not belong to the authenticated works by the famous philosopher [5,6]. Nevertheless, these quotations are of interest. They are probably the oldest citations which explain the name and the concept of myopia and the first ones which allude to presbyopia:

> There are two kinds of weak eyes. The one is the myope and the other one occurs in old people. The first one will hold objects close in order to see sharply while the other one will hold them far away.
>
> The vision of old people is opposite to that of myopes: the first do not see clearly what is close, but see well at distance.
>
> Why does the myope hold everything close and the old man everything far away?

Some hints about myopia and hyperopia can be found in the authentic works by Aristotle, however. We find an allusion to presbyopia there as well. He says that old people do not see sharply because the transparent membrane in front of the pupil becomes wrinkled and casts a shadow. He had apparently already observed an elongation of the visual axis in myopic eyes (*Origin of Animals*) [7]. In these works he also asks:

> Why do myopes write in such small letters?
>
> Why do the myopes [those who squint their eyes] have a tendency to squint their lids?

This is the first time the word *myops* is encountered in the literature, a word which even today, 2000 years later, is used in the same sense. *Myein* means to close, especially the eye or the mouth; *myops* means to close or blink the eye. The same word also signifies the condition of myopia; only the later authors substitute for this term myopia. Before that the term *myopiasis* was used [8]. It aptly describes the facial expression of the uncorrected myope trying desperately to clarify the world. Until the general introduction of spectacles for the myope, squinting the lids, with the resulting production of a horizontal stenopeic slit, was the only practical means whereby clear distance vision could be achieved.

According to Hirschberg:

> *Presbys* means the old man or venerable man; *presbytes* is the senile man. This is also the meaning of the word in the original Greek quotation above; the meaning is obvious because in general old people will hold a book farther away, though exceptions exist. The meaning of this word as "poor vision in old age" was only acquired in modern times [6].

As to vision itself, the emanation hypothesis of vision, propounded by Pythagoras, held sway [9]. Accepted in one form or another with its many obscurities by such philosophers as Epicuros (341–270 BC), Euclid, Hipparchos (second century BC), and eventually by Ptolemy (AD second century) in Alexandria, and propagated to Arabic and thence to western medicine by the writings of Galen (AD 130–200), it claimed that vision was accomplished by the emission of a subtle "visual spirit" or "pneuma." This originated in the brain, the center of sensation and the seat of the ruling soul (probably located in the ventricles), circulated constantly through the hollow optic nerves (which were considered to be extensions of the brain itself) into the eye, and filled the crystalline lens from which it emanated in linear rays resembling sunlight (in the form of a cone) into space. In this view, the lens was the essential organ of vision, and the retina, a thinned expansion of the optic nerve, acted as a guide to enable the visual spirit to reach this vital organ and with its blood vessels also served as a means of nourishment to the vitreous and thus to the lens (Figure 2.6).

The alternative and rival view of Democrites (500 BC), accepted and elaborated by Aristotle, that light was an activity of an external ethereal substance originating from luminous or illuminated bodies, was largely ignored, although an attempt was made by Plato (429–327 BC) to combine the two opposing views in his somewhat vague concept that the rays of "inner light" emanating from the

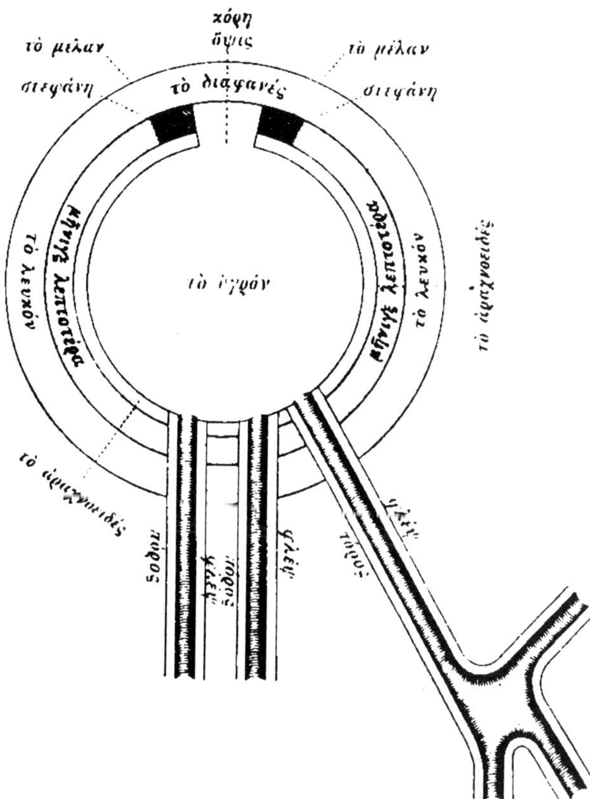

Fig. 2.6 The eye as understood in Hippocrates' time.

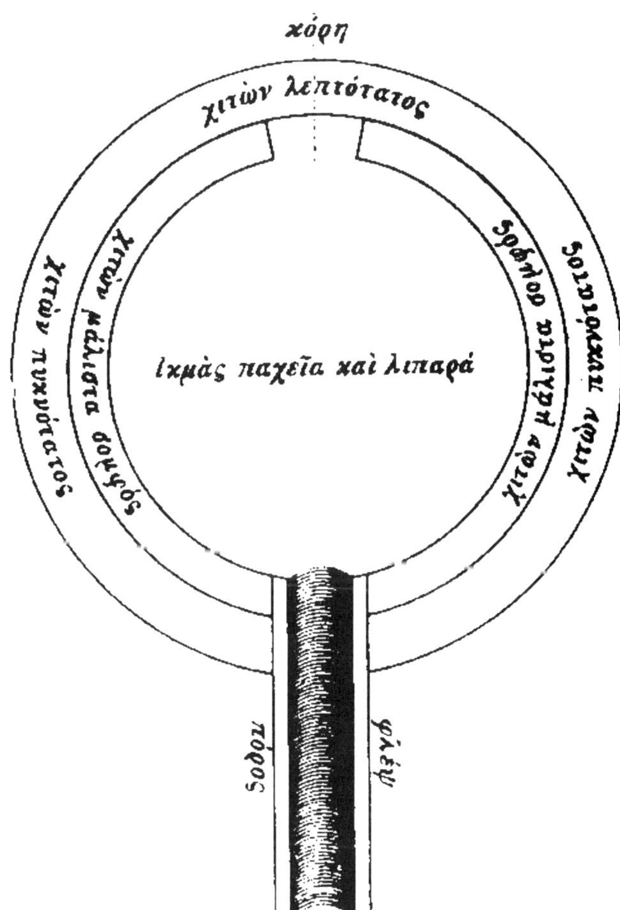

Fig. 2.7 The eye according to Democrites and as understood by Aristotle.

eye united with the rays of "outer light" emitted by the luminous object to accomplish the visual act. In this theory, if the corpuscles of inner light were sufficiently large to split up the outer light, the eye saw black; if they were small enough to be split up themselves, the eye saw white; colors emerged by different reactions of the two streams, and dazzling when the process of splitting occurred close to the eye. In either case vision centered upon the lens which acted as the essential organ of photoreception, a function conferred upon it by the circulating visual spirits (Figure 2.7).

Regardless that they may have differed in their opinions as to the nature of vision, the Alexandrian scholars seem to have agreed that light traveled in a straight line and at high speed. The major part of their knowledge of optics, however, concerned itself with catoptrics—the optics of mirrors or reflection (see also Chapter 4). It will suffice at present to say that the ancient scholars were hampered in their understanding of optics by their almost complete misunderstanding of vision and refraction, not to mention anatomy. Consequently, spectacles were also unknown to the Greeks.

The Roman period

In 30 BC, upon the death of the last of the Ptolemaic rulers—Cleopatra—Rome took over control of Egypt and the curtain fell on one of the glorious periods of medicine's history. Very little of Roman medicine was indigenous or original. All that was worthy of the name was Greek, practiced only by slaves, recently emancipated slaves or foreigners (Greeks or Egyptians), until the time of Julius Caesar. It was he who conferred Roman citizenship upon physicians resident in the Imperial City.

There were public lectures about medicine, but medical education was not regulated. There were no examinations, nor were the practicing physicians burdened with heavy responsibilities. Therefore many untrained and unskilled tried to practice the art. The income of well-known physicians was rather high. Not everything was always ethical. However, one should not believe everything that Pliny wrote—he hated *medici.*

It was Pliny who started the rumor that "the Emperor Nero used to observe the fights of the gladiators in an emerald." The much discussed paragraph in Pliny discusses only reflection, however. Nevertheless, emeralds are transparent and while some authors would have us believe that Nero viewed a reflection of the fights in the emerald with his back turned, as paranoid as he seemed to be, it is highly unlikely that he would sit with his back to armed men. The jury is still out on this but the emeralds were cut concave so that they acted like a mirror and produced an erect image—just what myopes need. If it was used in this dubious way then the episode represents the first known use of an optical aid to improve distance vision.

The most influential practitioner and writer of the Roman period was Claudius Galenus (Galen) of Pergamon (AD 130–200). Though the importance of his contribution to medicine can hardly be exaggerated, unfortunately it was not all to the good. His system was based on anatomic physiologic foundations, but permeated with the Hippocratic dogmas—especially those of humoral pathology—freely leavened with sophistry. To Hippocrates medicine was factual and what was unknown to him was freely acknowledged. Galen had no use for doubt and, where knowledge was lacking, metaphysics was called in as substitute. Everything was imbued with a divine purpose and each experimental observation had to be submitted to teleological analysis. This may seem naive but this view is still held subconsciously today. As von Bruecke put it: "teleology is a lady without whom no biologist can live; yet he is ashamed to show himself in public with her." Whereas Hippocrates had freed medicine from religious superstition, Galen, solving all problems and answering all questions, left it bound to dogma.

In Galen's view the retina was an expansion of the optic nerve which nourished the vitreous which in turn nourished the lens (Figure 2.8) [8]. This last—a tissue considered to be divine (*divinum oculi*)—was the essential organ of vision. From it visual emanations were emitted into outer space in the form of a cone to touch the objects seen; and from it also visual sensations were dispatched up the optic nerves to the mysterious third ventricle of the brain, the abode of the soul. To Galen the myope possessed a clear visual spirit but in too small a quantity to reach a distant object.

These two misconceptions—the sensory function of the lens and the emission hypothesis of vision dating from Pythagoras—although denied by Aristotle in the classical Greek period and later by Al-Hazen in the Middle Ages, dominated ophthalmologic thought and retarded the progress of the subject up to the time of Johannes Kepler in the 17th century [10]. Just as Galen himself idolized Hippocrates, so also was his system accepted throughout the medical world without question for nearly 15 centuries, partly because its theistic implications suited both Islam and Christendom and partly because his comprehensive works were available at a time when books were scarce. Of the 500 or so known works of Galen, 83 medical treatises have survived to this day (Figure 2.9). The unsettled conditions of the Middle Ages provided a fertile ground for his concepts to thrive. Unrest produced a longing for certainty and authority—an attitude especially prevalent in the Muslim East and the Christian West. Galen's dogmatic style, leaving no question unanswered, satisfied the desire for absolutes and his teleologic reasoning made his ideas easy for the Christian Church to embrace.

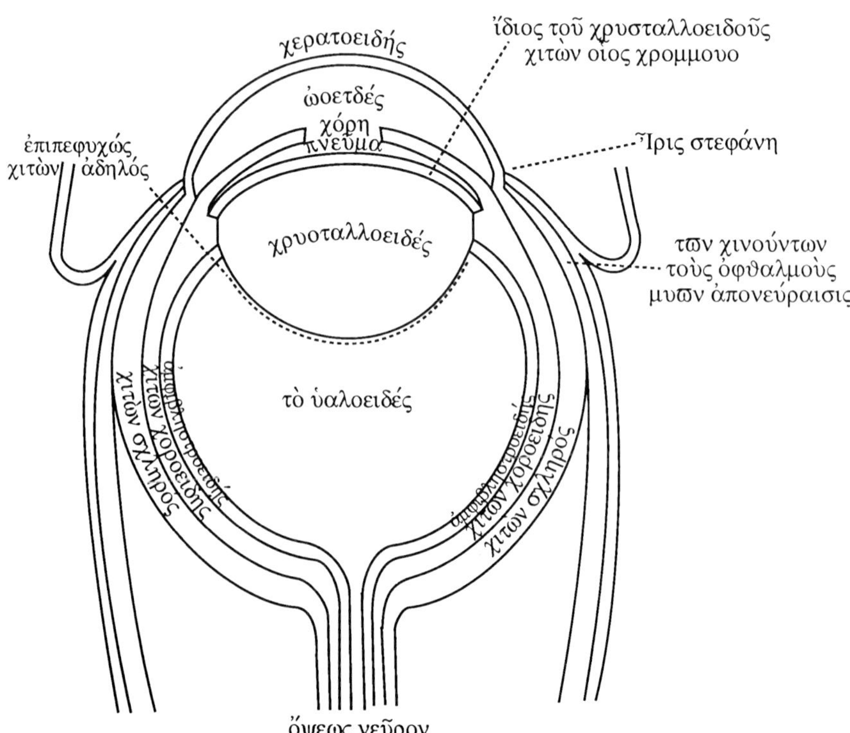

Fig. 2.8 The eye in the time of Galen.

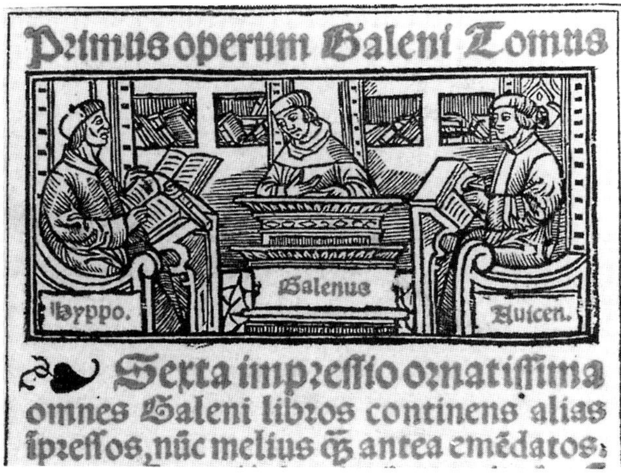

Fig. 2.9 Manuscript illustration showing Galen flanked by Hippocrates and Avicenna from an edition of the works of Galen published in 1528 (National Library of Medicine, Washington).

In the paralyzing atmosphere of clerical obscurantism which pervaded the Eastern Empire, all scientific investigation ceased. Little was added to ophthalmology and nothing at all to ocular anatomy. Finally, with the moral, economic, and physical decay of Rome and its fall to the barbarians in AD 455, the Dark Ages engulfed the west, lasting from the 5th to the 10th centuries.

It is possible, indeed, that much which had been gained to that point would have been lost had not the fanatical followers of Mohammed embraced science with the same enthusiasm with which they waged their religious wars. However, this Arabian renaissance of learning was preservative rather than creative, revering authority rather than observing and experimenting. Had not the Koran prohibited dissection, Mohammedan medicine might have been very different. Nevertheless, though largely borrowed from Greek sources, these Arabic writings were not by any means always uncritical and several new observations were made in that period.

Al-Hazen (Ibn Al-Hytham Al Basri), among his many varied writings, transformed this science in *The Book of Optics (Opticae Thesaurus)* and *De Luce*. The oldest extant diagram illustrating the eye and its central nervous connections is found in the latter book. Adopted by Al-Hazen's Persian commentator Kamal al-Din al-Farisi in 1316, it received wide publicity. In Al-Hazen's diagram the lens is more or less central and since it was considered the essential organ of vision the optic nerves ran directly to it (Figure 2.10).

Al-Hazen conducted experiments with plane, spherical, cylindrical and parabolic mirrors. Additionally, his studies of magnifying glasses brought him close to a rational theory of convex lenses. Of more importance, however, was the philosophical theory he presented on the nature of light; he discarded the emanation hypothesis and adopted the Aristotelian view that rays of light traveled from external objects into the eye (although Al-Razi had rejected the Pythagorian theory 100 years earlier) [11]:

> However, those who are convinced that vision consists in the formation of an image of the object which is produced within the eye have to assume that rays are propogated on a straight line from the object toward the center of the eye . . . The straight lines which extend from the center of the eye toward the viewed object are those which are used by the light beam [12].

However, he still placed the formation of the image on the anterior surface of the lens.

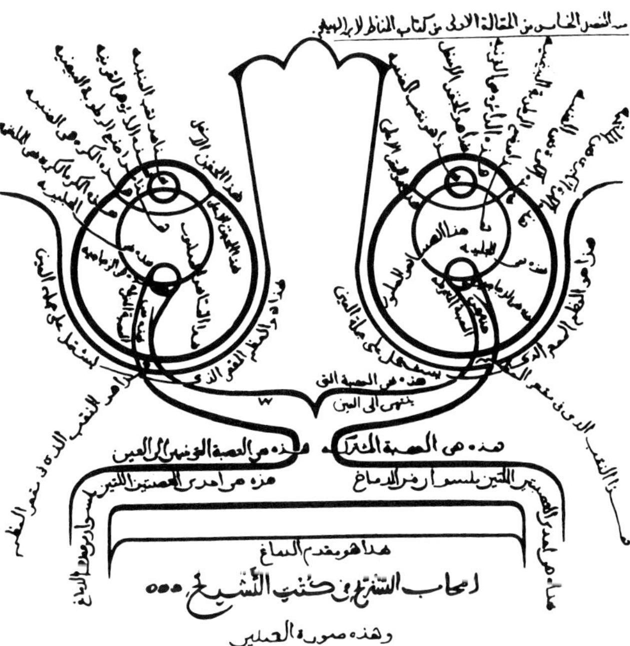

Fig. 2.10 The eye, from Al-Hazen's *Opticae Thesaurus*—AD 1038.

As to glasses and the treatment of refractive disorders, they had nothing to add. Even within the complete textbook of ophthalmology by Ali Bin Isa there is not the slightest mention of any concave or convex lenses but of ametropia there is a hint:

> A patient who sees well at distance but not at near (an affection which usually occurs in old patients) should keep a healthy lifestyle and should put styptic medication into his eye. A patient who sees well at near but not at distance should take liquid food and should sometimes use a salving medication into his eye [11].

Neither mirrors nor specially cut gemstones or glass are mentioned in the Arabic literature for the treatment of refractive disorders—certainly spectacles are not described.

The best that can be said for that period in medical history from the fall of the Byzantine Empire to the Renaissance is that it was a holy mess, quite literally. The traditional seat and focus of learning—the clergy (priests)—

were caught up in ecclesiastical pursuits of relics of the true cross or fragments of a saint's bones. The philosophical discussions, if any, concerned the pressing question of whether angels were male or female and how many could stand on the head of a pin. The medieval Christian God was portrayed as a rigid, nonphilosophic, gloomy, and intolerant God. The body was looked upon not as a temple for the soul and a manifestation of God's grace—it was rather an object of scorn not worth knowing nor saving. Disease was once again a punishment for sin, real or imaginary. Nature was overwhelmed by a supernaturalism which had in it no place for scientific observation; miracles were expected rather than reasoned therapeutics, fables credited before facts. Thus Galen fit right in—the main reason for his influence over the centuries: his was "right" thinking.

Physicians of the time were forced to rely on works which were poor copies of the Arabic references. Typically slavishly copied by ignorant and probably lazy scribes working under conditions of poor lighting and poorer health, they abounded in mistakes. The crude drawings of the Arabic literature—transliterated from Greek texts—were reduced to meaningless circles and lines (Figure 2.11). Knowledge of the function of the eye was stagnated by the persistent belief that the lens was the visual receptor and by the Pythagorean concept that visual rays emanated from the eye itself. Anatomic studies which would eventually lead to decipherment of this mysterious organ were stymied by the interdiction of dissection. In an age which featured the Inquisition and encouraged death and torture in God's name, there was an absolute horror of the anatomist's knife.

The church was not totally successful in stamping out the rational spirit however. Within the maelstrom there appeared, over time, small islands of enlightenment and reason which withstood the assault of conformity. Ironically, but not surprisingly, some of the first chinks in the wall were created by members of the establishment itself—the clergy—representing as they typically do the most educated of the prevailing society. Through these cracks began a trickle of rationality which enlarged into a torrent and which eventually led to that second golden period of human existence—the Renaissance.

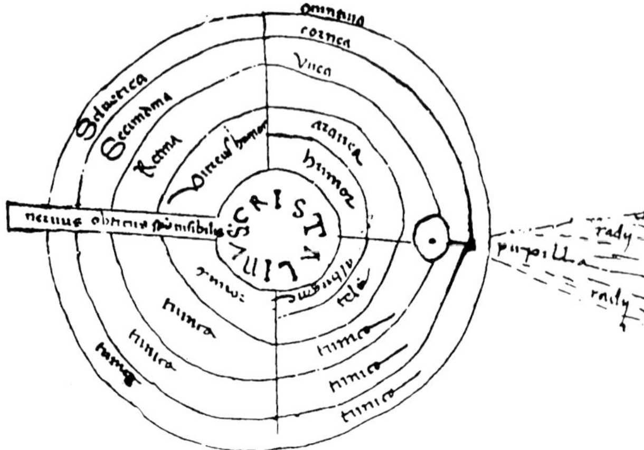

Fig. 2.11 The eye at the beginning of the Renaissance. Redrawn from the *Codex Trivultanius* (14th century).

Roger Bacon

Roger Bacon (1214–1294)—*doctor mirabilis*—a Franciscan friar and philosopher at Oxford was one of the most notable of the early writers who swam against the mainstream. A product of an aristocratic family, he studied philosophy and science at the University at Oxford and then in Paris, joining the Franciscan order where in 1250 he became a monk. That was bad judgment for he was temperamentally unsuited for the contemplative life of a friar. His fractiousness, particularly with respect to educational reform within the Franciscan order, led to his censure and eventual incarceration where he was provided with ample time to contemplate his sins. He took advantage of the opportunity to compile a reference work on scientific knowledge. Upon his release by Pope Clemens in 1267, he dedicated his *Opus Majus* (as well as his *Minus* and *Tertium*) to his benefactor. In this work he commented upon the phenomenon of magnification as gleaned from the writings of Al-Hazen. He suggested that the difficulty experienced by the aged in seeing near objects was due to an increase of moisture in the eye and a wrinkling of the cornea resembling the wrinkling in the aged skin. He suggested as a remedy the magnification given by a segment of a sphere of glass or crystal when laid upon the letters to be read; by such means, he said, the "smallest particles of sand or dust could be seen."

> If anyone examine letters or other minute objects through the medium of crystal or glass or other transparent substance, if it be shaped like the lesser segment of a sphere, with the convex side towards the eye, and the eye being in the air, he will see the letters far better, and they will seem larger to him. For according to our canon concerning a spherical medium beneath which the object is placed, the centre being beyond the object, the convexity being towards the eye, all causes agree to increase the size, for the angle in which it is seen in greater, the image is greater, and the position of the image is nearer, because the object is between the eye and the centre. For this reason such an instrument is useful to old persons and to those with weak eyes, for they can see any letter, however small, if magnified enough.
>
> For we can so form glasses and so arrange them with regard to our sight and to objects that the rays are refracted and deflected to any place we wish, so that we see the object near at hand or far away beneath whatever angle we desire. And so we can read the smallest letters or count grains of sand or

> dust from an incredible distance owing to the magnitude of the angle beneath which we see them, and again the largest objects close at hand might be scarcely visible owing to the smallness of the angle beneath which we see them; for it is on the size of the angle on which this kind of vision depends, and it is independent of distance save per accidens. So a boy can appear a giant, a man seem a mountain, and in any size of angle whatever, for we can see a man under as large an angle as though he were a mountain and make him appear as near as we desire. So a small army might seem very large, and though far away appear near, and conversely: so, too, we could make sun, moon and stars apparently descend here below, and similarly appear above the heads of our enemies, and many other similar marvels could be brought to pass, that the ignorant mortal mind could not endure the truth (*Opus Majus,* Part V).

Bacon's idea of a "glass" was a handled, segmented sphere to be used as a reading aid. He sent such a glass to Pope Clemens in 1267. This does not make Bacon the inventor of spectacles as some claim, however, because other than the reading glass mentioned (which does not qualify as a spectacle) he apparently never carried out any practical experiments of his ideas (Figure 2.12).

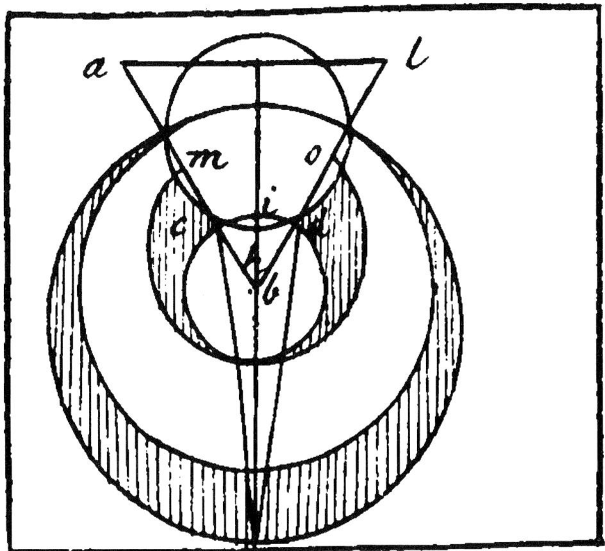

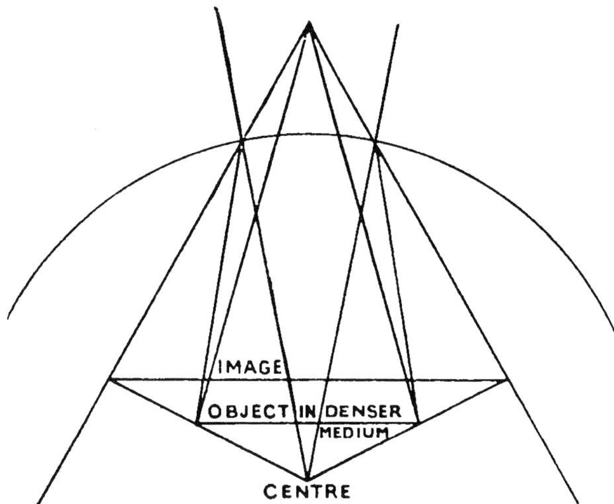

Fig. 2.12 (a) Roger Bacon's drawing of the eye from his *Opus Majus*, 1268. (b) Roger Bacon's diagram of a planoconvex lens. The diagram is wrong, but the idea is there.

Spectacles

Spectacles as we know them did not make an appearance until sometime around 1276 in Venice, Italy. It is possible that Bacon's idea made its way to the glass capital of Europe but the exact inventor is not known with certainty. The premise that Europeans learned of spectacles from the Chinese, however, is not tenable even though they are supposed to have been mentioned in the memoirs of Marco Polo. Polo's ventures lasted from 1271 to 1295 but the *Travels* were not dictated until 3 years later and were revised 9 years after that; by that time spectacles had been in use in Europe for several years [11]. In any case, nowhere in Polo's original writings are spectacles mentioned [13].

The first authenticated mention of spectacles is in a collection of minstrel's ballads dating from 1280. In 1305, according to Francesco Redi, Brother Giordano da Rivalto, of the Order of St Dominic stated in a sermon: "Not even 20 years have passed since the art to make spectacles has been invented. These help us to see and this is one of the greatest and most necessary inventions the world has seen" [14]. Redi also mentions in one of his letters not the inventor, but the reinventor of spectacles:

> In the library of the Dominican Monastery of Santa Caterina in Pisa there is an old manuscript which represents the chronicle of this monastery. Within this manuscript, the following comments are found: "Brother Alexander de Spina of Pisa could make with his hands whatever he wanted to. He preached charity to others. When somebody invented the glasses and it was proven to be a useful invention nobody could make other spectacles. Then our good brother started making spectacles without a teacher and taught this procedure to others who wanted to learn it" [11,14].

Whoever the inventor may really have been, the following interesting inscription is found on a grave stone from the churchyard of Santa Maria Maggiore (Figure 2.13):

> Here lies Salvino d'Armato of the Armati of Florence
> Inventor of the spectacles.
> God pardon him for his sins.
> AD 1317

QUI DIACE
SALVINO D ARMATO DEGLI ARMATI
DI FIRENZE
ANNO D MCCCXVII

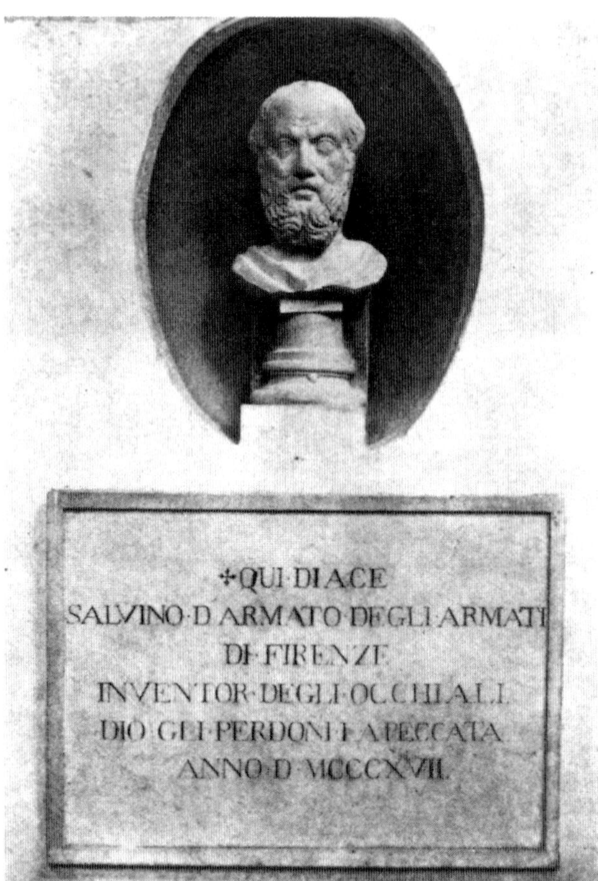

Fig. 2.13 Tombstone of Salvino d'Armato, inventor of spectacles—1317.

Certainly spectacles were well known by 1300 although still expensive and somewhat of a novelty, not becoming popular until the 15th century—the advent of printing. Medical manuscripts mention spectacles only from this time on (Figure 2.14). Even then they were not widely prescribed by physicians. In the *Lilium Medicinae* (1305) of Bernard of Gordon, he described the use of a collyrium of such strength "that it makes old people read the smallest print again without that they need to use spectacles (*oculus berrelerius*)" [15]. Guy de Chauliac (1300–1368) of Lyons mentions in his *Chirurgie* of 1363 first some good medications against poor vision and then adds, less cynically: "If this does not work one has to turn to the spectacles" [16,17].

Furthermore, such spectacles as existed were only available for presbyopia (hyperopia was confused with presbyopia and thought only to occur in the aged—the myope was doomed to suffer for some 200–300 years more (Figure 2.15). They were also prescribed for aphakic patients but the problem was still considered to be presbyopia. Hollerius, the famous French professor (1553), was supposedly the first physician who prescribed them for myopes [11]. However, it has only been since the

Linea der biſchoff
Zaraya

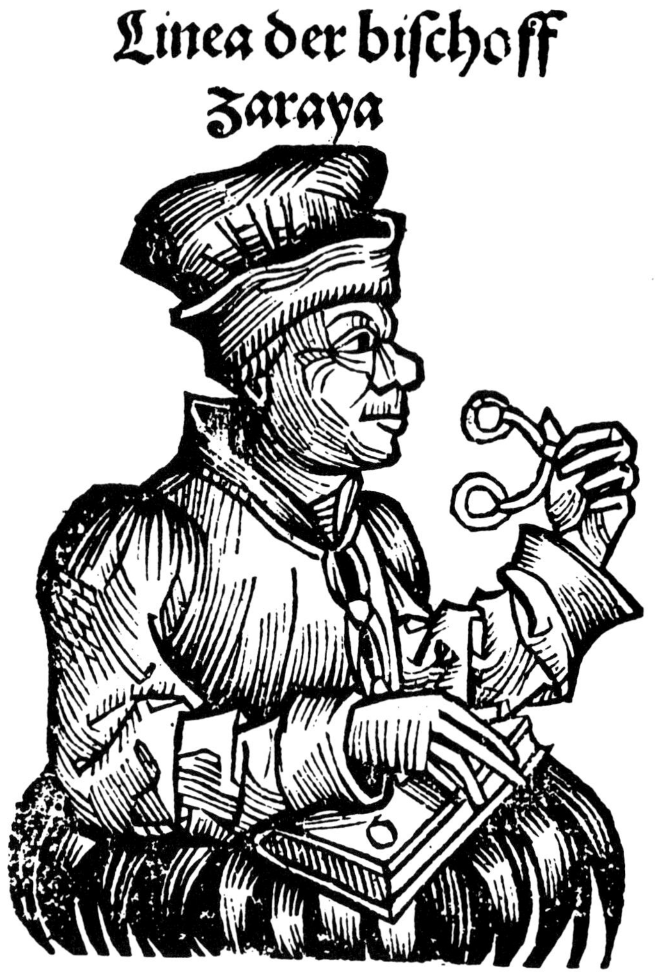

Fig. 2.14 The first printed illustration of spectacles—Schedel, *Liber Chronicarum*—Nürnburg, 1493 (Countway Library, Harvard School of Medicine).

middle of the 19th century that ophthalmologists have seriously involved themselves in the selection and calculation of lenses. Moreover, cylindric lenses were only produced in the 19th century—probably because of an incomplete understanding of the optics of the eye which still prevailed.

Felix Platter

Felix Platter (1539–1614) altered the whole of the theory of ophthalmic optics by advancing the revolutionary view, already suggested four centuries previously by Ibn Rushd, that the retina and not the lens was the visual receptor. Platter proved his thesis by showing that vision was still possible after severing the zonule through which the visual impulses were supposed to pass from the lens to the retina and optic nerve [18]. For the first time the lens was thus accurately described as the dioptric mechanism and the retina as the photoreceptor. This view was

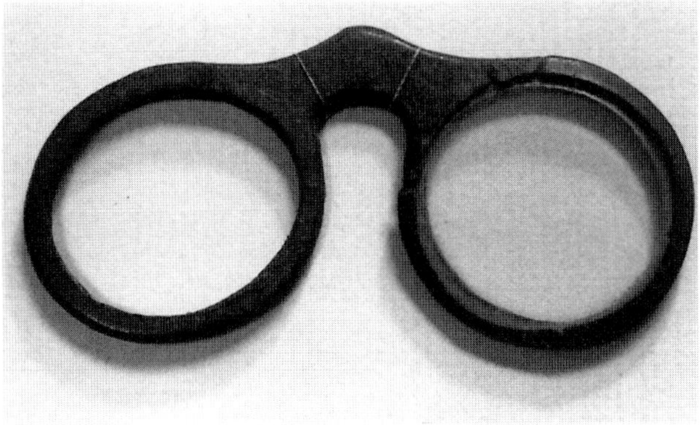

Fig. 2.15 Leather spectacle frames, circa 1400 (American Academy of Ophthalmology).

proved by Christopher Scheiner, by the simple expedient of observing an image formation after the sclera and choroid had been removed from an eye. Descartes repeated this experiment by cutting off the back of an ox eye and observing the image on a piece of paper [19].

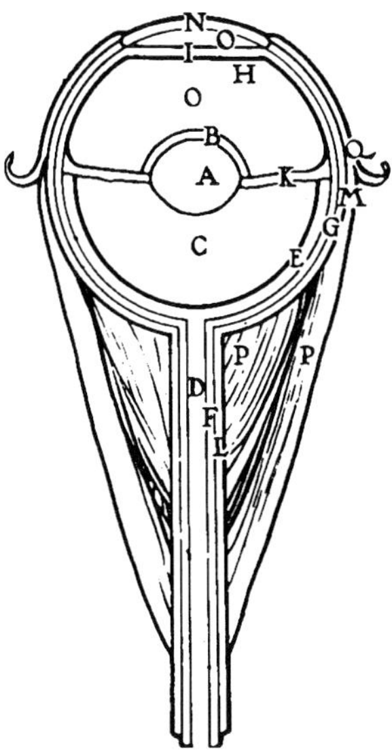

Fig. 2.17 The eye at the time of Kepler. From Vesalius' *De humani Corpus Fabrica*, 1543, Basel.

Johannes Kepler

The optics of myopia, however, were not clearly explained until the 17th century by Johannes Kepler (the founder of dioptrics) in his classical works, *Ad Vitellionem Paralipomena* (A Supplement to Vitello, 1604) and *Dioptrice* (1611) [20–23]. In the first treatise, Kepler applied his vast optical and mathematical skills to the problem, demonstrating the role of both the lens and the cornea in vision and again placing the inverted image on to the retina where it belonged (Figure 2.16). Kepler's anatomy of the eye, however, was drawn from Platter and Aquapendente and is quite similar to that of Vesalius and thus adheres to the Galenic view (Figure 2.17). He described the curvature of an image cast by a lens secondary to the stronger refractive power of its periphery than its center—220 years before Airy. He defined the action of concave and convex lenses upon this system, although he only approximated the laws of refraction which were finally codified by Snell.

In the second treatise—a mere 80 pages in length—he revolutionized contemporary thinking on optics. In his initial clarification of ophthalmic dioptrics he correctly assumed that in myopia, the incident light was brought to a focus in front of the retina, a view subsequently accepted by Isaac Newton 100 years later. Both of these pioneers in optics also considered myopia and presbyopia to be antitheses.

> Those who see clearly at distance but indistinctly at near are helped by convex spectacles, and those who see poorly at distance but well at near are helped by concave spectacles. How amazing that while the practical use of this fact is so widespread, its scientific cause remained obscure.

Kepler, himself myopic, also wrote about accommodation but did not identify it as such. In this area of his writings there is a considerable degree of confusion as a result of his inability to appreciate the fact that presbyopia occurred in both myopia and hyperopia. Kepler attributed the ability to see clearly at both distance and near to alterations in the shape of the eye, proposing that the lens moved backwards and forwards (through changes in the length of the eye) to provide clear near and far vision.

> It is impossible for the retina, which is fixed within the eye, to perceive clear images simultaneously from near and far. Some see well at distance, some at near. Those who see everything confused have imperfect eyes due to faulty structure. In those who see everything distinctly, either the retina or the lens must change its position relative to one another.
>
> It is probable that in young and healthy eyes the globe is alternately compressed and dilated at the equator when vision shifts to different distances.

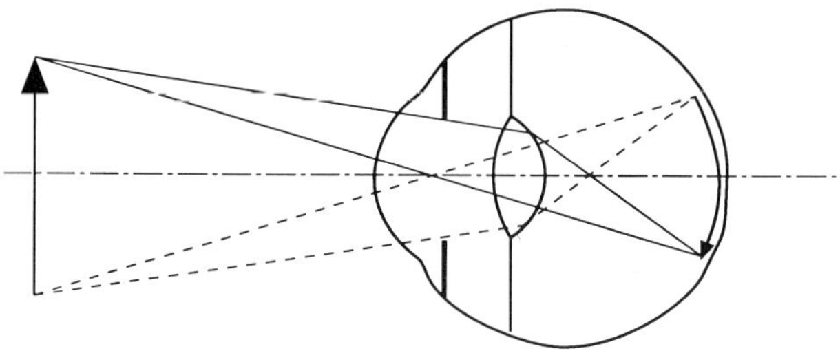

Fig. 2.16 Kepler's refraction of the eye—from his *Ad Vitellionem Paralipomena*, 1604.

Kepler attributed this action to the ciliary processes which act like a muscle. When they contract the equator is pulled inward and the eye becomes elongated, as happens in encirclage for retinal detachments. In this case Kepler deduced that the retina had to be moved back in order for a near object to be seen clearly. Kepler made all his observations through deduction only—as he told a friend: "I am no empiricist concerned with the accumulation of observed data" [20]. Hence he could probably never get his work published in today's journals which require original data and documented facts. But as Dewey wrote: "Every great advance in science has issued from a new audacity of imagination" (John Dewey—*The Quest for Certainty*).

He went on to propound the "near-work" hypothesis for myopia by stating that study and fine work in childhood rapidly accustom the eye to near objects. According to Kepler, with advancing years this adaptive mechanism produces a permanent, finite far point such that distant objects are seen poorly:

> It is false that only old people see poorly at near and the young at distance. Both conditions may occur at all ages [here is an important observation and a clue to hyperopia—which he missed]. With age, however, the power of changing the view from distance to near weakens, and hence those with healthy eyes at youth see well only at distance. Furthermore, it is more natural and less tiring to hold the eyes parallel rather than converged on near objects. Therefore, too, tired old eyes remain focused for distance. Those who do much close work in their youth become myopic.

This theory led to the formation of "myopia schools" in later years and is still very much in evidence today.

Plempius

Vopiscus Fortunatus Plempius, professor of therapeutics at Loewen in Holland, described anatomically the unusual distance between the lens and the retina in myopic eyes [24]. This view was confirmed by Georg Albert Hamberger, professor of mathematics at Jena who also correctly described the phenomenon of "second sight" in the aged with an early cataract—100 years before it was rediscovered by Demours and others [25].

Boerhaave

Hermann Boerhaave of Leyden, who was the first university professor to teach the correct concept of vision as well as Kepler's explanation of myopia and hyperopia, attributed the defect of myopia to either an increased convexity of the cornea or the undue length of the globe. This latter cause was factually confirmed by Morgagni and Scarpa among others [26,27]. Still other causes that were postulated were an increase in the thickness of the lens, an increase in its refractive index, and a change in its position. Boerhaave's picture is shown here (Figure 2.18), though for quite another reason. In 1708 he made the observation that since after cataract surgery, myopes see quite clearly without lenses, it seemed reasonable to treat myopia by extracting the clear lens: "This will allow the eye to focus the rays onto the retina, whereas, before the operation the focus was in front of the retina" [28]. This is the earliest reference to this technique that the author could find. Clearly, Fukala did not invent this technique—of which we will have more to say in Chapter 13.

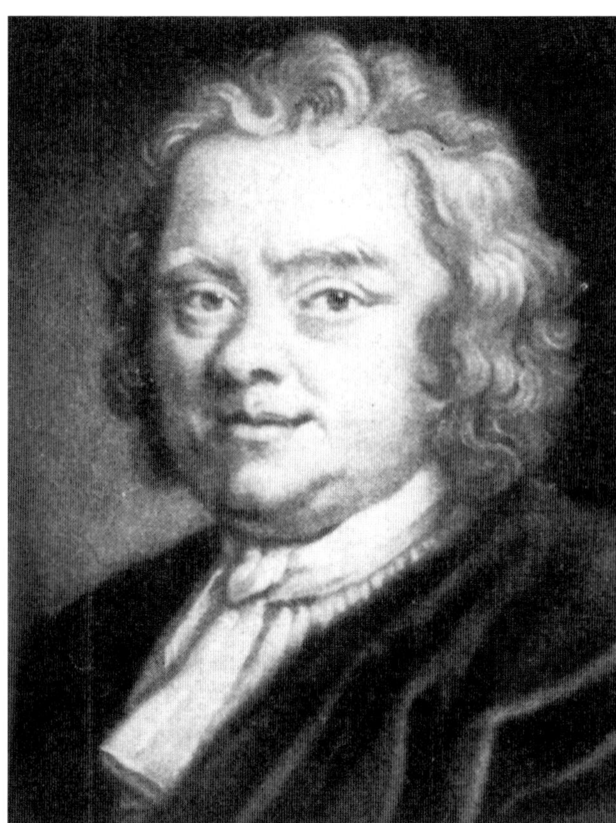

Fig. 2.18 Hermann Boerhaave (1708)—the first to suggest clear lens extraction for myopia (Mary & Edward Norton Library, Bascom Palmer Eye Institute).

Hyperopia

Since the refractive power of the cornea is largely abolished when it is immersed in water, divers become so hyperopic that clear vision is impossible. This is, in fact, the method whereby Young discovered his astigmatism. Benito Daza de Valdes prescribed convex lenses for distant as well as for near vision in the aged—in fact, such use was described in his book *Uso de los Antojos y Comentarios a Propósito del Mismo* (Figure 2.19) [29]. The first optical explanation of the anomaly, however, was not made until 1696 by Hamberger who described the phenomenon

VSO
DE LOS ANTOIOS
PARA TODO GENERO DE VISTAS:
En que se enseña a conocer los grados que a cada vno le faltan de su vista, y los que tienen qualesquier antojos.

Y ASSI MISMO A QVE TIEMPO SE AN de vsar, y como se pediran en ausencia, con otros auisos importantes, a la vtilidad y conseruacion de la vista.

POR EL L. BENITO DAÇA DE VALDES, Notario de el Santo Oficio de la Ciudad de Sevilla.

DEDICADO A NVESTRA SEÑORA de la Fuensanta de la Ciudad de Cordoua.

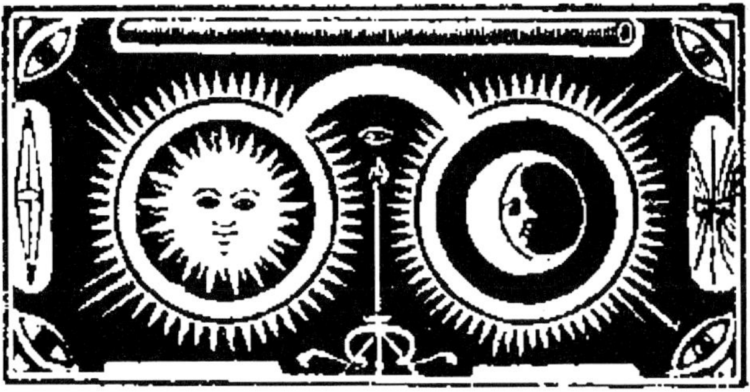

CON PRIVILEGIO
Impresso en Seuilla, por Diego Perez. Año de 1623.

Fig. 2.19 Title page of Valdes' book on the use of spectacles to treat far-sight (1623).

as occurring sometimes in the young as well as congenitally [30]. However, long-sight was still considered identical with presbyopia. The latter was thus explained by Newton:

> If the Humours of the eye by old age decay, so as by shrinking to make the Cornea and the Coat of the Crystalline Humour grow flatter than before, the Light will not be refracted enough, and for want of a sufficient Refraction will not converge to the bottom of the Eye but to some place beyond it . . . This is the reason for the decay of sight in old Men and shews why their Sight is mended by Spectacles. For their Convex glasses supply the defect of plumpness in the Eye, and by increasing the Refraction make the Rays converge sooner, so as to convene at the bottom of the Eye if the Glass have a due degree of convexity. And the contrary happens in short-sighted Men whose Eyes are too plump. For the Refraction being now too great, the Rays converge and convene in the eyes before they come to the bottom . . . unless the Object be brought so near to the Eye as that the place where the converging Rays convene may be removed to the bottom . . . or the Refraction is diminished by a Concave-glass of a due degree of concavity [31].

With Newton's concept of hyperopia as a condition due to parallel rays of light converging *behind* the retina, the stage was set for the acceptance of the axial length of the eye as the sole determinant of refraction, thereby opening a floodgate of speculation.

The same theme was described and illustrated by the great mathematician of Cambridge, Robert Smith [32]. Kastner, professor of mathematics at Leipzig, in his annotated translation of Smith's book, called the optical state in long-sighted individuals *hyperpresbytas* [33]. The general outline of the optics of long-sight, still described as presbyopia, also was understood by Thomas Young, who stated clearly:

> A convex lens is necessary for far-sighted or presbyopic eyes. And it often happens that the rays must be made not only to diverge less than before, but even to converge towards a focus behind such an eye, in order to make its vision distinct.

This is probably the first unequivocal description of hyperopia. From the clinical point of view Janin distinguished three types of sight—normal, short-sight, and long-sight, "the first two occurring naturally and the third fortuitous and occurring only in old people" [34].

Many investigators conducted studies on the axial length during that period. Morgagni [26], Guerin, Geudron, and Pichter [35] and some—Scarpa [27] and von Ammon [36]—noted posterior staphylomas but did not associate them particularly with myopia. It wasn't until 1856, in an excellent monograph by von Arlt [37], that a convincing association was made, though it had been suggested 2 years before by von Graefe [38] in a combined ophthalmoscopic and anatomical study of two eyes measuring 29 mm and 30.5 mm in length.

As a consequence of these studies, the greatest efforts of the ophthalmologic community were concentrated on a search for the causes of the increased axial length of the eye. That this search became indiscriminate and almost absurd can be appreciated by a review of the early theories of the etiology of myopia. It is interesting to read the medical papers of that era and note the plethora of treatises on the causes and nature of myopia. It resembles, in some ways, the feeding frenzy of sharks in its irrationality, ferocity, and redundancy of attack. It has its parallels even today, in a more "enlightened" time.

In 1793, Young had described the mechanism of accommodation in which he posited that the lens was a muscular organ. In this same paper, while discussing the fibers within an ox lens, he declared that sclerosis of these fibers with age explains, at least partially, presbyopia [39]. Young retracted his muscular lens theory in his next publication but stated that the lens did have the ability to change its shape [40]. He proved this by using his optometer with aphakic patients, finding that the refractive power remained absolutely stationary.

In 1813, Ware made it clear that long-sight was not necessarily associated with presbyopia. He described "young persons who have so disproportionate a convexity of the cornea or crystalline, or of both, to the distance of these parts of the retina, that a glass of considerable convexity is required to enable them to see distinctly, not only near objects, but also those that are distant" [41]. Such an idea, however, was not well understood, and some ascribed such a visual defect to asthenopia until Stellwag von Carion gave a relatively clear account along with an optical explanation in 1855 [42,43]. Nevertheless, it was left to Franz Donders to establish the optical nature and frequent occurrence of hyperopia and point out its differentiation from presbyopia [44].

Astigmatism

While the optics of astigmatism were briefly described by Kepler in 1604, the first clinical description of this problem was made by Young in 1801 (Figure 2.20), by practicing Scheiner's experiment (see below) and finding that he had 3.94 D of myopia in the vertical meridian and 5.62 D in the horizontal [19,40]. Curiously, he did nothing to follow up his discovery. Young, a Quaker, was one of those singular human phenomena that occur sporadically through time. After qualifying in medicine, he went on to make major contributions in physiologic optics, the theory of light, and the deciphering of Egyptian hieroglyphics and the Rosetta Stone. At the age of 19 he read his first paper, on the accommodation of the eye, to the Royal Society [39]. In a course of lectures given while professor of natural philosophy at the Royal Institution, the definition of the familiar Young's modulus of elasticity was given as well as the wave theory of light.

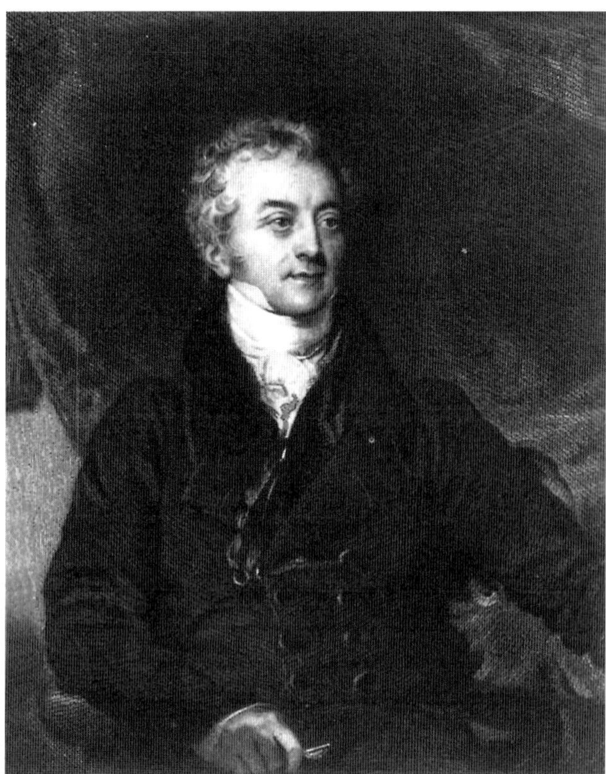

Fig. 2.20 Thomas Young, ophthalmologist and natural philosopher (Countway Library, Harvard School of Medicine).

The introduction of astigmatic lenses, however, had to wait until Sir George Biddell Airy. Airy, 24 years after Young, described the astigmatic change that had occurred in his own eyes, and to correct it designed and had made an astigmatic spectacle lens [45]. The name astigmatism itself was suggested to Airy in 1849 by the Reverend Whewall, who was then professor of mathematics and philosophy at Cambridge.

In those days, astigmatism was considered an oddity and worthy of notice and report. Several such cases were reported in 1847 by Sir William Hamilton of Dublin, visually characterized by the distinctness of horizontal and the indistinctness of vertical lines, and also by Henry Goode the same year. One case was reported from Europe by Schnyder [46] in 1849, who corrected the error in his own eyes by astigmatic lenses, and three by Isaac Hays in the American edition of *Lawrence's: A Treatise on Diseases of the Eye* [47]. One of the cases described by Hays is of particular interest because it represents the first instance of astigmatism treated by spectacles in the New World. A Reverend Goodrich managed to figure out the cause of his weakened sight and had lenses ground to correct it [48].

The optics and the importance of the defect were clearly defined by Donders in 1864 [44]. Generally speaking, very little was done to deal with the problem until the beginning of the 20th century when Jackson fitted the first spherocylinder spectacles. Prior to these attempts, astigmatism was compensated for by fitting spherical spectacles alone—a compromise at best. In 1869, Snellen, in an article published in the German literature, discussed the possibilities of surgically correcting corneal astigmatism. Bates, in 1894 [49], detailed a surgical technique for such modification and reported a number of cases, as did Lans in 1898 [50]. We will have more to say about these gentlemen when we examine more thoroughly the subject of the surgical correction of astigmatism in Chapter 9.

Ametropia

The nature of ametropia is an extensive subject, and complete coverage would require an entire book—something not in my mandate. The reader is referred to the section on further reading for assistance in that regard. It is within my mandate, however, to discuss ametropia in some detail in order to more completely understand attempts to correct it. Thus I will hit the high points, defining ametropia as well as presenting a sketch of its prevalence and development and how it impacts on the human condition. An understanding of the nature of ametropia is an essential precursor to any attempt to correct it, be it by surgery or any other method.

In the physiologically normal eye, parallel light rays converge to form a principal focus on the retina; when these ideal optical conditions occur with the eye in a state of rest, the condition is termed *emmetropia*. Since the principal focus is of a size approximating a point and lies in one plane, such a system is also called *stigmatic* (from the Greek meaning point or mark). Since this requires a rather precise correspondence of all the optical components of the eye, it would, as so aptly expressed by Duke-Elder,

> . . . be strange indeed if this were a common state of affairs, for its attainment depends on an almost perfect correlation of such measurements as the length of the eye and the shape of the cornea and the lens. Such regularity and conformity to optical perfection necessitates a mathematical accuracy which is nowhere realized in the constitution of living organisms. Emmetropia may be optically normal, but it is no more biologically normal than would be the universal attainment of a uniform height of 5 feet 6 inches [51].

In fact, its opposite condition, *ametropia*, wherein light rays are not focused exactly on to a single point at rest, is by far the more common. With more exact means of measuring, emmetropia is found to be very rare indeed. However, if small errors in refraction are neglected (up to 0.25 D), most people are emmetropic or very nearly so. An examination of a large series of patients reveals that emmetropic cases are more prevalent than would be predicted and that the incidence of myopia is disproportionately excessive. The relative incidence of refractive errors is shown in Figure 2.21.

Complicating this picture is the fact that the refracting components of the eye are not symmetrically arranged around a common axis, and even if a reasonable facsimile of one could be constructed, the fovea would not be on it. Furthermore, the refracting surfaces are highly aspheric. In any event, even in the best of circumstances, the focus of the eye is not a discrete point but rather a diffusion circle of measurable diameter. Considering the imperfections that exist within the optical components of the eye, it is no wonder that von Helmholtz stated:

> If an optician should try to sell me an instrument possessing the faults mentioned above, it seems to me—without overstressing the matter—that I should think myself wholly justified in using the most severe language with regard to the carelessness of his work and returning the instrument under protest [52].

Classification of ametropia

Ametropia has three main subdivisions or types: hyperopia, myopia, and astigmatism. In *hyperopia* (or *hypermetropia*), the rays of light come to a focus behind the retina. The eye is said to be relatively too short (see section on hyperopia, below). In the opposite case, the eye is relatively too long, and the focus occurs in front of the retina. Such a condition is termed *myopia* and is by far the greatest part of ametropia (see section on myopia, below). In the event that conditions are such that the rays of light converge to not one but several foci, such a condition is nonstigmatic or, as commonly termed, *astigmatic*. The various foci may, in turn, lie entirely before the retina—compound myopic astigmatism; wholly behind the retina—compound hyperopic astigmatism; or partly before and partly behind—mixed astigmatism (see sec-

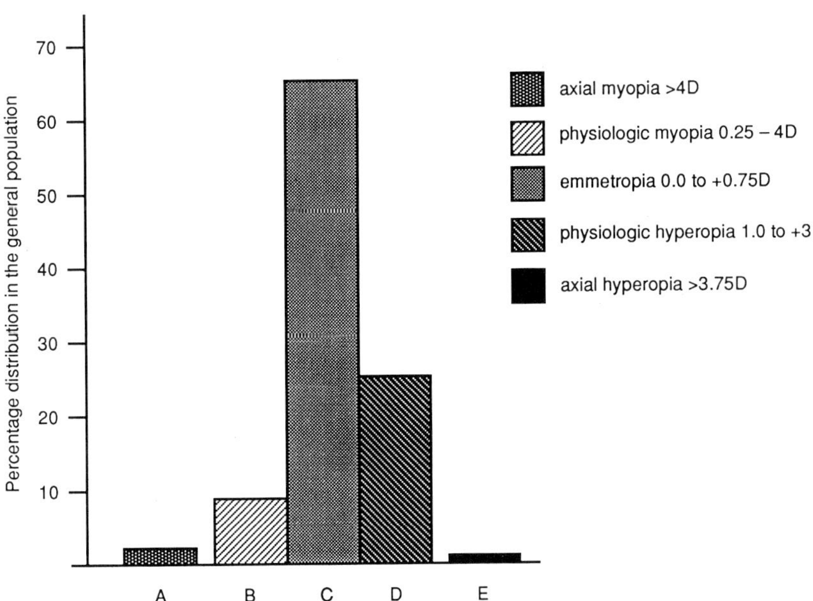

Fig. 2.21 Percentage incidence of ametropia in the general population (from Stromberg. Refraction and axial length of human eyes. Acta Ophthalmol, 1936).

tion on astigmatism, below). There can be a number of different causes for any one of these conditions to exist, or in some instances, all three may occur in a single eye. The following classification is after Duke-Elder and will serve to introduce the reader to the subject [51]. It will be expanded on in the individual sections that follow.

Ametropia due to positional anomalies

The eye may be of a length which does not correlate with the corneal curvature or the lens may be malpositioned.
1 If the axial length of the eye is too long relative to the power of the cornea and lens, the resulting myopia is said to be of the *axial type*. In this case, the corneal curvature is relatively too steep.
2 Conversely, if the eye is too short, the corneal curvature is said to be relatively too flat and axial hyperopia exists.
3 If the lens is dislocated forward, the principal focus is also moved forward of the retina, and myopia will result; if backward, hyperopia results. This can occur in a traumatic recessed angle.

Anomalies of the refractive surfaces

The curvature of the cornea or of the lens may be too steep, giving a curvature myopia, or too flat, giving a curvature hyperopia, or be toroidal (toric surfaces are discussed more thoroughly in Chapter 3), varying in different meridians, giving astigmatism. Typically, a greater and (relatively) lesser curvature of the surface can be identified (major and minor meridians) simultaneously (see section on astigmatism, below).
1 If the major and minor meridians are at right angles to one another, the condition is called *regular astigmatism* and the refractive surface has the properties of a regular toroidal lens.
2 If they are not so related, the astigmatism may be called *bioblique* [53]. I term this condition *asymmetrical astigmatism*, preferring to confine the term *oblique* to describe astigmatic axes other than at 90 or 180°.
3 In some cases there may be no symmetry whatsoever in the system. In these instances, the rays may form foci at different positions which may not be aligned on the optic axis nor lie in a single plane. This occurs, for example, in the cornea after corneal ulceration or in the lens in developing cataract. The astigmatism is termed *irregular*, and the surface possesses the characteristics of an irregular toroidal lens.

Since the latter two are asymmetric toroidal surfaces not easily corrected by spectacle lenses, they are usually grouped together as *irregular astigmatism*.

Obliquity of the system elements

The refractive elements may not be aligned with the optic center or may be rotated.

Lenticular obliquity. If the lens is placed obliquely or subluxated, astigmatism will result.

Retinal obliquity. The posterior pole of the eye may be placed obliquely, as when it bulges backwards in a staphyloma in high myopia, and if the summit of the staphyloma does not correspond to the fovea the rays do not fall upon this region perpendicularly. If the focus were a point this would be without effect, but since it is a diffusion circle the obliquity will deform and increase it, thus diminishing visual acuity.

It is likely, as well, that the latter two conditions will produce astigmatism of the irregular variety. In these cases, compensation by either spectacles or contact lenses may not be possible.

Anomalies of the refractive index

The refractive index of the transparent media may be abnormal.
1 If the refractive index of the aqueous humor is too low, or that of the vitreous humor is too high, there will be an index hyperopia. This can happen when silicone oil is used to replace vitreous during retinal detachment surgery. Conversely, if the refractive index of the aqueous is too high, as in certain types of iridocyclitis (this has also been postulated as one of the reasons for induced myopia in the uncontrolled diabetic) or that of the vitreous too low (gas replacement in retinal detachment surgery or liquefaction of the vitreous gel), there will be an index myopia.
2 If the refractive index of the lens as a whole is too low, the light is bent less, and there will be index hyperopia. If the index of the cortex increases relatively and approximates that of the nucleus, as it does normally with age, the lens tends to act as a single refractive element with flatter refractive surfaces, and consequently has less converging power than normal; the eye therefore becomes hyperopic. Conversely, if the refractive power of the nucleus increases, as frequently occurs in early cataract, index myopia is produced. Such induced myopia offsets the normal presbyopia and produces the phenomenon called in the laity "second sight." In this case the patient finds that he or she is able to read much better without spectacles than before—in fact, may be able to dispense with them entirely. If the increase in the refractive index of the nucleus is very marked a false lenticonus may be produced wherein the central part of the pupil is myopic and the periphery hyperopic. In these cases the patient may find that both near and distant vision is relatively clear and may be able to function—for a time at least—without bifocals.

Absence of system element

The absence of the lens produces extreme hyperopia. Astigmatism of the against-the-rule variety is almost always present following wide incision cataract surgery as well but is reported less and less as the incisions have become smaller [54,55].

Many of the definitions just given in this classification of refractive anomalies are much too simplistic and require qualification. The concept of an eye which is too long or too curved or has any other physical or geometric abnormality of optical significance leads by implication to the notion that normal values can be established. This is not the case. The range of variability of the optical components of the eye can be considerable. Small errors of total refraction can be associated with extreme variation of the refractive constituents. In fact these deviations can be much greater than those occurring in conditions considered pathologic.

The axial length of an eye with emmetropia can, in some instances, be found to be greater than that of one with progressive myopia. A typical case showing progressive changes in the fundus may have an axial length shorter than normal (mean 22.39 mm). Nevertheless, it is useful to retain the distinction between axial ametropia wherein an alteration in axial length is the main factor, and refractive ametropia wherein the anomaly lies principally in the curvature or indices of the refracting media.

Myopia

In myopia, parallel rays of light entering the eye are brought to a focus anterior to the retina (Figure 2.22). That is, the total refraction is greater than that required for emmetropia. If they are to be brought to a focus upon the retina, parallel rays coming from distant objects must be rendered more divergent at the cornea, and this can only be done by placing a concave lens in front of the eye (Figure 2.23). It follows that distant objects cannot be seen clearly without artificial aid; only divergent rays will meet at the retina, and thus, in order to be seen clearly, an object must be brought close to the eye, so that the rays coming from it are rendered sufficiently divergent. This point, the furthest at which objects can be seen distinctly, is called the far point (*punctum remotum*). In the emmetrope it is at infinity; in the hyperope it is behind the eye and therefore virtual; in the myope it is a finite distance in front of the eye and therefore real, and the higher the myopia, the shorter is this distance.

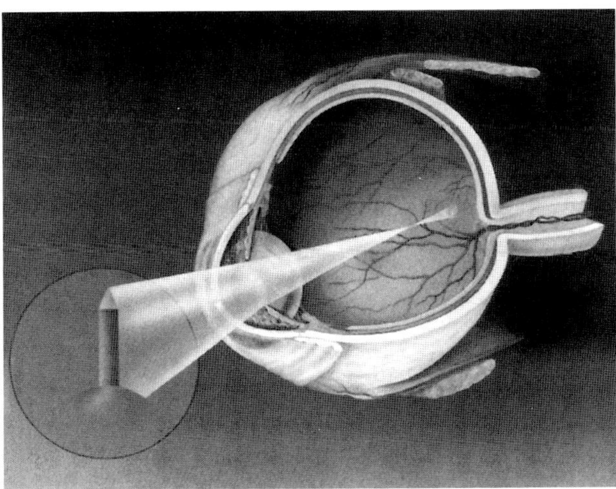

Fig. 2.22 The myopic eye.

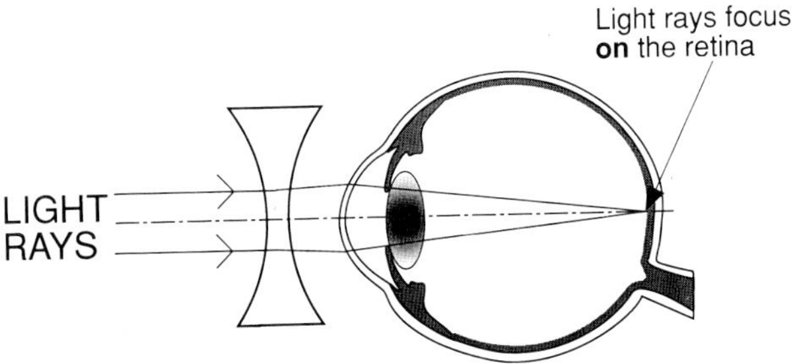

Fig. 2.23 A corrected myopic eye.

It is important, at this point, to note that the symptom of blurred distance vision and the diagnosis of myopia are common denominators of what have been described as two different clinical entities: physiologic myopia and pathologic myopia.

Physiologic myopia

Physiologic (simple, school, low, benign) myopia is an optical condition of the eye in which a chance combination of normal refractive components renders the eye nearsighted. An increase in curvature of the surfaces of the cornea or lens (decrease in radius of curvature) and an increased axial diameter of the eye attained by normal growth are factors which are both capable of producing myopia unless proportional compensatory changes are present in the other components. The axial length of the eye as well as the corneal and lens power are within the normal limits for the population, but are mismatched, so the image does not fall on the fovea.

Pathologic myopia

Pathologic (degenerative, progressive, malignant) myopia is a direct consequence of an abnormal component of refraction. In its general usage and as a strict diagnostic term, it indicates those cases associated with an abnormal lengthening of the eye. The condition may be generalized and involve the entire posterior sclera as far forward as the insertions of the recti muscles. This diffuse process is usually associated with a herniation of an area of the posterior pole, which yields the dramatic picture of a posterior staphyloma (Figure 2.24). This is generally

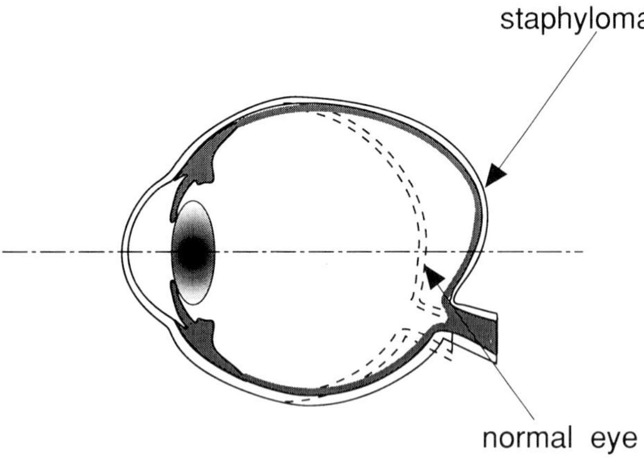

Fig. 2.24 Staphyloma in pathologic myopia.

attributed to the stretching of the scleral wall. In pathologic myopia, the total refraction of the cornea and lens falls within normal limits and the myopia state is produced by excessive axial elongation; the axial diameter of the eye lies outside the normal binomial curve [56]. Ectatic and degenerative changes are often present in the posterior globe (Figure 2.25).

The differential diagnosis between physiologic and pathologic myopia is not discrete [57]. As a general rule, we separate the two by:

Degree of myopia. Pathologic myopia usually has -6 D or more of refractive error.

The axial diameter of the eye. Adult eyes of more than 26.5 mm show an increased incidence of degenerative fundus changes.

History. Pathologic myopia is a congenital (or neonatal) disease, whereas physiologic myopia has its onset anywhere from 5 to 12 years of age.

Ophthalmoscopic findings. This is by far the best differential point. The posterior fundus of the physiologic myopia eye has a normal appearance, although a small temporal crescent (0.3 disk diameter or less) is compatible with this diagnosis. Pathologic myopia, on the other hand, almost always has changes in the retinal pigment epithelium that are present at the earliest age and appear as a localized or generalized pallor and tessellation of the posterior fundus. Stereoscopic fundus examination will reveal an ectasia of the posterior globe that begins in the second decade and expands in the third. The scleral crescent is also present at earliest examination, is usually large (greater than 0.5 disk diameter), and often encircles the disk. The degenerative changes of small punched-out areas of focal chorioretinal atrophy within the staphyloma confirm the pathologic nature of the myopia (see Chapter 14 for a classification of pathologic myopia fundi).

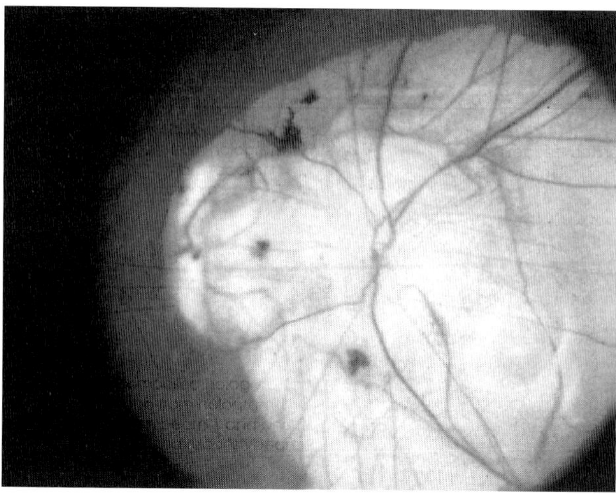

Fig. 2.25 The fundus in pathologic myopia.

Progression. Physiologic myopia progresses during childhood, slows during the second decade, and is stable by the third decade, whereas pathologic myopia usually becomes worse during the second decade and may progress in the fifth decade.

Technically, the term *pathologic myopia*, in its broadest sense, can be applied to such myopias as those found in keratoconus and spherophakia. To avoid confusion, these entities are probably best termed *curvature myopias*. In this book, the term *pathologic myopia* will be used only in the strict sense to mean a myopia due to abnormal axial lengthening of the eye accompanied by staphyloma formation. There is clearly, however, a large group of myopic eyes that cannot be classified as physiologic because they show evidence of abnormally increased axial lengths. On the other hand, they should not be classified as pathologic because they do not display the classic degenerative fundus changes of this disease. These eyes should be classified as intermediate in type, as suggested by Curtin [35].

Hyperopia

I have said that in the emmetropic eye parallel rays of light are brought to a focus on the retina, but with hyperopia (hypermetropia or far-sight), parallel rays come to a focus behind the retina, and the diffusion circles which are formed result in a blurred and indistinct image (Figure 2.26). It follows that with the emmetropic eye objects theoretically at infinity are seen distinctly when the eye is at rest, while in hyperopia the formation of a clear image of any kind is impossible unless the converging power of the optical system is increased either by placing a convex lens in front of the eye or by an effort of accommodation (Figure 2.27).

This condition is the normal state in the newborn and persists in 50% of the population in most of the countries of the world. The normally 2 to 3 D of hyperopia present at birth usually decreases rapidly in the early years and is all but gone by the age of puberty. In some hyperopes it may actually increase between the ages of

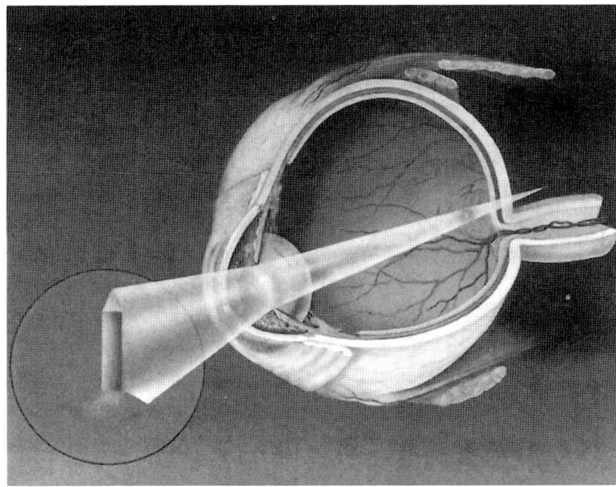
Fig. 2.26 The hyperopic eye.

5 and 14 years [58]. Any residual hyperopia will tend to remain stable until middle life, where it again reappears due to lens changes (so-called senile hypermetropia of Straub). The vast majority of simple hyperopia is under 3 D but in the presence of ocular malformations or pathology can reach 20 D or more.

The structure of the hyperopic eye

These eyes are typically small, not just axially, but in all dimensions. The cornea is small as well. Since the human lens appears to vary little, if any, in size—it is relatively large leading to a shallowed anterior chamber—this carries with it the increased likelihood of angle closure glaucoma. Additionally, the macula is situated farther from the disk than in emmetropes and the cornea is likewise decentered, typically showing a large angle α (see Chapter 3).

Axial hyperopia is due to abnormal shortening of the globe; each millimeter of change is equal to 3 D. This condition is typically developmental, as in microphthalmos (where in some cases the refraction may even be normal). Progressive hyperopia can be seen in certain diseases such as orbital tumors or retinal exudates. Rarely the

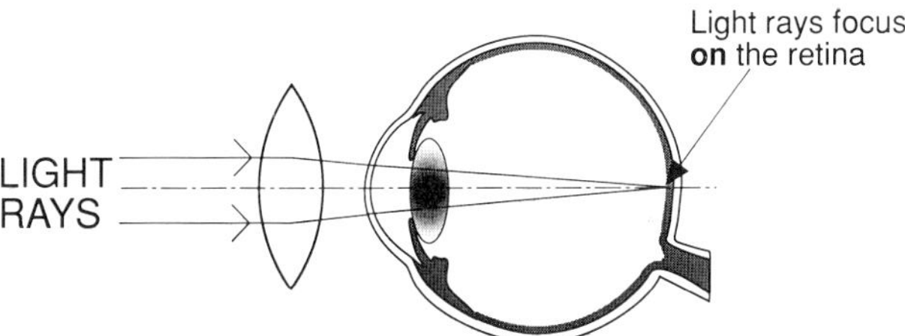

Fig. 2.27 The corrected hyperopic eye.

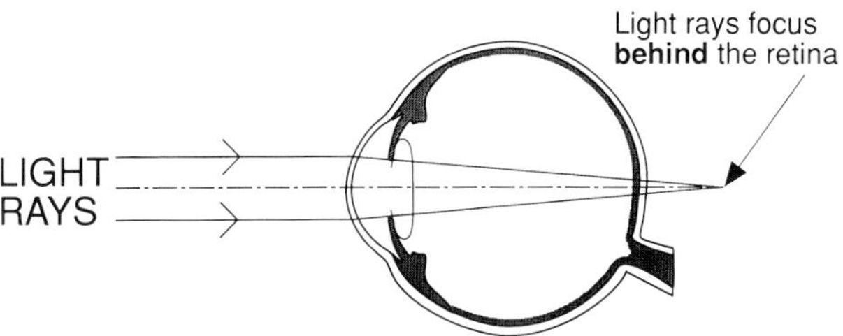

Fig. 2.28 The aphakic eye.

cornea can be found to be markedly flattened—as flat as 29 D—cornea plana. In some of these cases the total hyperopia may not be high at all (2–3 D), whereas in others it could be considerable. The latter are usually associated with high degrees of astigmatism as well.

The best-known form of acquired hyperopia is, of course, aphakia (Figure 2.28). Here the absence of nearly +19 D of refractive power pushes the focal point as far back as 31 mm behind the retina. This necessitates strong convex lenses being placed before the eye to compensate—typically +10 to +11 D in power. Such lenses were supposedly first advocated by Benito Daza de Valdes, though the first mention of such usage is to be found in the writings of Nicholas Cusanus (1401–1464) in his work, *De Beryllo* (Spectacles) [59,60]. Writing one of the earliest works on spectacles, not only did Valdes suggest such use in aphakes but recommended concave spectacles for myopes and convex lenses for hyperopes. In that period such lenses were only prescribed for presbyopes (Figure 2.29), and it wasn't until 1725 that their use in aphakia was finally put into practice by Heister. It was to be another 225 years before the suggestion of Tadini to re-

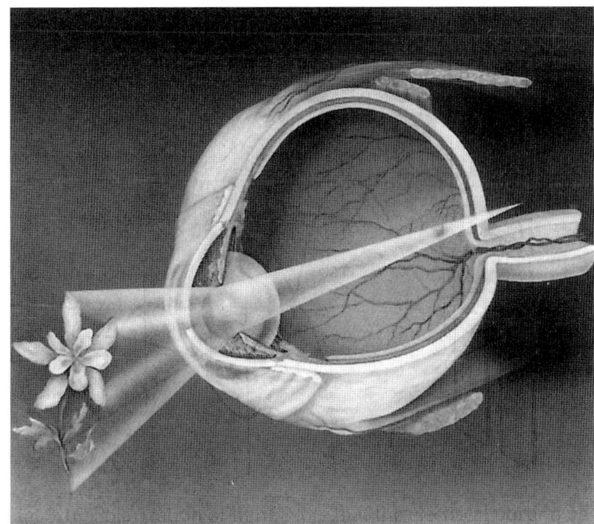
Fig. 2.29 Presbyopia.

place the cataractous lens was successfully carried out by Ridley [61] (see also Chapter 13).

Characteristics of hyperopia

Hyperopia is called far-sight because the near point is at a considerable distance in front of the eye, making far vision more comfortable and clearer than near vision. In some cases, this deficit can be overcome by the act of accommodation. However, while this might suffice to clarify objects at a distance, sufficient accommodative amplitude may not exist to produce clear images at near.

The amount of hyperopia compensated for by normal tonus of the ciliary muscle is called *latent*, while any remaining is termed *manifest*. Taken together, the two constitute *total hyperopia*. It follows that the amount of latent hyperopia decreases over time as the lens becomes less flexible until presbyopia results, at which time all the hyperopia becomes manifest. Manifest hyperopia is further made up of facultative hyperopia, which is that amount that can be compensated for by the act of accommodating. That remaining uncompensated is termed *absolute hyperopia*. Since accommodative amplitude varies from individual to individual as well as by age, it follows that cycloplegic examination of the hyperope (occasionally into the 50s) is necessary to uncover the total hyperopia present.

Frequently, fogging techniques are insufficient to uncover the latent and/or facultative hyperopia. In fact, the amount of unsuspected facultative hyperopia can be astonishing. I once examined a 36-year-old naval supply officer who was complaining of asthenopia (his commanding officer also was complaining about this man's surly disposition). Uncorrected, and with no obvious effort, his visual acuity was 20/20 on the Snellen chart, both for near and far. On manifest examination, his refraction was +1 D OU, while on cycloplegic his refraction was +4.00 D! He was unable to tolerate any plus correction until we adopted the expedient of administering cycloplegia and ordering him to wear his glasses while the drop was wearing off. That ploy worked, and he was finally able to wear +3 D comfortably, banishing his asthenopic complaints. Interestingly, his disposition improved markedly as well.

The neglected hyperope

In the literature concerning ametropia, myopia has received most of the attention, and hyperopia has been all but ignored. In a review of references listed in the huge database compiled by the National Medical Library (from 1966 to the present), 3411 articles exist dealing with myopia and only 773 with hyperopia (4:1). Within that enduring "bible" of ophthalmology, *System of Ophthalmology* by Sir Stewart Duke-Elder, 72 pages are devoted to myopia and only 14 to hyperopia (5:1). Refractive surgery too is about myopia and astigmatism, or so it seems. In a review of extant literature, less than 10% of the articles dealing with the surgical treatment of ametropia, excluding aphakia, are about hyperopia. Yet hyperopia appears to be more prevalent than myopia by at least 2:1. Thus hyperopia would seem to be a poor relative indeed. Why should this be? After all, the first spectacles were prescribed—in 1290—for hyperopia (actually for presbyopia), not myopia. It wasn't until almost 300 years later that myopes had some relief from their affliction.

Perhaps it is because myopes need a correction most of the time, or perhaps it is because myopia is perceived as more threatening [62–64]. Probably the main reason for this emphasis is that being associated with poor vision, myopia alone seems to hold the threat of blindness. In fact, throughout the world myopia is listed as one of the leading causes of visual loss—hyperopia is not on that list. Interestingly, the first schools for partially sighted children, established in London, were called myopia schools and designed for the express purpose of enabling high myopes to avoid eyestrain and thereby prevent further progression of the myopia. Whatever the reason, myopia has received the lion's share of attention. Many methods have been devised for the prevention or control of myopia but little or no effort has been expended for a like process with hyperopia.

Yet a significant number of the world's population (almost 50% in most countries) are hyperopic de novo, not to mention those cases iatrogenically produced through one means or another. If Grosvenor is correct, hyperopia per se represents a significant impediment to the learning process [65]. Evidence exists connecting it with behavioral problems as well as low academic standing among elementary school children (see section on ametropia, intelligence, and scholastic standing, below). Still and all, hyperopia does not seem to be regarded as a problem of pressing proportions. In fact, hyperopia among adults is not often discussed, perhaps because the malady is dealt with (most of the time) behind closed doors where the afflicted can wear their "grannies" or bifocals in secret. Also most hyperopes are of such degree that they can "muddle through" the day without exposing their "weakness." Broekema showed that normal visual acuity occurred in 82% of the hyperopes in his study whose refractive error was 1 to 2 D; in 64% from 3 to 4 D; in 44% from 5 to 6 D; and in only about 15% from 7 to 10 D [66].

Many vision practitioners, as well as the general public, still consider myopia a weakness and all the more so because the myope displays his or her weakness in public by wearing spectacles. For despite efforts at destigmatization, the wearing of spectacles still carries with it significant social penalty. Even in this age of "enlightenment" the wearing of glasses, especially by a child, tends to set one apart. In contrast, many hyperopes find that they can conceal their anomaly by only wearing glasses in the privacy of their homes or offices—at least for a while—for close work. The wearing of glasses is also perceived as being a sign of intelligence—a paradox to be sure. It's very likely that we are more concerned about the appearance of weakness than in the malady itself, however. This is underscored by the fact that optometrists, once heavily involved in attempts to control or prevent myopia by visual training, undercorrection, or plus lenses for reading, have almost completely abandoned these attempts and have turned instead to the fitting of contact lenses. Of course, some of the impetus to this trend may stem from the demonstrated failure of these methodologies to make more than a token dent in the problem.

Whatever may be the *casus omissus* of the situation, considerable evidence exists in the literature pointing to the relationship of ametropia to intelligence test scores, reading ability, and school achievement. It is apparent that at least some hyperopes are having problems in that regard. Grosvenor reviewed the situation and suggested that more attention be paid to this sector of the population [65]. He presents some compelling arguments to support his thesis.

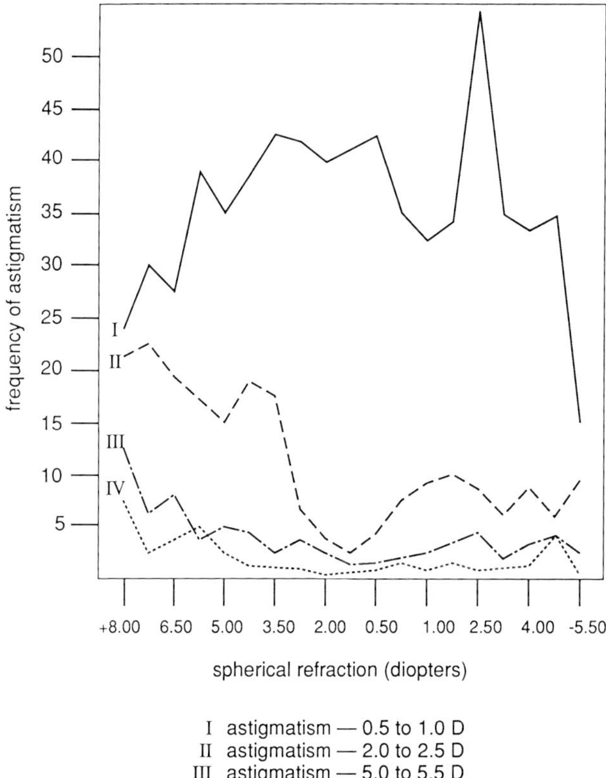

Fig. 2.31 The variation in frequency of various degrees of corneal astigmatism associated with different refractive states (from Kronfeld and Devney. The frequency of astigmatism. Arch Ophthalmol, 1930).

Astigmatism

We have said previously that in the eye when light rays converge on, behind, or in front of the retina, and the principal focus approximates a point lying in one plane, such a system is termed *stigmatic* (pointlike). This condition also can be termed *anastigmatic* (without astigmatism). When the principal focus lies not within one plane but in many planes, no one principal focus is formed, and the condition is termed *astigmatic* (Figure 2.30). Ocular astigmatism is physiologic and almost invariable but usually small in degree and of little visual effect (Figure 2.31).

Astigmatism ordinarily depends on the presence of toroidal instead of spherical curvatures of the refracting surfaces of the eye. The refractive power as a whole, therefore, instead of being equal in all meridians, changes gradually from one meridian to the next by uniform increments, and each meridian generally has a uniform type of curve. If the axes showing the greatest difference in curvature are at right angles to one another, the condition is called regular astigmatism and is correctable by a cylindrical lens. If they are not so related, the astigmatism may be called *bioblique* and can be treated by a cross cylinder. Typically, the major and minor axes are oriented such that one of them is at or near 90°. If they are not so oriented, the astigmatism is said to be *oblique*. When, however, as in cases of corneal disease such as keratoconus or in lenticular sclerosis, there are irregularities in the curvature of the meridians, the condition is called *irregular astigmatism*. Unless such a defect is corneal, it cannot be compensated for by spectacle lenses but sometimes can be by contact lenses (Figure 2.32).

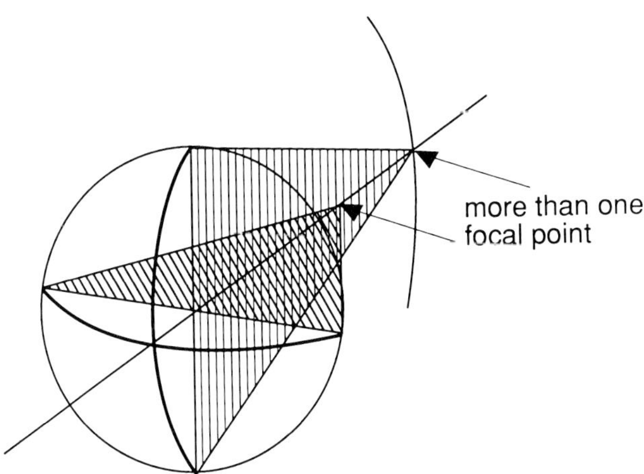

Fig. 2.30 The astigmatic eye.

Types of astigmatism

I have already noted that astigmatism can be regular or irregular, oblique or bioblique. Additionally, the curvatures producing the astigmatism can cause the foci to vary in their anteroposterior relationship to the fovea. Thus,

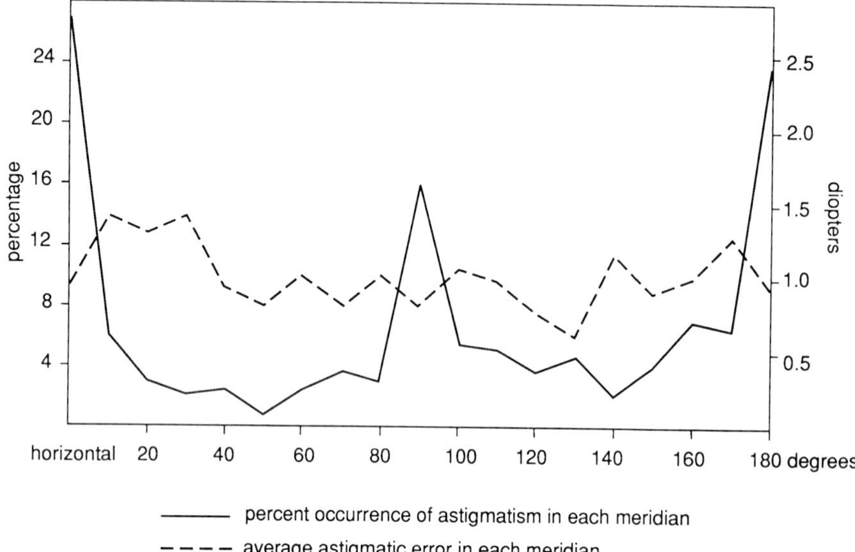

Fig. 2.32 The percentage incidence of the direction of the axis of astigmatism. (from Lang. Incidence of astigmatism axis in myopia. Br J Ophthalmol, 1920).

in hyperopic astigmatism, for example, the curvatures of both axes are unequal and too flat (large radii). In myopic astigmatism they are both unequal and too steep (small radii). If both foci lie either before or behind the retina, the condition is termed *compound astigmatism* (Figures 2.33 and 2.34). When the two conditions are combined so that one axis is hypermetropic and the other myopic—that is, the principal foci lie both before and behind the retina—the condition is termed *mixed astigmatism* (Figure 2.35). If one focus lies on the retina and the other before or behind it, the astigmatism is considered *simple astigmatism* (Figures 2.36 and 2.37).

Regardless of whether the astigmatism is simple, mixed, or compound, there is more than one focal point strung out along the visual axis. The interval between the anterior and posterior focus is called the *interval of Sturm* and varies in its extent depending on the amount of astigmatism present in the optical system (Figure 2.38). The diffusion "circles" formed at these points are typically elliptical in shape. There is one point between the most anterior and the most posterior focus where the focal spot is circular, however. This circle is called the *circle of least confusion* and is located approximately one-third of the way from the anterior-most focus. At this point in

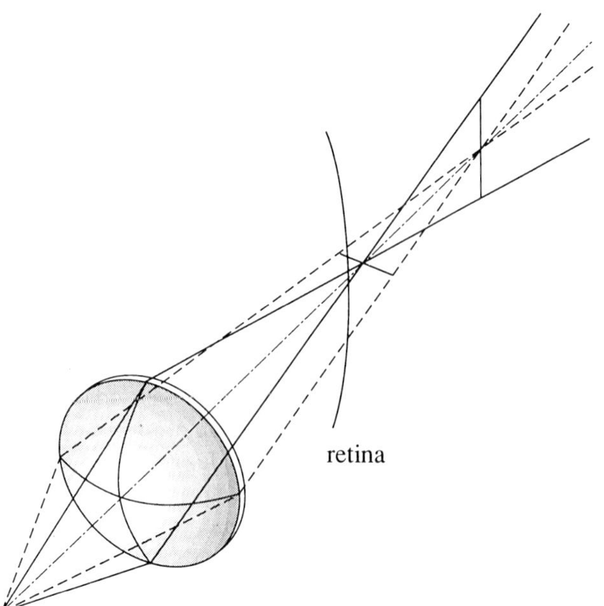

Fig. 2.33 Compound hyperopic astigmatism.

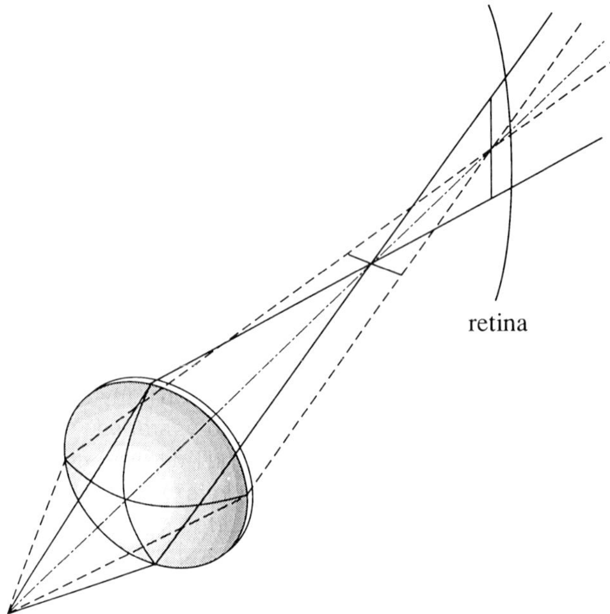

Fig. 2.34 Compound myopic astigmatism.

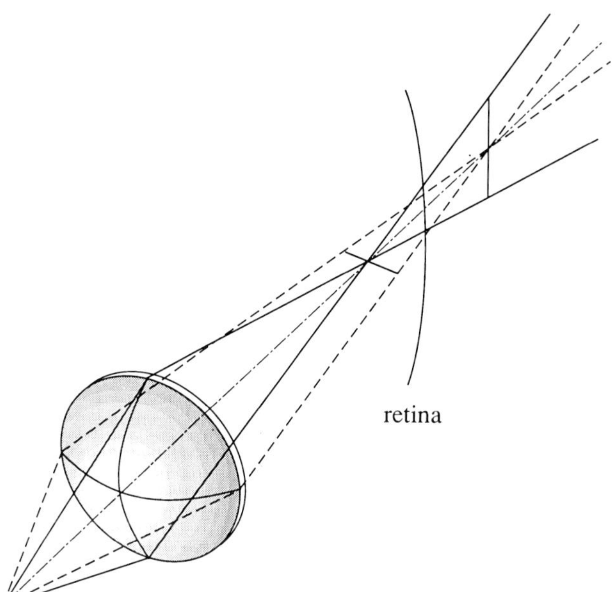

Fig. 2.35 Mixed astigmatism.

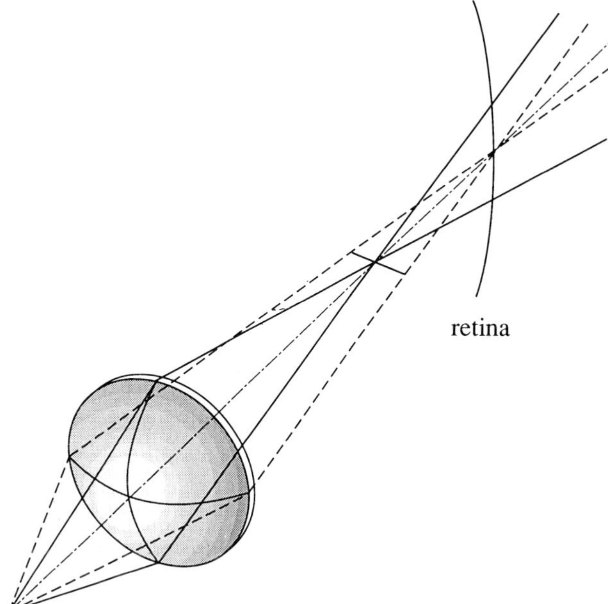

Fig. 2.37 Simple myopic astigmatism.

space, in the absence of any optical correction, the image formed by the system is the best possible. Before the advent of spherocylindric spectacle lenses, physicians compensated for astigmatism by choosing a spherical lens which basically moved the circle of least confusion on to the retina. Typically this power corresponds to the so-called spherical equivalent of the refractive system; that is, a spherical lens of that power will produce a circle of least confusion on the retina similar to that of the astigmatic system alone.

The components of total astigmatism

Curvature variation of the anterior surface of the cornea occurs physiologically and is thus responsible for the majority of cases of astigmatism. The average difference be-

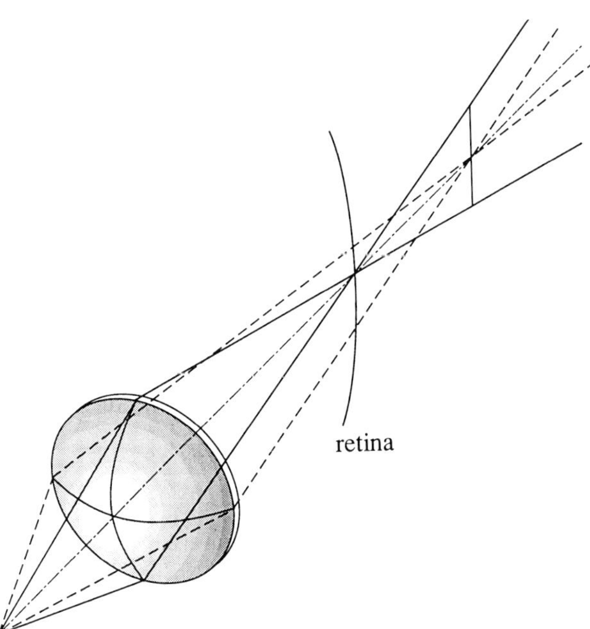

Fig. 2.36 Simple hyperopic astigmatism.

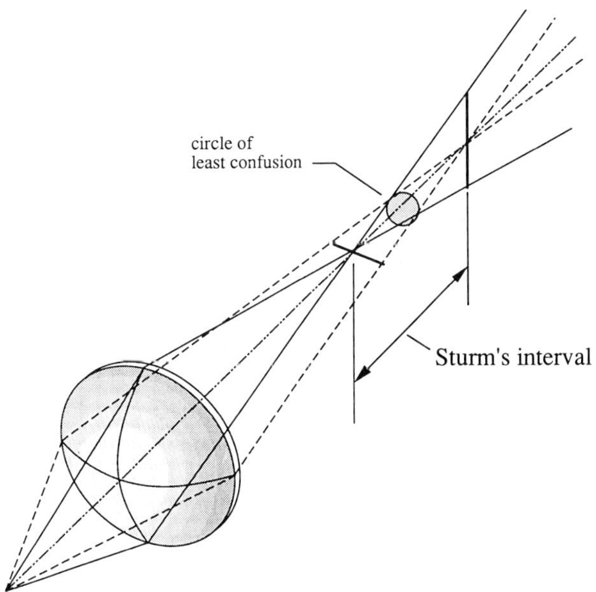

Fig. 2.38 Astigmatism and the interval of Sturm.

tween the refractive powers of the two corneal meridians lies between 0.5 and 0.75 D. Donders [44] gave a mean value of 1 D, Pfalz [67] of 0.75 D, Sorensen [68] of 0.75 to 0.5 D, Steiger [69] and Gullstrand [70] of 0.5 D, while Kronfeld and Devney [71] suggested that any value over 1 D should be regarded as pathologic. I prefer to consider any astigmatism over 1 D as significant and any over 4 D as pathologic. Furthermore, I consider any astigmatism that equals or exceeds 20% of the associated spherical component as significant and an indication for surgical intervention. In about 90% of these cases the meridian of least curvature (flattest) is horizontal (Figure 2.39). If that meridian lies within 30° of the horizontal plane, the astigmatism is said to be *direct* or *with the rule* (W-T-R). If it makes such an angle with the vertical plane so that the horizontal curvature is greater, it is said to be *inverse* or *against the rule* (A-T-R).

This tendency toward W-T-R astigmatism has never been adequately explained, although Snellen associated it with pressure on the globe from the eyelids [72]. This view has had considerable support from other investigators and may be true to some degree. In keratoconus, where the cornea is extremely malleable, W-T-R astigmatism is quite frequent. This also occurs if external ocular pressure is increased by forceful lid closure or by increased weight of the eyelid, as with lid tumors. It may be thought that increased intraocular pressure alone, as in glaucoma, may have the effect of producing inverse astigmatism. However, while this may occur in experimental animal models, it does not seem to be of clinical significance. It seems more likely that since the corneal curvature is an extension of the same general curvature as the sclera, the cause is more a defect in growth of the eye. This view is substantiated by the common occurrence of

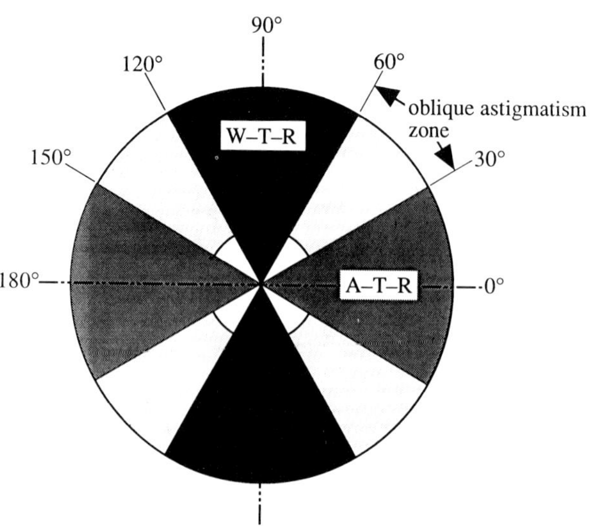

Fig. 2.39 Astigmatism axes.

high astigmatism in deformities of the globe—even of the posterior segment. Inverse astigmatism often follows the healing of a large horizontal scar such as is seen in large-incision cataract surgery (see also Chapter 13).

The posterior surface of the cornea also shows an astigmatic curvature which typically ranges from 0.25 to 0.5 D, sometimes reaching 1.0 D [73]. It is usually inverse in type neutralizing that of the external surface. In some cases, it may be the cause of so-called residual astigmatism encountered in contact lens fitting and can also account for that seen after refractive surgery in the presence of a spherical anterior surface.

Curvature astigmatism of both lens surfaces is also a normal occurrence and is typically less than that of the cornea and in the opposite direction. For example, Tscherning's measurements for the radii of the anterior lens surface were 10.2 mm horizontal and 10.1 mm vertical and of the posterior surface 6.17 and 6.13 mm, respectively [73]. Typically, such asphericity is small in degree—0.50 D. In an otherwise normal eye, it is assumed that most, if not all, astigmatism is corneal in origin. However, many patients do, in fact, possess considerable degrees of lenticular astigmatism. This is of particular importance in refractive surgery. It is essential to compare the net refractive error with that of the corneal curvature when evaluating a patient for this type of surgery. The presence of A-T-R astigmatism in a young individual should alert the examiner to the possibility of significant lenticular astigmatism. Only occasionally will the cornea be steeper horizontally; it typically shows direct or vertical astigmatism.

Astigmatism from decentration of the optical system is also physiologic and invariable since the refracting surfaces are neither geometrically centered nor concentric to the anatomic axis. Thus the optic axis intersects the cornea as much as 0.25 mm below and nasal to the corneal apex. This is a small deviation and tends to neutralize physiologic direct astigmatism. Additionally, the fovea is not on the optic axis but some 1.25 mm down and temporal. The pupillary axis is somewhat eccentric as well, lying to the nasal side of the corneal center. Thus, if we accept Gullstrand's usual 5° angle between the pupillary and optic axes, the resultant astigmatism is 0.1 D for a pupil of 2.0 mm [74].

The total astigmatism of the ocular system is made up primarily by that of the corneal surface with the rest (the residual astigmatism contributed by the surfaces of the posterior cornea, lens, and component decentration) tending to neutralize this effect. This residual astigmatism, while usually of small degree, cannot be totally ignored. Jackson examined a large number of young adults and found the average corneal astigmatism to be 1.04 D while the residual averaged 0.61 D—a not inconsiderable amount [75]. The extremes were 8.0 D of corneal, 4.25 D of lenticular, and 6.0 D of total astigmatism. It seems evident from these figures that it is not possible nor rational to attempt to correct astigmatism through keratometry readings alone. Thus it would be unwise to rely on Javal's rule [51], especially in refractive surgery. Javal's rule gives an empirical relationship between total or subjective astigmatism (AST) and the keratometric (corneal) astigmatism (ASC) but is prone to too many exceptions:

$$AST = k + 1.25\ ASC$$

where $k = 0.25$ D against the rule. It is interesting to note that while the total astigmatism of one eye may be quite different from its fellow, the residual astigmatism is similar [76].

Astigmatism and age

Regular astigmatism is age-variable with a small degree of W-T-R astigmatism occurring early in life. This astigmatism may not be present at birth, however—the neonate cornea is usually spherical—but develops somewhat later in life and changes little during the school years. During early adulthood on, there is a slight tendency for the W-T-R astigmatism to decrease or even reverse, with changes occurring more usually in men than women [77,78]. Jackson's figures [75] are illustrated in Table 2.1.

Table 2.1 Astigmatism and age. From Jackson E. Norms of refraction. JAMA 1932; 98:132

	Nil	Horizontal	Vertical	Oblique
Corneal astigmatism				
Before 25 years	52	24	910	32
After 50 years	84	118	737	86
Residual astigmatism				
Before 25 years	62	817	61	52
After 50 years	72	726	63	163

Accommodation

Accommodation is not ametropia per se, but this would appear to be the most appropriate place to discuss it, particularly as it applies to the postoperative course in refractive surgery. The existence of accommodation was proved by the classic but little appreciated experiment of Scheiner in 1619 (Figure 2.40) [19]. Alteration of ocular length was, for 150 years, the most popular theory by which this phenomenon occurred. Kepler described accommodation as occurring through elongation and shortening of the globe through the action of the ciliary processes [22,23]. This mechanism was elegantly disproved by Young in 1801 [40]. Having prominent eyes, he was able to place, after strong convergence, a ring, both at the inner orbital angle and at the outer, which pressed against the eye, the latter over the macula. Pressure on the rings produced bright circular spots in the field of vision called *phosphenes*. On strong accommodation, neither of the images was displaced nor altered, thus showing that elongation of the eye did not occur in accommodation. In the same paper he dispelled the theory of Lobé that changes in the corneal curvature occurred to produce clear near vision. This was accomplished by showing that accommodation was unimpaired if corneal refraction was eliminated by attaching a glass lens to his cornea (one of the first, if not the first, examples of a contact lens) and filling the space between with water. Interestingly, it was while conducting this experiment that he discovered that he had astigmatism (see also section on astigmatism, above).

It is also interesting to note that corneal curvature changes actually do occur during accommodation, but not the radius change from 8.0 to 6.8 mm needed to accomplish clear near vision in the normal eye [52]. These changes in the normal have been attributed to convergence by some investigators [79,80]. That the accommodative mechanism is capable of altering corneal shape was demonstrated in a study of post-radial keratotomy patients with mild presbyopia [81].

This left only the lens which, it was suggested, moved backward and forward during accommodation [23]. However, it would require a total movement of 10 mm to produce the effects seen. Thus it remained that perhaps accommodation did occur—in the manner originally suggested by Descartes [82] (Figure 2.41), demonstrated by Porterfield, and corroborated by Young—due to a change in lens shape [83]. Helmholtz demonstrated that accommodation resulted from increased curvature of both the

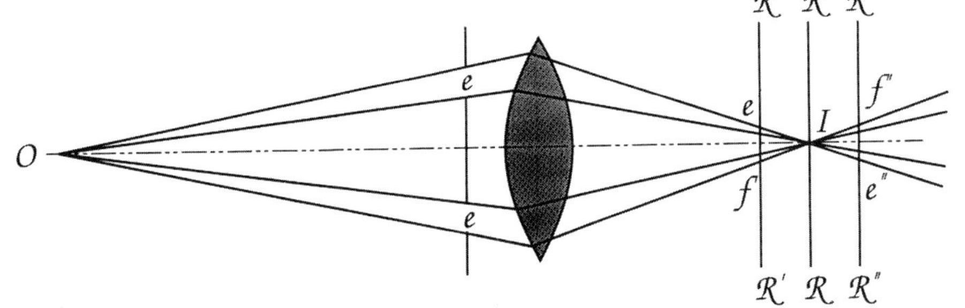

Fig. 2.40 Scheiner's classic experiment. If two holes are made in a card (*e–e′*), the object *O* is brought to a focus on the screen *R* where one image, *I*, will appear. If the screen is held at *R′* or *R″*, two images will appear (*e′f′* and *e″f″*). The experiment proves that there is a focusing mechanism within the eye (from Scheiner C. *Occulus Hoc est: Fundamentum Opticum*. Innsbruck, 1619).

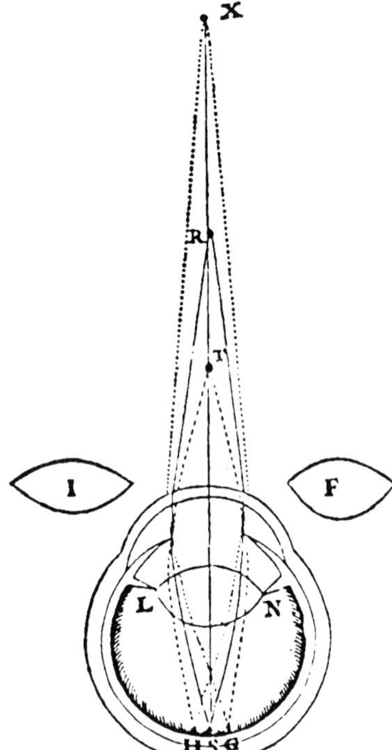

Fig. 2.41 Descartes' theory of accommodation. "In order to represent the point *X* distinctly it is necessary that the whole shape of the humor *NL* be changed and that it becomes a little flatter as that which is marked *I*, and to represent the point *T* it is necessary to become a little more convex like that which is marked *F*" (from Descartes R. *Traité de l'Homme*. Paris, 1677).

anterior and posterior capsules of the lens, commenting on the conoidal shape of the postero-central part of the lens when accommodated [52]. Fincham explained this singular shape change by the molding capacity of the peculiar configuration of the lens capsule (Figure 2.42) [84]. In this he was in opposition to the view of Helmholtz who suggested that this shape was due to some elasticity of the lens itself which opposed that of the capsule. This latter view was shown to have some validity in the work of Kikawa and Sato [85] as well as Fisher [86]. Despite this hard evidence, Bates insisted that the lens was unnecessary in accommodation and persisted in his teaching that he, and he alone, was correct [87]. I will have more to say about William Bates in Chapter 10.

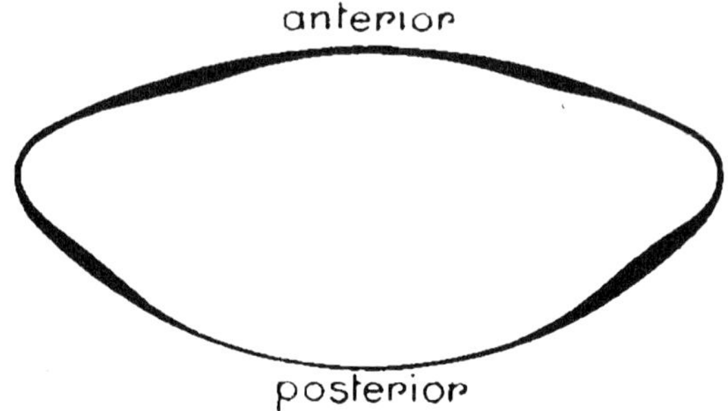

Fig. 2.42 Fincham's diagram of the lens capsule (from Fincham EF. The changes in the form of the crystalline lens in accommodation. Trans Opt Soc Lond 1925; 26:239–269).

The significance of accommodation

The farthest point at which an object can be seen clearly is called the far point. When maximum accommodative effort is exercised, the closest point at which an object can be seen clearly is the near point. Range of accommodation is defined as the distance from the far point to the near point and represents the distance over which the near focus is effective. Amplitude of accommodation is defined as the difference in the refraction of the eye between these two values expressed in diopters, thus it is an expression of work done or to be done. Typically, the range of accommodation for an uncorrected myope decreases in nonlinear proportion to the degree of myopia, whereas the reverse is true in the hyperope (Figure 2.43). In the myope, full spectacle correction increases the accommodative demand, that is, the fully corrected eye must exert more accommodative effort to discern near objects clearly—the reverse is true for the hyperope. The demand is more for a myope than for a hyperope due to the relative inefficiency of spectacle lens for divergent as opposed to parallel light rays. This difference is typically on the order of 0.9 D and depends on the vertex distance. This is especially evident in contact lens wearers, who may find that their demand increases as much as 50% [88]. This explains the middle-aged myopic contact lens wearer who finds that in giving up his or her spectacles he or she has attained the dubious advantage of having clear vision for distance but now requires spectacles with which to read. This fact also may mean the necessity of prescribing reading correction for presbyopia sooner than in the hyperope.

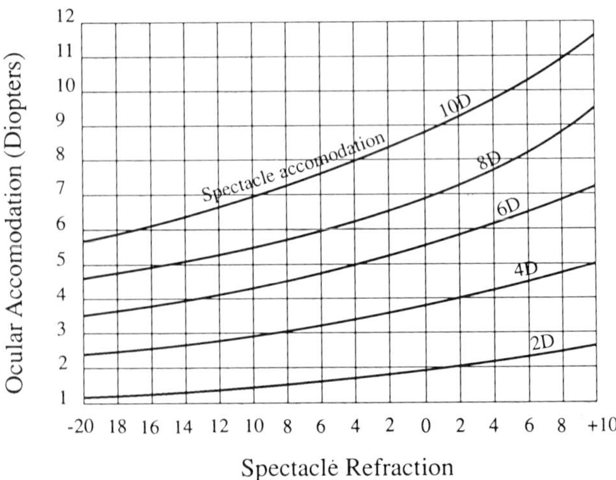

Fig. 2.43 Spectacle accommodation (from Bennett. *Optics of Contact Lenses*, 4th ed. Association of Dispensing Opticians, 1966).

This phenomenon is especially evident after refractive surgery, even in young individuals, who often complain of difficulty with reading which was never experienced before. In some cases this is also seen in contact lens wearers who had not experienced this problem while wearing contacts prior to surgery. The fact of increased demand has encouraged some clinicians to advocate the undercorrection of the myope or even to prescribe plus lenses for near to offset the need for increased accommodation. Articles advocating such an approach were prevalent in the literature (including in the United States) from the middle 19th century through the early 20th [89,90]. Today, most advocacy seems to be centered in the Japanese and Russian literature [91,92]. It is of interest that the wearing of contacts to increase accommodative demand is advocated to reduce progression of myopia by the most ardent proponents of the theory of environmental myopigenesis, particularly the role played by the malignant effects of accommodation and convergence.

The natural history of ametropia

My discussion will begin by considering the condition (for want of a better, more universal description) of myopia—by far the greater portion of the problem of ametropia.

Ametropia—affliction or disease?

It seems somehow ironic that a condition, considered by many authorities [35,44] to be one of the leading causes of visual impairment in this country (as well as in others), is described by some others not even as a disease [93,94]. Yet myopia meets the definition of a disease in *Webster's International Dictionary*, namely: "an impairment of the normal state of the living animal or plant body or any of its components that interrupts or modifies the performance of the vital functions." Would anyone argue that vision is not one of the vital functions? Not to put too fine a point on it, but I submit that vision has survival value and that any impairment of it reduces one's chances in an increasingly hostile world.

The evolution of our knowledge of myopia has been marked by occasional giant strides based on careful investigations and their impartial analysis. All too often, however, the contributions to this subject have been bewildering in their protocols, their results, and their conclusions. A tendency toward advocacy rather than investigatory curiosity can especially be seen to permeate the early literature.

Regardless of the somewhat blurred data representing the prevalence of myopia among the world's population, there is no doubt that myopia (except in its milder forms) and, to a lesser extent hyperopia, inflict a grave socioeconomic burden upon the individual. This burden has not been truly appreciated by some and has been deprecated by many. We can make a beginning in our assessment of the question by considering that the cost of optical aids amounts to something in excess of $4 billion annually in the United States alone! This burden starts early and continues for a lifetime. In a survey conducted by the Department of Health, Education, and Welfare in 1974, it was found that 34% of individuals between ages 12 and 17 years were wearing correcting lenses. Myopic corrections accounted for an increasing proportion of these wearers—72% at age 12 to 87% at age 17 [95].

If myopia only caused a significant reliance upon optical corrections, it would be a problem of major proportions. Unfortunately it has been found to be the fifth most frequent specific cause of impaired vision in the United States; the seventh most frequent cause of legal blindness and the eighth most frequent cause of severe visual impairment (Table 2.2)

Curtin feels that these data may be somewhat misleading, however. He points out that pathologic myopia

Table 2.2 Estimates of prevalence of impairment from vision disorders, in thousands. From *Support for Vision Research.* Publication no. [NIM] 76-1098. Department of Health, Education, and Welfare, Washington, DC, 1976

Type of eye affection	Impaired vision	Severe visual impairment	Legal blindness
Glaucoma	1,070	207	56
Cataract (prenatal, other)	1,711	217	64
Retinal disorder (prenatal, diabetic, other)	815	392	118
Retrolental fibroplasia	19	19	10
Myopia	715	36	14
Cornea or sclera	294	67	22
Uveitis	285	67	23
Optic nerve disease	121	107	41
Multiple affections	90	90	23
Refractive errors with lesser disability	1,662	0	0
Other affections	3,656	103	45
Unknown	221	179	53
Total (all affections)	10,699	1,483	468

is a single disease entity, and in these tabulations it is ranked behind such disease groupings as cornea or sclera, uveitis, optic nerve disease, prenatal, vascular, and the like [35]. It is apparent that as a single cause of visual loss, pathologic myopia is underestimated to a significant extent by some of these surveys. An equally important aspect in the consideration of the visual loss produced by myopia is its relatively early onset.

A recent investigation in the United States attributes 5.6% of blindness among school children to myopia, making it the fifth most frequent cause of blindness after retrolental fibroplasia, cataract, optic nerve atrophy, and the combined category of anophthalmia-microphthalmia [96]. The prevalence of world blindness in general and myopic blindness in particular varies widely with the parameters used in different surveys (Table 2.3).

The Model Reporting Area studies on blindness conducted by the U.S. Department of Health, Education, and Welfare indicate that, in addition to ranking seventh as a cause of blindness (1969–1970), the incidence of myopic blindness increased from 0.1% in children under 5 years of age to 0.6% in the aged [97]. The sharpest increase was noted to occur in the middle of the fifth decade. This, unfortunately, coincides with that period of life in which the talents and productivity of those affected are at a maximum, as well as with that time at which there is a peak in financial responsibility; thus the impact of this blindness on the family is particularly severe (Figure 2.44).

In Europe, a large number of such studies have been conducted. The data from the United Kingdom are of particular note because of Sorsby's interest in myopia [98]. In an early survey of blindness in England and Wales, he found myopia to be the second most frequent cause of blindness in persons between the ages of 30 and 49 years. In the next age group (50–69 years) it ranked second only to cataract. Overall, myopia was ranked as the third most prevalent cause behind cataract and glaucoma. In a more recent study of the same population, Sorsby found myopic atrophy and retinal detachment to be the cause of 14% of blindness in all age groups behind diabetic retinopathy and cataract. It would appear that in Scotland the problem of myopic blindness is even more grave. Here it has been found as the single greatest cause in persons in the fifth decade of life. According to surveys conducted in 1942 and 1946, it was ranked second only to cataract among all age groups. The combination of these data revealed a significantly earlier onset of blindness among myopic persons (mean 52.1 years) as compared with persons with blindness due to other causes.

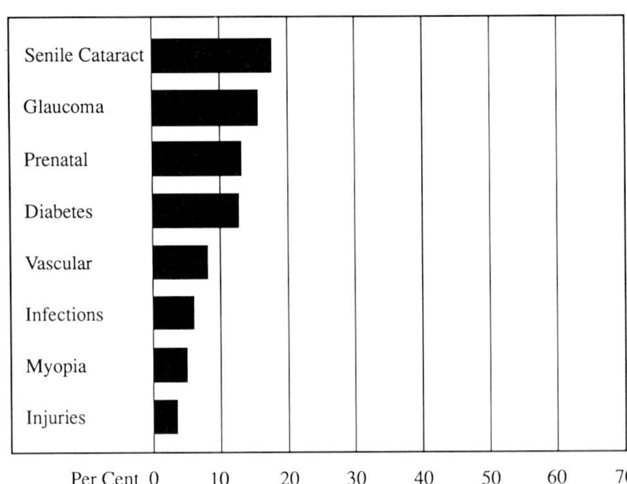

Fig. 2.44 The eight major causes of blindness in the United States: population 20 years of age and above (from *Estimated Statistics on Blindness and Visual Problems.* National Society for the Prevention of Blindness, New York, 1966).

Table 2.3 The world's major blinding conditions. From Lim AS, Jones BR. World's major blinding conditions. Vision 1981; 1:101

Country or territory	Ranking as cause of blindness	Percentage of population affected
United States	7th	3
Hong Kong	5th	8
Japan	5th	8.4
Sri Lanka	5th	Not reported
Denmark	3rd	Not reported
German Democratic Republic	1st or 3rd	14.7 or 13.9
German Federal Republic	7th	6.6
Malta	1st	19.4
Poland	3rd	11
USSR	2nd	Not reported

Unfortunately, there has been wide variance in the definition of blindness and, specifically, myopic blindness. In some surveys, the blindness of a myopic eye due to glaucoma, for example, may be reported as myopic in nature. Conversely, blindness due to retinal detachment in eyes with substantial degrees of myopia is reported as due to retinal and not myopic causes. In some surveys blindness secondary to cataract as well as retinal detachment in myopic eyes was reported as myopic in nature. The inclusion of the former is of questionable validity however, and a somewhat exaggerated picture of the importance of myopia emerges from this review.

The development of ametropia

It is apparent, in retrospect, that this central canon of the old school would eventually be challenged. That axial length was not the sole determinant of refraction was appreciated by Donders [44]. Schnabel and Herrnheiser [99] had found axial diameters varying from 22.25 to 26.24 mm in 23 emmetropic eyes and postulated that emmetropia was determined by the relation between axial length and total refraction. It was, however, Steiger's

Table 2.4 Range and mean values of the four components of refraction obtained by three major studies. From Curtin BJ. *The Myopias: Basic Science and Clinical Management.* Harper & Row, New York, 1985

	Tron		Stenstrom		Sorsby	
	Range	Mean	Range	Mean	Range	Mean
Corneal power (D)	37–49	43.41	39.2–48.5	42.84	39–47	43.14
Anterior chamber depth (mm)	2.16–5.05	3.27	2.8–4.55	3.68	2.6–4.4	3.47
Lens power (D)	15–29	20.44	12.5–22	17.35	17–26	20.71
Axial diameter (mm)	21–38	25.14	20–29.5	24.00	21–37	23.94

See text for details.

work in 1913 [69] on 5000 juvenile eyes that finally de-emphasized the role of axial length as the sole contributor to the myopic condition. Despite defects in his methodology, especially in assuming lens power as a constant, his work ushered in a new era in the study of myopia. The variability of lens power had been alluded to as early as 1575 by Maurolycus [100], and variations in lens thickness, refractive index, and position had been enumerated as possible causes of myopia prior to Donder's time. Furthermore, actual lens power measurements, albeit in small samples, had been demonstrated by von Reuss [101,102] and Awerbach [103] as showing considerable variations (Table 2.4).

Tron confirmed most of Steiger's earlier work (avoiding its pitfalls) and in addition showed that axial length was a determinant in ametropia only in ranges beyond +4 and –6 D [104, 105]. Stenstrom [64] elaborated on some earlier work by Rushton [106] on determining the axial length using x-rays. In a series of 1000 eyes he confirmed Tron's earlier data showing essentially normal distribution curves for corneal power, depth of anterior chamber, lens power, and total refraction. It was also noted by Stenstrom that the distribution curve of refraction had basically the same pattern as that of axial length, featuring both a positive excess at emmetropia and a skewness toward myopia. This deviation in the population refraction curve had been noted previously by Scheerer [107, 108] and Betsch [109] (Figure 2.45), who had attributed this to the incorporation of eyes with crescent formation at the optic nerve.

When these eyes were deleted from the data, a symmetric curve was obtained for the distribution of refraction. In the analysis of these data it was pointed out that a positive excess still persisted in the corrected curve. Stenstrom's refractive curve after the removal of eyes with crescents also demonstrated an excess. This central peaking was attributed to two factors: the first was the effect of component correlation in the emmetropic range as postulated by Wibaut [110] and Berg [111] and the second was the direct effect of axial length distribution on the curve of refraction.

Sorsby's work in 1957 and again in 1961 [112,113] stands as the model and framework for our current understanding of the evolution of ametropia, particularly myopia. Sorsby and coworkers demonstrated conclusively in their study of 341 eyes that an "emmetropization" effect was noted in distribution curves of refraction as a result of a correlation of corneal power and axial length. In ametropias of ±4 D and above, this correlation appeared to break down, however. Their study also indicated that neither the lens nor the anterior chamber depth was an effective emmetropizing factor. In all of their investigations, the dominant finding was the high correlation of total refraction with axial length. This is true especially in the emmetropic range of refraction (–0.75 to +1.50 D) in which the correlation of corneal power diminishes the impact of axial length upon the refraction. The latter remains, for the most part, as the primary determinant even in this range of refraction. The question then arises, what is the natural history of physiologic myopia?

By and large myopia illustrates marked changes at three periods of development: newborn, childhood, and adult. From premature infant to about 6 months of age,

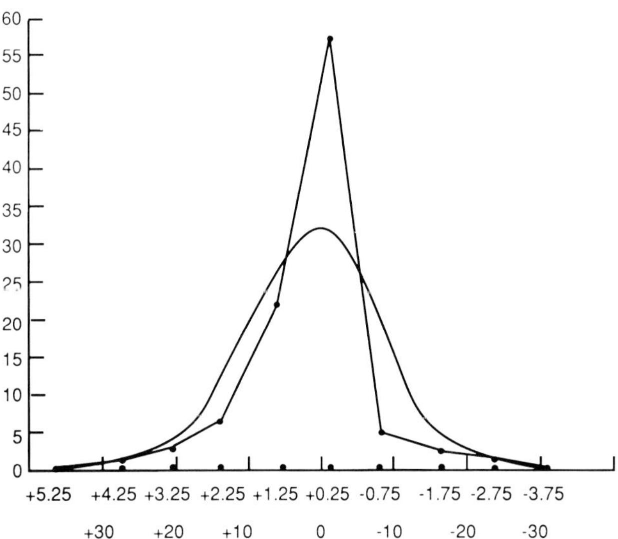

Fig. 2.45 Refraction curves of Scheerer and Betsch compared with a theoretical binomial curve.

the trend in myopia is downward, showing a marked rise from age 5 to 13 years. Following this period, until age 20, a gradual decline in the degree of myopia is seen.

In a classic paper, Brown performed atropine refractions at least 1 year apart on 1203 eyes, from birth to age 51, for a total of 8820 comparative measurements (Figure 2.46) [114]. He concluded that

> myopia increases and hyperopia decreases rapidly from age 8 to 13 years. From 14 to 20 years, this increase in myopia continues each year, but at a rate barely half that of the previous period. Puberty possibly tends to bring about an *emmetropization.* [This concept makes some investigators uncomfortable. Acceptance of the fact of this mechanism, however, does not mean the phenomenon is teleologic in nature.] Increase of myopia after the age of 20 is practically negligible . . . between 20 and 33 years the increase continues at a very low average yearly rate (0.04 diopter). Between 34 and 42 years, the refraction shifts to the low yearly decrease in each successive year, averaging only 0.03 diopter.

Lepard [115] performed 797 examinations on 55 patients aged 1 to 28 years and found that his "data indicate that eyes with normal visual acuity become progressively more myopic with growth and development until 25 years of age, and are in excellent agreement with the data of Brown." On the basis of these studies, we can conclude that changes in refraction after radial keratotomy in individuals aged 21 or older are most likely due to the surgery, since spontaneous regression of myopia is virtually unheard of and since the progression of myopia after this age is very small compared to the effect induced by the surgery.

Ocular growth manifests in two distinct phases: the first or rapid phase occurs from birth to 3 years and the second or slow phase is from age 3 to 13. The different refractions and axial lengths are not related to bodily stature and weight, nor does there appear to be a spurt in growth at puberty. Furthermore there is no sexual predilection—the growth of the eye appears to be completed by the age of 13 or 14 in both boys and girls [112]. This latter observation is in line with the growth pattern of the central nervous system in general, of which the eye is, of course, an integral part.

The corneal diameter attains its full adult size (mean 11.7 mm) by 5 years of age, and may possibly reach it by age 1 year. This was well demonstrated in Priestley Smith's classic study [116] and substantiated by others [117]. The remainder of the eye does not show the same degree of stability—particularly the weight and axial length [118]. In the full-term infant, ocular length ranges

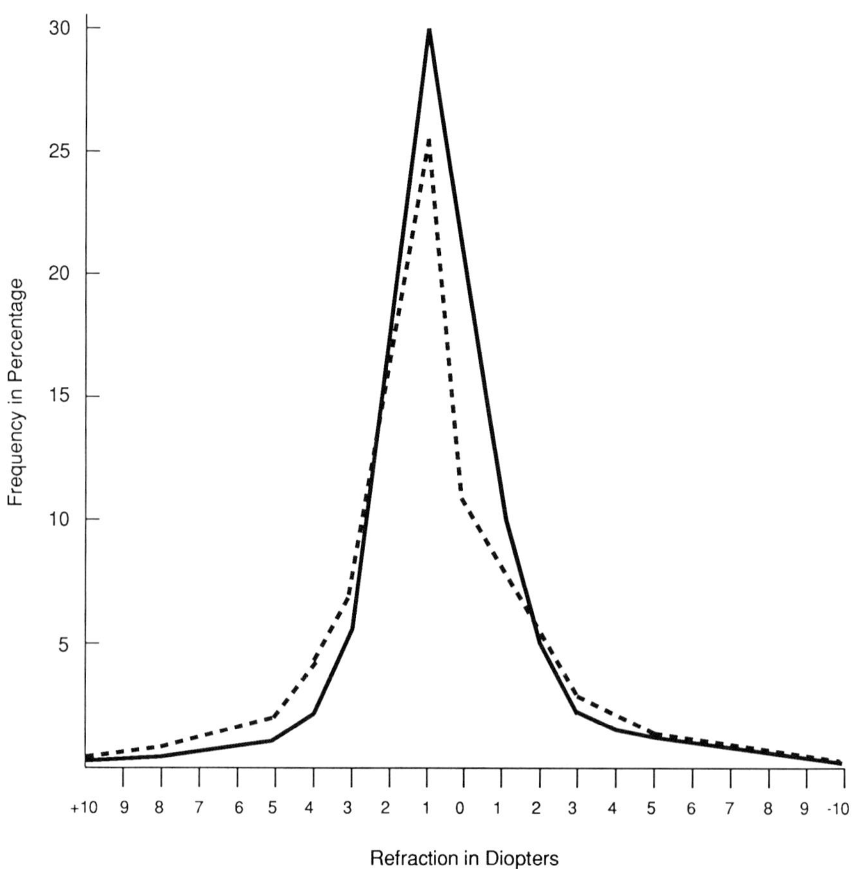

Fig. 2.46 Relative incidence of refractive errors in adolescents under 25 (from Brown, Kronfeld. The refraction curve in the U.S. with special reference to the first two decades. Thirteenth Council Ophthalmol 1929; 1:86.

from 17.5 to 18.5 mm. Since the mean adult length lies between 23 and 25 mm, 6 mm would seem to be the usual increase in ocular size during childhood. This growth is neither uniform nor marked but still necessitates considerable change in the dioptric powers of the lens and cornea (to a lesser extent the anterior chamber depth) in order to compensate.

The eye grows most of the remaining 6 mm (an additional 5 mm) between birth and age 3 years [113]. The lens and/or the cornea must therefore undergo almost 20 D of compensatory change during this period, for there is no drastic change in the refraction of the eye during this time. Whether the cornea and lens are equally concerned in this compensation is uncertain; it has been shown that changes in corneal power in the order of 20 D do occur in the rabbit but comparable changes have not been satisfactorily demonstrated in humans. It follows that the changes must therefore occur mostly in the lens during infancy but evidence for these changes is not clearcut.

During the next 10 years there is a gradual elongation of the eye by approximately 1.0 mm. Consequently, less change is required of either the cornea or the lens. The increase in axial length represents a potential reduction of some 3 D of hyperopia, but the actual reduction is less since flattening of the lens reduces its power by about 1.5 D, and there is also some flattening of the cornea. It is apparently the shortfall of such changes that results in ametropia. That is, it is the failure to compensate for axial growth that produces myopia and it is the failure of ocular growth itself that produces hyperopia. That these changes do occur is evident by the fact that the percentage of eyes showing axial elongation is greater than those eventually showing myopia. This correlation of increasing ocular elongation and decreasing power of the lens and cornea is the normal pattern in childhood. Sorsby [113] was able to demonstrate flattening of the corneal curvature associated with increasing ocular elongation. Therefore, the main trend is toward emmetropia; marked reduction in hyperopia or the breakdown of this correlation leading to myopia is uncommon.

That a slight increase in hyperopia was the rule during the first 7 years of life was found by Brown in his study [119]. This rather surprising finding was confirmed by Slataper, but his figures for refraction in the early years of life were restricted and he included Brown's figures in his own series [120]. On the other hand, the longitudinal studies of Hirsch and Weymouth on a slightly older age group appear to indicate that while an increase of hyperopia is found in a small proportion of children, a decrease is the rule [121].

The more rapid changes in axial length as well as the capacity to compensate are greater in the younger age groups. The slower rate of growth as seen in the older age groups along with a diminished capacity to compensate correlates well with the greater incidence of myopia in those older age groups. This phenomenon must be kept in mind when evaluating studies that purport to show that myopia increases during later school and college years and that therefore near-work produces the impetus for such change. The temptation to conclude that *post hoc, ergo propter hoc,* while tempting must be resisted.

Component coordination

How this coordinated growth is achieved is uncertain. In an earlier study it has been shown that the eye is a coordinated organ and not a haphazard association of optical components [112]. It was therefore suggested that the axial length is the determining factor in the dioptric architecture of the globe, and that normally the curvatures of the cornea and of the lens are determined by axial length. In the case of the cornea this followed from the fact that a larger globe had flatter surfaces; in the case of the lens the physical basis was not so obvious. Full coordination and automatic adjustment gave emmetropic eyes, and less full coordination resulted in errors falling within the range of ±4.0 D. It appears that all but some 3% to 4% of eyes in the general population have full or fairly full coordination.

Sorsby and his associates amplified these findings in showing that the process of coordination is active throughout childhood (Figure 2.47). Here the adaptation of the cornea and of the lens to axial elongation is seen in operation. It was also shown that compensation by flattening of the cornea and lens tends to lag behind the axial elongation, so that during growth the optical components are not only coordinated, but so keyed that some reduction in refraction follows: this is the process of emmetropization in action. Since growth of the eye implies increase in axial length and decrease of the curvature of the lens—and to a lesser extent of the cornea—it follows not only that the child's eye is smaller but that the quotient of axial length to the curvature of the lens is lower than in the adult.

Sorsby and his group invoked embryonic organization as the factor responsible for the negative correlation between the power of the lens and the axial length. Simple mechanical factors, however, may provide a partial explanation as well. As an example, the ring into which the outer extremity of the suspensory ligament is inserted increases in diameter with the growth of the globe and so will tend to flatten the lens, and it has been suggested that the tone of the ciliary muscle may itself affect the axial length of the globe [56,122,123].

This latter concept has led to an exploration of the role accommodation may have in promoting the progression of myopia [124]. Various authors have advocated the use of atropine drops to suspend accommodation, claiming a slowing or arresting of the growth of the eye [125–128]. Atropine is a dangerous drug, however, and its potential side effects must be weighed against its potential benefits, because the evidence of its efficacy is not clearcut. However, Curtin feels that the possible risk of atropine

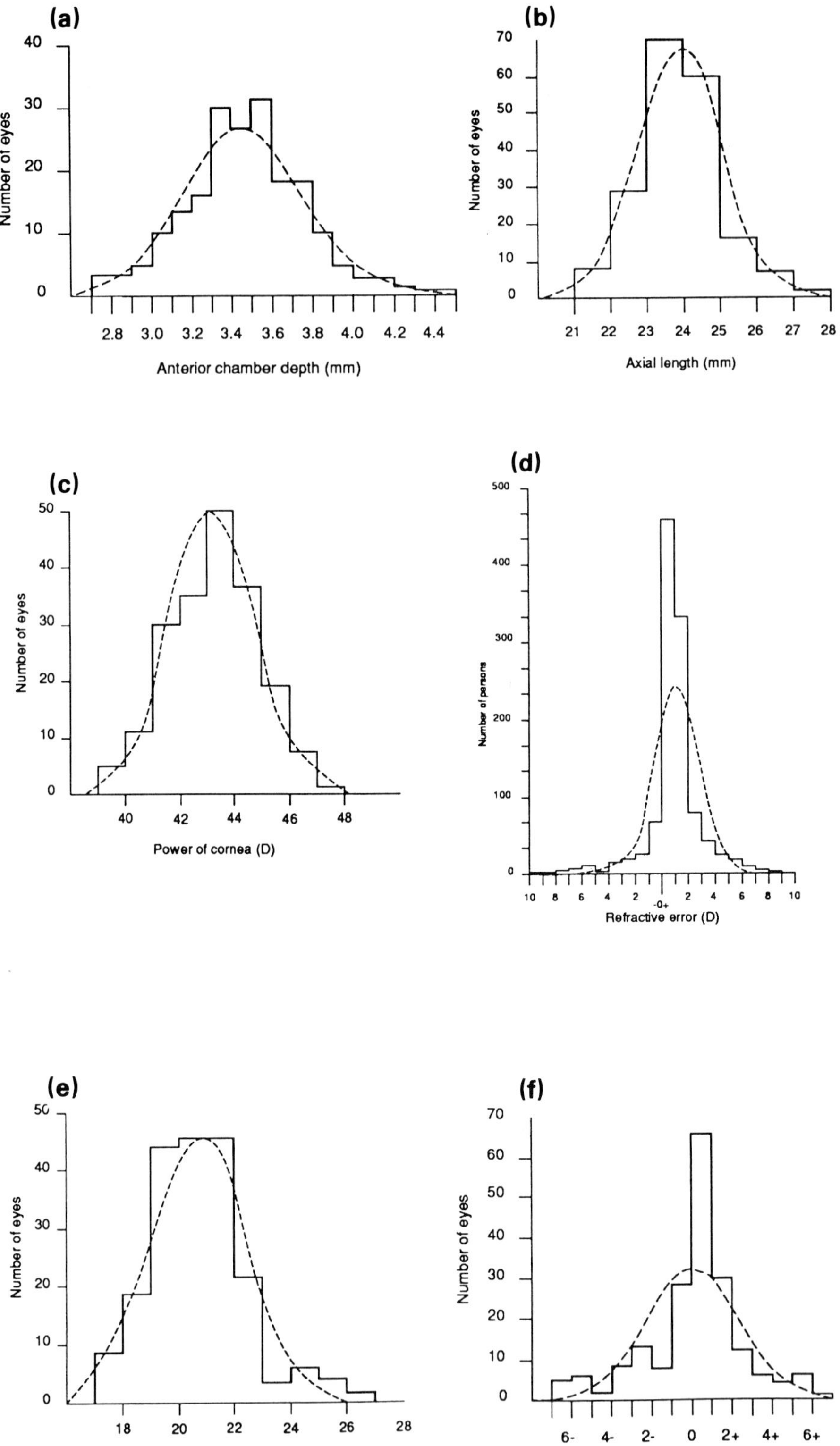

Fig. 2.47 (a,b) Ocular component dimensions in children: AC depth/axial length. (c,d) Cornealpower/distribution of refractive error. (e,f) Lens power/total refraction (from Sorsby A, Benjamin B, Davey J. *Emmetropia and Its Aberrations*. Medical Research Council, London, 1937).

therapy in intermediate myopia is outweighed by the real morbidity of an increase in myopia from 3 to 5 D, for example, which might otherwise occur [35].

Ocular development between the ages of 3 and 14 years is both slow and slight compared with the rapid and marked changes that occur in the infant under 3 years of age. Of this infantile phase we know little beyond the fact that it does occur. It is tempting to postulate that just as there are individual variations in development after the age of 3, so there are individual variations before that age. It is possible that in some eyes axial elongation falls short of the usual 5 mm or so, and that in consequence the infants enter on the second phase of ocular growth—the definitive phase—with globes considerably shorter than normal. Such adjustments that take place during the definitive stage would not be enough to carry these eyes into the normal range, and thus it is these that remain markedly hyperopic. Such a hypothesis recalls the older view that the hyperopic eye is an undeveloped one and it is probably true that the highly hyperopic eye is structurally abnormal. Similarly, while low degrees of myopia can be precipitated by the breakdown of coordination of the ocular components at the end of the definitive phase of growth, the highly myopic eyes, like the highly hypermetropic ones, fall outside the range of the changes that are part of normal growth.

The individual variations in axial elongation and in reduction of corneal and lens powers are such that it is impossible to forecast the refraction of a child who is, for example, emmetropic at the age of 8. The axial length may remain stationary and the refraction unchanged; there may be axial elongation which will be fully compensated for and so leave emmetropia, or there may be axial elongation only partially compensated for, giving myopia. Each of these three patterns was observed by Sorsby in his short follow-up study, as were similar patterns for hyperopic eyes. It seems clear that there is much to be learned from an adequate follow-up study of a substantial number of children throughout growth (Figures 2.48 to 2.50, Tables 2.5 and 2.6).

Changes in the refractive state in the adult

We have seen that it is probable that significant growth of the eye proceeds only until early puberty; thereafter in the majority of subjects the axial length of the globe remains practically unaltered. Nevertheless, after ocular growth has ceased, the evidence indicates that refractive changes still occur with age. Thus Slataper found that there was a slight but steady increase in hyperopia from the third to the seventh decade, and it is generally recognized that this process, although mild in degree, is the rule after the age of 40 [58,77]. Thus an eye which was emmetropic at 30 years of age will show 0.25 D of hyperopia at 55, an addition of 0.75 D may be evident at 60, of 1 D at 70, and at 80 years this may increase to about 2.5 D.

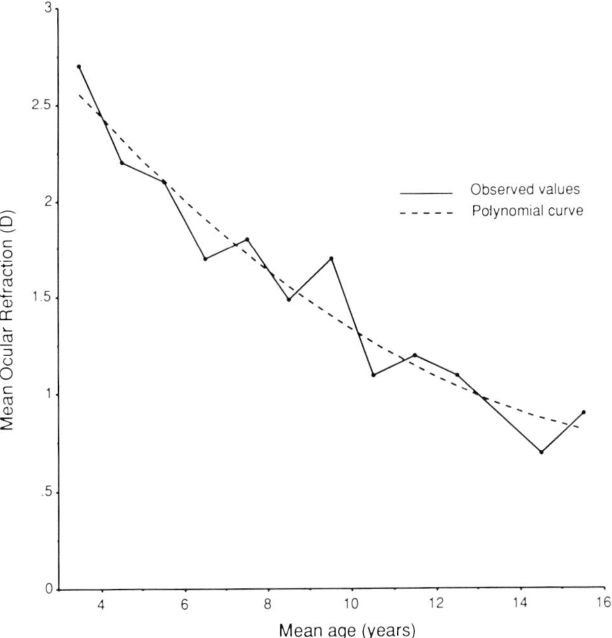

Fig. 2.48 Mean ocular refraction in diopters (from Sorsby M, Benjamin B, Sheridan M. *Refraction and Its Components During the Growth of the Eye from the Age of Three.* Medical Research Council Special Report series no. 301. Her Majesty's Stationery Office, London, 1961).

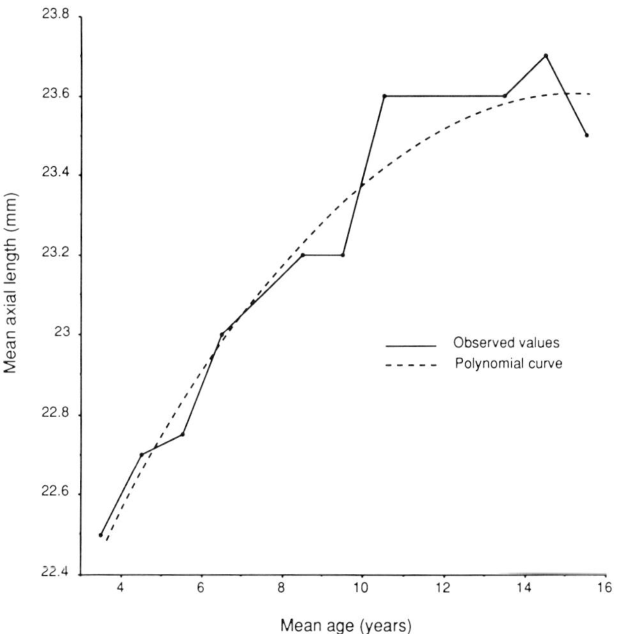

Fig. 2.49 Mean axial length in millimeters (from Sorsby M, Benjamin B, Sheridan M. *Refraction and Its Components During the Growth of the Eye from the Age of Three.* Medical Council Special Report series no. 301. Her Majesty's Stationery Office, London, 1961).

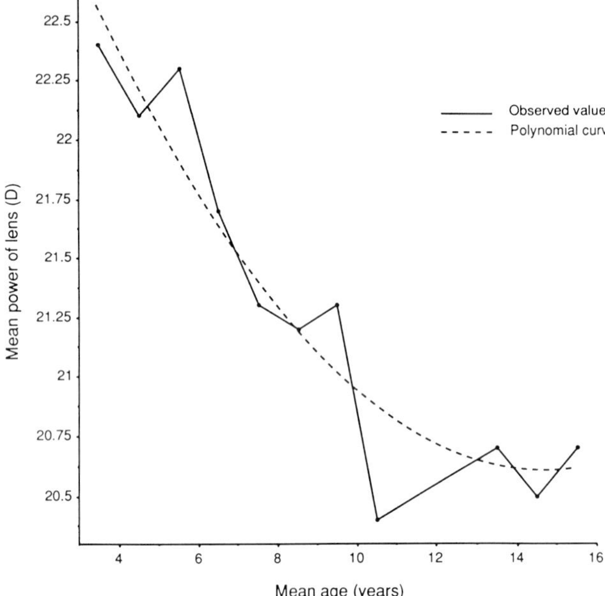

Fig. 2.50 Mean power of lens in D (from Sorsby M, Benjamin B, Sheridan M. *Refraction and Its Components During the Growth of the Eye from the Age of Three.* Medical Council Special Report series no. 301. Her Majesty's Stationery Office, London, 1961).

Hyperopia of this origin is frequently designated as acquired hyperopia (senile hypermetropia of Straub). On the other hand, in extreme old age, a trend toward myopia may develop but this change is probably due to the presence of nuclear sclerosis. Slataper, in an examination of 1404 subjects in the eighth decade, found that only 18% had clear lenses [120].

The cause of these variations in refraction originates from changes in the lens. The decreasing curvature of its surfaces as it continues to grow throughout life is probably of importance, while it has been suggested that changes in the refractive index involving an increase in optical density of the cortex, thus making the lens more uniformly refractive, could also contribute to a decrease of its optical power [129]. However, it is by no means certain that the refractive index of the nucleus of the normal lens or cortex alters with age. Possibly the relative or absolute size of the nucleus may decrease with advancing years, thereby reducing the lenticular power.

Table 2.5 Mean values of ocular refraction during growth in 1432 children. From Sorsby A, Benjamin B, Sheridan M. *Refraction and Its Components during the Growth of the Eye from the Age of Three.* Medical Council Special Report series no. 301. Her Majesty's Stationery Office, London, 1961

	Boys			Girls		
Age (years)	No.	Mean ocular refraction (D)	Standard error of mean	No.	Mean ocular refraction (D)	Standard error of mean
3	56	+2.33	±0.24	39	+2.96	±0.19
4	54	+2.24	±0.12	51	+2.33	±0.15
5	56	+2.21	±0.16	58	+2.20	±0.17
6	56	+1.71	±0.16	54	+1.83	±0.19
7	64	+1.92	±0.20	57	+1.98	±0.20
8	60	+1.76	±0.19	60	+1.63	±0.15
9	50	+1.52	±0.24	56	+2.03	±0.24
10	51	+1.43	±0.22	63	+1.33	±0.20
11	57	+1.63	±0.23	85	+1.50	±0.20
12	67	+1.19	±0.23	60	+1.04	±0.19
13	58	+1.38	±0.20	61	+0.96	±0.13
14	42	+0.93	±0.38	80	+0.62	±0.26
15				37	+0.64	±0.18
	671			761		

Table 2.6 Comparison of correlation coefficients for five refraction variables. From van Alphen GWHM: On emmetropia and ametropia. Ophthalmologica 1961; 142 (suppl):7

For refractions between column	Stenstrom ±10 D I	British ±8 D II	Stenstrom ±3 D III	British ±3 D IV
12	−0.75	−0.77	−0.45	−0.59
13	−0.34	−0.46	−0.40	−0.50
14	−0.19	−0.30	−0.21	−0.26
15	−0.02	+0.28	+0.13	+0.42
23	+0.44	+0.46	+0.45	+0.39
24	−0.31	−0.28	−0.52	−0.51
25	−0.39	−0.49	−0.60	−0.60
34	+0.09	+0.19	+0.09	+0.14
35	−0.26	−0.46	−0.32	−0.44
45	−0.10	−0.10	−0.09	−0.09
Number of right eyes	1000	96	886	78

Prevalence of ametropia

The question that invariably arises during the course of any discussion of refractive surgery is: just how prevalent is ametropia anyway? Figure 2.51 shows a combined graph for the prevalence of myopia as reported by several authors [62,75,130].

There are any number of monographs and treatises dealing with this subject which have been printed over the years. The problem lies in separating the wheat from the chaff, as it were. Authors have faulted their own studies by poor sampling or restricted or too broad interpretation of the term ametropia. In some studies of myopia, cases with astigmatism were eliminated, in others such cases were retained. In others such cases were included but only the spherical equivalents recorded. In still others cycloplegia was used in the examinations, in others not.

Coupled with those variants is the apparent inherent variable incidence of myopia among certain racial and

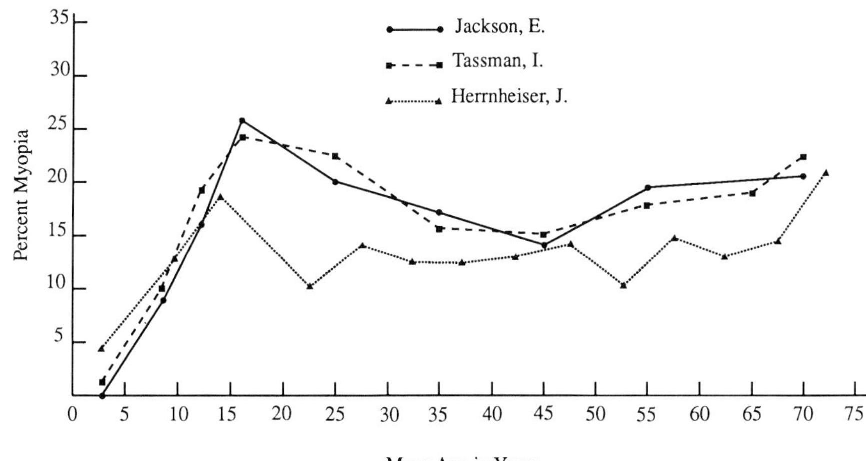

Fig. 2.51 Prevalence of myopia (derived from Jackson, Herrnheiser, and Tassman).

ethnic groups associated with the influence of the environment. For example, a study of 120,000 rural Chinese undertaken in 1912 has no real bearing on the incidence of myopia amongst urban Britons nor, for that matter, on contemporary rural Chinese. The prevalence of myopia demonstrates considerable changes with age as well. Then too, some studies examine a specific population in cross section while others examine a smaller group at regular intervals over time.

The classic example of this variability is the relatively homogeneous population of Germany. Reports from the Federal Republic of Germany find myopia to be the seventh most frequent cause of blindness (6.6% of cases) [131]. The neighboring Democratic Republic to the east finds myopia to be either the first or second most frequent cause in two surveys (14.7% and 13.9% of cases, respectively) [131]. More reliable data will be forthcoming when international health agencies can standardize such reportage. In spite of the obvious shortcomings of these surveys at the present, the prevalence of myopia as a blinding disease is most impressive.

There is evidence that the incidence of myopia may be even higher in Orientals. Blacks seem to show a lower incidence of myopia than do nonblacks and there is a slight skewing toward a higher incidence among urban populations. Some studies show as much as a 2:1 ratio of occurrences in Jews as opposed to non-Jews; others show it to be 33% more among persons of Jewish extraction. This was not shown in Sorsby's work, however (Figure 2.52).

The prevalence of ametropia also varies with age. The typical incidence of myopia at age 6 months is 4% to 6%. The overall incidence of myopia among school children ranges from 4% in ages 4 to 14 in England to 25% in the same age group in Japan. In the United States, the large HANES study examined the incidence of myopia among youths aged 12 to 17 and found that the incidence rose from 29.3% at age 12 to 33.2% at age 17 [132]. Curtin's study, conducted during the early part of this century, aptly demonstrates the changes in myopia during rapid childhood development. Among children in the 1st through 4th grades, the frequency of myopia was 10%, in grades 5 through 8, 11%; and in grades 9 through 12, 16.35%. Sorsby found a gradual decrease in hyperopia for the same age groups: +2.65 D at age 3, +1.77 D at age 6 [133]. Later he demonstrated a change from +2.33 D to +0.93 D in boys aged 3 to 14 years. Girls showed a similar, slightly larger change in the same age group. In a group of 231 hyperopic school children followed over a 3- to 8-year period, Sorsby showed that 6% had an increase in their hyperopia, 60% were stable, and the remainder became less hyperopic. In a parallel study of 130 myopic school children, 65% showed an increase in their myopia from −0.75 D to more than −4.00 D [134]. Most showed an increase in the range of −1.25 to −2.00 D. A somewhat later study demonstrated a change of −1.00 to −2.00 D in 72% of the students [135]. This gradual reduction in hyperopia during childhood has also been found in the studies of Herrnheiser [130], and Hirsch [136, 137]. Cross-sectional studies will occasionally show an increase in average hyperopia during an isolated 1-year interval depending on how the sample is obtained. Three such shifts are exhibited for both boys and girls in Sorsby's data [113] and one at age 6 (male) is demonstrated in Hirsch's data [121], but these changes can be attributed to the nature of cross-sectional sampling rather than to actual longitudinal increases in hyperopic refractions. In view of the general agreement regarding the behavior of refraction during childhood, the data of Brown and Slataper (see above), for example, must be taken with reservations. Their data showed an increase in mean hyperopic refraction through the 7th year, then a gradual decrease in hyperopia was found. This variation can probably be attributed to the population sampled since, of those children below age 8 in Brown's population sample, over 50% had strabismus. Because Slataper incorporated Brown's population in his study, the unusual incidence of high hyperopia in this

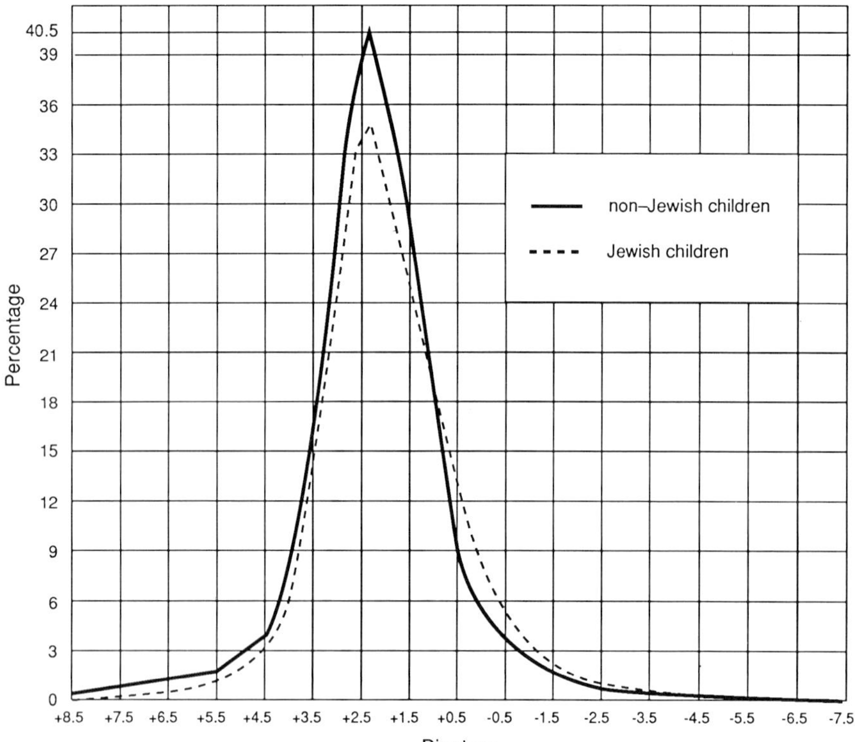

Fig. 2.52 Relative incidence of refractive errors in children aged 4 to 8 (Sorsby).

group could affect the findings of both studies. This shows the importance of longitudinal studies in interpreting data gleaned from cross-sectional investigations.

Ametropia and personality

Much has been written about the personality characteristics of the myope, less about the hyperope. Schapero and Hirsch refer to the inhibited disposition and overcontrolling nature of the myope as opposed to the happy-go-lucky, carefree affect of hyperopic brethren [138]. Other studies have reported similar findings.

The psychologic effects of myopia are operative, for the most part, during the crucial periods in the development of personality. The gradual loss of efficient distance vision tends to concentrate the interest and energies of these patients more and more on near tasks. This obligatory shift to near is capable of producing subtle as well as striking changes in the attitudes and aptitudes of the individual. Justly or not, the myope has always been considered the introverted, bookish, nonathlete who is the academic bane of more outgoing emmetropic and hyperopic fellows. Rice stressed the tendency of the myope to become finicky, painstaking, and scrupulous. These characterizations were more the impressions of the author and were unsupported by scientific data, however. There is, nevertheless, more than fragmentary evidence that this impression is true, at least to a limited extent. Rice also observed that the use of correcting lenses, as in the case of Theodore Roosevelt, could prevent the development of such an intolerant personality (how much that helped in this case is debatable) [139].

In an early study of college students, it was found that myopes did indeed show a slight but consistent tendency toward introversion when compared with normally sighted colleagues [140]. The average difference as measured by the Bernreuter Personality Inventory was not statistically significant and, in addition, was unaffected by the degree of myopia and the duration of the use of corrective lenses. A number of other tests consistently show differences in the mental makeup and attitudes of the myope. Schapero and Hirsch [138], using the Guilford-Martin Temperament Test, found myopes to be more prone to emotional inhibition and disinclined toward motor activity. These authors noted that the myope was inclined toward social leadership—somewhat at odds with introverted personality traits, one would think.

A later study by Stevens and Wolff using a test for the evaluation of leveling-sharpening mentation, showed a significant correlation with refraction [141]. Myopia was associated with highly differentiated memories as a result of minimal perceptual interaction. In 1967 Young used the Edwards Personal Preference Schedule and found that myopes scored higher than nonmyopes in achievement, introspection, abasement, heterosexuality, and aggression needs [142]. Nonmyopes scored higher in deference, order, exhibitionism, dominance, and change. Statistical significance was achieved only in abasement (guilt feelings, willingness to accept blame), exhibitionism (need to be noticed), and change (the desire to vary or avoid routine).

Using the Rorschach test, Rosanes compared the myope with the emmetrope and hyperope and presented the hypothesis that myopia might be a protective or adaptive mechanism, a reaction pattern to anxiety [143]. She theorized that myopia might be one of a series or constellation of tendencies or reactions to stress by a certain type of personality configuration—a somewhat teleological explanation of myopia. The cock crows and the sun rises; therefore, it is the crowing of the cock that causes the sun to rise. To propose that myopia is a *result* of a personality disorder is a novel concept indeed. This study concluded that myopes have a statistically significant increase in covert anxiety, with a decrease in motor activity compared with other refractive groups ($p < 0.01$). Rosanes also noted the fact that both hyperopes and myopes demonstrate less variability in exhibiting anxiety than do emmetropes ($p < 0.01$). These two groups also showed less variability in exhibiting hostility compared with those who were emmetropic ($p < 0.01$). She further concluded that myopes have a high tolerance for anxiety and exhibit excessive control. They are less likely to place themselves in a situation where they can be attacked. They are innately cautious and use compromise generously. She found that the typical attitude of the hyperope could be characterized as "fight" and that of the myopes as "fright"—understandable in any sentient who finds himself or herself "hemmed in" by a blurred and uncertain environment.

An earlier Rorschach test survey conducted by van Alphen had found that myopes demonstrated a unique system of abstract thinking but had a deep-seated anxiety pattern [56]. From these results it would appear that myopia is associated with certain differences in cerebration that are accompanied by distinguishing personality traits. Guilt feelings, anxiety, and introversion are frequently cited in this regard, and these emotions may have much to do with the greater achievements of the myope.

Ametropia, intelligence, and scholastic standing

The earliest and most extensive reports on this subject were those of Cohn in Germany [144]. He found 1.4% of children in the primary grades to be nearsighted. This increased to 26.2% at the university level. Cohn compiled an extensive, international survey of the relationship between myopia and academic achievement. In Japan this same phenomenon has been seen. A very large 1937 study found that myopia increased in the school population from 27% in the elementary grades to about 46% in middle grades to a high of 67% in high schools [145, 146]. Myopes seem to cluster among the high achievers as well, whereas hyperopes seem to be scattered through the ability groups at random. Goldschmidt made a careful survey of school children in the Danish population in 1968 [147]. He noted a significant plurality of myopes in the academic groups as compared with the other two, intellectually less rigorous, comprehensive and general groups. He also noted that whereas the frequency of this condition was about the same in the normal school populations and in schools for emotionally disturbed children and those for the deaf, the frequency of myopia was significantly less among retarded children.

The remarkable academic success of the myopic population has naturally raised questions regarding the association of myopia and intelligence. Various studies relating ametropia to intelligence scores have been reported in the literature [80,148–150]. A number of tests have demonstrated a measurable difference in the intelligence quotient (IQ) of persons with various refractive states. The myope usually scores perceptibly higher than the emmetrope and hyperope. All these studies indicate that, on average, hyperopes achieve lower intelligence scores than do myopes (Table 2.7).

Although numerous studies have found the IQ of the myope to be somewhat higher than that of nonmyopes, statistical significance has not been established. At this time there is no body of scientific evidence to support or refute this concept. Hirsch's study of 14- to 17-year-olds is of interest because it showed that IQ scores increased in proportion to the degree of myopia, while a reverse relationship was shown in hyperopes; this was especially apparent when reading was used as a basis for the score [80]. Taken together, the indicators are that hyperopes are not necessarily less intelligent than myopes but that their average reading scores on such tests are lower.

Table 2.7 Reading scores and ametropia. From Angle J, Wissmann DA. The epidemiology of myopia. Am J Epidemiol 1980; 111:220–228. Roberts J, Slaby D. Refraction Status of Youths 12–17 Years. United States Vital Health Statistics Series 11, No. 148. (HRA) 75:1630, 1974

	Myopic (%)
Reading test (deciles)	
1 (low)	19.7
2	24.9
3	27.6
4	30.9
5	31.3
6	32.4
7	31.0
8	38.1
9	37.5
10 (high)	45.3
Time spent reading in a typical day	
<1 hour	27.7
1–3 hours	32.8
>3 hours	34.6

Still, there is very little unequivocal evidence that overall, hyperopes have a greater reading disability than do myopes. Most studies purporting to show this relationship often neglect to indicate the spread of refractive error and frequently neglect to use cycloplegia. One of the most widely quoted studies on this subject is the one by Eames [151]. In this study, refraction without cycloplegia was done in 1000 children who were judged reading failures. Of this group 43% were found to be hyperopic as opposed to only 13% in a group selected at random. Unfortunately, no distribution of the hyperopia is given. Thus the 30% differential between the two groups is meaningless. It is likely that these data are skewed by the high incidence of hyperopia in the general school population.

In the United States, Dunphy et al. in 1968, found a disproportionately high frequency of myopia in 200 graduate students attending the Harvard schools of business and law [152]. The implication is that the level of education affected the degree of myopia. This study is flawed, however, in the manner of establishing the cohort and many students failed to return for follow-up examinations.

Nadell et al., administering the California Test of Mental Maturity (CTMM) to 414 students, demonstrated a data trend that indicated that myopes were generally more intelligent, but not to a significant degree [148]. One year later Hirsch published the results of another study in which he administered the Stanford-Binet test to children 6 to 7 years of age and the CTMM to older pupils: 544 students were tested in all [80]. He found no statistical difference in scores among youngsters 6 to 9 years of age, but among those aged 10 to 13, myopes scored higher ($p < 0.001$). In these data there was an almost linear increase in IQ from students with hyperopia of greater than +2 D to myopic students of greater than –2 D. These results were seen as being the result of several possible mechanisms: an overdeveloped eye associated with greater cerebral development; the effect on test scores of reading experience and proficiency; the tendency of intelligent children to read more and thereby become myopic; and the superior reading ability of myopes leading to an increase in their scores.

Young later studied 251 students using both the Stanford-Binet and the CTMM. All correlations were low and negative. The larger differences favoring myopes were contained in the results of the CTMM, which requires greater reading ability. Young then tested the reading ability of 117 students and found that myopes were significantly better readers than the emmetropes [149].

In summary, it may be said that myopes generally score higher on intelligence tests, although not to a significant degree. Part of this, but not all, can be attributed to their demonstrably superior reading ability and their personality traits. Given the hereditary background of myopia, scholarship reinforcement is also more likely to be present at home. The myopic student more often has a similarly affected parent, often of academic achievement, who would stress intellectual pursuits and academic hobbies. Even the very wearing of spectacles may play a small part in the tendency to regard myopes as more intelligent.

Thornton found that merely wearing glasses can give the impression of intelligence [118]. Additional observations of those with short sight have included the allegation that they are essentially night people who like to stay up late. This is said to be related possibly to the greater security felt by the myopic child at night, at which time the darkness neutralizes the handicap to some degree. If dimness of the external world of the myope retards the development of an extroverted, gregarious personality, it appears to be a superb catalyst for the development of artistic skills. Or as Curtin put it:

> It has been said that "success dwells in the silences." It is conceivable that myopia provides just such a "silence" for the young it afflicts [35].

References

1 Ferry AP. "Professor" Charles Tyrell and His Ideal Sight Restorer. Ophthalmology 1986; 93(9):1246–1257.

2 Breasted J. *The Edwin Smith Surgical Papyrus.* University of Chicago Press, Chicago, 1930.

3 Ebers G. *Papyrus Ebers, das hermetische Buch über die Arzeneimittel der alten Ägypter in hieratischer Schrift.* Leipzig, 1875.

4 Bryan CP. *The Papyrus Ebers.* Geoffrey Bles, London, 1930.

5 Aristotle. *Problems,* 2 volumes. WS Hett (transl). Harvard University Press, Cambridge, Mass, 1961.

6 Hirschberg J. *Antiquity, vol. 1. The History of Ophthalmology,* FC Blodi (ed). Wayenborgh Verlag, Bonn, 1982.

7 Aristotle. *Parts of Animals,* 1 volume. WS Hett (transl). Harvard University Press, Cambridge, Mass, 1961.

8 Galen C. *On the Use of the Parts of the Body,* 2 volumes. MT May (transl). Ithaca, 1968.

9 Moon RO. The influence of Pythagoras on Greek medicine. In Proceedings of the Seventeenth International Congress of Medicine, Sect 23, London, 1913.

10 Duke-Elder S, Abrams D. Historical development. In: *System of Ophthalmology. II. The Anatomy of the Visual System,* SS Duke-Elder (ed). C.V. Mosby, St. Louis, 1970.

11 Hirschberg J. *The Middle Ages,* vol 2: *The History of Ophthalmology,* F Blodi (ed). Wayenborgh Verlag, Bonn, 1982.

12 Al-Haytham I. *Opticae Thesaurus Alhezeni libri VII.* F Risner, Basel, 1572.

13 Polo M. *The Travels of Marco Polo.* Yule, London, 1875.

14 Manni D. Lettera intorno all'invenzione deglie occhiali. In: *Degli occhiali da naso inventati da salvino Armatis, Gentiluomo Florentino.* Accademico Florentino, Florence, 1738.

15 Gordon B. *Practica su Lilium Medicinae, Particula III: De passionibus oculorum.* J & G DeGregoriis, Venice, 1496.

16 Cooper S. The Medical School of Montpellier in the fourteenth century. Ann Med Hist 1930; 2:163.

17 Chauliac G. *Chirurgia magna.* Venice, 1553.

18 Platter F. *De corporis humani structura et usu.* Officinia Ionnis Oporinus, Basel, 1583.

19 Scheiner C. *Occulus Hoc est: fundamentum opticum.* Daniel Agricolam, Innsbruck, 1619.

20 Mark HH. Johannes Kepler on the eye and vision. Am J Ophthalmol 1971; 72:869–878.

21 Nutton V. *From Democedes to Harvey: Studies in the History of Medicine.* Variorum Reprints, London, 1988.

22 Pliny the Elder. *Natural History*, 10 volumes. H Rackham, WHS Jones and DE Eicholz (transl). Loeb Classic Library, Harvard University Press, Cambridge, Mass, 1942.
23 Rogers S. *Primitive Surgery: Skills Before Science.* Thomas, Springfield, 1985.
24 Plempius V. *Ophthalmologica.* Henrici Laurentii, Amsterdam, 1632.
25 Hamberger G. *Optica Oculorum.* Literis Gollnerianis, Jena, 1696.
26 Morgagni GB. *De Sedibus et Causis Morborum per Anatomen Indiaatis.* Remenainiana, Venice, 1761.
27 Scarpa AA. *A Treatise on the Principal Diseases of the Eye.* J Bregg, London, 1818.
28 Boerhaave H. *Praelectiones Publicae, de Morbis Oculorum.* A Vandenhoek, Göttingen, 1746.
29 Valdes BD. *Uso de los antojos y comentarios a propósito del mismo.* Diego Perez, Seville, 1623.
30 Hirschberg J. *The Renaissance of Ophthalmology in the Eighteenth Century*, part 2, vol 4: *The History of Ophthalmology*, F Blodi (ed). Wayenborgh Verlag, Bonn, 1982.
31 Newton I. *Opticks.* Smith and Walford, London, 1704.
32 Smith R. *A Compleat System of Opticks.* Cornelius Crownfield, Cambridge, 1738.
33 Kästner AG. *Vollständiger Lehrbegriff des Optick.* Altenberg, 1755.
34 Janin de Combe-Blanche J. *Mémoires et Observations Anatomiques, Physiologiques et Physiques sur l'Oeil.* Didot, Paris, 1772.
35 Curtin BJ. *The Myopias. Basic Science and Clinical Management.* Harper & Row, New York, 1985.
36 von Ammon FA. Uber die angebornen Spaltungen in der Iris, Chorioidea and Retina des menschlichen Auges. (About congenital colobomas of the iris, choroid and retina in the human eye.) Ophthalmologie 1831; 1:55.
37 von Arlt CF. *Ueber die Ursachsen und die Entsehung der Kurzichtigkeit.* Wilhelm Braumuller, Vienna, 1856.
38 von Graefe A. Zwei Sektionbefunde von Scleratio-Chronivites posterior und Bermerbegen uber diese Krankeit. Arch Ophthalmol 1854; 1:390.
39 Young T. Observations on vision. Phil Trans R Soc Lond 1793; 83:169.
40 Young T. On the mechanism of the eye; the Bakerian lecture. Phil Trans R Soc Lond 1801; 91:23–88.
41 Ware J. Aberrations relative to the near and distant sight of different persons. Phil Trans Lond 1813; 1:31.
42 MacKenzie W. *A Practical Treatise on the Diseases of the Eye.* Longman, London, 1830.
43 Stellwag von Carion K. Refractive anomalies. S B Akad Wiss Wein, Math Klasse 1855; 16:187.
44 Donders FC. *On the Anomalies of Accommodation and Refraction of the Eye*, WD Moore (transl). Hatton Press, London, 1864.
45 Airy G. On a peculiar defect in the eye, and a mode of correcting it. Trans Camb Phil Soc 1827; 2:267–273.
46 Schnyder. Ann Oculist (Paris) 1849;21:222.
47 Hays I. Ocular Astigmatism. In: *Lawrence's: A Treatise on Diseases of the Eye*, I Hays (ed). Lea & Blanchard, Philadelphia, 1854.
48 Noyes HD. Cylindrical glasses in astigmatism. Am J Med Sci 1872; 63:355–359.
49 Bates WH. A suggestion of an operation to correct astigmatism Arch Ophthalmol 1894; 23:9–13.
50 Lans L. Experimentelle Untersuchungen uber die Entstehung von Astigmatismus durch nicht Perforirende Corneawunden. (Experimental studies of the treatment of astigmatism with nonperforating corneal incisions.) Albrecht von Graefes Arch Klin Exp Ophthalmol 1898; 45:117–152.
51 Duke-Elder S, Abrams D. Anomalies of the optical system: Types of ametropia. In: *System of Ophthalmology. V. Ophthalmic Optics and Refraction*, SS Duke-Elder (ed). C.V. Mosby, St. Louis, 1970.
52 Helmholtz H. *Treatise on Physiological Optics*, vol 1, J Southall (transl). Opt Soc Am, New York, 1924.
53 Roure MF. Deux problèmes sur la correction de l'astigmatisme cornéen par les verres cylindriques. Ann Oculist (Paris) 1896; 115:99–107.
54 Brint S, Ostrick D, Bryan J. Keratometric cylinder and visual performance following phacoemulsification and implantation with silicone small-incision or poly (methyl methacrylate) intraocular lenses. J Cataract Refract Surg 1991; 17:32–36.
55 Parker W, Clorfeine G. Long-term evolution of astigmatism following planned extracapsular cataract extraction. Arch Ophthalmol 1989; 107:353–357.
56 van Alphen G. On emmetropia and ametropia. Ophthalmologica 1961; 142:33.
57 Curtin BJ. Physiopathology and therapy of the myopias. Trans Can Ophthalmol Otolaryngol 1966; 5:331–339.
58 Hirsch MJ. The longitudinal study of refraction. Am J Optom 1964; 41:137.
59 Cusanus N. *Opscula*, Part II: *De Beryllo.* Nuremberg, 1441.
60 Duke-Elder S, Abrams D. Spectacles. In: *System of Ophthalmology. V. Ophthalmic Optics and Refraction.*, SS Duke-Elder (ed). C.V. Mosby, St. Louis, 1970.
61 Ridley H. Intraocular acrylic lenses. Trans Ophthalmol Soc UK 1951; 71:617.
62 Tassman I. Frequency of the various kinds of refractive errors. Am J Ophthalmol 1932; 15:1044.
63 Tenner AS. Refraction in school children: 4800 refractions tabulated according to age, sex and nationality. NY Med J 1915; 102:611.
64 Stenstrom S. Untersuchungen uber die Variation und Kovariation der optischen Elemente des menschlichen Auges. Acta Ophthalmol (suppl) 1946; 26:7.
65 Grosvenor T. The neglected hyperope. Am J Optom 1971; 48: 376–382.
66 Broekema O. Bijdrage tot de kennis der hypermetropie. Thesis. Amsterdam, 1909.
67 Pfalz G. Ophthalmometrische untersuchungen ubër cornealastigmatismus; mit dem ophthalmometer von Javal und Sciötz. Graefes Arch Klin Exp Ophthalmol 1885; 31:201.
68 Sorensen SK. L'astigmatisme du cristallin, déterminé comme la différence entre l'astigmatisme cornéen et l'astigmatisme total, illustré par l'examen de ses variations d'apres l'âge. Acta Ophthalmol (Kbh) 1944; 22:341.
69 Steiger A. *Die Entstehung der Sparischen Refraktionen des menschlichen Auges.* Karger, Berlin, 1913.
70 Gullstrand A. Beitrag zur Theorie des Astigmatismus. Scand Arch Ophthalmol 1890; 2:269–359.
71 Kronfeld PC, Devney C. The frequency of astigmatism. Arch Ophthalmol 1930; 4:873–884.
72 Snellen H. Die Richtunge des Hauptmeridiane des Astigmatischen Auges. (The axis of the major meridians of the astigmatic eye.) Albrecht von Graefes Arch Klin Ophthalmol 1869; 15: 199–207.
73 Tscherning M. Physiological optics. Encycl Franc Ophthalmol (Paris) 1904; 3:105.
74 Gullstrand A. *Einfuhrung in die Methoden die Dioptrik des Auges.* Leipzig, 1911.
75 Jackson E. Norms of refraction. JAMA 1932; 98:132.
76 Hofstetter HW, Baldwin W. Bilateral correlation of residual astigmatism. Am J Optom 1957; 34:388–391.
77 Exford J. A longitudinal study of refractive trends after age forty. Am J Optom 1965; 42:685–692.
78 Forsius H, Eriksson AW, Fellman J. Corneal refraction according to age and sex in an isolated population and the heredity of the trait. Acta Ophthalmol (Kbh) 1964; 42:224.
79 Steiger A. Beitrage zur Physiologie und Pathologie der Hornhautrefaction. Arch Augenheilkd 1894; 29:98.
80 Hirsch M. The relationship between refractive state and intelligence test scores. Am J Optom Arch Am Acad Optom 1959; 36:12–21.

81 Bores L. *Pseudo-accommodation Following Radial Keratotomy.* Quintum Forum, Bogota, Columbia, 1987.

82 Descartes R. *Tractatus de Homine.* Elsevier, Amsterdam, 1977.

83 Porterfield W. *Treatise on the Eye, the Manner and Phenomena of Vision.* Hamilton & Balfour, Edinburgh, 1759.

84 Fincham EF. The changes in the form of the crystalline lens in accommodation. Trans Opt Soc Lond 1925; 26:239–269.

85 Kikawa N, Sato T. Lenticular elasticity. Exp Eye Res 1963; 2:210.

86 Fisher RF. The significance of the shape of the lens and capsular energy changes in accommodation. J Physiol 1969; 201:21–47.

87 Bates WH. *Cure of Imperfect Sight by Treatment Without Glasses.* Central Fixation, New York, 1920.

88 Kuster A. Myopieprogression bei Kontaktlinsen und bei Brillentragern in 400 Fallen. (The progression of myopia in wearers of contact lenses and spectacles. 400 cases.) Klin Monatsbl Augenheilkd 1971; 159:213–219.

89 Warren GT. Myopia control and abatement. Opt J Rev Optom 1955; 92:33.

90 Takemura T. The influence of the use of glasses on the progress of myopia. Acta Ophthalmol (Jpn) 1943; 47:906.

91 Savolyuk MM. Optical correction and progressive myopia. Vestn Oftalmol 1968, 1:82.

92 Takamaya H. The effects of glass correcting corneal astigmatism on refractive components. Acta Soc Ophthalmol (Jpn) 1974; 78:220.

93 Rubin ML, Milder B. Myopia—a treatable "disease"? Surv Ophthalmol 1976; 21:65–69.

94 Safir A. Orthokeratology: II. A risky and unpredictable "treatment" for a benign condition. Surv Ophthalmol 1980; 24:291, 298–302.

95 Roberts J, Slaby D. Refraction status of youths 12–17 years. United States Vital Health Statistics Series 11, No. 148 (HRA) 75:1630, 1974.

96 Hatfield E. Why are they blind? Sight Sav Rev 1975; 45:3.

97 Kahn H, Moorhead U. Statistics on blindness in the model reporting area. (NIM) 73–427 1970.

98 Sorsby A. The incidence and causes of blindness: an international survey. Br J Ophthalmol 1950; 34(suppl):13–14.

99 Schnabel I, Herrnheiser J. Uber Staphyloma posticum, Conus und Myopie. Z Augenheilkd 1895; 16:1.

100 Maurolycus F. *Photismi de lumine et umbra.* Venice, 1597.

101 von Reuss A. Augen-Untersuchungen an zwei Weiner Volksschulen. (Eye examinations in two Viennese public schools.) 1881; 22:200.

102 von Reuss A. Untersuchungen uber die optischen Constanten ametropischer Augen. Albrecht Von Graefes Arch Ophthalmol 1880; 23:183.

103 Awerbach M. The dioptrics of refraction (in Russian). Thesis, Moscow, 1900.

104 Tron E. Variationsstatistiche untersuchungen uber Refraction. Graefes Arch Ophthalmol 1929; 122:1–34.

105 Tron E. Ein Beitrage zur Kenntnis der Refractionskurve. Graefes Arch Ophthalmol 1930; 124:544–565.

106 Rushton RH. The clinical measurement of the axial length of the living eye. Applied Optics 1938; 58:136–142.

107 Scheerer R. Zur entwicklungsgeschlechtlichen Auffassung der Brechzustande des Auges. Ber Zusammenkunft. Dtsch Ophthalmol Ges 1928; 47:118.

108 Scheerer R, Seitzer A. Ueber das Auftreten von sogennanten myopischen Veranderungen am Augenhintergrund bei den verscheidenen Brechungzustanden des Auges. Klin Monatsbl Augenheilkd 1929; 82:511.

109 Betsch A. Ueber die menschliche Refraktionskurve. (Regarding the human refraction curve.) Klin Monatsbl Augenheilkd 1929; 82:365.

110 Wibaut F. Uber die Emmetropisation und den Ursprung der Spharischen Refraktionsanomalien. Albrecht von Graefes Arch Ophthalmol 1925; 116:596.

111 Berg F. Uber Variabilitat und Korrelation bei den verscheidenen Abmessungen des Auges. Albrecht von Graefes Arch Ophthalmol 1931; 127:606.

112 Sorsby A, Benjamin B, Davey J, Tanner JM. Emmetropia and its aberrations. Med Res Counc Spec Rep Ser (London) 1957; 293.

113 Sorsby A, Benjamin B, Sheridan M. Refraction and its Components during the Growth of the Eye from the Age of Three. Medical Research Council Special Report Series No. 301. Medical Research Council, London, 1961.

114 Brown EVL. Net average yearly changes in refraction in atropinized eyes from birth to beyond middle life. Arch Ophthalmol 1938; 19:719.

115 Lepard C. Comparative changes in the error of refraction between fixing and amblyopic eyes during growth and development. Am J Ophthalmol 1975; 80:485–490.

116 Smith P. On the size of the cornea in relation to age, sex, refraction, and primary glaucoma. Trans Ophthalmol Soc UK 1890; 10:68.

117 Peter R. Ueber die Corneagrosse und ihre Vererbung. Albrecht von Graefes Arch Ophthalmol 1924; 115:29.

118 Thornton G. The effect of judgment of personality traits of varying a simple factor in a photograph. J Appl Psychol 1944; 28:203.

119 Brown EVL, Kronfeld PC. The refraction curve in the US with special reference to the first two decades. Thirteenth Council of Ophthalmology 1929; 1:86.

120 Slataper F. Age norms of refraction and vision. Arch Ophthalmol 1950; 43:466.

121 Hirsch M, Weymouth F. A longitudinal study of refractive state of children during the first six years of school. Am J Optom Arch Am Acad Optom 1961; 38:564.

122 Collins ET. Lectures on the anatomy of the eye. Lancet 1890; 2:1329.

123 Weale RA. *The Aging Eye.* Harper & Row, London, 1963.

124 Armaly M, Burian H. Changes in the tonogram during accommodation. Arch Ophthalmol 1958; 60:60.

125 Kelly TS, Chatfield C, Tustin G. Clinical assessment of the arrest of myopia. Br J Ophthalmol 1975; 59:529–538.

126 Young F. The nature and control of myopia. J Am Optom Assoc 1977; 48:451–457.

127 Dyer J. Role of cycloplegics in progressive myopia. Ophthalmology 1979; 86:692–694.

128 Bedrossian RH. The treatment of myopia with atropine and bifocals: A long-term prospective study. Ophthalmology 1985; 92:716.

129 Parsons JH. The pathology of the eye. Br J Ophthalmol 1906; 3:929.

130 Herrnheiser J. Die Refraktionsentwicklung des menschlichen Auges. (The refraction development of the human eye.) Z Augenheilkd 1892; 13:342.

131 Lim A, Jones B. World's major blinding conditions. Vision 1981; 1:101.

132 Sperduto R, Seigel D, Roberts J, Rowland M. Prevalence of myopia in the United States. Arch Ophthalmol 1983; 101:405–407.

133 Sorsby A. Normal refraction in infants and its bearing on development of myopia. London Co Council Rep 1933; 4(3):55.

134 Sorsby A, Leary GA. A longitudinal study of refraction and its components during growth. Med Res Counc Spec Rep Ser (London) 1969; 309:1–41.

135 Sorsby A. *Epidemiology of Refraction. Historical: A Qualitative Approach.* Little, Brown, Boston, 1971.

136 Hirsch MJ. The changes in refraction between the ages of five and fourteen: Theoretical and practical considerations. Am J Optom 1952; 29:445.

137 Hirsch ND. Sex differences in the incidence of various grades of myopia. Am J Optom 1953; 30:135.

138 Schapero M, Hirsch M. The relationship of refractive error and Guilford-Martin temperament test scores. Am J Optom 1952; 29:32.

139 Rice T. Physical defects and character: II. Nearsightedness and astigmatism. Hygeia 1930; 8:644.

140 Mull H. Myopia and introversion. Am J Psychol 1948; 61:575.

141 Stevens D, Wolff H. The relationship of myopia to performance on a test of leveling-sharpening. Percept Motor Skills 1965; 21:399–403.

142 Young F. Myopia and personality. Am J Optom 1967; 44: 192–201.

143 Rosanes M. Psychological correlates to myopia compared to hyperopia and emmetropia. J Proj Tech Pers Assess 1967; 31: 31–35.

144 Cohn H. *Hygiene of the Eye in Schools.* Simpkin, Marshall, London, 1886.

145 Sato T. *The Causes and Prevention of Acquired Myopia.* 1957.

146 Otsuka J. Research on the etiology and treatment of myopia. Nippon Ganka Gakki Zasshi 1967; 71:1–212.

147 Goldschmidt E. On the etiology of myopia. An epidemiological study. Acta Ophthalmol (Copenh) 1968; 98:1.

148 Nadell M, Hirsch M. The relationship between intelligence and the refractive state in a selected high school sample. Am J Optom 1958; 35:321–326.

149 Young E. Reading, measures of intelligence and refractive errors. Am J Optom 1963; 47:257.

150 Grosvenor T. Refractive state, intelligence test scores, and academic ability. Am J Optom 1970; 47:355–361.

151 Eames T. Visual problems of poor readers. In: *Clinical Studies in Reading*, H Robinson (ed). University of Chicago Press, Chicago, 1953.

152 Dunphy E, Stoll M, King S. Myopia among American male graduate students. Am J Ophthalmol 1968; 65:518–521.

Further reading

Badawi A. Kom-Ombo sanctuaries. Inst Fr d'Arch Or, XXXII, Cairo, 1921.

Biedermann H. *Medicina Magica: Metaphysical Healing Methods in Late-antique and Medieval Manuscripts with Thirty Facsimile Plates.* Classics of Medicine Library, Birmingham, 1986.

Biggs R. Medicine in Ancient Mesopotamia. In *History of Science*, A Crombie and M Hoskins (eds). Heffer, Cambridge, 1969.

Breasted J. *The Edwin Smith Surgical Papyrus.* University of Chicago Press, Chicago, 1930.

Breasted J. *A History of Egypt.* 2d ed. Hodder and Stoughton, London, 1950.

Castiglioni A. *A History of Medicine.* New York, 1958.

Celsus. *De Medicina*, 3 vols, W Spencer (transl). Loeb Classic Library, London, 1935.

Cockburn A, Cockburn E. *Mummies, Disease and Ancient Cultures.* Cambridge University Press, Cambridge, 1968.

Davis A. *Medicine and its Technology.* Greenwood Press, Wesport, 1981.

Dawson WR. The Egyptian medical papyri. In *Science, Medicine and History*, EA Underwood (ed). Oxford University Press, London, 1953.

Estes JW. *The Medical Skills of Ancient Egypt.* Science History Publications, Canton, 1989.

Galen C. *On the Use of the Parts of the Body*, 2 vols, MT May (transl). Ithaca, 1968.

Garrison F, Morton L. *A Medical Bibliography.* J.B. Lippincott, New York, 1970.

Harper R. *The Code of Hammurabi King of Babylon about 2200 BC.* University of Chicago Press, Chicago, 1904.

Hippocrates. *The Genuine Works of Hippocrates*, 2 vols, F Adams (transl). Sydenham Society, London, 1849.

Jackson R. *Doctors and Disease in the Roman Empire.* University of Oklahoma Press, Norman, 1988.

Jastrow M Jr. Babylonian-Assyrian medicine. Ann Med Hist 1917; 1:231–257.

Kramer SN. *History Begins at Sumer.* The Falcon's Wing Press, Garden City, 1959.

Levey M. Some objective factors of Babylonian medi-cine in the light of new evidence. Bull Hist Med 1961; 35:61–70

Lyons AS, Petrucelli RJ. *Medicine: An Illustrated History.* Harry N Abrams, New York, 1987.

Nutton V. *From Democedes to Harvey: Studies in the History of Medicine.* Variorum Reprints, London, 1988.

Pliny the Elder. *Natural History*, 10 vols, H Rackham, WHS Jones and DE Eicholz (transl). Loeb Classic Library, Harvard University Press, Cambridge, 1942.

Rogers S. *Primitive Surgery: Skills Before Science.* Thomas, Springfield, 1985.

Sandison AT. Diseases of the eyes. In: *Diseases in Antiquity*, D Bothwell and AT Sandison (eds). Thomas, Springfield, 1967.

Saunders JB. *The Transitions from Ancient Egyptian to Greek Medicine.* University of Kansas Press, Lawrence, 1963.

Scarborough J. *Roman Medicine.* Cornell University Press, Ithaca, 1969.

Sigerist HE. *A History of Medicine.* Oxford University Press, London, 1951.

Waterman L. *Royal Correspondence of the Assyrian Empire.* University of Michigan, Ann Arbor, 1930.

Wells C. *Bones, Bodies and Disease.* Thames & Hudson, London, 1964.

Whipple AO. Role of the Nestorians as the connecting link between Greek and Arabic medicine. Ann Med Hist 1936; 8:313–323.

3
Light, Optics, and Refractive Surgery

He who does not imagine in stronger and better lineaments and in stronger and better light than his perishing mortal eye can see, does not imagine at all. [William Blake]

While complete elucidation of the subject of light and optics lies beyond the scope of this work, some elaboration on the topic is in order. I am keenly aware of the anathema with which the subject of optics is greeted by most ophthalmologists—still, we must acknowledge that optics plays a vital role in our specialty. To paraphrase a familiar expression: Without optics, the eye is nothing. That's because the eye serves to focus light on to the prime receptor organ of the brain—the retina—via its optical properties. That's what optics do—focus that light. Of course we all know what light is, or at least we think we do. Actually, no one knows for certain what light is—not really. It seems to be two things, or at least acts as though it were two things, or one thing with two properties. Whatever, nobody really knows, although we can make some reasonable assumptions based on its properties and its actions. Nevertheless, despite our relative ignorance, let us review what we think we know about light and then move on.

The nature of light

Light is a form of energy. Not to put too fine a point on it, light is therefore us: We too are energy, as are all things in the universe. It's just that we are more sedate than other forms of energy—except for rocks. Some energy forms move along in a more sprightly manner. Light moves very snappily indeed—some 186,000 miles per second—which makes light the fastest thing in the universe. Light is, furthermore, a special kind of energy—electromagnetic energy. That is, it possesses both electric and magnetic characteristics. More specifically, light is only a small portion of the total spectrum of electromagnetic energy. This portion is the relatively narrow band from 400 to 700 nm (a nanometer equals 10^{-9} m or 10^{-6} mm) and is called the *visual spectrum* because these wavelengths can be perceived by the human retina (Figure 3.1).

Sources of light

Before we can talk more about what light is, it will probably be a good idea to discuss from whence light comes. Basically it comes from hot matter—so-called thermal and spectral emitters. Thermal emitters are characterized by producing light as a portion of the continuous electromagnetic spectrum; an example is a light bulb. In classic pre-Planckian physics, electromagnetic waves are said to be induced by vibrating charged particles whose frequency of vibration decreases as their energy is removed by the induced electromagnetic waves; this results in a continuous energy spectrum. Max Planck forever modified this view by demonstrating that electromagnetic energy could be emitted only in discrete amounts or packets which he termed *quanta*. The energy of these quanta is proportional to a fundamental constant and the frequency of the light:

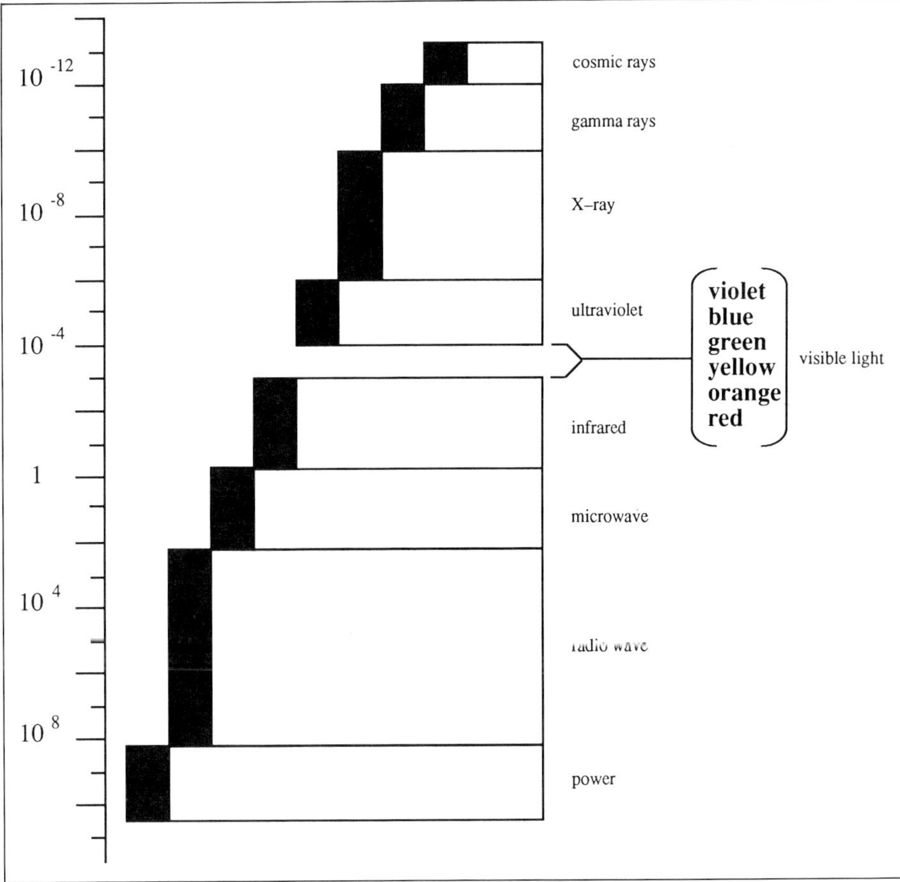

Fig. 3.1 The electromagnetic spectrum.

$E = \hbar f$

where E is the energy of the electromagnetic wave, $\hbar$ is Planck's constant, and f is the frequency of the emitted wave and therefore of the vibrating charged particle.

Prior to Planck, classic theory predicted that every object with a temperature above absolute zero continuously emitted an infinite amount of very high frequency energy, which was decidedly contrary to experience—after all, the stars still shone. This prediction was called the *ultraviolet catastrophe* and was obviously erroneous because any object that radiates an infinite amount of energy would destroy the universe in short order (Figure 3.2). However, Planck's theorem, which led to the creation of quantum mechanics and modern physics, correctly predicted the emission spectrum of hot objects. So the classic viewpoint gave way, grudgingly, to the new.

The laws of physics for hot objects were derived originally for so-called black bodies. A black body absorbs all energy striking it and reradiates that absorbed energy until it goes into thermal equilibrium with its surroundings. Under a steady-state condition, it would be the same temperature as its surroundings. At room temperature, a lump of charcoal (or other black object) is a reasonably good example of this. At higher temperatures, the same charcoal lump heated to glowing is another. Figure 3.3 represents the various spectra of black bodies at different temperatures. Note that the higher the temperature the higher the frequency (shorter wavelength) at which the maximum energy is radiated. This explains why objects at higher temperatures feel hotter (they radiate more energy) and are therefore bluer in color (more of their radiation is at higher frequencies, or the blue end of the spectrum).

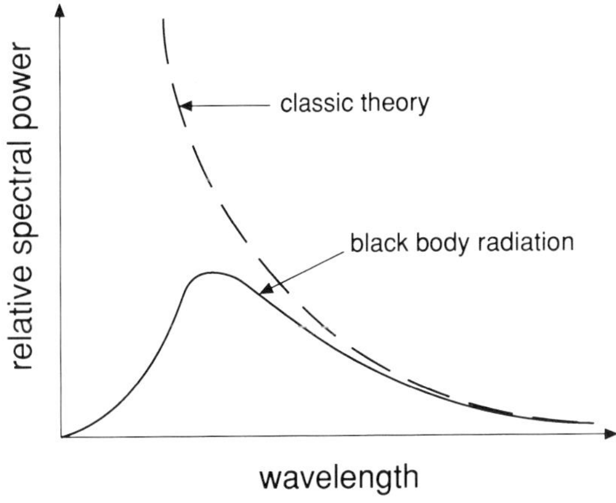

Fig. 3.2 The emission spectrum of black bodies.

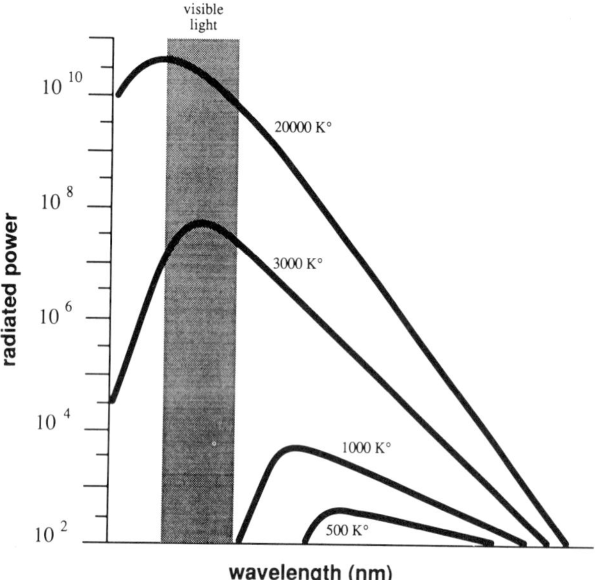

Fig. 3.3 Radiation power curves of black bodies.

Wien's displacement law, which predicts the wavelength at which the black body emits at maximum power, is

$$\lambda_m T = 0.2867 \text{ cm deg}$$

where λ_m is the wavelength of maximum emission in centimeters and T is the temperature of the black body in degrees Kelvin; thus the emission of a black body depends only on its temperature.

The energy radiated per unit area of a black body is proportional to the fourth power of its temperature. Raising an object to twice its original temperature will cause it to radiate 16 times as much energy ($2^4 = 16$). This is the reason why it is difficult to get objects to very high temperatures. The hotter an object gets, the more efficiently it radiates its energy, and the harder it is to get it hotter.

The other most common source of light is the discrete spectral emitter, which emits light at discrete frequencies rather than as a continuous spectrum. The spectrum of a black body (thermal emitter) in a spectrograph is a continuous blur between red and blue, whereas the spectrum of a discrete emitter consists of numerous distinctly colored lines, called a *line spectrum*. A line spectrum also can be produced through dispersion (see below). These discrete lines derive from the fact that the electrons which create the light are restricted to certain orbits in their atoms according to the rules of quantum mechanics. The orbit depends on the angular momentum of the electron—thus its energy. The orbital angular momentum can only be an integer multiple of $\hbar$, Planck's constant, that is:

$$\text{Orbital angular momentum} = n\hbar$$

where $n = 1, 2, 3, \ldots$, and so on. Because of various angular momenta and spins, there may be no more than $2n^2$ electrons in any orbit; therefore, two electrons for $n = 1$, eight for $n = 2$, etc. The lower the orbit, the less energetic an electron is in the orbit. If all the electrons in the atom are in their lowest possible orbits, the atom is said to be in a *ground state*. If one of the electrons somehow absorbs energy, it can be pushed into a higher orbit, but it may not stay there. According to quantum theory, the electron can give its energy away in the form of an electromagnetic wave or photon. Since the energy of the orbits is quantized, when an electron drops into a lower orbit, the energy it gives off to the photon is equal to the energy difference of the two orbits. The various transitions between different orbits therefore result in different and discrete wavelengths of light. In general, the more complex an atom, the more possible are transitions and the more allowable are frequencies (or colors or lines) in the spectrum. Hydrogen, for example, has only four lines in the visible spectrum, while iron has thousands.

According to the laws of quantum mechanics, there are some transitions that an electron is likely to undergo—the so-called allowed transitions—and some transitions that are unlikely—the so-called forbidden transitions. Einstein's transition probability states that there are two ways in which an electron can drop from a higher to a lower state. The first is by spontaneous emission, that is, the electron in an excited state has a certain probability to drop into a particular lower level just by chance. The probability of a particular transition occurring depends on the similarity of the various separate quantum numbers of the upper and lower levels. The second way for a transition to occur is by induced emission. If an electron is in an upper state and is hit by a photon of exactly the energy difference of a given transition to a lower orbit, the photon will induce the electron to make the transition, thus radiating a photon of exactly the same frequency and polarization of the original photon. Because of this interaction, there are now two identical photons and one atom in the ground state, where there were originally one photon and one atom in the excited state. This phenomenon is important and will be discussed in Chapter 11—which is the whole point of the preceding discussion.

Wave property of light

As stated in the beginning of this chapter, light has a dual nature, acting both as a particle and as a wave. When discussing its creation or destruction, the particle nature fits best. When discussing the propagation of light through space, the wave model, as enunciated by Thomas Young in 1801, is more apt [1]. This theory was probably first proposed by Aristotle around 360 BC. Actually, all matter can be described in terms of waves and particles, although the wavelike nature of matter is more significant for particles the size of electrons or smaller. All wave motion consists of a disturbance moving through a medium. The medium itself does not move along with the wave (this is easily demonstrated by floating a cork on water). In the case of a water wave, the surface of the water moves up and down as the wave passes. The same thing happens with a wave propagating along a rope. This wave motion is usually described as a relatively small back-and-forth, or up-and-down, motion of the particles of the medium as the wave passes through the medium.

Two types of waves can be described: longitudinal and transverse. Longitudinal waves—such as sound makes—require a medium through which to travel. In this case, condensation and rarefaction of the particles of the medium occur. Transverse waves need no medium in order to propagate. The disturbance caused by the wave is perpendicular to the direction of the wave. Thus light takes the form of a transverse wave. Furthermore, for the purposes of our discussion on optics, we will agree that a light wave has the properties of a simple vertical sine wave, even if it doesn't.

A light wave actually is two waves having two different properties. The electronic portion of light moves along the direction of travel or propagation and is our simple vertical sine wave. At the same time, the magnetic portion of the light vibrates at right angles to the line of propagation, again in the form of a sine wave (Figure 3.4). Light tends to move along in a straight line unless acted upon by an external force. One of the forces that acts on light is gravity, but since it is a relatively weak force we mere mortals do not notice its effect on light here on Earth. We have, however, observed the effect of gravity on light in space in the form of a galactic lens and the displacement of star images near the sun.

The maximum displacement of a particular wave (crest to midpoint) is termed *amplitude* (Figure 3.5). The crest of any such wave is called the *maxima*, and the trough, the *minima*. The distance between two successive maxima or any other two successive corresponding points describes one cycle of the wave and is called the *wavelength*. A fraction of a complete cycle is called the *phase*. The phase difference between two waves traveling in the same direction is the fraction of a wavelength by which one wave leads the other. If an imaginary particle passes through a complete cycle, it is conventionally denoted as having a phase change of 360°. The *period* of the wave is the time necessary for an imaginary particle to travel one complete cycle. Distances along a wave may be measured in units of length, such as meters, or in units of angle, such that one cycle is equal to 2π rad, or 360°.

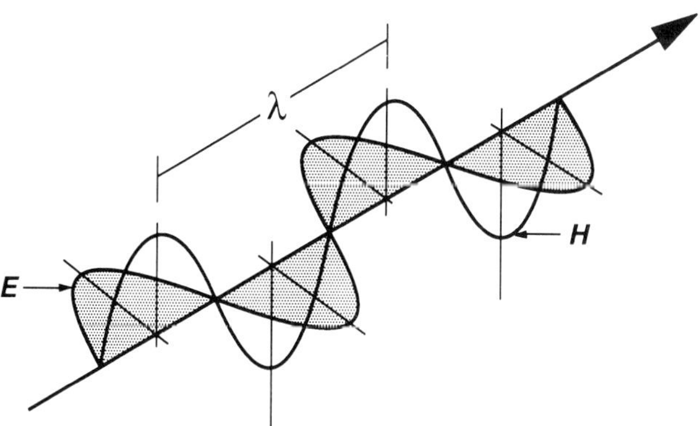

Fig. 3.4 Schematic of an electromagnetic wave—light. A light wave has a magnetic as well as an electronic part.

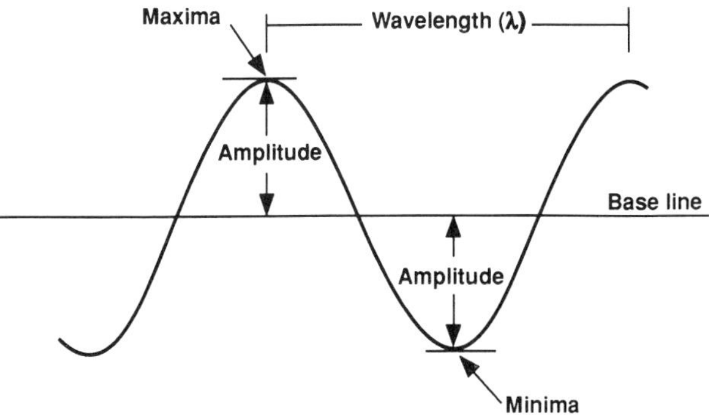

Fig. 3.5 The anatomy of a light wave.

The length of any given wave of light is inversely related to just how energetic the photons are in the wave. That is, the more energetic, the shorter the wavelength. This relationship is classically described in terms of a weight attached to a spring which is set into oscillation—ignoring the effects of friction. The number of complete excursions (maxima to maxima) within a given time period is the *frequency* of oscillation of the weight—the number of vibrations per unit time. If one were to attach a pen to the weight such that it could inscribe a mark on a moving piece of paper, the line drawn would be in the shape of the sine wave previously described. If the paper were to be moved at a constant rate, it follows that the peak-to-peak dimension of a wave (the wavelength) would depend on the speed with which the weight is oscillating. Since (as far as we know) the speed of light is constant, wavelength is therefore inversely related to frequency.

Both the electric and magnetic portions of the light wave are related to each other in time and share the energy of the wave, which is proportional to the square of its amplitude. Physically, electric and magnetic fields are force fields that act on charged particles. An electric field pulls in a positively charged particle and repels a negatively charged particle. A magnetic field acts only on moving charges, which are deflected at right angles to both the direction of motion of the charge and the direction of the magnetic field. Being force fields, they are described by vectors—that is, with magnitude and direction—and can be resolved into perpendicular components. This property will be important later in the discussion of polarization.

Color of light

Color is determined by the frequency of the light wave. Red light falls at the low-frequency or long-wavelength end of the spectrum, while blue light falls at the high-frequency or short-wavelength end of the spectrum. All other colors occur in between these limits. The visual spectrum is bordered on the long-wavelength side by infrared and on the short-wavelength side by ultraviolet. By convention, infrared and ultraviolet are called light, although, strictly speaking, since they are not visible to the human eye, they are not light.

Refractive index

I have said that light moves along at 186,000 miles per second, and so it does—in a vacuum, at least. However, when light travels through another transparent medium, it interacts with the atoms of that medium and slows up, just a little. The slowing occurs because the photons produce an oscillation in the electrons of the medium. The energy produced is released in the form of heat. Since heat is also a form of electromagnetic energy, it would seem that if the induced oscillations were of sufficient frequency, the energy released could reach the visual spectrum or higher. This is, in fact, similar to what happens in a laser (see Chapter 11). This property of light was first postulated by Pierre Fermat in his "principle of natural economy" and confirmed by Roemer (who also had established that light moved at a constant and finite velocity) in 1676 [2,3].

If the light enters such a medium at an angle, its path is changed, sometimes profoundly (Figure 3.6). We can express the ratio of that slowing and hence the bending by dividing the speed of light (c) in a vacuum, or in air, by its speed within the medium (c_m). This ratio is always larger than 1 and is called the *index of refraction*. The index of refraction of the human cornea is approximately 1.3776. The importance of this index will be discussed more thoroughly in the section on geometric optics, below.

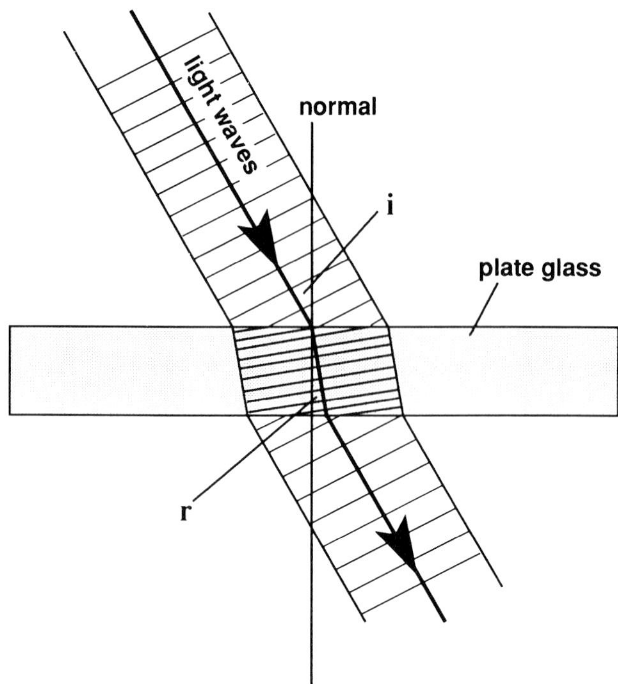

Fig. 3.6 Path of light from one medium to another.

Dispersion

The actual amount of deflection that occurs is related to the wavelength or frequency of the light itself for any given medium. That is, the shorter, more energetic wavelengths are slowed more than the longer, less energetic waves. This phenomenon is termed *dispersion*. Dispersion is related to index of refraction in that the higher the index, the greater is the dispersion of the light. It is dispersion that produces chromatic aberration in uncorrected lens systems. The spectrograph uses the property of dispersion to separate light into its various wavelengths. Combining a prism with a slit aperture, this device breaks a light source down into discrete bands of color called a *line spectrum*. Various elements produce different kinds of light when heated; thus a spectrograph can be used to analyze the content of unknown substances or even to detect such substances in outer space. The relative intensity of the lines also can be used to determine the temperature of an object.

Interference

Because of the wave nature of light, it seems logical that it might be possible for two or more light waves to collide or otherwise interfere with one another, and so they can, if the light is coherent. That is, if the waves have the same polarization and wavelength and are of constant phase difference, then the resulting amplitudes at that point remain constant and a pattern of light and dark bands will be produced. However, if the two waves are not coherent, the resulting amplitudes change from one instant to the next, depending on the differences in the relative phases, no collisions occur, and thus no pattern emerges. This is the principle of Young's classic experiment, which was one of the first to prove that light acts as a wave [4]. In Young's experiment, light from a small source is filtered to make it monochromatic and is then allowed to pass through two narrow slits separated by a few tenths of a millimeter. When the light waves that have passed through the two slits illuminate a screen, a pattern of light spots and dark spots is seen (Figure 3.7). The light spots correspond to places where the waves arrive with the same phase, and the dark spots are places where the waves from the two slits have opposite phases and so cancel each other.

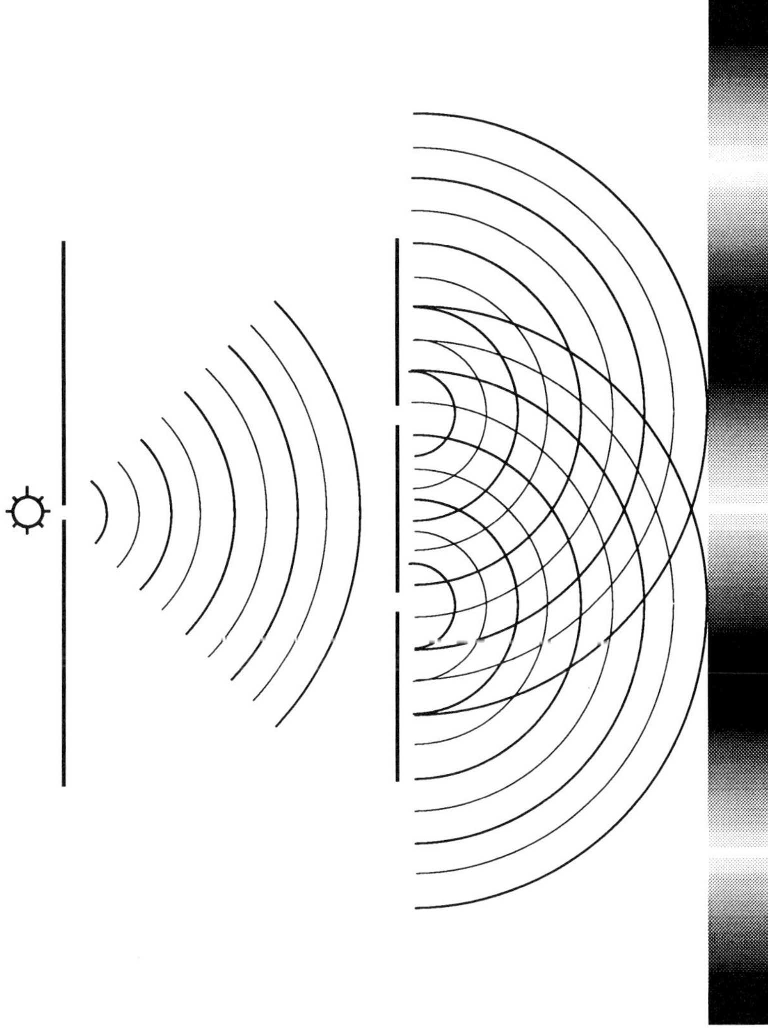

Fig. 3.7 Thomas Young's experiment showing the interference phenomenon.

The results of Young's experiment follow directly from the wave nature of light. Nevertheless, it is quite contrary to all our ordinary experience for two light waves to combine and produce darkness. This is so because ordinary light sources are not coherent, and there is no fixed relationship between the phases of waves from different places on the source. Since so many different, independent atoms are involved, the relative phases fluctuate rapidly, and the intensity at places on the illuminated screen is some average value. Interference is therefore a phenomenon associated with coherent light except in certain circumstances when it can occur in white light. They may be observed when two nearly parallel glass surfaces are in close proximity (Figure 3.8). This is the problem sometimes encountered in microscopy when there is air between a slide and its cover glass. Waves are partially reflected from the glass-air surface and from the air-glass surface. Interference occurs between these two waves of light, and the result is a fringe pattern. In this illustration, light is depicted as rays so that the sites of reflection may be more clearly indicated. The optical path between the reflections from each of the two surfaces determines the phase difference between the waves, which in turn determines the final fringe pattern. The fringe pattern is thus an indication of the physical distance between the two surfaces. When a spherical transparent surface is in contact with a plane reflecting surface, a phenomenon called

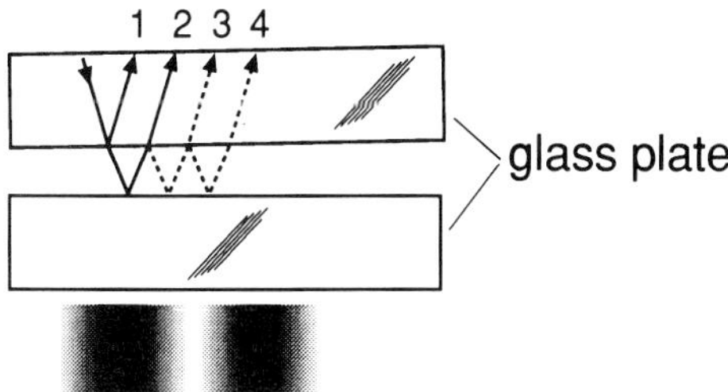

Fig. 3.8 Rays reflecting from two almost parallel glass surfaces. When the optical path traversed by ray 2 is one-half wavelength greater than the path for ray 1, destructive interference occurs. A dark band (fringe) is seen at that point.

Newton's rings occurs which is a bull's-eye-shaped pattern of alternating white and dark rings (Figure 3.9). Finally, the rainbow colors seen in the surface of a soap bubble or in a thin oil film on water are interference patterns. In each of the preceding three cases, reflections from the interfaces partially polarize the light rays, which in turn produce the phase differences resulting in interference patterns.

The result of such interference depends on whether the waves are in or out of phase—that is, whether the troughs and crests correspond or overlap. If the troughs and crests exactly overlap—their phase difference is zero—then the maxima will add to maxima and minima to minima. The intensity of the light therefore increases. Since the intensity of light is proportional to the square of the amplitude, if two waves are in phase, the intensity will increase fourfold. This is called *constructive interference* (Figure 3.10).

If the waves are 180° out of phase so that troughs match crests, then the maxima add to minima and the sum is zero—no light is present; that is, the intensity is zero (Figure 3.11). In between these two conditions the light intensity will vary (Figure 3.12). This is *destructive interference.* Thus there will be seen an alternating series of bright and dark lines; the bright areas correspond to superimposition of two maxima or two minima and the dark areas to the superimposition of waves 180° out of phase with each other. The alternating bright and dark lines obtained on a screen are known as an *interference fringe pattern* (Figure 3.13).

Just because there is no light does not mean that the light was destroyed, however. In coherent light, the energy gained at the interference maxima because of constructive interference is exactly matched by the energy lost elsewhere as a result of destructive interference. The same total amount of energy is present whether or not the waves are coherent, but the energy falls into a sort of large blur.

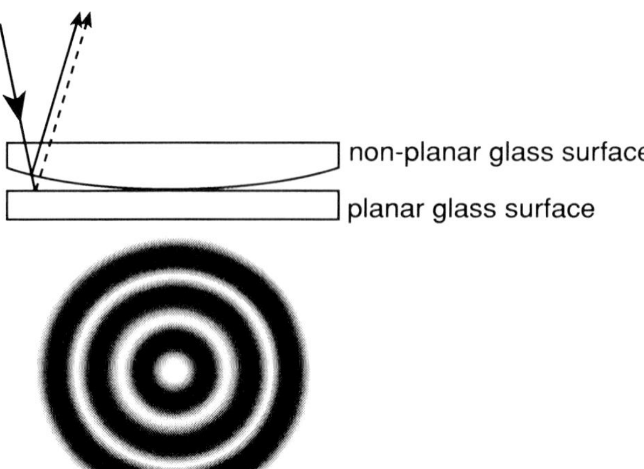

Fig. 3.9 Newton's rings.

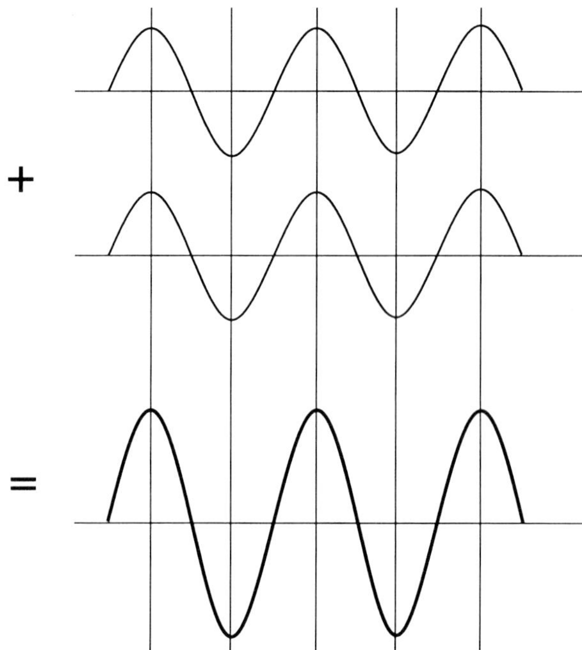

Fig. 3.10 The interaction of coherent light. Constructive interference.

The distance traveled by the light going between two points is called the *optical path;* in the illustration in Figure 3.13, this is the distance from the source of light to the screen. If the optical path from one source were changed slightly, as by a curved reflecting surface, the result would be a change in the location of the maxima

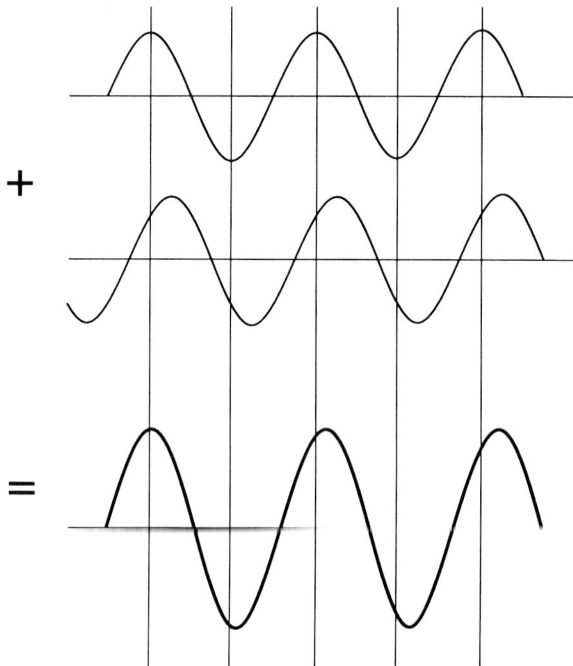

Fig. 3.11 Waves slightly out of phase.

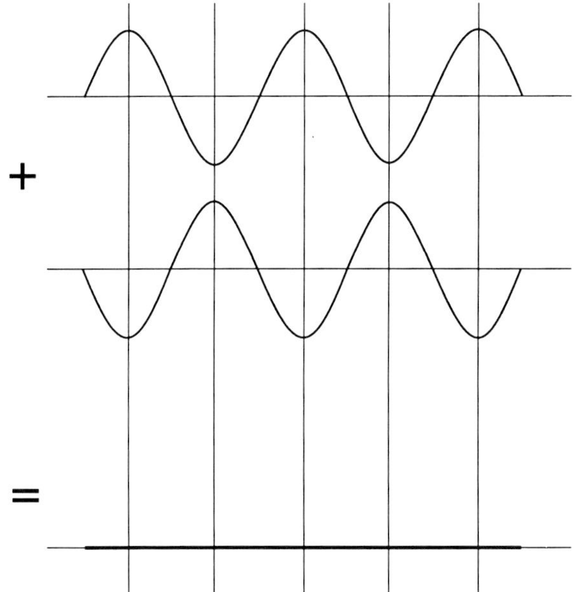

Fig. 3.12 Destructive interference.

from that source. This in turn would alter the location of the bright and dark fringes, since the intersection site of the maxima and the minima would be similarly altered. The change in optical path would be manifested as a shift in the interference pattern. The extent of this shift can be used to gain information about the reflecting surface.

If the location of the sources of light in Figure 3.13 is unchanged but the color of light (i.e., the wavelength) is changed, the fringe pattern also would be altered. Shortening the wavelength causes the maxima to be closer together, and in the resulting fringe pattern, the bright and dark fringes are also closer together. Longer wavelengths would produce a fringe pattern in which the bright and dark fringes are separated by a greater distance.

The phenomenon of interference is used to design lens coatings to reduce unwanted reflections. These coatings are typically made from dielectric (nonconductive) materials that have been vacuum-deposited on to a lens surface to a thickness of one-fourth wave. Some of the light striking the surface will be reflected at the air-material interface and some at the material-glass interface, while the rest will be transmitted. If the index of refraction of the coating has been chosen to equal that of the lens material, exactly the same amount of light will be reflected from each interface. Since the light from the second reflection has to pass through the coating twice, it will be 180° out of phase with that of the first reflection and hence each cancels the other out. The result is 0% reflection and 100% transmission. The rub is that the coating can only be made to match one-fourth of one particular wavelength—which is not too effective in white light. Also, no one material has been found that is equal in refractive index to that of spectacle crown glass. The problem can be partially solved by depositing multiple coating layers, each

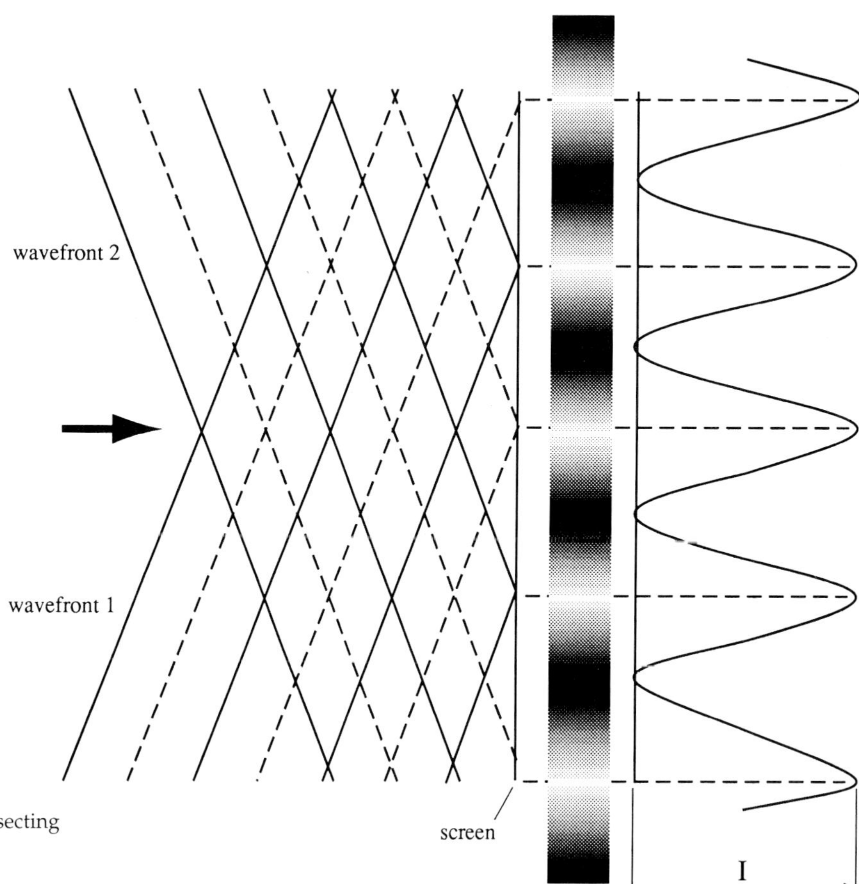

Fig. 3.13 Interference produced by two intersecting waves.

one of which is turned to a different frequency and related to one another with respect to their indices of refraction.

The phenomenon of interference has become of increasing importance, especially as regards refractive surgery. This special property of electromagnetic radiation gives us an extremely sensitive tool to measure with. This property is also important in measuring the efficiency of an optical system by means of the modulation transfer function. This function is discussed under the section on geometric optics, below. The most familiar form of such a device is the laser visual acuity tester. In this device, two pinpoint beams of a low-wattage laser are directed into the eye. As the light waves traverse the eye, they interfere with one another, producing alternating light and dark bands which can be perceived by the patient. It is possible to adjust the separation of these bands so as to correspond to dimensions equal to that of a standard vision chart letter form. In practice, the beams are adjusted until the banding can no longer be detected. The acuity is taken as the next highest setting. As long as the medium has some ability to transmit light, the use of this device can give both the surgeon and the patient some practical assessment of the vision to be expected after cataract extraction.

Another application, of more immediate concern in refractive surgery, is holography. Anyone who has visited Disneyland has been exposed to one or more holograms, particularly some of the ghostlike images in the Haunted Mansion. A hologram is made using laser light that has been split into two beams, a reference beam and an object beam (Figure 3.14). The reference beam is directed onto the photographic (or other) recording medium without being focused. The object beam is directed onto the subject, and the reflected light is allowed to strike the recording medium, again without being focused.

Since the two beams of light are coherent and parts of the object beam will be out of phase with the reference, an interference pattern will be produced on the recording medium. When the film is developed, no recognizable image will be seen. However, if the negative is illuminated with the reference beam and then viewed, that light will react with the pattern to form an exact replica of the object beam and hence an image of the object will be clearly visible. Since all the data present in the original object have been duplicated by the object beam, the image will appear to be fully dimensional.

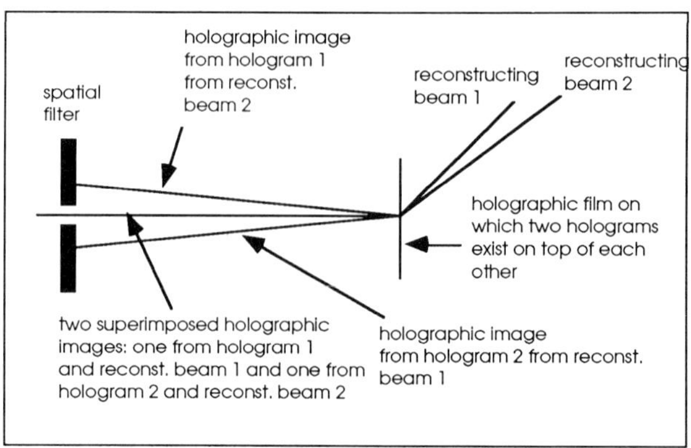

Fig. 3.14 Schematic of two-beam holographic system.

Outside of its amusement value, the same principle can be used to construct a two-dimensional image of the corneal surface which can then be manipulated and its curvature measured. Because we know the exact wavelength of the light used to construct the image, we can reproduce the corneal elevations exactly as well (see also Chapter 6).

Scattering

I have described how light is slowed when it passes through a medium other than a vacuum by interacting with the atoms within that medium. If those particles are larger than atoms—perhaps molecules—the light will be reflected and diffused. If the particles are even larger, such as large dust grains or ice crystals in the sky, all wavelengths of light will be affected. In this case the intensity of the light will be less and more diffuse, causing gray skies and soft shadows. If, however, the particles are smaller than the wavelength of light, the proportion of the light scattered will be inversely related to the fourth power of the wavelength. Thus blue light, whose wavelength is approximately $\frac{4}{7}$ that of red, is scattered $(\frac{4}{7})^4$ or 10 times as much, which gives the sky its blue color and makes the sun appear much redder than it actually is. In the evening, when the low level of the sun causes light to travel a much greater distance, the sun appears redder still.

Diffraction

When light is projected through an aperture, secondary wavelengths will be formed at the edge of the aperture which interfere with the main wavefront. This phenomenon is called *diffraction*. As the aperture is made smaller, the more important this edge effect becomes and the larger the bull's-eye-like diffraction pattern that results. The size of the "x-ring" of the bull's-eye—the central bright spot—is called the *Airy disk* and is given by the formula

$$R = \frac{1.22\lambda F}{d}$$

where R is the radius of the disk, F is the distance from the aperture to the screen, λ is the wavelength, and d is the diameter of the aperture. About 83% of the energy of the point source will be found within the Airy disk (Figure 3.15). Since this disk is an image of the source, the smaller this disk, the sharper is the image and therefore the greater is the resolving power of the system. The *resolution* of a lens is the smallest possible distance between

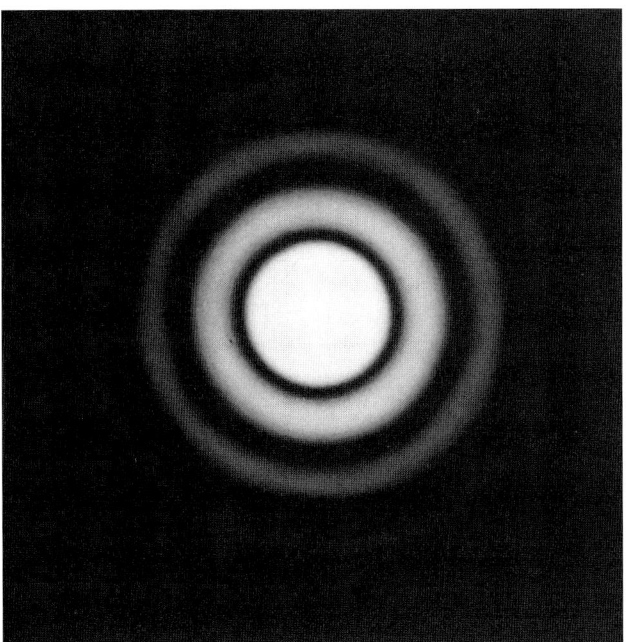

Fig. 3.15 An Airy disk at the limit of resolution.

two point sources at which their images can be recognized as distinct. This distance is typically the point where the minimum of the Airy pattern of one source falls on the maximum of the second source; thus the absolute limit to resolving power is set by the laws of diffraction (see the section on resolving power, below).

Since diffraction occurs at every obstacle to a wave motion or aperture, the effect is always present in optical systems, including the eye. An ideal lens with no aberrations when imaging a point source will still form a diffraction pattern instead of a point image, as predicted by the theory of geometric optics. An image can be improved by reducing the size of the aperture, which reduces or eliminates aberrations in the system. The size of the imaging aperture is limiting, however. There is a size aperture beyond which the edge effects become dominant and the image becomes degraded or blurred. Such a system is described as *diffraction-limited.*

If one considers the human eye, the most efficient diameter of the pupil is 2.5 mm. Above this, various refractive aberrations limit the resolution, and below this, diffraction effects limit the resolution. Because of these diffraction effects, the typical pinhole used to estimate latent visual acuity will not improve that acuity to better than 20/25. I will have more to say about this phenomenon when I discuss the optics of the human eye in the following section on geometric optics.

Polarization

If light waves are traveling in the same direction, their electric fields may or may not be parallel to one another but will instead be randomly related. Such light is said to be *nonpolarized* (unpolarized)—the condition of almost all light sources. Polarized light can be created from unpolarized light by one of three methods—transmission, reflection, or scattering.

If unpolarized light passes through a medium containing asymmetrically charged molecules that are oriented in the same direction, these molecules will absorb the electric field of the light in the same direction—thus causing the wavefront to collapse—and transmit the remainder. This phenomenon is typically described by using the analogy of a rope being wriggled through a picket fence, the idea being that only when the waves (wriggles) are parallel to the pickets will they be passed through. That's a lovely analogy but for the fact that reality is exactly the reverse of this picture. The electrical component is perpendicular to the magnetic portion (Figure 3.16). Since the molecules within the polarizing material absorb the electrical portion, they only pass the light that is perpendicular to their arrangement. This is the type of polarization that exists naturally in crystals.

Artificial polarizing materials were created 40 years ago by spraying iodide crystals on plastic and then stretching the plastic so that all the crystals would line up in the same direction. Since then, more sophisticated techniques have been found, but the basic principle remains the same.

An interesting experiment that shows some of the physical properties of polarized light consists of taking a linear polarizer and putting it in the path of a white light source. A second linear polarizer is placed perpendicular to the first, also in the path of the light. This is known as crossed polaroids. Light that passes through the first polarizer is polarized 90° to the plane of the other polarizer so that no light will get through the combination of

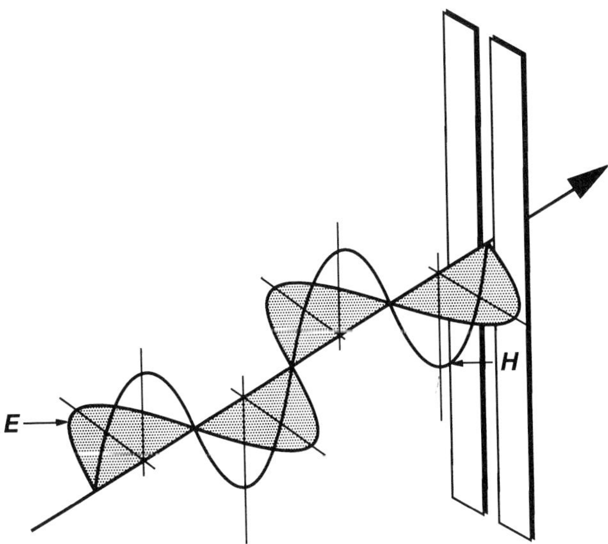

Fig. 3.16 Polarization of light. Note that the electrical portion of the light wave (*E*) is perpendicular to the pickets; hence this light wave is not passed through.

crossed polaroids. However, if we interject yet a third polarizer between the first two at 45°, some light will get through. This happens because light is a vector. When the unpolarized light reaches the first polaroid, it is oriented parallel to this polaroid. When it strikes the second polaroid, it is at 45° to the plane of that polaroid, which means it can be resolved into components perpendicular and parallel to the second polaroid. The perpendicular component is absorbed but the parallel component is transmitted, which then strikes the third polaroid, which is now 45° to the plane of polarization of the light. This can then be resolved once more into light polarized perpendicular to the polaroid. Again, the parallel light will get through. Only about an eighth of the light actually gets through the system, as half was absorbed at the first polaroid and half again was absorbed at the second polaroid.

Polarization also can be created if the light falls on a partially transmitting material at an oblique angle. Some of the light will be reflected and some will be transmitted. The light will be bent according to Snell's law:

$$n_1 \text{ sine } a_1 = n_2 \text{ sine } a_2$$

where n_1 is the index of refraction of the first medium, and n_2 is the index of refraction of the second medium. The two angles, a_1 and a_2, are the angles that the light makes with the component perpendicular to the surface of the interface of the first and second media, respectively. The law of reflection says that the angle of incidence is equal to the angle of reflection. As the light strikes the interface at an oblique angle, it is bent by the medium to a new angle, as given by Snell's law. In general, it bends toward the normal (a normal in optics is a line drawn perpendicular to a surface) in going from a less dense to a more dense medium. Likewise, some of the light is reflected by the molecules of the second medium at an angle, as given by the law of reflection. The reflected angle cannot be perpendicular to the angle of refraction, however, because then the electric field of the light in the molecules would be parallel to the direction of the propagation of the reflected light. This is impossible because light is a transverse wave. Therefore, at this angle only light with an electric field parallel to the direction of propagation may be reflected; thus the light is polarized (Figure 3.17). This is important because glare is reflected light and therefore polarized to some extent; thus polarized sunglasses reduce reflected glare more than the background illumination, which is unpolarized light.

Light is polarized by scattering molecules in the atmosphere in a very similar way. This scattering of sky light can be easily verified by looking at a clear sky 90° to the direction of the sun while wearing polarized sunglasses. If one's head is rotated somewhat while looking in this direction, the light of the sky will be diminished considerably, but any clouds in that area will remain fairly constant in brightness. This is so because the light from the atmosphere reaches the eye exclusively from scattering

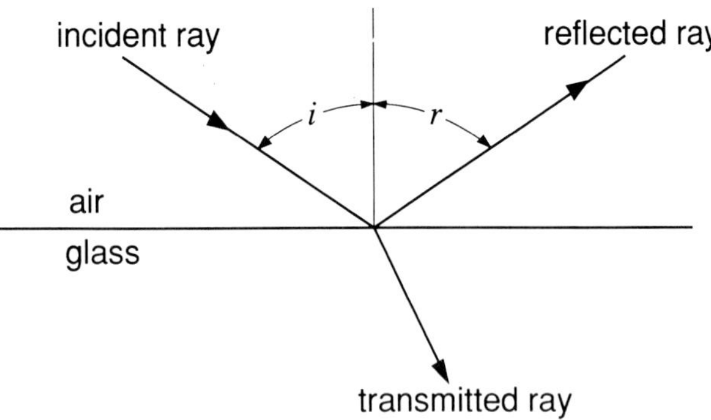

Fig. 3.17 Polarizing angle. The reflected light is polarized.

by relatively few air molecules and is thus polarized. Light from the clouds reaches the eye from scattering by many, much larger water droplets in the cloud, which destroys the polarization.

Fluorescence

Light may be absorbed by an electron in the ground state, raising the electron into an excited state. The excited electron may then decay to a lower level. If the electron decays to a state higher than the ground state, it will emit a photon that is less energetic than the absorbed photon and therefore of a longer wavelength. This process is called *fluorescence.* A commonly used dye in ophthalmology, fluorescein, absorbs light at 490 nm in the blue and reradiates it at 530 nm in the green when stimulated by white light.

Absorbance

When light falls on an object, it may be transmitted, reflected, absorbed, or more usually, undergo some combination of the aforementioned. A number of optical devices such as light filters and sunglasses make use of absorption. If light of intensity I_0 falls on a partially transparent plate, the intensity of the transmitted light would be $I = TI_0$, where T, called the *transmittance*, is a unitless number between 0 and 1. If several plates are stacked, the total transmittance of the stack is the product of the individual transmittances. It is sometimes more useful to add terms than to multiply them, so another term, called the *density*, was invented:

$$D = \frac{\log I}{T} = 10^{-D}$$

where D is the density. Since numbers can be multiplied by adding their logarithms, the density of a series of plates is the sum of the densities of the individual plates. Absorbed light is usually converted into heat by the absorbing electrons, but it may be used to excite an electron into a higher level and be reradiated, as in the case of fluorescence.

Photometry

Photometry is concerned with the measurement of light in a system and the effect that the light has on the visual sensation. Light that differs only in wavelength can be distinguished by the eye because of two properties—color and apparent intensity. The eye is more sensitive to some parts of the spectrum than to others, so the apparent intensities of the different parts of the spectrum will be different, even if the incident light intensity is the same at all wavelengths. There are four characteristics of the eye that determine its response to light.

Spectral sensitivity. From an inspection of the luminosity curve, one can see that an eye is very sensitive to green light and rather insensitive to red and violet light. If violet illumination is to give the same sensation of brightness as a green source, much more power is needed.

Range of sensitivity. The human eye can detect energies of a few photons per second up to bright sunlight, a difference in sensitivity of 10^{15}.

Fechner's law. The relative sensation of an increase in sensitivity is proportional to the log of the change, so by increasing the intensity of a lamp from 1 to 10 foot-candles, the same sensation of change as from 10 to 100 foot-candles is given. This law applies for four orders of magnitude.

Weber's law. The change of brightness necessary to be noticed is proportional to the original brightness, that is, $DL = KL$, where DL is the least amount of change of intensity noticeable, K is a constant, and L is the brightness of the light. Therefore, the change necessary before a difference is noticed in a bright light source is larger than in a dim one.

Geometric optics

The process of discovery and furtherance of knowledge is often a painful process, resembling the ebb and flow of the tides. Low water alternates with high, with the occasional neap or excessively high tidal flow. So it was with the optics of the eye. While myopia and hyperopia were recognized and described in Aristotle's time, the possibility of definite treatment beyond medicinal awaited the more complete understanding of the optical nature of the human eye. Much of the progress in this was stymied by the prevailing notions of the time regarding sight itself.

The manner in which vision works has been the subject of much philosophic discussion down through the ages. Nothing, however, exists in the extant ancient Egyptian or Sumerian writings alluding to vision or the phenomenon of sight, though a practical knowledge of refraction existed among the Assyrians (see also Chapter 2). The first such writing comes from the time of Pythagoras, in 600 BC, referring to his "emanation theory" of vision. Vision was supposed to result from the emission of a subtle "visual spirit" or pneuma originating in the brain, traveling down the hollow optic nerves and filling the lens from whence it emanated in rays similar to those of sunlight. How this concept persisted in the face of the fact that vision is impaired in the absence of light is a mystery.

This thesis was denied by Aristotle (360 BC), who adopted and expanded on an original proposal of Democrites (500 BC). Sixty years later, Plato tried without success to reconcile both views. The Arabic writers Al-Hazen and Ibn Rushd also supported this concept of Aristotle, expanding it to include the retina as the seat of visual reception, to no avail. Leonardo Da Vinci attempted and failed to combine both views as well. The "consecration" of the Pythagorean view by Galen centuries before had insured its acceptance for 2500 years, practically unchallenged. This hypothesis held sway until the time of Felix Platter in 1583, when it was finally put to rest.

The durability of this thesis is surprising in view of the knowledge of optics possessed by the Greeks. Although something of optics must have been known to the Babylonians and Egyptians before then, it would seem likely that it was limited to deductions from ordinary observable phenomena. The first optical treatise (*Optics*) was written by Euclid in 300 BC. This work was followed shortly thereafter by that of Aristarchus; next by the *Catoptrics* of Heron in the first century AD; and finally by the *Optics Thesaurus* of Claudius Ptolemeus (Ptolemy) in AD 100. Ptolemy was described as the father of optical science, and his work remained the essential source of knowledge until the 1600s. The sum of this knowledge concerned itself with catoptrics or the optics of reflecting surfaces, however; of dioptrics little was known. Ptolemy's construction of an object AB, as seen under water, is shown in Figure 3.18. The rays from the eye, OM and ON, are refracted at the surface and reach the object along paths MA and NB. Ptolemy knew that a normal ray was not refracted and concluded that the virtual image, $A'B'$ is

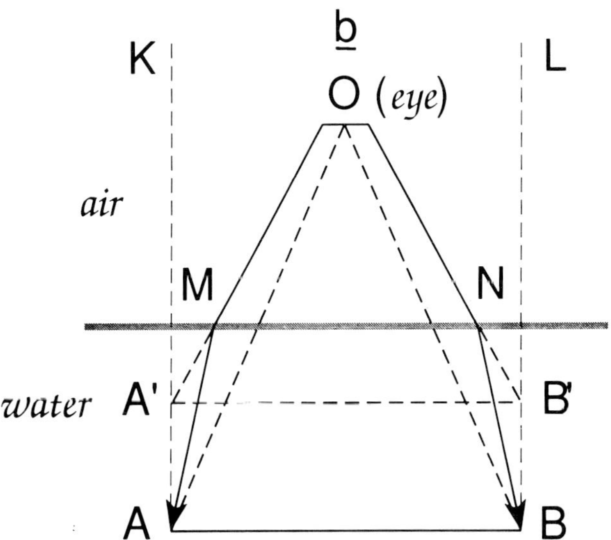

Fig. 3.18 Refractive concepts of Ptolemy.

located by protracting the rays, *OM* and *ON* until they reach the perpendiculars, *AK* and *BL*. He postulated that the image was magnified because the visual angle, *A'OB'*, was greater than the angle *AOB*, through which it would be seen if in air.

The ancients had observed the magnifying qualities of a water-filled flask, as well as its ability to concentrate the sun's rays. Though the Roman physician Heliodorus described this as a refractive phenomenon, its nature was apparently not understood. Ptolemy's construction remained the standard explanation for centuries—it was even copied by Roger Bacon—and remained so until corrected by Barrow in 1674. This understanding was undoubtedly hampered by the inability of such philosophers to break the bonds of dogma and theocratic meddling. It takes great moral courage and not a little *chutzpah* to fly in the face of established precedent—it is safer to "go along." It would have helped had not the authorities stymied the science of anatomy by interdicting human dissection. Nevertheless, even when dissection was allowed, the study of the eye continued to be hampered by the difficulty in preserving it intact for study.

Newton (Figure 3.19), in his *Opticks* (Figure 3.20), consolidated the entire system of optics, reflection, refraction, image formation, and dioptric system of the eye and included the rudiments of color theory. He did it so thoroughly that nothing more was added for nearly a century. In 1841 Gauss (a prodigy ranked with Archimedes and Newton) produced the elegant mathematic construction that solved the problem of complex optical systems, which essentials are still accepted today. Listing, Gauss' student, devised a very accurate theoretical schematic eye which culminated in the simplified, but still elegant, schematic eye of Allvar Gullstrand [5].

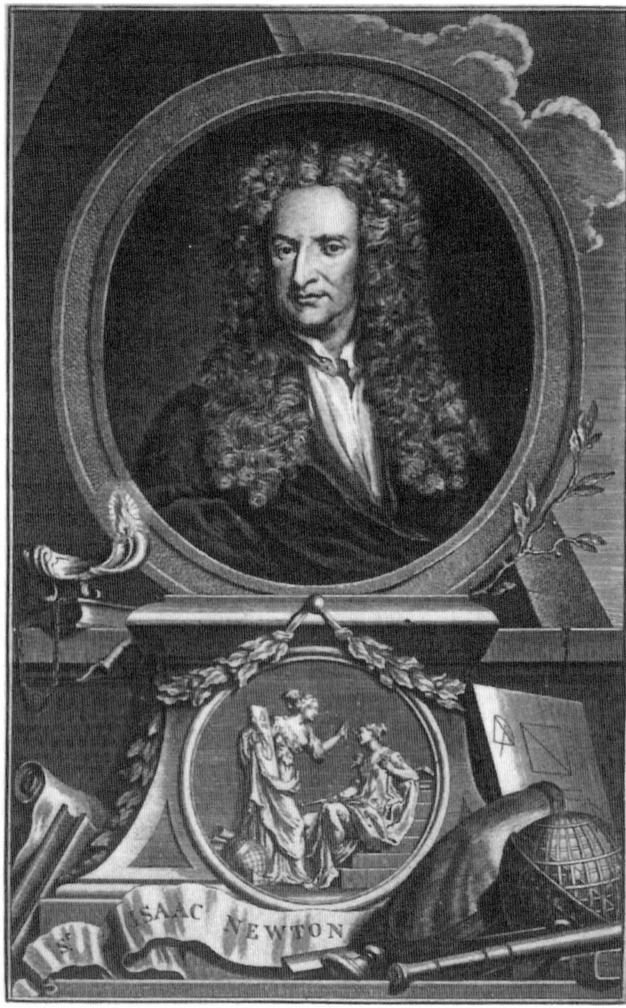

Fig. 3.19 Sir Isaac Newton.

Geometric optics deals with light as rays and the formation of images using optical devices such as lenses, prisms, and mirrors and the physical laws governing the characteristics of such images. It concerns itself with three aspects:

1 The size of the image.
2 The distance of the image from the optical surface.
3 The characteristics of the image: inverted or erect; real or virtual.

We are interested in such things because we are choosing to meddle with the mechanism by which we see—the eye—and the eye is, of course, an optical device. Our discussion will touch upon some aspects of the science of optics. The reader is referred to the section on further reading for more detailed coverage. To deal more adequately with this subject, however, we must define some terms of usage.

Object. This is a source of light or the origin of rays directed toward an optical system. An object may be real or tangible or it may be virtual or intangible, formed by projection of the rays through an optical system to a location where it cannot be imaged on to a screen.

Image. An image is a concentration of rays from an object by an optical system to produce a likeness of the object. As in the case of an object, the image may be virtual or real.

Optical axis. This is an imaginary line, about which the components of an optical system are centered.

Infinity. In the classic sense this term has no dimension and refers to the location of an object or image. In the sense in which we will use it in our discussion, this distance refers to that which is greater than that of the optical system itself.

Focal length. This is the distance between a lens or mirror and the image of an object located at infinity and is abbreviated *f*. The position of the image is the point at which the parallel rays from an object are brought to a focus by the optic. The designation of this point is *F*. Focal length is commonly employed as an expression of optical power.

Diopter. This term is also used to express optical power. It is expressed in this manner:

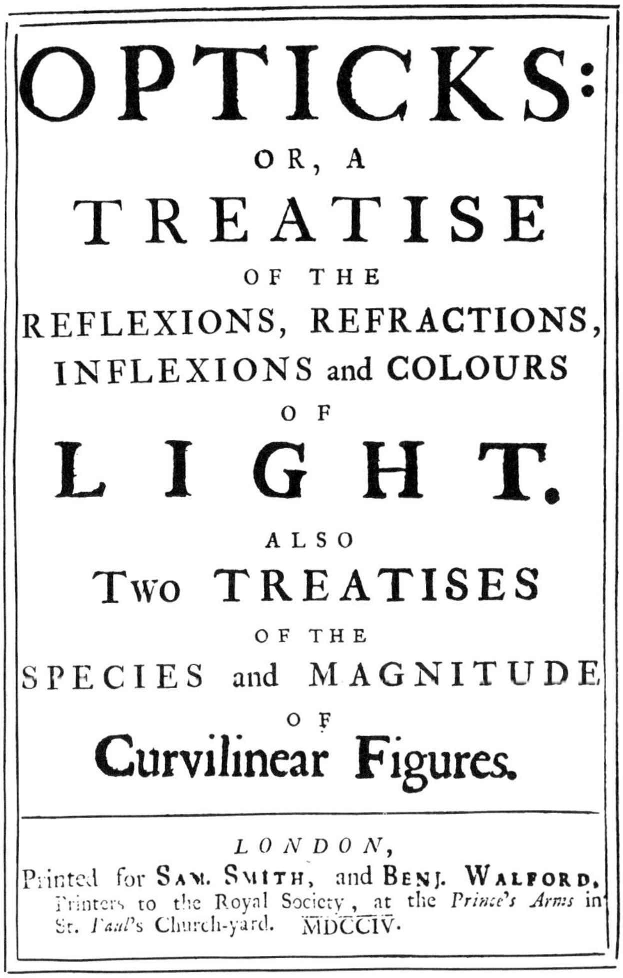

OPTICKS:
OR, A
TREATISE
OF THE
REFLEXIONS, REFRACTIONS,
INFLEXIONS and COLOURS
OF
LIGHT.
ALSO
Two TREATISES
OF THE
SPECIES and MAGNITUDE
OF
Curvilinear Figures.

LONDON,
Printed for SAM. SMITH, and BENJ. WALFORD,
Printers to the Royal Society, at the *Prince's Arms* in
St. *Paul's* Church-yard. MDCCIV.

Fig. 3.20 The title page of Newton's *Opticks*.

$$D = \frac{1}{f \text{ (in meters)}}$$

Thus a 1-D lens would deviate a ray 1 cm at a distance of 1 m. If such a lens (or mirror) causes a ray to be deviated toward the optic axis of the system (converge), that lens is said to have plus power. In this case the lens would be described as +1 D. If the lens (or mirror) were to cause the ray to deviate away from the optic center (diverge), it is said to have minus power. By convention, an unsigned diopter is considered to be of plus power.

Magnification. The relationship between the size of the object and the size of the image is expressed thus:

$$M = \frac{\text{image size}}{\text{object size}}$$

Transparent. This is an optical medium that transmits light with minimal attenuation. These substances (or media) are typically clear, such as glass, water, and air.

Opaque. Opaque is the opposite of transparent and either reflects or absorbs the light.

Incident. In the discussion the term is used to describe a ray of light striking a surface. Thus the ray was incident to the surface of the mirror. Dropping the mirror would also be an incident but of a different category and consequence.

Interface phenomenon

An *interface* is the junction of two optical media. For a lens in air, the interface is located at the surface of the lens. This interface is thus an optical surface. Three things can happen to a ray of light when it strikes such a surface:

Reflection. The light is bounced back into the initial medium. Depending on the quality of the surface the reflection can be specular (from a mirrorlike surface) or diffuse (as from a flat painted surface) or a combination of both.

Absorption. The light is so attenuated by the medium that it is converted to heat. Sometimes the absorption is not obvious, as in a shallow pan of clear water which becomes heated if left in sunlight.

Refraction or transmission. Refraction is the bending of a ray as it passes (is transmitted) from one medium to another.

Optical surfaces

The optical interface or surface can take many shapes. It can be flat or plano. It may also be convex, in which case the surface is curved toward the object (or thicker at the optic axis) or it may be concave, the opposite condition. If the surface has an even curvature overall as if sliced from a round ball, such a surface is said to be spherical. If the curvature is not so shaped it is called aspherical. A regular aspherical surface has a curvature which deviates from a single radius of curvature from center to the periphery in the same manner in all meridians. It should be obvious that such a surface would not have a single point of focus, although the defocus spot would be a circle.

The corneal surface is highly aspherical and cannot be described in simple geometric terms. This fact has serious implications when attempts are made to measure the curvature of this surface. These implications will be discussed more thoroughly in the section on corneal topography (see Chapter 6). Wavefront analysis techniques are more appropriate for the study of surfaces of this nature.

An aspherical surface can have other properties. In Chapter 2 I discussed how such a surface can have astigmatism. In an astigmatic system the surface curvature can vary in a regular fashion from one meridian to another such that the extreme deviations lie at 90° to one another. Such a condition is termed regular astigmatism. Astigmatism is usually considered to be a deviation from the underlying spherical surface, hence the surface is termed *spherocylindric*—a cylinder lens superimposed on to a spherical lens. A cylinder lens is one in which the refracting power is directed along one axis only, as if the lens were a slice from a glass rod or cylinder, hence its name. Such a surface would not have a single point of focus either, but in contradistinction to a regular asphere, the focal spot would be an ellipsoid (oval).

Astigmatism also can result from misalignment of an optic. Thus, if a lens deviates from the vertical (or horizontal) plane, if it is tilted, astigmatism due to tilt results. If the lens is not so tilted but is slightly off-center, a type of astigmatism results called *coma* (pronounced "comma"). The eye encompasses all these aberrations within its optical system, some of which tend to cancel or neutralize each other. Tilt and coma are not usually considered in corneal surface analysis using current techniques (since they are not easily measured with photokeratoscopic methods) but are important when dealing with the corneal surface, particularly when attempting ray tracing (see also Chapter 6).

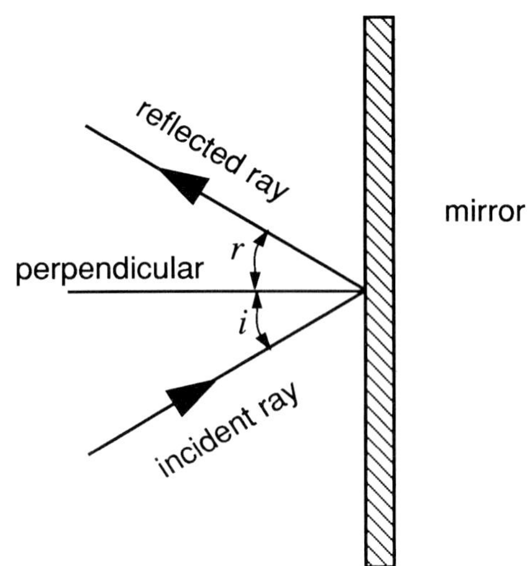

Fig. 3.21 The law of reflection applied to a plane surface.

Index of refraction

This is one of the most important characteristics of an optical medium. It is expressed mathematically as follows:

$$n = \frac{c}{c_m}$$

where c is the speed of light in a vacuum (or air), and c_m is the speed of light in the medium. The indices for some ocular media are

Saline	1.33
Cornea	1.3775
Air	1.0003

Certain laws govern the behavior of single rays at an optical surface. These are the law of reflection and the law of refraction (Snell's law).

The law of reflection

This rule or law applies when a ray is reflected back into the initial medium after striking an optical surface. It basically states that the angle of reflection is equal to the angle of incidence and is expressed thus (Figures 3.21 and 3.22):

Angle i = angle r

It is true for all optical surfaces.

The law of refraction (Snell's law)

When a ray is transmitted rather than reflected, Snell's law (derived in 1621) applies (Figure 3.23). This rule states that the angle of refraction at an optical surface is proportional to the sine of the angle of incidence and the ratio of the refractive indices. It is written algebraically as follows (Figure 3.24):

n sine $I = n'$ sine I'

In small angles of incidence (under 6°), the sine of the angle is almost equal to the angle; thus Snell's law is greatly simplified:

$$I' = \frac{n}{n'} I$$

Selected ray imaging is another technique for determining the size, location, and characteristics of an image in any optical system. This technique employs only two rays. To use this technique, we must assume that no aberrations exist in the optical system—all rays emanating from a single object will converge at a single point. The two rays selected for this purpose are these:

1 Any incident ray parallel to the optic axis must pass through the focal point after refraction or reflection.

2 A ray passing through the center of rotation of the surface is not refracted or is reflected back on itself. Thus the

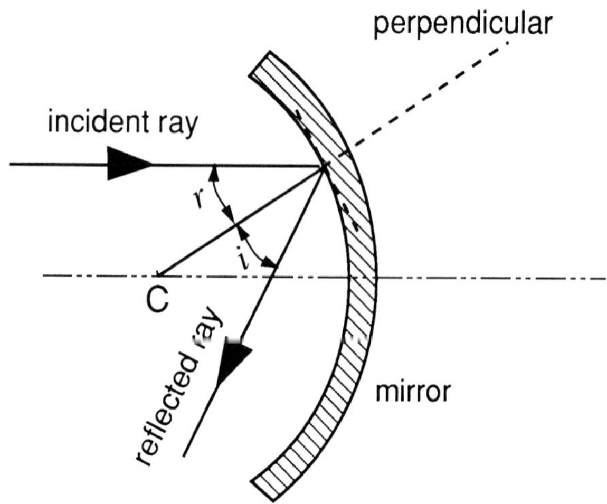

Fig. 3.22 The law of reflection applied to a curved surface.

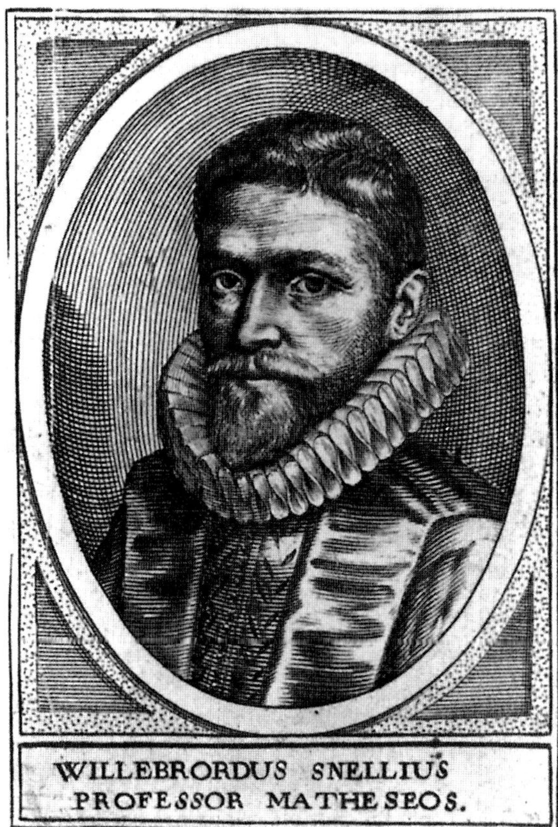

Fig. 3.23 Willebrord Snell.

angle of incidence is zero. In a lens this would only be true if it were infinitely thin but is close enough when dealing with the cornea.

The reflecting characteristics of the cornea are of special interest to us when measuring its curvature. The refracting characteristics must also be understood when calculating the effect that any surgical procedure on this

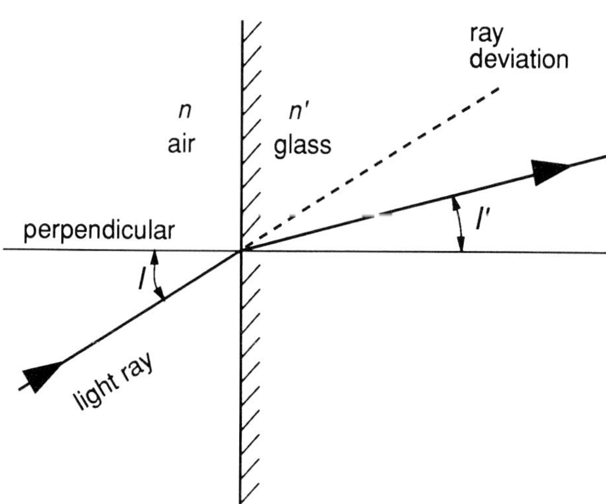

Fig. 3.24 Basic principle of Snell's law of refraction.

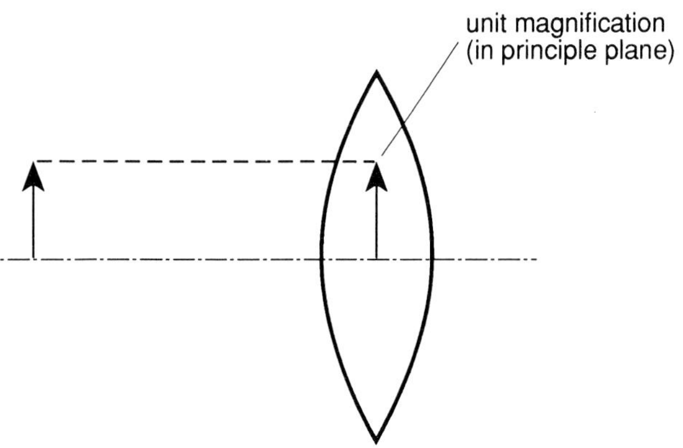

Fig. 3.25 Definition of principal plane.

surface has on total refraction of the eye. In the latter case, the cornea is treated like a thin meniscus lens.

Cardinal points and planes

Cardinal points and planes are constructions located to permit the use of two-ray procedures in thick lenses. The use of these constructs will result in greater precision, but the thin-lens alternative is adequate for most ophthalmic purposes. There are three pairs of cardinal points on the optic axis. The cardinal planes, which correspond to these points, are planes perpendicular to these points. The points and planes commonly encountered are the principal planes, nodal points, and focal points.

Principal plane

The formal definition of this plane is that it is a plane of unit magnification (Figure 3.25).

Focal point

The focal point is located on the optic axis at the point where rays from an object at infinity cross (are focused). The focal length is that distance from the principal plane to the focal point (Figures 3.26 and 3.27).

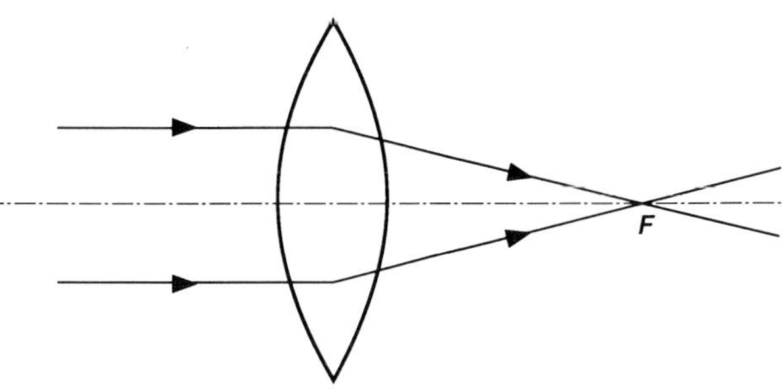

Fig. 3.26 The focal point.

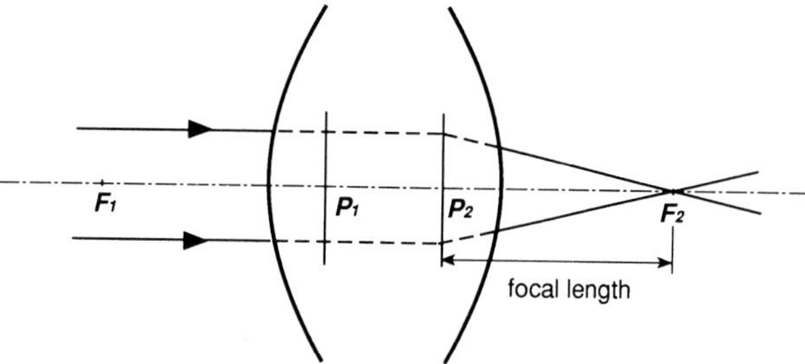

Fig. 3.27 The focal length of a lens defined.

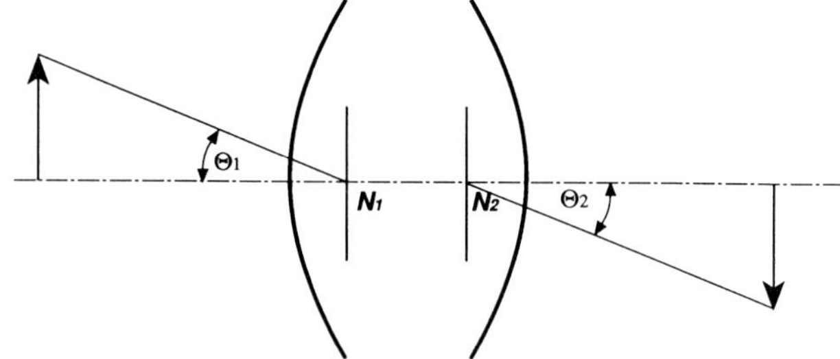

Fig. 3.29 Nodal points—thick lens.

Nodal point

The nodal point of a thin lens is characterized by no deviation from the initial to the final media of a refracted ray passing through the point (Figure 3.28). The angle of incidence of the ray passing through the nodal point is therefore equal to the angle of refraction. Thick lenses have two nodal points. A ray of light directed toward the first nodal point will appear to be coming from the second (Figure 3.29). In most situations, the indices of refraction of the media in which both the object and image are located are equal. In the case where this medium is air, the nodal points are superimposed on the principal planes (Figure 3.30).

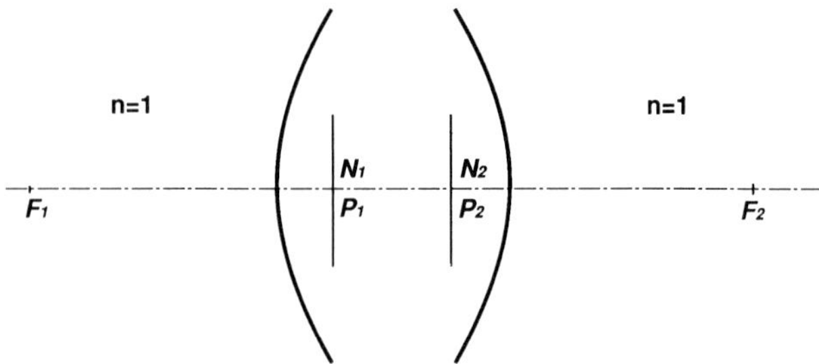

Fig. 3.30 In air, the nodal points and principal planes coincide.

Single refracting surfaces

A single refracting surface is one in which refraction occurs at one surface with the image located in a medium whose index of refraction differs from that in which the object is located. The behavior of cardinal points is as follows:

1 There is only one nodal point, one principal plane, and one focal point (Figure 3.31).
2 The principal point is located at the refracting surface.
3 The focal length is proportional to the index of refraction (Figure 3.32); therefore:

$$F_2 = n'F_1$$

4 The nodal point is not located at the principal plane. It is shifted toward the second focal point at the center

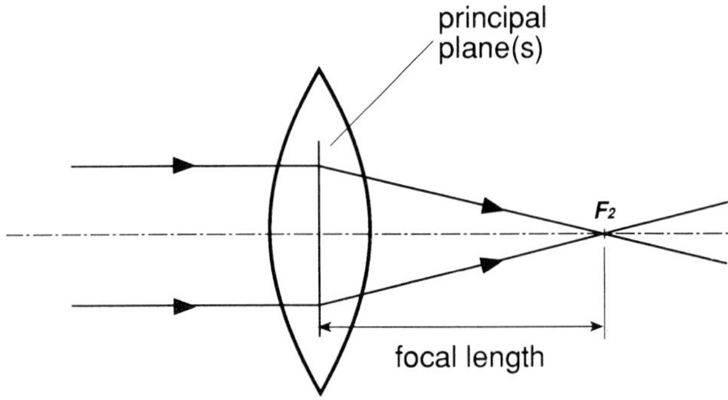

Fig. 3.31 Single refracting surface. There is only one principal plane and one focal point.

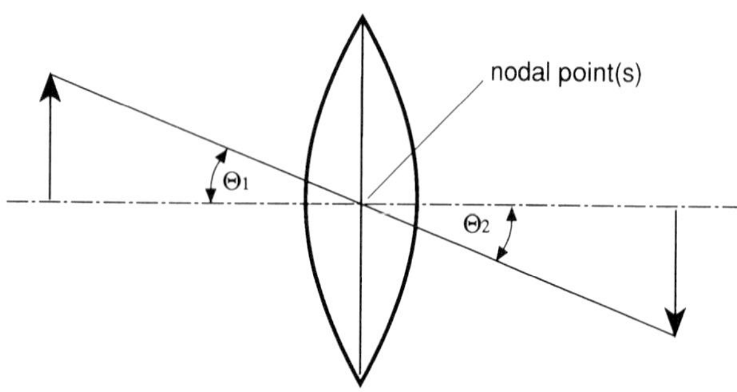

Fig. 3.28 Nodal points—thin lens.

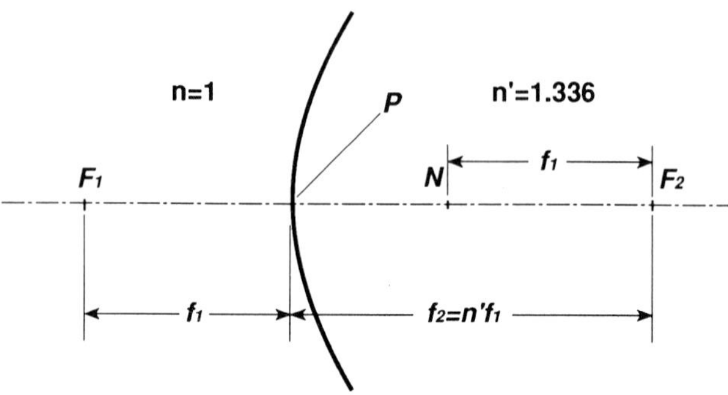

Fig. 3.32 In a single refracting surface, the focal length is proportional to the index of refraction.

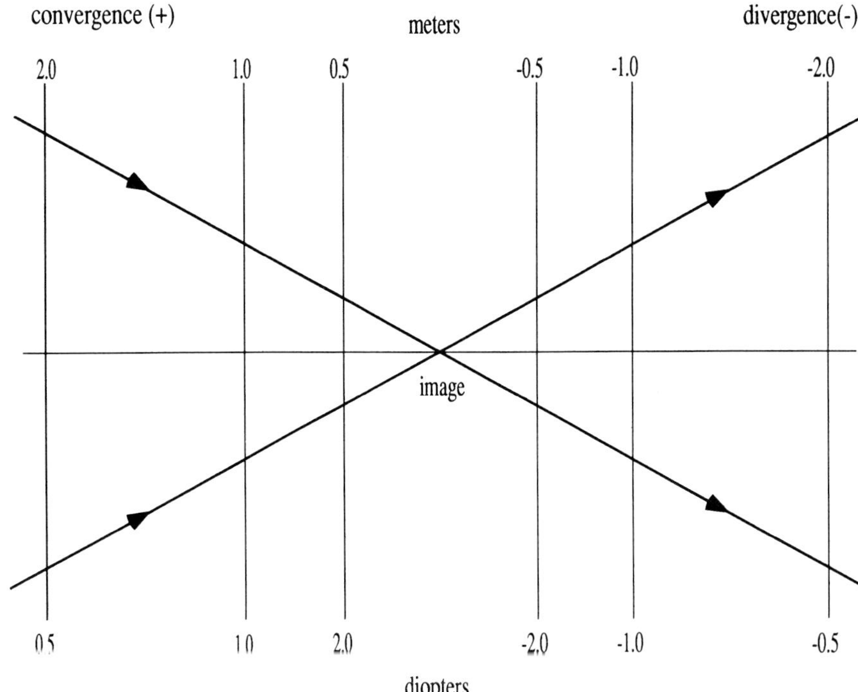

Fig. 3.33 Vergence of light rays. Converging light rays are plus and diverging beams are minus. The power of the ray is determined by its distance from the image.

of curvature of the surface (Figure 3.32). Thus the distance from the first focal point to the principal plane is equal to the distance from the nodal point to the second focal point.

Vergence

One other method employed to determine image characteristics is vergence, used with the two-ray trace procedure (Figure 3.33). Most problems should be solved using both methods. The application of vergence requires the use of five rules:

1 Distances of the object and image have dioptric value. This is expressed as the reciprocal of those dimensions, in meters.

2 Divergent beams have minus power.

3 Convergent beams have plus power.

4 The power of each element is expressed in diopters.

5 The ray, mirror, and lens powers are added algebraically.

Figure 3.34 shows a reduced eye using this method.

Magnification

Magnification refers only to the relationship between the image and object size, as expressed by

$$M = I/O$$

It is evident that magnification can also be expressed in terms of object and image distance (Figure 3.35):

$$M = \frac{\text{image distance}}{\text{object distance}} = \frac{D'}{D}$$

Greatest magnification occurs when the object is located at the first focal point of the lens. Changing the distance from the lens to the eye only alters the size of the field of view through the magnifying lens, not the size of the resulting image. Telescopes are two-stage magnifiers in which the object lens (objective) forms an image of the object. This image is further imaged by the much stronger magnifying power of the second lens, the ocular (Figure 3.36).

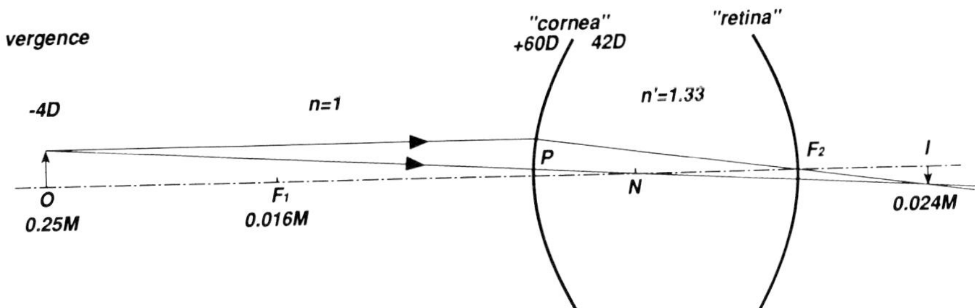

Fig. 3.34 A single-surface schematic eye demonstrating the use of vergence.

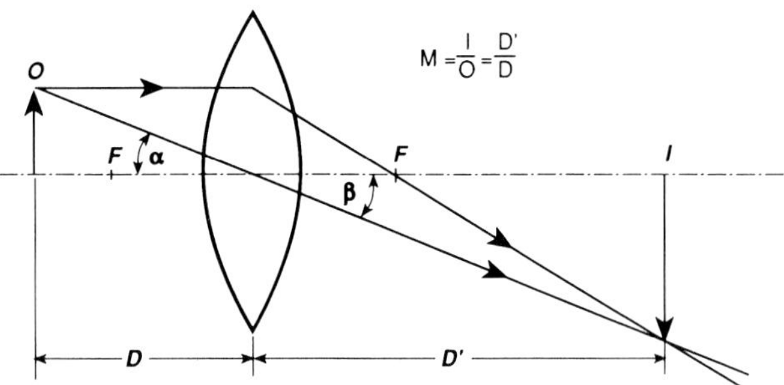

Fig. 3.35 Magnification.

Optical aberrations

In all the foregoing I have assumed a perfect optical system—that is, every ray of light passing through the system must converge to or diverge from a single point on the image. The image also must lie in a plane perpendicular to the optic axis and must be a symmetric copy of the object, whether erect, inverted, larger, or smaller. However, no optical system is ever perfect, nor are all the light rays identical. If Snell's law is applied to various parts of a spherical lens, it will be discovered that greater refraction occurs at the periphery than at the center. Unless incoming rays are paraxial, the rays of light will not come to a point focus; instead, the image will take the shape of a blurred circle (Figures 3.37 and 3.38). Lord Rayleigh suggested that the image does not deteriorate appreciably as long as the maximum difference in equivalent optical path at best focus does not exceed a quarter wavelength of light—the Rayleigh limit. Thus it can be expected that some abnormalities will exist in the image formed by any system. These deviations or aberrations are divided into two main groups:

1 Aberrations due to the multi-wavelength nature of light—chromatic aberrations.

2 System aberrations:
  (a) occurring on the optic axis—spherical aberrations.
  (b) occurring off axis—astigmatism, coma, distortion, field curvature, tilt.

Chromatic aberration

Chromatic aberration is not negligible, but neither is it considerable. The eye is not achromatic, as once believed (Figure 3.39). The magnitude of this phenomenon was first measured by the Astronomer Royal, Nevil Maskelyne, in 1789. He found a difference in focal length of the eye for red and violet light of 0.535 mm—quite close to more modern averages. While there is some variability, it is low and the average amount of this difference is 0.9 D. With a 2-mm-diameter pupil, 70% of the light falls on an area 0.005 mm in diameter, and thus the effects of chromatic aberration fall within the same magnitude as diffraction. As the pupil widens, the effects of increased chromatic aberration are offset by increasing diffractive effects. The net result is that image definition is practically unchanged.

Spherical aberration

The effects of spherical aberration in the eye are small (Figure 3.40). This is partly due to the relative flatness of

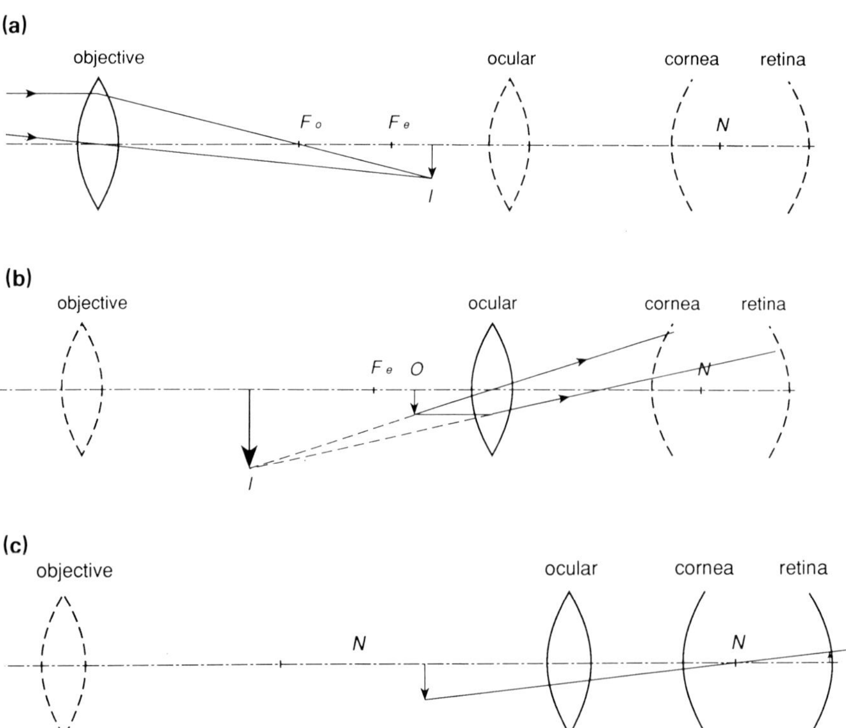

Fig. 3.36 (a–c) Telescopic magnification.

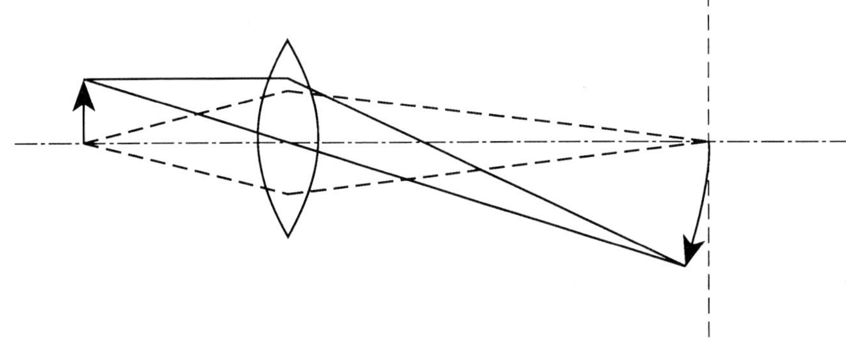

Fig. 3.37 Field curvature from a thick lens. Note that rays striking the periphery of the lens undergo more refraction.

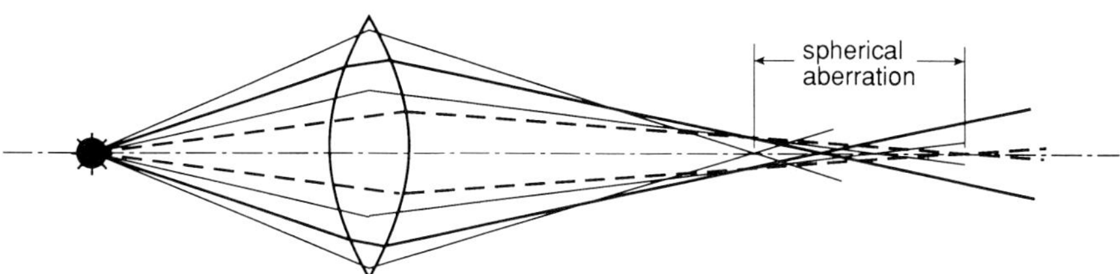

Fig. 3.38 Spherical aberration showing the resultant caustic or shape of the bundle at the putative focal point.

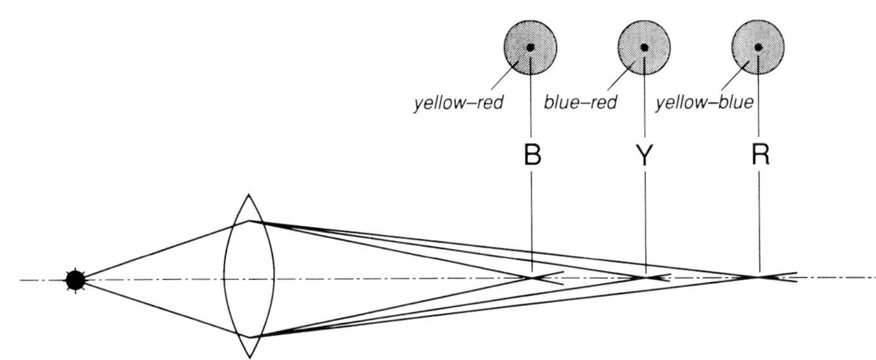

Fig. 3.39 Chromatic aberration.

the cornea in the periphery. However, most of the correction occurs because the lens nucleus is more dense than the periphery, refracting the axial rays more strongly than the marginal ones. It might be expected that the act of accommodation would affect the aberration present. It can be seen that during accommodation, the aberration becomes overcorrected and is least when 1 to 2 D of accommodation is exerted (Figure 3.41).

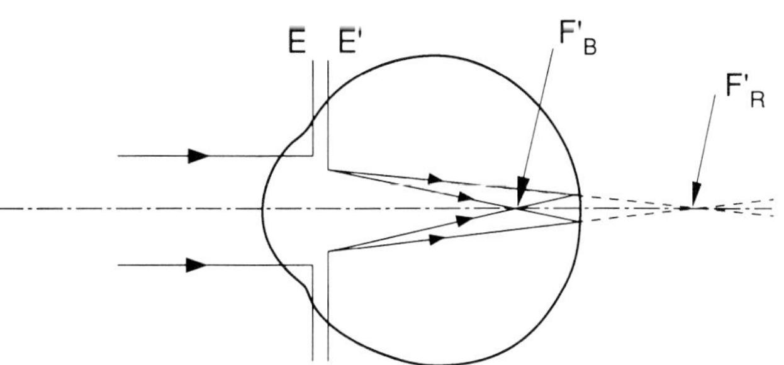

Fig. 3.40 Aberration in the human eye is small.

Other types of aberrations typically found in optical systems are negligibly small in the eye. Thus, although some obliquity of the light rays striking the retina occurs (because the optics are not coincident with the visual axis), the angle is usually very small. Therefore, as far as central vision is concerned, the effects of oblique astigmatism, lateral spherical aberration, tilt, and coma are not operative to any significant degree. However, any or all of these factors can take on more significance after the corneal surface shape has been altered through surgical, or other means.

Image curvature

One of the factors affecting image quality is image curvature. This occurs because the periphery of any lens has greater refracting power resulting from the greater obliquity of its surface there; thus peripheral rays are brought to a focus sooner (see Figure 3.37). This phenomenon was clearly described by Kepler in 1604 [6,7]. Although first elucidated mathematically by George Biddle Airy in 1827,

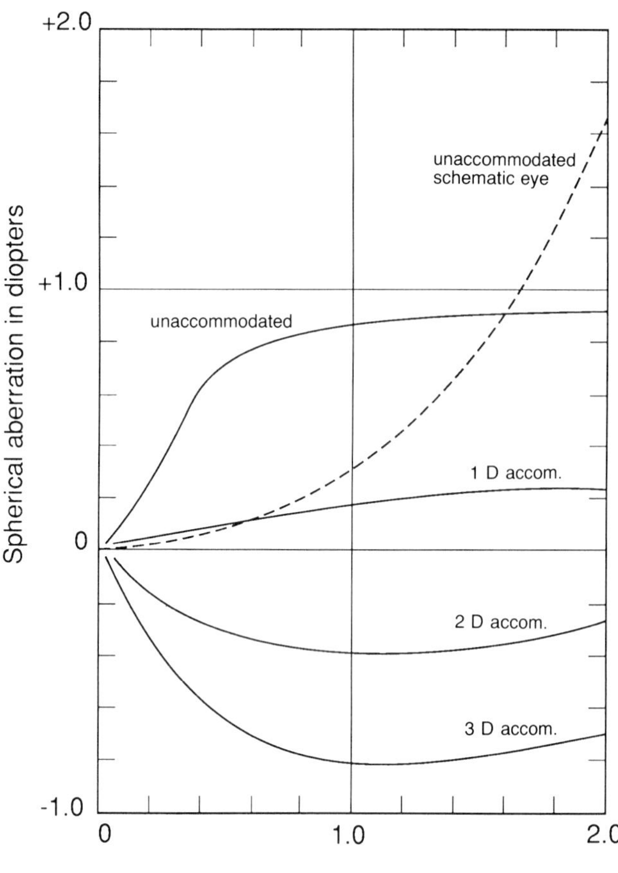

Fig. 3.41 Spherical aberration in the human eye is modified by accommodation.

this curvature is generally known as *Petzval's curvature* or *surface*. Airy's formula for the curvature is

$$\frac{1}{r} = -\frac{1}{n_1 f_1'}$$

Two factors lessen the effect of such aberrations in the periphery. The first of these is the fact that the back surface of the eye is curved. Thus the image shells approximate the true shape of the retina (Figure 3.42). The second point is that the resolving power of the peripheral retina is much less than that of the center, therefore more aberration can be tolerated without notice.

Astigmatism

Astigmatism is a characteristic of spherical surfaces in that the aberration results in more than one point of focus along the optic axis. This is true only in the sense that, typically, the major and minor meridians are spheres whose radius of curvature differ. However, astigmatism also can occur in surfaces that are regular aspheres (such as the cornea). The interval between the anterior and posterior focus is called the *interval of Sturm* and varies in its extent depending on the amount of astigmatism present in the optical system (Figure 3.43). Anterior to the first focal plane, the vertical rays converge more rapidly than the horizontal, and consequently, the bundle's cross section will be that of a horizontal ellipse. At the first focal plane, all the vertical rays have come to a focus and the bundle now takes the shape of a horizontal line. Beyond this point, the vertical rays begin to diverge while the horizontal rays are still converging, and the ellipse begins to shorten. At the posterior (second) focal plane, the condition is such that the horizontal rays have all come to a focus as a vertical line. Beyond that point the bundle again takes on the appearance of a vertical ellipse. There is one point between the anterior and posterior focus where the bundle's cross section is circular, however. This circle is called the *circle of least confusion* and is located approximately one-third of the way from the anterior-most focus (Figure 3.43). At this point in space, in the absence of any

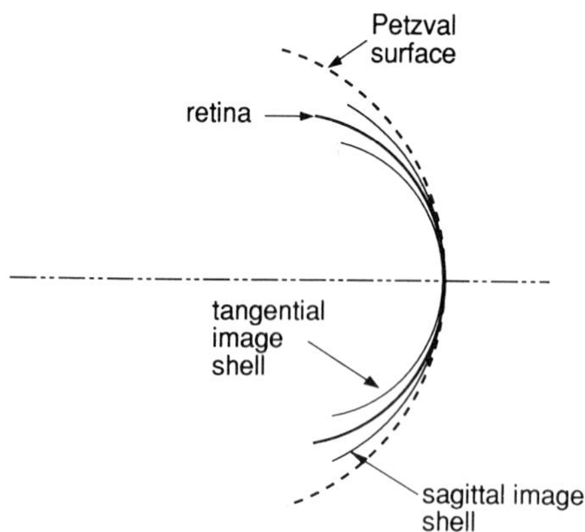

Fig. 3.42 Petzval's curvature or natural plane of focus for a thick lens, as in the human eye. Note that the image shells approximate the curve of the retina.

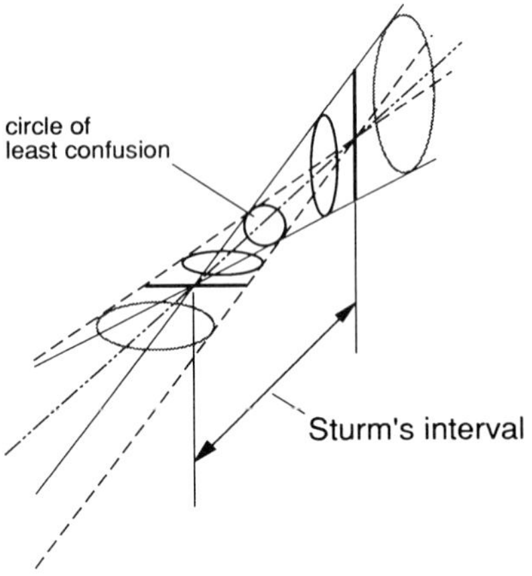

Fig. 3.43 An astigmatic system showing the shape of the light bundle making up Sturm's conoid.

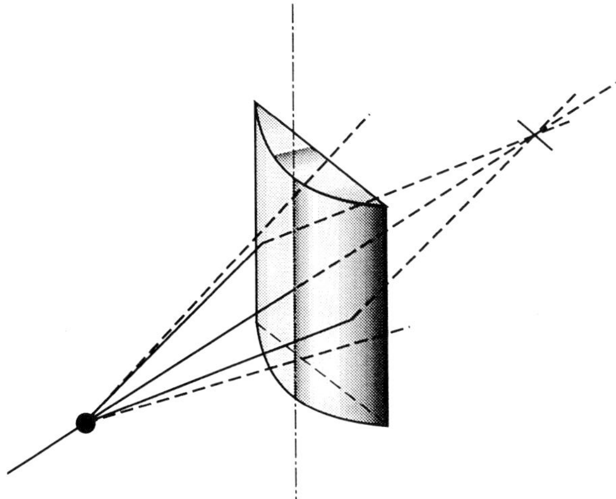

Fig. 3.44 A cylindric lens. Note that the image is a line perpendicular to the long axis of the lens.

optical correction, the image formed by the system is the best possible. Typically this power corresponds to the so-called spherical equivalent of the refractive system; that is, a spherical lens of that power will produce a circle of least confusion on the retina similar to that of the astigmatic system alone.

The simplest form of astigmatic system is one in which the curvature exists in only one direction (Figure 3.44). In this event, the image of a circle would be a straight line whose direction would depend on the angle of rotation of the surface (Figure 3.45). Thus we see that astigmatic lenses possess a direction or axis. An astigmatism occurring in a spherical system could be thought of as a cylinder lens superimposed on a spherical lens (Figure 3.46).

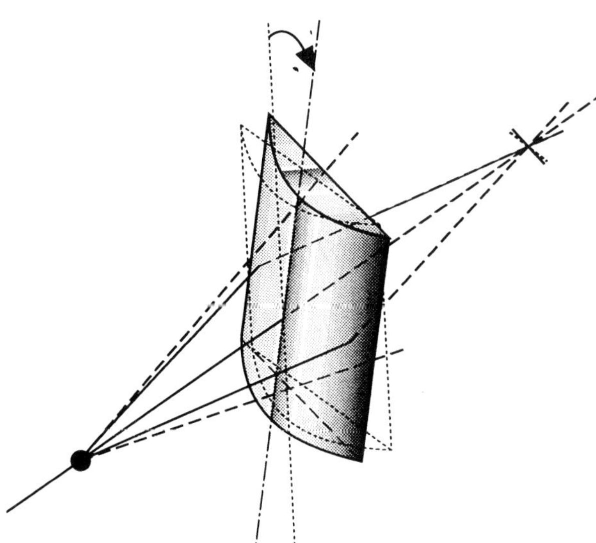

Fig. 3.45 When a cylinder lens is rotated, the image also rotates. Thus a cylinder lens has direction.

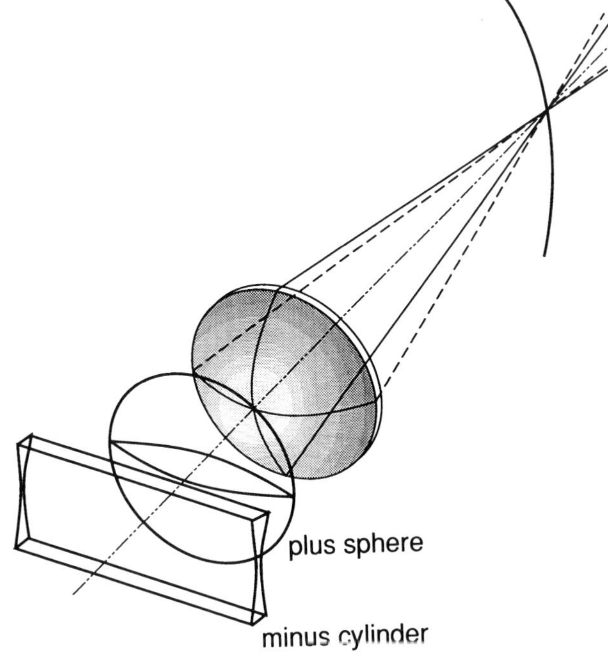

Fig. 3.46 A regular toroidal astigmatic refracting surface is corrected by applying both spherical and cylindric lenses of appropriate power.

Such a surface would be called *spherocylindric* or *toroidal.* An example of an extreme toroid would be a doughnut.

Coma and tilt

Coma and tilt are special forms of astigmatism. Coma occurs in images of objects located off the optic axis (Figure 3.47). The resulting image is characteristic, having a bright center with a less bright tail; hence its name. Less discrete objects will appear to be smeared. Tilt occurs when an element is rotated around a plane perpendicular to the axis (Figure 3.48). The resulting image is also smeared but in two or more directions. Such aberrations have less effect in the eye due to the fact that the asymmetry of the ocular system corrects part of these

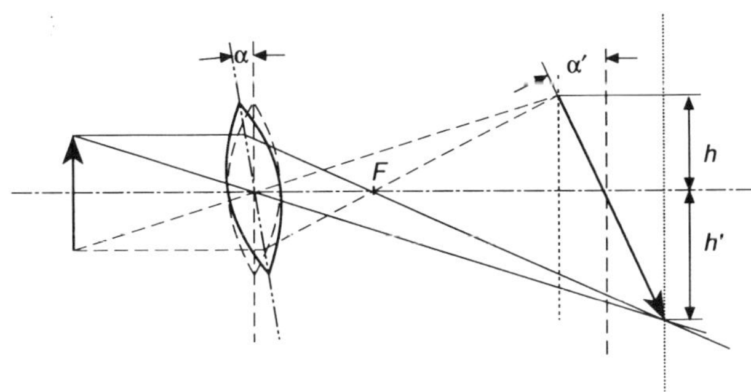

Fig. 3.47 Tilt in an optical system. Tilt is axisymmetric whereas coma is not.

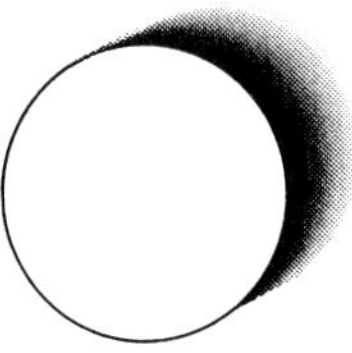

Fig. 3.48 Characteristic appearance of coma.

aberrations and also because the image falls on to a curved surface (the retina).

Resolving power

To distinguish two luminous points, two cones must be stimulated with the one between unstimulated. The smallest resolvable image therefore has a diameter just slightly larger than a macular cone cell. This distance has been shown to be around 0.002 mm. Therefore, the minimal visual angle possible is

$$\tan aNb = \frac{ab}{bN} = \frac{0.002}{17.054} = \tan 24.14 \text{ s}$$

However, the ultimate resolving power of the eye is really determined by Rayleigh criterion. Here we must return to the wave nature of light and the subject of wavefronts. It must be remembered that a circular aperture such as the iris produces a diffraction effect resulting in an image that is made up of alternate dark and light rings surrounding a bright central disk (see Figure 3.15). The size of this disk is usually expressed as the angular radius of the first dark ring. In order to distinguish (resolve) two points, Lord Rayleigh suggested that a separation of the Airy disks by this magnitude is necessary (Figure 3.49). Thus the resolving power of the eye can be measured by calculating the size of the Airy disk using the formula

$$\phi = \frac{1.22\lambda}{d}$$

where λ is the wavelength and d is the diameter of the pupil. Thus, for yellow light and a pupillary diameter of 6.0 mm, the visual efficiency would be 0.3 min of arc; for a 2.0 mm pupil, 1.22 min (in blue light, 1.05 min).

We are used to estimating the efficiency of an optical system such as the eye by its resolving power. Today, however, we are hearing about a more sophisticated methodology of measurement—the modulation transfer function—applied to optics and the eye. This concept is borrowed from the study of electricity and works because of the similarity of optical and electric systems. It is important for the reader to grasp this concept because it applies not only to light transmitted through the optical system of the eye but also to that reflected from its surface. Since it is the reflecting (or catadioptric) nature of the cornea which allows us to study its surface changes, a working knowledge of the concept of modulation transfer functions will assist in the interpretation and understanding of modern topographic mapping devices.

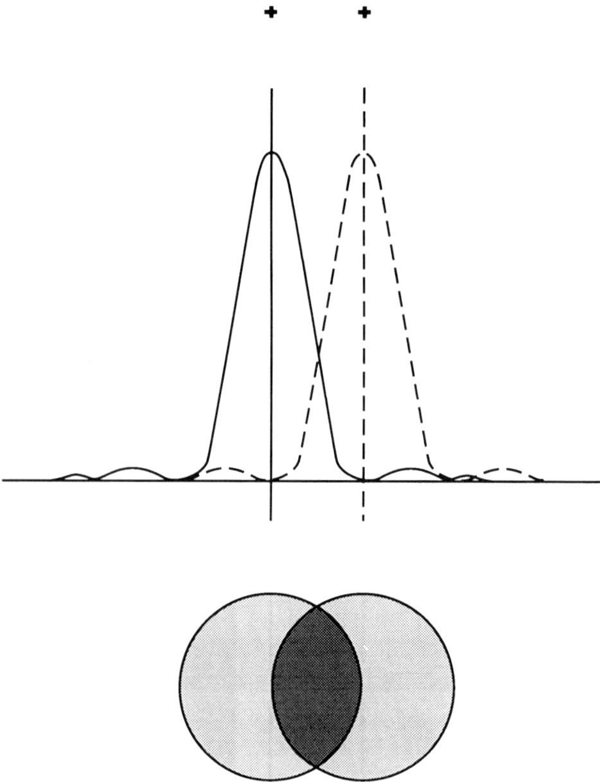

Fig. 3.49 Superimposed Airy disks demonstrating the principle of Rayleigh's criterion for resolving discrete objects. Only the central, bright spot is represented.

Any signal entering an electric system can be considered as a series of sinusoidal waveforms by means of Fourier analysis. According to Fourier's theorem, any wave, regardless of its complexity, can be reproduced by combining a number of waves of different amplitudes, frequencies, and phases. The emerging signal can be treated in the same manner, but the waves will differ among themselves depending on how they have been attenuated by the system through which they have passed. The curve of attenuation against frequency is called the frequency response function.

The optical analog to this system lies in considering the light as a series of spatial frequencies, each representing an imaginary grating. The curve of amplitude against the spatial frequency is the optical transfer function. In both cases we are concerned with the change in frequency or phase, in other words, the modulation of the signal. Hence the term *modulation transfer function*. Above a certain critical frequency, the "noise" from diffraction cancels out the response; thus the frequency is dependent on the aperture. For 100% modulation, the absolute sensitivity of the eye with a 2.0 mm pupil is 0.5 min of arc.

It is possible to use this method to measure the contrast sensitivity of the retina alone because the production of

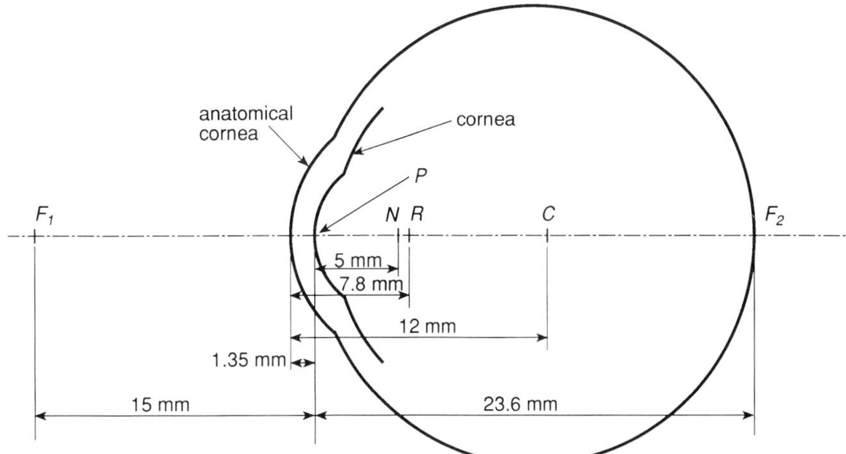

Fig. 3.50 The schematic eye of Listing.

interference fringes is largely unaffected by the focusing mechanism of the eye (I will have more to say about interference fringes in my discussion on corneal topography in Chapter 6). The relationship of this measurement and that of the visual apparatus as a whole is the transfer function of the dioptric apparatus.

The optics of the eye

It should be evident by now (see also Chapter 2) that the optics of the eye is a complex subject. It is made more so by the fact that a large part of the refraction occurs at a single surface, yet the eye must be considered as a thick-lens system. Despite the confusing behavior of the cardinal and nodal points of the eye, their locations are the result of a logical application of the optical rules discussed in the previous section. Thus

1 The eye cannot be considered a thin-lens system. Thus P_1, P_2, N_1, and N_2 are not superimposed in one position.

2 The eye has characteristics of a single refracting surface. Thus the anterior focal length is shorter than the posterior focal length. This means that the nodal points are shifted posteriorly. The distance between the first nodal point and the first principal point is equal to the distance between the second nodal point and the second focal point.

3 The eye is not optically homogeneous—there are several surfaces where refraction occurs because the eye is made up of various structures all having different indices of refraction. This fact also separates each of the principal and nodal points.

4 The eye is a variable optic. That is, accommodation can shift the overall refractive power of the eye toward the center of the lens.

Optical constants

Because of the complexity of the human optical system, ray tracing using the two-ray method becomes tedious. It has proved useful, therefore, to employ a schematic representation of the eye taking into account the various factors and replacing them with approximations. Several such schematic eyes have been devised. Listing was one of the first to do so, but most students of the human eye use the reduced eye of Gullstrand.

Reduced eye of Listing

This is somewhat more complex than that of Gullstrand. Figure 3.50 is derived from the modification by Donders.

Gullstrand's eye

The groups of ocular constants in Tables 3.1 through 3.4 are derived from Helmholtz and refer to Figure 3.51, the schematic eye of Gullstrand.

Those of particular concern to us are the anterior and posterior surfaces of the cornea and lens. Pertinent

Table 3.1 Power of optical elements. Adapted from Helmholtz H. *Treatise on Physiological Optics*, JPC Southall (transl). Optical Society of America, New York, 1924

	Far	Near
Cornea	43	43
Lens	20	33
Total	60	71

Table 3.2 Indices of refraction. Adapted from Helmholtz H. *Treatise on Physiological Optics*, JPC Southall (transl). Optical Society of America, New York, 1924

Air	1.00
Cornea	1.37
Aqueous	1.33
Lens cortex	1.38
Lens nucleus	1.40
Vitreous	1.33

Table 3.3 Refracting surfaces. Adapted from Helmholtz H. *Treatise on Physiological Optics,* JPC Southall (transl). Optical Society of America, New York, 1924

	Radius (mm)	
	Far	Near
Anterior cornea	7.8	7.8
Anterior lens	10.0	5.3
Posterior lens	6.0	5.3

Table 3.4 Cardinal points. Adapted from Helmholtz H. *Treatise on Physiological Optics,* JPC Southall (transl). Optical Society of America, New York, 1924

	Distance from vertex of cornea (mm)	
	Far	Near
First principal point, P_1	1.5	1.8
Second principal point, P_2	1.6	2.0
First focal point, F_1	15.2	12.3
Second focal point, F_2	22.3	18.9
First nodal point, N_1	6.9	6.5
Second nodal point, N_2	7.3	6.9
First focal length	16.7	14.1
Second focal length	22.3	18.9
Position of near point		100.8

indices of refraction are those of the cornea, aqueous, lens, and vitreous. The axial length is also important in ray tracing and determines, many times, the optical state of the eye [8]. This schema can be even further simplified, but the constants given will provide sufficient information and accuracy to use with any ray tracing computer program; among these, I recommend BEAM4. The methods by which these constants were, are, or can be derived are many but are not germane to our discussion. The reader is referred to the appropriate literature for that information.

Angles and axes of the eye

As I have already pointed out in Chapter 2, the optical complexity of the eye is compounded by the fact that the ocular components are not symmetrically aligned along a common axis. This fact has led to a veritable stew of angles and axes which are defined as follows:

1 The visual axis is an imaginary line passing through the macula, the nodal point, and the object (fixation) point (Figure 3.52).

2 The optic axis (a real imaginary line—the stuff of fantasy) passes through the anterior and posterior poles of the eye and through the nodal point (Figure 3.53). As in any optic system, it is the line along which all the optical components of the eye are, theoretically, aligned. The operative word here is theoretically.

3 Angle α, typically 5°, is formed between the optic and visual axes at the nodal point (Figure 3.54).

4 The pupillary line (or axis) is drawn through the apparent center of the pupil, perpendicular to the corneal surface (Figure 3.55). It is not symmetric to the remainder of the optic system because the pupil is usually displaced nasally.

5 The principal line of vision is the axis from the apparent center of the pupil to the object (Figure 3.56). Note that this is not the same as the pupillary axis.

6 Angle κ is the angle formed between the visual and the pupillary axis (extended posteriorly) at the nodal point (Figure 3.57). It also has been defined as the angle between the pupillary axis and the principal line of vision

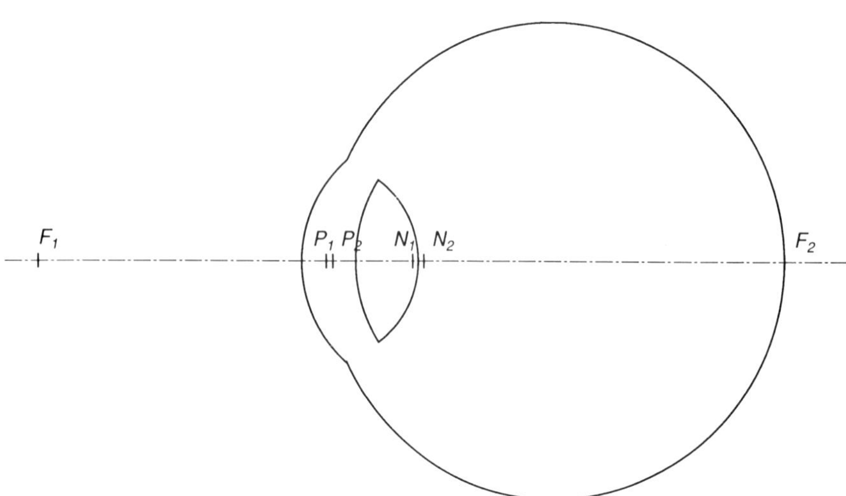

Fig. 3.51 The schematic eye of Gullstrand.

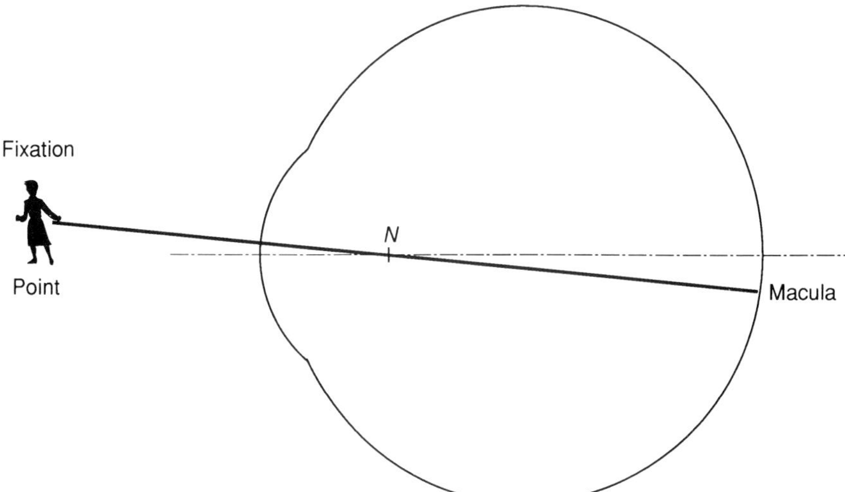

Fig. 3.52 The visual axis. It does not correspond to the geometric axis.

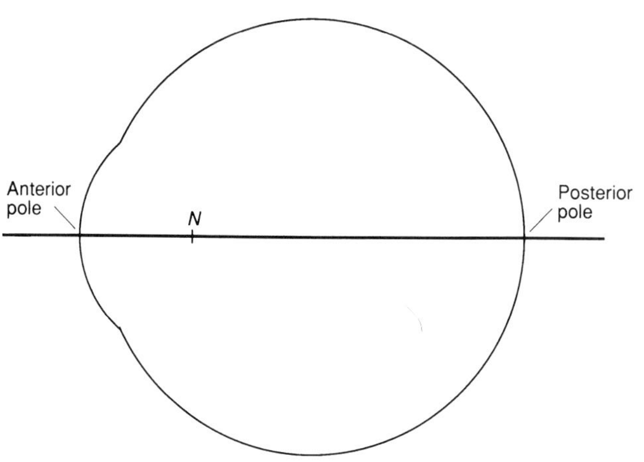

Fig. 3.53 Optic or geometric axis.

(Figure 3.58). The difference between the two definitions is very small and can be ignored.

7 The fixation axis is the line joining the object with the center of rotation of the eye. The rotation point is usually located on the optic axis 13 mm posterior to the corneal surface (Figure 3.59).

8 Angle γ is the angle formed by the fixation and optic axes at the center of rotation (Figure 3.60).

Visual acuity

The current method of deriving the visual acuity uses various-sized letters (called *optotypes*) printed or projected in a high-contrast setting (Figure 3.61). The acuity is recorded in terms of Snellen's fraction, where the numerator is the distance (typically 20 ft or 6 m) at which the letter is viewed and the denominator is the relative distance

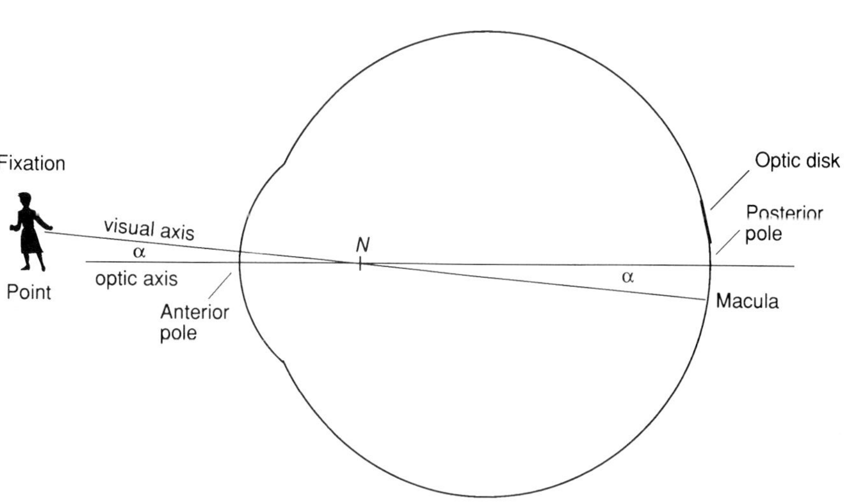

Fig. 3.54 Angle alpha.

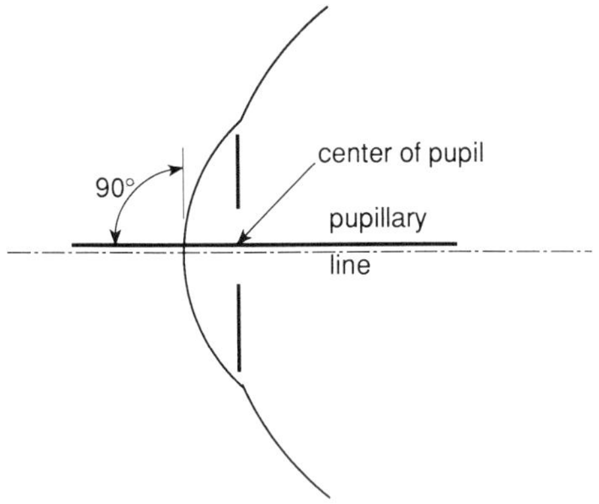

Fig. 3.55 Pupillary line.

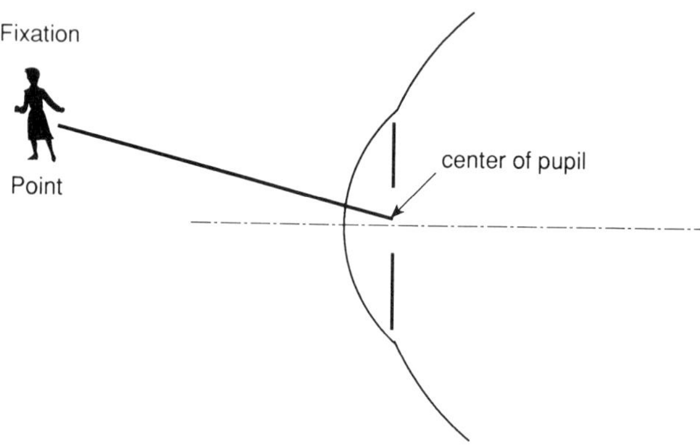

Fig. 3.56 The principal line of vision.

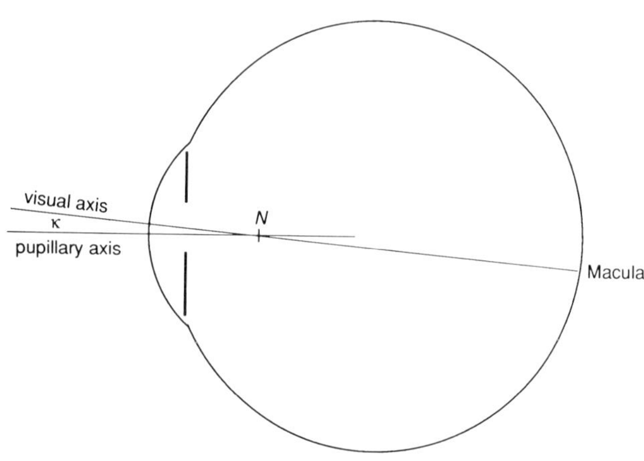

Fig. 3.57 Angle kappa—defined as the angle between the visual and pupillary axis at the nodal point.

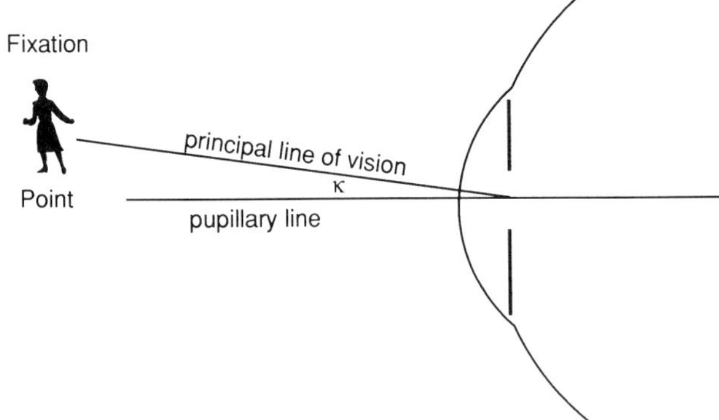

Fig. 3.58 Angle kappa—defined as the angle between the pupillary axis and the principal line of vision.

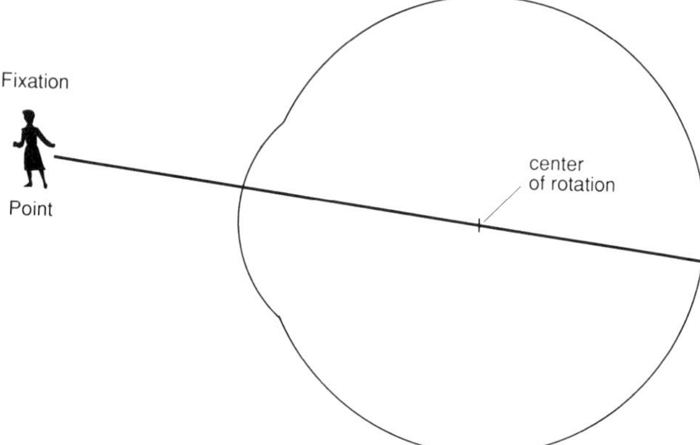

Fig. 3.59 The fixation axis passes through the center of rotation of the eye.

(also in feet or meters) at which the letter will subtend an angle of 1 min on the retina. Other ways of expressing the fraction are in decimal notation or as a percentage. Thus 20/20 = 1.0 (or 100%), 20/40 = 0.5 (50%), 20/200 = 0.1 (10%), and so on. This method, in use for around 125 years, is a way to record ocular resolution in an artificial environment. The acuity measurement very much depends on the contrast of the letter with the background. Unfortunately, the technique has few counterparts in the real world and equally unfortunate is the fact that it is firmly entrenched in society. It is well known in clinical practice that the visual acuity as measured by the Snellen chart is often in no way indicative of the existence of a visual handicap. Many individuals with increased lenticular turbidity can discern 20/40 or better and yet are unable to recognize a face in normal lighting or drive safely at night. Contrast sensitivity methods are probably a more realistic test of visual efficiency but a standard has not yet been established for their use.

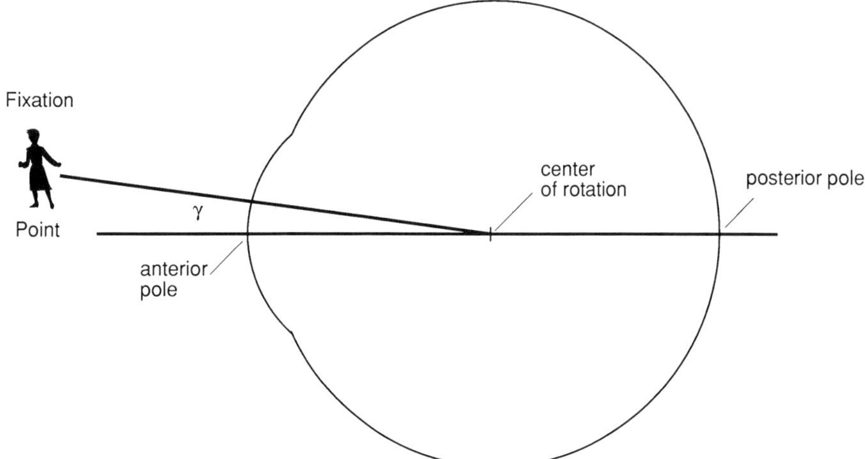

Fig. 3.60 Angle gamma.

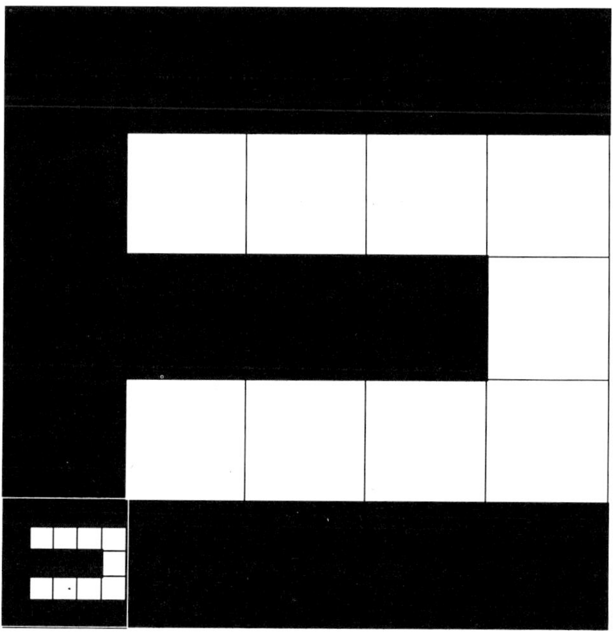

Fig. 3.61 The Snellen optotype showing the relationship between a 20/20 and a 20/200 letter.

In any event this subject completes our brief discussion of light and optics, for the moment. Do not despair, however; we will encounter certain of the principles reviewed here from time to time in other parts of this treatise.

References

1 Young T. *A Course of Lectures on Natural Philosophy and the Mechanical Arts.* Royal Society, London, 1807.

2 Taton R. Roemer et la vitesse de la lumiere. In: *Proceedings of the Centre National Reserche Scientifique.* Paris, 1976.

3 Fermat P. *Varia Opera Mathematica.* Joannem Pech, Tolosa, 1679.

4 Young T. On the theory of light and colours. Phil Trans R Soc Lond 1802; 92.

5 Gullstrand A. *Einfuhrung in die Methoden die Dioptrik des Auges.* Leipzig, 1911.

6 Kepler J. *Ad Vitellionem Paraliponema.* Frankfurt, 1604.

7 Kepler J. *Dioptrice.* Frankfurt, 1611.

8 Helmholtz H. *Treatise on Physiological Optics,* vol 1, JPC Southall (transl). Optical Society of America, New York, 1924.

Further reading

Born M, Wolf E. *Principles of Optics.* Macmillan, New York, 1964.

Donders FC. *On the Anomalies of Accommodation and Refraction of the Eye,* WD Moore (transl). Hatton Press, London, 1864.

Hardy AC, Perrin FH. *The Principles of Optics.* McGraw-Hill, New York, 1982.

von Helmholtz H. *Treatise on Physiological Optics,* vol 1, J southall (transl). Optical Society of America, New York, 1924.

Jenkins F, White H. *Fundamentals of Optics,* 3d ed. McGraw-Hill, New York, 1957.

Ogle K. *Optics: An Introduction for Ophthalmologists.* Thomas, Springfield, Ill., 1961.

Sears FW. Optics. In: *Principles of Physics,* vol III, 3d ed. Addison-Wesley, Reading, Mass., 1948.

Tscherning M. *Physiological Optics,* C Weiland (transl). Philadelphia, 1904.

4

Anatomy and Physiology of Corneal Wound Healing

IAGO: . . . *How poor are they that have not patience!*
What wound didst ever heal but by degrees?
Thou knowest we work by wit and not by witchcraft?
And wit depends on dilatory time.
[Othello, Act II, Scene iii]

Corneal anatomy and physiology

The healing of corneal wounds is of vital concern to all ophthalmic surgeons. The advent of refractive surgery has created entirely new potential healing problems. Proper management of postoperative care enhances tissue repair, which plays a pivotal role in the end results. To optimize results, it is important to consider the complex sequence of events that take place during corneal healing. An understanding of corneal anatomy and physiology is critical for understanding the processes that influence corneal wound healing.

Anatomy

The cellular components of the cornea are limited to the epithelium, keratocytes, and endothelium, which account for only 15% of the total corneal thickness. The bulk of the cornea consists of the extracellular matrix that is largely collagen but also contains glycosaminoglycans, glycoproteins, and a variety of complex molecules that are likely important in maintenance and healing. The cornea classically is divided into five layers that include epithelium, Bowman's membrane, stroma, Descemet's membrane, and endothelium (Figure 4.1).

Corneal epithelium

The corneal epithelium (Figure 4.2) is composed of five to eight layers of stratified squamous cells. The cells of the basal layer are regularly aligned and attached to their secreted basal lamina by hemidesmosomes (Figure 4.3b). These latter structures are responsible for integrity of the epithelial sheet; defects in hemidesmosome formation are responsible for recurrent erosions, which may present problems in healing of refractive surgical procedures. Mitotic activity takes place in the basal layer. As new cells are produced, they become flattened and gradually move to the surface, eventually being cast off in the tear film. Multiple fine, unmyelinated branches of the trigeminal nerve insinuate themselves between the cells of the basal layer and provide corneal sensation.

The lateral cell membranes of the corneal epithelium are characterized by complex interdigitations that, along with fine filaments (tonofibrils), contribute intercellular adhesion (Figure 4.3). The surface cell membranes are also folded, forming microplicae and microvilli. This folding increases the effective epithelial surface and is critical to adhesion of the tear film.

Unlike the skin, the normal cornea does not become cornified. It is important to be aware that the limbal conjunctiva is the source of stem cells for renewal of the corneal epithelium [1] and that there are also specific areas of stem cell renewal for the conjunctiva [2,3]. In some instances, corneal stem cells play a vital role in corneal

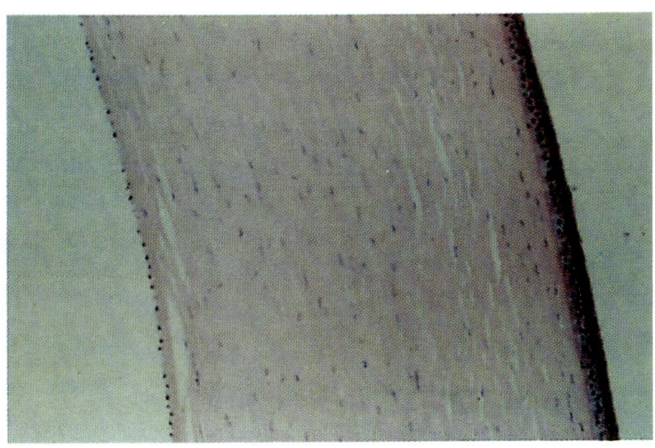

Fig. 4.1 Normal cornea (H&E stain; ×10).

wound healing (see below), which is critically dependent on corneal epithelial healing. Many of the clinical problems that occur in corneal surface disease are related to the extent of unhealthy corneal epithelium and the presence of damage to corneal stem cells [4,5].

Bowman's layer lies directly beneath the corneal epithelium. It varies in thickness between 8 and 14 μ. It is composed almost entirely of loosely packed dispersed collagen with small amounts of glycosaminoglycans and glycoproteins, similar to those found in the corneal stroma. The periodicity of the collagen is less evident than in the corneal stroma, with which Bowman's membrane imperceptibly blends.

The corneal stroma comprises over 90% of the normal corneal thickness. The bulk of the stroma is composed of types I and V collagen, which are arranged in highly ordered lamellae [6] (Figures 4.4 and 4.5). The corneal lamellae have an average thickness of 2 μ, and each extends across the entire cornea. This regular arrangement of the lamellae and the collagen fibers they contain plays a central role in corneal transparency. In addition to types I and V collagen, special techniques allow visualization of type VI collagen, with its longer spacing of 80 to 100 nm [7]. Type VI fibers are intimately associated with type I and V fibers. Further, it has been suggested that this association is based on binding by dermatan sulfate proteoglycans (especially decorin) that may serve to stabilize the collagen lamellae [7]. The remaining extracellular matrix is composed of glycosaminoglycans, glycoproteins, and allied compounds and constitutes about 1%

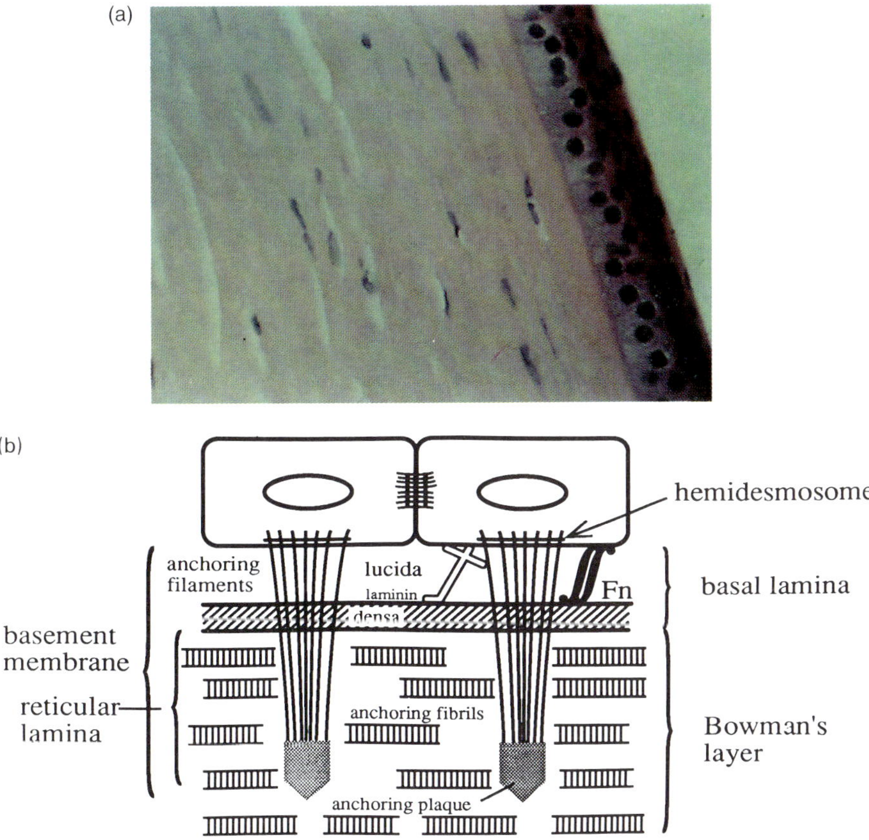

Fig. 4.2 (a) Corneal epithelium, Bowman's membrane, and anterior stroma (H&E stain; ×80). (b) Schematic of the relationship of the basal columnar cells to Bowman's layer (from Beuerman RW, Crosson CE, Kaufman HE. *Healing Processes in the Cornea*, vol. 1, p 243. Gulf, Houston, 1989, with permission).

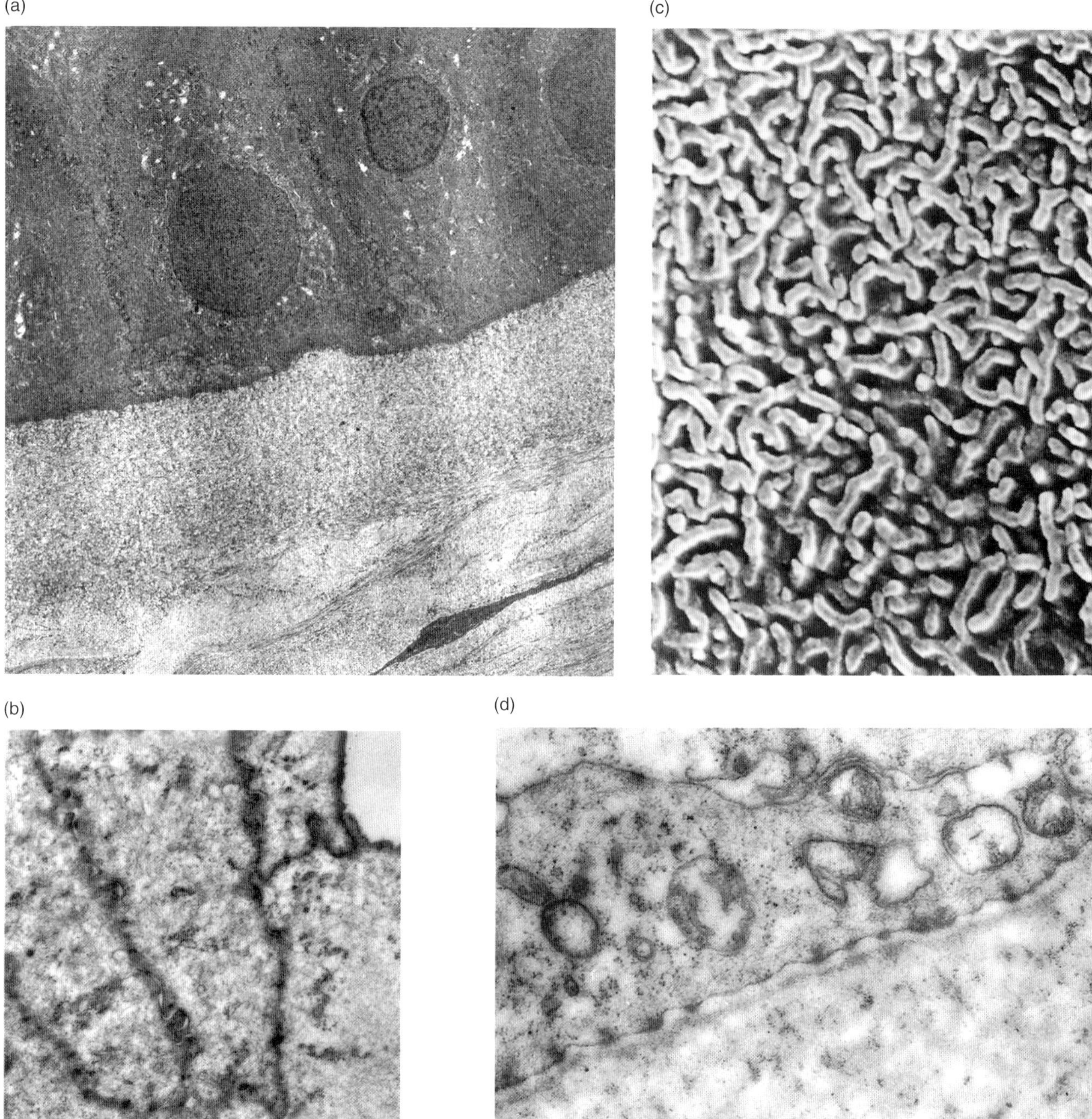

Fig. 4.3 (a) Corneal section at Bowman's layer showing columnar basal cells and basal lamella. Note Bowman's layer blends into the underlying stroma (×15,200). (b) Corneal epithelium, showing the numerous sites of attachment along adjacent cell membranes (×27,400). (c) Microvillae (×15,000). (d) Basal layer of corneal epithelium. Numerous hemidesmosomes attach to a thin basal lamina that merges with Bowman's membrane (×31,800).

of corneal wet weight (see below). The keratocytes are modified fibroblasts, which are few in number and show little activity in normal cornea.

The collagens are a complex family of structural proteins that form highly organized supramolecular complexes [8,9]. There are over 19 different collagen types, composed of as many as 33 different gene products. The common critical feature of all collagens is their basic building block of three polypeptide pro-α chains that wind together to form a triple helix [8,9]. From their origin in the endoplasmic reticulum of fibroblasts, the procollagen undergoes a series of complex modifications that require many other enzymes and proteins before final collagen structure is completed [8,9].

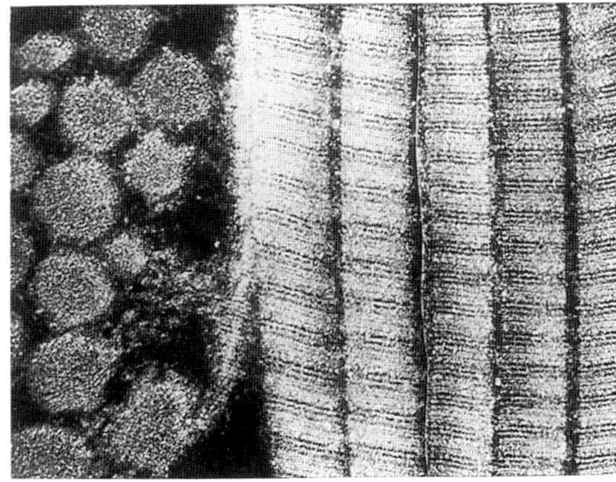

Fig. 4.4 Characteristic banding seen in collagen fibrils (×50,000).

Glycosaminoglycans

Glycosaminoglycans (GAGs) are macromolecules of the class proteoglycans (in the past called *mucopolysaccharides*). Proteoglycans are large, complex molecules that consist of a core protein with one or several covalently bound GAG chains [10]. Because of the numerous active groups available on the different GAGs, they can bind to a variety of other compounds. This binding is important in cellular interactions, cell adhesion, cell migration, cell growth, and assembly of the extracellular matrix [10]. Proteoglycans are present in all ocular compartments, and their composition varies with the tissue involved [10]. Proteoglycans are water-soluble molecules that carry a high negative charge (anionic glycosaminoglycans, AGAGs) and thus tend to repel each other. This latter feature causes them to form stiff chains and is directly responsible for corneal swelling pressure (see below) [11]. AGAGs form fibril-to-fibril bridges that link across as many as four collagen fibers. As such, the AGAGs play a direct role in maintaining the controlled distance between adjacent collagen fibers that is critical for creating corneal transparency [11,12].

The bulk of corneal GAGs are keratan sulfate, and its abundance in the stroma suggests a tissue-specific function. Second in abundance is dermatan sulfate, which differs from the same compound in other connective tissues in being less sulfated and having a lower level of iduronic acid (reviewed in [13]). GAGs fill the space between collagen fibers and stromal keratocytes. It is remarkable that the cornea is as clear as it is considering that it is made up of layers of fiber bundles all of which can produce diffraction and scattering of light [14]. However, as discussed in Chapter 3, if such differences in indices are less than half the wavelength of light apart (or about 200 nm), transparency is preserved. The ability of proteoglycans to bind and separate collagen, as discussed earlier, is the key to corneal transparency. If the distance increases as it does in stromal edema, the corneal fibers act as a sinusoidal grating, the modulation transfer function of the stroma is altered, and scattering is increased, much as happens at sunset on a dusty day [15,16]. GAGs are also responsible for the imbibition (swelling) pressure that draws water into the cornea [17].

Collagen

Collagen is composed of complex glycoproteins including mucins. Collagen accounts for approximately 71% of dry

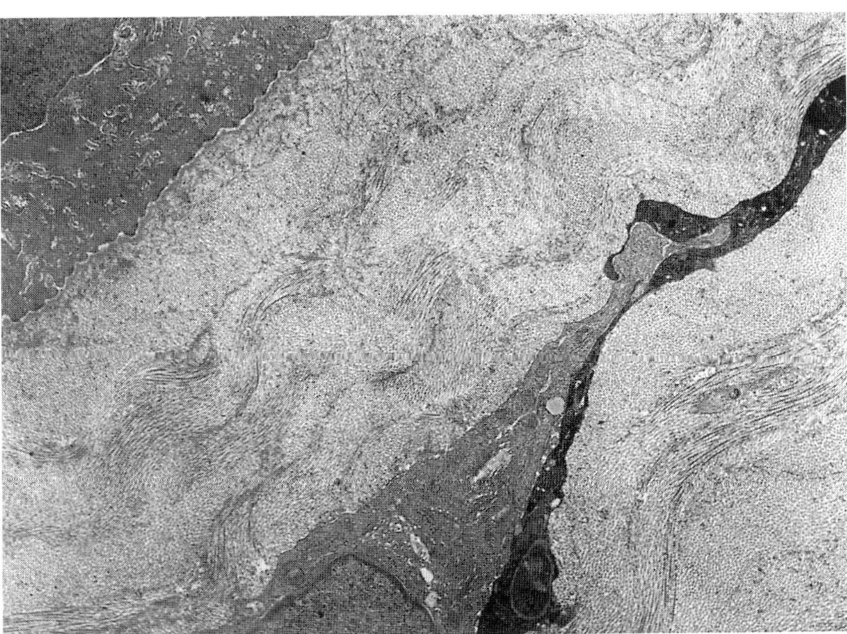

Fig. 4.5 Corneal stroma demonstrating the interlacing of collagen fibers surrounding a keratocyte. Note the layered nature of the stroma (×10,500).

corneal weight and is the most abundant protein in the body [18]. In the cornea, collagen is present in the subepithelial basement membrane, the fibrils of Bowman's layer, the stromal lamellae, and Descemet's membrane.

Production of collagen begins intracellularly with the synthesis of precursor forms in the rough endoplasmic reticulum, followed by secretion through the Golgi apparatus. Production of sub-units called *pro-α chains* occurs first with linking of amino acid chains. Hydroxylation and glycosylation of these chains occurs, which causes the maturing pro-α chains to twist into individual helices. A helical α chain joins together with two other chains to form procollagen, which is secreted from the cell. Further maturation of the collagen fibers continues extracellularly, where the nonhelical peptide ends are enzymatically trimmed, leaving the basic unit of collagen—tropocollagen. Collagen fibrils in their native state consist of tropocollagen molecules (approximately 300 nm in length) arranged in a staggered manner with about a 25% overlap. The characteristic banding pattern of approximately 67 nm (see Figure 4.4) is produced by this overlapping.

Five collagen types are defined by the variety of α chains present: $\alpha 1$, $\alpha 2$, αA, and αB, and they are the result of heterogeneity in location of specific amino acids within the chains. Thus there is a type I $\alpha 1$ chain [denoted as $\alpha 1(I)$] that is found primarily in skin, for example. Bowman's layer contains type I collagen. Type I collagen consists of two $\alpha 1(I)$ chains and one $\alpha 2$ chain and is designated as $\alpha 1(I)_2\ \alpha 2$. Type II collagen, found in cartilage is designated as $\alpha 1(II)_3$. Type III, which is frequently found in association with type I in skin, blood vessels, and smooth muscle, is designated as $\alpha 1(III)_3$. There is also basement membrane collagen (type IV), whose exact α chain composition has not been completely worked out, and type AB (type V), probably consisting of two αB and one αA chains [19,20].

Descemet's membrane is the acellular basal lamina of the corneal endothelium. Compared with other basal laminae, it is unusually thick, reaching 10 to 12 µ by adult life (Figure 4.6). It is composed of fine filaments of collagen that merge with the corneal stroma (Figure 4.7). This is probably type IV collagen in large part. It is unusual in that it has a high carbohydrate content and is amorphous. Although Bowman's layer does not undergo repair if damaged, overlying endothelial cells can heal small gaps in Descemet's membrane. Descemet's membrane may undergo a variety of pathologic changes during life and in various disease states. The most common is cornea guttata due to diffuse or focal thickening.

The corneal endothelium (see Figure 4.7) is a monolayer of cells that do not proliferate during adult life in humans. This results in a progressive decline in cell density with age. Spreading of adjacent cells covers focal defects in the endothelial sheet; as a consequence, individual cells become larger, and the cell count drops.

(a)

(b)

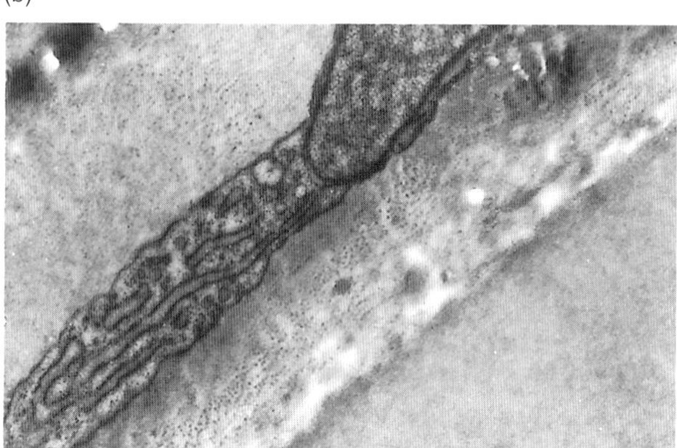

Fig. 4.6 (a) Corneal endothelium, Descemet's membrane, and the posterior corneal stroma (H&E stain; ×100). (b) Next to the stroma, Descemet's membrane is a heterogeneous layer of larger collagen filaments (×16,600).

Accidental or surgical trauma may produce a precipitous decline in the endothelial cell population. Because the endothelium is responsible for normal corneal deturgescence, a significant loss of endothelial cells may produce corneal decompensation and edema (see also Chapter 7). The intercellular space between adjacent cells is closed at the apex (facing the anterior chamber) by serial gap and tight junctions that impede the flow of some substances. Mitochondria are abundant in endothelial cells, reflecting their vigorous metabolic activity [21]. The endothelium actively transports bicarbonate and is capable of moving fluid at 6.5 mL/cm^2 per hour against normal hydrostatic pressure [22–24].

Physiology

We have already suggested the importance of GAGs in corneal transparency. It should be apparent that control of corneal hydration is crucial to maintenance of transparency. The corneal stroma ordinarily has a higher water content than connective tissue elsewhere in the body, a finding related to the water-binding capacity of GAGs.

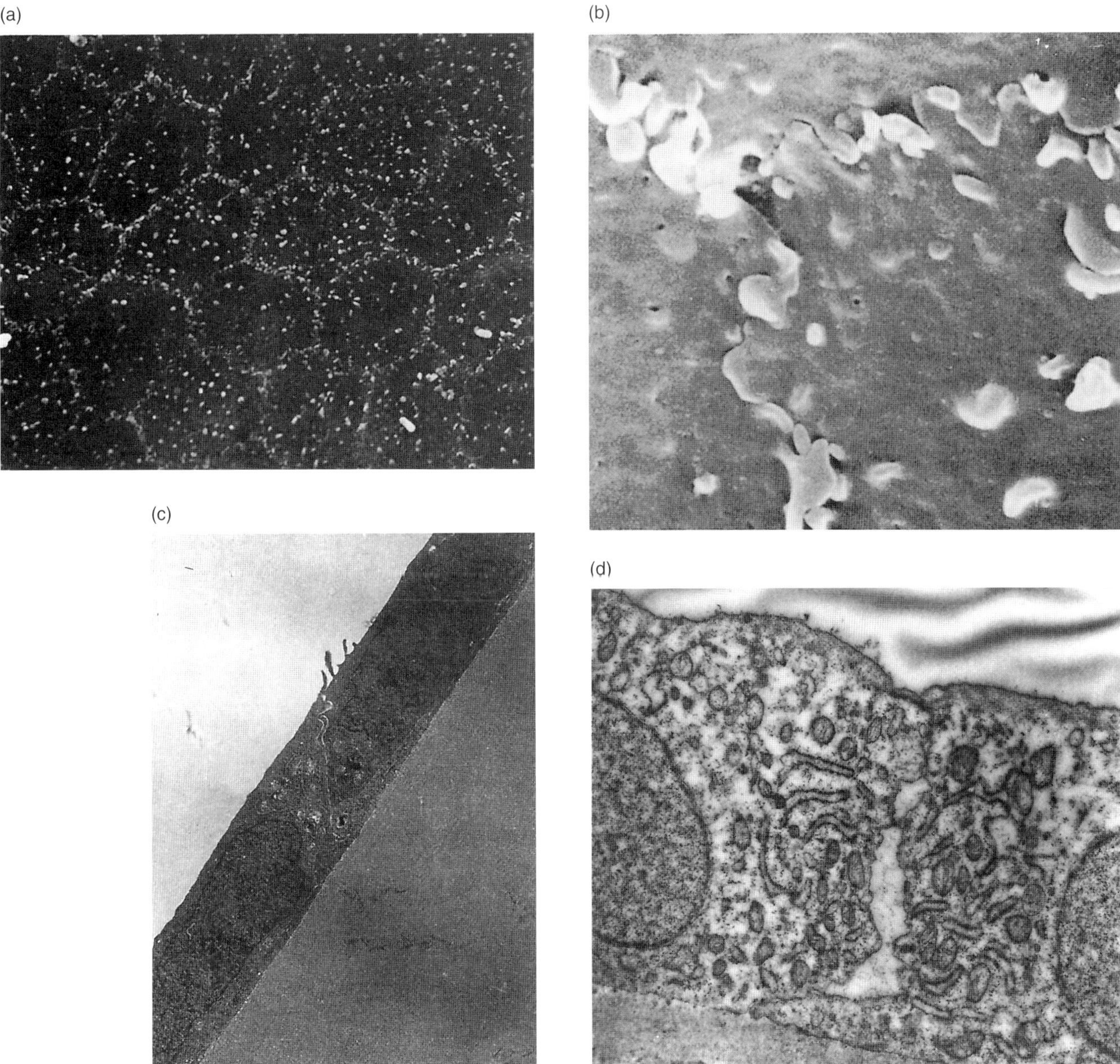

Fig. 4.7 (a) Scanning electron micrograph of corneal endothelium, showing the hexagonal pattern of the cells and their complex interdigitations (×2250). (b) Higher-power view of the endothelium (×30,000). (c) Side view of the endothelium showing how the interdigitation lies in two planes (×10,250). (d) The corneal endothelium lies on Descemet's membrane. The cells are joined on the anterior chamber side by short flap junctions (×26,100).

This affinity for water is responsible for the stromal swelling pressure (SP) (Figure 4.8 and 4.9). This pressure is considerable—amounting to 40 to 50 mm Hg at normal corneal thickness—thus variations in intra-ocular pressure (IOP) up to 50 mm Hg will have virtually no effect on corneal thickness [25,26]. However, pressure decreases as the cornea swells, so when the cornea is twice normal thickness, the SP drops by about a third (see Figure 4.9). This mechanism also works in the opposite direction: If the cornea becomes dehydrated, the tendency to swell (by imbibition) is greatly increased.

Both the epithelium and the endothelium act as barriers to the rapid influx of water into the stroma, although some leakage occurs. The corneal epithelium is 2000 times more resistant to fluid transfer than the stroma and 200 times more than the endothelium. This osmotic gradient tends to cause retention of fluid within the stroma, and an active pumping mechanism to remove it is necessary [27]. The epithelium acts as a semi-permeable membrane but is highly vulnerable to damage.

Evaporation of water from the corneal surface is a constant process. This results in hypertonicity of the tear

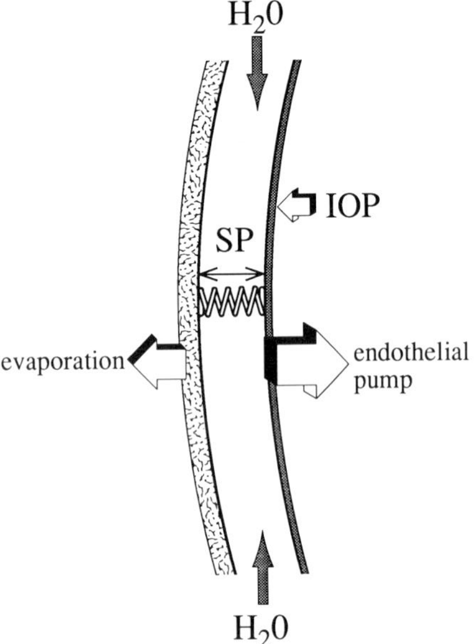

Fig. 4.8 Factors affecting hydration of the cornea. The tendency of the stroma to swell (*swelling pressure* [SP]) is balanced by the barriers imposed by the epithelium and endothelium, as well as by the endothelial pump. Evaporation plays a minor role, and intraocular pressure (IOP) has almost no effect over a wide range of pressures.

film layer, which produces an osmotic gradient causing fluid to be pulled out of the corneal stroma. In the normal cornea this results in a slight thinning during the day—increasing in the afternoon when the blink rate decreases [28]. This mechanism has an effect on epithelial edema and explains why many patients with early epithelial edema experience poor vision immediately on awakening that gradually clears during the day. Sometimes edema will persist in the upper part of the cornea hidden by the upper lid—which is not exposed to the effects of evaporation. In a cornea that undergoes progressive decompensation, edema eventually becomes so severe that evaporation cannot overcome the fluid influx.

Corneal thickness (percentage normal)

Swelling pressure (mm Hg)

Hydration (gm H_20/gm dry tissue wgt)

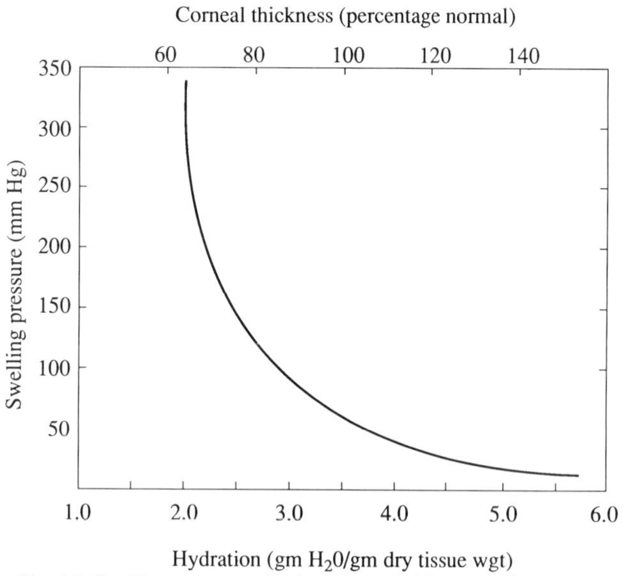

Fig. 4.9 Swelling pressure, hydration, and thickness of the cornea. As corneal thickness and hydration increase, the tendency to swell decreases (from Dohlman CH. Physiology of the cornea; corneal edema. In: *The Cornea: Scientific Foundations and Clinical Practice*, G Smolin and RA Thoft (eds). Little, Brown, Boston, 1983).

It is remarkable how thick the cornea can become from edema before there is a noticeable effect on vision. For example, in bovine cornea, a transparency equivalent of 20/30 was maintained with as much as a 60% increase in thickness [29]. Temporary corneal swelling is a nearly universal finding after radial keratotomy. Simple incisions through Bowman's layer that extend deep into the stroma are always accompanied by an increase in corneal thickness without noticeable changes in corneal clarity. This swelling occurs immediately and is likely responsible for incision depth irregularity that was seen in early cases (see also Chapter 8). Swelling may be persistent. The author has recorded significant increases in corneal thickness (20 to 30 μm) lasting in excess of 22 months; this also has been reported elsewhere [30]. In a cornea with a pre-operative central thickness of 500 μm, such an increase would amount to 6% of the total. This is a significant amount and must be considered when doing repeat incisional refractive surgery (see also Chapter 8).

Epithelial edema may affect vision sooner and to a greater extent even when swelling can only be seen at the slit lamp. This occurs because of light scattering within and between cells and as a result of increased microscopic irregularity of the corneal surface.

The tear film

The tear film is often referred to as the sixth corneal layer, because the cornea functions poorly without it and because it is more than a mere aqueous layer (Figure 4.10). Classically, the tear film was described as a three-layered structure composed of lipid, aqueous, and mucous layers from top to bottom. It is better thought of as a two-layer structure—a thin lipid layer (0.1 mm) overlying a thick aqueous lake—because the mucous layer is intimately attached to the epithelial cells [31,32]. The tear film including the mucous layer is about 7 μm in thickness.

The lipid layer is secreted by the Meibomian glands and is compressed on a blink, after which it rapidly spreads over the corneal surface after the lids open. The lipid layer covers the aqueous tear layer and retards its evaporation and prevents overflow of tears. As the lipid spreads over the aqueous layer, it drags liquid with it, thickening the tear film—the Marangoni effect (Figure 4.11). This of course presupposes a relatively smooth corneal surface—something that may not be present immediately following corneal refractive surgery.

Table 4.1 summarizes information on the content of the aqueous layer [32]. At one time it was thought that

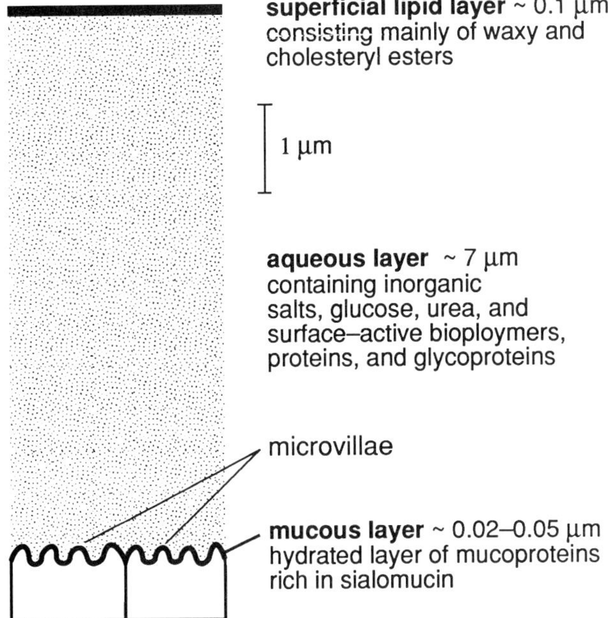

Fig. 4.10 The three layers of the tear film (from Holly FJ, Lemp MA. Tear physiology and dry eyes. Surv Ophthalmol 1977; 22(2):69–87).

Table 4.1 Composition of tears. From Lamberts DW. Physiology of the cornea: physiology of the tear film. In: *The Cornea. Scientific Foundations and Clinical Practice,* G Smolin and RA Thoft (eds). Little, Brown, Boston, 1983

Component	Concentration
Water	98.2%
Sodium	145 mmol/l
Potassium	20 mmol/l
Chloride	128 mmol/l
Bicarbonate	26 mmol/l
Calcium	2.11 mg/dl
Magnesium	Trace
Zinc	Trace
Glucose	3 mg/100 ml
Amino acids	8 mg/100 ml
Urea	7–20 mg urea N/100 ml
Oxygen	155 mm Hg (eyes open)
Total protein	0.9 ± 0.1%
Lysozyme	1.3 ± 0.6 mg/ml
Complement	Present
Mucus secretory substance	Present
Lysosomal hydrolases	Present
Lysosomal enzymes	Present
Lactate and pyruvate	Present

the cornea obtained nutrients from the tear layer, but this is not true [33]. However, the corneal oxygen supply is derived from the tear layer. Another important tear film component is lysozyme, which is produced and secreted by the lacrimal gland [34]. Lysozyme destroys bacterial cell wall integrity and likely aids in maintaining a sterile corneal surface. The entire immunoglobulin-complement pathway is also present within the tears, as well as specific antibodies against such things as *Chlamydia trachomatis* and herpes simplex and influenza viruses [32].

The hydrophilic mucous layer makes the hydrophobic epithelial cells wettable both by coating their surfaces and by resisting lipid contamination. This layer is secreted by the goblet cells of the conjunctiva and helps stabilize the tear film. The tear film mucus functions as a surfactant, lowering its surface tension and promoting wetting of the corneal surface.

An understanding of tear film dynamics is important (see Figure 4.11). During blinking, upper lid motion and pressure wipes the cornea and resurfaces it with mucus. At rest, the mucous layer is separated from the lipid layer

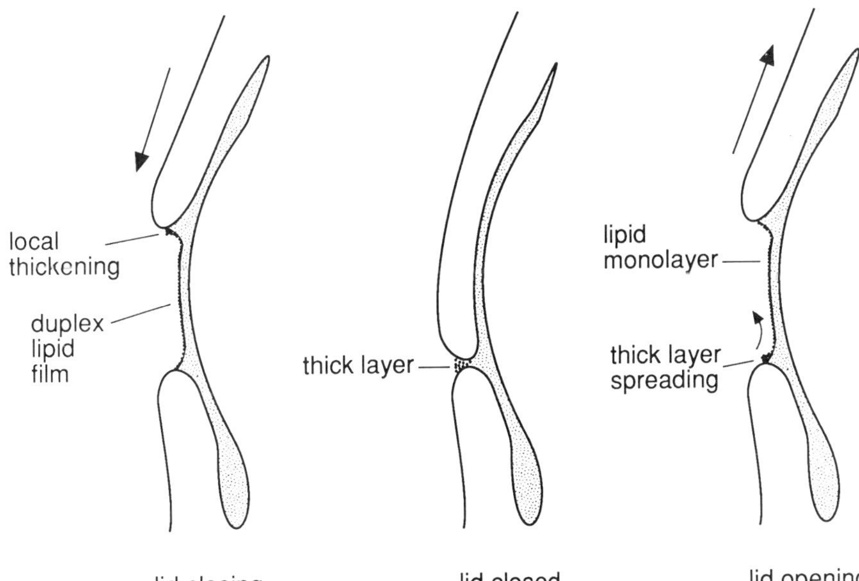

Fig. 4.11 The dynamics of the tear film during a blink.

by the aqueous phase of the tear film. After a blink, however, the lipid becomes somewhat admixed with the aqueous layer, eventually reaching the mucus. The lipid binds to the mucus, and eventually, lipid contamination causes the mucus to become hydrophobic. The tear film may then rupture, forming dry spots on the cornea (Figure 4.12). Sufficient mucus must be present to resist lipid contamination until the next blink occurs—which is what happens in a normal eye—blinking occurs before a dry spot appears [35].

Rose Bengal dye is a vital stain that marks not only injured epithelium but also lipid-contaminated mucus and corneal filaments. The more commonly used fluorescein dye only marks epithelial defects, so more frequent use of Rose Bengal testing may provide additional information regarding the health of the tear film and ocular surface. Recently, a phenol red-impregnated cotton thread placed into the inferior cul-de-sac has been employed to differentiate between normal, aqueous-deficient, and non–aqueous-deficient dry eyes [36].

Another useful tool in assessing corneal surface status is the tear breakup time (BUT), a measure of the stability of the tear film and, indirectly, the health of the goblet cells and the lacrimal apparatus (although there can be many causes for a shortened BUT). The test is conducted by placing a drop or two of fluorescein dye on the eye and having the patient blink several times. Without touching the lids, the time in seconds from the blink to the appearance of a dark spot on the surface (where there is no wetting) is measured. This event should be recorded several times and averaged. The dark spots should appear in random areas for the test to be accurate. While the test itself has been subject to criticism, it is easily done and provides useful information on the state of the tear film. It is recommended as part of the preoperative workup for corneal refractive surgery patients. A subnormal BUT, while not contraindicating surgery, may serve as a harbinger of possible problems in the post-operative period. Sufficient irregularity may exist in the corneal surface following refractive surgery to make a marginal case of inadequate tearing the pre-operative acquire the propositions of a major post-operative problem.

Corneal wound healing

It is useful to compare corneal wound healing with similar events in other tissues. Wound healing throughout the body is the end result of a sequence of events, controlled and modulated by many factors. When a wound occurs elsewhere in the body, there is bleeding, the clotting cascade is activated, and bleeding ceases. Necrosis and apoptosis eliminate injured cells. Concurrently, proteolysis may alter the extracellular matrix (ECM), local cells are activated and proliferate, and there is an acute inflammatory response. Phagocytosis of devitalized tissue is followed by fibroblastic and vascular proliferation. When collagen synthesis is complete, there is contraction and remodeling of the scar, which concludes the process.

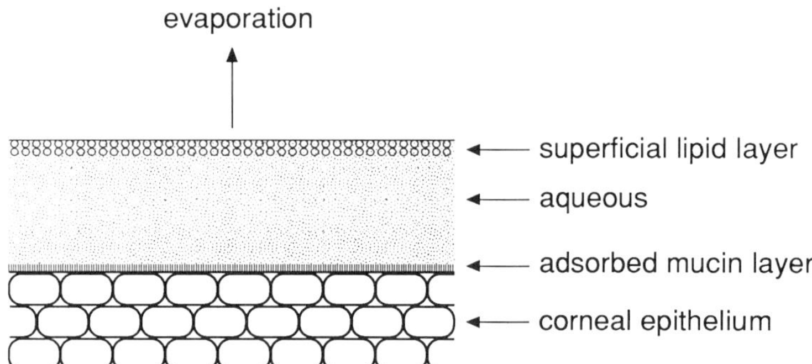

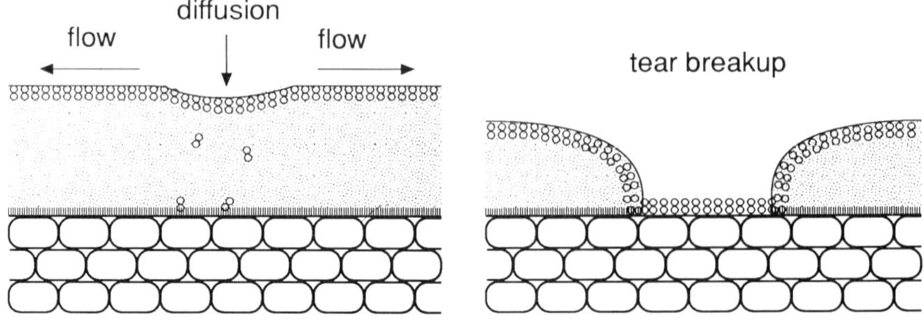

Fig. 4.12 The mechanism of tear breakup. Lipid contaminates the mucin layer from the mixing that occurs during the blink. Eventually, the hydrophilic mucin layer becomes hydrophobic.

It is pertinent to note that while much attention has been paid to the processes that initiate healing, relatively little is known about how it ceases. In the cornea, for example, vessels will grow in response to a stimulus but stop growing when the stimulus is removed. The control mechanism for this phenomenon is unknown. Elements of the clotting cascade, growth factors, cytokines, and angiogenic factors are all likely important in control of corneal wound healing and vascularization.

Compared with cutaneous healing, corneal wound repair is more complicated. The cornea is more differentiated than the dermis. Bowman's and Descemet's membranes and their healing patterns are unique. The vital role played by the corneal endothelium has no exact parallel elsewhere in the body. The absence of a vascular system in the normal cornea leaves the immune system out of the healing loop in many instances, which results in a slower rate of healing.

It would be easy to conclude that the hemostatic system plays no role in corneal wound healing. However, plasminogen activator has been detected in clear cornea [37,38], and free fibrin is found in the tissues during the critical period of endothelial mitosis, when corneal vascularization is often induced [39]. Indeed, fibrin appears at the earliest stages of neovascularization and then disappears when new vessel growth is complete. This suggests a relationship of this clotting product to the process of new vessel formation, a hypothesis that deserves additional study.

Formation and contraction of scar tissue usually signals a successful conclusion to wound healing elsewhere but may be a functional disaster in the cornea, leading to loss of vision, irregular astigmatism, or corneal ectasia. Control of scar tissue formation and vascularization is essential for proper healing of corneal wounds. The purpose of this section is to review the pathophysiology of corneal wound healing and to provide a basis for the following section, which deals with histology and wound healing in refractive surgery.

Epithelial healing

When an epithelial wound is made without damage to other corneal structures, the healing process is relatively simple. Two steps are involved: migration of existing cells and proliferation of those cells to restore the normal thickness of the epithelial sheet. Soon after occurrence of an epithelial defect, the basal epithelial cells at the wound margin become flatter and close the defect by lateral movement [40,41] (Figure 4.13), which is mediated by intercellular actin filament formation and contraction. The process is inhibited by exposure to cytochalasin B, which blocks assembly of actin filaments within the cytoplasm of epithelial cells. In contrast, colchicine, which inhibits microtubule formation, has no effect on epithelial migration [42].

(a)

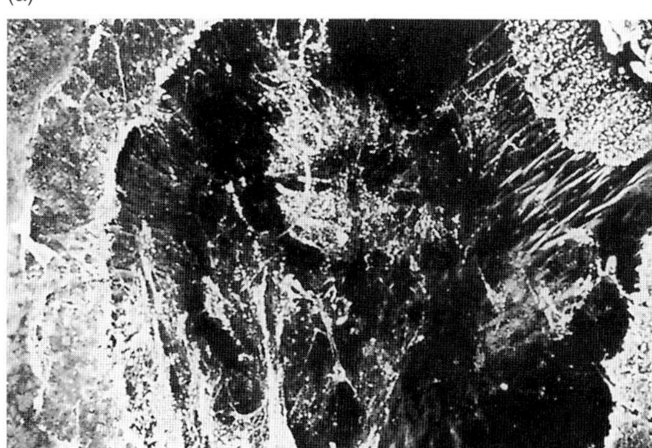

(b)

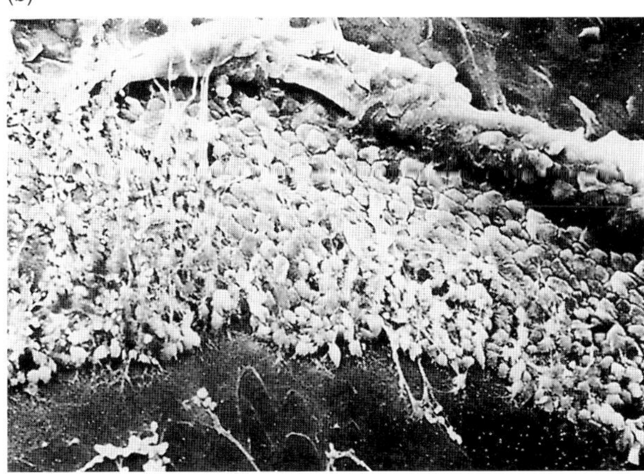

Fig. 4.13 (a) Scanning electron micrograph of healing corneal abrasion (×1000). (b) Epithelium sliding to cover bare stroma (×4000).

A second essential component for epithelial migration is fibronectin. Both in tissue culture and in living animals, fibronectin is important in epithelial resurfacing. Cell surface receptors for fibronectin are present in the cornea. These receptors help the corneal epithelial cells bind to fibronectin by way of the intercellular actin filaments. Contraction of the actin filaments helps the cell move across the epithelial defect. When corneal healing is complete, fibronectin disappears [43].

The next steps in healing an epithelial defect are epithelial cell mitosis and proliferation, which serve to return the epithelium to its original thickness [44]. There is increasing evidence that these changes are mediated by growth factors. In 1953, Levi-Montalcini discovered nerve growth factor (NGF) and demonstrated its ability to stimulate nerve cells to growth [45]. In 1962, Cohen isolated epidermal growth factor (EGF—the name is derived from the stimulatory effect this agent has on epithelial growth and differentiation) from the submaxillary glands of mice [46]. Subsequently, a host of other growth factors have been isolated and characterized. Many of these factors may exert an influence on corneal wound healing.

EGF is a strong mitogen for corneal epithelium in the presence of stroma but does not have this effect on isolated epithelial cells in tissue culture. This is a good example of the interaction of different corneal tissues, discussed later in this chapter. The effect is so strong that in some experimental situations the epithelium becomes hyperplastic and thicker than normal [47,48]. In contrast, the use of EGF in clinical situations has been disappointing. It is hypothesized that this may be due to saturation of the system. In other words, all receptor sites are occupied by naturally occurring EGF, and the system is being driven at maximum speed [49]. Fibroblast growth factor (FGF) is also a mitogen for corneal epithelium. Its effect varies with the dosage, unlike EGF. Its role in normal healing remains to be defined [50]. It is highly likely that other growth factors modulate wound healing. It would be helpful if a growth factor succeeded in stabilizing the corneal curvature fluctuations that occur following radial keratotomy. If, instead, progression of the scarring mechanism was stimulated, there could be negative effects. For example, some radial keratotomy (RK) patients demonstrate spontaneous and progressive corneal flattening. Additionally, some of the effect of RK develops over time—thus timing of the application of growth factors could be critical.

The basal cells of the corneal epithelium are attached to their basement membrane and Bowman's layer by filamentous hemidesmosomes. These attachment bodies are absent in epithelium migrating over a debrided surface and during the proliferative phase of healing. When healing is complete, they re-form, at which point the corneal epithelium returns to a resting state and becomes securely attached. Failure of hemidesmosome formation is the proximate cause of recurrent epithelial erosion syndrome.

Since damage inflicted on the corneal epithelium usually is accompanied by damage to the epithelial basal lamina (basement membrane), it is not surprising that reconstitution of the basal lamina is important in healing of the epithelium. Although very thin, the basal lamina is a complex structure that includes laminin, heparan sulfate, proteoglycan, type IV collagen, and entactin (reviewed in [51]). Members of the transforming growth factor (TGF) family of cytokines are important in basal lamina healing. TGF-α is structurally similar to EGF, binds to the EGF receptor, and performs several EGF functions [51]. TGF-β regulates cell proliferation and differentiation and promotes deposition of ECM [51]. It would appear that TGF-α and TGF-β act in opposition and at different stages of the epithelial wound-healing process. For example, TGF-α inhibits adhesion complex formation, enhancing lateral cell migration early in wound healing. In contrast, TGF-β promotes adhesion complex formation and epithelial-ECM adhesion [51]. The rapidly growing knowledge base of the molecular mechanisms involved in development, growth, differentiation, and wound healing suggests that what was described above is merely the tip of the iceberg! It is known that numerous protein gene products that interact control these processes and are up- and down-regulated as tissue demands change.

The situation is more complex if a wound extends into Bowman's layer or the stroma. With a small wound in Bowman's, the defect is filled by epithelium to form an epithelial facet (Figures 4.14 to 4.16). Bowman's layer does not regenerate. If damage to Bowman's layer and the basement membrane of the epithelium is severe, epithelial healing is often slowed. The absence of basement membrane may interfere with formation of hemidesmosomes by the basal cells. Failure of attachment of the basal cells can lead to repeated epithelial breakdown—a finding characteristic of a number of corneal problems, such as recurrent erosion, Cogan's microcystic dystrophy, and other anterior membrane dystrophies [52,53]. Destruction of Bowman's layer in laser ablative techniques suggests a potential risk of recurrent corneal erosions.

In deep stromal wounds, the healing process demonstrates interaction between the epithelium and stroma. When there is a superficial epithelial injury, as would

(a)

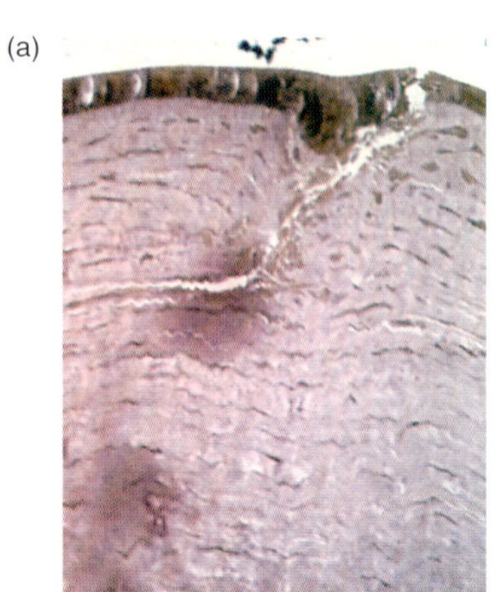

(b)

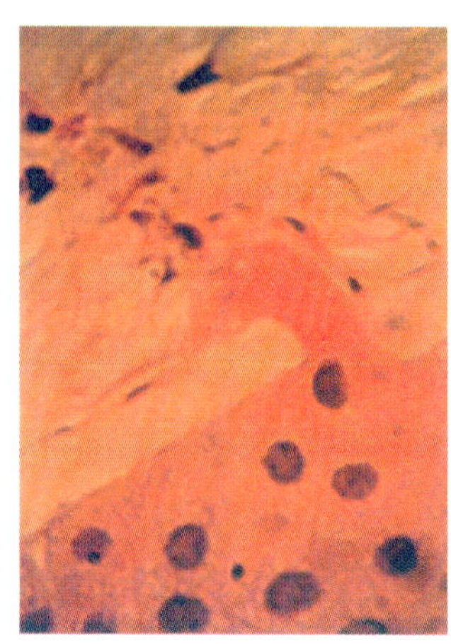

Fig. 4.14 (a) Epithelial facet formation following experimental stromal incision (paraphenylene-diamine stain; ×80). (b) Break in Bowman's layer (H&E stain; ×80).

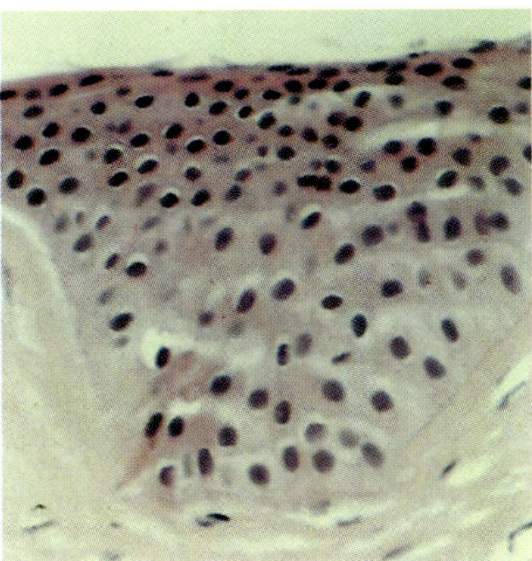

Fig. 4.15 Epithelial plug filling wound after radial keratotomy (H&E stain; ×80).

occur with excimer laser keratectomy, there is rapid disappearance of keratocytes in the superficial corneal stoma [54]. In controlled experimental situations, the keratocytes disappear, absent any acute inflammatory response. The lack of inflammation in this process suggests that it takes place by apoptosis (programmed cell death) [55–57]. Recent work has established that keratocyte loss associated with epithelial injury is indeed due to apoptosis [58,59] and that keratocyte apoptosis may play a role in wound healing after PRK or LASIK [58,60,61]. Inflammatory cells from the tear film are attracted to the injured tissue and carry with them a variety of cytokines, proteases, and growth factors that make the healing process highly complex.

The tendency of epithelium to cover a bare surface leads to migration of epithelial cells into the stromal wound. Epithelial proliferation fills the gap and forms an epithelial plug (see Figures 4.14 and 4.15). This chain of events is typical of an early RK wound. In the normal course of events, stromal healing occurs. Formation of new collagen and scar tissue "pushes" the epithelial plug out with a return to more normal appearance (see Figure 4.16). With broad, irregular stromal wounds, this may be a prolonged process. Persistence of the epithelial plug for a year or more has been documented in RK patients. A wound bridged by epithelium is obviously not as strong as one closed by collagen. Fibroblast [50] and mesodermal growth factors can accelerate stromal healing, although their potential therapeutic value has yet to be realized [62].

It is important to consider both physical and biochemical factors that affect wound healing. Without doubt, the most important physical factor in epithelial healing is the quality and integrity of the tear film. The corneal epithelium provides the major barrier to infection. When there is a tear deficiency, the ability of the epithelium to cover a defect is compromised and the possibility of invasion by micro-organisms is enhanced [63]. Tear deficiency can lead to chronic epithelial defects that may be associated with stromal inflammation and scarring [2]. Chronic epithelial defects are often associated with production of collagenase, which can produce stromal melting and necrosis [64]. This melting process, which can be rapid or slow, eventually may lead to corneal perforation. A failure of proper epithelialization is a known risk factor for stromal melting in epikeratophakia (Figure 4.17).

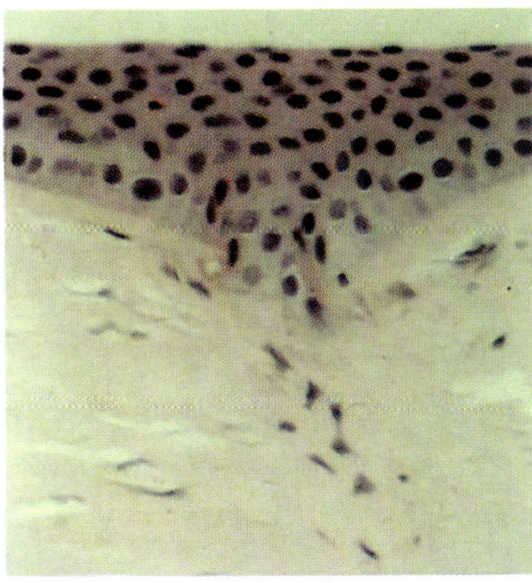

Fig. 4.16 Regressing epithelium and stromal scar following radial keratotomy (H&E stain; ×80).

Abnormal corneal wound healing

In the context of refractive surgery, it is important to review abnormalities of corneal wound healing because they may play a significant role in postoperative problems. The importance of an intact tear film and epithelial surface has been noted from the point of view of resistance to infection. Of even greater importance in refractive surgery, the epithelial sheet must be smooth and regular for best-quality vision [6].

Pharmaceutical agents

Many commonly used ophthalmic pharmaceutical agents interfere with epithelial healing. These include topical anesthetics, antivirals, corticosteroids, and aminoglycoside antibiotics [65]. Excessive use of any of these drugs can cause superficial punctate keratitis (Figures 4.18 and 4.19). Breakdown of the epithelial barrier increases the risk of secondary infection with bacteria or fungi. While this most often occurs as a consequence of non-surgical treatment, it also may occur in refractive surgery patients. There is particular risk with lamellar procedures, since the tear film is disturbed at the same time that drug therapy is intense (see "The tear film," above). Superficial punctate keratitis, always present initially, may progress to persistent epithelial defects that could lead to eventual corneal melting.

(a)

(b)

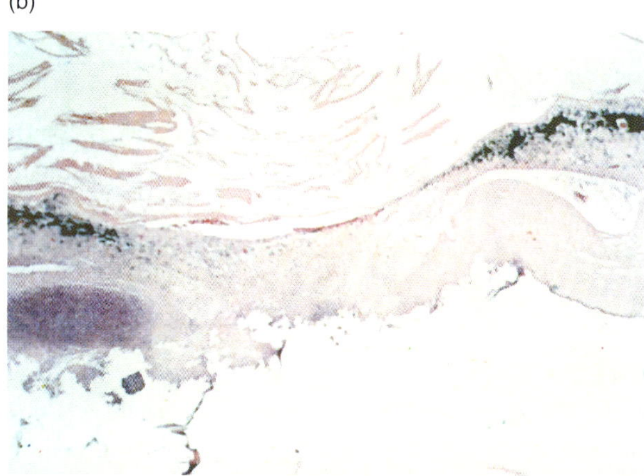

Fig. 4.17 (a) Corneal melting at graft margin with descemetocoele formation. (b) Marked stromal loss from corneal melting (H&E stain; ×10).

Anterior membrane dystrophies

Abnormal epithelial healing is a hallmark of the anterior membrane dystrophies. These include microcystic dystrophy, Meeseman's dystrophy, macular dystrophy, and lattice dystrophy [52]. All these conditions are characterized by abnormalities of the epithelial basement membrane, and all may be associated with a recurrent erosion syndrome. The mechanism is the same as that following a traumatic corneal abrasion in that the hemidesmosomes of the basal epithelium do not form properly and fail to attach the epithelium to the basement membrane. The presence of any of these conditions may be a contraindication to refractive surgery.

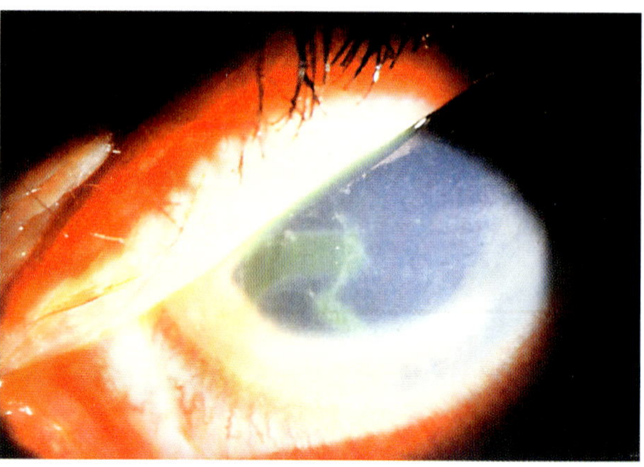

Fig. 4.18 Persistent epithelial defect in an anesthetic abuser.

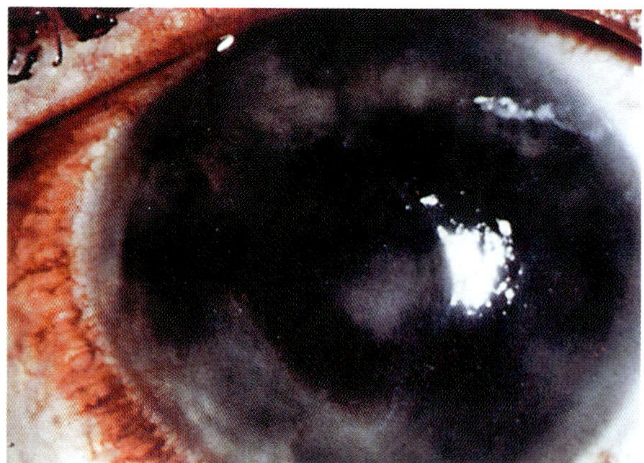

Fig. 4.19 Indolent ulcer in a patient with chronic stromal herpes keratitis.

Epithelial downgrowth

Another example of abnormal epithelial wound healing is epithelial downgrowth (Figures 4.20 to 4.22). This problem has been reported after penetrating keratoplasty and cataract and glaucoma filtration surgery, as well as after trauma [66]. While the risk of this complication is low in refractive surgery, an inadvertent perforation during refractive surgery, especially RK or epikeratophakia, could provide an avenue for classic epithelial downgrowth.

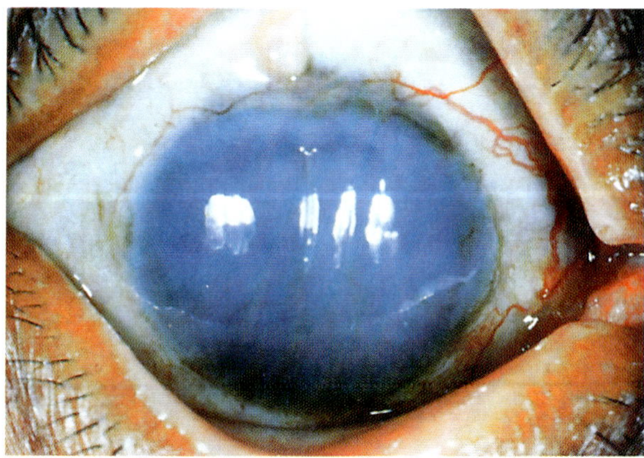

Fig. 4.20 Epithelial downgrowth following cataract surgery. A small filtering bleb above indicates the point of entry. Note the scalloped white border inferiorly, marking the advancing epithelium. The overlying cornea shows marked edema.

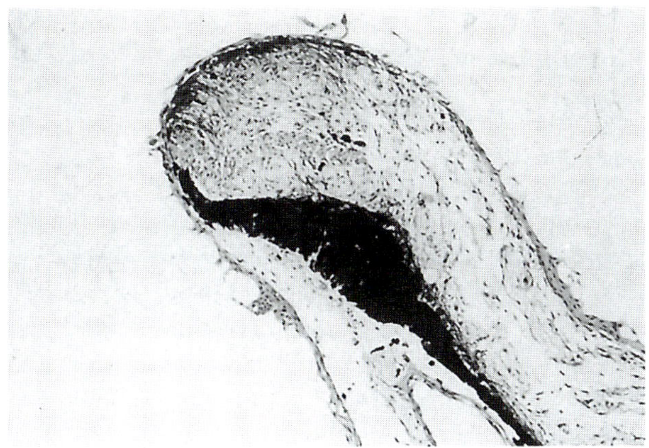

Fig. 4.21 Epithelium growing on the anterior iris surface has produced a prominent ectopion uveae (H&E stain; ×60).

Although unlikely to occur in refractive surgery, epithelial downgrowth is a major clinical disaster. Any wound that remains open for a period of time provides a pathway for epithelium to grow through the wound and into the eye [67]. The epithelium continues to grow and eventually may totally cover the endothelial surface of the cornea as well as the iris and other intraocular structures. This leads to endothelial death and corneal decompensation and often produces an intractable glaucoma [68]. If caught at an early stage, a 50% cure rate has been reported. The treatment is drastic, requiring double freezing of the involved cornea, excision of all affected intraocular tissue, and extensive vitrectomy. Patients with more advanced cases may lose all useful vision. It is appropriate to emphasize that while the corneal epithelium is only fulfilling its role of covering bare surfaces, the results may be destructive.

Ingrowth of epithelium beneath donor lenticules has been reported in epikeratophakia (Figure 4.23) and could well occur with intrastromal alloplastic implants or with any keratomileusis-based procedure. In both instances, the mechanism is similar. The natural tendency of epithelium to cover a bare surface—which works to our advantage in corneal abrasions—can cause serious problems in refractive surgery. Ingrowth of epithelium beneath a homologous or heterologous lenticule may lead to opacification of the lenticule-recipient interface [69]. In the case of epikeratoplasty, such ingrowth might result in unsatisfactory wound healing at the interface with loss of the lenticule.

The interaction of the corneal epithelium with the rest of the cornea is well illustrated by indolent ulcers. In patients with herpes simplex or other chronic stromal inflammation, portions of the epithelium may slough off and resist efforts at healing for many weeks (see Figure 4.19). Chronic inflammation, combined with damage to Bowman's layer and the epithelial basement membrane, prevents re-formation of the epithelial sheet [70]. Tear film abnormalities potentiate this problem.

Inflammation can stimulate growth of fibrovascular tissue from the limbus (Figures 4.24 and 4.25) in patients with repeated epithelial disruption, as seen in bullous keratopathy. This degenerative pannus contributes to loss of vision [71]. The potential for a similar occurrence is present with refractive surgery in the presence of chronic and recurrent epithelial defects.

Stromal healing

Although epithelial wound healing appears much faster than stromal healing, laboratory research has demonstrated that there are dual effects on keratocytes within a few hours of stromal wounding. The most superficial keratocytes undergo apoptosis and disappear within 24 to 48 hours after significant epithelial injury [58–60,72]. More deeply placed keratocytes develop phagocytic activity and proliferation of cytoplasmic organelles. DNA synthesis and mitotic activity occurs within 24 hours. In addition, macrophages enter the stromal wound from the tear

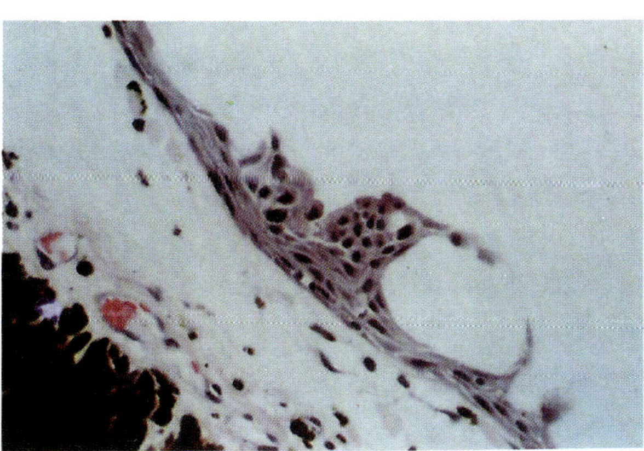

Fig. 4.22 High-power view of Fig. 4.21 showing a part of the epithelial sheet from the iris surface (H&E stain; ×100).

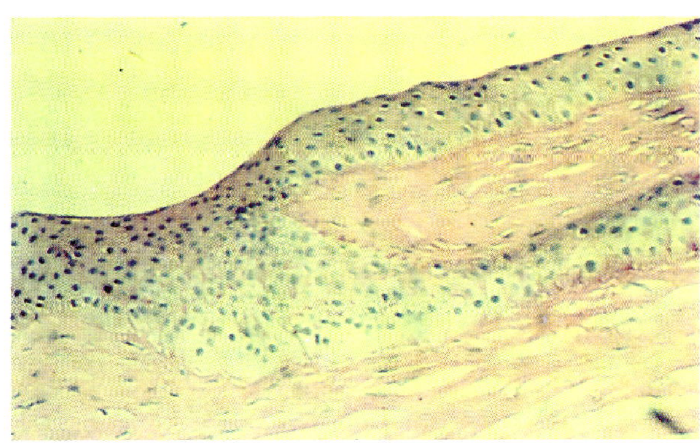

Fig. 4.23 Epithelium infiltrated beneath an epikeratophakia lenticule (H&E stain; ×100).

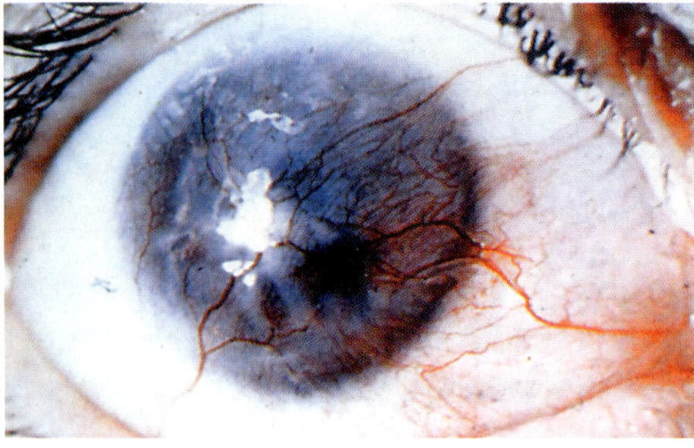

Fig. 4.24 Corneal vascularization in a patient with chronic aphakic bullous keratopathy.

film and undergo fibroblastic transformation [73]. Initially, there is a breakdown of damaged collagen. Within a few days, the wound shows uptake of radio-labeled hydroxylysine, hydroxyproline, and sulfur that is followed by formation of new collagen and glycosaminoglycans [74]. Over a period of several weeks, collagen synthesis occurs, and amino acid uptake ceases.

In excimer laser keratectomy, the epithelium must grow and heal over bare corneal stroma in the absence of Bowman's layer. This is exactly the situation in which recurrent erosions and indolent ulcers occur. Early studies of excimer keratectomy suggested that this was not a problem [75]. However, injury to Bowman's layer and epithelial healing problems may relate to the problem of prolonged corneal haze observed after laser keratectomy [6].

In a dermal wound, the final change in the sequence of wound healing is contraction of the scar tissue. Fibroblasts develop actin filaments and are transformed into myofibroblasts. It is the contraction of these cells that are associated with collagen bundles that produces shrinkage of the wound [76]. The role of this process in the cornea is less clear. Nevertheless, the opacity of corneal scars is clear evidence that the orderly array of stromal collagen has been lost (see Figures 4.19 and 4.20).

Scarring with proliferation is more likely to occur with penetrating wounds. Retrocorneal membranes after keratoplasty and stromal ingrowth after cataract surgery are examples of proliferative scarring. Similar problems potentially may occur with perforations during refractive surgery (Figures 4.26 to 4.29). When a retrocorneal membrane covers Descemet's membrane, the endothelium is destroyed. The loss of this fluid barrier causes corneal edema and further visual loss.

There are several mechanisms to explain the visual loss. Irregular astigmatism may develop as the result of severe surface irregularity. There also may be light scattering due to scar tissue, since corneal transparency depends on uniform collagen fiber diameter and spacing. This spacing should be less than half the wavelength of light, or about 200 nm. Unfortunately, the response to wounding produces collagen fibers that vary in diameter considerably—from 20 to 120 nm. Because the response is chaotic, the new collagen fibers never become organized in the normal lamellar arrangement. Some of the spacing differential is due to edema that follows wounding. Additionally, the collagen fibers themselves differ in GAG content from normal and hence have different indices of refraction.

Corneal vascularization

Because of the primary involvement of the stroma, it is appropriate to consider corneal vascularization in a discussion of stromal healing. This process has fascinated researchers for many years. Cogan was the first to suggest that corneal vascularization was related to a loss of stromal compactness. He demonstrated that stromal swelling always preceded the ingrowth of new vessels [77]. That this is not the sole factor in vascularization is shown

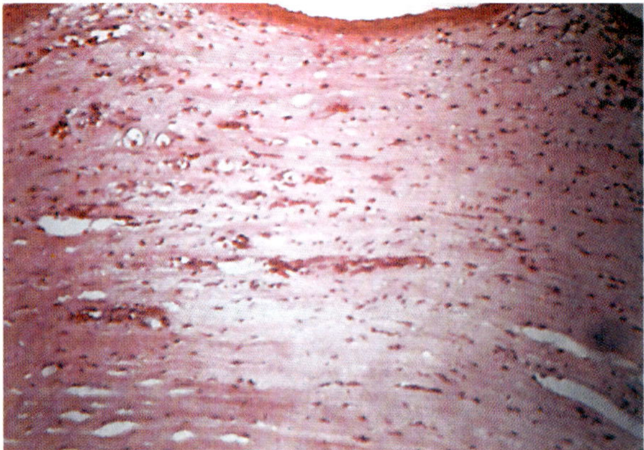

Fig. 4.25 Anterior and midstromal corneal vascularization in a corneal button from a patient with bullous keratopathy (H&E stain; ×80).

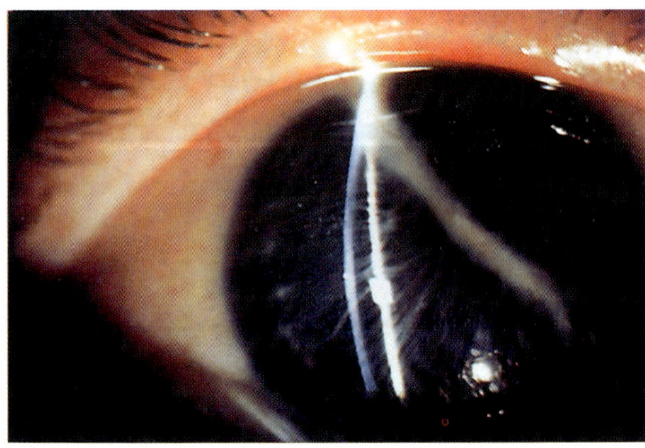

Fig. 4.26 Corneal scar following accidental penetrating wound.

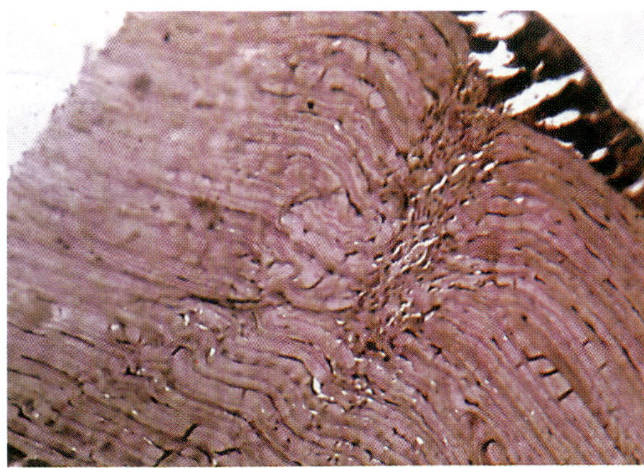

Fig. 4.27 Irregular stromal scar following a penetrating corneal wound (paraphenylene-diamine stain; ×60).

Fig. 4.29 Sub-endothelial fibrous proliferation following a microperforation.

by the avascularity of many eyes with severe stromal edema in bullous keratopathy.

An alternate hypothesis suggests that vascularization is due to loss of an inhibitor of vascularization or to the release of an angiogenic substance [78,79]. The latter theory was supported by studies of tumor angiogenesis factor. Tumor cells injected into the anterior chamber proliferate to form a cell clump about 1 mm in diameter. Growth ceases unless the cell mass settles on the iris and establishes a blood supply. Tumor growth accelerates when this happens. Tumor extract or a fragment of tumor tissue implanted in the cornea is associated with ingrowth of vessels from the limbus. Tumor angiogenic factor acts as a growth factor [80] and has been isolated and characterized [81,82].

In recent years, there has been considerable interest in the subject of ocular neovascularization because of its potentially serious effects on vision [83]. Despite the apparent lack of a role for tumor angiogenic factor in normal corneas, a host of other angiogenic proteins likely take part in corneal wound healing. In particular, vascular endothelial growth factor (VEGF) appears to play a prominent role in corneal, retinal, and choroidal neovascularization [83–85]. In addition to VEGF, a considerable number of other growth factors have been linked to corneal neovascularization, including basic fibroblast growth factor (bFGF) [86], thrombospondin [86,87], members of the interleukin family [59,87,88], tumor necrosis factor α (TNF-α) [89], eicosanoids [90], pigment epithelium-derived growth factor [91], CXC chemokines [92], and prolactin [93]. In addition, some angiogenic pathways interact with other proteins, such as p53 [94–96]. It is highly likely that the information in this paragraph is only a small part of the extremely complex processes involved in development of neovascularization in corneal wound healing.

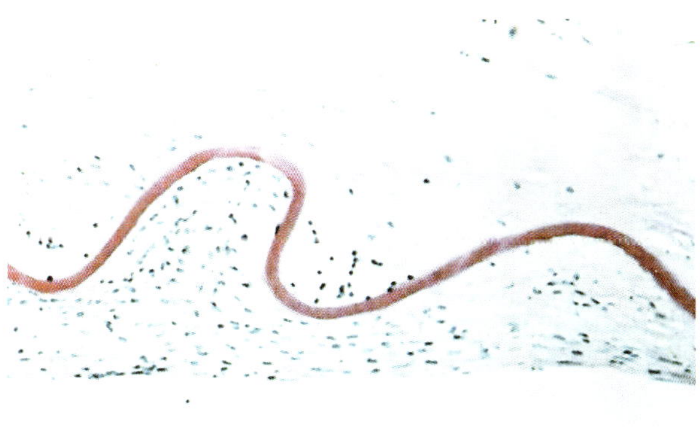

Fig. 4.28 Retrocorneal membrane after failed keratoplasty. Note the fixed folds in Descemet's membrane (PAS stain; ×60).

Descemet's membrane and the endothelial cell layer

Changes in Descemet's membrane and the corneal endothelium may occur with refractive surgery, but the need for primary healing of these structures is present only when there is a full-thickness corneal wound. The endothelium is able to regenerate short stretches of Descemet's membrane, although there are limits to this ability (Figure 4.30). Endothelial mitosis does not occur to an appreciable degree in human eyes [97]. Defects in the endothelial layer are covered by the spreading of adjacent cells, which results in lower endothelial cell counts. Both migration and spreading are mediated by changes in intracellular actin filament organization [98].

Accidental perforation of the cornea in refractive surgery, as may occur during RK, causes focal injury to Descemet's membrane and the endothelium that is often not functionally significant. The endothelial cell loss that occurs following RK is acute, nonprogressive, and limited to between 5% and 7% [99,100]. On the other hand, it

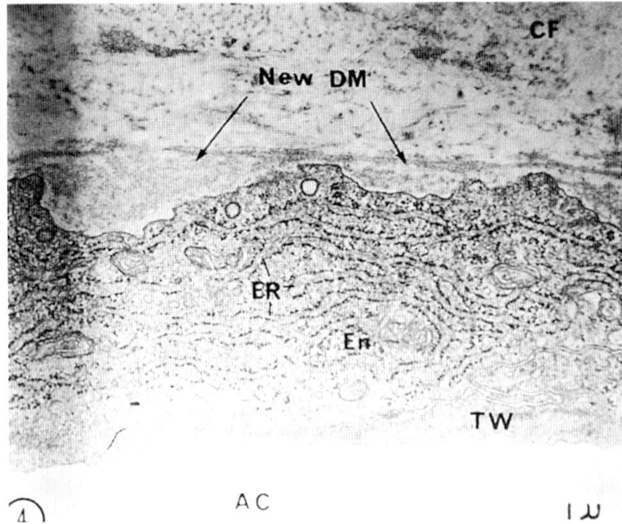

Fig. 4.30 Healed Descemet's membrane following injury (×22,500).

is possible that an unhealthy endothelium may respond with greater cell loss after refractive surgery.

Corneal wound healing and its sequelae are complex processes that may result in uneventful recovery of visual function or which may produce permanent visual loss. While much remains to be learned about the events that occur in this process, it is important for the refractive surgeon to understand the known mechanisms and use them to achieve a successful surgical result. The next section will deal with specific problems of healing related to refractive surgery.

Healing of the cornea in refractive surgery

The preceding section emphasized the interaction of the various layers of the cornea during the healing process. In all refractive surgery, a successful result depends on proper healing of the corneal surface and control of stromal scarring. Defects in either process may produce serious complications such as infection or stromal melting.

The intact corneal epithelium, and more specifically, the overlying tear film, provides the primary refractive interface of the cornea and is also the major barrier to invasion by micro-organisms. Most refractive surgical procedures discussed in this chapter cause an initial loss of some or all of the surface epithelium. The epithelium that remains must slide over the bare corneal surface, attach to the basement membrane, and undergo proliferation to return to normal. Basement membrane damage retards effective healing, since hemidesmosomes may fail to re-form. Faulty hemidesmosome formation is associated with recurrent erosion and persistent epithelial defects. The repercussions of a failure of epithelial resurfacing also may include infection [101], increased stromal scarring [102,103], and corneal melting.

The transparency of the cornea depends on the highly regular arrangement of the collagen fibers that form the stromal lamellae. An opaque scar may lead to a visual failure of the refractive surgery. In some procedures, such as RK, the scarring plays a role in production of the optical effect of the procedure. However, scarring in the visual axis leads inevitably to a variable and permanent loss in visual acuity.

Aberrant healing of the epithelium may contribute in a negative way with secondary inadequate stromal healing or enhanced stromal scarring. With incisional refractive surgery, epithelium may invade the incision and persist for long periods. Because the epithelium has little tensile strength, these areas of the cornea are weakened. Epithelial cysts may form beneath the stroma in lamellar procedures and cause interface opacity. Finally, if there is accidental corneal perforation during surgery, epithelium may migrate through the perforation and produce epithelial downgrowth. The serious consequences to the eye caused by this downgrowth were outlined in the preceding section (see "Epithelial downgrowth").

Failure of the epithelium to reestablish its integrity can be associated with corneal melting. It is well established that persistent epithelial defects may encourage collagenase production from invading neutrophils or from the injured epithelium [64]. Persistence of collagenase leads to stromal liquefaction and may progress to perforation and loss of the eye.

The normal eye with intact corneal epithelium is highly resistant to micro-organisms. An epithelial defect is a potential portal of entry for bacteria, fungi, viruses, and *Acanthamoeba*. Corneal ulcers from these pathogens often occur in contact lens wearers and also may follow refractive surgical procedures. The end result of a corneal ulcer is stromal scarring and loss of vision [102,104,105].

Incisional procedures

Radial keratotomy

Wound-healing problems in RK take two forms: those related to faulty production of the incisions at the time of surgery and those related to abnormal wound healing (Tables 4.2 and 4.3). Accurate knowledge of corneal thickness and precise calibration of the cutting instrument are critical factors in all forms of keratotomy surgery. Effectiveness of the surgery is related directly to the depth of cut. An incision that is too deep will result in a micro- or macro-perforation. After healing of a micro-perforation, there is a focal loss of endothelial cells from direct trauma as well as localized proliferation of fibrous tissue. A micro-perforation also presents the possibility of invasion by micro-organisms or by epithelium to cause a downgrowth.

A macro-perforation usually causes termination of the procedure and may require suturing of the wound to maintain the anterior chamber. All the possible compli-

Table 4.2 Radial keratotomy. From Binder PS. What we have learned about corneal wound healing from refractive surgery (Barraquer lecture). Refract Corneal Surg 1989; 5(2):98–120

Acute surface features
Rupture/loss of cells within 50–100 μm of either side of wound
Debridement of epithelium in a triangular pattern with apex toward optical clear zone (concordes)
Inadvertent epithelial implantation into wounds
Focal fractures in Bowman's layer and basement membrane when grasped with forceps or with attempted re-entry of wounds with the blade
Blade entry site smaller and more sharply demarcated than blade exit
Acute stromal and endothelial features
Loss of keratocytes within 200–300 μm of wound
Jagged wound edge with fragmented collagen fibers
Posterior bowing of Descemet's membrane toward anterior chamber
Ruptured endothelial cells along posterior Descemet's folds

Table 4.3 Radial keratotomy. From Binder PS. What we have learned about corneal wound healing from refractive surgery (Barraquer lecture). Refract Corneal Surg 1989; 5(2):98–120

Chronic features
Epithelium
Abnormal surface cells over wounds
Epithelial ridges over wounds
Map-dot-fingerprint dystrophy changes affecting basal lamina
Iron deposition
Bowman's layer
Focal fractures
Inward bowing at incision sites
Stroma
Viable epithelium in wounds (cysts, plugs)
Epithelial degenerative products in wounds
Neovascularization proximal to limbus
Non-aligned collagen lamellae/fibers
Activated keratocytes under incisions
Bowing of lamellae toward anterior chamber
Variable incision depths within the same wounds and between wounds in the same specimen
Non-perpendicular incisions in the same corneal specimen
Descemet's membrane
Bowing of Descemet's membrane toward anterior chamber
Normal endothelial morphology over incisions except at micro-perforation sites

cations of micro-perforations must be entertained in this event. Additionally, the full-thickness wound and its repair may cause irregular stromal scarring that may interfere with visual rehabilitation. Deep wounds also tend to exert pressure on Descemet's membrane, causing focal raised endothelial surfaces, the "log under a rug" phenomenon (Figure 4.31a). In some cases, endothelial cells can be destroyed (Figure 4.31b). Severe regular or irregular astigmatism may result, as with any healed corneal scar. This is more likely with wounds made with steel blades, which typically cause jagged wound edges.

Nearly all RK patients report glare after surgery, which may last from 1 to 3 months. The glare results from the scattering of light by incisional edema and scar tissue. The ideal incision should be made perpendicular to a tangent to the cornea. An oblique incision (Figure 4.32) produces a broader base for light scattering and aggravates the glare. If scarring is sufficiently severe, disabling glare may be a permanent problem.

As noted previously, stromal wounds usually are sealed with an epithelial plug that disappears as the wound heals. The way in which the wound is produced may alter the sequence of events. For example, RK wounds show a relatively simple form of healing. Following the acute surgical incision, the corneal epithelium migrates

(a)

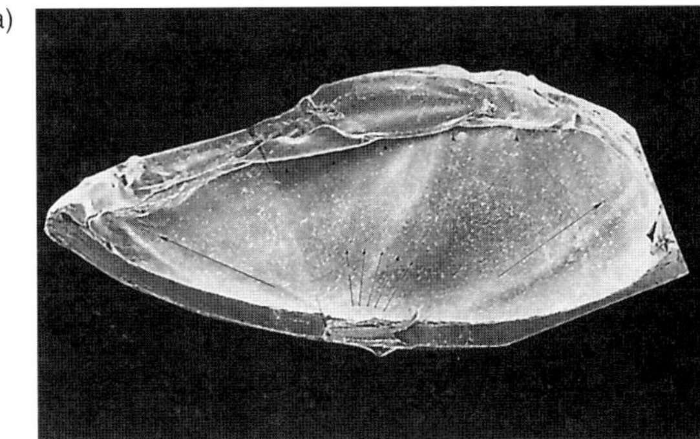

(b)

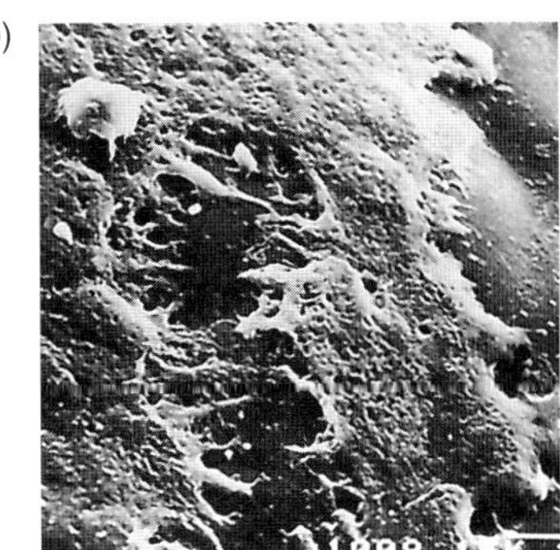

Fig. 4.31 (a) Scanning electron micrograph of a trephined section showing the "log under a rug" effect beneath RK incisions. (b) Endothelial damage following RK in a rabbit (×15,000). (Figure 4.31b from Yamaguchi T, Polack FM, Valenti J, Kaufman HE. Endothelial damage after anterior radial keratotomy: An electron microscopic study of rabbit cornea. Arch Ophthalmol 1981; 99(12):2151–2158).

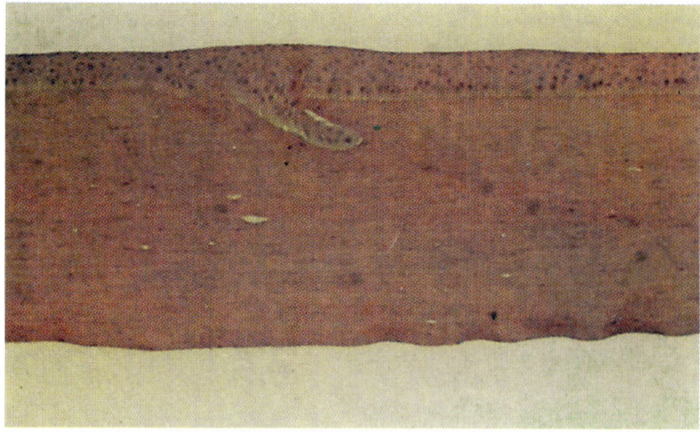

Fig. 4.32 A healed RK scar is marked by a small epithelial plug that extends obliquely across the cornea for two-thirds stromal thickness. Such a scar is associated with severe and persistent glare (H&E stain; ×50).

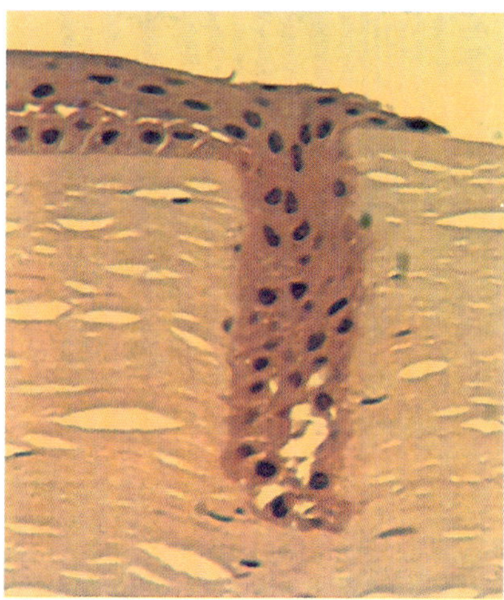

Fig. 4.33 An early RK incision is filled by an epithelial plug (H&E stain; ×100).

(Figure 4.33) down the lateral walls of the incision and then proliferates, forming an epithelial plug [106]. In the normal sequence of events, fibroblastic repair and proliferation gradually push the plug out of the wound with formation of an avascular scar (Figure 4.34). Unlike a single isolated stromal wound, final healing of an RK wound and expulsion of epithelium may be prolonged in some patients. In some cases, the epithelial plug persists for many months or years [107]. In fact, small inclusions of epithelium can become implanted within the scar, which causes incomplete or prolonged healing. It has been suggested that prolonged healing is due to flexure of the multiple stromal wounds, which prevents normal healing—although there has not been good correlation with pathology [108]. The situation is different in epikeratophakia, where healing must take place between the stroma of the lenticule and the host Bowman's layer, in addition to epithelial healing.

Marsupialization also can occur, especially if wound gape is excessive [109]. If epithelial cells are implanted within the incision, they may proliferate to form cystic structures—sometimes of considerable size (Figure 4.35). Talcum from incompletely washed gloves and other foreign bodies can lodge in these incisions. Red blood cells, if not irrigated from the wound, can be converted by the keratocytes into lipid deposits—sometimes of impressive dimensions (see also Chapter 15).

It has been suggested that corneas of myopes may respond in a unique fashion. Kurasova has noted that wound appearance correlates with result and has defined four different types of wounds seen after RK [110]. "Feathering" of the wound margins has been described by the author and others [111], but the clinical appearance has not been correlated histologically [112]. It is possible that we are dealing with different types of collagen in these cases; certainly there appears to be something different about the healing processes in RK [113,114].

Map-dot changes have been reported following RK [115] (see also Chapter 15). Binder attributes these to

(a)

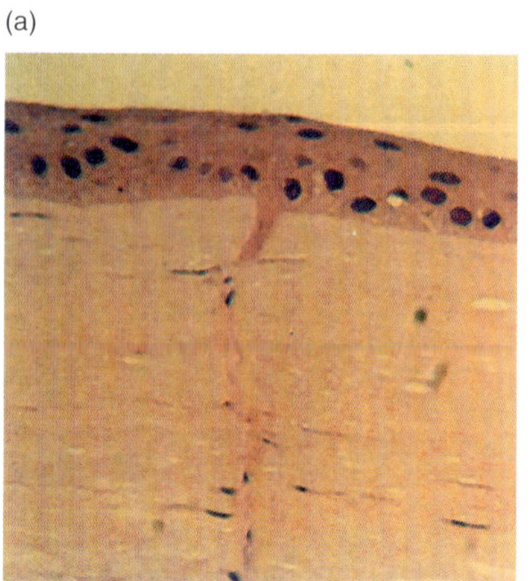

(b)

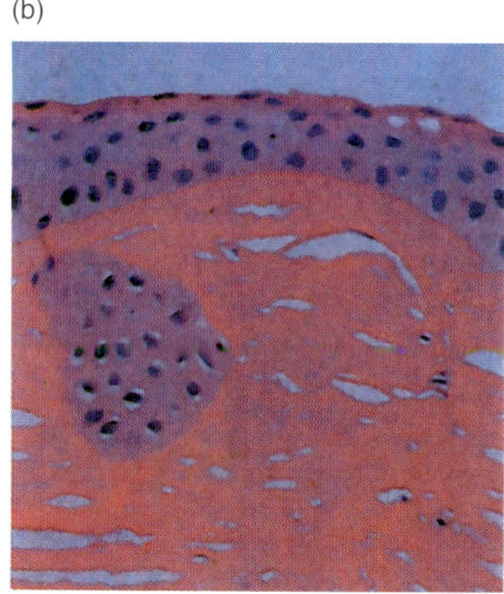

Fig. 4.34 (a) A late RK scar. The incision is marked by a break in Bowman's membrane and a well-healed stromal scar (H&E stain; ×100). (b) Epithelial island or cord trapped within corneal stroma (H&E stain; ×100).

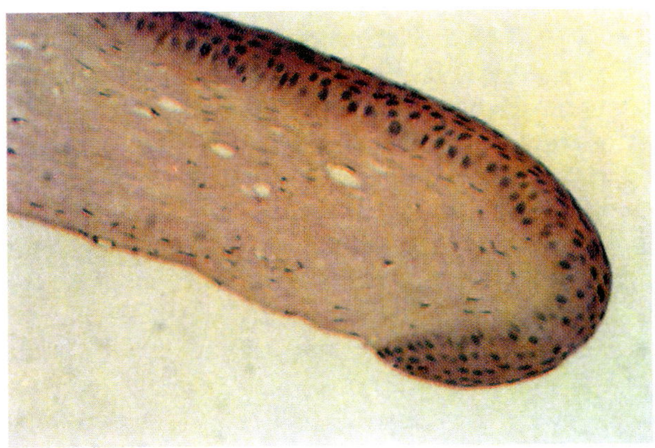

Fig. 4.35 A persistent stromal defect lined by epithelium is seen after a Ruiz procedure with intersecting incisions. An elevated stromal flap has resulted from the improper healing (H&E stain; ×50).

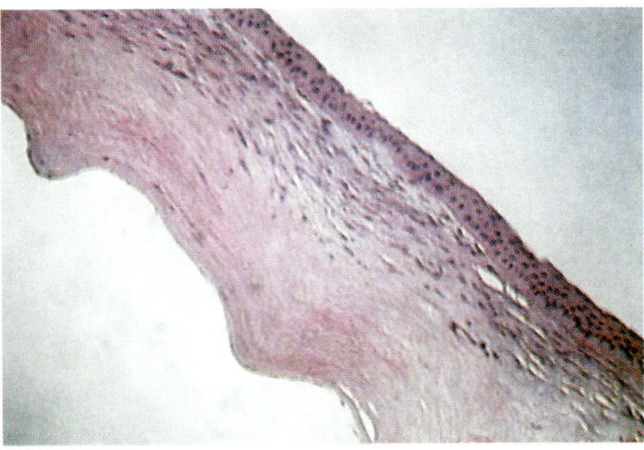

Fig. 4.36 Cornea following thermokeratoplasty. Bowman's membrane is absent, and there is irregular anterior stromal scarring (H&E stain; ×50).

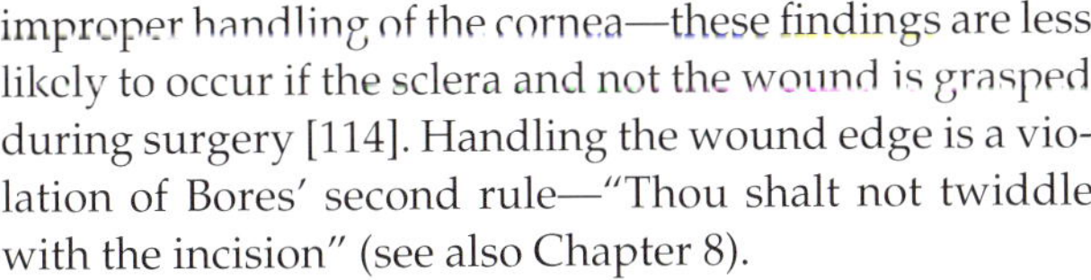

improper handling of the cornea—these findings are less likely to occur if the sclera and not the wound is grasped during surgery [114]. Handling the wound edge is a violation of Bores' second rule—"Thou shalt not twiddle with the incision" (see also Chapter 8).

Astigmatic keratotomy

In addition to all the preceding problems, astigmatic keratotomy has other complications. At one time, it was customary to connect the transverse cuts with the radial cuts performed in a Ruiz procedure. Many patients were found to have one or more V-shaped corneal flaps at the incisional crossings after this procedure. The flaps (see Figure 4.35) became edematous and elevated above the surface of the remainder of the cornea. Chronic epithelial defects, corneal melting, and irregular scarring are possible complications—which cannot be avoided completely even in the best of hands [116].

Thermal procedures

Thermal (planiform) keratoplasty

Collagen undergoes shrinkage when heated, a fact that suggested a potential application in refractive surgery (see also Chapters 8 and 15). At one time it was felt that thermal shrinkage could be used in patients with keratoconus to alter corneal curvature, improve contact lens fitting, and avoid the need for keratoplasty. Thermokeratoplasty was attempted with a number of instruments, all of which caused similar complications. Regardless of the method of heat production, the procedure damages Bowman's layer, which in turn interferes with reestablishment of the epithelial sheet and can cause stromal scarring (Figure 4.36). Heat often destroys stromal keratocytes as well (Figure 4.37), which may lead to additional stromal scarring. The persistent epithelial defect can potentiate production of collagenase, leading to corneal necrosis and melting (Figure 4.38). These were observed in several patients [117]. Binder has observed that severe corneal damage can occur with as few as four burns. Hyperopic thermokeratoplasty (HTK) employs 12 to 96 deep stromal burns—a sobering fact and one to ponder in light of the potential complications.

Hyperopic (punctiform) thermal keratotomy

Fyodorov in Russia and Neumann in this country proposed a radial thermal pattern for the treatment of hyperopia (see also Chapter 14). No animal studies were published, but one might predict irregular astigmatism, persistent epithelial defects, and perhaps some of the problems associated with planiform thermokeratoplasty.

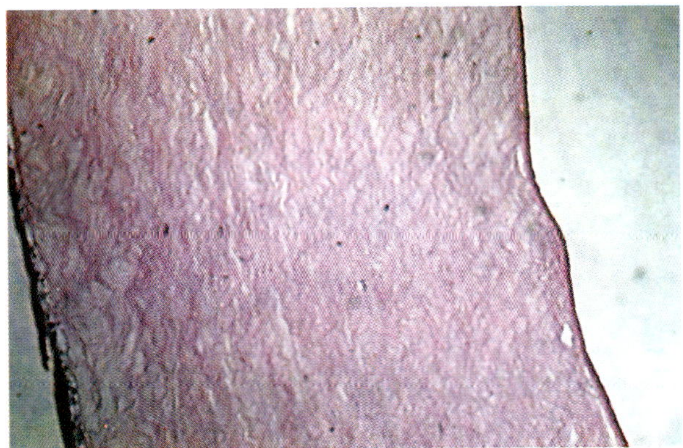

Fig. 4.37 Cornea following thermokeratoplasty. Basilar epithelial edema is present, and there is epithelial thinning related to poor healing. Corneal edema is prominent, and there is a marked decreased in the number of keratocytes (H&E stain; ×100).

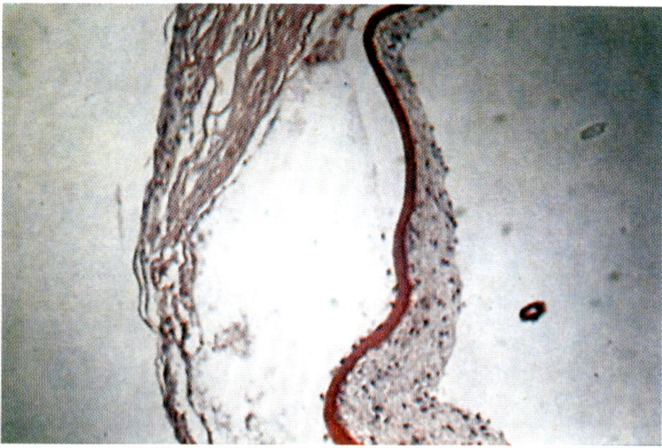

Fig. 4.38 The corneal epithelium is absent following thermokeratoplasty. There is marked central stromal melting resulting in a descemetocoele. A fibrin plaque is present on the posterior surface of Descemet's membrane (H&E stain; ×50).

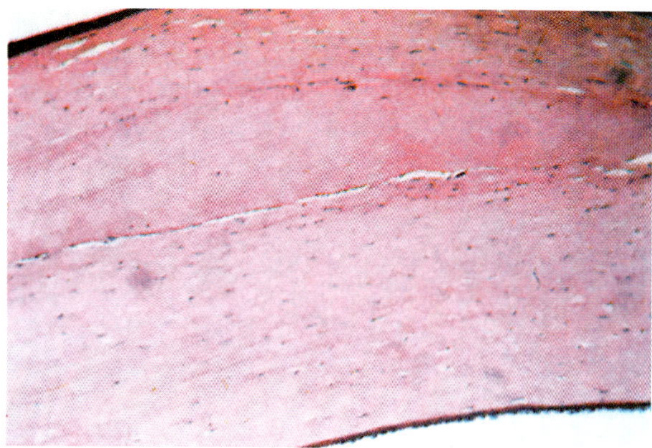

Fig. 4.39 In keratophakia, keratocytes are absent in the lenticular stroma (H&E stain; ×100).

Lathed tissue procedures

Barraquer is the father of corneal lathing as a method of altering the anterior curvature of the cornea. Keratophakia, keratomileusis, and epikeratophakia all make use of this general concept. Because the operative techniques vary, there are specific abnormalities of wound healing associated with each procedure. For example, epikeratophakia uses a lathed donor button of either frozen or fresh tissue that is placed directly on the recipient Bowman's layer.

Keratophakia

In keratophakia, a donor lamellar disc is cryolathed and then placed within the patient's cornea in a previously prepared lamellar bed. Since the donor lenticule is frozen prior to being implanted, there are no viable keratocytes within it. Collagen and GAGs, by light microscopy, are apparently undisturbed by the freeze-processing other than distortion of the lamellae. Electron microscopy, however, demonstrates distorted and occasionally fractured collagen along with reduced ground substance. Unlike keratomileusis, the donor button shows little repopulation by keratocytes (Figure 4.39), even up to a year after surgery [118,119]. It has been suggested that this failure of keratocyte invasion is due to interface pressure or lack of horizontal edge alignment. Irregular healing in this and the other lathed tissue procedures often results in irregular astigmatism. The most frequent reason for removal of a keratophakia lenticule, however, is inappropriate optical correction.

Keratomileusis

In keratomileusis, a lamellar button from the patient's own cornea is frozen, lathed to a new shape, and placed back into the corneal bed. Both hyperopic and myopic correction may be achieved by this procedure. Epithelial vacuolization and intraepithelial cyst formation may occur, perhaps related to freezing damage (see also Chapters 11 and 15). In some cases, the epithelium separates from Bowman's layer due to fibrocellular proliferation. Despite the fact that the lenticule is frozen, it is rapidly repopulated by keratocytes [118,119]. The lamellar arrangement of collagen is undisturbed. Fractures of Bowman's layer (Figure 4.40), however, are particularly likely to occur in myopic keratomileusis [119]. This is due to physical distortion of the very thin central portion of the lenticule during surgical manipulation. Damage of the epithelial basement membrane results in fewer hemidesmosomes that can lead to persistent epithelial defects, as well as the potential risk of infection and scarring. To avoid this, the central lenticular thickness is held to a minimum of 0.015 mm. When this is done, cracking of Bowman's layer and scarring, in my experience, rarely occurs.

Additional interference with vision may result from epithelial invasion of the interface between the lenticule and the underlying stroma (Figures 4.41 and 4.42). This also can occur in the nonfreeze forms of keratomileusis, but the incidence is low. This is probably related to the fact that the donor epithelium is undamaged in the nonfreeze method; thus the area to be covered by epithelial cells is less, and consequently, so is the collagenase activity [120]. Table 4.4 summarizes the histologic features of keratophakia and both freeze and nonfreeze keratomileusis.

Epikeratophakia

The original epikeratophakia buttons were prepared by cryolathing eye bank donor tissue designed to produce the desired refractive effect. Both hyperopic and myopic lenticules can be produced and, in the commercial lenticules, are lyophilized for storage. The patient's epithelium

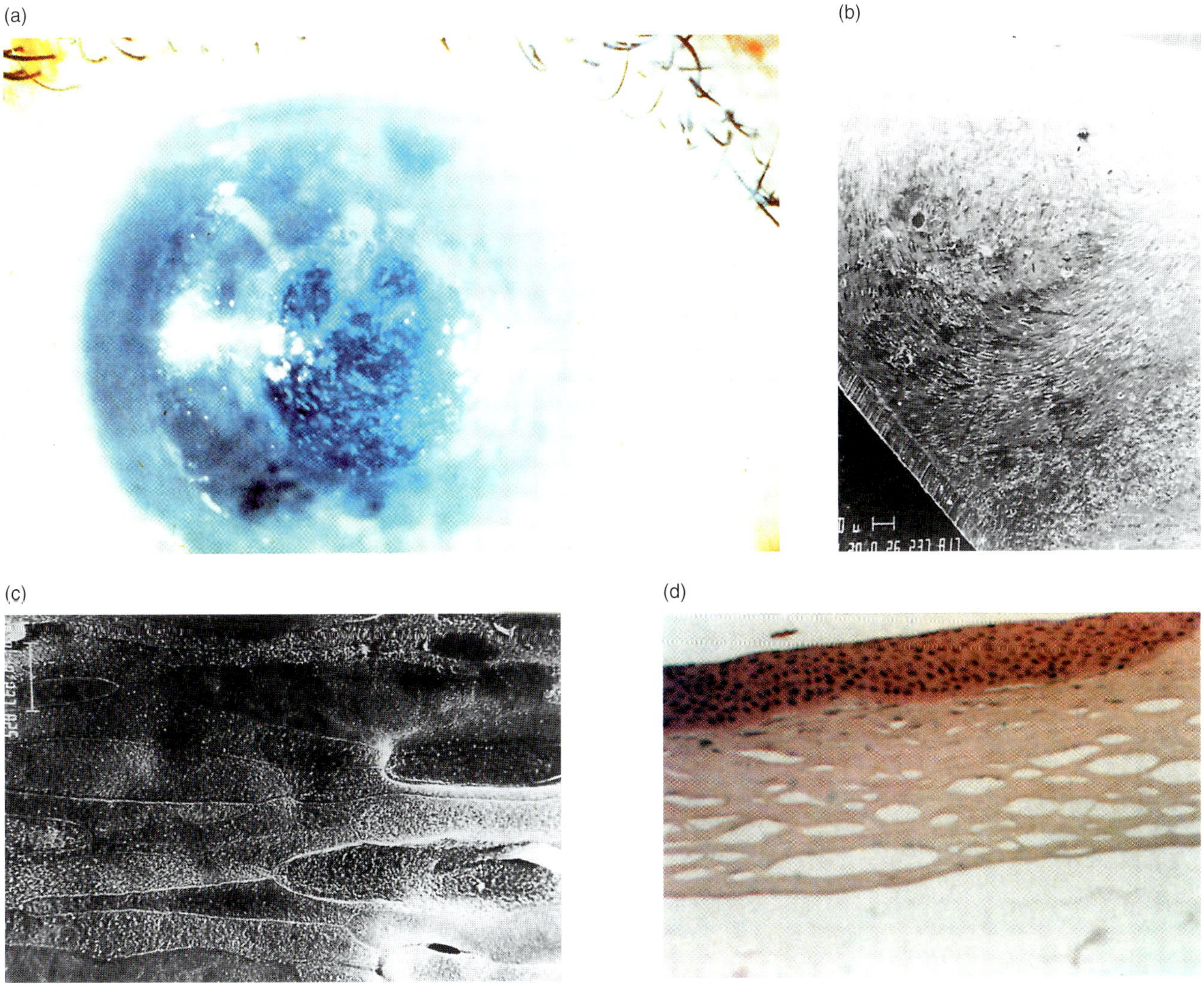

Fig. 4.40 (a) Spiral epithelialopathy following myopic keratomileusis. (b) Scanning electron micrograph of the surface of the failed lenticule (×2250). (c) Higher-power view showing the peculiar nature of the epithelium (×10,500). (d) Bowman's membrane is absent, and there is anterior stromal scarring following failed myopic keratomileusis (H&E stain; ×100).

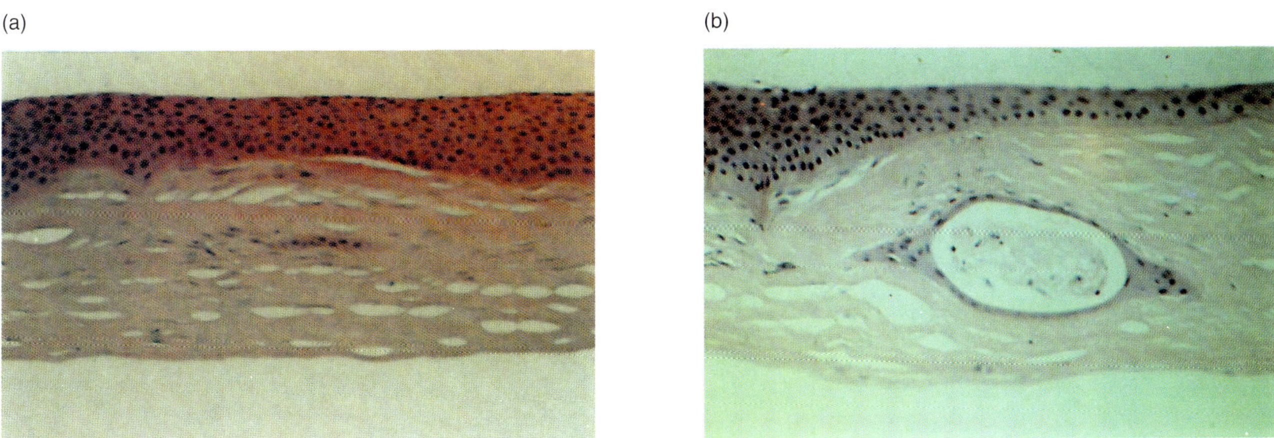

Fig. 4.41 (a) Epithelial inclusion at the interface between lathed tissue and deep stroma following myopic keratomileusis. Superficial stromal irregularity and thickened epithelium also are evident (H&E stain; ×100). (b) Epithelial cyst following myopic keratomileusis. Note bulging of Descemet's membrane (H&E stain; ×100).

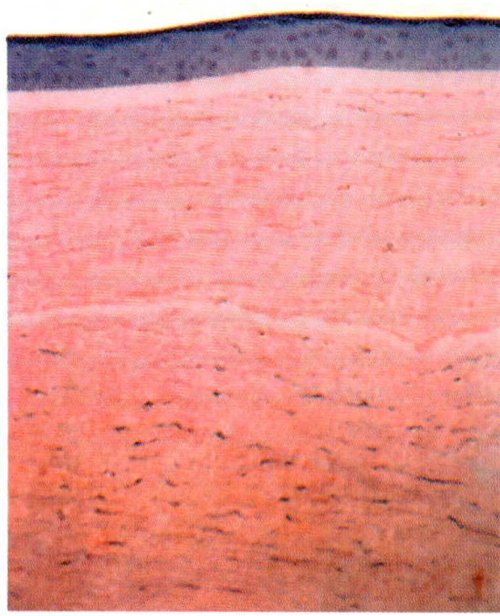

Fig. 4.42 Penetrating keratoplasty button after epikeratoplasty. The interface between the epikeratoplasty lenticule and the recipient is shown (H&E stain; ×50).

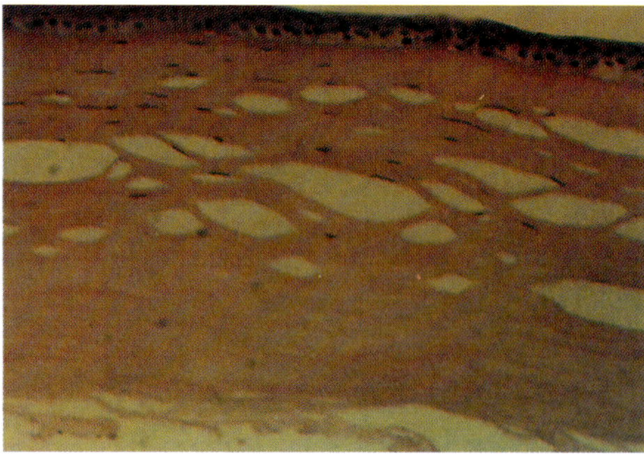

Fig. 4.43 Failed epikeratoplasty. Keratocytes are absent (H&E stain; ×100).

is removed prior to placement of the donor tissue onto the recipient's Bowman's layer. The prepared lenticule is sewn into a circular keratotomy of varying diameter. The practice of annular keratectomy—removal of a ring of corneal stroma, the source of irregular healing and astigmatism—has been abandoned. Although little histopathology is available, there has been a recent interest in lathing fresh, unfrozen tissue, a technique that avoids death of donor keratocytes [121–129] (see also Chapter 11). In the frozen lenticules, the keratocytes are destroyed, as they are in keratophakia and keratomileusis. In lenticules that have been studied some time after surgery, keratocytes usually are present anteriorly and peripherally but are sparse or absent in the posterior aspects of the lenticule (Figure 4.43). Some have ascribed this irregular keratocyte repopulation to interference with diffusion of nutrients by the host Bowman's layer [130].

A major problem in epikeratophakia relates to resurfacing of the donor lenticule with host epithelium [131]. Re-epithelialization plays a role in lenticular clarity—the faster this occurs, the clearer are the final results. Persistent epithelial defects are common in epikeratophakia (Figure 4.44)—the epithelial basement membrane may be abnormal in some cases; fractures and folds can occur [132]. As in other procedures, such defects may provide an entry for infectious agents or may be associated with corneal melting of both host and donor cornea at the interface, forcing removal of the lenticule. Subsequent scarring may

Table 4.4 Histologic features of lamellar surgery. From Binder PS. What we have learned about corneal wound healing from refractive surgery (Barraquer lecture). Refract Corneal Surg 1989; 5(2):98–120

Keratophakia	Keratomileusis	Nonfreeze keratomileusis
Acute features		
Killed keratocytes	Killed keratocytes	Viable keratocytes
Distorted lamellae	Normal lamellae	Normal lamellae
Stromal edema	Minimal edema	No edema
—	Dead epithelium	Normal epithelium
—	Bowman's fractures	Bowman's fractures —peripheral
Chronic features		
Stromal edema	Bowman's fractures	Intact Bowman's
—	Normal epithelium	Normal epithelium
Distorted lamellae	Thin central stroma	Normal thickness
Interface epithelium	Interface epithelium	Interface collagen
Anterior cap pannus	Normal keratocytes	Interface keratocytes
Neovascularization	Interface keratocytes	—

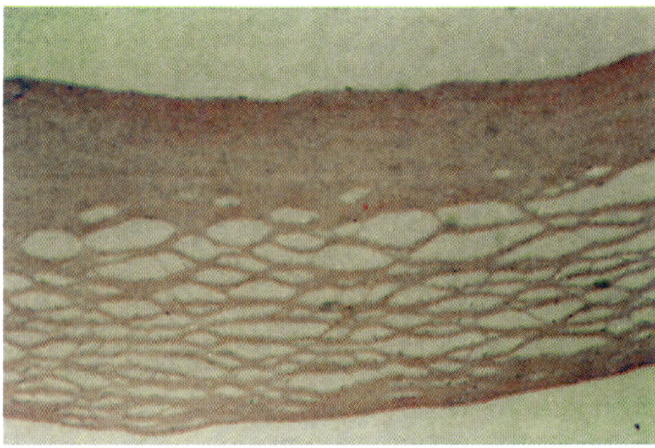

Fig. 4.44 Failed epikeratoplasty. The corneal epithelium is absent. The artifactual clefting of the stroma suggests edema. Keratocytes are absent (H&E stain; ×50).

interfere with visual function and necessitate a penetrating keratoplasty [133,134]. Epithelial cells pile up at the host–graft edge. While this tends to smooth out the change in corneal curvature, thickened epithelium may prove to be unstable in the long run.

The edge of the lenticule may provide a route for epithelium to grow downward and between the lenticule and donor cornea (Figures 4.45 to 4.50)—although more likely in keratomileusis. This will produce an interface opacity if not removed and sometimes even if it is removed. Such opacities also may result from scarring (see also Chapter 15 for a discussion on complications occurring with lamellar refractive procedures). An additional cause of interface opacification is seen in keratoconus patients. Epikeratophakia has been used in keratoconus to flatten the cone and to provide an improved optical surface [135] (see also Chapter 11). If central scarring is present in the host, vision is not improved by the clear epikeratophakia button (Figure 4.51). The tension exerted by the tightly sewn epikeratophakia button also can produce wrinkling of Bowman's layer (Figure 4.52), which also may contribute to a reduction in visual acuity. Tables 4.5 and 4.6 summarize problems leading to lenticule removal in epikeratophakia and their histologic features.

Implantation procedures

Intrastromal lenses

Another approach to refractive surgery is to implant a plastic material of appropriate refractive index to alter the patient's underlying refractive error (see Chapter 11 for a discussion on allopathic intrastromal inlays). Early experience with methyl methacrylate and other water-impermeable substances failed because nutrients were blocked from the portions of the cornea anterior to the implant. This often resulted in necrosis, melting, and extrusion of the implant. Subsequently, water- and oxygen-permeable plastics such as HEMA and polysulfone have been somewhat more successful [114].

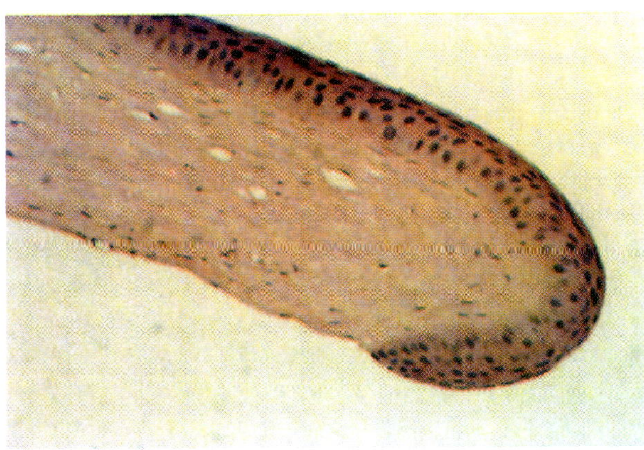

Fig. 4.45 At the edge of a failed epikeratoplasty, epithelium is growing around the edge of the lenticule. This resulted in improper healing and ectasia of the lenticule (H&E stain; ×100).

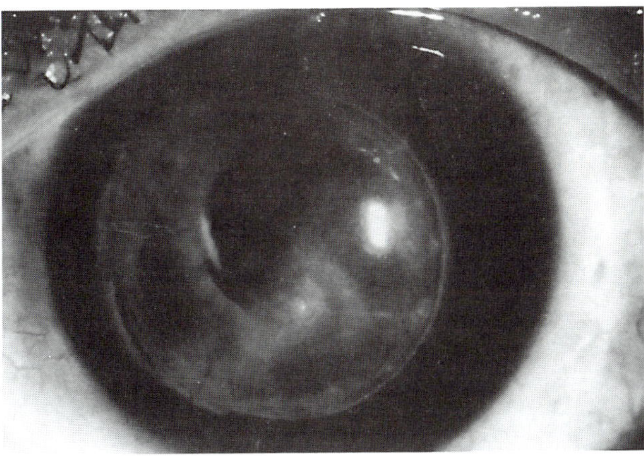

Fig. 4.46 Patient received lyophilized (AMO) lenticule but had a persistent epithelial defect not responsive to therapy. Clinical appearance 4 months after surgery with scarring of the epikeratoplasty lenticule (from Grossniklaus HE, Lass JH, Jacobs G, Margo CE, McAuliffe AM. Light microscopic and ultrastructural findings in failed epikeratoplasty. Refract Corneal Surg 1989; 5(5):296–301).

Polysulfone lenses

These lenses are inserted through a superior corneal incision into a pocket created by an intrastromal dissection—

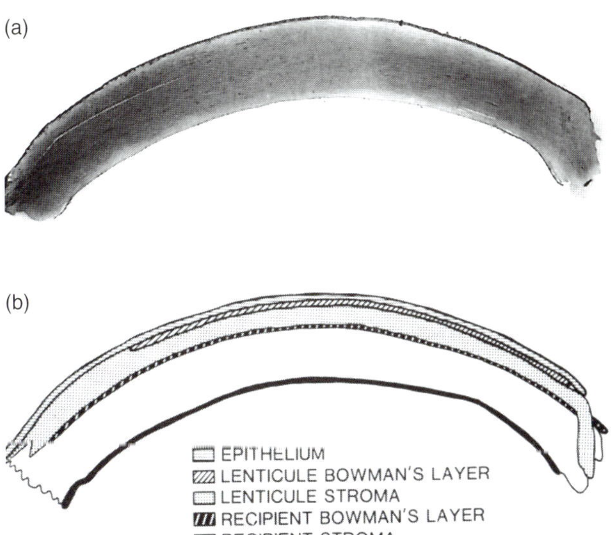

Fig. 4.47 (a) Corneal button (Masson's trichrome, original magnification ×4). (b) Corresponding diagram (from Grossniklaus HE, Lass JH, Jacobs G, Margo CE, McAuliffe AM. Light microscopic and ultrastructural findings in failed epikeratoplasty. Refract Corneal Surg 1989; 5(5):296–301).

(a)

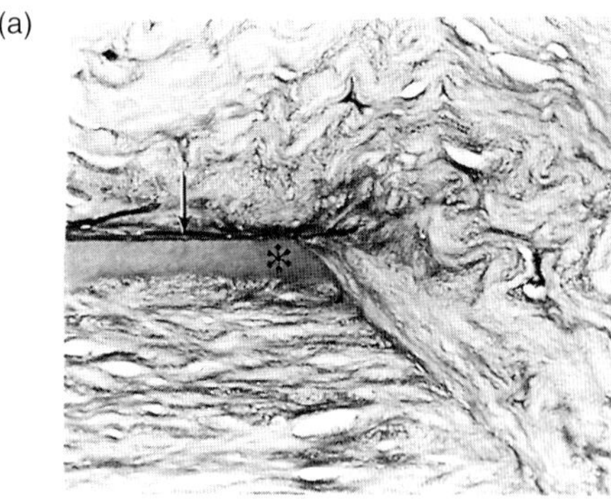

(b)

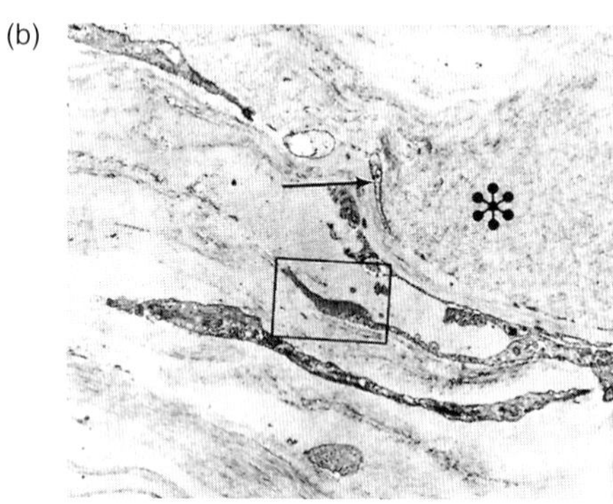

(c)

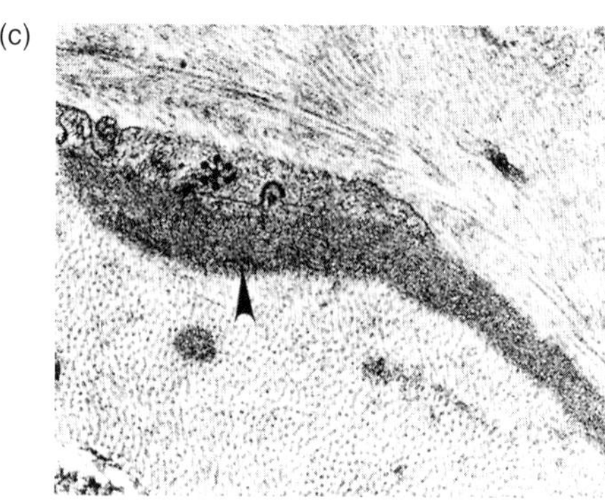

Fig. 4.48 (a) Keratocytes (arrow) are present anterior to cut margin of recipient Bowman's layer (arrowhead). Lenticule stroma contains relatively more keratocytes than recipient in this particular field; however, there was an overall decrease in the number of keratocytes in the lenticule as compared with the recipient stroma (PAS stain; original magnification ×700). (b) Electron micrograph of cut edge of recipient Bowman's layer (asterisk) corresponding with part a. Lenticular keratocytes (arrow) are draped over the edge of Bowman's layer. Electron-dense material is associated with a lenticule keratocyte (bracketed area) (original magnification ×1700). (c) Higher magnification of bracketed area shown in part b demonstrates fibrillogranular material (arrowhead) associated with a lenticule keratocyte (asterisk) in surrounding collagen matrix (original magnification ×35,000) (from Grossniklaus HE, Lass JH, Jacobs G, Margo CE, McAuliffe AM. Light microscopic and ultrastructural findings in failed epikeratoplasty. Refract Corneal Surg 1989; 5(5):296–301).

sometimes aided by sodium hyaluronic acid. As with the lamellar procedures, debris and epithelial cells may be implanted accidentally into the pocket along with the lens. Opacities similar to those seen with epikeratophakia may result. Animal studies have shown that the epithelium and endothelium generally remain intact over these lenses [114].

These lenses are able to correct large refractive errors, but acute failures occur because of edema and severe stromal inflammation. Late effects include epithelial thinning, anterior stromal melting with implant extrusion, gray anterior interface deposits, and neovascularization. Evidence of chronic keratocyte damage—such as vacuolization and lipid degeneration—is also seen. The anterior stroma typically shows a significant decrease in keratocytes. These changes seem to indicate interference with normal corneal nutrition [136], and to avoid this possibility, lenses were fenestrated [137] (Figure 4.53). This procedure decreases the severe complications, but collagen invades the fenestrations with localized opacification. Lipid deposits also have been reported beneath the unfenestrated areas [114]. Although these lenses are easy to insert, it seems apparent that new materials must be developed before this class of plastic shows clinical usefulness.

Hydrogel lenses

These lenses are inserted either into a free-hand stromal pocket or preferably into a space created by a microkeratome. As with all lamellar procedures, the implantation of epithelial cells and debris can cause problems because of localized opacification. In contrast to the polysulfone lenses, hydrogel lenses are well tolerated. The typical cornea is optically clear both in front of and behind the lens (Figure 4.54). The corneal endothelium is normal. There is a remarkable absence of inflammation and stromal scarring. In a few eyes there has been anterior stromal melting, but the majority of cases show a healthy Bowman's layer and corneal epithelium [114,138]. In lenses inserted into free-hand pockets, there may be consequent wrinkling of Bowman's and Descemet's membranes, which can cause interference with visual acuity; this is avoided by removing the upper layer with a microkeratome. Fibrosis also may occur around the implant because of faulty edge design that leaves an unfilled space.

With all lamellar procedures, there is always a risk of infection in the postoperative period or if there is erosion of the anterior stroma and epithelium. The results are predictably disastrous, with peri-implant abscess formation and permanent loss of vision. Table 4.7 lists the acute and chronic histologic changes with allopathic stromal implants.

Laser ablative procedures

Laser radiation in the far ultraviolet region (150 to 200 nm) can be produced by a number of different lasers using halogens or noble gases. Extensive animal studies have shown that the argon fluoride excimer laser, operating at 193 nm, has the optimal effect on corneal tissue. The effect

(a)

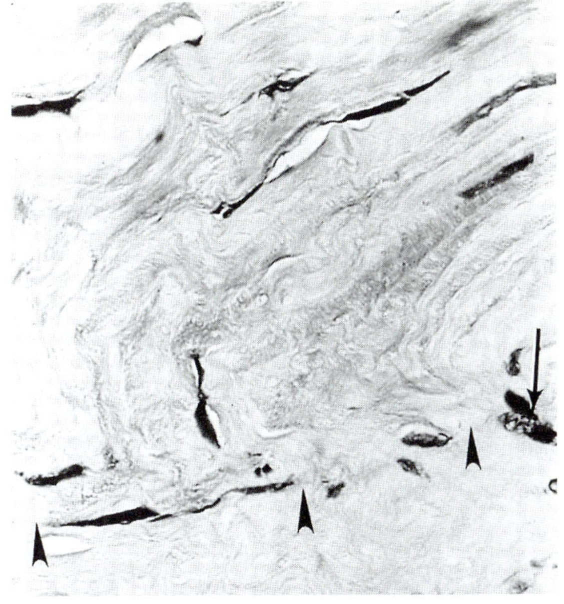

(c)

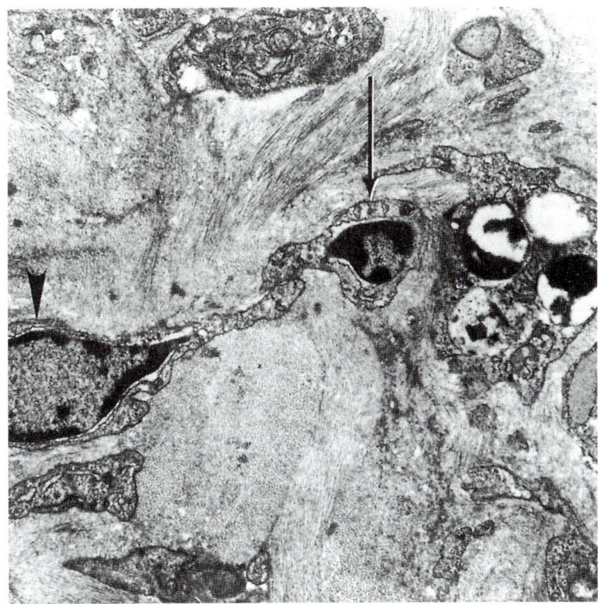

(b)

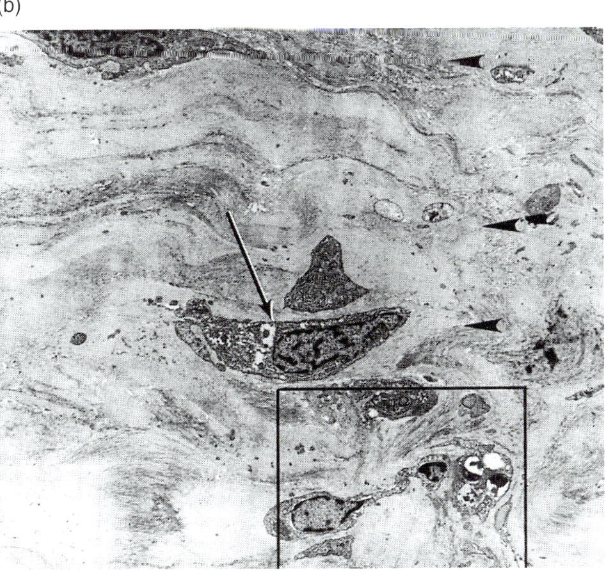

Fig. 4.49 (a) Trephination wound (arrowheads) interface of recipient stroma on left and donor stroma on right. Note apparent migration of plump keratocytes (arrow) between recipient and lenticule (Masson's trichrome stain; original magnification ×700). (b) Election micrograph of recipient–lenticule interface (arrowheads corresponding to area shown in part a. Note plump keratocyte (arrow) and apparent migration between recipient keratocyte on left and lenticule keratocyte on right (bracketed area) (original magnification ×7500). (c) Higher magnification of bracketed area shown in part b shows that keratocyte in recipient (arrowhead) is in contact with a keratocyte in the lenticule (arrow) via an opening in the collagen lamellae (original magnification ×24,000) (from Grossniklaus HE, Lass JH, Jacobs G, Margo CE, McAuliffe AM. Light microscopic and ultrastructural findings in failed epikeratoplasty. Refract Corneal Surg 1989; 5(5):296–301).

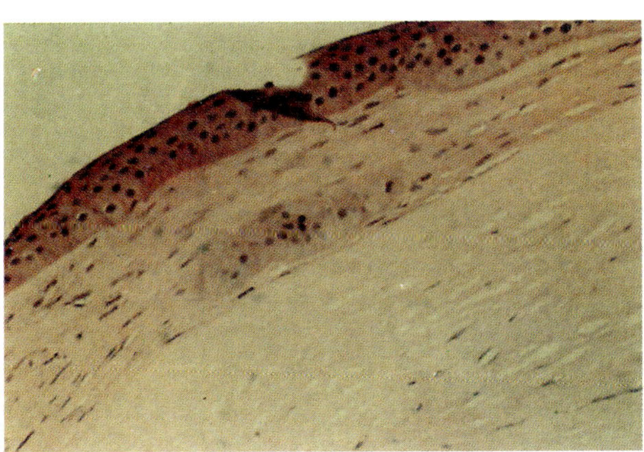

Fig. 4.50 An isolated island of epithelium is present centrally at the interface between the epikeratoplasty lenticule and the host. This produces a local opacification that interferes with vision (H&E stain; ×100).

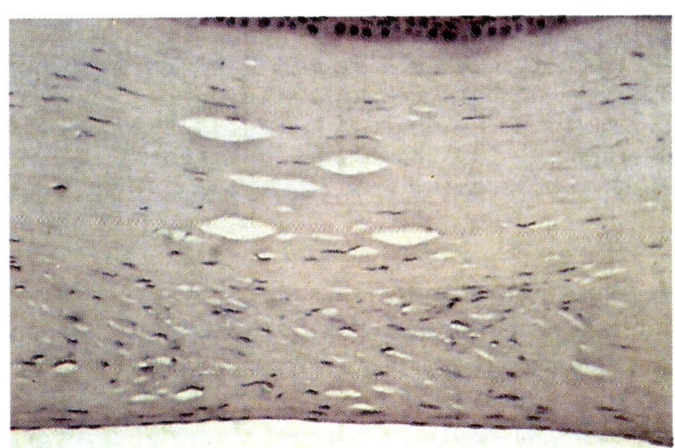

Fig. 4.51 Although the epikeratoplasty lenticule is clear, host stroma scarring persists in this keratoconus patient (H&E stain; ×100).

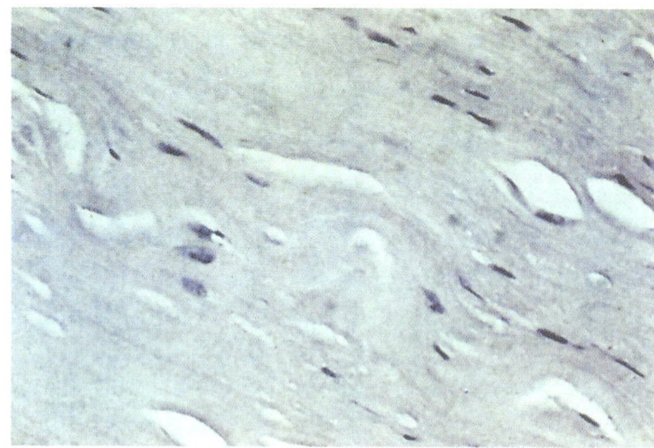

Fig. 4.52 There is marked wrinkling of the host Bowman's membrane in this keratoconic epikeratoplasty (H&E stain; ×200).

Table 4.5 Epikeratophakia. Indications for lenticule removal. From Binder PS. What we have learned about corneal wound healing from refractive surgery (Barraquer lecture). Refract Corneal Surg 1989; 5(2):98–120

Loss of best corrected acuity for no apparent reason
Loss of best acuity due to irregular astigmatism, epithelial ingrowth, Bowman's scarring, or particulate material
Significant under- or overcorrection
Lack of lenticular clarity in the absence of an infective process
Chronic nonhealing epithelial defect with or without stromal melting
Infection within cornea or lenticule
Progression of keratoconus under lenticule

Table 4.6 Epikeratophakia. Histologic features from failed specimens. From Binder PS. What we have learned about corneal wound healing from refractive surgery (Barraquer lecture). Refract Corneal Surg 1989; 5(2):98–120

Epithelial ulceration
Stromal tissue loss (melting)
Increased collagen interfibrillar distance
Loss of ground substance GAGs with stromal edema
Abnormal epithelium covering lenticule (too thin or too thick)
Focal epithelial cyst formation within stromal wounds
Scars in recipient Bowman's layer
Absent to decreased keratocyte re-population of lenticule
Neovascularization and/or epithelium, collagen, keratocytes in interface
Frank bacterial ulceration

(a)

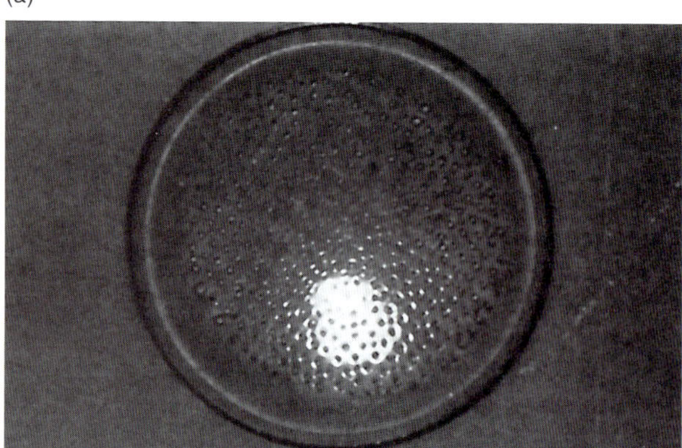

(b)

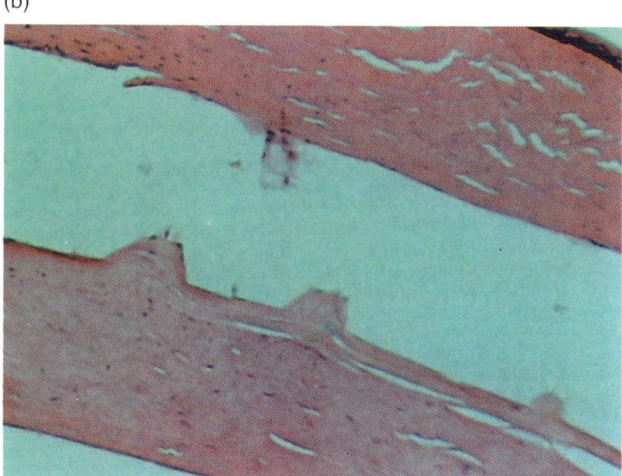

(c)

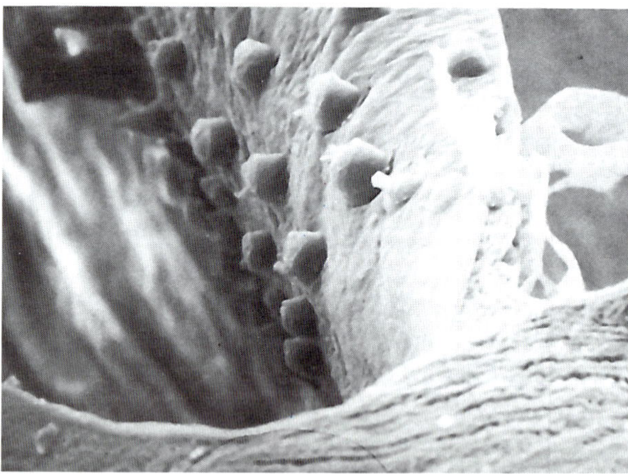

Fig. 4.53 (a) Fenestrated polysulfone lenticule. (b) Histologic section of intralamellar pocket following removal of a fenestrated lens. Note normal keratocytes within pegs of corneal stroma growing through the fenestrations (H&E stain; ×10) (c) Scanning electron micrograph demonstrating corneal stromal pegs and smooth intralamellar pocket (×22) (from Lane SS, Lindstrom RL. Polysulfone intracorneal lenses. Int Ophthalmol Clin 1991; 31(1):37–46).

(a)

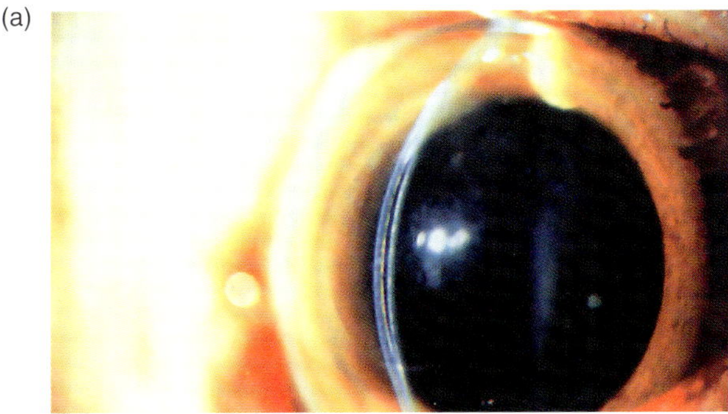

(b)

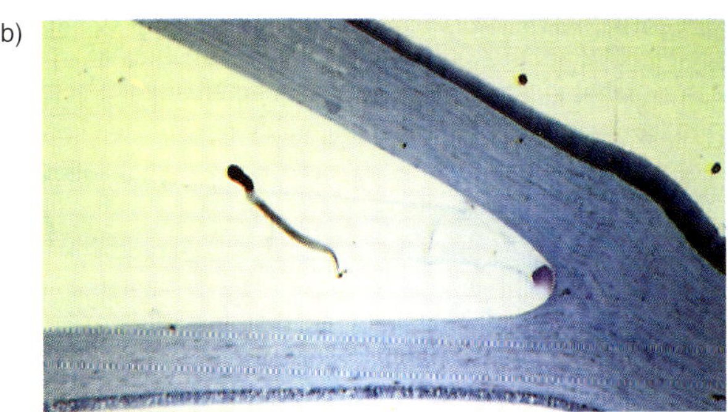

Fig. 4.54 (a) Intrastromal hydrophilic (KeratoGel) implant. (b) Intrastromal alloplastic implant. Inflammation and stromal scarring are absent (toluidine blue stain; ×100) (courtesy of Bernard McCarey, PhD).

of these lasers is produced by ablative photodecomposition in which the irradiated tissue is broken down into volatile fragments without heat effects in the adjacent tissues [139].

The excimer laser may be used for refractive surgery either in a cutting mode, to produce an RK wound, or in a broad ablative mode, to alter the curvature of a central

Table 4.7 Histologic features of alloplastic stromal implants. From Binder PS. What we have learned about corneal wound healing from refractive surgery (Barraquer lecture). Refract Corneal Surg 1989; 5(2):98–120

Hydrogel implants	Polysulfone implants
Acute features	
Lamellar separation	Lamellar separation
Interface epithelium	Interface epithelium
Microkeratome damage to Bowman's	Descemet's perforation
Chronic features	
Thinned epithelium	Thinned epithelium
Interface collagen	Absent/decreased keratocytes
Interface keratocytes	Interface keratocytes, epithelium
	Anterior lipoid degeneration
	Epithelial ulceration
	Anterior stromal melting
	Descemet's scarring

optical zone. Most of the RK studies have been limited to the laboratory. In experimental animals, the excimer laser can make a sharp vertical cut with good depth control. Light microscopic studies show no damage to the adjacent tissues and no inflammatory reaction other than a thin pseudomembrane on the stromal edge [139] (Figure 4.55). Incisions that approach Descemet's membrane show endothelial cell rupture immediately over the excision site [140]. These wide excision sites (wherein the beam acts like a trenching tool—or Ditch Witch) provide a formidable obstacle for the epithelium to cross. These sites accumulate a large epithelial plug similar to that seen in wide gaping RK incisions or where such incisions cross. Marsupialization of such wounds is a distinct possibility but has not been reported to date [141].

Clinical studies of excimer laser photorefractive keratectomy have been reported [142]. Animal studies in rhesus monkeys demonstrate that corneal changes are limited to the area of laser treatment [143,144]. Immediately after ablation, a marked reduction in the numbers of keratocytes in the anterior stroma was seen. Damaged keratocytes were present within a week of treatment; epithelium had grown over the bare stroma and was thicker than

(a)

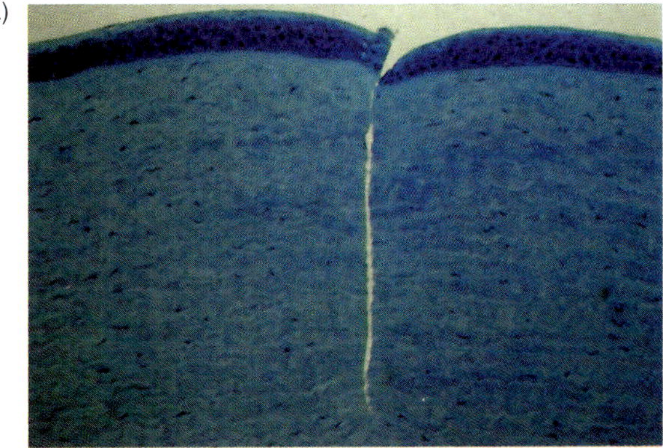

(b)

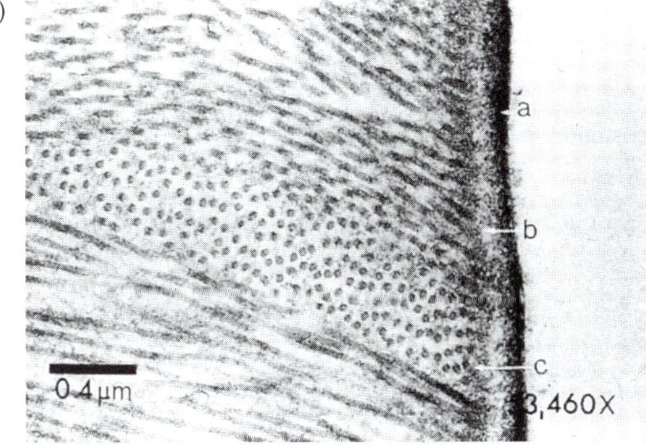

Fig. 4.55 (a) Incision made in rabbit cornea using 193-nm ultraviolet laser (excimer). (b) Edges are smooth, and the typical stromal edema and destruction seen in thermal burns are absent (from Puliafito CA, Steinert RF, Deutsch TF, Hillenkamp F, Dehm EJ, Adler CM. Excimer laser ablation of the cornea and lens: Experimental studies. Ophthalmology 1985; 92(6):741–748).

normal. Focal production of basement membrane and hemidesmosomes was seen. Marshall and coworkers hypothesize that a pseudo-Bowman's layer is created by the ablation process—supporting the establishment of a normal epithelial layer [145]. Fibroblasts were present in the anterior stroma.

By 3 weeks, there was a further increase in the number of fibroblasts in the anterior stroma. Electron microscopy of these cells showed intense metabolic activity, suggesting protein synthesis. The anterior stromal lamellae were irregular. Clumps of extracellular matrix were present adjacent to the fibroblasts [143,144]. Because ultraviolet (UV) light is known to be mutagenic, concern has been raised over the effect on tissue from far UV exposure. Nuss and colleagues demonstrated unscheduled DNA (a marker indicating chromosome damage) synthesis in corneal tissue subjected to both 193- and 248-nm radiation. The rate was much higher for 248-nm laser light [146]. Trentacoste found no increased incidence of anaplastic changes in fibroblast cell culture after exposure to 193-nm radiation [147].

Some of these animals showed a dense anterior stromal haze at 3 months. Microscopic study revealed dark basal cells with vacuolization at the stromal–epithelial junction. The basement membrane remained fragmented in these animals. Numerous fibroblasts and abundant ECM persisted. However, these features were absent in the animals that showed only minimal or absent corneal haze [143,144].

At 6 and 9 months after surgery, the severe changes had disappeared in most animals. Those with persistent haze continued to show some fragmentation of the basement membrane as well as a few active fibroblasts. Throughout the time periods, the posterior stroma, Descemet's membrane, and the corneal endothelium appeared within normal limits. Despite the changes noted in the basement membrane, recurrent epithelial erosions were not observed. The lack of uniformity in histopathology and clinical appearance was felt to be due to individual variation in response to the phototic injury [143,144].

Intraocular procedures

The effects on the cornea of implantation of an intraocular lens have been well documented [148–151]. Certain of these have been reduced by the advent of folding lens technology and small incisions, but they have not been eliminated completely. The possibility of corneal decompensation, while less, is still there—thus the concern with the implantation of intraocular lenses (IOLs) into phakic eyes. The poor results obtained by Strampelli and Barraquer cannot be ignored [152–154]. Some of these newer lenses are similar to the design of Kelman and rely on scleral angle fixation—with all that implies. Baikoff has reported endothelial cell loss in some of his cases—two severely [155,156]. At least one case of cataract formation has been reported with the angle-supported myopic lens [156]. While mild uveitis also has been reported, no cases of the uveitis-glaucoma-hyphema (UGH) syndrome have been reported to date. No clinical reports of the "collar button" lens advocated and implanted by Fyodorov's group are, as yet, available. It remains to be seen how well the crystalline lens tolerates these types of lenses. We will have somewhat more to say on these implants in Chapter 13.

Scleral procedures

The reader is referred to standard texts on ophthalmic pathology and retinal detachment surgery for a thorough discussion of the histology of these procedures (see also Chapter 14).

Principles of wound healing as applied to refractive surgery

The following is excerpted from Binder's excellent work [114] on healing in refractive surgery:

1. Permanent corneal curvature changes occur when Bowman's layer is severed.
2. Fewer radial incisions and a standard surgical approach to radial keratotomy may improve the safety, predictability, and stability of the procedure.
3. Optical interfaces tend to degrade the visual image. The potential space that is created can serve as a location for foreign material, keratocytes, and epithelium, which collectively have the potential to further degrade the visual image.
4. Freezing and lyophilization produce severe morphologic changes in the cornea. Refractive procedures that use fresh tissue appear safer.
5. Water-impermeable (bioincompatible) intrastromal implants cannot be used for refractive surgery.
6. All thermal collagen shrinkage procedures produce severe and permanent stromal damage and only temporarily produce collagen shrinkage.
7. The wound healing response of the cornea needs to be controlled if photorefractive keratectomy is to be successful.

The preceding pretty much encapsulates the current thinking in refractive surgery. The reader is advised to take note and heed these observations.

References

1 Schermer, A., S. Galvin, and T.T. Sun, Differentiation-related expression of a major 64K corneal keratin in vivo and in culture suggest limbal location for corneal epithelial stem cells. J Cell Biol 1986; 103:49–62.

2 Tseng, S. and K. Tsubota, Important concepts for treating ocular surface and tear disorders. Am J Ophthalmol 1997; 124:825–35.

3 Wirtschafter, J.D., J.M. Ketcham, R.J. Weinstock, *et al.*, Mucocutaneous junction as the major source of replacement conjunctival epithelial cells. Invest Ophthalmol Vis Sci 1999:40:3138–46.

4 Smith, R.S., N.L. Hawes, S.D. Kuhlmann, *et al.*, Corn1: A mouse model for corneal surface disease and neovascularization. Invest Ophthalmol Vis Sci 1996; 37:397–404.

5 Wagoner, M.D., Chemical injuries of the eye: current concepts in pathophysiology and therapy. Surv Ophthalmol 1997; 41: 275–313.

6 Assil, K.K. and A.J. Quantock, Wound healing in response to keratorefractive surgery. Surv Ophthalmol 1993; 38:289–302.

7 Nakamura, M., M. Kobayashi, K. Hirano, *et al.*, Glycosaminoglycan and collagen fibrillar interactions in the mouse corneal stroma. Matrix Biol 1994; 14:283–86.

8 Lamonde, S.R. and J.F. Bateman, Procollagen folding and assembly: The role of endoplasmic reticulum enzymes and molecular chaperones. Cell Develop Biol 1997; 10:455–64.

9 Chan, D., S.R. Lamande, D.J. McQuillan, *et al.*, In vitro expression analysis of collagen biosynthesis and assembly. J Biochem Biophys Methods 1997; 36:11–29.

10 Goes, R.M., E.M. Laicine, M.A. Porcionatto, *et al.*, Glycosaminoglycans in components of the rabbit eye: synthesis and characterization. Curr Eye Res 1999; 19:146–53.

11 Scott, J.E., Extracellular matrix, supramolecular organization and shape. J Anat 1995; 187:259–69.

12 Freegard, T.J., The physical basis of the transparency of the normal cornea. Eye 1997; 11:465–71.

13 Funderburgh, J.L., N.D. Hevelone, M.R. Roth, *et al.*, Decorin and biglycan of normal and pathologic human corneas. Invest Ophthalmol Vis Sci 1998; 39:1957–64.

14 Miller, D. and G. Benedek, *Intraocular Light Scattering*. Springfield CT: Thomas. 38,53–67; 1973.

15 Goldman, J., G. Benedek, C. Dohlman, *et al.*, Structural alterations affecting transparency in swollen human corneas. Invest Ophthalmol 1968; 7(5):501–519.

16 Farrell, R.A., R.L. McCalley, and P.E.R. Tatham, *Wavelength dependencies of light scattering in normal and cold swollen corneas and their structural implications*. J Physiol (London) 1976; 233:589.

17 Hedbys, B.O., The role of polysaccharides in corneal swelling. Exp Eye Res 1961; 1:81.

18 Newsome, D.A., J. Gross, and J.R. Hassell, Human corneal stroma contains three distinct collagens. Invest Ophthalmol Vis Sci 1981; 22:376.

19 Miller, E.J. and S. Gay, Collagen: an overview. Mthods Enzymol 1982; 82:3.

20 Piez, K.A. and A. Miller, The structure of collagen fibrils. J Supramol Struct 1974; 2:121.

21 Hogan, M.I., J.A. Alvarado, and J.E. Weddell, *Histology of the Human Eye*. W.B. Saunders Company. Philadelphia: 64–111; 1971.

22 Hodson, S. and S. Miller, The bicarbonate ion pump in the endothelium which regulates the hydration of the rabbit cornea. J Physiol (London) 1977; 203:563.

23 Hull, D.S., Corneal endothelial bicarbonate transport and the effect of carbonic anhydrase inhibitors on endothelial permiability and fluxes and corneal thickness. Invest Ophthalmol 1977; 16:883.

24 Baum, J.P., D.M. Maurice, and B.E. McCarey, The active and passive transport of water across the corneal endothelium. Exp Eye Res 1984; 39(3):335–342.

25 Dohlman, C.H., B. Wortman, B.O. Hedbys, *et al.*, The swelling pressure of the corneal stroma. Invest Ophthalmol Vis Sci 1963; 1:158.

26 Dohlman, C.H., *Physiology of the Cornea: Corneal Edema, in The Cornea. Scientific Foundations and Clinical Practice*, G. Smolin and R.A. Thoft, Editors. 1983, Little, Brown and Co: Boston/Toronto, 3–17.

27 Klyce, S.D., Electric profiles in the corneal epithelium. J Physiol (London) 1972; 226:407.

28 Manchester, P.T., Hydration of the cornea. Trans Am Ophthalmol Soc 1970; 68:425.

29 Zucker, B.B., Hydration and transparency of the corneal stroma. Arch Ophthalmol 1966; 75(2):228–31.

30 Fyodorov, S.N. and A. Agronovsky, Long Term results of anterior radial keratotomy. J Ocul Ther Surg 1982; 1:217.

31 Holly, F.J., Formation and rupture of the tear film. Exp Eye Res 1973; 15:515.

32 Lamberts, D.W., *Physiology of the cornea: Physiology of the tear film, in The Cornea. Scientific Foundations and Clinical Practice*, G. Smolin and R.A. Thoft, Editors. 1983, Little, Brown and Co: Boston/Toronto, 31–42.

33 Thoft, R.A. and J. Friend, Corneal epithelial glucose utilization. Arch Ophthalmol 1972; 88:58.

34 Gillette, T.E., J.V. Greiner, and M.R. Allansmith, Immunochemical localization of human tear lysozyme. Arch Ophthalmol 1981; 99:298.

35 Holly, F.J., The precorneal tear film. Contact Intraocular Lens Med J 1978; 4:134.

36 Patel, S., J. Farrell, K.J. Blades, *et al.*, The value of a phenol red impregnated thread for differentiating between the aqueous and non aqueous deficient dry eye. Ophthalmic Physiol Opt 1998; 18(6):471–6.

37 Tripathi, B.J., J.D. Geanon, and R.C. Tripathi, Distribution of tissue plasminogen activator in human and monkey eyes. An immunohistochemical study. Ophthalmology 1987; 94(11): 1434–8.

38 Geanon, J.D., B.J. Tripathi, R.C. Tripathi, *et al.*, Tissue plasminogen activator in avascular tissues of the eye: a quantitative study of its activity in the cornea, lens, and aqueous and vitreous humors of dog, calf, and monkey. Exp Eye Res 1987; 44(1):55–63.

39 McCracken, J.S., P.C. Burger, and G.K. Klintworth, Morphologic observations on experimental corneal vascularization in the rat. Lab Invest 1979; 41:519–530.

40 Buck, R.C., Cell migration in repair of corneal epithelium. Invest Ophthal Vis Sci 1979; 18:767–784.

41 Crosson, C.E., S.D. Klyce, and R.W. Beuerman, Epithelial wound closure in the rabbit cornea. Invest Ophthal Vis Sci 1986; 27: 464–473.

42 Soong, H. and B. McClenic, EGF Does not enhance corneal epithelial cell motility. Invest Ophthal Vis Sci 1989; 30:1808–1812.

43 Ding, M. and N.L. Burstein, Review: fibronectin in corneal wound healing. J Ocular Pharmacol 1988; 4:75–91.

44 Jumblatt, M.M. and A.H. Neufeld, A tissue culture assay of corneal epithelial wound closure. Invest Ophthal Vis Sci 1986; 27:8–13.

45 Levi–Montalcini, R. and V. Hamburger, A diffusable agent of mouse sarcoma producnig hyperplasia of sympathetic ganglia and hyperneurotization of viscera in the chick embryo. J Exp Zool 1953; 123:233–288.

46 Cohen, S., Isolation of a mouse submaxillary gland protein accelerating incisor eruption and eyelid opening in the new-born animal. J Biol Chem 1962; 237:1555–1562.

47 Baudouin, C., D. Fredj–Reygrobellet, and J. Caruelle, Acidic fibroblast growth factor distribution in normal human eye and possible implications in ocular pathogenesis. Ophthalmic Res 1990; 22:73–81.

48 Kitizawa, T., S. Kinoshita, and K. Fujita, The mechanism of accelerated corneal epithelial healing by human epidermal growth factor. Invest Ophthal Vis Sci 1990; 31:1773–1778.

49 Leibowitz, H.M., S.J. Morello, M. Stern, *et al.*, Effect of topically administered epidermal growth factor on corneal wound strength. Arch Ophthalmol 1990; 108(5):734–7.

50 Soubrane, G., J. Jerdoln, and I. Karpouzis, Binding of fibroblast growth factor to normal and neovascularized cornea. Invest Ophthal Vis Sci 1990; 31:323–333.

51 Gassner, H.L., M. Esco, M.W. Smithson, *et al.*, Differential effects of transforming growth factors on localization of adhesion complex proteins following corneal epithelial wounding. Curr Eye Res 1997; 16:387–95.

52 Fogle, J.A., K.R. Kenyon, W.J. Stark, *et al.*, Defective epithelial adhesion in anterior corneal dystrophies. Am J Ophthalmol 1975; 79:925–940.

53 Werblin, T.P., L.W. Hirst, W.J. Stark, *et al.*, Prevalence of map–dot–fingerprint changes in the cornea. Brit J Ophthalmol 1981; 79:925–940.

54 Campos, M., K. Szerenyi, M. Lee, *et al.*, Keratocyte loss after corneal deepithelialization in primates and rabbits. Arch Ophthalmol 1994; 112:254–60.

55 Thatte, U. and S. Dahanukar, Apoptosis: clinical relevance and pharmacological manipulation. Drugs 1997; 54:511–32.

56 Ashkenazi, A. and V.M. Dixit, Death receptors: signaling and modulation. Science 1998; 281:1305–8.

57 Evan, G. and T. Littlewood, A matter of life and cell death. Science 1998; 281:1317–22.

58 Wilson, S.E., Molecular cell biology for the refractive corneal surgeon: Programmed cell death and wound healing. J Refr Surg 1997; 13:171–75.

59 Wilson, S.E., Y. He, J. Weng, *et al.*, Epithelial injury induces keratocyte apoptosis: hypothesized role for the interleukin-1 system in the modulation of corneal tissue organization and wound healing. Exp Eye Res 1996; 62:325–37.

60 Wilson, S.E., Keratocyte apoptosis in refractive surgery. CLAO J 1998; 24:181–85.

61 Wilson, S.E., Stimulus-Specific and cell type-specific cascades: Emerging principles relating to control of apoptosis in the eye. Exp Eye Res 1999; 69:255–66.

62 Smith, R.S., L.A. Smith, L.F. Rich, *et al.*, Effects of growth factors on corneal wound healing. Invest Ophthal Vis Sci 1981; 20: 222–229.

63 Musch, D.C., A. Sugar, and R.F. Meyer, Demographic and predisposing factors in corneal ulceration. Arch Ophthalmol 1983; 101:1545–1548.

64 Berman, M., C.H. Dohlman, M. Gnadinger, *et al.*, Characterization of collagenolytic activity in the ulcerating cornea. Exp Eye Res 1971; 11(2):255–257.

65 Fraunfelder, F.T. and S.M. Meyer, *Drug Induced Ocular Side Effects and Drug Interactions.* Lea and Febiger; Philadelphia: 1989

66 Smith, R.S., *Clinical Diagnosis and Management,* in *Corneal Disorders,* H.M. Leibowitz, Editor. 1984, W.B. Saunders Company: Philadelphia. 499–509.

67 Claoue, C., S. Lewkowicz-Moss, and D. Easty, Epithelial cyst in the anterior chamber after penetrating keratoplasty: a rare complication. Br J Ophthalmol 1988; 72(1):36–40.

68 Stark, W.J. and R.G. Michels, A. Maumenee, *et al.*, Surgical management of epithelial ingrowth. Am J Ophthalmol 1970; 85; 772–780.

69 Yee, R.D. and T.H. Pettit, Corneal intrastromal cyst following lamellar keratoplasty. Ann Ophthalmol 1975; 7(5):644–646.

70 Kenyon, K.R., Decision–making in the therapy of external disease: non–infected corneal ulcers. Ophthalmology 1982;89:44–51.

71 Waring, G.O., M.M. Rodrigues, and P.A. Laibson, Corneal dystrophies. II. endothelial dystrophies. Surv Ophthalmol 1978; 23:147–168.

72 Wilson, S.E. and W. Kim, Keratocyte apoptosis: implications on corneal wound healing, tissue organization and disease. Invest Ophthalmol Vis Sci 1998; 39:220–26.

73 Weimar, V. and M. Fellman, Connective tissue cell mobilization and migration following wounding. I. inhibition of mobilization by chloroquine and inhibition of migration by colchicine. Exp Eye Res 1970; 9:12.

74 Cintron, A.C., H. Schneider, and C. Kublin, Corneal scar formation. Exp Eye Res 1973; 17:251–259.

75 McDonald, M.B., J.M. Frantz, S.D. Klyce, *et al.*, One-year refractive results of central photorefractive keratectomy for myopia in the nonhuman primate cornea. Arch Ophthalmol 1990; 108(1): 40–7.

76 Welch, M.P., G.F. Odland, and R.A. Clark, Temporal relationships of F–Actin bundle formation, collagen and fibronectin matrix assembly, and fibronectin receptor expression to wound contraction. J Cell Biol 1990; 110:133–145.

77 Cogan, D.G., Vascularization of the cornea. Its functional induction by small lesions and a new theory of its pathogenesis. Arch Ophthalmol 1949; 41:406–416.

78 Klintworth, G.K., The contribution of morphology to our understanding of the pathogenesis of experimentally produced corneal vascularhation. Invest Ophthal Vis Sci 1977; 16:281–284.

79 Furcht, L.T., Editorial: critical factors controlling angiogenesis: cell products, cell matrix and growth factors. Lab Invest 1986; 55:505–509.

80 Folkman, J. and M. Klagsbrun, Angiogenic factors. Science 1987; 235:442–447.

81 Folkman, J., Angiogenesis in cancer, vascular, rheumatoid and other disease. Nat Genet 1995; 1:27–31.

82 Folkman, J. and P.A. D'Amore, Blood vessel formation: what is its molecular basis. Cell 1996; 87:1153–55.

83 Miller, J.W., Vascular endothelial growth factor and ocular neovascularization. Am J Pathol 1997; 151:13–23.

84 Okamoto, N., T. Tobe, S.F. Hackett, *et al.*, Transgenic mice with increased expression of vascular endothelial growth factor in the retina. Am J Pathol 1997; 151:281–91.

85 Amano, S., R. Roban, M. Kuroki, *et al.*, Requirement for vascular endothelial growth factor in wound- and inflammation-related corneal neovascularization. Invest Ophthalmol Vis Sci 1998; 39:18–22.

86 BenEzra, D., B.W. Griffin, G. Maftzir, *et al.*, Thrombospondin and in vivo angiogenesis induced by basic fibroblast growth factor or lipopolysaccharide. Invest Ophthalmol Vis Sci 1993; 34:3601–08.

87 Jimenez, B., O.V. Volpert, S.E. Crawford, *et al.*, Signals leading to apoptosis-dependent inhibition of neovascularization by thrombospondin-1. Nature Med. 2000; 6:41–48.

88 Strieter, R.M., S.L. Kunkel, V.M. Einer, *et al.*, Interleukin-8: A corneal factor that induces neovascularization. Am J Pathol 1992; 141:1279–84.

89 Sunderkotter, C., J. Roth, and C. Sorg, Immunohistochemical detection of bFGF and TNF-α in the course of inflammatory angiogenesis in the mouse cornea. Am J Pathol 1990; 137:511–15.

90 Stoltz, R.A., M.S. Conners, M.E. Gerritsen, *et al.*, Direct stimulation of limbal microvessel endothelial cell proliferation and capillary formation in vitro by a corneal-derived eicosanoid. Am J Pathol 1996; 148:129–39.

91 Dawson, D.W., O.V. Volpert, P. Gillis, *et al.*, Pigment epithelium-derived factor: A potent inhibitor of angiogenesis. Science 199; 285:245–48.

92 Strieter, R.M., P. Polverini, D.A. Arenberg, *et al.*, The role of CXC chemokines as regulators of angiogenesis. Shock 1995; 4:155–60.

93 Duenas, Z., L. Torner, A.M. Corbacho, *et al.*, Inhibition of rat corneal angiogenesis by 16-kDa prolactin and by endogenous prolactin-like molecules. Invest Ophthalmol Vis Sci 1999; 40: 2498–2405.

94 Dameron, K.M., O.V. Volpert, M.A. Tainsky, *et al.*, Control of angiogenesis in fibroblasts by p53 regulation of thrombospondin-1. Science 1994; 265:1582–84.

95 Stellmach, V., O.V. Volpert, S.E. Crawford, *et al.*, Tumor suppressor genes and angiogenesis: the role of TP53 in fibroblasts. Eur J Cancer 1996; 32A:2394–2400.

96 Rak, J., J. Filmus, and R.S. Kerbel, Reciprocal paracrine interactions between tumor cells and endothelial cells: The 'angiogenesis progression' hypothesis. Eur J Cancer 1996; 32A: 2438–50.

97 Laing, R.A., L. Neubauer, and S.S. Oak, Evidence for mitosis in the adult corneal endothelium. Ophthalmology 1984; 91: 1129–1134.

98 Joyce, N.C., B. Meklir, and A.H. Neufeld, In vitro pharmacologic separation of corneal endothelial migration and spreading responses. Invest Ophthal Vis Sci 1990; 31:1816–1826.

99 Smith, R.S. and J. Cutro, Computer analysis of radial keratotomy. CLAO J 1984; 10(3):241–8.

100 MacRae, S.M., M. Matsuda, and L.F. Rich, The effect of radial keratotomy on the corneal endothelium. Am J Ophthalmol 1985; 100:538–542.

101 Read, R.W., R. Chuck, N.A. Rao, *et al.*, Traumatic acremonium atrogriseum keratitis following Laser-assisted in situ keratomileusis. Arch Ophthalmol 2000; 118:418–21.

102 Smith, R.J. and R.K. Maloney, Diffuse lamellar keratitis. Ophthalmology 1998; 105:1721–26.

103 Vesaluoma, M., J. Perez-Santonja, W.M. Petroll, *et al.*, Corneal stromal changes induced by myopic LASIK. Invest Ophthalmol Vis Sci 2000; 41:369–76.

104 Ormerod, L.D. and R.E. Smith, Contract lens-associated microbial keratitis. Arch Ophthalmol 1986; 104 (1):79–83.

105 Schein, O.D., R.J. Glynn, and E.C. Poggio, The relative risk of ulcerative keratitis among users of daily–wear and extended–wear soft contact lenses. New Eng J Med 1989; 321:773–778.

106 Ingraham, H.J., D. Guber, and W.R. Green, Radial keratotomy. Clinicopathologic case report. Arch Ophthalmol 1985; 103 (5): 683–8.

107 Binder, P.S., S.K. Nayak, J.K. Deg. *et al.*, An ultrastructural and histochemical study of long-term wound healing after radial keratotomy. Am J Ophthalmol 1987; 103(3 Pt 2):432–40.

108 Yamaguchi, T., H.E. Kaufman, A. Fukushima, *et al.*, Histologic and electron microscopic assessment of endothelial damage produced by anterior radial keratotomy in the monkey cornea. Am J Ophthalmol 1981; 92(3):313–327.

109 Jester, J.V., R.A. Villasenor, and J. Miyashiro, Epithelial inclusion cysts following radial keratotomy. Arch Ophthalmol 1983; 101 (4):611–615.

110 Kurasova, T.P., *Klinicheskoe techenie posleoperatzionnovo perioda pri keratotomii (Clinical course of the postoperative period following keratotomy), in Surgery of Refractive Anomalies of the Eye,* A.I. Ivashina and S.A. Kolmanovskii, Editors. 1981, Moscow Scientific Research Institute for Eye Microsurgery: Moscow. 27–32.

111 Waring, G.O., E.B. Steinberg, and L.A. Wilson, Slit lamp microscopic appearance of corneal wound healing after radial keratotomy. Am J Ophthalmol 1985; 100:218–224.

112 Coalwell, K. and P.S. Binder, High voltage electron microscopic evaluation of human radial keratotomy. Invest Ophthalmol Vis Sci (AMA Abstract) 1988; 29:280.

113 Davison, P.S. and E.J. Galbavy, Connective tissue remodeling in corneal and scleral wounds. Invest Ophthalmol Vis Sci 1986; 27:1478–1484.

114 Binder, P.S., What we have learned about corneal wound healing from refractive surgery (Barraquer Lecture). Refract and Corneal Surg 1989; 5(2):98–120.

115 Nelson, J.D., P. Williams, R.L. Lindstrom, *et al.*, Map-fingerprint-dot changes in the corneal epithelial basement membrane following radial keratotomy. Ophthalmology 1985; 92 (2):199–205.

116 Deg, J.K. and P.S. Binder, Wound healing after astigmatic keratotomy in human eyes. Ophthalmol 1987; 94:1290–1298.

117 Aquavella, J.V., R.S. Smith, and E.L. Shaw, Alteration in corneal morphology following thermokeratoplasty. Arch Ophthalmol 1976; 94(12):2082–2085.

118 Barraquer, J.I., *Cirugia Refractiva de la Cornea: Queratofaquia.* Vol. 1. Bogota Columbia: Instituto Barraquer de America. 328–353; 1989.

119 Pokorny, K.S., K.R. Kenyon, C. Swinger, *et al.*, Histopathology of human keratorefractive lenticules. Cornea 1990 9(3):223–233.

120 Bores, L.D., Unpublished data, 1991.

121 Bores, L.D., Mechanical modulation of the corneal surface. Int Clinics Ophth 1991; 31(1):25–36.

122 Krumeich, J.H. and A. Knuelle, [Non-freeze epikeratophakia (Live epikeratophakia)]. Fortschr Ophthalmol 1990; 87(1):20–24.

123 Krumeich, J.H. and C.A. Swinger, Nonfreeze epikeratophakia for the correction of myopia. Am J Ophthalmol 1987; 103 (3 Pt 2): 397–403.

124 Lieurance, R.C., A.C. Patel, W.L. Wan, *et al.*, Excimer laser cut lenticules for epikeratophakia. Am J Ophthalmol 1987; 103 (3 Pt 2):475–476.

125 Maguen, K., S. Pinhas, and S.M. Verity, Keratophakia with lyophilized cornea lathed at room temperature: New techniques and experimental surgical results. Ophthalmic Surg 1983; 14:759–762.

126 Binder, P.S., J.H. Krumeich, and E.V. Zavala, Laboratory evaluation of freeze vs non-freeze lamellar refractive keratoplasty. Arch Ophthalmol 1987; 105(8):1125–1128.

127 Rostron, C.K., G.P. Brittain, D.B. Morton, *et al.*, Experimental epikeratophakia with biological adhesive. Arch Ophthalmol 1988; 106(8):1103–1106.

128 Zavala, E.Y., J. Krumeich, and P.S. Binder, Clinical pathology of non-freeze lamellar refractive keratoplasty. Cornea 1988; 7(3):223–230.

129 El Maghraby, M.A., E. Vitero, and L. Ruiz, Keratomileusis in situ to correct high myopia. Ophthalmology 1988; 95 (Suppl):145.

130 Jaeger, M.J., P. Berson, H.E. Kaufman, *et al.*, Epikeratoplasty for keratoconus. A clinicopathologic case report. Cornea 1987; 6 (2): 131–139.

131 Steinert, R.F. and R.B. Grene, Postoperative management of epikeratoplasty. J Cataract Refract Surg 1986; 14:225–264.

132 Binder, P.S., E.Y. Zavala, S.D. Baumgartner, *et al.*, Combined morphologic effects of cryolathing and lyophilization on epikeratoplasty lenticules. Arch Ophthalmol 1986; 104 (5):671–679.

133 Binder, P.S., J.P.J. Beal, and E.Y. Zavala, The histopathology of a case of keratophakia. Arch Ophthalmol 1982; 100 (1):101–105.

134 Binder, P.S., S.D. Baumgartner, and J.A. Fogle, Histopathology of a case of epikeratophakia (aphakic epikeratoplasty). Arch Ophthalmol 1985; 103 (9):1357–1363.

135 Dietze, T.R. and D.S. Durrie, Indications and treatment of keratoconus using epikeratophakia. Ophthalmology 1988; 95 (2): 236–246.

136 Climenhaga, H., J.M. Macdonald, B.E. McCarey, *et al.*, Effect of diameter and depth on the response to solid policysulfone intracorneal lenses in cats. Arch Ophthalmol 1988; 106(6):818–24.

137 Lane, S.S., R.L. Lindstrom, and J.D. Cameron, Fenestrated intracorneal lenses. Ophthalmology 1987; 94(Suppl):125.

138 Beekhuis, W.H., B.E. McCarey, G. van Rij, *et al.*, Complications of hydrogel intracorneal lenses in monkeys. Arch Ophthalmol 1987; 105(1):116–22.

139 Trokel, S.L., R. Srinivasan, and B. Braren, Excimer laser surgery of the cornea. Am J Ophthalmol 1983; 96(6):710–5.

140 Dehm, E.J., C.A. Puliafito, and C.M. Adler, Corneal endothelial injury in rabbits following excimer laser ablation of 193 and 248 nm. Arch Ophthalmol 1986; 104:1364–1368.

141 Fenzl, R.E., personal communication. 1991.

142 Taylor, D.M., F.A. L'Esperance, Jr., R.A. Del Pero, *et al.*, Human excimer laser lamellar keratectomy. A clinical study. Ophthalmology 1989; 96(5):654–64.

143 Fantes, F., K.D. Hanna, G.O. Waring, *et al.*, Wound healing after excimer laser keratomileusis (photorefractive keratectomy) in monkeys. Arch Ophthalmol 1990; 108:665–675.
144 SundarRaj, N., M.J. Geiss, F. Fantes, *et al.*, Healing of excimer laser ablated monkey corneas. An immunohistochemical evaluation. Arch Ophthalmol 1990; 108(11):1604–10.
145 Marshall, W.J., S.L. Trokel, and S. Rothery, Photoablation reprofiling of the cornea using an excimer laser photorefractive keratectomy. Lasers in Ophthalmology 1986; 1:21–48.
146 Nuss, R.C., C.A. Puliafito, and E. Dehm, Unscheduled DNA synthesis following excimer laser ablation of the cornea in vivo. Invest Ophthal & Vis Sci 1987; 28(2):287–294.
147 Trentacoste, J., K. Thompson, R.K. Parrish, *et al.*, Mutagenic potential of a 193-nm excimer laser on fibroblasts in tissue culture. Ophthalmology 1987; 94(2):125–9.
148 Castroviejo, R., Comments on cataract surgery. Usual and unusual procedures including an evaluation of cryoextraction. Am J Ophthalmol 1966; 61(5):1063–77.
149 Charlin, R., Peripheral corneal edema after cataract extraction. Am J Ophthalmol 1985; 99(3):298–303.
150 Cotlier, E. and M. Rose, Cataract extraction by the intracapsular methods and by phacoemulsification: the results of surgeons in training. Trans Am Acad Ophthalmol Otolaryngol 1976; 81 (1): 163–182.
151 Panariello, G.F. and J. Cooper, Complications in cataract surgery. J Am Optom Assoc 1983; 54 (8):713–718.
152 Strampelli, B., Lentilles camerulaires Après 6 années d'experiences. Acta Conc Ophtal Belgica (Brussels) 1958; 11:1692–1698.
153 Strampelli, B., Sopportabilita di lenti acriliche in camera anteriore nella afachia e nei vizi di refrazione. Atti Soc Oftal Lomb 1953; 8:292.
154 Barraquer, J., Anterior chamber plastic lenses. Results and conclusions from 5 year's experience. Trans Ophthalmol Soc (UK) 1959; 79:393–424.
155 Baikoff, G. and J. Colin, Damage to the corneal endothelium using anterior chamber intraocular lenses for myopia: letter. Refract Corneal Surg 1990; 6(5):383.
156 Baikoff, G., The refractive IOL in a phakic eye. Ophthalmic Practice 1991; 9(2):58–61.

5
Patient Workup

Science is facts, just as houses are made of stones, so is science made of facts; but a pile of stones is not a house and a collection of facts is not necessarily science.
[Henri Poincaré]

The proper evaluation of a candidate for refractive surgery includes a number of considerations. The following criteria are those currently used to screen candidates for refractive surgery within the author's clinic. These are subject to modification by circumstances that may arise from time to time.

- Any patient whose age is 18 or more and whose myopia is greater than 1.00 D and who has shown no progression of the myopia for the last 18 months. This does not preclude anisometropic children. However, no protocol for children has as yet been evolved. A change of ±0.50 D within a year is considered normal. A change of 1.0 D within a year is considered significant. In addition, any patient (as above) whose hyperopia is greater than 1.50 D.
- Patients with astigmatism greater than 1.00 D (or 20% of the spherical component) are also candidates but require special procedures (see Chapter 9).
- Patients with corneal curvatures of less than 40 D are not considered good candidates for most refractive surgery techniques unless they have low to moderate myopia.
- No evidence of corneal disease and/or dystrophic changes can be present.
- Any patient with an external ocular disease process should be off medication and clear for 3 months before scheduling surgery. Surgery on patients with a past history of actual or suspected herpes simplex keratitis is contraindicated.

Patient evaluation

The following workup procedure is offered as a guide to establishing your own specific schedule. Recommendations will be made as appropriate within this outline in order to establish those points I deem important. The general outline of the workup process will be followed by a more detailed description of the actual examination procedures.

Preliminary screening and intake

Patients will inquire of your receptionist to find out if indeed you do perform refractive surgery. The receptionist should be prepared to answer this question as well as those of a more general nature—briefly. It is suggested that patients be offered information about the surgery either by mail or by pickup. This information can take many forms.

To determine whether a patient is a possible candidate prior to making an appointment, the receptionist should request that the patient bring or mail in copies of his or her most current eyeglass and contact lens prescriptions (if available). This is particularly important for patients intending to travel long distances for this service. In such cases, this information is vitally important and may save the patient considerable time and expense.

Dealing with contact lenses

When making an appointment for a patient, the receptionist should ascertain if the caller is a contact lens wearer and what type lens is being worn. The patient is requested to remove any contact lenses for the period of time that you have determined adequate (Table 5.1). For example, hard contacts should be out for a minimum of 7 days—longer if possible. The length of time can be adjusted depending on the time duration of spectacle blur. At my clinic, I add 3 days for each 30 minutes of spectacle blur. As an example, a patient experiences 45 minutes of blur from the time she removes her contacts until she can see clearly with her current spectacles. The length of time that she should have her lenses out would be 7 + 4 = 11 days—minimum. Patients like this should be routed to your nurse or assistant to ensure that the response obtained is correct. Soft contacts should be removed for a minimum of 48 hours. On the other hand, if the patient is wearing "retainer lenses" for orthokeratology, these lenses must be out a minimum of 6 months! These lenses are known to produce long-standing corneal distortion [1–3].

An occasional patient will state that he or she does not have "fall-back" spectacles. In this situation, the nurse or assistant should become involved. The patient is requested to remove the lens from the nondominant eye for the duration specified. If coming from a distance, he or she should be advised to obtain an inexpensive pair of spectacles (or find an old pair) that can be worn in the interim.

Patients should bring with them any old optical aids that they have retained and that may have been worn in the last few years. These will be useful during the initial visit to determine how stable the patient's refraction and keratometry readings are. Old prescriptions are also requested to be brought.

Table 5.1 Length of time contact lenses should be removed before the initial visit

Lens type	Minimum time*
Hard	1 week
Soft	48 hours
Ortho-K	6 months

*See text.

The initial visit

Workup outline

1 Complete ocular history
2 Visual acuity—corrected/uncorrected (near and far)
3 Refraction—cycloplegic as warranted
4 Intra-ocular pressure
5 Keratometry
6 Slit-lamp examination
7 Measurement of corneal diameter
8 Determine dominant eye/handedness
9 Funduscopic examination
10 Viewing of informed consent videotape
11 Patient questions to be answered
12 Record patient expectations on chart

A patient intake form is to be supplemented through careful history taking by your nurse or assistant (Figure 5.1). Reading over this form and your nurse's notes is helpful prior to examining the patient yourself and may suggest some important avenues to explore further. After this form is filled out, it should be checked by the receptionist and any blanks filled in or marked "NA" by inquiry. Sometimes patients will prefer not to reveal some history to the receptionist. In this event, that fact should be noted or flagged to the attention of the doctor and/or nurse to be followed up. The receptionist should photocopy all submitted prescriptions, referral letters, etc., during this period and attach them to the chart. Any spectacles should be neutralized, the age of each noted, and this information affixed to the record as well.

Keratoconus

Although epikeratoplasty (see Chapter 10) has been more or less shelved as a primary procedure for routine use, it should be considered as an alternative to photoablative refractive keratectomy (PKP) in some keratoconus cases. I have had success in cases with small cones and in those with traumatic ectasia. Others have reported good results in such cases as well [4]. In some cases, the lenticule can be shaped on a cryolathe to assist in correcting any accompanying refractive error; cryolathing is not a dead art by any means. I have done this successfully in these cases, the only problem being to assess a representative power. A rigid contact lens can help here.

Dry eyes

Treatment

The usual treatment modality for dry eye is the administration of tear substitutes containing various wetting agents. While these work well for the milder forms of this problem, more severe cases may require punctual plugs. Even wetting drops and punctual occlusion may not solve the problem, however. This seems to be the case in dry eye occurring after laser in situ keratomileusis (LASIK; see also Chapter 15). Attempts at treating severe cases with cyclosporine in a 0.05% solution applied topically have shown promise [5,6]. Autologous serum also has shown promise in Sjögren's and other severe forms of keratitis sicca [7].

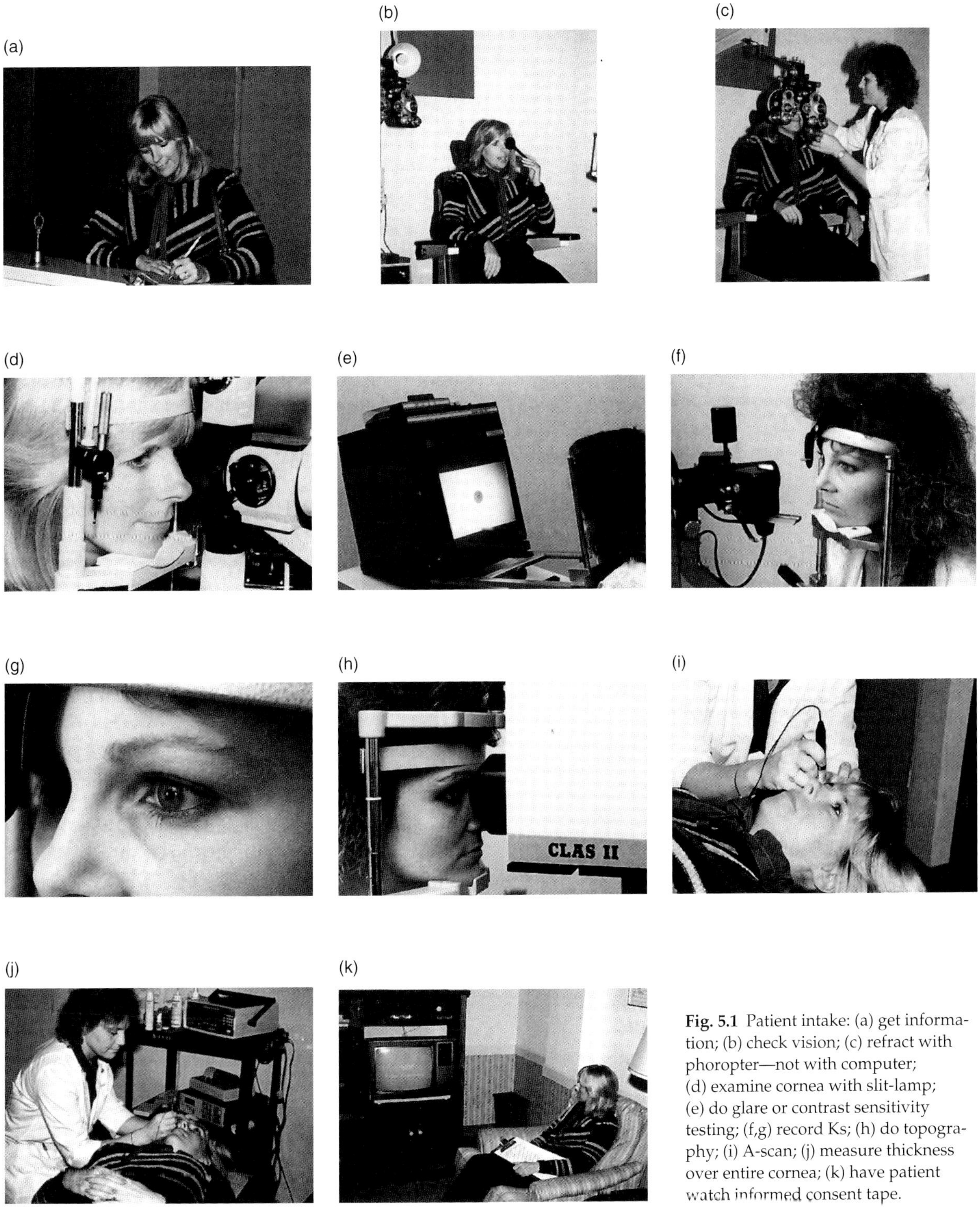

(a) (b) (c)

(d) (e) (f)

(g) (h) (i)

(j)

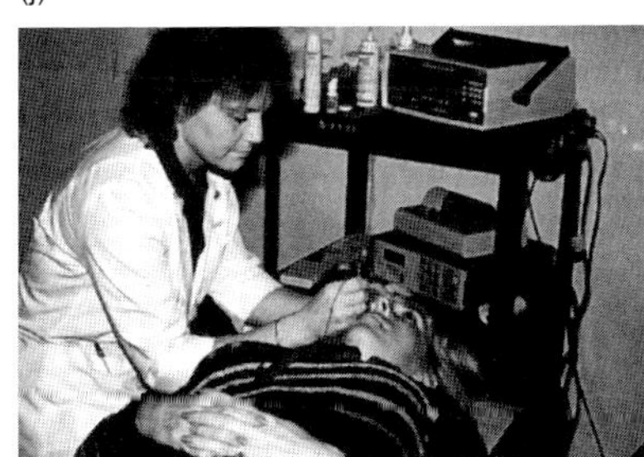

(k)

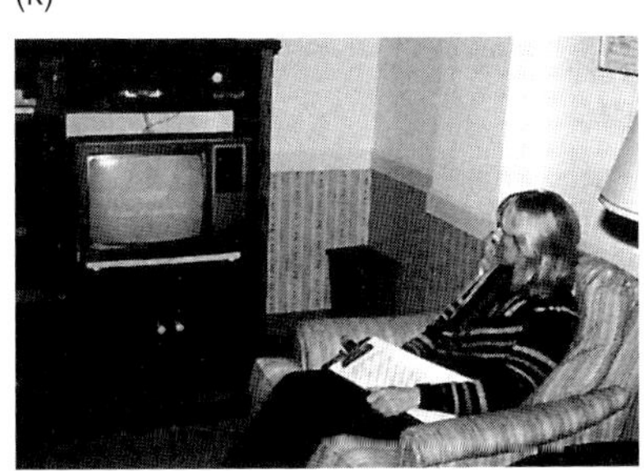

Fig. 5.1 Patient intake: (a) get information; (b) check vision; (c) refract with phoropter—not with computer; (d) examine cornea with slit-lamp; (e) do glare or contrast sensitivity testing; (f,g) record Ks; (h) do topography; (i) A-scan; (j) measure thickness over entire cornea; (k) have patient watch informed consent tape.

The refractive surgeon must maintain a high index of suspicion when contemplating corneal refractive surgery in middle-aged adults, particularly women, so as to avoid aggravating a preexisting problem or creating one. Sjögren's syndrome affects approximately 3 million people in the United States alone. Until recently, it has been thought to be the result of immune-related destruction of the lacrimal and salivary glands and associated nerves. It was thought that somehow the immune system invaded both the lacrimal and salivary glands and then started destroying tissue and that this also altered the enervation of tissue. Results from two studies, however, run counter to this theory. In the first of two studies done in a murine model, results indicated that the nerves of the lacrimal gland were still present but that tear secretion was being blocked by a problem in the signaling pathway. Cytokines originally secreted by the lymphocytes are probably regulating the secretions of the lacrimal acinar cells, also secreting that cytokine, preventing the release of neurotransmitters. Results of the second study showed that when an agonist was added to mimic the neurotransmitters, the nerves operated properly, indicating that they were still capable of functioning [8]. This could mean new therapy for Sjögren's sufferers as well as providing clues to the mechanism of a problem afflicting millions more.

The workup

The patient is placed into an examination room, where preliminary data are obtained. A careful recording of the patient's visual acuity both with and without correction is vital. If the patient is a contact lens wearer, the lens should be removed before the initial visit and must be kept out for a period of time corresponding to the type of lens and amount of spectacle blur experienced after removal (see above). In these cases, I recommend a pre-examination or acuity screening visit prior to the workup, if possible.

Contrast sensitivity and/or "glare" testing also should be performed, especially in contact lens wearers. There has been some discussion about the validity of devices such as the Miller-Nadler Contrast Tester (marketed by the Titmus Company). It has been said that devices such as these do not truly measure glare, but rather—flare. Since there is no general agreement as to the definition of *glare* and/or *flare,* it is difficult to decide this question unequivocally. Test results from these instruments do not correlate well with so-called contrast sensitivity testers—each appears to be measuring something different. Still, the results of such tests seem to relate to the real world much more closely than do high-contrast Snellen letter charts. Furthermore, the results of such tests may bear on the experience of the patient postoperatively.

The acuity measurement very much depends on the contrast of the letter with the background. Unfortunately, the technique has few counterparts in the real world, and equally unfortunate is the fact that it is firmly entrenched in society. It is well known in clinical practice that the visual acuity as measured by the Snellen chart is often in no way indicative of the existence of an actual visual handicap. Many individuals with increased lenticular turbidity can discern 20/40 or better and yet be unable to recognize a face in normal lighting or drive safely at night. Contrast sensitivity methods are probably a more realistic test of visual efficiency, but a standard has still not been established for their use.

It would be well to consider that the Snellen optotypes were invented over 125 years ago. They have been used universally and religiously ever since to record visual acuity. *Religiously* is not too strong a word to use in connection with the Snellen vision chart—mainly because its employment is almost a matter of Canonical Law. To suggest that it is time it was supplanted by a modern method that has more relevance to the real world is seemingly to commit an act of heresy, with all that act implies. Yet the Snellen chart measures only the ability of an eye to discern the shapes of high-contrast objects—not the actual efficiency of the visual system in a normal environment. It is not unusual for an individual to score 20/40 vision on a Snellen chart and yet be unable to recognize a familiar face at arm's length. This same individual may be found to fail a contrast sensitivity test altogether. Regardless, such a Snellen visual acuity score permits this individual to drive an automobile—day or night—regardless of the fact that his or her visual efficiency may be below par. However, until such time as these contrast sensitivity measuring devices are standardized, their results will not be universally accepted. That's the nice thing about glare "standards"—there are so many to choose from. Nonetheless, their employment in the evaluation of pre- and postoperative refractive surgery patients is highly recommended and in my clinic—mandatory.

Glare testing generally follows the recording of the visual acuity, after which the keratometry readings are also recorded. The sequence of events is arranged so as to produce the least possible alteration in the results of the following examination. In any case, pachymetry and the intraocular pressure (IOP) are the last measurements to be taken—after the informed consent.

The informed consent

The patient is then removed to the secondary waiting area, where, alone or with others, he or she views an informed consent videotape presentation. A short written examination follows this video presentation and is so arranged as to ensure that the essential material is understood by the viewer. The patient is then returned to the examination room and awaits refraction, slit-lamp examination, funduscopy, etc.

When the examination is completed, any questions that the patient may have are answered. Patients are then asked if there are any more questions that they would like answered—if the answer is yes, these additional questions are answered. If no other questions are pending, then the informed consent portion of the examination is ended. However, the patient is encouraged to write down any questions that inevitably come up after leaving the office so as to have them answered at a later time. Complete candor is essential at this point. If the patient is a candidate for surgery, his or her expectations are recorded, in his or her own words, into the record. If the patient agrees to have surgery performed, he or she is required to sign both the video test and the informed consent form—even though surgery may not yet be scheduled. Patients are assured that they are under no obligation when they do this and may change their minds—at any time. It is important to get the consent form signed while everything is fresh in the patient's mind and, more important, to avoid the possibility of the patient reaching the operating room with an unsigned consent form. Once the patient is premedicated, it is too late to get the consent form signed—postponing the surgery until a later day (at least a week hence) is the only alternative. In any case, at this point the patient is ready for the preoperative testing and is placed into the surgical workup queue. Photokeratometry and/or corneal surface topography needs to be done, and lastly, pachymetry, axial length, and the IOP are recorded.

One of the questions frequently asked by patients is their chance for success. The answer should be based on *your* percentage of success in cases similar to their own. Success is described as the achievement of 20/40 unaided visual acuity postoperatively. You can demonstrate varying degrees of refractive error reduction for a patient by adjusting his or her correction within the phoropter or trial frame and allowing the patient to observe the surroundings with and without this correction. You may find that, in some cases, uncorrected vision of less than 20/20 is acceptable to the patient. In this event, patients will express themselves, and this also should be recorded in the record. This process can help patients decide whether or not the surgery meets their needs. If a patient's expectations seem unreasonable or the patient insists on or expects "perfect" vision after surgery, gently but firmly suggest that the patient reconsider having any such surgery performed on his or her eyes and then dismiss this patient.

Gathering preoperative data

It should be evident by now that although the outcome of radial keratotomy (RK) surgery (for example) is inversely related to the size of the surgical optic zone (Figure 5.2), there are other factors that have been shown to modify this outcome as well. The "trick" in all of this is to combine these factors into a surgical plan that will produce a satisfactory result—satisfactory to the patient and the surgeon alike. This is also true of any of the various refractive surgical procedures. During the workup of the patient, you will be gathering the raw materials to determine the surgical parameters you will use. It will behoove you to make sure that the data obtained are as accurate and complete as possible and that no shortcuts are taken—either in the gathering of the data or, ultimately, in the performance of the surgery.

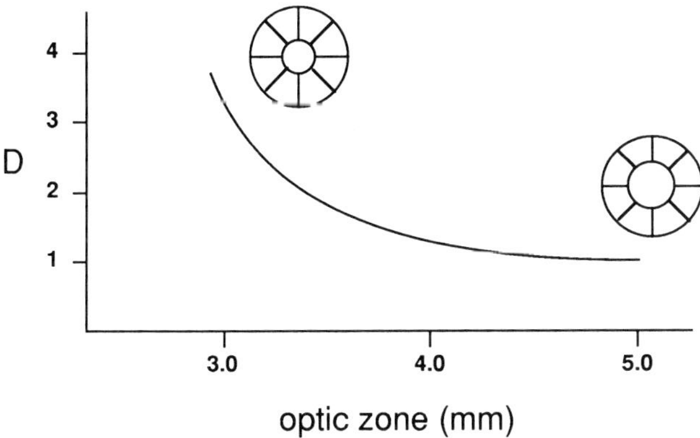

Fig. 5.2 Effect of optic zone size on surgical outcome.

Some of the tests suggested, such as A-scan, endothelial studies, AC depth, etc., may not seem to be strictly required for evaluation from a surgical standpoint. However, some of these measurements are essential in high myopia, and it is recommended that you make them, especially if you hope to obtain accurate predictions with the computer programs.

Visual acuity

Any method of determining the visual acuity is acceptable as long as the method is standardized for all patients. If you have more than one refraction lane, make sure that the projectors used are the same as well as the room lengths. If this cannot be done, perform the acuity testing in one specific room. Try to keep the room lighting at the same level for each examination and the methodology of testing the same as well. Record the acuity for each eye separately with and without correction both for near and distance, and then test binocular acuity as well. The recommended acuity chart is that promulgated by the National Eye Institute (NEI). A separate chart is used for each eye (to minimize chances for a patient memorizing the letters). It is possible to use the logarithm of the minimal angle of resolution (log MAR), which for the NEI chart changes 0.1 unit for each line. Each line has five letters; thus each letter can be assigned a value (0.02 log MAR), and the total of all the letters read correctly results in a visual acuity score. The 20/200 equivalent line is assigned a log MAR value of +1.0, whereas 20/20 is valued at 0.0 units. If an individual reads down to the 20/50 line (value +0.4) plus 2 letters from the 20/40 line ($0.02 \times 2 = 0.04$), the score would be $0.4 - 0.04 = 0.36$. The lower the score, the better is the vision (Table 5.2). If your clinic is performing outcome analyses, the ETDRS illuminated acuity chart available from Precision Vision is recommended for determining visual acuities.

Ocular dominance

An attempt should be made to determine which of the eyes is dominant. Typically this will correspond to the handedness of the patient—but not in all cases. It is crucial that surgical planning take this factor into account. The rationale for determining ocular dominance is simply to indicate which eye will have the surgery first. Experience

Table 5.2 Comparison of methods of Snellen visual acuity notation with logarithm of the minimal angle of resolution (log MAR) values. From Ferris FL, Kassoff A, Bresnick AH. New visual acuity charts for clinical research. Am J Ophthalmol 1982; 94:91–96

6 m	20 ft	Decimal equivalent	Log MAR
6/60	20/200	0.10	+1.0
6/48	20/160	0.125	+0.9
6/38	20/125	0.16	+0.8
6/30	20/100	0.20	+0.7
6/24	20/80	0.25	+0.6
6/20	20/63	0.32	+0.5
6/15	20/50	0.40	+0.4
6/12	20/40	0.50	+0.3
6/10	20/32	0.63	+0.2
6/7.5	20/25	0.80	+0.1
6/6	20/20	1.00	0.0
6/5	20/16	1.25	−0.1
6/3.75	20/12.5	1.60	−0.2
6/3	20/10	2.00	−0.3

has shown that the postoperative course of patients is much smoother when the nondominant eye is operated on first. There are compelling reasons for this approach—not the least of which is the relative unpredictability of the current surgical techniques. Since the two eyes can be assumed to have the same physical and healing characteristics (except in unusual cases of anisometropia), the first eye acts as the bellwether for the other, or "workhorse," eye.

Allowing sufficient time for the eye to react to surgery points up any potential over- or undershoot in the results of the first procedure, which knowledge can be applied to the second. This is of special significance if one is planning "monovision." It is simply not possible to know in advance the exact results of your surgical plan. Thus, if you are attempting to undercorrect one eye, it makes more sense to operate on the reading eye for the lesser amount first and find out where it ends up. Hence, if the patient is very undercorrected, allowances can be made for this in the other eye, and the first eye can be corrected further later. If there is an overcorrection (unlikely but possible), an unpleasant "surprise" is avoided. This is so because it can be used as a control for the fellow or dominant eye. Thus any "misses" can be corrected for in the dominant eye. In case of over- or undercorrection, the nondominant eye will cause fewer postoperative problems to the patient. In addition, the side effects of the surgery are better tolerated in this eye. By the time the patient is ready to have the other eye done, he or she will be better equipped to handle any postoperative sequelae.

Generally speaking, do not schedule surgery on the fellow eye until the first eye has achieved a vision of at least 20/40—with or without correction—or is at a level, at 1 week, that experience leads you to believe will come up to 20/40 or better within a reasonable period of time. This has been standard procedure at my clinic from the beginning, and I have never had cause to regret it. However, if the correction has been sufficiently successful so as to produce some degree of symptomatic anisometropia, it is better to continue with the second eye as soon as possible. This is true even if an overcorrection has occurred with the first surgery. It is unlikely that a similar overcorrection will occur in the second eye, but even if it should, the patient will be much better served by that condition than by one of major anisometropia that would result if the second eye were left untouched.

Regardless of any normal high score on the preoperative testing for glare, some patients may experience incapacitating glare postoperatively. This problem proves to be easier to cope with when it is the nondominant eye that is affected. A legitimate question then is: "What happens when it's the other eye's turn?" The answer is that patients seem to cope with the glare much more easily after they have experienced it and single vision the first time in the nondominant eye.

Many tests for determining ocular dominance depend on correspondence with handedness. A more objective method, proposed by Milder and Rubin, is recommended [9]. A 2.5 cm (approximately 1 in.) circular hole is cut in the center of an $8\frac{1}{2} \times 11$ in. white piece of cardboard. The patient, seated in the examining chair, is instructed to hold the paper in his or her lap with both hands and to observe a 20/100 letter on the screen. The following instruction is then given: "Keep both eyes on the letter, quickly lift the paper up with your arms extended in front of you, and observe the letter through the hole with both eyes. Keep the letter in view and slowly bring the card toward your face." The hole will be in front of the dominant eye. This procedure is repeated five times, and the eye that is dominant three or more times is recorded as the dominant eye. The number of times this eye appeared to be dominant out of five is recorded for future reference.

Near point of accommodation

Mount a Prince rule on a phoroptor, and place either a Rosenbaum pocket vision screener card or the standard Prince rule reading card in the clip. Place the patient's manifest refraction in the phoroptor before each eye. Slide the test card toward the patient, and have him or her read the 6-point (20/40) print. If the patient can see the print at 40 cm, continue to slide the test card toward the patient, instructing him or her to identify the point at which the print begins to blur. If it is difficult to tell this end point and the patient has 6/6 visual acuity, try the small 5 or 4 point print, which may detect the point of blur more precisely. If the patient cannot see the print at 40 cm, place a +1.50 D lens in front of each eye and increase the power of the lens until the patient can see the print at 40 cm. Then slide the test card toward the patient and detect the first point of blur. If the patient's best corrected visual acuity is worse than 6/6 (20/20), use a test type that is big enough that the patient can see it at 40 cm.

Record the results as follows:

- Print size (in point notation)
- Power of the additional plus lens in the phoroptor
- The location on the Prince rule where the first blur occurred, in both centimeters and diopters

Corneal diameter (Figure 5.3)

Note that there is space provided for "corneal diameter" on the biometry form as well as the evaluation form. While this is important in the final outcome (see Chapter 7), no one has as yet suggested a foolproof method of determining the exact diameter of the cornea—as those of you who have implanted anterior chamber lenses can attest. The use of a Castroviejo muscle caliper is recommended for this purpose. The cornea is measured from "white to white" at 90°, 180°, 45°, and 135°, and each measurement recorded. The average of these four readings is taken as the nominal corneal diameter.

Scleral rigidity

Scleral rigidity is an important measurement and must be derived either by using the Maklakov tonometer or by allowing the computer to calculate the statistical mean for you.

For years physicians in the former Soviet Union have been taking measurements of intraocular pressure using the Maklakov tonometer. This instrument consists of several "dumbbell" shaped weights held in a wire holder that allows the weights to slide freely. Argyrol (or similar silver solution) is applied in a thin coating to each end of the weights via a pad similar to a rubber stamp inkpad. The weights are applied to the anesthetized cornea of the supine patient in ascending order, with two applications made for each weight—one for each end. The imprint is then either transferred to paper using alcohol as a mordant or, better, the footplate is examined directly—a method used at the BEI. In either case, the small white center section is measured across its smaller diameter with the plastic nomogram supplied with the instrument. A deviation of 0.1 mm between successive readings (of the same weight) is cause for remeasurement.

It is a characteristic of this device that as the weights increase, so does the measured IOP. Since this results in a false-positive reading, tables have been constructed to compensate for this induced error. If the pressures are plotted on a graph against the weights, a straight line can be drawn between these points. The angle of the resulting slope gives a fair indication of the resistance of the cornea to flattening and thereby an indication of its "rigidity." The tangent of this angle is the coefficient of corneal rigidity (Figure 5.4). Such a coefficient is typically 0.95 for the average myope and gets smaller as the myopia increases and larger as it decreases. It also increases with the age of the patient and is somewhat less for females of the same age until approximately 45 years of age [10] (Figure 5.5).

The Maklakov tonometer, however, has been difficult to obtain in this country and requires a fair amount of expertise to produce repeatable readings. Consequently, few individuals have used this measurement in the calculations required to determine the surgical parameters for an individual case. Many have derived empirical age or age/sex factors to account for the relationship between rigidity and age, sex, and surgical outcome. Recently, the instrument has become available through Meditech (Bausch & Lomb). The Differential Tonomat, manufactured by Ocular Instruments of Redmond, Washington, is no longer available. It uses the same principles but requires that only two measurements be taken. It still has some of the disadvantages of the other instrument, however.

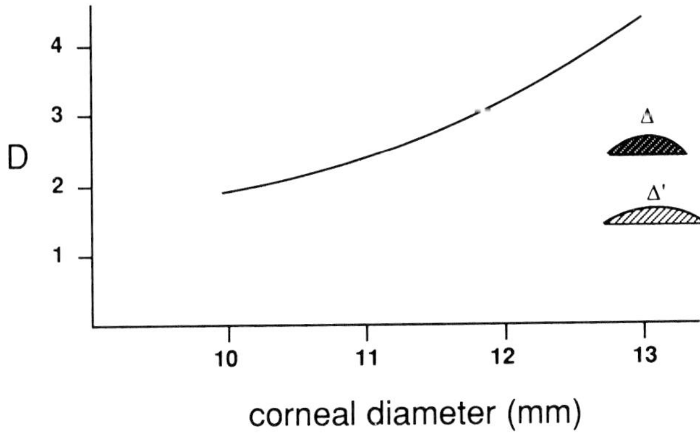

Fig. 5.3 Effect of corneal diameter on surgical outcome.

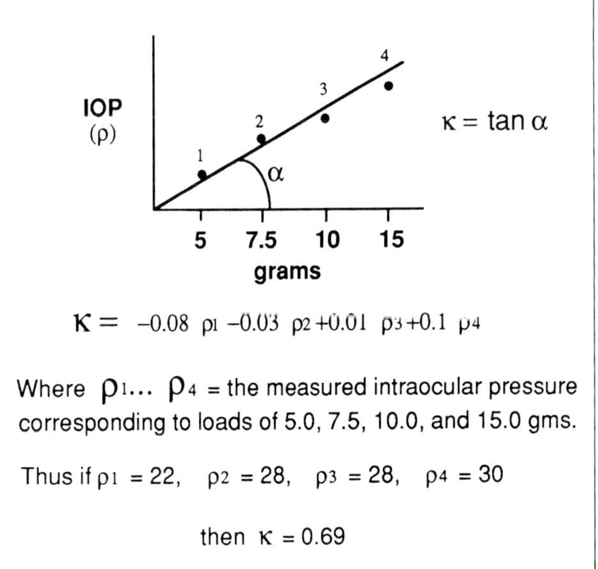

Fig. 5.4 Derivation of the rigidity coefficient.

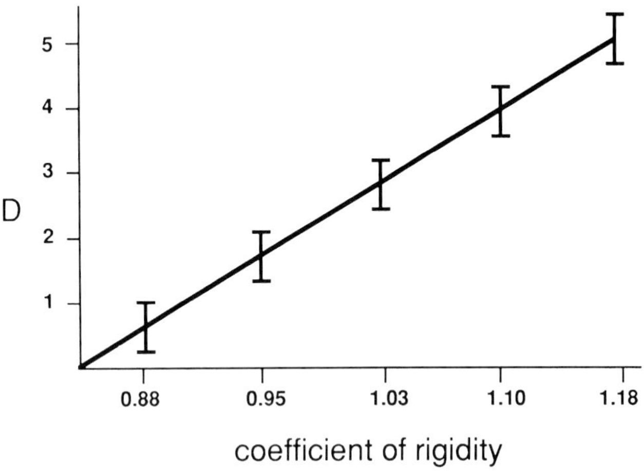

Fig. 5.5 Effect of corneal rigidity on surgical outcome.

It is impossible to state with assurance that such a factor represents the true corneal rigidity—other factors could be acting. The observer must make the assumption that the IOP remains constant during the measurement and that the sclera has the same factor of rigidity as the cornea. Regardless of the exact nature of this "factor," there is a positive correlation between it and the outcome of surgery. Therefore, until a better instrument is evolved, one of these devices will have to be used or some other means employed to account for this factor. The RK Datamaster computer program uses a statistically derived table built into the main calculation module to arrive at this factor. Other programs, such as the Deitz-Retzlaff-Sanders (DRS), use built-in factors based on the patient's age and are essentially accounting for the same thing (Figure 5.6).

Table 5.3 represents the average scleral rigidity for the various parameters illustrated. These figures were obtained through actual measurement of over 560 patients in six groups divided equally between males and females. The sex of the patient is also important and must be taken into account. There is sufficient evidence to show that women get significantly lower results for a given set of parameters than do men. Since both age and sex play a role in the outcome of the surgery, they have been integrated into this table. Besides helping select the size of the optical zone, this table can help weed out those patients who have an abnormally low rigidity and who do not seem to do well, statistically, with RK surgery.

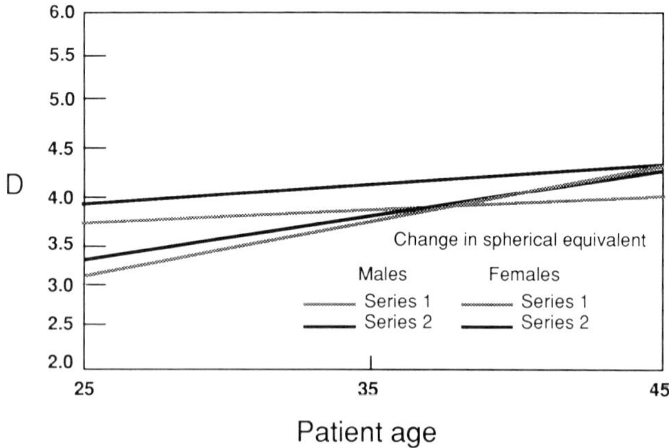

Fig. 5.6 Effect of age and sex (from Deitz M, Sanders D, Marks R. Radial keratotomy: an overview of the Kansas City study. Ophthalmology 1984; 91(5):467–478).

Table 5.3 Mean corneal rigidity

		Age (years)		
Myopia	Sex	25	35	45
1.5 D	Male	0.95	1.02	1.12
	Female	0.92	1.00	1.11
3.0 D	Male	0.90	0.95	1.04
	Female	0.88	0.90	1.03
5.0 D	Male	0.86	0.90	0.99
	Female	0.81	0.87	0.98
7.0 D	Male	0.80	0.82	0.96
	Female	0.70	0.78	0.95

Axial length

Axial length is not currently used in the computer programs to predict the outcome of refractive surgery. The omission of this reading will not significantly reduce the accuracy of the predictions for RK, but you are encouraged to obtain these measurements whenever possible. They are, of course, essential in clear lens extraction and in scleral reinforcement procedures.

Refraction

A careful manifest and/or cycloplegic refraction must be done. Autorefractor data should not be relied on. Do a manifest in addition if you are using this type of equipment. Cycloplegic refractions are performed routinely in the initial examination of all hyperopic patients and in the presence of mixed astigmatism. It is suggested that the duochrome (red-green) test be performed to avoid overminusing the myopic patient during the manifest refraction. In this test, the patient is shown a screen of grouped letters of varying size over which is superimposed a vertically split red-green screen. Spherical lenses are added or subtracted in 0.25 D increments until the patient's response to the question "Which color makes the letters darker? Red or green?" is answered "About the same" or the patient indicates a slight preference for the red. This will ensure that the image is focused on the retina without undue accommodative influence. The cylinder should be measured and recorded in plus cylinders (see Chapter 10).

Ophthalmometry (keratometry)

Keratometry is, in the author's view, the single most important preoperative measurement that must be obtained in refractive surgery. There has been some controversy over the exact role this factor played in RK surgery in the past—as far as surgical outcome is concerned. Some authors have suggested that the preoperative K-readings are not relevant to the result and need not be accounted for in the surgical plan [11]. Since the study referred to was done on cadaver eyes, it is difficult to take its conclusions seriously—especially in view of the published experience of other investigators, including myself [10,12–14]. Nonetheless, Barraquer's calculations for lathing procedures depend on these values, as do those for stromal implants and epikeratophakia [15–19]. Thus it is essential that this measurement be done. At the same time, the surgeon should be aware of the major shortcomings of this method of corneal curvature measurement (see Chapter 7).

Figure 5.7 is from Dietz and colleagues and represents the findings of a study of two groups of patients undergoing RK [20]. The influence of preoperative keratometry on the postoperative spherical equivalent is very evident. This relationship was noted early on in the history of RK surgery and, while remarked on frequently, was not given sufficient weight by many investigators. From the very beginning of this surgery, Fyodorov and the author have taken the preoperative K-readings into account in establishing the surgical parameters [10,21,22] (Figure 5.8). Figure 5.9 illustrates the results of surgery in a series of patients in whom the K-readings were integrated into the preoperative calculations used to establish the surgical optical (or free) zone size. The trend of this plot shows a definite slope upward to above the emmetropia line. If the K-readings did not have any appreciable effect on the surgical outcome, then the results of surgery in those groups whose corneal curvatures are the steepest should have had less effect from the surgery than those with flatter corneas. This should occur because the optic zones in the steeper cases were made larger to account for the increased corneal power and to prevent overcorrection. It is evident, in examining the plot, that the steeper cases are showing a slight tendency toward overcorrection—leading one to the conclusion that not enough weight has been given those K-readings. If the K-reading is not taken into consideration, as some have recommended, overcorrections are likely to occur. This could account for the cases of progressive corneal flattening that were reported in the PERK study [23].

These measurements are taken with a calibrated keratometer and for best results should be taken by the same person each time. The axis, while not needed in the calculations, should be recorded as well (see Chapter 9 for a discussion of the significance of the axis of keratometry). Be aware that routine measurements represent only

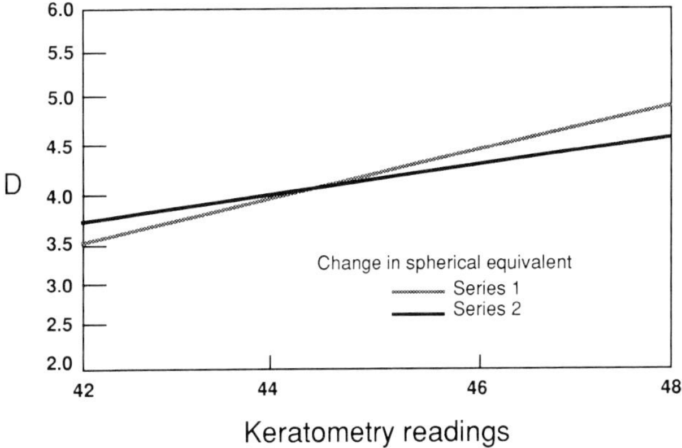

Fig. 5.8 The effect of preoperative K on surgical outcome (from Deitz M, Sanders D, Marks R. Radial keratotomy: an overview of the Kansas City study. Ophthalmology 1984; 91(5):467–478).

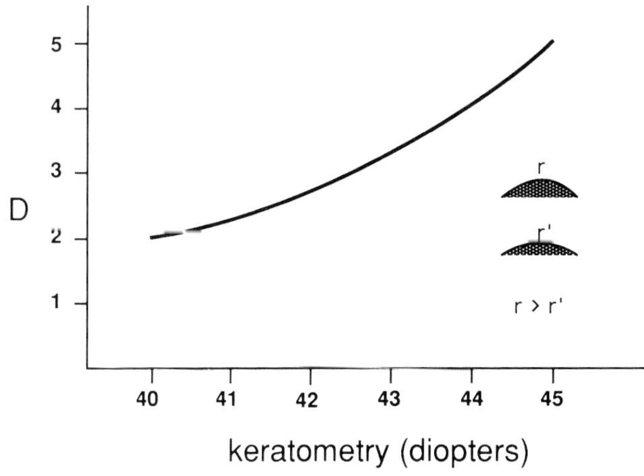

Fig. 5.7 The effect of preoperative K on surgical outcome (S.N. Fyodorov).

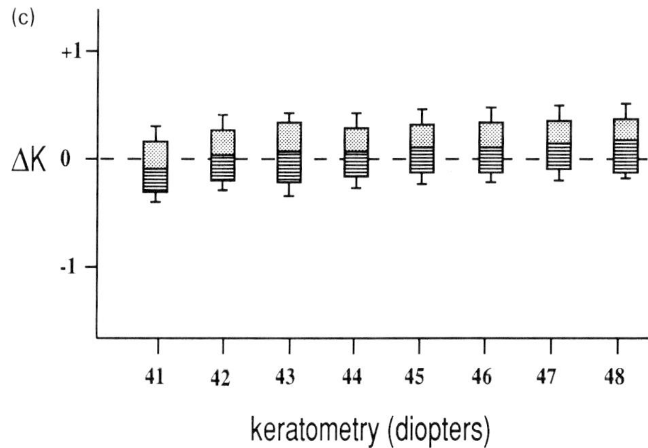

Fig. 5.9 Graph of results showing outcome related to preoperative keratometry.

the central 4.00 mm of the corneal surface and that keratometers are designed to be most accurate when measuring spherical surfaces. Furthermore, the keratometer assumes an average index of refraction for the cornea as a whole. The limitations of the keratometer are discussed further in Chapter 6.

The refractive power of the cornea, which is a curved surface, depends on a number of factors, some of which are constant and some variable. The ability of a curved surface to bend or refract light when situated between media of differing refractive indices is well known in optical physics.

The refractive power D of such a surface is given by the formula:

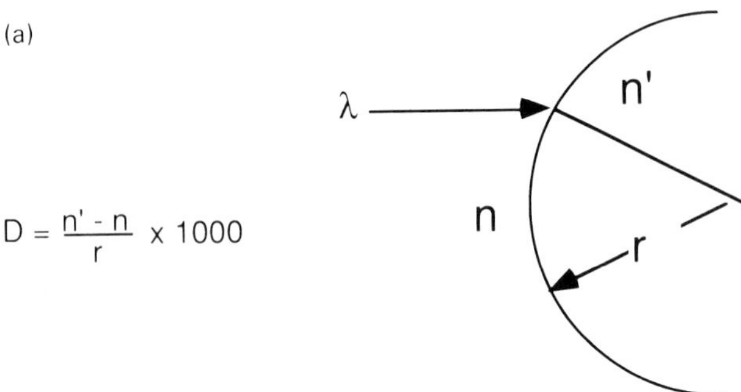

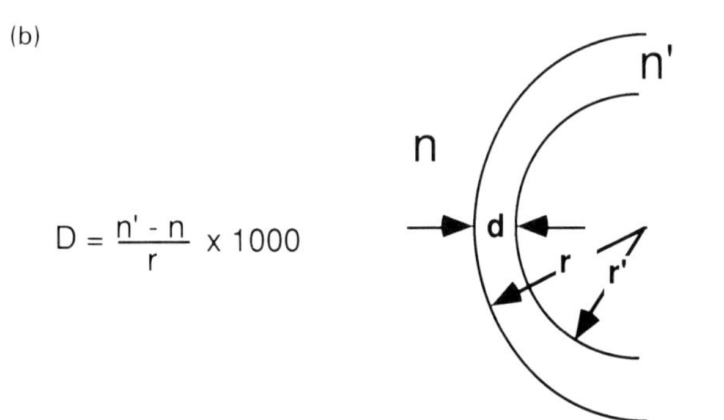

where D is the dioptric power; n' is the index of refraction of the second medium; n is the index of refraction of the first medium; and r is the radius of the refractive surface in millimeters.

Constants

Index of refraction of air 1.000
Index of refraction of the cornea........... 1.376
Index of refraction of the aqueous........ 1.336

For the cornea, the variables are

Radius of the anterior cornea................ 7.70 mm
Radius of the posterior cornea............. 6.80 mm
Corneal thickness................................... 0.50 mm

Then the refractive power at the anterior surface is

$$D = \frac{1.374 - 1.000}{7.70} \times 1000 = 48.83 \text{ D}$$

and the refractive power at the posterior surface is

$$D = \frac{1.334 - 1.376}{6.80} \times 1000 = -5.882 \text{ D}$$

The resulting corneal power is thus

$$D = 48.83 + (-5.882) = 42.95 \text{ D}$$

Because the cornea is comprised not merely of two surfaces but has a definite thickness, there is a small refractive power (0.1 D) due to this factor. Therefore, we can consider the dioptric power of the cornea as arising from three factors:

1	Anterior surface =	48.83
2	Posterior surface =	−5.88
3	Corneal thickness =	0.10
		43.05 D

The readings displayed by the typical keratometer are in diopters and represent the effective corneal power. This value for corneal power is derived by taking an arbitrarily low value for the corneal refractive index—1.3375—that takes into account the front and back surface powers of the cornea and its thickness. That this is effective corneal refractive power must be kept in mind when evaluating the output of some corneal topographers. These instruments typically give the actual corneal curvature and not the effective refracting power of the cornea. Hence a conversion must be made when trying to equate the resulting values with those of standard keratometers. Some instruments, such as the CLAS II, display the effective total corneal power, the front surface corneal power, and the true external corneal curvature.

It should be apparent that attempts to modify the refractive power of the eye would most effectively be applied to the anterior corneal surface, where there exists a variable factor of considerable magnitude. It is important to remember always that the keratometer is an instrument for directly measuring radius of curvature—not refractive power. Furthermore, certain assumptions are made about conditions that may not exist in a given eye. The power reading given by the keratometer assumes a given value for n' such that for a given radius of anterior corneal curvature, the net power displayed approximates that which would be obtained if one calculated the net power from both the anterior and posterior surfaces (as illustrated above). This assumption is reasonably valid over the range of curvatures normally found clinically—at least for the central 4.00 mm of the cornea.

However, a problem arises once we have modified the corneal thickness by the Barraquer procedures (MKM, KP, and HLK) or by epikeratophakia because now the anterior and posterior surfaces deviate considerably from parallel. For this reason, one must calculate the net corneal power by solving for both surfaces. In short, K-readings taken after such procedures will not represent the true corneal net power. No current topographer units are capable of accurately rendering both the anterior and posterior corneal curvatures to facilitate these types of measurements. Useful, if inaccurate, expressions of corneal power can still be obtained with standard keratometers, though, so do not get rid of your instrument yet. These devices come in handy for "quick and dirty" measurements when extreme accuracy is neither needed nor warranted—such as in current methods of contact lens fitting. Furthermore, until additional investigation and standardization of topography nomenclature and displays are effected—not to mention clinical work to establish the relationship between the shape of the cornea pre- and postoperatively—the K-readings will continue to be important (see Chapter 7).

Central keratometry

The standard clinical method to measure corneal shape is central keratometry. Accurate keratometric measurements are important in this surgery for three reasons:

- The preoperative keratometry readings have an effect on the amount of correction achieved with these techniques—the flatter the cornea, the less the effect.
- The change in central keratometry after surgery is a major response variable that indicates not only how flat the cornea has become but also whether the surgery has induced astigmatism, either regular or irregular.
- Although the keratometer measures the curvature of only the central 3.4 to 4.2 mm, the keratometric readings are analyzed and communicated easily.

To ensure that your results are in line with those of other surgeons, use instruments that are optically interchangeable, that is, the Bausch & Lomb, the Topcon, and the Haag-Streit devices. This uniformity is desirable because different types of keratometers assume different indices of refraction for the cornea to convert the radius of curvature measurements, which the keratometer reads directly, to power measurements in diopters. For example, the Haag-Streit and Bausch & Lomb instruments use an index of 1.3375, whereas the American Optical instrument uses 1.336 and the Gambs instrument uses 1.332—the true refractive index of the cornea is 1.376. In these three examples, a radius of 7.8 mm will read 43.27, 43.08, and 42.56 D, respectively.

Basic principles of keratometry are discussed in standard textbooks, and the procedures specified here for using the Bausch & Lomb instrument are modified from its instruction manual [24–27].

Keratometer setup

To calibrate the instrument, secure a steel test ball of known curvature (usually 45.00 D and supplied with the device) on the concave end of a magnetic rod that can be attached to the frame of the instrument. Position the steel ball in the optical axis of the keratometer, set both drums to 45.00 D, adjust the eyepiece (described below), and superimpose the crosses of the focusing circle and horizontal drum. If the reading on the horizontal drum is 45.00 D, the instrument is calibrated properly. If the reading differs from 45.00 D, readjust the eyepiece. If the reading is still inaccurate, the instrument must be calibrated properly by the manufacturer. Repeat this calibration check annually.

Eyepiece calibration

Particular attention must be given to adjustment of the eyepiece of the keratometer each time the instrument is used in order to ensure accuracy of readings for each patient. The first time the operator uses this instrument, he or she must adjust the eyepiece for his or her eye; otherwise, the readings taken will be erroneous. To adjust the eyepiece, proceed as follows:

- Position the white-backed occluder in the optical axis of the instrument (unless the steel calibration ball is used).
- Turn the eyepiece cap counterclockwise as far as possible.
- Turn the instrument lamp on, and look through the eyepiece—a blurred cross will be seen.
- Continue looking through the eyepiece and slowly turn the eyepiece in a clockwise direction, to come from the plus side and which avoids accommodation, to that position where the cross is in the sharpest focus. (*Note:* Do not turn the eyecap back and forth to focus the cross. This tends to stimulate accommodation and will result in erroneous readings.)
- When the cross is in the sharpest focus, note the reading on the outer periphery of the eyecap.
- Repeat the preceding three steps *at least three times*. If the results are approximately the same each time, the eyepiece is adjusted for your eye. Make sure that this setting is recorded somewhere for each person designated to perform this examination. If possible, assign one person to do all these readings.

The calibrated scale on the outer periphery of the eyecap is for the operator's convenience. Once the operator has ensured that the eyepiece is adjusted for his or her eye, he or she should note and remember or record the setting. The next time the instrument is used, the eyecap is turned to this setting, and it will be in adjustment for the operator's eye. However, this setting should be verified occasionally.

The patient's chin should fit snugly into the chin rest. For accurate results, it is necessary that the patient hold his or her head firmly against the head rest during the complete keratometer examination. For the patient with an extremely receding forehead or with deep-set eyes and a protruding forehead, it may be necessary to adjust the forehead or chin rest.

Grasp the grip that rotates the keratometer drum, and rotate the instrument so that the axial scale reads exactly

90° and 180° at the axis marks. Release the set screw so that the tube of the instrument can be moved to one side. Raise or lower the instrument until the pin on the side of the lamp housing and the white axis marker are aligned, like gunsights, with the patient's pupil or outer canthus. Cover the eye not under examination with the occluding shield.

After the patient's head has been lined up and leveled accurately, turn the instrument so that it points directly at the eye to be examined. Looking from the side, the observer will then see a tiny, bright ring in the center of the cornea (the corneal image of the circular mire). When the correct position has been found, the patient will see a reflection of his or her own eye in the tube of the instrument with an image of the mire in the center of his pupil. The patient should fixate on this image. If there is difficulty with this procedure, shine a penlight through the eyepiece to assist with alignment.

Technique of measurement

Looking through the eyepiece, the operator will see images of the target mire, perhaps very blurred (Figure 5.10). This may be cleared with the focusing knob. By swiveling the instrument slightly and by making fine adjustments of the elevator knob, the black crosshairs may be put near the center of the double circle. This doubled circle is called the *focusing circle*. When this is done, tighten the locking screw, and measure the corneal surfaces.

It is important that the crosshairs be near the center of the focusing circle, for when this condition is attained, the optical axis of the instrument will coincide with the visual axis of the patient's eye, as it should for accuracy. At the same time, the image of the patient's eye will be directly in front of the patient. These conditions constitute the *triple alignment* so necessary to precision measurements. When the instrument is out of focus, the central focusing circle and the plus and minus signs are doubled, but when the exact focus is located by turning the focusing knob, the focusing circle will appear single and sharp.

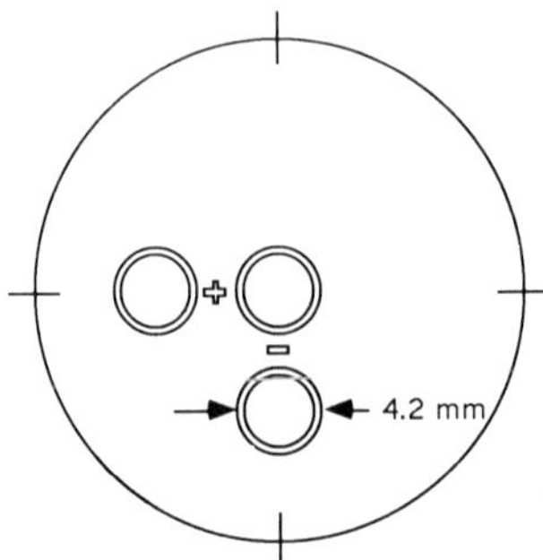

Fig. 5.10 Typical keratometry mires of Bausch & Lomb keratometer.

In an astigmatic cornea, all the central focusing circle will not appear exactly in focus at the same time. Therefore, for greater accuracy, the operator may direct his or her attention to the doubled plus sign and focus it sharply. The focus of the minus sign can be disregarded until a later step.

Locating the cylinder axis

Two plus signs will be seen between the left-hand and central focusing circles within the telescope. The axis of the cylinder can be found most easily when the tips of these plus signs just touch. Turn the horizontal measuring drum until the plus signs are barely separated. If the horizontal lines of the plus signs appear to be continuous and unbroken, the instrument is already set at the position of the axis of the astigmatism. If the horizontal lines appear discontinuous, the keratometer is not at the cylinder axis.

Grasp the keratometer at the rotating grip, and rotate the entire tube while looking into the eyepiece. At some position, which can be found readily by watching closely, the horizontal lines of the plus signs will appear continuous and unbroken. A further check on the accurate location of the axis may be obtained by throwing the instrument slightly out of focus. Then the plus sign of the central focusing circle will be doubled. If the axis is correct, the horizontal line in the plus sign of the left circle will be exactly midway between the double horizontal line of the other plus sign.

If it is not at the midpoint, a slight rotation of the instrument one way or another will move the line to the midpoint. The double cross should be focused next so that it becomes single. The two horizontal lines will then become continuous. This extra check on the corneal axis is particularly valuable in low astigmatic errors. When these horizontal white lines of the plus signs appear tip to tip and continuous, the keratometer is set so as to indicate the axis of the astigmatism.

Measuring the horizontal principal meridian

After the axis has been found, turn the horizontal measuring drum knob, and the left-hand plus sign will move to the right or left. Move this plus sign until it is exactly superimposed on the plus sign of the central focusing circle. This completes the setting for the rear horizontal meridian. The scale of the left-hand or horizontal measuring drum indicates the actual diopter power of the cornea in the horizontal or near-horizontal meridian.

Measuring the vertical meridian

You should use the crosses to measure the vertical meridian, since they are more accurate than the minus signs described by the manufacturer. To measure the curvature in the vertical meridian, rotate the drum so that the plus sign of the central focusing circle is vertical, and repeat the procedure followed for the horizontal meridian.

While measuring, one hand should be constantly on the focusing screw to keep the meridian being measured in sharp focus. The operator's judgment of focus in this instrument is very keen, thanks to the coincident method of focusing. This permits him or her to keep the mire, whose image in the cornea he or she measures, a constant distance from the eye despite the small movements that every eye constantly makes. Unless the object distance is a fixed one, the measurements of the image size will be erroneous.

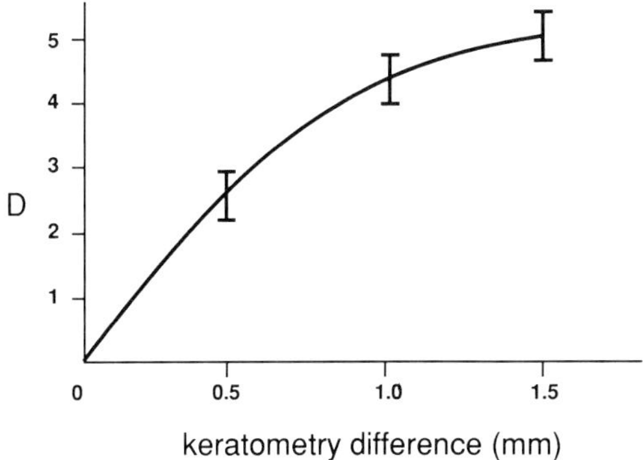

Fig. 5.11 Effect of corneal asphericity (Fyodorov).

Reading the amount of astigmatism

On the left, or horizontal, measuring drum, the power of the cornea in the meridians nearest to 0° to 180° is read. When the drum is rotated vertically, the difference between these two readings is the amount of corneal astigmatism. If the two readings are the same, there is no measurable corneal astigmatism.

Axis of astigmatism

The meridian indicators of the keratometer tube are engraved white lines on the body bearing facing the operator. The horizontal marks on each side indicate the meridian measured on the horizontal drum, and the vertical mark on top indicates the meridian measured when the drum is turned vertically. If the astigmatism is to be measured in a minus cylinder form, take for its axis that mark representing the drum having the lower dioptric reading. If the astigmatism is to be measured in a plus cylinder form, take for its axis the mark representing the drum having the higher dioptric reading. The two curvatures in diopters and the axis of each are recorded on the data forms.

Extended range for flat corneas

A loose trial frame lens may be used with the Bausch & Lomb keratometer to extend the range to read flatter corneas. If the keratometer drum is turned to its flattest extent and still cannot read the corneal curvature accurately, a −1.25 D lens is taped, convex side out, over the front aperture of the keratometer, the drum reading is obtained, and the supplied nomogram chart is used to determine the true keratometric reading.

Determining degree of corneal asphericity

There is a relationship between the successful outcome of RK surgery and the relative asphericity of the cornea (Figure 5.11). If the cornea is too spherical, that is, the peripheral corneal curvature approaches in degree that of the center, very little, if any, effect will result from the surgery. At first the myopia will be reduced, but within a short period of time the curvature will return to the same (or very nearly) as that of the preoperative state. For this reason, the peripheral corneal curvature should be measured in the horizontal and vertical meridians and compared with those of the center. In the author's experience, if the difference between the two readings is equal to the degree of myopia present, the result will be that predicted by the calculations. If the difference is equal to or less than half the myopia, it is very likely that no lasting change will occur in the corneal shape as a result of the surgery. It can be argued that given the nature of keratometers, measurements of the peripheral cornea with these instruments is completely inaccurate. While this is true, peripheral K-readings are of sufficient clinical reliability to recommend their use—as opposed to nothing—until something better comes along.

Take the measurements as in central K-readings, except that the patient is directed to fixate eccentrically. The patient should be encouraged to move his or her eyes sufficiently off axis so as to cast the mires onto the limbal zone. The mires inevitably will be distorted when this occurs. To reduce this distortion and to obtain a reading, have the patient blink several times in succession and have the patient rotate his or her eyes medially so as to move the mire somewhat closer to center. Use only one drum to make the measurement (preferably the plus), and rotate the tube as necessary to clarify the mire. Record both the horizontal (temporal) and vertical (6 o'clock) readings.

Glare or contrast sensitivity testing

There are three ways in which a retinal image may be degraded:

1 It may be out of focus, as in uncorrected ametropia.

2 It may be degraded by light scatter from opacities in the ocular media.

3 It may be affected by a combination of both factors. In patients having refractive surgery, both ametropia and glare from surgical scars may degrade the retinal image.

The standard visual acuity test projects a high-contrast black letter or number on a white background. The patient with glare may read all letters correctly but fail to comment that the letters actually appear as a washed-out faded gray. In the world outside the examining room, the person observes that delicate shades of gray and subtle color tones actually may be lost in a nondescript, hazy fusion and that image outlines are blurred. Thus the standard visual acuity chart gives no information about the quality of contrast and may be dangerously misleading regarding visual function under real-life conditions, particularly in bright light and at night.

Many researchers have sought ways to evaluate glare sensitivity by way of contrast measurements [28–34]. The Miller-Nadler Glare Tester (Titmus) is one of several such instruments available, enabling the clinician to quantify glare sensitivity. The instrument consists of a constant bright rectangular glare source that surrounds a series of randomly oriented, constant-sized, black Landolt rings positioned on a background that is progressively darkened until a contrast threshold is reached. The apparatus consists of a desktop slide projector that provides the constant glare source and a series of specially made 35-mm slides.

LeClaire, Nadler, Weiss, and Miller have proposed that glare sensitivity be graded by using a comparison method, as occurs in determination of Snellen acuity [35,36]. By this method, most normal individuals in the first three decades of life can see to a contrast level of 5%. This means that there is only 5% contrast between the Landolt ring and its immediate background. If a patient's glare contrast sensitivity is such that a 10% contrast between the Landolt ring and its surround is required before the Landolt ring can be seen, the increase in contrast compared with normal is 2x, still an excellent score.

Wolf found a clear division of glare sensitivity between patients below and above age 50 [31]. An increase in contrast of 3x or 4x (10% to 20% contrast) may be normal for patients above age 50 who have no obvious opacities in the ocular media. A glare contrast sensitivity of 11x to 15x (55% to 75% contrast) or more may indicate severe visual disability under bright-light conditions, even though a good Snellen acuity may be obtained in the refracting lane. Such patients can be visually crippled with an effective acuity as low as 20/800 outside on a bright day.

LeClaire and colleagues performed glare and visual acuity tests on 161 normal eyes, 144 eyes with cataracts, 100 eyes with intraocular lenses, and 26 eyes wearing aphakic spectacles. They found that the normal patients averaged 6% contrast level, those with Copeland intraocular lenses 15% contrast, those with Lynell intraocular lenses 20% contract, and those with aphakic spectacles 18% contrast. The glare readings of normal patients were significantly different from those of the corrected aphakic patients, regardless of the method of correction ($p < 0.001$). For management of glare, see Chapter 15.

Pachymetry

Until the advent of RK, it was assumed that the corneal thickness varied smoothly from a relatively thinner central portion to a relatively thicker peripheral portion. However, the occurrence of microperforations in areas of the cornea in which these were not anticipated spurred a search for the cause. These perforations generally occurred in the midperiphery and, for the most part, nonuniformly. In other words, they were happening where the cornea was supposed to be thicker and sometimes when incisions had already been made across this same midzone in other parts of the cornea with the same blade. This stimulated the author to begin mapping out the corneal thickness over its entire surface. The study was facilitated by the use of ultrasonic pachymetry. It was found that in approximately 11% of patients, small isolated areas of abrupt corneal thinning—dubbed *corneal dimples*—were found. While these appeared initially to occur at random, a pattern soon emerged such that they seemed to group primarily in the inferotemporal part of the cornea at the midperiphery (Figure 5.12). In addition, some older patients exhibited rather large areas of prelimbal corneal thinning—again mostly in the inferotemporal quadrant.

From this work, certain corneal thickness patterns have been recognized:

Type 1 (most common): Corneal thickness proceeds in a smooth, even transition from a thinner central section to a thicker peripheral section. Within this type, two subtypes occur:

Type 1a: In this type, the transition is smooth and gradual (Figure 5.13a).

Type 1b: Here the transition is smooth, but the thickening occurs more rapidly than type 1a in the prelimbal area

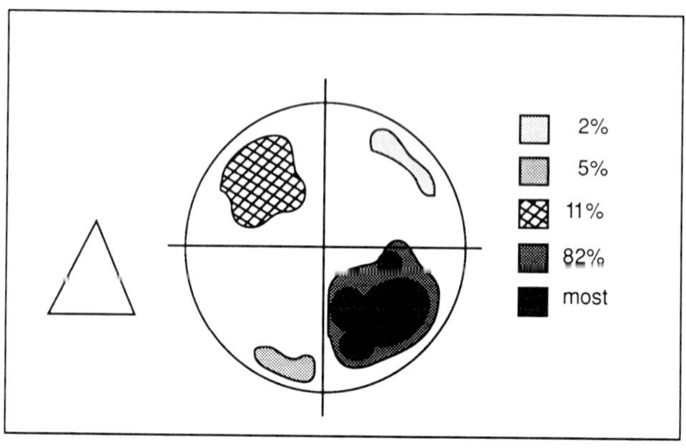

Fig. 5.12 Distribution of thin areas.

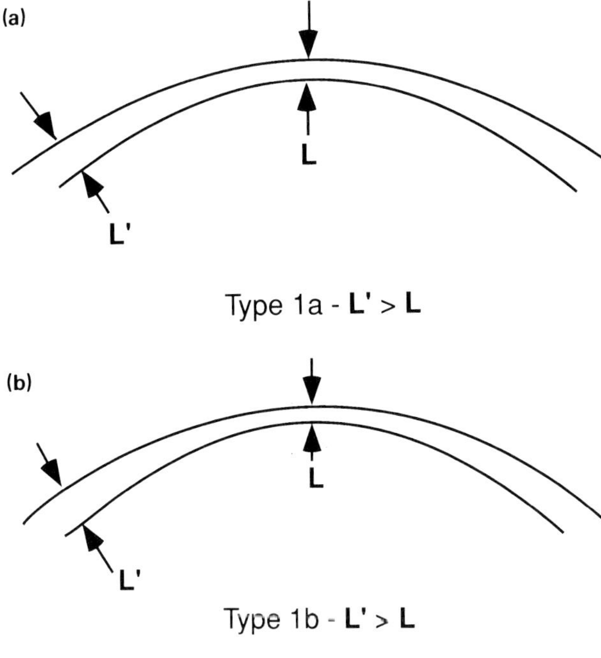

Fig. 5.13 Corneal thickness types: type 1 (most common)—corneal thickness proceeds in a smooth, even transition from a thinner central section to a thicker peripheral section. Within this type two subtypes occur: (a) type 1a; (b) type 1b.

(Figure 5.13b). The limbal cornea is typically thicker than in type 1a.

Type 2: In this type (sometimes called the *plateau cornea*), the corneal thickness varies very little from the central zone until somewhere near or just past the midperipheral point, whereupon it begins to thicken rapidly. This type of cornea is seen in higher myopes and the average peripheral pachymetry is typically thinner than in type 1.

Type 3: This is, for the most part, similar to type 1, with the added feature that the cornea becomes thinner again at the periphery in the inferotemporal quadrant. This type is seen most often in eyes over 50 years of age.

Type 4: This possesses the characteristics of type 1 with the addition of having small, well-circumscribed areas of abrupt corneal thinning—corneal dimples. Most of these occur in the inferotemporal quadrant, and there does not appear to be any association with age. However, no patient has been described with both type 3 and 4 in combination either in the same eye or in opposite eyes.

Instrumentation

Ultrasonic pachymetry is the recommended method for obtaining corneal thickness measurements [37]. None of the optical methods used previously (Haag-Streit, Zeiss, or Heyer-Schulte) have proven to be of sufficient accuracy or reproducibility for use in difficult cases or in aiding predictability. Also, as incisions have become deeper, more precise measurements are necessary to prevent or reduce the incidence of perforations.

Ultrasonic pachymetry possesses the advantages of

- Reproducibility
- Ability to take measurements anywhere on the cornea
- Not dependent on patient fixation
- High accuracy
- Ability to be used intraoperatively (not recommended)
- Ease of use by relatively unskilled personnel

All the available ultrasonic instruments represent a sizable investment. It is not possible, however, to perform this surgery with any degree of confidence without one. In a comparison of all the available pachymeters (done by an independent ophthalmologist), which were donated by the manufacturers, the one that tested out as the best was the DGH-1000/2000. This instrument embodies all the design characteristics that the author desired.

It has an integral printer; which lists out not only the readings but also where they were taken, plus a frontal map of the reading format or mode selected as well as a profile of corneal thickness across the cornea in up to four sections. There is an internal memory allowing for editing of the recorded data prior to printout, selection of multiple measurement modes with an incremental guide map, and two self-test modes—one for the device and one for the solid probe tip. Tip coupling is provided by the standard solid probe tip, which eliminates the usual ultrasound gel (filled once daily). Other features include a two-stage foot switch that is provided for obtaining and storing the measurements; a digital readout of data with a two-tone signal; rejection of nonperpendicular readings; provision to preset the "bias" for automatic blade-setting calculations; automatic gain control; provision to reset speed of sound (default—1640 m/s), and there is a port at the rear of the instrument to allow direct input into a computer and to allow it to interact with the other planned instruments in the series.

The 2000 series embodies all the preceding features with the addition of

- Automatic averaging of rings
- Programmable mapping
- An optional plug-in predictability module

Making the measurements

The following description applies particularly to the DGH-2000 Series Ultrasonic Pachymeter. Some differences exist with different manufacturers.

Prepare the instrument by switching it on. On power-up, the DGH-2000 will run through a short self-testing program to ensure that all systems are nominal. Next;

press the CLR button, followed by "PQT" (Probe Quality Test). The instrument will respond by producing a reading on the screen (e.g., PROBE EFFICIENCY = 81%). If there is not enough gel (in the older model probe), the socket is dry, or the probe is not plugged in, you will get a message telling you about the problem. In this case, remove the tip and refill the cavity, ensuring that no air bubbles are trapped in the gel. If the readout indicates an efficiency of 75% or greater, the probe is ready for use. Newer probes have a go-no go mode; thus, if the probe is defective, that message will appear. Otherwise, the system will cycle to the next step.

Press CLR again, and then press BIAS—it should be 100%. You can reset this using the keyboard if desired. If you make a mistake in entry, repeatedly pressing the CLR key will cause the reading to march off the screen digit by digit. When you are satisfied, press ENTR. Next, select the mode by pressing MODE, followed by a number from 1 to 9. The actual number does not matter because only the central corneal measurement is important. Corneal mapping is not absolutely necessary in HLK, KMK, and KMIS lamellar procedures such as LASIK. However, it is recommended that mapping be done in all refractive surgery cases and that all 33 points on the map be recorded (Figure 5.14). The left-hand group of LEDs will light up in a pattern specific to the number entered. In addition, the screen will display the characteristics of the readout, such as what each circle represents. When you are satisfied, press ENTR, and you are ready to take readings.

The patient is placed supine in a well-lighted room. An auxiliary floor lamp shining obliquely on the cornea will facilitate accurate placement of the transducer probe. Under these conditions, the pupil will be constricted to between 2.5 and 3.0 mm in most cases.

The operator sits at the right side of the patient's head with the foot switch so placed that the foot straddles the middle of the switch. By moving the foot slightly to the right, the measurement side of the switch is depressed—to the left, and the reading is stored. The instrument should be placed to the patient's left so that the entire front panel can be seen clearly by the operator.

Two drops of appropriate topical anesthetic are applied to each cornea. To begin the measurements, the operator depresses the right foot pedal once. This will cause the LEDs to go out and be replaced by a single blinking central red light. The position of the blinking light indicates where the next reading is to be taken. The readout on the screen also will spell out the two-letter code for that location.

The probe is now applied to the central cornea (Figure 5.15) within the pupil, slightly indenting the corneal surface. The right foot pedal is depressed once again. If the probe is perpendicular to the cornea, the instrument will respond with an immediate short beep. A reading also will appear on the screen. Press the left pedal once to store the reading. Note that the flashing light has now become a steady light, and the next position is flashing. If there is no immediate beep, the instrument will try to take more measurements and then will give you the raspberry and print NO READING POOR APPLANATION on the screen. If this happens, adjust the orientation of the probe and try again.

Next, move the probe so as to straddle the pupillary margin. Depress the right foot pedal to acquire a reading. This is the paracentral (PC) reading corresponding to the first or A circle (Figure 5.16). Press the left foot pedal to store the reading, and move the probe tip to a point that causes the tip to just butt against the edge of the epithelial imprint from the preceding reading.

This next reading is the midperipheral (MP) reading and corresponds to the B ring on the map (Figure 5.17). Store the reading. Note that again the blinking light

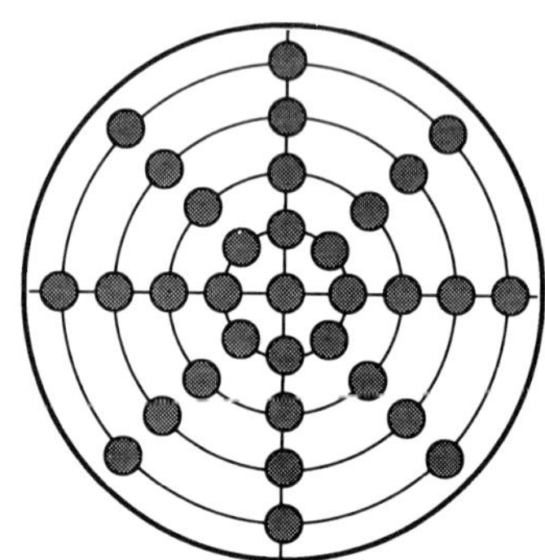

Fig. 5.14 Typical mapping pattern.

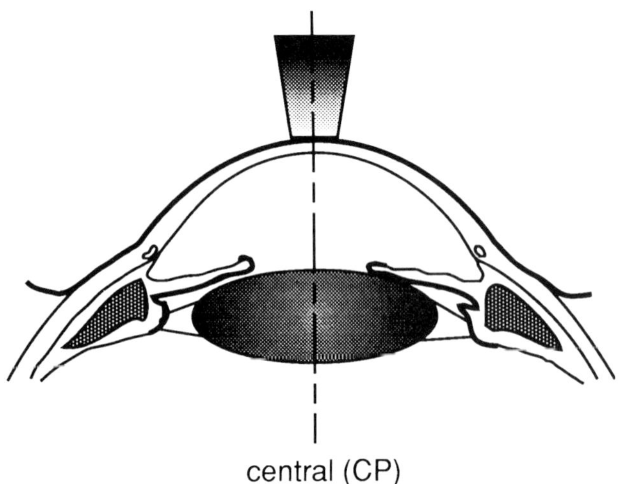

Fig. 5.15 Central pachymetry (CP).

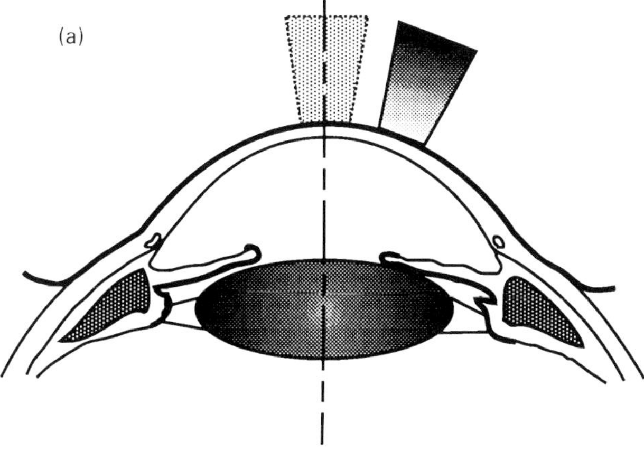

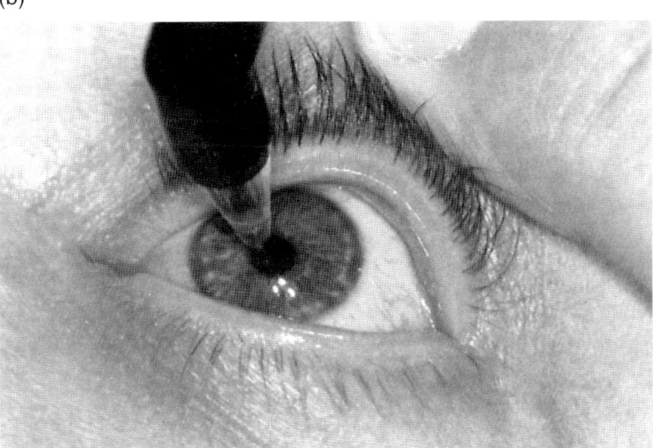

Fig. 5.16 (a,b) Paracentral pachymetry (PC).

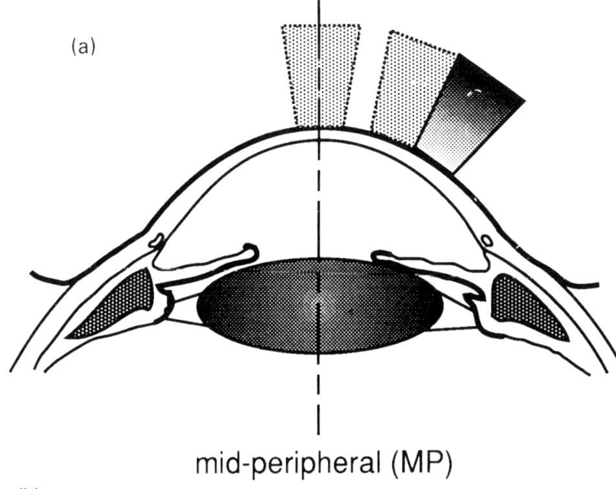

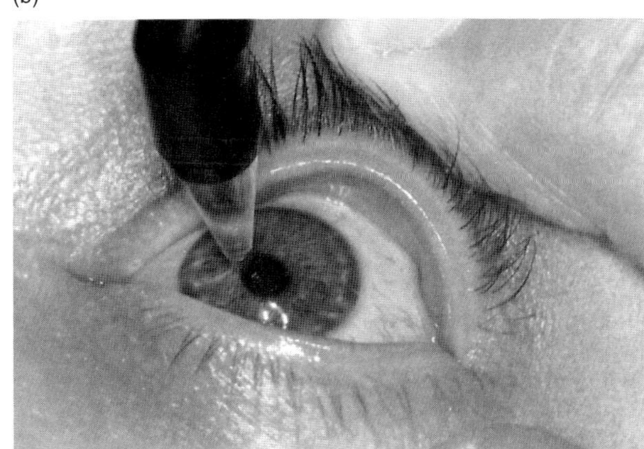

Fig. 5.17 (a,b) Midperipheral pachymetry (MP).

becomes steady, and the next lighted spot begins to blink.

The probe is now moved to a point halfway between the paracentral point and the limbus (Figure 5.18). This is the paraperipheral (PP) measurement point.

Acquire and record this reading. Finally, the probe is moved so as to straddle the transition between clear cornea and the limbus.

This is the far-peripheral (FP) reading and corresponds to the outer or D ring on the map. Acquire and store the reading as before (Figure 5.19).

Continue in this manner until all 33 points in the map are recorded. If you have difficulty with any particular reading, depress the left foot pedal to store a null or blank reading. This will cause the corresponding map light to turn off. When you have completed the mapping, use the UP/DOWN (arrows) buttons to move back to this point, and try again.

It helps if you seat yourself on the same side as the eye you are attempting to measure. With practice, a typical corneal mapping will take less than 5 minutes. It is not necessary to lift the probe between readings.

When you have completed the mapping process, pressing the PRINT button will cause the readings stored in memory to be printed out. When the printing is completed, it is a good idea to immediately record the eye measured and write the patient's name and the date on the printout. Press CLR, and reenter the desired mode to get ready for the left eye.

The probes can be used for intraoperative pachymetry by dry-gas sterilization or by soaking in CIDEX. However, CIDEX can leave a residue and has been implicated in causing postoperative keratitis, so take care that the tip is rinsed thoroughly before use. Do not autoclave any portion of the probe, and do not soak the plug portion of the probe. If soaking the older-model fillable probes, remove the probe tip beforehand. I prefer to gas the cord and transducer and soak the probe tip. Use sterile methylcellulose or A-scan gel as a coupling medium. *Do not use saline!*

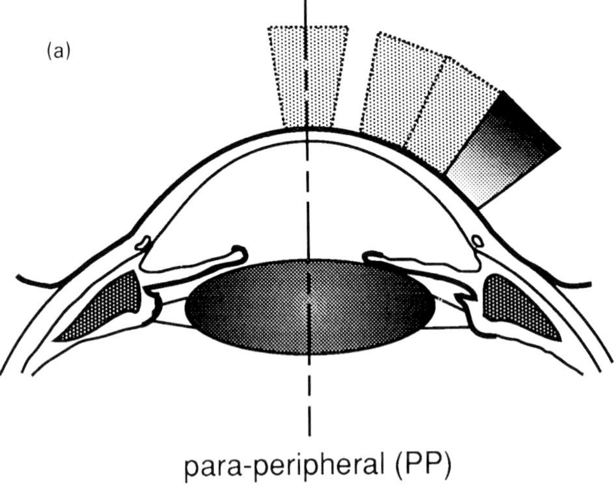

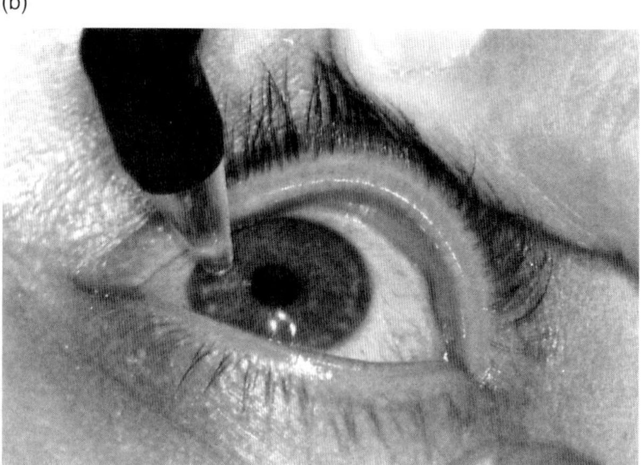

Fig. 5.18 (a,b) Paraperipheral pachymetry (PP).

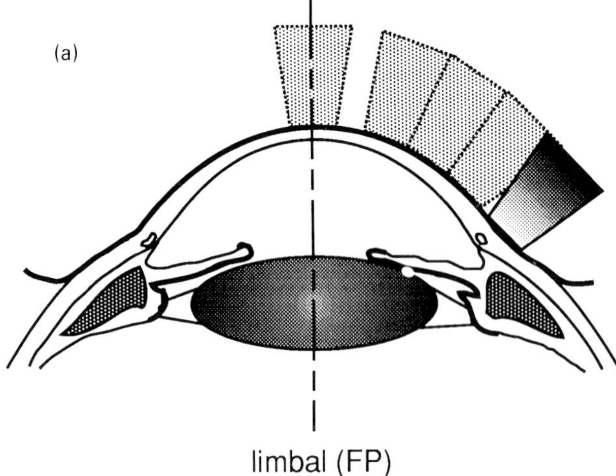

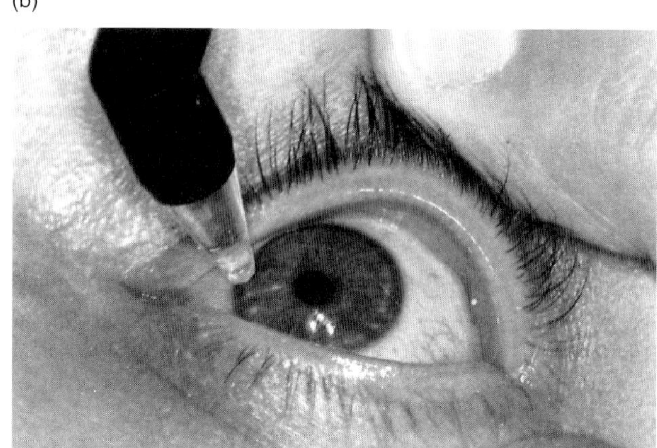

Fig. 5.19 (a,b) Limbal pachymetry: far peripheral (FP).

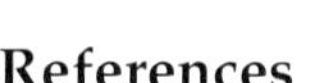

References

1 Binder, P.S., C.H. May, and S.C. Grant, An evaluation of orthokeratology. Ophthalmology 1980; 87 (8): p. 729–44.
2 Levy, B., Permanent corneal damage in a patient undergoing orthokeratology. Am J Optom Physiol Opt 1982; 59 (8): p. 697–9.
3 Polse, K.A., R.J. Brand, D.W. Vastine, *et al.*, Corneal change accompanying orthokeratology. Plastic or elastic? Results of a randomized controlled clinical trial. Arch Ophthalmol 1983; 101 (12): p. 1873–8.
4 Vajpayee, R.B., N. Sharma, R. Saxena, *et al.*, Epikeratoplasty for traumatic corneal ectasia. Cornea 1999; 18(2): p. 237–9.
5 Stern, M.E., R.W. Beuerman, R.I. Fox, *et al.*, The pathology of dry eye: the interaction between the ocular surface and lacrimal glands. Cornea 1998; 17(6): p. 584–9.
6 Tauber, J., A dose-ranging clinical trial to assess the safety and efficacy of cyclosporine ophthalmic emulsion in patients with keratoconjunctivitis sicca. The Cyclosporine Study Group. Adv Exp Med Biol 1998; 438: p. 969–72.
7 Tsubota, K., E. Goto, S. Shimmura, *et al.*, Treatment of persistent corneal epithelial defect by autologous serum application. Ophthalmology 1999; 106(10): p. 1984–9.
8 Zoukhri, D., R.R. Hodges, C. Sergheraert, *et al.*, Protein kinase C isoforms differentially control lacrimal gland functions. Adv Exp Med Biol 1998; 438: p. 181–6.
9 Milder, B. and M.L. Rubin, *Fine Art of Prescribing Glasses Without Making a Spectacle of Yourself*. Triad Scientific Publishers; Gainesville 1978.
10 Bores, L.D., Historical review and clinical results of radial keratotomy. Int Ophthalmol Clin 1983; 23(3): p. 93–118.
11 Salz, J., J.S. Lee, J.V. Jester, *et al.*, Radial keratotomy in fresh human cadaver eyes. Ophthalmology 1981; 88 (8): p. 742–6.
12 Bores, L.D., W. Myers, and J. Cowden, Radial keratotomy: an analysis of the American experience. Ann Ophthalmol 1981; 13(8): p. 941–8.
13 Cowden, J.W. and L.D. Bores, A clinical investigation of the surgical correction of myopia by the method of Fyodorov. Ophthalmology 1981; 88(8): p. 737–41.
14 Rowsey, J.J., H.D. Balyeat, B. Rabinovitch, *et al.*, Predicting the results of radial keratotomy. Ophthalmology 1983; 90 (6): p. 642–54.
15 Barraquer, J.I., *Terminologia y Calculos Basicos, in Cirugia Refractiva de la Cornea.* 1989, Instituto Barraquer de America, Bogota Columbia. p. 147–181.
16 Choyce, D.P., Intra-cameral and intra-corneal implants. A decade of personal experience. Trans Ophthalmol Soc UK 1966; 86: p. 507–25.
17 Werblin, T.P., J.E. Blaydes, A. Fryczkowski, *et al.*, Refractive corneal surgery: the use of implantable alloplastic lens material. Aust J Ophthalmol 1983; 11(4): p. 325–331.
18 Werblin, T.P., R.L. Peiffer, and A. Fryczkowski, Myopic hydrogel keratophakia: preliminary report. Cornea 1984; 3(3): p. 197–204.

19 Morgan, K.S., P.A. Asbell, and H.E. Kaufman, Cataracts in children: epikeratophakia for the correction of aphakia. J La State Med Soc 1983; 135 (2): p. 23–5.

20 Deitz, M.R., D.R. Sanders, and R.G. Marks, Radial keratotomy: an overview of the Kansas City study. Ophthalmology 1984; 91(5): p. 467–78.

21 Fyodorov, S.N. and V.V. Durnev, The use of anterior keratotomy method with the purpose of surgical correction of myopia, in *Practical Problems in Ophthalmic Surgery*, A.I. Ivashina, Editor. 1977, Minister of Health, U.S.S.R.: Moscow. p. 47–48.

22 Fyodorov, S.N. and V.V. Durnev, Operation of dosaged dissection of corneal circular ligament in cases of myopia of mild degree. Ann Ophthalmol 1979; 11(12): p. 1885–1890.

23 Waring, G.O., M.J. Lynn, W. Culbertson, *et al.*, Three-year results of the Prospective Evaluation of Radial Keratotomy (PERK) Study. Ophthalmology 1987; 94(10): p. 1339–1354.

24 Duke-Elder, S. and D. Abrams, Ophthalmic optics and refraction., in *System of Ophthalmology*, S.S. Duke-Elder, Editor. 1970, C.V. Mosby, St Louis.

25 Sampson, W.G., Keratometry, in *Corneal Contact Lens*, L.J. Girard, J.W. Soper, and W.G. Sampson, Editors. 1970, C.V. Mosby Company: St. Louis. p. 65–92.

26 Mohrman, R., The keratometer, in *Clinical Ophthalmology*, T.D. Duane, Editor. 1976, Harper and Row, Hagerstown. p. 1–3, 9–12.

27 Ruben, M., *Contact Lens Practice*. Baltimore, Williams and Wilkins; 1975.

28 Miller, D., M.S. Jernigan, and S. Molnar, Laboratory evaluation of a clinical glare tester. Arch Ophthalmol 1972; 87: p. 324.

29 Miller, D. and G. Benedek, *Intraocular Light Scattering*. Springfield CT, Thomas. 38,53–67; 1973.

30 Holladay, L.L., The fundamentals of glare and visibility. J Opt Soc Am 1926; 12: p. 492.

31 Wolf, E., Glare and age. Arch Ophthalmol 1960; 4: p. 502.

32 Hess, R. and G. Woo, Vision through cataracts. Invest Ophthalmol 1978; 17: p. 428.

33 Arden, G.B., Spatial contrast sensitivity [editorial]. Br J Ophthalmol 1978; 62(4): p. 197.

34 Paulson, L.E. and J. Sjorstand, Contrast sensitivity in the presence of a glare light. Invest Ophthalmol 1980; 19: p. 401.

35 Nadler, M.P., New glare tester [letter]. Arch Ophthalmol 1982; 100(10): p. 1676.

36 LeClaire, J., M.P. Nadler, S. Weiss, *et al.*, A new glare tester for clinical testing. Results comparing normal subjects and variously corrected aphakic patients. Arch Ophthalmol 1982; 100(1): p. 153–8.

37 Villasenor, R.A., V.R. Santos, K.C. Cox, *et al.*, Comparison of ultrasonic corneal thickness measurements before and during surgery in the prospective evaluation of Radial Keratotomy (PERK) Study. Ophthalmology 1986; 93(3): p. 327–30.

6 Topography—The Fine Art of Corneal Surface Measurement

The history of science in general has often been the story of scientists vigorously fighting an onslaught of new ideas. This is because it is difficult to relinquish the sense of security that comes from a long and rewarding acquaintance with a particular point of view.
[Gary Zukav, The Dancing Wu Lei Masters]

Philosophers and bards wax poetic about the eye being the "window of the soul," whereas iridologists claim to be able to diagnose disease from a study of the iris crypts. All lovely and romantic to be sure, but these notions stray far from the fact that the eye is an optical device—and a relatively poor one at that.

For example, *optical axis* is an oxymoron when applied to the human eye, and *symmetry* for the same organ is likened to the unicorn—a beast fabled of legend but nowhere to be seen on Earth. It was Helmholtz [1] who said—and rightly:

> If an optician should try to sell me an instrument possessing the faults mentioned, it seems to me—without overstressing the matter—that I should think myself wholly justified in using the most severe language with regard to the carelessness of his work and returning the instrument under protest.

How it is that the eye works as well as it does is a mystery. But perhaps the reason is because it is attached to the brain—a wonderful discriminator capable of making much of the imagery sent to it; much like the scientists who were able to glean valuable data from the malfunctioning Hubbell telescope. Without the brain, the eye is—quite literally—nothing. It is in fact this self-same brain that has created the confusion surrounding the optics of the eye—both directly and indirectly. It is the brain's wonderful ability to adjust reality—in the one case, the data stream flowing from the retina to the visual cortex to provide clear vision and, in the other, reality as presented to us by the world, which in turn causes us to come to understand that same world. It is remarkable that given the same facts in each case, over the centuries—nay, millennia—different conclusions and therefore different understandings have resulted. It should not be wondered at, then, that confusion reigns; Zukav is right.

Needs of the refractive surgeon

In refractive surgery we seek to modify the corneal surface in such a way as to compensate for deficiencies in the total optical system of the eye. The need for accurate and precise methods of evaluating the contour of the anterior corneal surface has paralleled the rapid development of keratorefractive surgery. Thus the suboptimal refractive predictability of procedures such as penetrating keratoplasty, astigmatic keratotomy, radial keratotomy, intracorneal inlays/implants, and laser in situ keratomileusis (LASIK) has provided impetus for the development of techniques for measuring and presenting corneal topography that are essential for understanding changes induced by surgical manipulations of the corneal surface.

Surgeons have realized that simple demonstrations of corneal topographic changes in corneal and keratorefractive procedures do not provide enough information; quantification of the topography of these frequently complex corneal surfaces is necessary. There can be no more compelling demonstration of the need and desirability for accurate corneal surface measurements than the patients described by Maguire and McDonnell [2–4]. These studies add further evidence to the hypothesis that a subset of patients who undergo refractive surgery are left with a postoperative topography characterized by a small central area of minimum power surrounded by concentric bands of increasingly higher power [5]. When these bands of higher power are located within or close to the entrance pupil, they have the ability to allow "good" visual acuity (as measured by standard visual acuity charts) to be maintained over a greater refractive range than is possible with normal corneal surface optics. For the radial keratotomy patient with –3.00 D of residual cycloplegic refractive error who is able to maintain good-quality 20/20 to 20/40 uncorrected vision, the "multifocal effect" of such an extremely aspheric corneal surface could hardly be deemed a complication [6]. Unfortunately, some post-refractive surgery patients may develop a pattern of corneal asphericity severe enough to cause a significant degradation in the quality of the visual image while still maintaining 20/20 visual acuity and a "multifocal lens effect" over an extended refractive range. One would be hard pressed to convince such a patient that he or she has not had a surgical complication. And this problem is just not confined to radial keratotomy. Practitioners of other modalities are reporting an uncomfortable number of patients with surface aberrations causing subnominal vision.

These findings concerning the relationship of corneal surface topography to visual performance and the hypothesis regarding the cause of this pattern of corneal irregularity leads to the following conclusion, expressed by Leo Maguire:

> Our knowledge of the effect preoperative topography has on postoperative results following refractive surgery is less than adequate. If patients are capable of maintaining excellent Snellen visual acuity in the presence of severe corneal irregularity after such surgery, is it not possible that a subset of the normal population demonstrates similar degrees of variable central corneal irregularity prior to surgery? It is increasingly obvious that our understanding of the topography of the postoperative corneal surface, its relation to multifocal effects in particular, and visual performance in general is still in its infancy [2,7].

This possibility is given weight by the appearance of suspicious steep areas of the cornea seen on such maps that bear a striking resemblance to keratoconus absent keratometric findings of nonsuperimposable mires, a normal ultrasonic pachymetry, as well as a history of a relatively stable refraction.

Today, with the increased interest in refractive eye surgery, suppositions and guesswork will no longer serve. Operations such as keratomileusis and LASIK, in which the central corneal cap or apex curvature is modified through tissue ablation, depend very much on the primary curvature of that same area. Empirical formulas have been employed to control the amount of tissue removed. While such empiricism works, predictability of the outcome is still elusive. The uncertainty of the ultimate corneal shape makes even more difficult modification of the external corneal curvature through employment of intrastromal allopathic lenticules, such as the hydrophilic implant. Peripheral modification of the cornea in an effort to alter the apex—the hallmark of the radial keratotomy procedure as well as radial implants (ICRS)—is also affected by the overall shape of the cornea. In this instance, the corneal surface need be moved only a few tens of microns to alter the refraction significantly. Laser tissue ablation (PRK) is even more problematic because reliance is placed on micron-level tissue layer removal. Progress in intraocular lens design, as well as the surgery of corneal transplantation and that of cataract, hinges on a more enlightened understanding of the surface that produces 90% of the refractive power of the eye.

The quality of vision greatly depends on the topography of the cornea. The keratometer is used routinely to measure the shape of the cornea in the clinical practice of ophthalmology, but this instrument measures corneal curvature from the reflection of mires at only four positions along two meridians at right angles. While this method can achieve an accuracy of better than 0.25 D in measuring steel balls, clinical keratometers cannot be used to measure irregular astigmatism or corneal asphericity. For example, the keratometer cannot be used to assess the size of the central zone of uniform power following radial keratotomy or any other technique.

Thus we have employed moiré keratometry, electronic keratometry, ultrasound, photogrammetry, profile photography, and interferometry to perform this task. Each has its own unique advantages and disadvantages, each of which will be discussed within this chapter. Underlying the eclecticism of evolving topographic instrumentation lies a very real and intensive attempt to understand and codify something that has proven to be a very slippery customer over the last century or so—the corneal surface shape.

The following is a synopsis of what is fittingly called the "state of the art" (emphasis on the last word). The term *art* aptly fits the mélange of brightly hued and occasionally abstract images facing the ophthalmologist seeking the Grail of refractive surgery.

Surface zones of the cornea

A useful simplification to understand the topography of the cornea is to consider the corneal curvature as a section of an ellipse. In most normal corneas, the central zone is steeper than the paracentral and peripheral zones, a configuration referred to as having a *positive shape factor* (positive because the radius of curvature becomes larger from the center to the periphery) and a *prolate shape*. A prolate shape is that shape taken across the narrow end of an ellipse or—better—the pointy end of an egg. The opposite topographic pattern rarely occurs in normal eyes but appears commonly after radial keratotomy: The central zone is flatter than the paracentral and peripheral zones, a configuration referred to as having a *negative shape factor* and an *oblate shape*—which is the section taken across the long axis of an ellipse (Figure 6.1).

A similar oversimplification takes place when the cornea is divided into surface zones (e.g., optical zone, apical zone). None of these areas is discrete, because the cornea forms continuous curves. Nevertheless, for practical optical and anatomic purposes, we can divide the surface of the cornea into two overall regions: the central optical zone and the remainder of the cornea (sometimes called the *periphery*) [8]. However, it appears that the arbitrary division of the cornea into the central and peripheral topographic regions is far too simplistic. Although these concepts may be useful when fitting contact lenses, in reality, one can only state with certainty that the normal cornea is steeper centrally and flatter in the periphery.

The *optical zone* forms the foveal image through the entrance pupil of the eye; its size, shape, and curvature vary among individuals. The rest of the cornea serves as a refracting surface for peripheral vision and for the foveal image when the pupil is widely dilated, as a mechanical structure, and as a source of cells during normal turnover and repair.

Apex of the cornea

Topographically, the central area of the cornea is generally referred to as the *apical zone*. The apical zone size differs among eyes, and its definition depends on who's describing it. This zone can be defined as the area surrounding the corneal apex that does not vary in curvature by more than 1 D. Various investigators have defined this zone differently [9]. Mandell defined the apical zone as being that area in which the central refraction differed by less than 0.25 D [10]. Others have defined it as the region around the apex where the radius of curvature differs by less than 0.05 mm [11–13].

Current evidence shows that the paraxial (optical) area is nearly spherical, but even in this region, the curvature seems to vary in different meridians (see above). In fact, this surface astigmatism is found, at least to some degree, in such a high proportion of the population that it should be considered a normal state of affairs. Thus—by definition—the central cornea is not spherical but is more properly described as *toroidal*. Dingeldein and Klyce found that the existence of a definable apical region could not be confirmed [14]. Their data suggest that a definitive apical area probably does not exist, but rather the central region blends homogeneously with the rest of the cornea. Suffice that for this discussion the apical zone is the central portion of the cornea that shows the least variation in dioptric power over its extent.

All studies to date, based on various methodologies, have indicated that the peripheral cornea is even more irregular and cannot be described in simple geometric terms. The general shape of the peripheral cornea is flatter than is the central portion, however, and this has led to a dividing of the corneal surface into zones (see below).

Conventionally, four concentric anatomic zones are recognized (Figure 6.2): central optical zone, paracentral

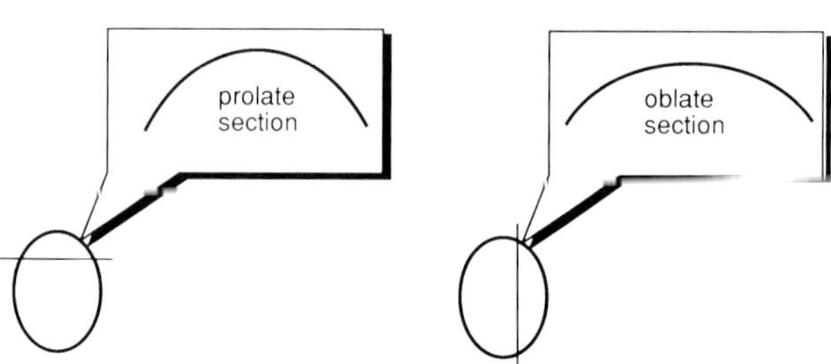

Fig. 6.1 Prolate and oblate curved sections.

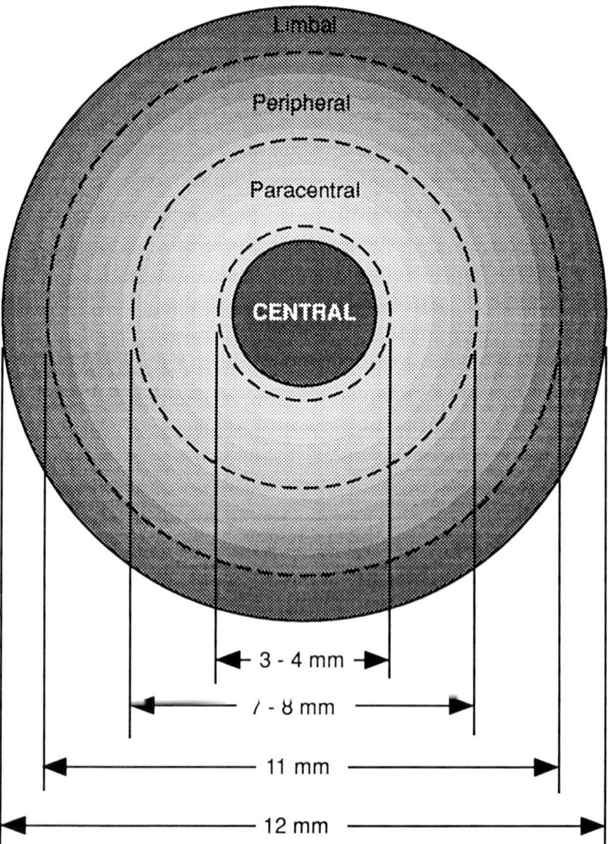

Fig. 6.2 Corneal zones.

intermediate zone, peripheral transitional zone, and limbal zone. It is important to distinguish these anatomic zones from those commonly associated with radial keratotomy so as to avoid confusion.

Central optical zone

The central zone is approximately 4 mm in diameter and has been called the *apical zone,* the *corneal cap,* the *optical zone,* and the *central spherical zone,* all terms intended to designate this region of the cornea as the more spherical, symmetrical, and optically important. The term *central zone* appears most apt. Now that corneal topography is requiring more careful definitions, we must distinguish among four designations:

- The anatomic central zone, which is 3 to 4 mm in diameter
- The functional optical zone, which is the area that overlies the entrance pupil and is smaller than the anatomic zone
- The "spherical" central part of the cornea, which is present in a minority of normal corneas
- The apex of the cornea, which is the highest spot on the cornea

The optical zone can be further defined in one of five ways depending on the optical circumstances:

- The anatomic center of the cornea, equidistant from the limbus and typically eccentric to the optic and visual axes
- The optical axis that connects the center of curvature of the cornea and centers of curvature of the crystalline lens (which also can be slightly eccentric to the visual axis)
- The pupillary axis that connects the center of the entrance pupil and the center of curvature of the cornea
- The line of sight that connects the fixation point with the center of the entrance pupil
- The visual axis that passes from the center of the fovea through the nodal points of the eye (Figure 6.3)

Detailed discussion of these often confusing axes can be found in Chapter 3. For practical purposes, the center of the optical zone should be considered the intersection of the pupillary axis with the cornea, because the entrance pupil determines the image-forming bundle of rays that reach the fovea. However that may be, this optical zone may not be coincident with the surgical optical or clear zone that is centered on the visual axis.

The term *optical zone* is used with four different meanings in the context of refractive surgery. The first meaning is that just defined: the central more spherical portion of the normal cornea overlying the entrance pupil. The second meaning refers to the portion of a keratomileusis or epikeratoplasty lenticule or excimer laser surface ablation that creates the major refractive change. The third meaning is the central uncut clear zone in radial keratotomy; *clear zone* is preferred by some but with no compelling reason. In the author's view, calling the area of the cornea most affected by the refractive surgical technique (the "business" part as opposed to the supportive part) the *optical zone* is apt and descriptive and should cause no confusion (except perhaps among purists). The fourth meaning is any circular mark on the cornea used to delineate or demarcate places where incisions begin or end—for example, a "7-mm optical zone" used for placement of transverse incisions. In this context, *optical zone* is

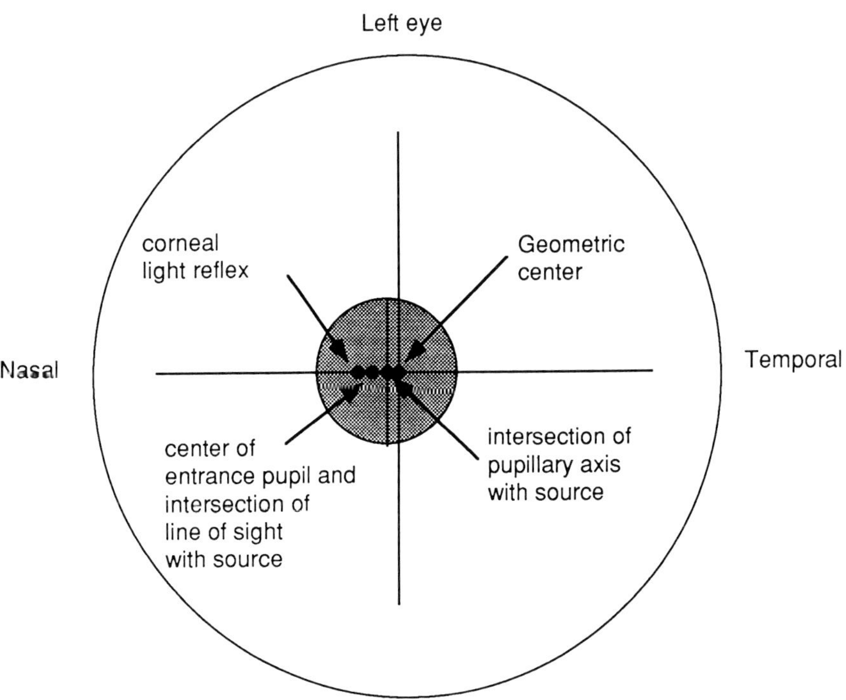

Fig. 6.3 Pupillary axes (see also Chapter 3).

truly a misnomer and should be replaced by the simple designation *surgical zone* or just *zone*, as in "the transverse incisions were placed at the 7-mm (surgical) zone."

Paracentral anatomic zone

The *paracentral anatomic zone* is an annulus approximately 4 to 7 mm in diameter and has been called the *mid, intermediate,* or *midperipheral cornea*. The term *midperipheral* is a misnomer because this zone does not occupy the middle of the periphery. A transverse incision made at the 6-mm zone would be "midperipheral" because while it is still within the central anatomic half of the cornea, it is partway into the peripheral zone and also at the midpoint of the cornea. The paracentral surgical zone in radial keratotomy is any zone mark from 3.0 to 5.0 mm in diameter and refers to the first or primary surgical zone. The central and paracentral zones together comprise what contact lens fitters call the apical zone.

Peripheral anatomic zone

The *peripheral anatomic zone* is an annulus from approximately 7 to 11 mm in diameter. This is the area in which the normal cornea flattens the most and becomes more aspheric. For this reason, it has been called the *transitional zone*. Note that this is not the same extent as described by Mandell [15]. In radial keratotomy, zones from 7 to 9 mm are called *paraperipheral* surgical zones.

Limbal anatomic zone

The *limbal anatomic zone* is the ring of cornea approximately 0.5 mm wide that abuts the sclera and contains the capillary arcade. The area from 9 mm to the limbus has been designated the *far-peripheral zone* by radial keratotomists.

Computerized keratoscopy also has revealed information about the topography of the normal peripheral cornea. Several investigators have found that peripheral flattening is asymmetrical in the majority of eyes [16–18].

A few other definitions need to be addressed. The *visual center* of the cornea is the point through which the visual axis passes. The *geometric center* is the point at which the longest horizontal and vertical surface arc lengths intersect [19]. The distance from the apical center to the visual center varies from person to person.

Optics and topography of the cornea

What I am describing here is the anatomy of the cornea in a somewhat general way, much like describing a scene that is spread out before an observer. It is possible to describe the undulations, the hills, the valleys, and the mountains. It is even possible to make some comments about the structure of the scenery by grubbing about in the dirt to see what the soil is made up of. However, this is all we can do until we get out our surveying instruments and get to work.

Many of the keratorefractive procedures directly involve the intermediate and peripheral zones of the cornea. Additionally, evaluating the refractive effect of these procedures involves assessing the topography of the cornea far beyond the central 3 to 4 mm covered by the keratometer.

General structure and function of the cornea

The cornea is a complex geometric structure. The basic anatomic components of the cornea account for its thickness, radius of curvature, and surface regularity, all of which play a role in its anterior topography. It is appropriate to begin any discussion of corneal topography with an analysis of these structural characteristics.

The cornea is not uniformly thick throughout. It is typically thinnest centrally, measuring about 0.5 mm, with a general trend of increasing thickness as the limbus is approached. The average thickness at the limbus measures about 1.2 mm.

Anterior and posterior corneal curvature

The difference in thickness from the center to the periphery determines, in large measure, the difference in radius of curvature between these two regions, with the average radius of curvature of the anterior surface of the cornea being about 7.8 mm and that of the posterior surface about 6.7 mm [20]. The difference between the anterior and posterior radii of curvature yields an average of 43 D of convergence, with the anterior surface contributing 49 D of convergence and the posterior surface 6 D of divergence. In actuality, the air–tear film interface, the interface having the greatest change in index of refraction in the eye's optical system, is responsible for the majority of this 43 D of convergence.

Because the tear film assumes the shape of the anterior corneal surface, for all practical purposes, the curvature of the anterior tear film is that of the anterior cornea. Since the crystalline lens only contributes about 20 D of convergence, the anterior surface of the cornea is the major topographic determinant of the eye's optical system and is thus a critical factor in proper visual function [21].

Surface smoothness

The anterior surface of the cornea is lined with an epithelial layer that is five to eight cells thick and approximately 50 to 100 μm in depth. The superficial cells of this epithelial layer are polyhedral in shape and, under normal circumstances, do not keratinize. Their nuclei are flat and are projected posteriorly. These qualities combine to create a very smooth anterior surface, an essential component for pinpoint refraction of light rays onto the fovea and thus for maximal visual acuity [22].

Disorders of these three basic components—thickness, radius of curvature, and surface regularity—can directly affect the topography of the cornea.

Normal variations in corneal topography

Corneal topography, although relatively stable with respect to maintaining accurate visual acuity, appears to undergo diurnal fluctuations. These changes appear to depend on a number of physiologic and anatomic conditions, including eyelid pressure, time of day, tear film tonicity, and hormonal levels.

When the eyelids are retracted, there is a shift toward "against-the-rule" astigmatism, suggesting that the pressure of the eyelids causes a "with-the-rule" astigmatism. Wilson and colleagues found not only that was there a shift toward against-the-rule astigmatism but also that the shift was a result of a steepening in the horizontal axis and not a flattening in the vertical axis [23,24].

In addition to the long-term influence of the eyelids on corneal topography, there are a variety of diurnal corneal changes that can alter normal topography. The most common of these occurs nightly during sleep. Most investigators have found that during sleep, there is a 3% to 8% increase in anterior corneal thickness. Following exposure during waking hours, the increased thickness returns to base line within 1 to 12 hours. About 75% of this process occurs within the first 2 h, with a gradual thinning over the rest of the day. The reason for increased corneal thickness during sleep is not completely understood.

Other factors that may influence the topography of the normal cornea seem to be hormonal in origin. Some data suggest that fluctuations in corneal topography may occur during the menstrual cycle. Keratometric steepening of both the horizontal and vertical meridians was found to occur at the beginning of the cycle, with a tendency toward flattening after ovulation. The changes in corneal thickness during menstruation tended to be quite variable throughout the cycle [25–27]. It is these variations which mitigate against performing refractive surgery during pregnancy or when a patient is coming off or going on birth-control medications.

The problem

So what's the problem? We've got "gizmos" that map the corneal surface in all kinds of pretty patterns and colors. What more do you want? The problem is that much of what we want cannot be obtained with today's crop of topographers. And why not? To answer this question, it must be said at the outset—and it must be understood thoroughly—that the cornea is not spherical. Without this understanding, nothing about what I am going to tell you will make the least sense.

It is a fact that the cornea is not spherical, yet we insist, many of us, that it be treated as if it were; too many people continue to believe that it is spherical despite evidence to the contrary. Devices have been designed and constructed that have measured something of its surface properties. But the exact shape of the corneal surface has, like the dark side of the moon, until recently remained out of sight and out of reach and, like the dark side of the moon, has been described rather fancifully. Those measurements which have been taken have, unfortunately, muddied the waters by creating certain mind-sets and preconceptions that are difficult to overcome. Much money has been spent and much time wasted on this fiction, and it is all Scheiner's fault.

Christopherus Scheiner, a Jesuit instructor in Hebrew and mathematics—and by all accounts a man of insatiable investigative zeal—has been given the credit for, in 1619, the first attempts to measure the curvature of the cornea. He did this by arranging glass beads of varying diameters in front of a multipaned window and comparing the reflected images in each with that of a human eye facing the same window. By this means he was able to estimate the corneal curvature [28]. By this means he is also entitled to much of the blame for the misconceptions that have existed since then about that same curvature.

This is not to say that our *knowledge* of how to measure the surface has not advanced—it has. It is just that we have not used the knowledge. We still insist that the eye is a spherical refracting surface; we attempt to measure its curvature using methods that only work with spheres, and we wonder why it is that none of the results of our measurements make any sense. While we know better now, many people still believe (without any supporting evidence) that some small portion of the cornea, perhaps the apical part, does indeed exist as a sphere. Would that this were truly the case—it would make measuring the surface curvature all the more simple. It is good that it is not, however, because were it so, the eye would be a worse optical device than it is, and our surgical attempts to modify the cornea would be less successful and perhaps even ineffectual.

The cornea is not spherical, and yet most of the current instrumentation that purports to measure the curvature of the human cornea is based on the assumption that it is. This assumption continues to be supported despite the fact that we have known it to be wrong since the inception of the first keratometer. The reasons for this are manifold:

1 It is easy to implement a sphere-based curvature measurement methodology. It is also easy to drive from Scottsdale to Tempe in order to get to Cleveland. Unfortunately, when you arrive—you're not in Cleveland!

2 It is believed that the deviation from spherical of the human cornea is regular and of small degree

Before launching into a discussion of the corneal shape, let's consider the problem we are facing, and we will see very quickly why many have tried to take the easy way out. We shall start by dealing with a certain perception, namely: *If it were so important, someone would already have done something about it.* This seems fair; after all, physicians have concerned themselves with the nature of the curvature of the cornea since 1619—almost 400 years now.

Timing is everything

Let's look at the situation. Kepler wrote his *Supplement to Vitello* (*Ad Vitellionem Paraliponema*) in 1604, and his *Dioptrice* did not see print until 1611 [29,30]. These works probably mark the beginning of the field known as *geometric optics* and represent a huge advance over what had gone before: a horrible mishmash of misunderstanding stretching back to the time of Euclid in 300 BC—a *mere* 2000 years. Kepler had nothing special going for him at that time—and he conducted no experiments whatsoever; these were mind problems—and although he was in print, books were rare, and people who could afford to buy them, let alone read them, were scarce. Thus, while it is possible that Scheiner knew of Kepler's work, it probably played no heavy role in his own.

Snell's law was propounded in 1621. Simply stated, it is

$$n \text{ sine } I = n' \text{ sine } I$$

that is, the angle of refraction at an optical surface is proportional to the sine of the angle of incidence and the ratio of the refractive indices. Newton published his *Opticks* in 1704 [31]. Since he was somewhat better known, his book created a larger sensation, but still it was not wholeheartedly accepted at the time.

It wasn't until 1841 that Gauss, a prodigy ranked with Archimedes and Newton, produced the elegant mathematical construction that solved the problem of complex optical systems. It was his student, Lister, who developed a very accurate, theoretical schematic eye. Allvar Gullstrand, himself a towering genius and recipient of a Nobel prize, could do no better than produce a simplified, but still elegant, copy of Lister's model eye [32]. As to astigmatism, nothing much was heard except as a curiosity worthy of discussion in such halls as The Royal Philosophic Society by none other than Thomas Young, who discovered it in himself [33]. It was not until the turn of the 19th century, that spherocylinder spectacles were prescribed regularly to the afflicted.

The concept of refractive surgery—altering an eye for the sole purpose of improving its refractive state—while first suggested by Boerhaave in 1708 [34], was not entertained seriously until 1896. Then, and almost simultaneously, Lans in Holland and Bates in the United States assayed to treat astigmatism—the former in rabbits and the latter in humans. But it was not until 1962 with Barraquer's work in keratomileusis that modulation of corneal shape began to become seriously noticed, and it was not until the author's work in 1978–1979 that the floodgates opened wide and refractive surgery as an ophthalmic surgical subspecialty took root and flourished. Never mind that Sato had done some important but flawed work in 1939 or that Fyodorov was toiling in obscurity in the Soviet Union in 1973. Thus it is that only within the last 20 or so years has there been a serious need for the data we are attempting to gather.

Solving the problem

What of the nature of the problem itself? Consider the issue posed: You are given a convex mirror—roughly the diameter of a nickel. Your task is to accurately produce a map of its surface. Straightforward enough, you say. Now come the disclaimers—we call them *constraints*. You are constrained by certain truths and requirements.

The truths are

1 The surface is *not* a section of a marble—hence spherical; rather, it is a section of an ellipsoid—egg-shaped—therefore aspherical and an asphere whose eccentricity is unknown and inconstant in the bargain.

2 The optic axis is statistically *not* coincident with the apex of the mirror surface—the apex being defined as the intersection of the longest arcs of the surface. It is known, through experiment, that the axis is off to one side of the apex in the majority of cases, but the actual displacement is not correlated with the surface arc. No help there (see Figure 6.3 and also Chapter 3).

3 The surface is asymmetrical. That is, knowing the curve of one semimeridian does not give you the opposite curve, nor does it supply you with any clue to its shape.

4 The target is not fixed in space but has a tendency to move about and at will and despite entreaty or beseechment.

5 Access to the surface is semirestricted by its environment.

The requirements are

1 The surface may not be touched in any way by any manifest instrument or device—therefore, no calipers, rulers, etc., may be employed, and small use they would be at this scale in any event.

2 The object must be dealt with in situ; it cannot be removed or detached from its situation.

3 The accuracy of measurement must be on the order of equal to (or greater than) ±0.25 D (the accuracy probably should be down in the micron range for laser guidance).

4 The data must be presented representationally in such a manner that study by reasonably intelligent users, trained in interpretation, can make practical sense of it.

5 The results of testing must be repeatable within certain bounds and conditions. That is, all else being equal, the output from the measurement process should be equal or nearly so from one measurement to the next.

Now that you know what you have to do—how will you go about it?

Solution 1

If your answer is that since the surface is a mirror, you will reflect an image of some geometric object of known dimension off the eye and measure that image, you will be doing what Scheiner did in 1619. And you will have violated one of the truths, namely, that the measured object is not spherical, and you will have progressed no further than Scheiner did 381 years ago. But at least you would have chosen a tool—*light*—that could be used to solve your problem. The rub is—how shall the tool be used? Before you get too wound up with Solution 1, let's see how others fared with this idea over the years.

Scheiner's idea was not totally illogical or unusable. The fact is that Javal and Helmholtz expanded on the basic principle by creating devices that quantitated the measurements of the central cornea [35,36].

Ophthalmometry

The concept of determining the curvature of a surface by measuring the size of the reflected image is well established in optics. However, measuring such a reflection on the eye is made difficult by the fact that the eye is constantly in motion. Almost four centuries have passed since the first attempt to measure the anterior surface curvature of the cornea, yet the exact form of this surface is still not well understood. While the methods of measurement have been diverse, nearly all the corneal measurements realized so far have been based on one optical property of the cornea—that it is a convex reflecting surface, that is, a mirror. In general, previous measuring devices were based on the assumption that the cornea was a conic section, that is, a sphere, an ellipse, a parabola, or a hyperbola. In reality, the living cornea is none of these but rather is an aspheric section with great individual variation—a toroidal asphere.

Ramsden, in 1796, adopted the concept of the heliograph and visual doubling to ocular surface measurement. Kohlraush measured the reflected image of an object on the cornea using a Kepler telescope [37]. Helmholtz perfected this device in 1856, and his design serves as the basis for many instruments in use today. While Helmholtz's modifications made a device that was accurate for scientific work, some further adjustment was necessary to adapt the instrument to use in clinical practice, particularly for the measurement of astigmatism. Helmholtz was the first to introduce the doubling device into an ophthalmometer [1]. Coccius [38], Landolt [39], Javal and Schiøtz [35], Sutcliffe [40], and Hartinger [41] followed with other measuring devices. The incorporation into a Wollaston prism (two rectangular prisms cemented back to back) by Javal and Schiøtz produced a doubling refracting system that created two complete light cones rather than one [35]. Fincham was the first to measure directly the corneal periphery using an autocollimation microscope [42]. Berg modified the Javal-Schiøtz ophthalmometer by placing a set of two lenses in front of it, forming an afocal system of magnification [43,44]. With this device he was able to explore a zone about 1 mm in diameter at various points over the cornea.

Current evidence shows that the paraxial (optical) area is nearly spherical, but even in this region the curvature seems to vary in different meridians. In fact, this surface astigmatism is found, at least to some degree, in such a high proportion of the population that it should be considered a normal state of affairs. Thus—by definition—the central cornea is not spherical but is more properly described as toroidal. All studies to date, based on various methodologies, have indicated that the peripheral cornea is even more irregular and cannot be described in simple geometric terms. The general shape of the peripheral cornea is flatter than is the central portion, however, and this has led to a dividing of the corneal surface into zones.

Traditionally, the corneal surface has been divided into two zones. The center, or corneal cap (apical zone), is the spherical or toroidal part, extending 4 to 5 mm in diameter. The peripheral, or annular part, extends to the limbus and is progressively flatter in contour (Figure 6.4). It is possible to define the cap as the central area having the maximum and most constant curvature. However, an annoying feature of the subject of corneal topography is the difficulty in deciding which point of the cornea to take as the apex of the cap. The center of the apical zone is not easily defined because the zone itself may be of indefinite size and extent. Defining the apex as the point of maximum curvature may result in this point not corresponding with the visual axis. Furthermore, it may be that major curvature in the toroidal form of the cornea is less marked at the apex than at the visual axis (Figure 6.5). Measurement in the latter instance may be a situation in which true toricity combines with an effect caused by tilt of an

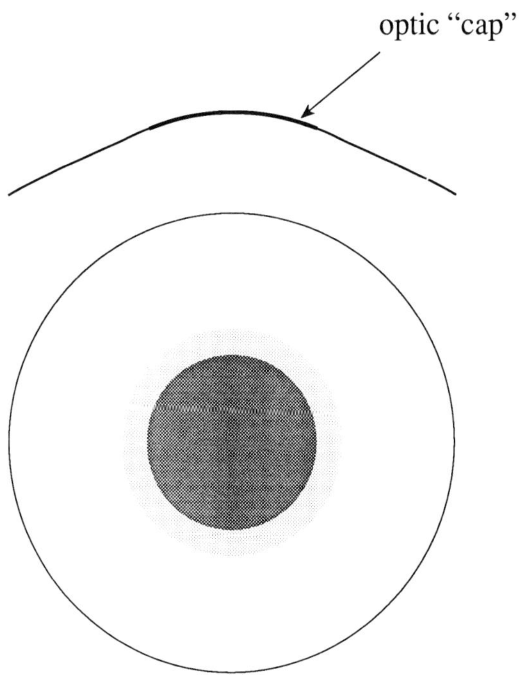

Fig. 6.4 Corneal apex or "cap."

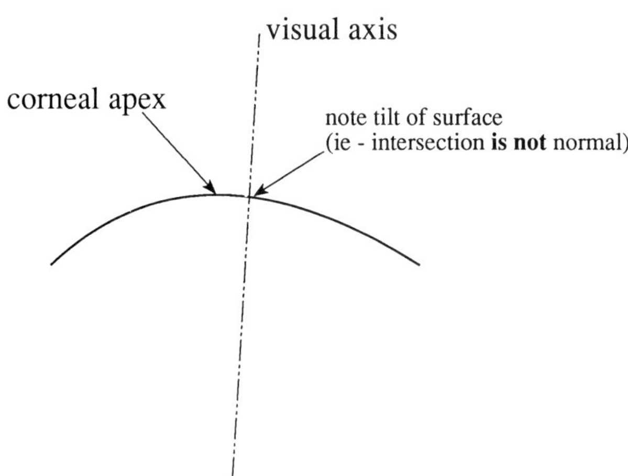

Fig. 6.5 The apex may not correspond with the optical axis or may be tilted.

aspheric surface. Additionally, no good data exist clearly defining either the size of the apical zone or where it ends and the peripheral zone begins. The limit or edge of this zone has been described by Mandell as the point where the radius of curvature increases by more than 0.05 mm (0.63 D) [45]. Thus the radius of curvature of the apex would lie between 7.2 and 8.7 mm—averaging 7.9 mm (46.62 to 38.62 and 42.50 D, respectively).

This division originally was proposed by Aubert, who described the cornea as having an optic part and a basilar part—on the basis of four measurements in six subjects—not exactly a statistically relevant sample [46]. Ericksen, using a Javal-Schiøtz type of ophthalmometer, described the cap as having a diameter of 4.0 mm delineated by a change in power of 1.0 D [47]. Gullstrand supported this early work in his studies using photokeratoscopy [48]. He, too, found the central zone to be spherical. Other investigators later found the cap to be less spherical and more conical in shape with no definite boundaries—hence the borders of the so-called corneal cap are arbitrary, depending on one's criteria.

For the purpose of our discussion, we will accept the boundary to be that place where the corneal curvature flattens by more than 1.0 D, even though this may not be entirely valid. Thus the average cap will have a diameter of 4.0 mm. If a 2.0-D flattening is used, the cap has a diameter of 6.0 mm—an interesting fact that I will touch on later. As measuring methods have become more precise, however, it is apparent that *constant corneal curvature* is an oxymoron and that only the very central part of the cornea has an instantaneous spherical shape. The student of such things may be moved to ask, "So what?" So what indeed. Probably "So nothing," except that it is difficult to abandon the notion that there must exist some sort of central zone of whatever stripe; otherwise, what is it that produces the reflex during skiaoscopy, and what are we correcting with our spectacles and other optical appliances?

Adding to the dilemma posed by such an uncooperative surface is the observation—reported by Reynolds and Kratt—that the cornea changes shape during the day, being flatter, and thus more hyperopic, in the morning as a rule [49]. This observation is separate from the even greater changes reported following radial keratotomy (RK) [50,51]. The act of accommodation itself (focusing for near) has been shown to affect the corneal curvature by 1.5 D in the horizontal and 0.5 D in the vertical meridians in normal individuals and by as much as 2 D in all meridians after RK [52]

I have mentioned a visual axis as if all the optical components of the eye were somehow symmetrically aligned along a common axis. Strictly speaking, such a condition does not exist. In fact, the best-derived optic axis that can be conceived—assuming such an alignment—does not strike the center of vision, the fovea, at all.

Another complicating factor, which becomes more manifest as the methods of measurement become more refined, is the fact that the corneal surface is wet—a con-

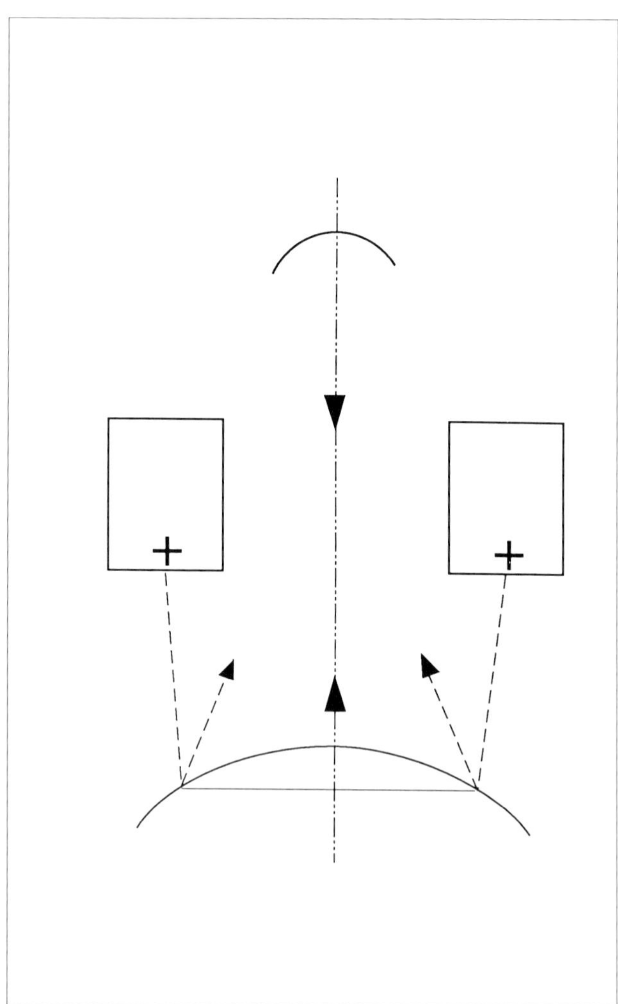

Fig. 6.6 Principle of ophthalmometry. Objects of known size are reflected by a curved surface forming the first Purkinje image. The size of this image is related to the degree of curvature.

dition that has important implications, as Bonnett found when he sprinkled talcum powder on the surface as a reflectant [53].

The keratometer is used routinely to measure the shape of the cornea in the clinical practice of ophthalmology, but this instrument measures corneal curvature using the reflected mires from only four positions along two meridians at right angles (Figure 6.6). In ophthalmometry, it is the spatial relationship between points before the cornea and the reflected image of these points that is used to calculate the average curvature between these reflected points on the cornea. To some extent, the smaller the area between these points on the cornea, the more representative of the actual surface contour the average can be.

The mire size is fixed by the manufacturer but is generally too large to be considered to be reflecting paraxial rays from the cornea; thus optical mirror formulas cannot be used where high accuracy is needed. The keratometer does not need to actually measure the mire size, however. It is enough to know the relative sizes of the images for various radii hence simple paraxial formulas can be used without concern for serious error. The derivation of this formula is based on an approximation—this is important in understanding the limitations of keratometry. Figure 6.7 illustrates the basics of keratometer optics using two-ray construction. The size of the virtual image can be found by using the relationship of similar triangles:

$$\frac{h}{h'} = \frac{f'}{x} = \frac{r/2}{x}$$

To simplify matters, the object (mire) is considered to be sufficiently far from the cornea that the virtual image is formed very near the focal point of the cornea. Thus the distance from the mire to the focal point is very slightly different from the actual distance d between the mire and its image. Hence

$$r \cong \frac{2dh'}{h}$$

The mires in the Bausch & Lomb instrument are shaped like pluses and minuses. The distance between the two "plus" mires represents the size of the object in the horizontal meridian, whereas the two "minus" mires perform the same function for the vertical meridian. This distance is typically 64 mm. The distance from the mires to the cornea (when properly focused) is 75 mm—3 in. The circle included in the mire target is for the purpose of showing any surface irregularities or asphericity (Figure 6.8).

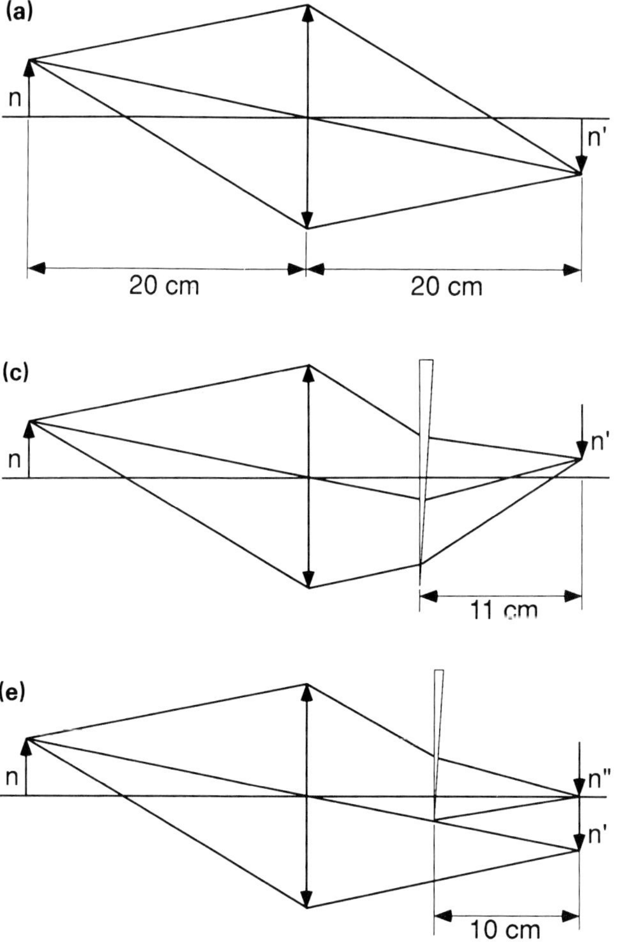

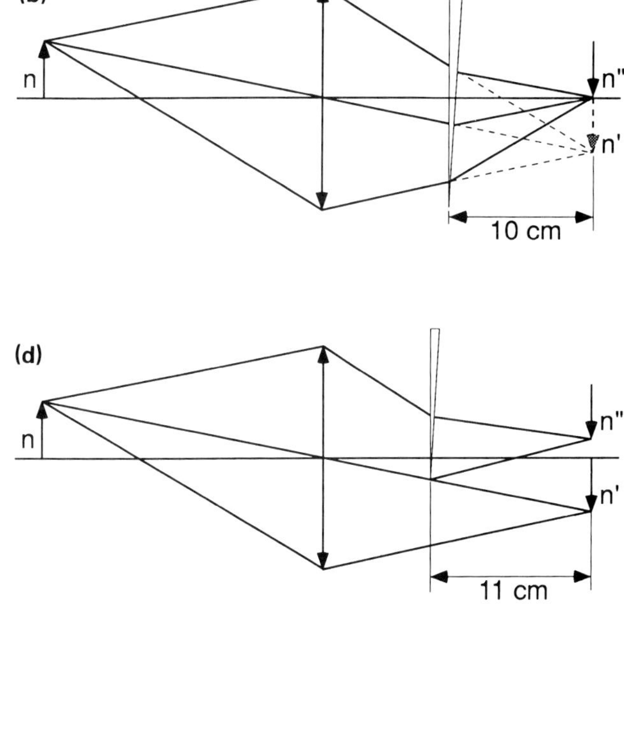

Fig. 6.7 (a) The relationship between object and image. (b) Introducing a prism displaces the image. (c) Moving the focal point displaces the image. (d) The prism can be situated so as to produce two images. (e) The separation of the images at a fixed distance is proportional to the image size.

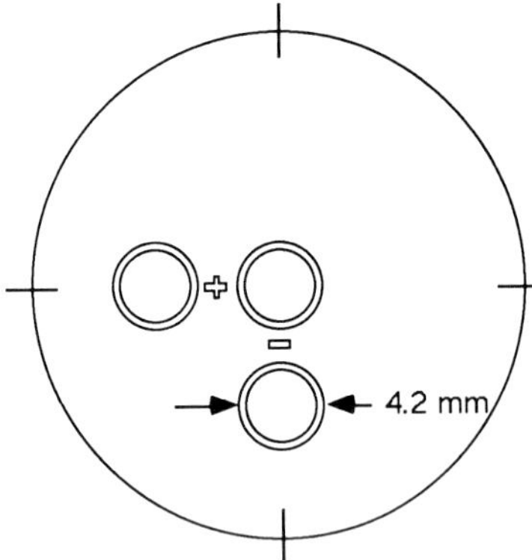

Fig. 6.8 B&L Keratometer mires.

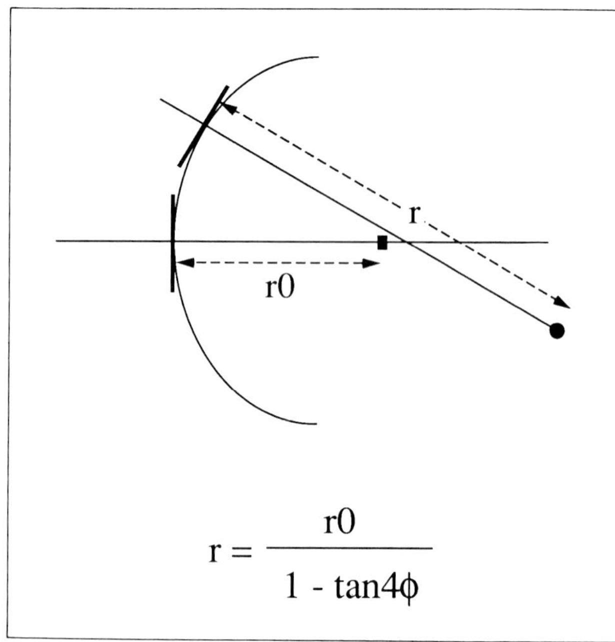

Fig. 6.9 Berg's formula to calculate peripheral corneal curvature.

Current instruments of either the Helmholtz "variable doubling" (B&L Keratometer) or the Javal "fixed doubling" (Haag-Streit Keratometer) type are so calibrated as to read directly the central corneal radius (in millimeters or in diopters). The latter figure is derived through incorporation of a deliberately chosen low value for the refractive index of the cornea (1.3375) as well as an arbitrary value for the corneal back-surface power—typically –5.85 D [20]. Thus the net power of the central cornea is read out. However, the numbers obtained are really *global* values for the portion of the central cornea ranging from 3.8 to 4.2 mm—and only the periphery of these areas at that. The entire center, where presumably the important part of refraction is going on, is missed. As to the peripheral cornea, the area beyond that 4.2 mm (92% of the corneal surface)—out here in *terra incognita*—here it can truly be said: "There be dragons."

Keratometry has several good points in its favor: 1) it is easy to do, and 2) it is a familiar methodology—beyond this, it is a rubber yardstick. The measurements made with an ophthalmometer are confined to a very limited paracentral portion of the cornea and have no relationship whatever to the rest of the cornea. Despite attempts to do so, it is not feasible to use this method for determining the curvature of the peripheral cornea (Figure 6.9). The only portions of the cornea actually measured are four in number, two vertical and two horizontal. Depending on the design of the instrument, the mires used for this measurement are separated by a distance ranging from 3.1 (B&L) to 2.6 (AO) mm. Thus a spherical area having a width of at least 3.0 mm can be measured accurately. This can be verified by examining calibrated steel balls of varying radii of curvature. The degree of accuracy on such surfaces is very high indeed, probably on the order of 0.25 D or less. It is assumed, therefore, that the same accuracy can be translated to measurements of the corneal surface. Since the corneal curvature is, except in rare instances, nowhere constant—this assumption is in vain and has led to many false premises.

Now, it is a sad commentary on the human species that its members tend to believe anything that is written down—especially if it is set down elegantly, illuminated by illustrations, and pressed between hard cardboard covers adorned with gilt lettering. Surely, I digress, but anyone experienced with lawyers will know the truth of my statement. Nevertheless, numbers could be extracted from these machines and written down, entered on a record of each eye for further study and comparison, and marveled at, one supposes. Surely they could not have been pondered on to any degree—except by a few—for the simple reason that the results obtained seemed to make sense and tallied with experience. This experience was that spheres and later spherocylinders seemed to afford excellent vision in patients whose corneas were afflicted with ametropia. The fact that Ptolemaic (pre-Copernican) theory of planetary movement also accorded with experience and later proved to be totally erroneous did not seem to weigh much with the workers of the time—or since. Pity, that. Pity forsooth because much time was wasted pursuing—what? Truth? Expediency? Money? The latter two surely, for the truth was known—the cornea is not spherical.

Solution 1b

We'll take Placido's disk, substitute a camera for the eye, and measure the rings! Fine, let's look at how others did just this.

Photokeratoscopy

I have said that almost 90% of corneal dioptric power arises from refraction at the anterior corneal surface.

Hence the quality of vision greatly depends on the topography of the cornea. The keratometer is used routinely to measure the shape of the cornea in the clinical practice of ophthalmology, but this instrument measures corneal curvature from the reflection of mires at only four positions along two meridians at right angles. While this method can achieve an accuracy of better than 0.25 D in measuring steel balls, clinical keratometers cannot be used to measure irregular astigmatism or corneal asphericity. For example, the keratometer cannot be used to assess the size of the central zone of uniform power following RK.

It is not easy (nor accurate) to obtain readings sufficiently peripheral with standard keratometers, nor do these instruments afford the physician any real appreciation of the corneal surface shape or topography. Furthermore, these devices are only accurate for spherical surfaces, which the human eye, most decidedly, is not. Brewster, as early as 1827, suggested a practical means whereby this measurement might be accomplished [54]. Goode, in 1847, was the first to establish a method to do so [55]. His attempts were further refined by Placido, resulting in the well-known Placido's disk [56–59]. This device consists of a centrally perforated flat black disk on which are painted evenly spaced white concentric bands. When held in front of the patient's eye (while the physician looks through the hole at the reflected rings), the rings take on the shape of the cornea and reflect any aberrations thereon. If the cornea is spherical, the rings will appear round and concentric; if astigmatic, the rings will appear elliptical (Figure 6.10). The steeper the cor-

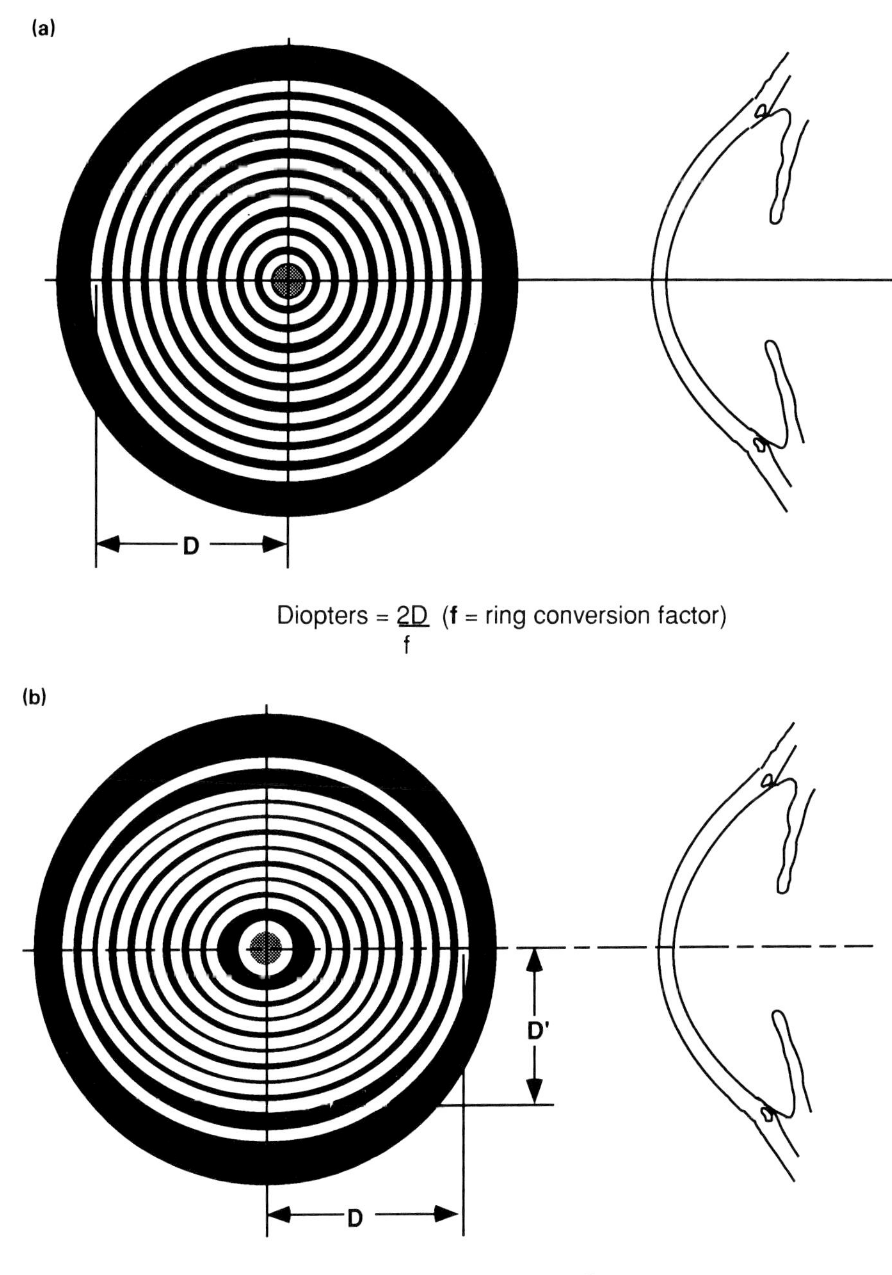

Fig. 6.10 Corneal contour map. (a) Spherical cornea (nine-ring instrument). (b) Astigmatic cornea (nine-ring instrument).

nea in a given meridian, the closer the rings are to one another—although it takes an astute observer indeed to note all the subtleties. In fact, the instrument provides only a very crude approximation of the actual corneal distortion. Placido expanded on his original idea by devising a method of photographically recording the appearance of the rings. He was followed shortly by Javal and Nordensen [35,60]. It was Gullstrand, however, in 1896, who introduced quantitative photokeratoscopy to measure corneal contour (Figure 6.11). Using this device, he was able to roughly map out the variability of the corneal curvature in all meridians [48] (Figure 6.12).

Qualitative estimates of the regularity of corneal curvature can be obtained by using Placido's disk, and these estimates can be quantitated by photographing the reflected image and measuring the distances between the concentric circles, much like one measures the distances between contour lines to determine altitudes on a topographic map. Gullstrand's original device has changed considerably over the years but still remains useful within its limitations (Figure 6.13).

The importance of measuring corneal contour was discussed in Chapter 5 and cannot be minimized. While the keratometer measures approximately the central 4.00 mm of the cornea (about 8% of the corneal surface), major changes in corneal shape after refractive surgery also occur in the paracentral and peripheral cornea. Measurement of the shape changes will give information about how the refractive surgical procedures worked, will help document the stability of the cornea, and will form a basis for future contact lens fitting—if needed. Thus these measurements must be precise.

Ophthalmometers measure an area ranging from 3.8 to 4.2 mm in diameter around the visual axis. If the cornea were spherical, this measurement would be adequate. However, it is widely understood that the cornea is not spherical but is, rather, aspheric. Various researchers have described it as paraboloid, ellipsoid, and conical. Regardless of which general shape one chooses to assign to it, the fact remains that until recently, the only accurate measurements of the cornea obtainable have been the sagittal height and the diameter. Between any three measurable points (Figure 6.14), the corneal surface can take any

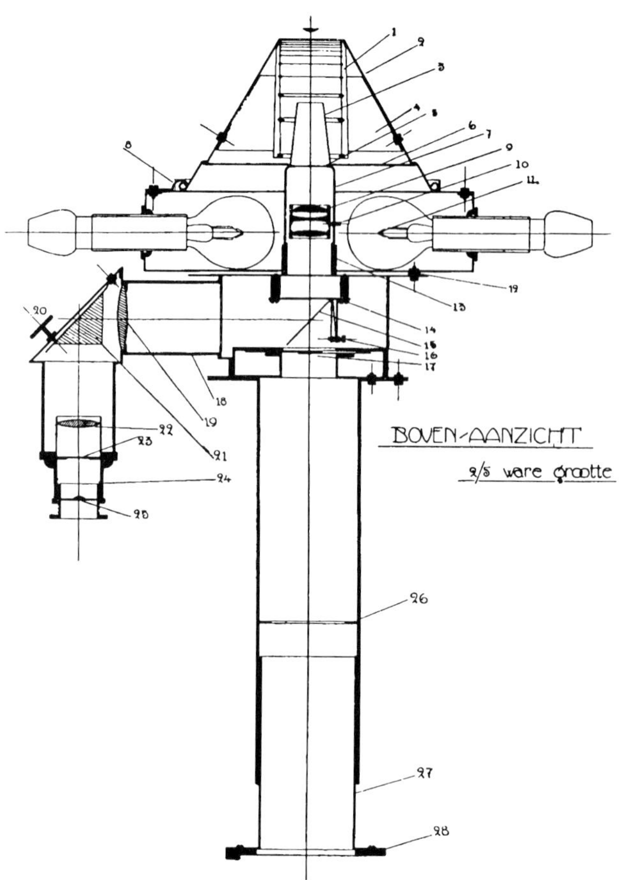

Fig. 6.11 Early model photokeratoscope (Corneoscope) (from Dekking H. Fotografic der cornea, opperwlakte Assen. Groninque th. med. 1930 No. 2, Van Gorcum in Bcm, 91, 360 (1930) no. 271, 1930).

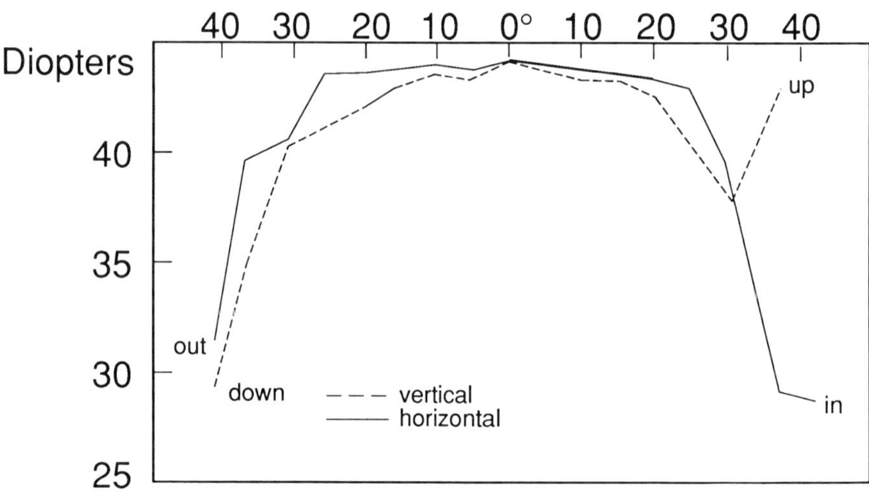

Fig. 6.12 Corneal curvature over 360° (from Gullstrand A. Photographisch-ophthalmometrische und klinishe untersuchungen uber die Hornhautrefraktion. Kongl Svenska Vet Akad Handl 1896; 28).

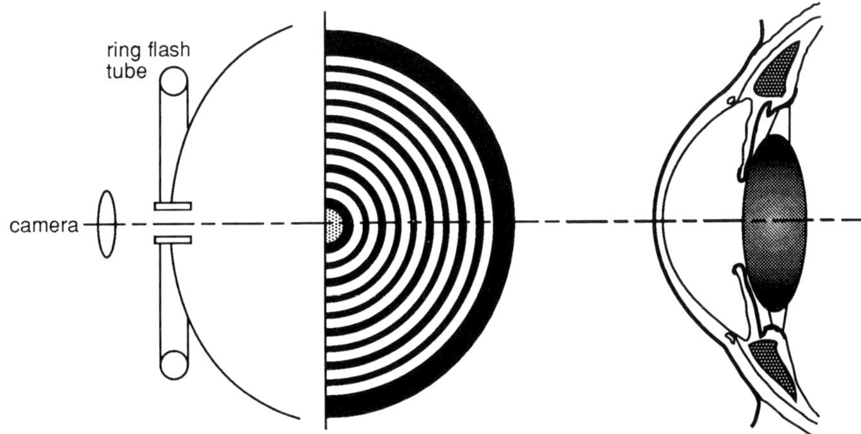

Fig. 6.13 Scheme of a typical modern photokeratoscope.

shape. It should be obvious that the keratometer cannot possibly measure such a surface.

The keratometer has a fixed focal distance between the apex of the cornea and its lens. The images of the mires are reflected off the cornea at a constant apical depth of 0.30 mm (Figure 6.15). The distance between the two reflected images is compared with the same images reflected off spheres of known radii of curvature. Since this measurement is only made in the center, K-readings give no information in the paracentral, midperipheral, or peripheral region. A photokeratoscope attempts to solve this problem by producing successive mires that take the chord length at increasing apical depth. In the case of the Corneometer, each ring represents an increasing apical depth of 0.1 mm. The first ring is at a depth of 0.2 mm, however, because of the need to provide space for the photographic element. The second ring is therefore at 0.3 mm, the third at 0.4 mm, etc. (Figure 6.16).

It would be helpful to have a photokeratoscope that measured the entire corneal surface, but the anatomy of the human face, with the corneal surface recessed behind the nasal and orbital bony protuberances, makes it all but impossible to get consistent ring reflections from the peripheral cornea. The photokeratoscope used most com-

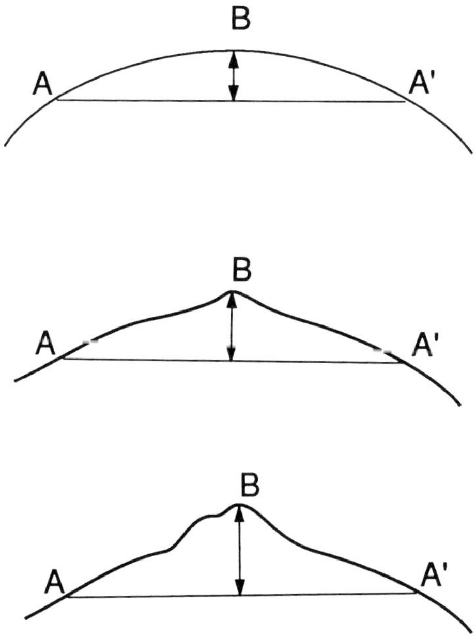

Fig. 6.14 Inherent weakness in the photokeratoscope.

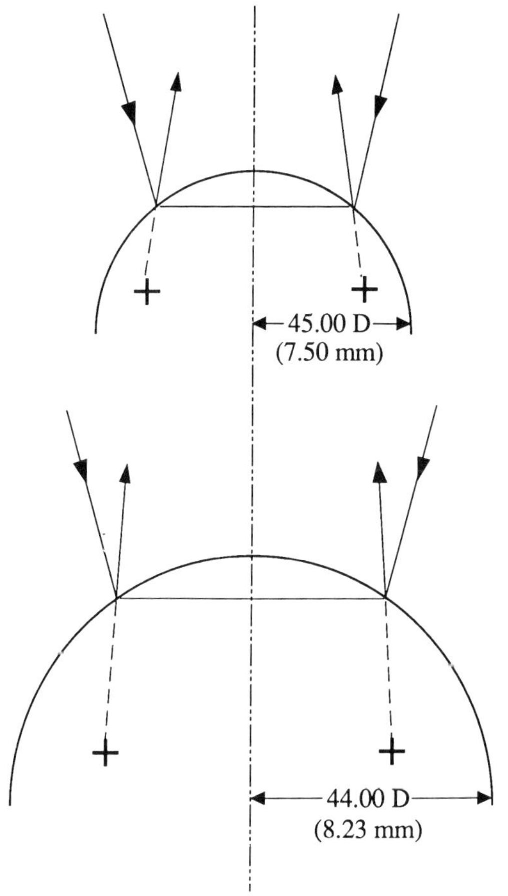

Fig. 6.15 The sagittal depth of the mires is kept constant in the keratometer.

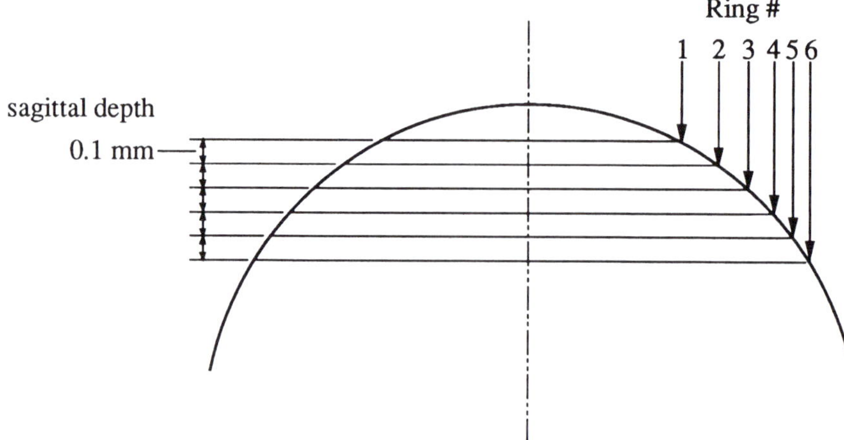

Fig. 6.16 Each ring (mire) in the photokeratoscope has a fixed sagittal depth much like a keratoscope.

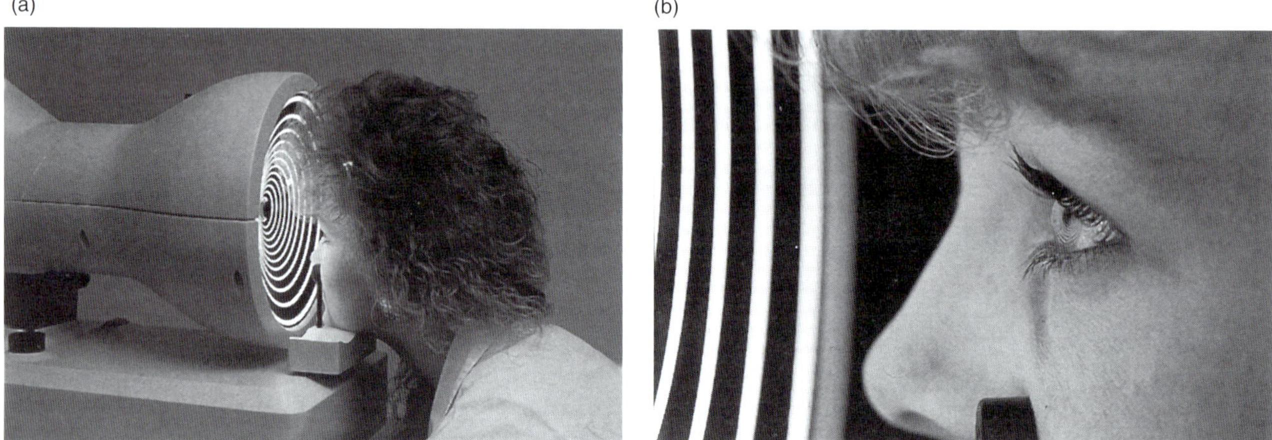

Fig. 6.17 (a) The Corneoscope. (b) Note reflected rings on the subject's cornea.

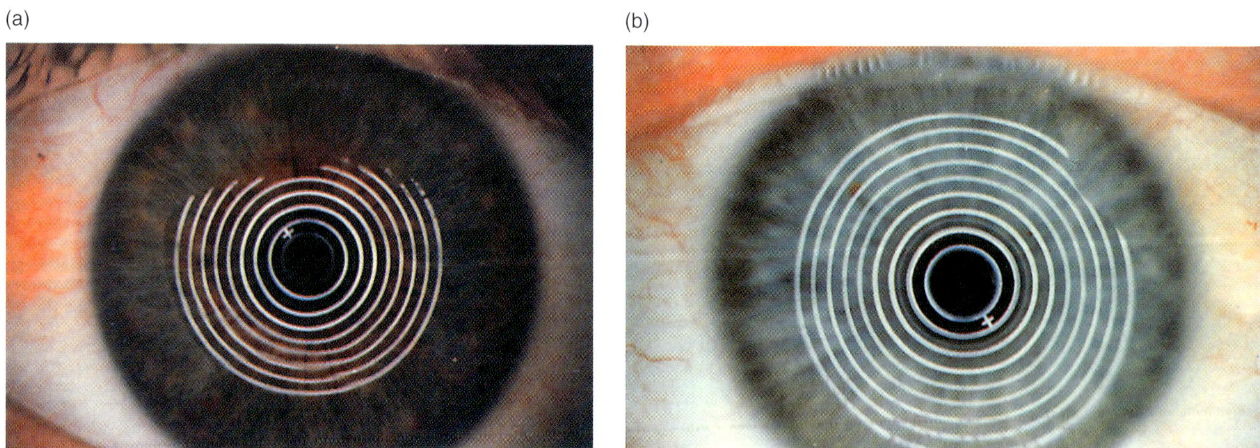

Fig. 6.18 (a) Characteristic nine-ring photokeratograph of a spherical cornea. (b) Subtle astigmatism exists on this corneal surface—against-the-rule at 15°. This cornea has low-grade keratoconus that is not demonstrated with this instrument (the patient can read 20/25 with low-power spectacles). Figure 6.19, taken with the CMS unit, is more revealing. This is borne out by the color-coded surface map in the next figure (Fig. 6.20).

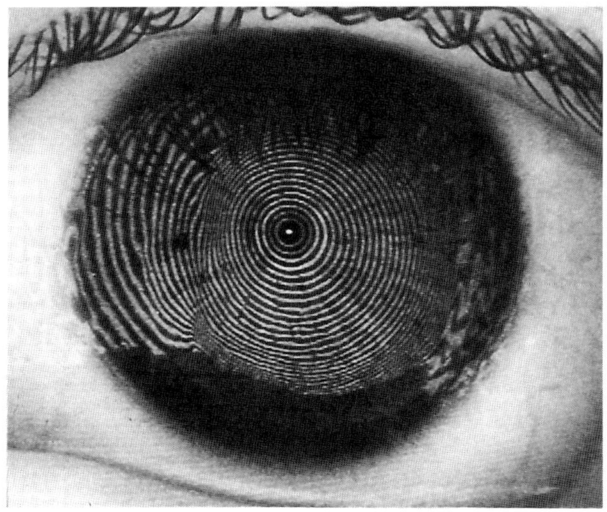

Fig. 6.19 CMS videokeratograph. (Courtesy of Computerized Anatomy.)

monly currently has 12 rings spaced 1 mm apart. The area of the cornea covered by the rings is inversely related to the corneal power. On a 40.00-D cornea, the ninth ring has a chord length of 8.3 mm, whereas on a 50.00-D cornea, the ninth ring has a chord length of 6.7 mm. Using these nine rings, the Corneoscope measures the curvature of approximately 55% of the corneal surface (Figure 6.17). The use of twelve rings extends the range only a little more. Automated reflection keratography, as is used by the Tomey photokeratoscope, for example, uses 32 rings (Figures 6.18 to 6.20).

The dioptric power of the cornea at any point along a ring is determined by measuring the distance from the center of the image to the middle of the ring. This becomes a problem when astigmatism is involved. The problem of imaging the cornea with this instrument is compounded by keratoconus.

Figure 6.21 shows a fairly regular form of keratoconus. Because of the limits in resolution of this type of instrument, much of the data about the cone is lost. Some increase in accuracy is obtained by using more rings. However, with present technology, Placido's disk–type instruments have inherent limitations due not only (as noted before) to the structure of the human face and orbit but also to the increased aberration of the image as the disk becomes larger and the limits set by a Petzval's surface are exceeded. Special curved film holders (as in a Schmidt camera) have been tried but found wanting.

Some units have only 9 rings. The Topcon unit uses 25 rings, and the Tomey unit uses 32 rings. Even with this number, the best resolution is still only about 0.5 D. The Tomey unit overcomes some of the difficulties with this type of imaging by using monochromatic laser light. However, the problems inherent to such optical imaging remain, even though the unit purports to measure all but the central 2.0 mm and the peripheral 11%.

Neither the keratometer nor the photokeratoscope provide an accurate or complete measurement of the entire corneal surface. In addition, neither of these methods can determine the curvature of the inner surface of the cornea.

The keratometer provides an averaged radius of curvature pericentrally and cannot be used with confidence peripherally or off-axis, even if fitted with a Soper topogonometer. The typical photokeratoscope ignores the critical central area entirely and cannot measure the peripheral 30% of the cornea. Despite the 1.0-mm ring spacing, the maximum measurement accuracy of this device is about 0.5 D in the center, with accuracy falling off rapidly toward the periphery. Another shortcoming of these types of instruments is in not providing a corneal profile measurement. Despite these inherent limitations,

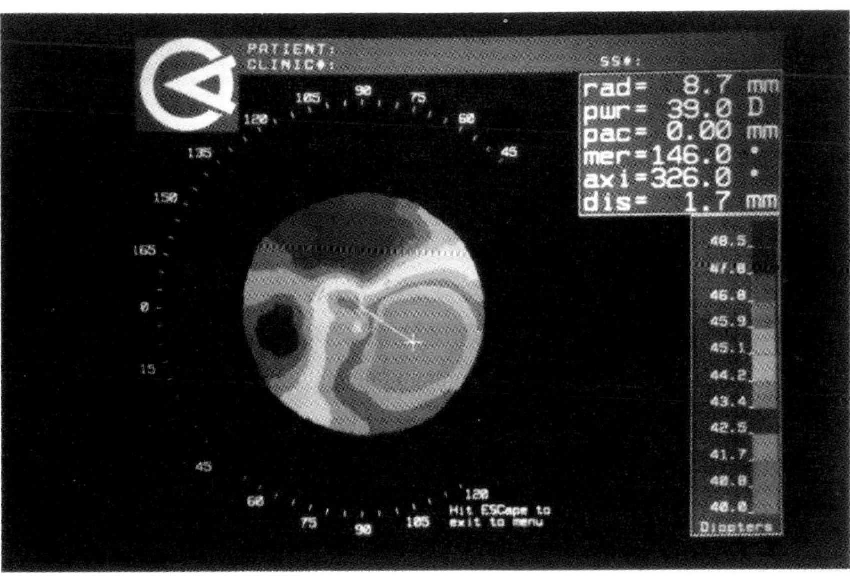

Fig. 6.20 CMS contour map of Fig. 6.19. (Courtesy of Computerized Anatomy.)

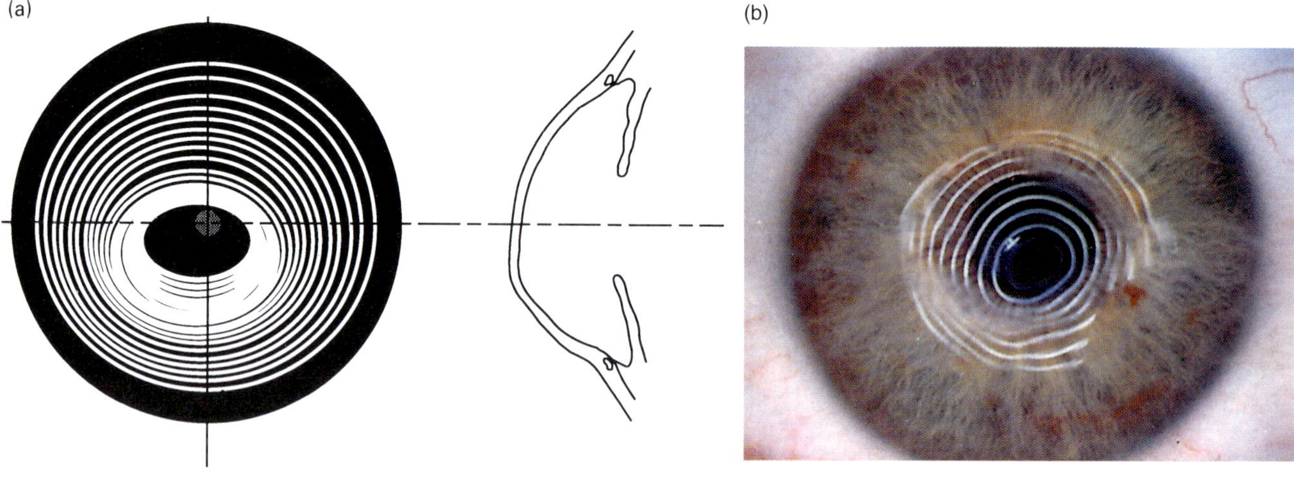

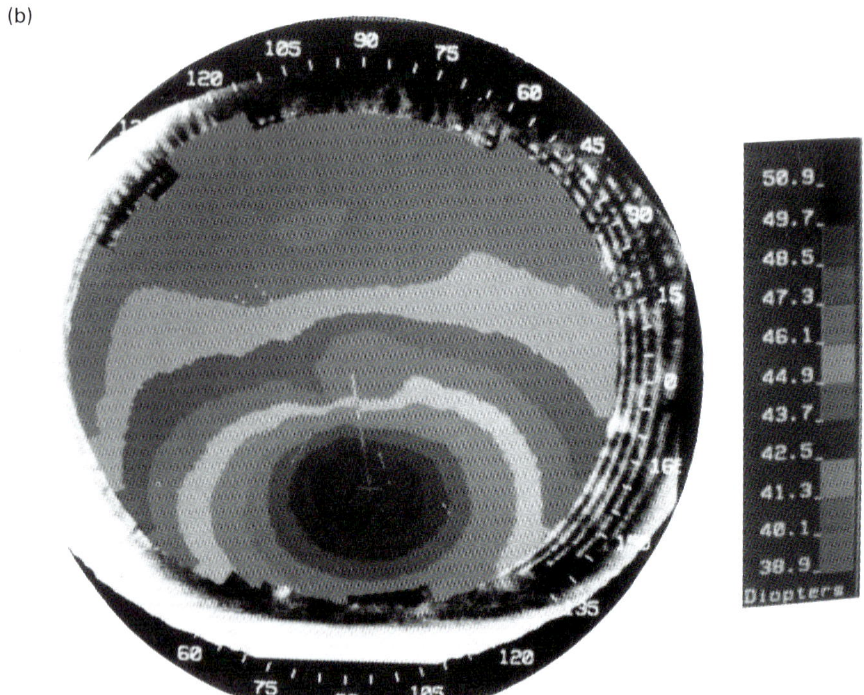

Fig. 6.21 (a) Corneal contour map—keratoconus (nine-ring instrument). This drawing is optimistic. (b) This photograph demonstrates a more typical appearance of the distortion produced by an irregular corneal surface; (c) and/or profile of the cone (from Camp J, Maguire L, Cameron B, Robb R. A computer model for the evaluation of the effect of corneal topography on optical performance. Am J Ophthalmol 1990; 109(4):379–386).

however, these devices still provide a qualitative view of the corneal surface obtainable in no other way.

Generally, keratoscope photographs (keratographs) have been interpreted by visual inspection of the mires [61]. With keratoscopy, it is possible to detect and diagnose many forms of corneal distortion, and relatively inexpensive hand-held keratoscopes can be used intraoperatively to correct gross amounts of astigmatism. However, direct reading or visual inspection of keratographs takes a great deal of training, and even seasoned topography experts cannot detect low-amplitude or complex corneal surface distortions (see below). Help in the form of computer transformation of the keratographs to amplify corneal distortions can be used to overcome this deficiency.

Despite improvements in depicting the corneal surface through photokeratoscopy, the fundamental deficiencies in this system remain. Mere ring patterns do not convey sufficient appreciation of the corneal surface shape, nor do measurements of inconstant ring diameters provide an unequivocal measurement of corneal curvature. Digitization of the keratographs either by hand or automatically through video capture with computer analysis using surface reconstruction algorithms provides more information but no increase in accuracy. Moreover, the critical central portion and the elusive peripheral cornea remain

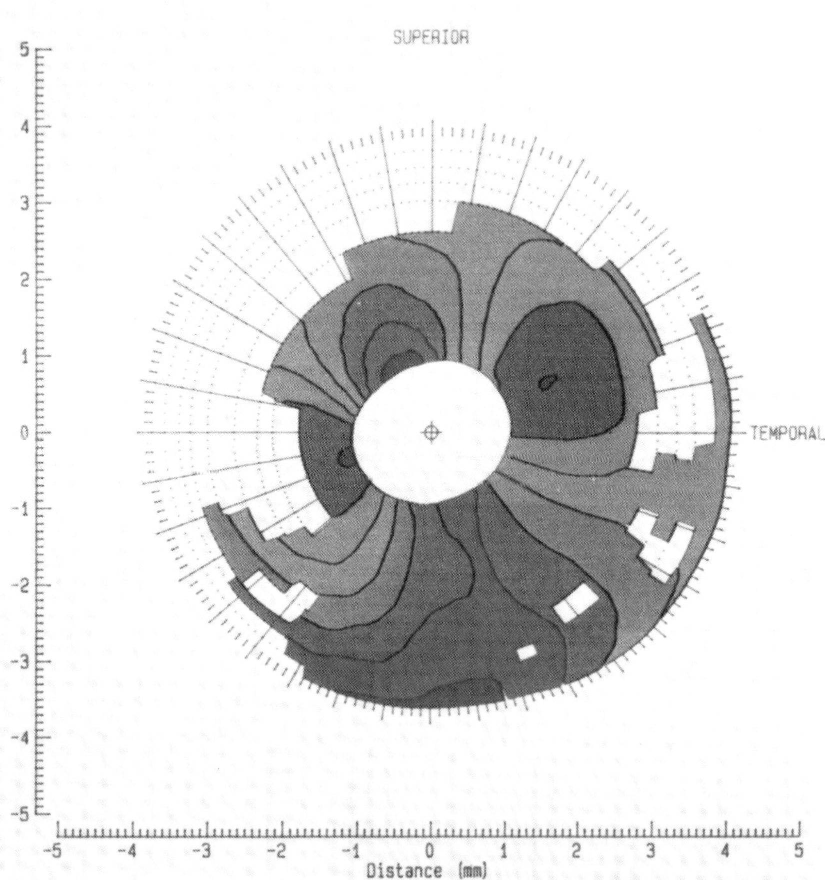

Fig. 6.22 A topographic map constructed from the LSU computer program. Note missing central data. (Courtesy of S. Klyce.)

unrecorded (Figure 6.22). Often, portions of the surface are obscured by the nose, brows, or lids (Figure 6.23). Some devices employ dithering techniques to "fill in" the data gaps left by these obscurations. However, this dithering process is accomplished by making assumptions about these gaps that may not be warranted. Moreover, since these devices depend on the reflective property of the corneal surface, any abnormality here reduces the quality of the image obtained. Epithelial defects, stromal ulcers, or scarring prevents or limits analysis. Highly irregular corneal surfaces can cause the reflected rings to run together, making it difficult or impossible to perform quantitative analysis (see Figure 6.23). To fully understand the shape changes the cornea undergoes following anterior segment surgery, trauma, and contact lens wear, there is a need for methods and instruments that can be used for the accurate and high-resolution measurement of corneal shape.

Thus, if Scheiner's idea is not good, how then shall we solve the problem? The answer has been, so far, to continue to apply spherical methods and somehow account for the deviations from spherical by various mathematical gyrations. All current topographers are mere expansions of the basic idea of Scheiner—sphere-based. Countless authors have come at the problem as moths to a candle flame—with little to show for it aside from singed wings and bruised egos. The aspherical cornea continues to resist attempts to sphericize it.

Does it matter that the cornea is not spherical? In the practical scheme of things, does it make any real difference? I submit that it does from several points of view. First, such an attitude perpetuates the myth that somehow curvature equals power. A compelling myth it is to be sure, because everyone *knows* that the more curved a surface, the shorter is the focus and therefore the more "power" the surface demonstrates. In point of fact, such a notion works—*for the paraxial portion of a lens,* those points on its surface very near its axis. Nevertheless, the mere fact that it works is not proof of the validity of the premise—after all, under certain unique circumstances, it is possi-

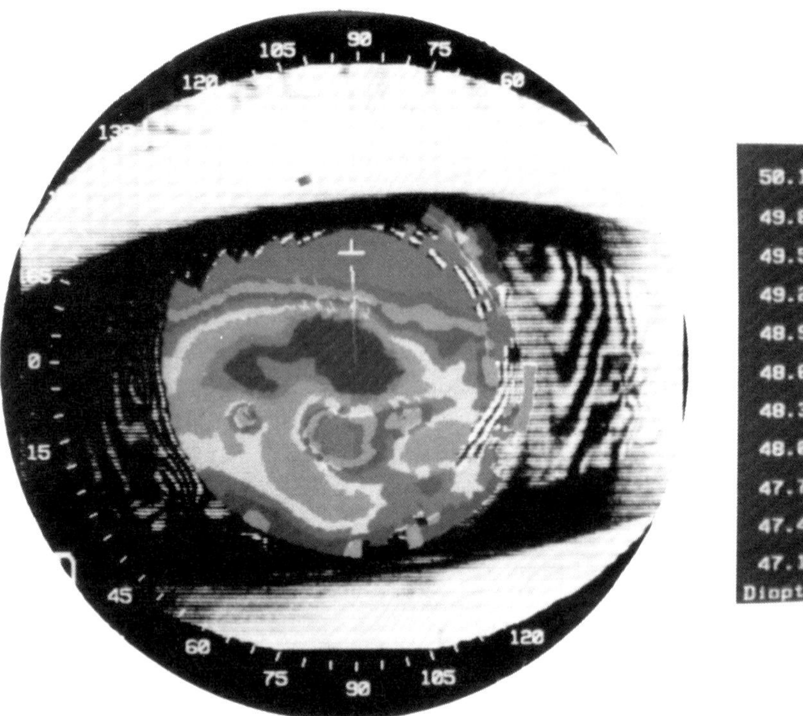

Fig. 6.23 Contour map of a highly irregular surface from a CMS unit. Note the shape of the "rings" on the right. Measurements under these circumstances cannot be relied on. As long as the surface being examined is smooth and regular, a Placido disk apparatus has no difficulty measuring the curvature changes. Surface irregularities, however, can be missed or be unmeasurable. This fact destroys the utility of such systems in studying corneal shape postoperatively. (Courtesy of S. Klyce.)

ble to fit a square peg into a round hole. Also, when the cock crows, the sun rises; *ergo* it is the crowing of the cock that causes the sun to rise. However, the sun also will rise should one barbeque the cock.

You can't get there from here

Depending on the steepness of the slope, the projected ray from the point of intersection of the incident ray to the point of intersection with the optic axis will be the optical path or the adjusted radius. Hence a slope may well have a nominal angle that corresponds to a radius of, say, 7.8 mm (43.26 D) but whose actual radius is 8.03 mm, and therefore, the power is really 42.02 D. What this illustrates is that the power is related to the optical path, whose direction is controlled by the instantaneous slope at the point of incidence—independent of the nominal radius of curvature of said slope. Part of the problem lies in insisting on attaching one's conceptualization of the corneal curvature to the idea of radius with its inevitable association with

$$F = n - 1/r'$$

or more familiarly:

$$D = 337.5/r'$$

This is not to say that the relationship is wrong—only that its use on the nonspherical cornea outside the paraxial region is wrong.

When the rays move out from center, beyond a specific distance that is a function of the slope (on the human cornea, this distance is about 1.0 mm from the apex), then the relationship of curvature to power breaks down. It is no longer possible to connect a curvature to a certain refractive power. This was shown convincingly in Roberts' examination of sphere-based topography mappers [62–64].

Two major conclusions result from this study. First, areas of similar curvature do not correspond to areas of similar refractive power in the peripheral regions, as previously assumed. Second, paraxial power approximations are not valid outside the central corneal region and may produce erroneous patterns that lead to clinical misinterpretation of the image-forming properties of the cornea. The more surprising results of this study indicate that not only is the error significant, the paraxial power approximations actually produce a completely opposite pattern from the corneal refractive power. In both ellipsoids studied, where the paraxial approximations show decreasing values, the corneal refractive power actually was increasing! Because the maps produced have different, opposing patterns, the results of the paraxial approximations may not even be interpreted qualitatively as power in a clinical environment. For example, in the 0.5 ellipsoid at $x = 2.25$ mm, the true refractive power is 45.66 D, paraxial approximation 1 is 44.50, and paraxial approximation 2 is 43.54 D, with paraxial errors of 1.16 and 2.12 D, respectively. The paraxial error becomes even more profound, however, if one considers the difference from the central value rather than just the absolute numerical values. The corneal refractive power increases 0.66 D from the apical value of 45 D, whereas paraxial approximation

1 decreases 0.5 D and paraxial approximation 2 decreases 1.46 D. This can have an extremely important impact in clinical interpretation because the human cornea is known to be approximately ellipsoidal in shape.

Well, darn! What else can we do?

Solution 2—Use light itself as a ruler

Underlying the eclecticism of evolving topography instrumentation and obscured by the smoke blown by rival gangs of "detail people" out to sell the "hottest of the hot"—tangible or ephemeral—lies a very real and intensive attempt to understand and codify something that has proven to be a very slippery customer over the last century or so—the corneal surface shape. The following is a synopsis of what is fittingly called the "state of the art" (emphasis on the last word). The term *art* aptly fits the mélange of brightly hued and occasionally abstract images facing the ophthalmologist seeking the Grail of refractive surgery.

Interferometry and holography

It is a given, by many authorities within the field of corneal and refractive surgery, that the technique of interferometry (or wavefront analysis using a Shack-Hartmann device) holds the answer to obtaining a precise modeling of the corneal surface shape. The use of a coherent and monochromatic light source (i.e., a laser) has extended the usefulness of different forms of interferometry, including holographic interferometry. The most fundamental of these forms are the Twyman-Green and Fizeau interferometers. The basic configuration of these two interferometers provides a foundation for other useful testing tools. Both these instruments are used extensively in optical surface testing (as is the S-H device). In point of fact, Placido's disk (sphere-based) analyzers are not to be found in any serious optics laboratory.

The imaging of the corneal contour must provide the means to measure large-scale events without sacrificing accuracy. The requirements for precision are in the range of longer-wavelength optical testing (10.6-μm source) with the ability to define the contour event to 1 μm or less. Using interference techniques, accuracies of a fraction of a wavelength can be obtained. The optical path differences (OPDs) can be measured to less than 0.10 μm, depending on the wavelength and the analysis of the wavefront interference using an appropriate algorithm.

The surface of the cornea is measured in terms of OPD, with the calibration and reference being the output spherical wavefront of the optical system. The surface elevations are arrived at by summing the OPDs with the average radius of curvature of the cornea at the center. While any point on the cornea can be referenced, the central or apical part has been chosen to relate the output to a more familiar mode of measurement—that is, keratometry. The use of any of these techniques for the measurement of a convex aspheric surface requires auxiliary optics commonly referred to as *null optics*. The purpose of this approach is to create a closely matching wavefront to impinge on the convex corneal surface and reflect the difference from the curvature of the aspheric.

A laser source that is in the visible, such as a helium-neon laser, has a sensitivity that is, at worst, submicron, and any large mismatch between null lens optics and the aspheric that is being tested will result in a large number of interference fringes. Holographic techniques are capable of reproducing minuscule aberrations in surface contour. That sensitivity, however, is one of this method's inherent problems. Too much sensitivity produces "noise" that tends to degrade performance in the system. Besides, what constitutes practical sensitivity? That is, how accurate is accurate enough?

In the case of a cornea with moderate astigmatism—2 D of refractive power—the surface radius change would be 0.4018 mm. This would be 633.931 waves at 0.6328 μm and 1267.86 fringes at the interference plane of the interferometer. The resulting pattern on a typical video format would result in having a fringe every 0.1 mm for a 5-in. frame. The fringe pattern (i.e., closed-form or circular fringes) also would have a form that is not easily fit using standard wavefront-reducing algorithms; Zernike polynomials, adapted to the shape of the fringe pattern, are required. (Figures 6.24, 6.25).

With this in mind, the measurement of a variable aspheric surface such as the anterior cornea requires the instrument to allow for strong irregular unknown curvatures to be imaged and to create an interference event that can be analyzed easily to produce accurate (>1-μm) surface contouring of the cornea.

The extreme amount of curvature variation on the corneal surface requires the use of an extremely fast lens system in the F/0.6 to F/0.7 range. The lens system must be able to function with at least a degree of field angle to allow for off-axis events and to be able to bring enough of the direct reflection back to the imaging system [65].

The surface of the cornea is in constant motion either from saccadic or volitional movement, requiring fast acquisition (0.1 s) of the direct reflection to avoid loss of information and to maintain high contrast of the interference event. The returning full reflection from the corneal surface will then have its own wavefront signature from every detail that has reflected enough light to be detected by the video camera. Figures 6.24 and 6.25 show contour maps resulting from a first-generation fringe analyzer. These maps show how the shape of the corneal surface differs from the shape of the spherical wavefronts created by the focusing lens [66].

Solution 2 therefore meets all the constraints placed on us and supplies the vital information that we require. However, before we go further, we must pause for a primer on the terms used in describing corneal topography in particular and optical systems in general.

(a)

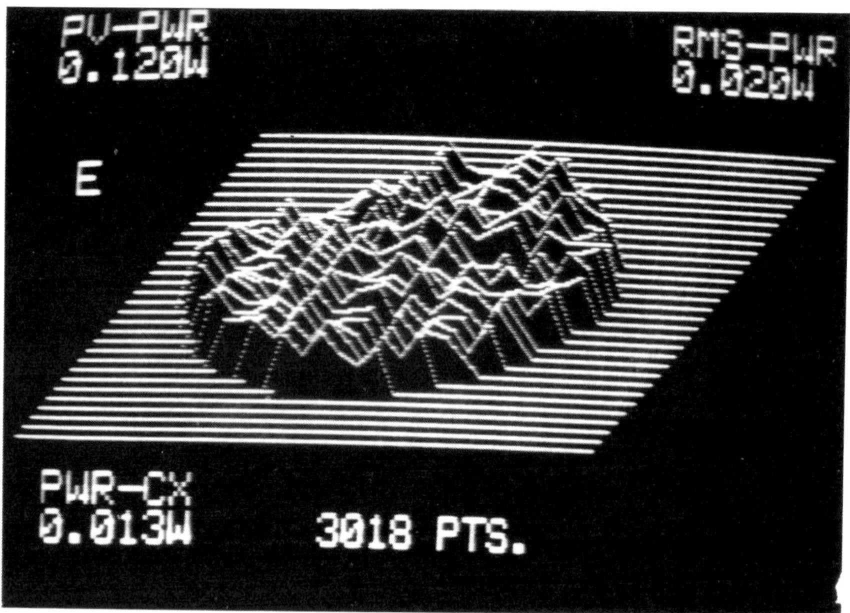

(b)

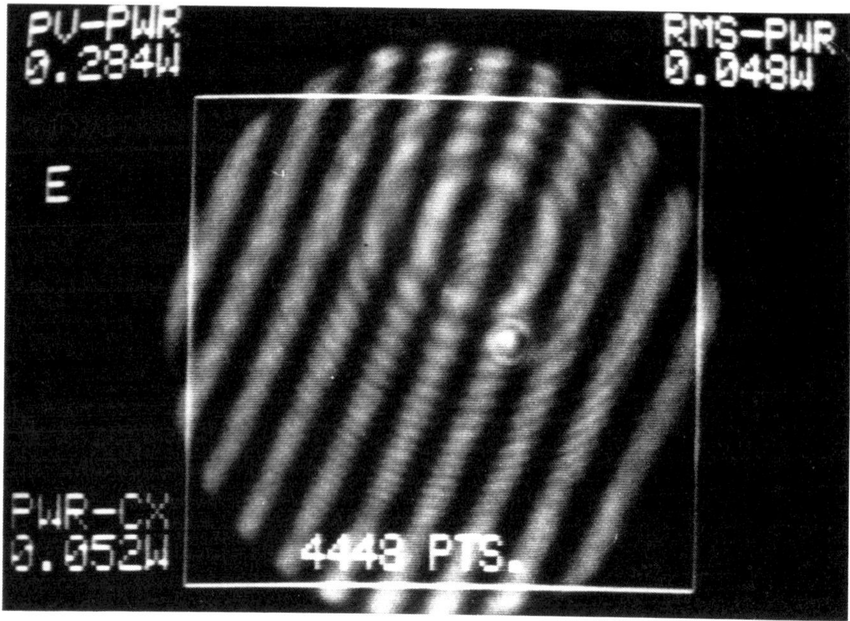

Fig. 6.24 Isometric surface map (a) and the hologram from whence it was constructed (b) This map was made by the author in 1983 using a ZYGO unit and represents the first actual curvature measurement of the human cornea—holographically.

Acquisition of the corneal image

Because of the extreme changes in curvature that occur on the corneal surface, conventional holographic methods were modified to fit the peculiar requirements of this clinical modality. Happily, these requirements allowed use of a single laser beam and a much more compact, folded optical system [67] (Figure 6.26). The current unit produces high-resolution holographic images of the entire corneal surface (limbus to limbus) within 1/60 of a second, essentially eliminating problems associated with normal ocular movement. The working distance is quite close to the eye, necessitating a very fast lens system, and this excludes shadows created by the nose and brow that plague other methodologies. The images are captured by a high-resolution charge-coupled-device (CCD) array camera and relayed to a high-speed full-frame two-page video frame grabber. The holograms in Figure 6.27 are a set of such images of a human cornea taken with a second-generation device.

The images are then digitized, and the OPDs are calculated using sophisticated Zernike polynomials. While digitization is essentially automatic, the operator, who controls all operations from the keyboard, can adjust or

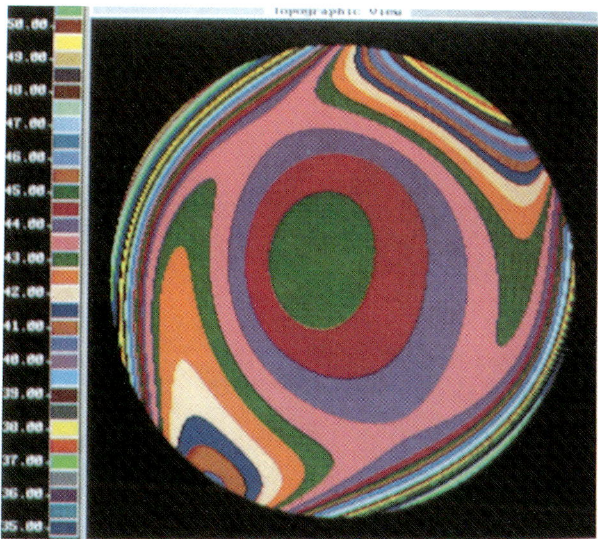

Fig. 6.25 This is the wavefront (Zernike polynomial) contour map of the interferogram in Fig. 6.24. This patient is showing a with-the-rule-astigmatism of low order (see also Fig. 6.31c).

add data points directly onto the displayed high-contrast fringe pattern. The resulting topographic coordinates are displayed in false editable colors in high resolution on a color monitor.

Corneal image feature extraction

The interference measurements used in this work are quite different from those of the Placido's disk photographic technique. This technique requires interpretation of a complex phase and interference pattern that has been stored in a holographic medium as a diffraction pattern. Reconstruction of the complex multiple-wavelength diffraction pattern yields the phase and interference information that can be digitized to produce the wavefront of the object under test.

The wavefront map is illustrated in Figure 6.28. This represents the errors in the interferograms shown in Figure 6.27. The irregularities on this map are a function of the OPDs recorded between the actual surface and a reference sphere (Figure 6.29). The reference sphere is obtained from an optical measurement of the corneal surface. It also can be derived from a real measurement of the limbal-to-limbal reflection of the cornea with the instrument. The value of the contour is established by the value of the equivalent wavelength. The resulting measured aberrations are in units of microns, which can be converted readily to dioptric equivalents.

The various aberration terms that result from the fitting of the digitized points define the optical characteristics of the measured surface. The varying degrees of astigmatism, coma, sphericity, tilt, and focus that emanate from

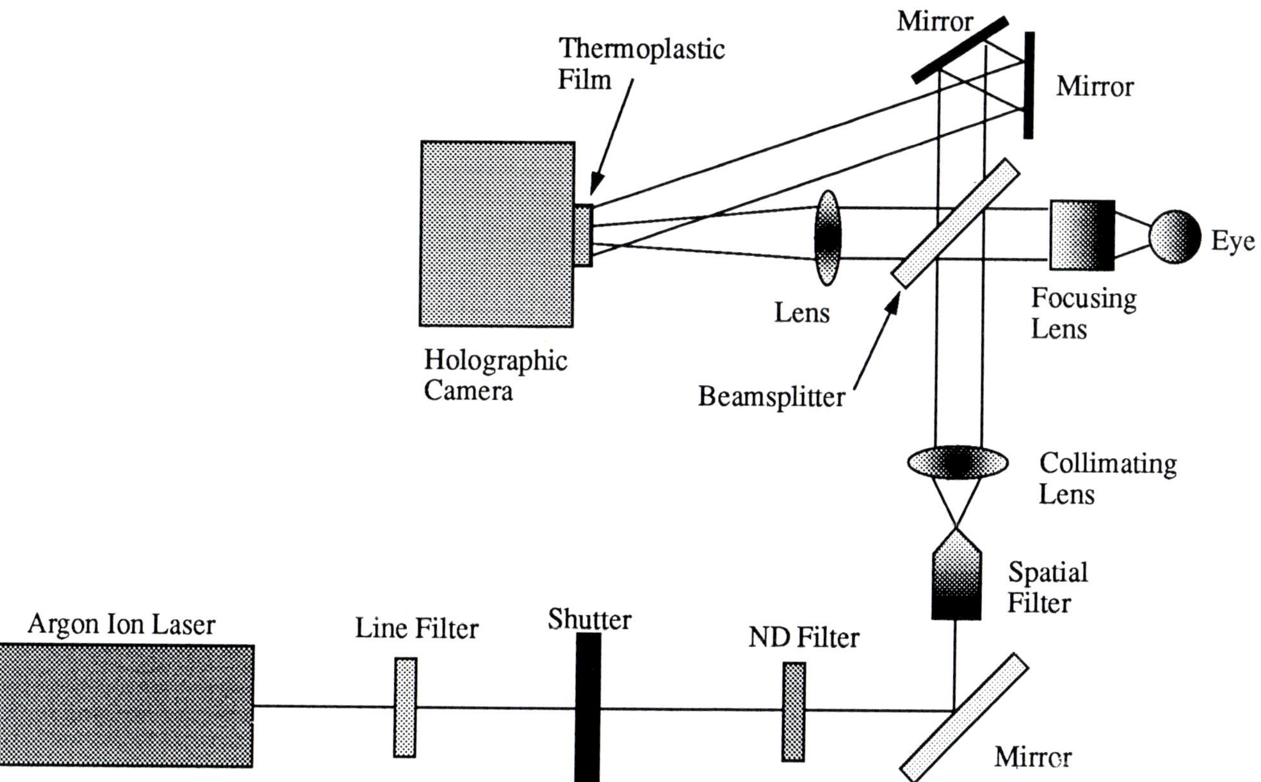

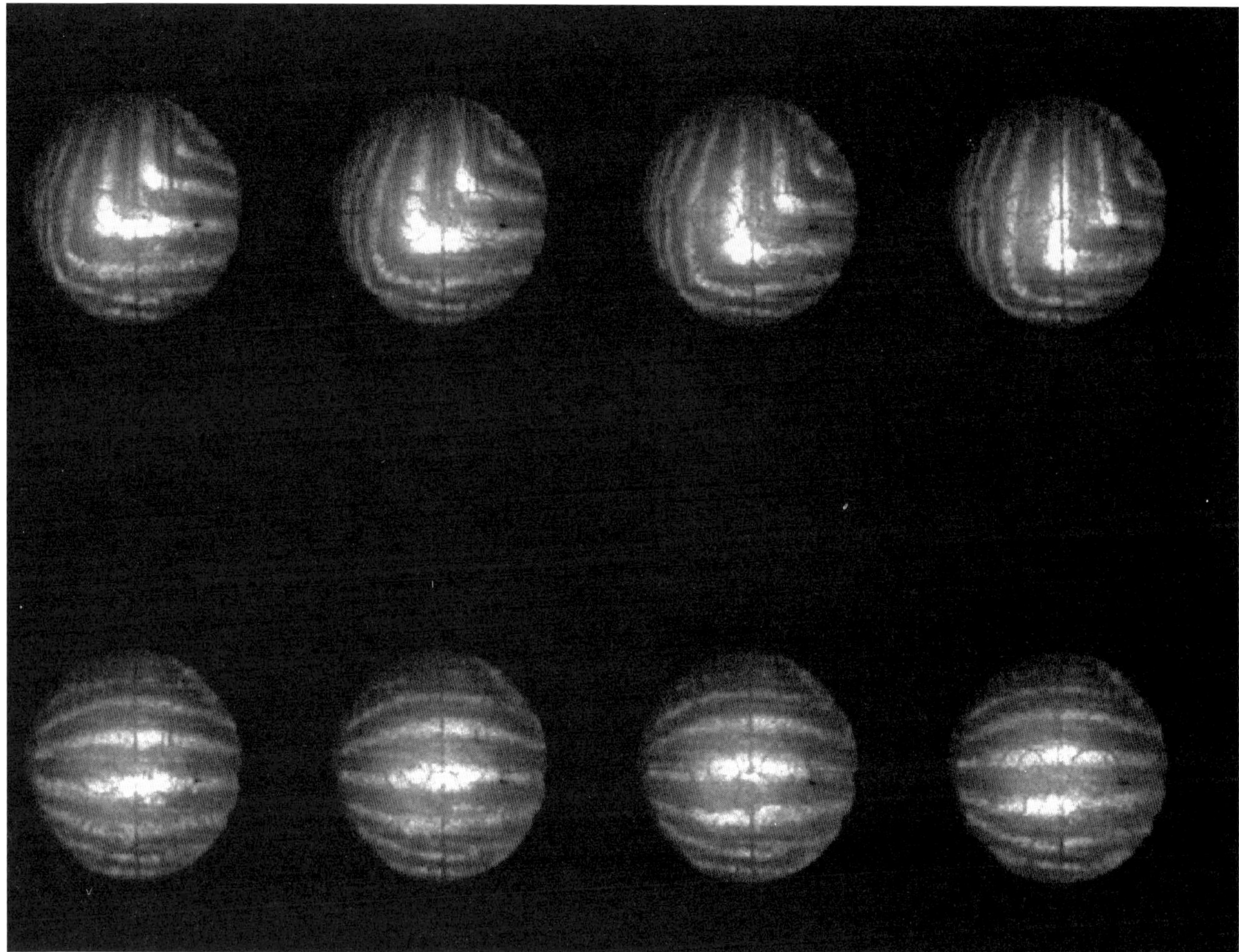

Fig. 6.27 This is a typical interferogram taken by a second-generation single-sideband, phase-modulated interferometer (CLAS II) of a postoperative RK patient. Eight frames are taken in one pass, and all eight frames are combined to produce the coefficients that are operated on by a Zernike polynomial subroutine.

the surface being measured are converted to real surface elevations as a function of the actual value of the aberration.

The aberrations of an optical surface can be obtained from the digitized coordinates of an interference pattern that has been fit to a monomial expression:

$$W(x, y) = \sum_{i=0}^{k} \sum_{j=0}^{i} B_{ij} x^j y^{i-j} \quad \mathbf{1}$$

The polynomial is of degree k, with $N = (k + 1)(k + 2)/2$ terms. The data that have been obtained during digitization and least-squares fit to the polynomial are then transformed to a linear combination of Zernike polynomials. The angular function that has been used to convert each Zernike polynomial to its corresponding monomial form can be found by substituting this angular expression into the U_{nm} of the Zernike polynomial as follows:

$$\left(\begin{matrix}\{\cos\}\\ \{\sin\}\end{matrix}\right)(n - 2m)0 = p^{-(n-2m)} \sum_{j=0}^{q} (-1\gamma \binom{n - 2m}{2i - p} x^{2j+p} y^{n-2m-j-p} \quad \mathbf{2}$$

This is valid only for $n - 2m > 0$. The parameters for p and q are:

		n(even)	n(odd)
Sine	{p	1	1
	{q	$n - 2m/2(-1)$	$n - 2m - 1/2$
Cosine	{p	0	0
	{q	$n - 2m/2$	$n - 2m - 1/2$

3

After solving for p and substituting in terms of x and y using the following expressions:

Equation 4 determines the radial polynomials over the $n - 2m > 0$ in terms of p

$$R^{n-2m}{}_{n}(p) = \sum_{s=0}^{m} (-1)^s \frac{(n - s)!}{s!\ (m - s)!\ (n - m - s)!} p^{n-2s} \quad \mathbf{4}$$

$$p^{2j} = \sum_{k=0}^{q} \binom{j}{k} x^{2k} y^{2(j-k)} \quad \mathbf{5}$$

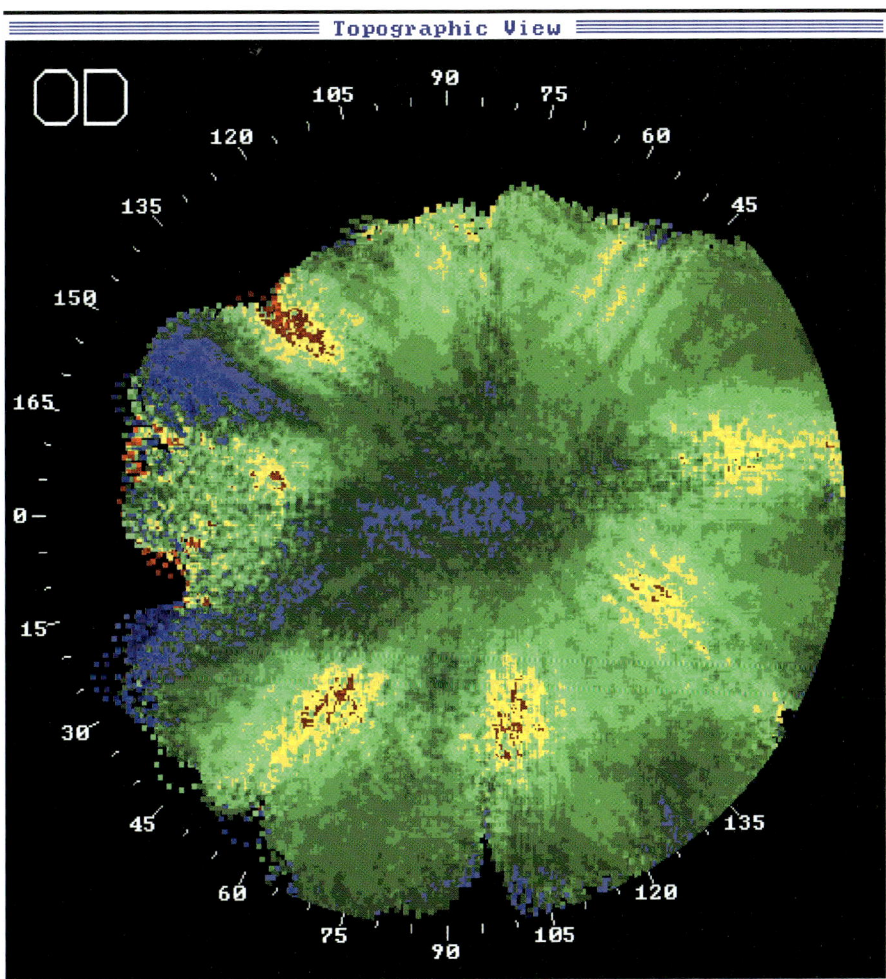

Fig. 6.28 This is a wavefront map of the interferogram in Fig. 6.27 converted to curvature values. The corneal elevations caused by tissue swelling can be readily seen around all eight of the radial incisions.

The final expression for the Zernike polynomials U_{nm} in terms of powers of x and y is:

$$U_{nm} = R^{n-2m_n} \begin{Bmatrix} \cos \\ \sin \end{Bmatrix} (n - 2m)0$$

$$= \sum_{i=0}^{q} \sum_{j=0}^{m} \sum_{k=0}^{m-j} (-1)^{i+j} \binom{n-2m}{2i+p} \binom{m-j}{k} \times \frac{(n-j)}{!(m-j)!(m-m-j)!} x^{2(i+k)+p} y^{n-2(i+j+k)-p} \qquad 6$$

The wavefront fitting that is being done is based on the fringe position caused by the reflected ray interference. This interference occurs from actual changes on the surface that perturb the return light path from the incoming normal position. The light-path position that has been altered due to surface changes sets up interference with the reference plane indicating a phase change in the interfering beams. The phase change is a physical difference in the distance traveled by the light reflected from the object as compared with the distance traveled by the reference beam. The total distance from the normal to the surface at any given point is the algebraic sum of the reference distance and the object distance. The path traveled by the object reflection has a value that is real with respect to the virtual image of a convex mirror or surface; this value is, however, normal to the surface and is not a value from a flat plane to a position on the corneal surface.

The surface that is constructed from the digitized points converted to wavefront monomials and then fit to circular Zernike polynomials can be treated as a real three-dimensional (3D) representation of the object with values in microns, millimeters, or other units. This 3D isometric representation of the object can be operated on to present the data in required forms.

The sheared diffraction pattern produces interference fringes that could be measured as a function of the grating spacing of the holographic pattern. The shear fringes could then be analyzed for the various aberrations, that is,

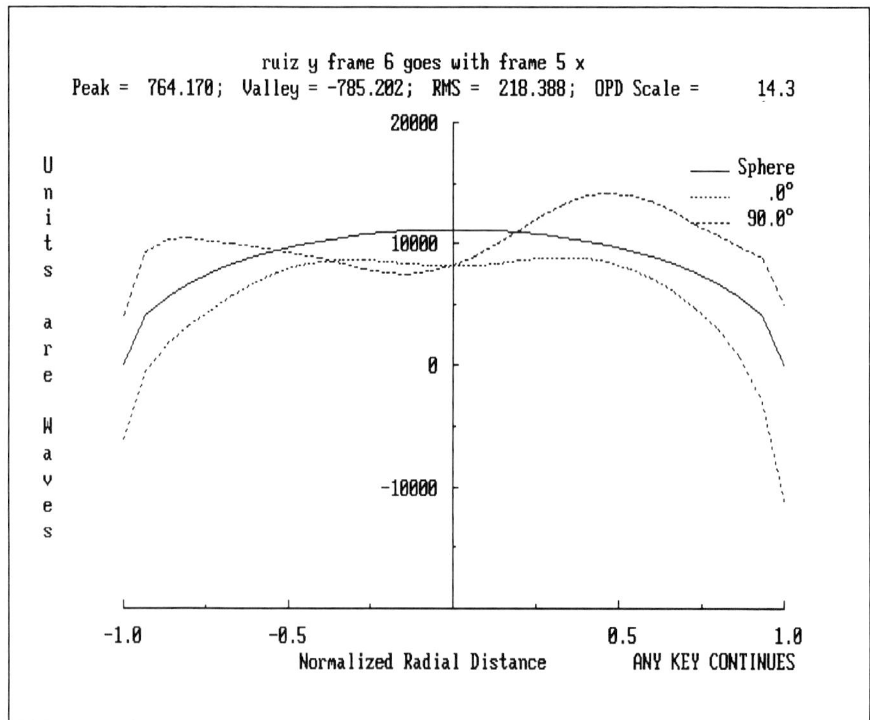

Fig. 6.29 Profile plot after a Ruiz procedure. Note how the surface major/minor meridians (dotted line) dip below (are flatter) and extend above (are steeper) the reference sphere (solid line).

sphericity focus, astigmatism, coma, etc. The use of shear fringes requires that two orthogonal patterns be analyzed in order to measure a nonsymmetrical object such as the cornea. The value of astigmatism is determined from the difference in the focus of the orthogonal patterns. The amount of spherical aberration is determined by the nonlinear shape of the shear fringe with the order of the fringes (number of fringes).

By adjusting the working distance and/or the lens system, measurements of the inside curvature of the cornea can and have been made. Further modifications have produced images of both the front and back lens surfaces. The most exciting aspect of this state-of-the-art technology is the ability to manipulate the laser light beam. By polarizing the beam in a certain way, corneal surface stress patterns can be seen. This opens the door to a whole new way of looking at postoperative results and inevitably will lead to changes in the way that all anterior segment ocular surgery is performed and complications (such as post–PKP astigmatism) are treated (see below and Chapter 11).

Interpreting the reconstruction of the corneal surface

The use of any new measuring system brings with it problems—I have just described some. Another is overcoming the hurdle of data interpretation. This is especially apt in the case of holography—the output is not in a form that encourages intuitive interpretation. The interference fringes look like nothing the average ophthalmologist has seen before. However, if we are to describe the "dark side of the moon" (corneal topography) correctly, we needs must do so from a fresh perspective. Just as we cannot see the dark side of the moon from our current vantage point, so it is that our traditional viewpoint must be altered to discover and examine the true shape of the cornea. We had to leave our comfortable, familiar, and solid observation platform—the Earth—and move out into the unknown, unfamiliar, and unsteady platform of space to see the far side of the moon. Thus it is that we must abandon our outmoded, comfortable, and treasured—albeit erroneous—notions of the shape of the cornea we have held dear for more than 300 years. Therein lies the rub—we have relied on keratometry and its ilk for too long to discard the methodology out of hand. Nor need we. We just have to adjust our thinking to place our reliance on more accurate means while still using the older (and more familiar) techniques to help bridge the gap.

While it is difficult to decipher a photo- or videokeratograph, with practice, an astute observer can glean considerable information about the quality of the corneal surface as well as its shape from such an image. Not so with images produced by holographic surface measuring devices such as the CLAS II. Here, the physician is confronted with a keratograph that more closely resembles a picket fence or latticework than an eye (see Figure 6.27). Except for some optical engineers, making sense of the image is all but impossible. The translation of image to a 3D shape is not intuitive. Compounding this problem is the way in which these devices actually measure surfaces. Whereas in Placido's disk-type devices the local corneal curvature is related to the diameter of the reflected ring—the chord of the arc—holograms record images through light-wave interference—hence the reason such images are called *interferograms* and the dark bands produced by this interference are called *fringes*. The image seen represents the pattern of this interference—not the shape of the cornea. In fact, except in extreme cases, the pattern may not even seem to be perturbed. Although the intervals between the dark-dark (or light-light) bands are important, they are not critical to the measurement of the surface shape because of the nature of the hologram. The corneal curve or Z-height at any point is not derived from the spacing of these bands, even though the actual number of such bands may vary somewhat from one patient to another and one meridian to another. The number of bands is more a function of the deviation of the measured surface from the control or reference shape (sphere) and does not represent "tick" marks on a ruler. With practice, a trained and experienced observer can make reasonable assumptions about the surface by virtue of the shape of the bands and whether they are straight, curved, or sinusoidal—but the actual surface profile has to be derived mathematically (Figures 6.30 through 6.33).

Corneal surface topography is a useful adjunct in assisting the clinician in assessing the visual status of the eye.

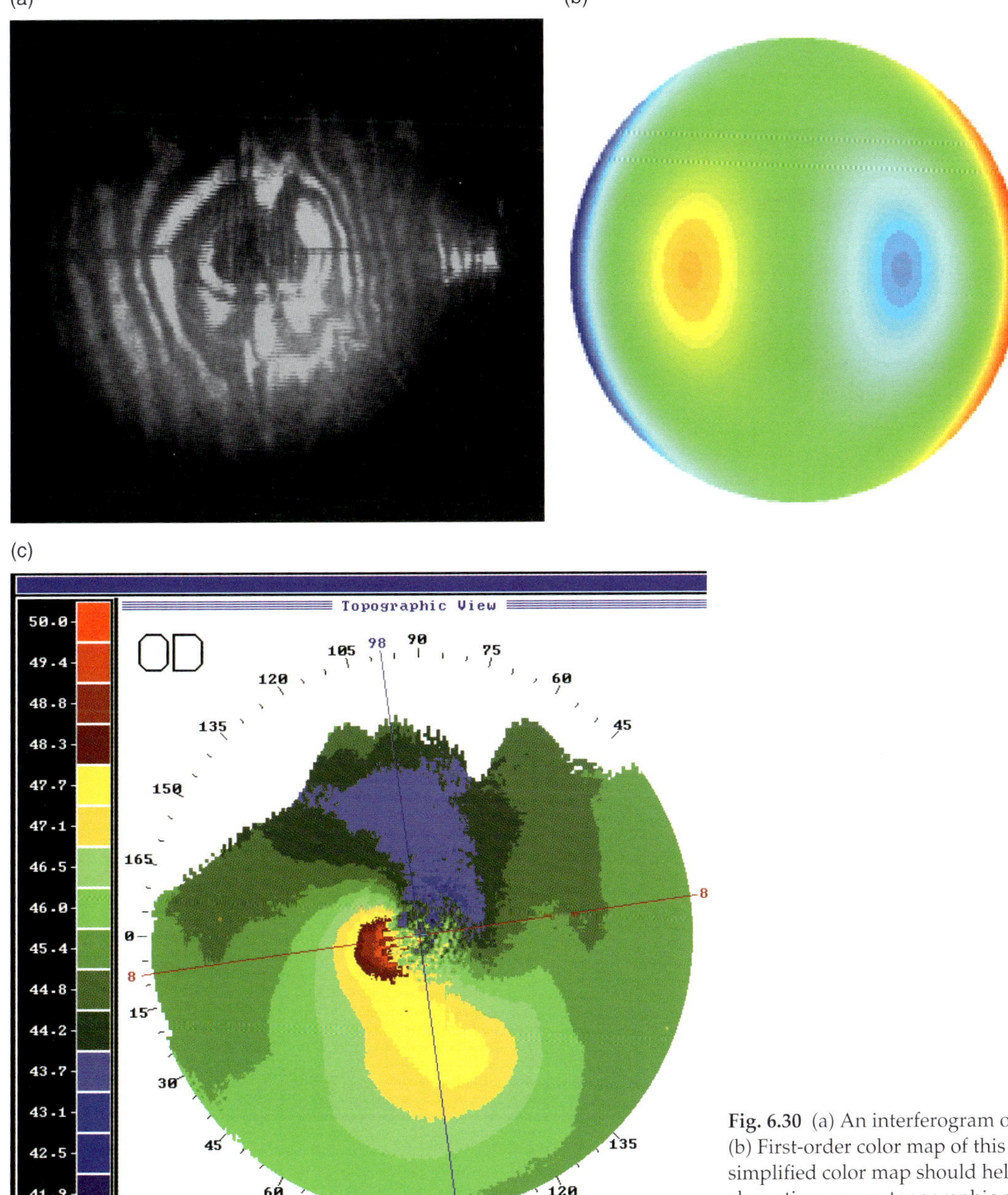

Fig. 6.30 (a) An interferogram of a surface showing *coma*. (b) First-order color map of this type of aberration. This simplified color map should help the surgeon identify this aberration on any topographic rendering. (c) Higher-order topographic map of an actual cornea showing coma.

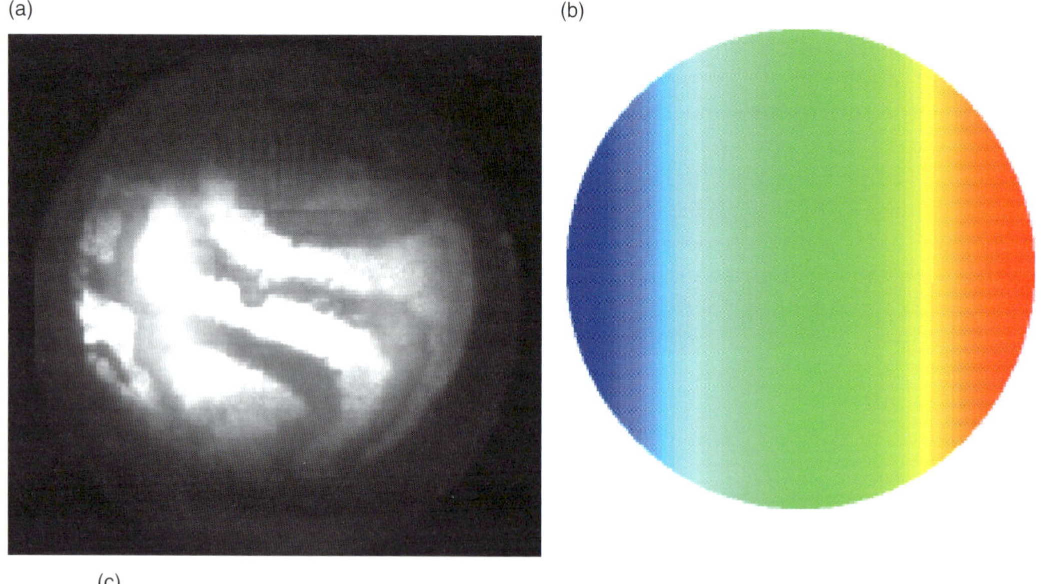

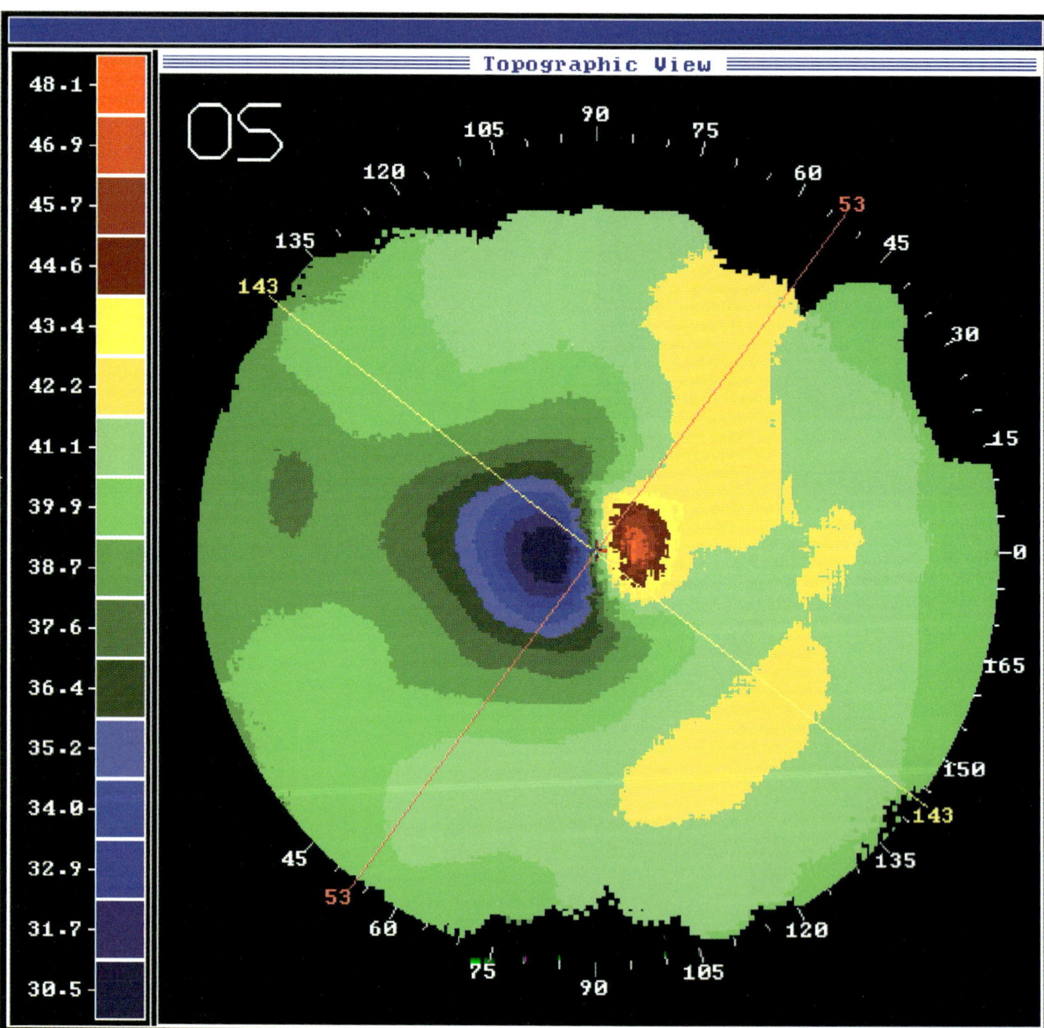

Fig. 6.31 (a) An interferogram of a surface demonstrating *tilt*. (b) First-order color map of this type of aberration. This simplified color map should help the surgeon identify this aberration on any topographic rendering. (c) Higher-order topographic map of an actual cornea showing tilt.

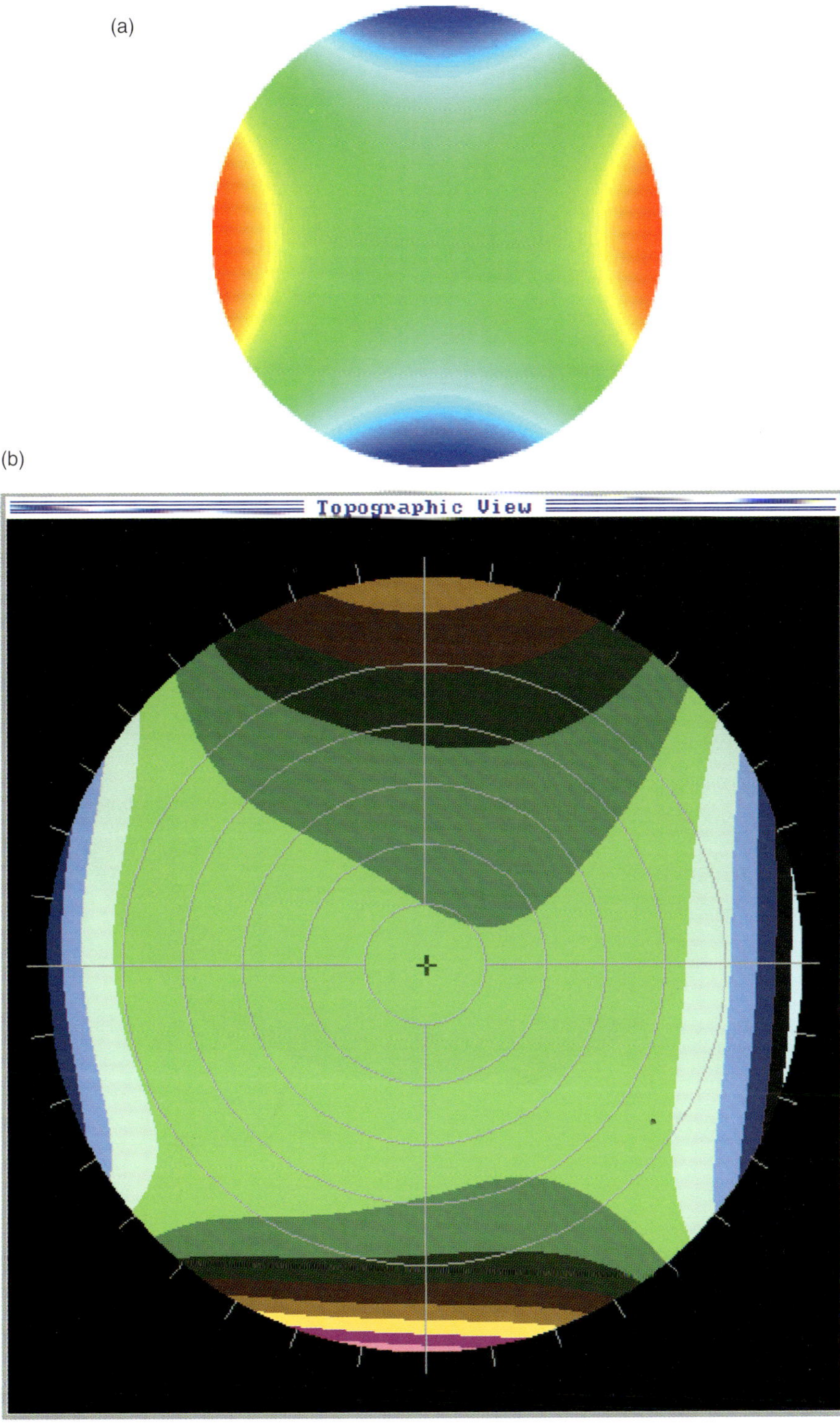

Fig. 6.32 (a) *Astigmatism.* First-order color map of this type of aberration. This simplified color map should help the surgeon identify this aberration on any topographic rendering. (b) A wavefront (optical efficiency) map of an actual cornea showing regular, orthogonal corneal astigmatism—unusual in the human. Most corneal astigmatism shows some obliquity of the opposing axes.

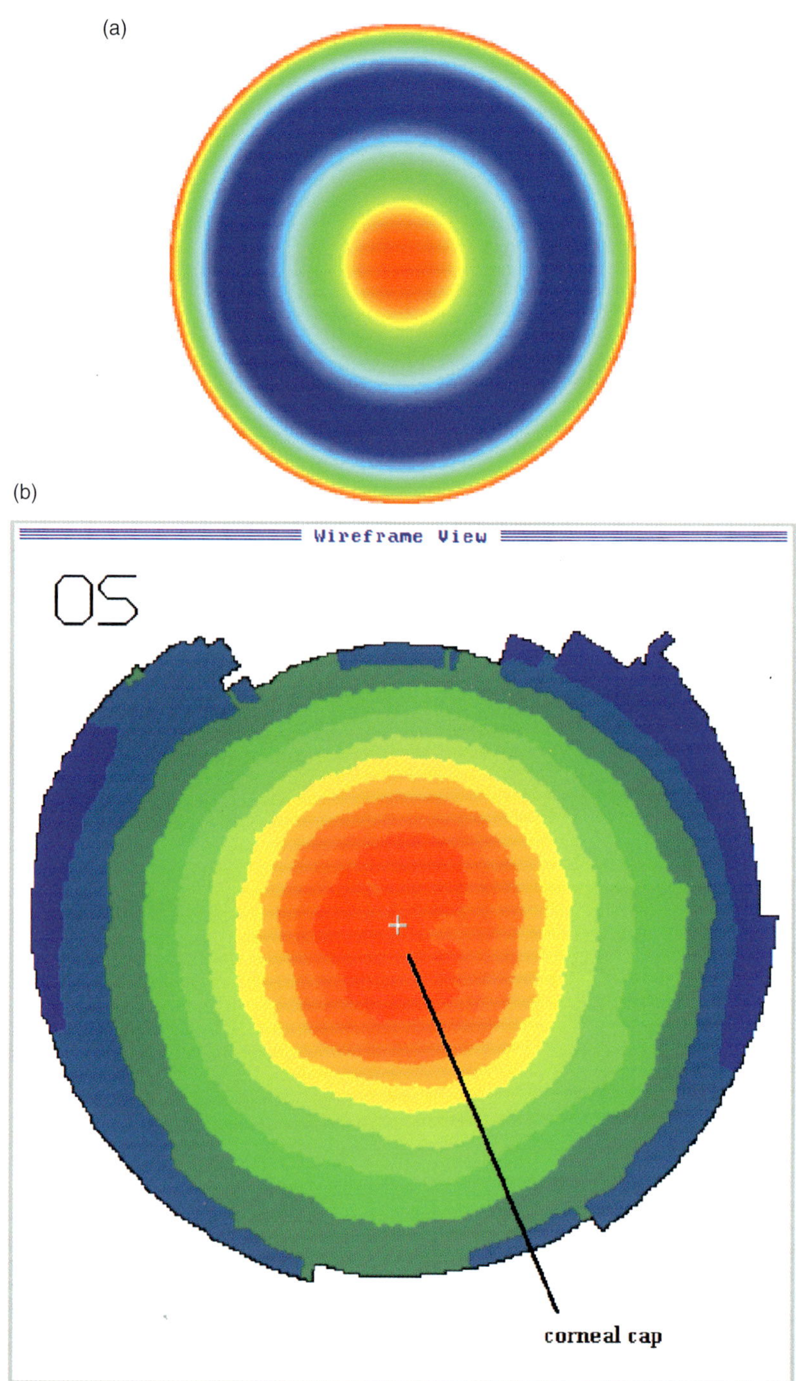

Fig. 6.33 (a) First-order color map of an aspheric surface. This simplified color map should help the surgeon identify this aberration on any topographic rendering. However, be sure that you know what the colors represent. If they represent Z-heights, this could be a map of a spherical surface. (b) Higher-order topographic map of an actual cornea showing a normal aspheric surface contour. The irregularities in the margins of the zones are also typical. It is unclear if these represent actual surface aberrations or aberrations due to tear evaporation irregularities.

However, topography is only the first step. Mere surface mapping of corneal curvature alteration, despite the heavy role of such changes, does not stand alone in determining vision. Intervening factors such as internal corneal curvature, natural lens surface curvatures, and axial length play an important role. Alignment of intermediate surfaces is also important. Using the information gained through high-resolution interferometry of the cornea and with the aid of a high-speed desktop computer, even more information can be obtained. The focal spot size and shape (Strell ratio), as well as the modulation transfer function (MTF), give more exact data pertaining to the actual visual state and answer the question *"Why can't my patient see?"*

Holographic interferometry of the corneal surface or total eye aberration technology, by using a Zernike polynomial fit of the corneal curvature data, results in an optical performance map that can explain why some patients with otherwise "rough" corneas can see, whereas some with "smooth" corneas cannot. New data suggest that corneal astigmatism often may be biaxial and that this condition is aggravated by tilt and coma. Such astigmatism is poorly defined by sphere-based systems.

Keratoconus

Keratoconus is a case in point. *Keratoconus* is an aberrant type of progressive myopic astigmatism that is usually irregular. In its manifest form, it is fairly obvious to the practitioner. However, mild cases of conus can be missed because they show very little or no surface irregularity and are easily corrected with spectacles. These cases may be described as *subclinical*. Manifest and subclinical forms can be expected to progress and usually do. Operating on such corneas (other than keratoplasty) is contraindicated.

Another form, called *forme fruste keratoconus,* has been described whose only manifestation is a steepening of the inferior corneal curvature, which steepening is found only on a topographic map—as if conus started and then stopped [68]. It is not known how many such cases progress—if any—nor is it known what percentage of the myopic population may possess the defect in this form. It would be nice to know if a patient has this peculiarity before surgery is performed and also to follow the pattern of corneal changes over time.

Approximately 8% of submitting myopes are shown to have corneal topographic changes suggestive of keratoconus using sphere-based or Placido's disk topographic mapping systems. That these changes are inherent in the design limitations of the method used to gather the data is suggested by the fact that only one of eight suspicious corneas in my experience is shown to have true keratoconus, either overt or forme fruste, using interferometric analysis—a much more sensitive method of measurement and one that yields true surface curvature data.

Corneal optics

The cornea is normally tilted to the so-called optical axis of the eye and is invariably decentered on that same axis. In conventional optics, such a configuration leads to distorted imagery. It must be understood, however, that the eye is not a conventional optical device and that such a situation does not lead to distorted imagery because of certain compensating factors within the system. Nonetheless, we need to know the degree to which such tilt and decentration exist preoperatively if we are to understand what is happening postoperatively. It is only in this manner that we can

1 Avoid patients in whom such tilt and decentration have been shown to produce bad results in retrospect (such as excimer laser corneal photoablation).

2 Weed out patients who have coma (coma is a form of astigmatism caused by decentration of an optic).

Accurate corneal maps can help us control postoperative astigmatism in transplant patients by helping us decide where to cut sutures.

Astigmatism—Extent and direction

The exact location of orthogonal axes of astigmatism assists in predicting the result of spectacle fitting and in comparing surgical nomograms. It also aids in the transition from placing incisions based on spherocylinder coordinates to placing them based on actual location. The latter cannot be attempted realistically until ray tracing can show the true state of the entire optical system of the eye. Accurate ray tracing cannot be performed with confidence using sphere-based systems.

We expect also that by knowing exactly what the corneal surface is and how it reacts to surgery we will be better able to plan and refine our surgical approach.

Determination of mean keratometry (power)

Reference sphere A concept used in making holographic surface measurements is that of the reference sphere (Figure 6.34); this troubles some people. They are concerned that somehow relating the actual surface to such an artificial construct may distort the rendering of that surface. This does not happen. It is, in fact, exactly what cartographers do when measuring elevations on the Earth's surface—they do so by relating such measurements to sea level. The reference sphere is the cornea's "sea level," or *eigenvalue*, and we can use the central corneal K-reading as the reference against which the OPDs detected by the holographer are plotted. Thus the elevations displayed are related to some measurement in which we have inherent faith—keratometry—because we know that that measurement is a reasonably accurate representative of some particular portion of the cornea. This should not be troubling either, because the K-reading is only a reference value. Deviations from this reference (in terms of actual corneal curvature) are plotted in relationship to this known. Thus steeper points will appear above this surface and flatter points below (Figure 6.35).

Moreover, we practitioners are used to seeing the astigmatism displayed in terms of *meridional values*. That is, we are used to values for a slope that are two-dimensional and which rotate around a common point or axis. In short, we are used to seeing sphere-based representations of the meridian of astigmatism—like a keratometer. An inter-

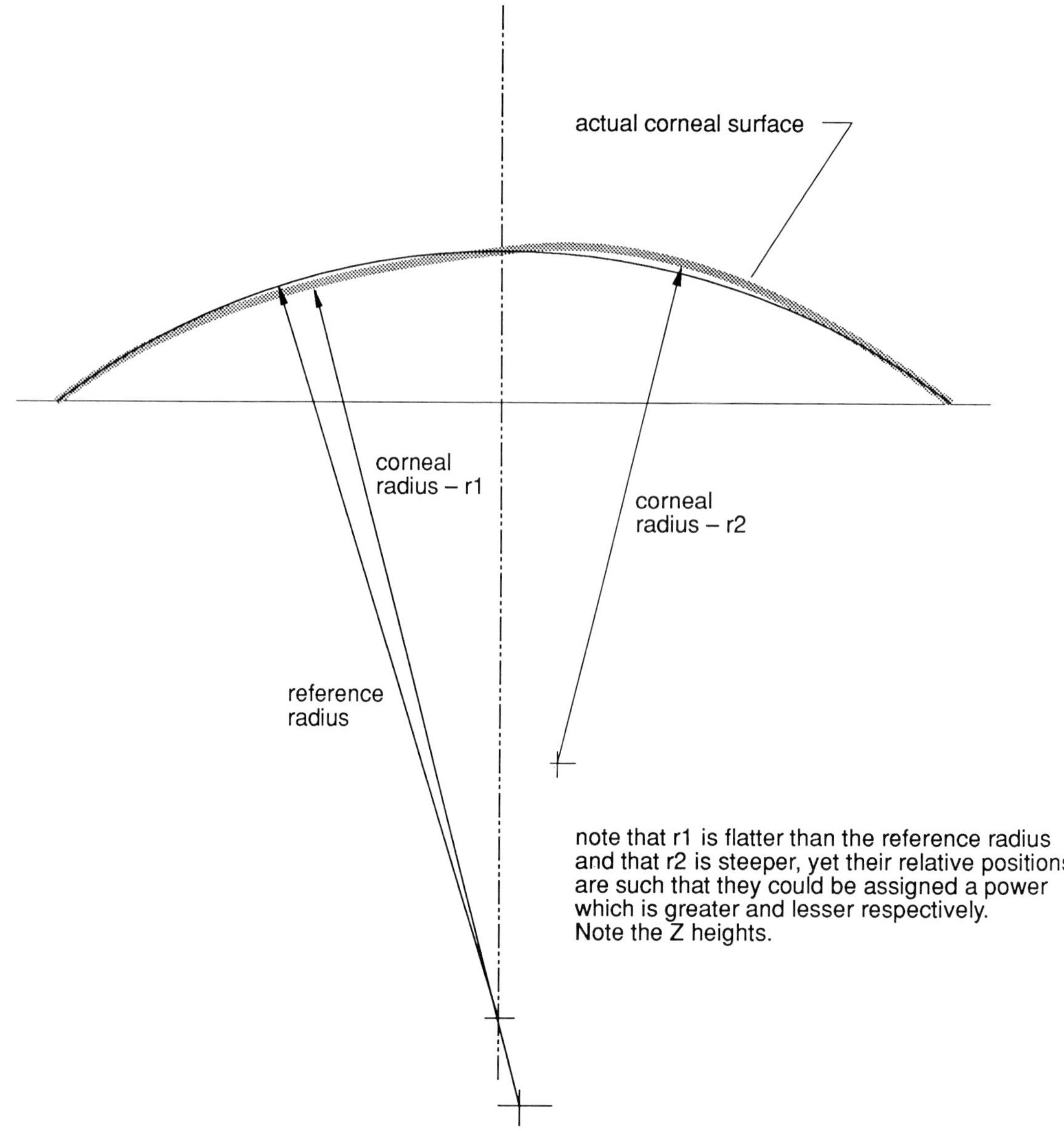

Fig. 6.34 Reference sphere–surface contour relationship.

ferometer expresses the OPD between a reference radius and the measured radius. The eye's slope data do not rotate around a common point—because an aspheric surface does not have a single point of origin. Hence maps rendered by non-sphere-based systems *look* different and *are* different—for this reason and for the fact that they are mapping only the "errors" or deviations from the reference sphere.

Corneal slope information

Sphere-based (Placido's disk) systems are mapping *power* by equating curvature with focal length. They are producing maps that, to the ophthalmologist, look like he or she thinks the cornea ought to look. However, all agree that no one expects a patient to be able to see through the characteristic hourglass shape (the hallmark of a sphere-based system), and most understand that it is an artifact.

There is considerable interest in the relationship of the corneal apex (highest point on the cornea) to the true visual axis. The exact location of the geographic corneal apex also has been a subject of much investigation over the years. With the emergence of refractive surgery, the location of the geographic apex and its relationship to the visual axis have acquired greater clinical importance. Using photoelectric keratometry to locate the corneal apex in a population of normal patients, about 63% had apices located on the temporal side of the vertical meridian of the cornea, 16.3% had apices that were nasal to the vertical meridian, and 21% had apices precisely on the vertical meridian [69]. With respect to the horizontal meridian, there was approximately an equal distribution

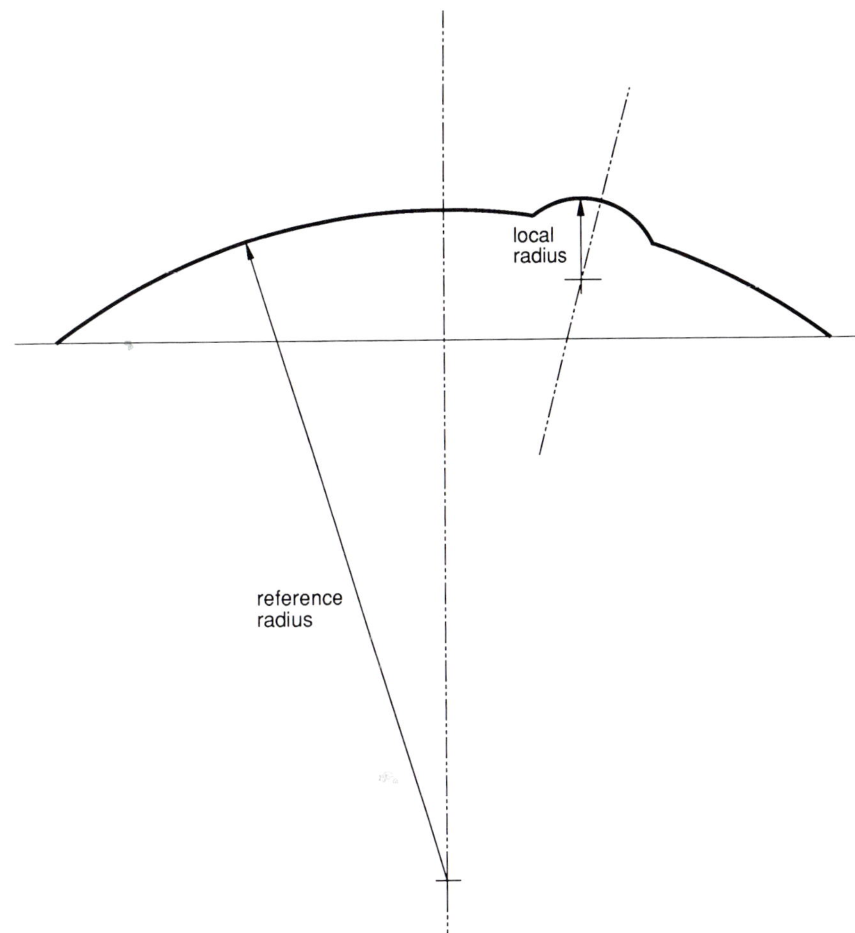

Fig. 6.35 Surface is drawn in relation to a reference sphere.

of the apices above, below, and on the horizontal meridian. It was four times more likely for the apex to be displaced nasally. However, the corneal apex was within 0.5 mm of the visual axis in 62% of eyes. Other authors have found similar temporal displacement of the corneal apex [45,70]. Dingeldein and Klyce, although they did not attempt to locate the corneal apex precisely, found that the area of greatest dioptric power (i.e., steepest corneal curvature) was at the central visual axis in 52% of eyes but in a significant percentage often was displaced temporally with respect to visual line of sight—that is, the visual axis was nasal to the apex [71]. This puts the visual axis on the side of the mountain, as it were. This also means that in the majority of eyes the optic is tilted—think about it. Better yet—do the math. Both tilt and coma are poorly measured with sphere-based systems.

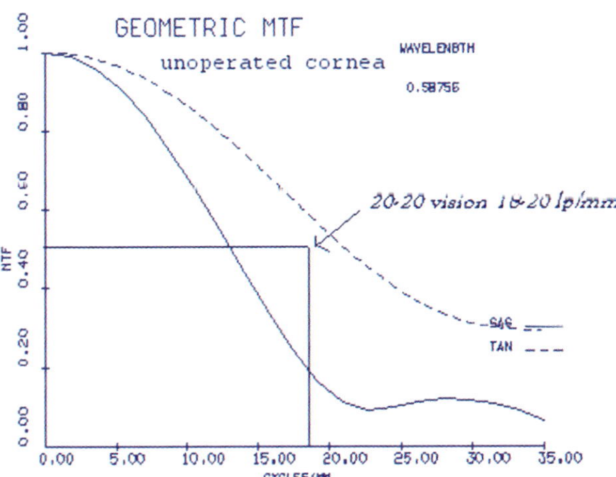

Fig. 6.36 Plot of modulation transfer function (MTF) of an eye.

Although the locations of the visual center and the apical centers are rarely identical, most instruments that measure the corneal surface make this assumption and center their measurements about the patient's visual axis. This central position can be calculated conveniently as the *centroid* of the corneal surface area enclosed by the first 1.0-mm² area surrounding the fixation point [72]. A more rigorous approximation involves a repetitive computational procedure that determines the geometrically averaged center of the innermost 0.5 mm from center coordinates of best-fitting circles for individual 10° arcs around the innermost mire.

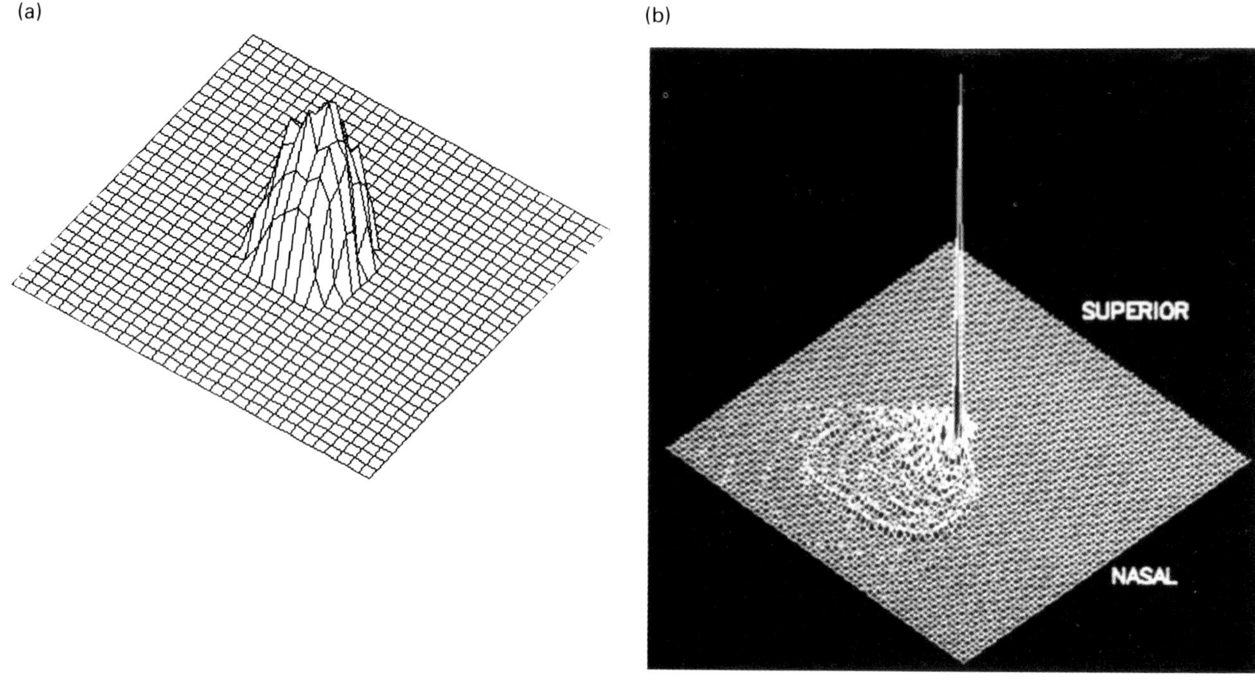

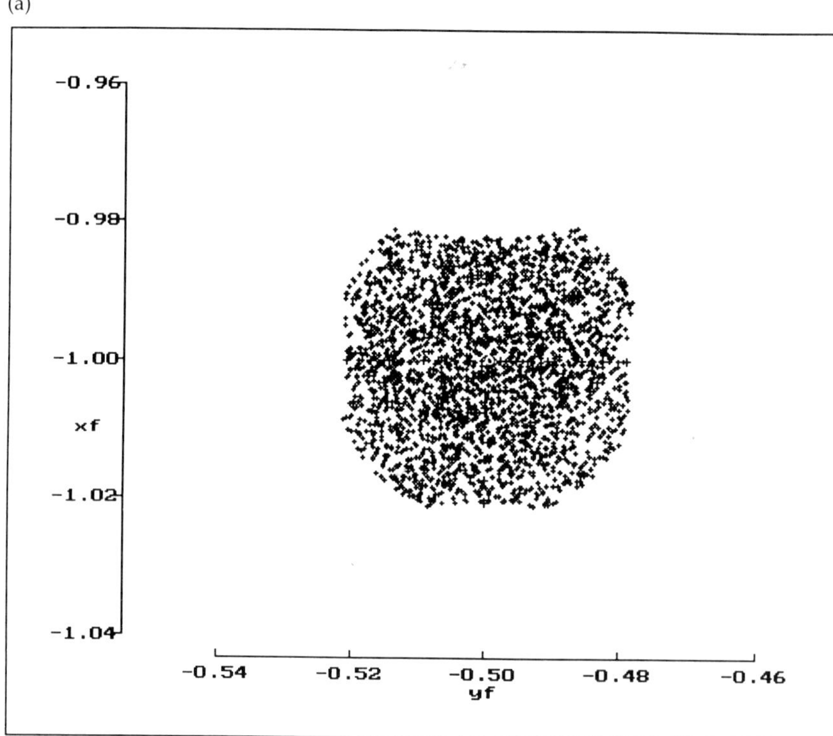

Fig. 6.37 (a) Airy disk of an eye constructed from a surface hologram using a ray tracing program (BEAM4). Such an analysis can provide information as to the optical efficiency of the eye because basically it is the Strehl ratio (S_r) that is being mapped. S_r is a measure of the size and relative brightness of the central Airy disk. (b) An Airy disk from a patient with keratoconus. Note the distortion of the pattern (Maquire). (c) Preoperative focal spot. (d) Post-Ruiz focal spot. Note coma. By plotting the shape and size of the focal spot, tilt and coma can be detected and measured. (Courtesy of L. Maguire.)

Modulation transfer function

This function is the ratio of resolution to contrast and is the most accurate reflection of the eye's ability to see. It is akin to the contrast sensitivity we have all heard about except that it is derived from the optical coefficients. It is therefore an objective measurement of true visual efficiency. Figure 6.36 shows a modulation transfer function (MTF) of a normal cornea using data obtained from the CLAS II device using optical bench software—in this case BEAM4.

Focal spot diagram and/or Strehl ratio (Airy disk)

The advent of holographic techniques has ushered in the use of more sophisticated and technical ways of examining not only the surface contour of the cornea but also

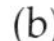

(b)

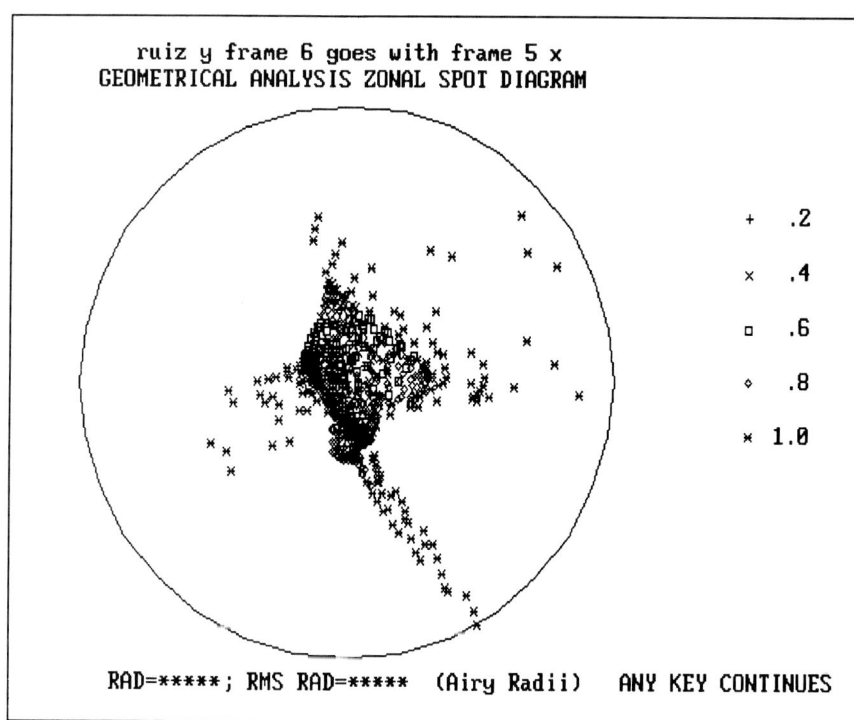

Fig. 6.37 *(Continued)*

its effect on the light bundle traversing the eye and the resulting image. For example, one means of evaluating the quality of a refracting system is the focal spot. The size and shape of the focal spot present the user with gobs of information about the condition of the central cornea. It answers the question *"Why can't my patient see better?"*

A spot diagram is generated by feeding the surface information into a ray-tracing algorithm. This algorithm projects or traces the path of single rays of light going through a transparent medium to a target—in this case the retina. This can take the form of an Airy disk (see Figure 3.15) or focal spot shape—also known as a *Strell definition* or *ratio* (the ratio of the light intensity at the peak of the diffraction pattern of the aberrated image to that at the peak of an aberration-free image) [73]. I have included a figure to illustrate the utility of spot diagrams (Figure 6.37a, b).

Figure 6.37c shows the focal spot of an unexcised cornea. Figure 6.37d shows the focal spot after a cornea has undergone a relaxing incision procedure for astigmatism (Ruiz technique). The patient has poor unaided vision and corrects to only 20/40 in that eye—therefore, I would predict clinically that the patient has irregular astigmatism. This patient experiences "ghosting of images" at 2 months postoperatively. Note that the focal spot is relatively compact but has a "tail" emanating from the center. This tail tells us that the patient has coma, a special type of astigmatism due largely to tilt and decentration of the surface. I would predict that a contact lens would not improve this person's vision, and it does not. Figure 6.29a shows this patient's corneal profile plotted against the reference sphere.

Figure 6.38 is an isometric surface map more familiar to optical engineers. However, the irregularities in the corneal surface can be seen readily, even though the irregularities are of small magnitude and require data scaling to reveal. A contour map is a *global* view of the cornea showing gross deviations—like observing the Earth from space. The isometric map is a *local* view with enhanced data—like observing the Grand Canyon from a low-flying aircraft.

As discussed in the next section, there are three other pieces of information that are useful to the refractive surgeon and obtainable from topography.

Surface asymmetry index (SAI)/surface regularity index (SRI)

SAI is the localized surface regularity within the central area of the cornea. It is, of course, a meridian-based calculation. It has significant value in predicting the best spectacle-corrected visual acuity but has been superseded by the SRI.

SRI seems to have a higher correlation with best spectacle vision than does the SAI. This value is representative of the smoothness of the virtual visual aperture. This aperture is taken to have a value of 4.5 mm (corresponding to ring 10 on the Tomey unit). Data points are measured at six equal (~0.25-mm) intervals from the

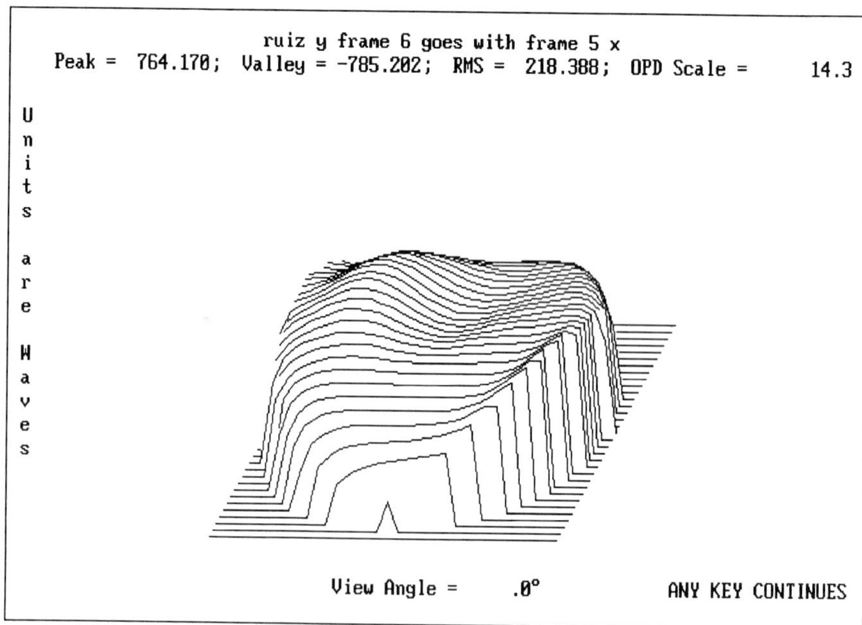

Fig. 6.38 Isometric surface plot after a Ruiz procedure.

1.0-mm ring (ring 2) to a distance of 4.5 mm (ring 10) for a total of at least 256 semimeridians. The powers on a given semimeridian for three successive points are examined.

If the powers of the three successive points are found to be irregular (other than steadily increasing, decreasing, or staying the same), this irregularity was summed into the final SRI as a positive number. In mathematical terms, any difference in power gradient between successive data pairs was assigned a positive value and added to the running sum. This process is continued for all data sets for each semimeridian and for all surface powers that fit in a ±1.0-D window of the most frequently occurring surface power within the area measured. The formula is

$$SRI = ln\left[A\cdot\frac{\sum_{i=1,256}^{j=1,6}\left|P_{i,j}\ \frac{(P_{i,j-1}+P_{i,j+1})}{2}\right|}{N}\right]-B$$

where A and B are scaling constants, $P_{i,j}$ is the matrix of corneal surface powers, i is the semimeridional index, j is the data-point index (keratoscope ring number), and N is the total number of powers within the ±1.0-D window.

ISR The ratio of the mean curvature difference of the superior to the inferior cornea can be useful in helping to make the diagnosis of keratoconus. The readings are taken at approximately the 4-mm zone. Any ratio equal to or greater than 3 is indicative of keratoconus. Thus, if the superior steep K is 41 and the lower is 45, the ratio 1:4 is greater than 3. The actual cones are always shown clearly on wavefront maps.

Sim K This is basically a synthesized K-reading designed to provide a comparative link between topography and keratometry. This value is derived in sphere-based systems by taking three readings along 128 separate meridians from the seventh to ninth rings. These correspond to the 3- to 4-mm zones or distances of 1.5, 1.75, and 2.00 mm from the center. The power of each meridian is the average of the six data points.

The steepest meridian (plus cylinder axis) is defined as the meridian with the highest mean power. The power and location of the orthogonal (90° away) to the steepest determines the flattest (minus cylinder axis) meridian. The sim K is derived from the mean of these two values.

Case studies

The time has come to "put up or shut up," as they say. I have been singing the praises of a more detailed (and sensible) way to examine the corneal surface, and what follows is a practical demonstration of the utility of a true corneal surface profile. You have already been exposed to some interferometry-generated maps (see above).

Case 1

Figure 6.39a is a photokeratoscope photograph taken with an EyeSys eight-ring instrument. Careful examination of this photograph demonstrates very subtle perturbations of an occasional ring out in the middle and far periphery that you would expect after an RK. This appearance was verified with a 32-ring CMS (Tomey) unit. This photograph shows a nice and smooth cornea, as would be expected 18 months postoperatively. Figure 6.39b is a sphere-based map generated from this keratoscopic image. Although I did not pick it up from the photograph, the device is telling us that this patient has some (1.0 D) residual with-the-rule astigmatism at 87°. Predicted visual acuity is 20/25. However, on a good day, this patient has a BC visual acuity of 20/50. She fares no better with a contact lens either. *Why can't this patient see?*

Figure 6.39c shows a slope map generated by a phase-modulated single-sideband interferometer. It is immediately obvious that this surface is not regular at all. Not only is the patient showing an exaggerated *tilt*, but there is an irregular disturbance over the visual axis characterized by a tiny area of steepening, a *microconus,* except that there is no corneal ectasia there. Figure 6.39d is an isometric of this cornea looking down from 12 o'clock with a 10° viewing angle from a flat plane. The tilt is obvious. Her right eye is no better and shows the same sorts of distortions. This patient had a bilateral RK performed 18 months previously with 1.5-mm optic zones.

Case 2

Figure 6.40a is a photokeratoscopic view of an eye that demonstrates frank astigmatism 18 months postoperatively. One of the strengths of sphere-based keratoscopes is that they show corneal distortions (at least for the most part; see above) on the photograph. I would not be without one in my clinic. Figure 6.40b is a sphere-based map that nicely shows this astigmatism as well as the typical inferior steepening often seen in post-RK patients. The astigmatism is well defined and reasonably regular. This patient started out with a refraction of $-7.50 + 0.50 \times 106$ with a BC visual acuity of 20/20 + 1. Her postoperative refraction is $-1.50 + 1.50 \times 125$—a nice result. She should have a good BC visual acuity (predicted BU visual acuity 20/25), but she does not. Her BC visual acuity is 20/40 – 2 with a Snellen chart; she fails a contrast sensitivity (modulation transfer test) test at 20/100 – (Figure 6.40c) and has to wear a GPCL to obtain functional vision. Figure 6.40d shows why this patient cannot see. The patient has a deep furrow right along the axis of cylinder; not only that, but the true cylinder is against the rule—90° away from its representation on the sphere-based map. This is a problem with the algorithm used in such systems: It has difficulty with steep events. Figure 6.40e is a higher-resolution map of the same surface in 0.50-D steps. By selecting the curvature (Z-height) view, it is possible to see an elevation map (Figure 6.40f). Not only is the generalized elevation of the midperiphery easily seen, but so also are some of the incisions. Figure 6.40g is an isometric of the same eye demonstrating the severe distortion. This patient's surgical OZ was 1.0 mm in diameter.

Case 3

Here is something that should be right up the sphere-based system's alley (Figure 6.41a). The distortion on the surface is plainly seen. However, the map of this surface (see Figure 6.41b) shows a well-defined residual astigmatism and again predicts good vision. Figure 6.41c, an interferometric map, is much more representative of the actual surface conditions on this cornea. Not only is there a large tilt, but the slope also cuts through the visual axis. This does not explain the patient's monocular diplopia, however. The isometric (Figure 6.41d) demonstrates the tilt much more graphically but does not explain the diplopia either. The Zernike-generated wavefront (or optical efficiency) map clearly shows the two well-defined apices (Figure 6.41e). Another subnominal OZ (1.0-mm) post-RK patient, this patient required a penetrating keratoplasty to recover useful vision.

Case 4

Sphere-based systems are all prone to misinterpreting surface profile. The next three images should clearly demonstrate the point (Figure 6.42a-c). Neither the slit-scanner (a) nor the Placido system (b) with a step-walking algorithm agrees with the actual surface topography (c). Figure 6.42d shows the curvature map of this post-Ruiz patient in whom both the radial and transverse incisions (T-cuts) can be seen clearly. Figure 6.42e shows the wavefront map and the iatrogenic kerectasia (keratoconus). This patient required a PKP to restore useful vision, but the operation was complicated by the presence of the T-cuts. The patient is doing well with a GPCL.

Case 5

Figure 6.43 shows one of the reasons ALK was abandoned. The sharp break at the margins of the second stromal cut, especially in higher myopes, produced a considerable decrease in visual efficiency. The visual aberration was exacerbated by any misalignment of the first and second cuts and by the abrupt transition at the margin of the second cut.

Case 6

Figure 6.44 is for the laser crowd, lest they get too smug. This shows a high-resolution rendering of a 20-week post-LASIK patient done with a Summit excimer laser. Despite that the surgery was done with a laser, the demarcation of the ablation is seen clearly. This patient had some problem with glare but recovered 20/25 UC visual acuity postoperatively. If nothing else, this map should demonstrate why precise centration of the ablation is so important. The reversed curvature clearly seen at the mar-

(a)

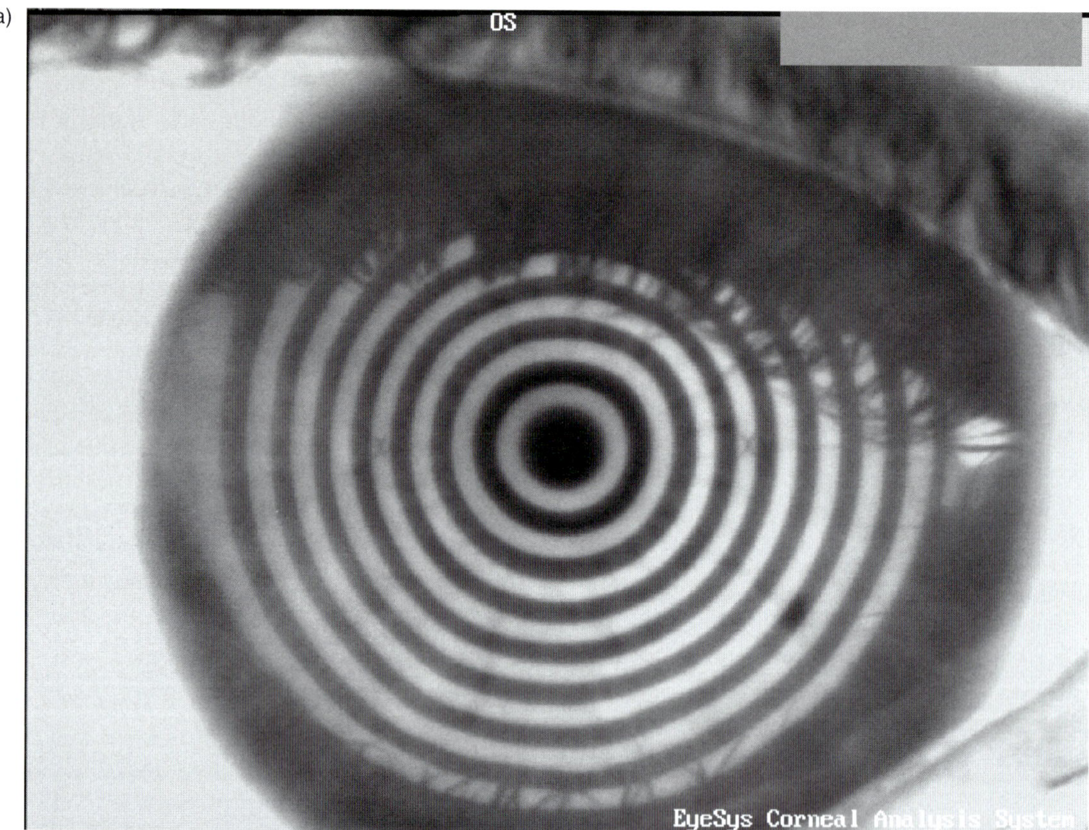

(b)

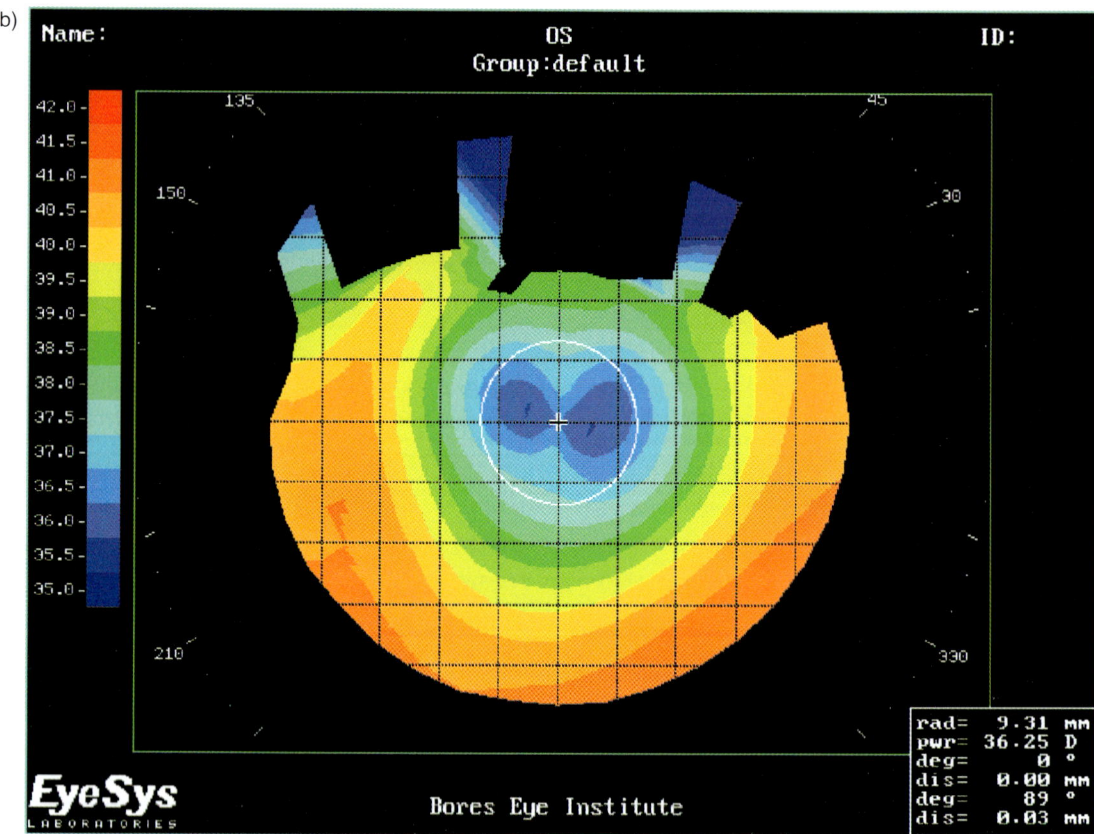

Fig. 6.39 (a) Photokeratoscope photo taken with an 8-ring videokeratoscope. This appearance was verified with a 32-ring CMS unit. (b) Sphere-based map generated from this keratoscopic image. This patient has some (1.0 D) residual with-the-rule astigmatism at 87°. Predicted visual acuity is 20/25. Actual best-corrected visual acuity is 20/50⁻. (c) Slope map generated by a phase-modulated, single-sideband interferometer. It is immediately obvious that this surface is not regular at all. Not only is the patient showing an exaggerated tilt, but there is an irregular disturbance over the visual axis characterized by a tiny area of steepening—a microconus, except that there is no corneal ectasis there. (d) An isometric of this cornea looking down from 12 o'clock with a 10° viewing angle from a flat plane. The exaggerated tilt of this refracting surface is obvious.

(c)

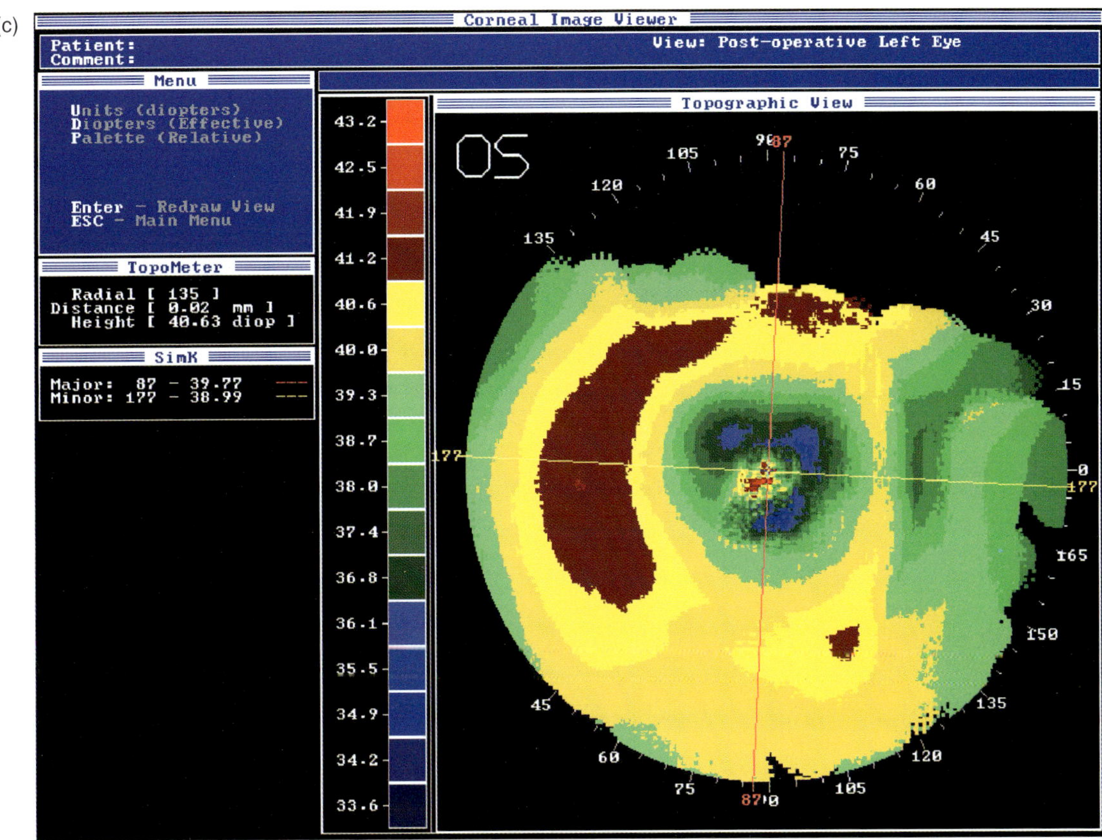

(d)

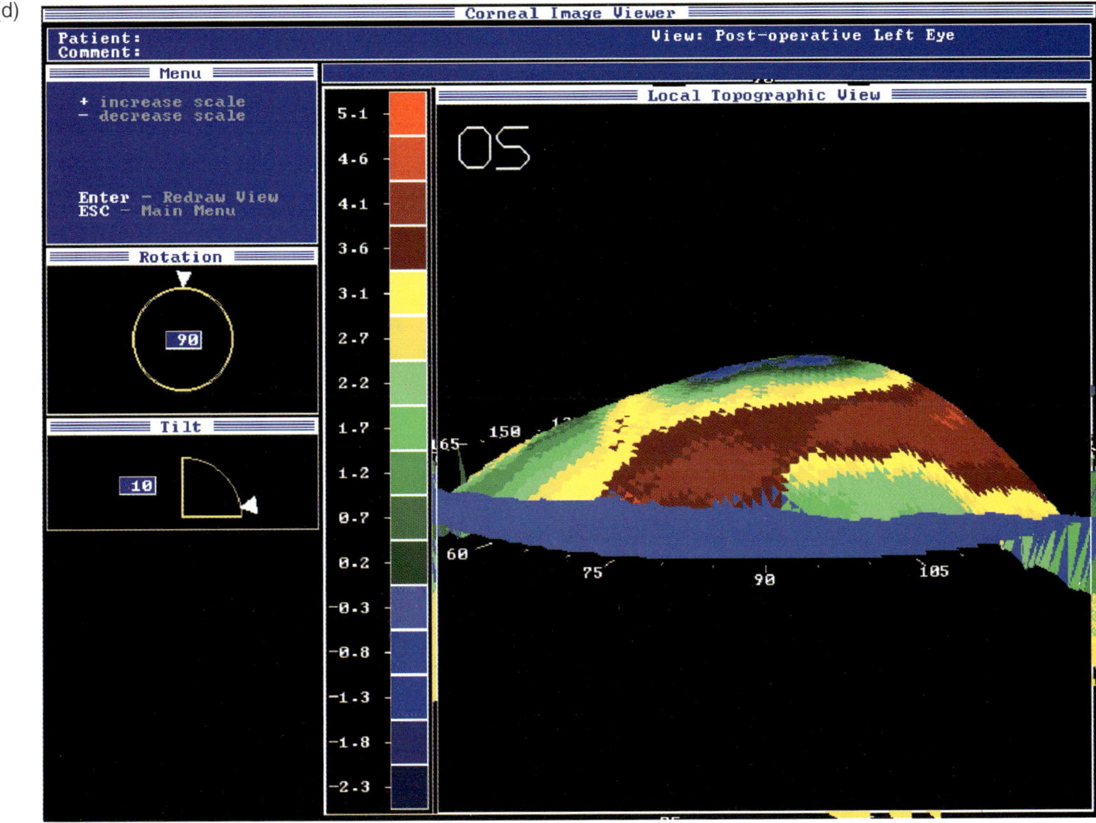

Fig. 6.39 (*Continued*)

(a)

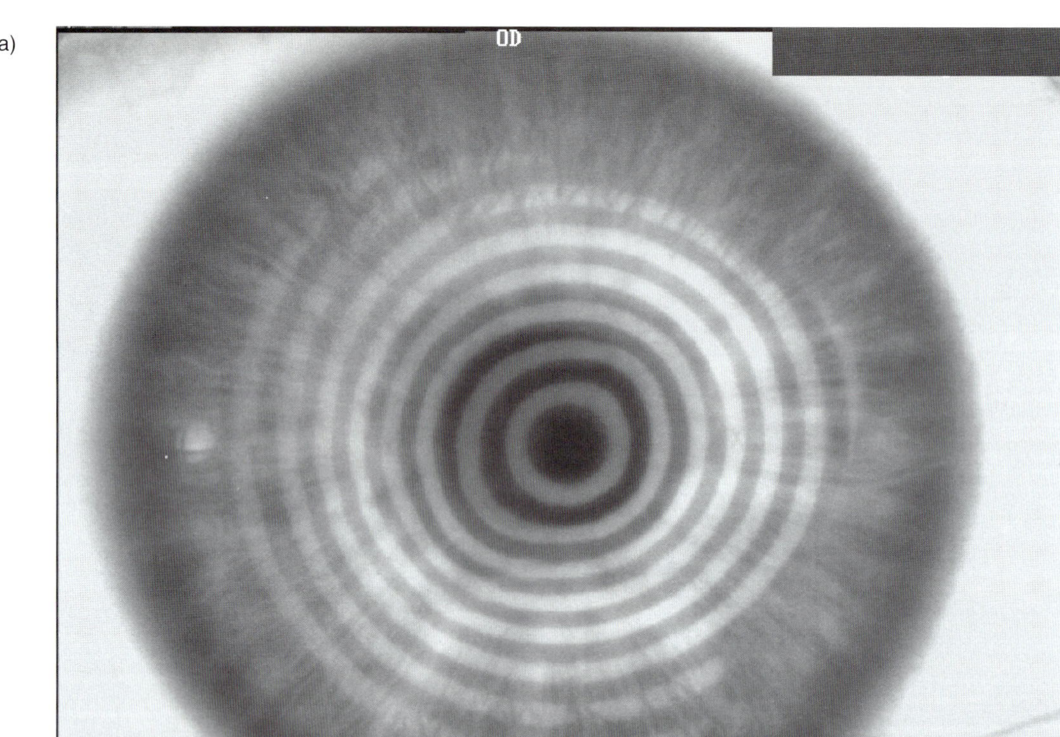

(b)

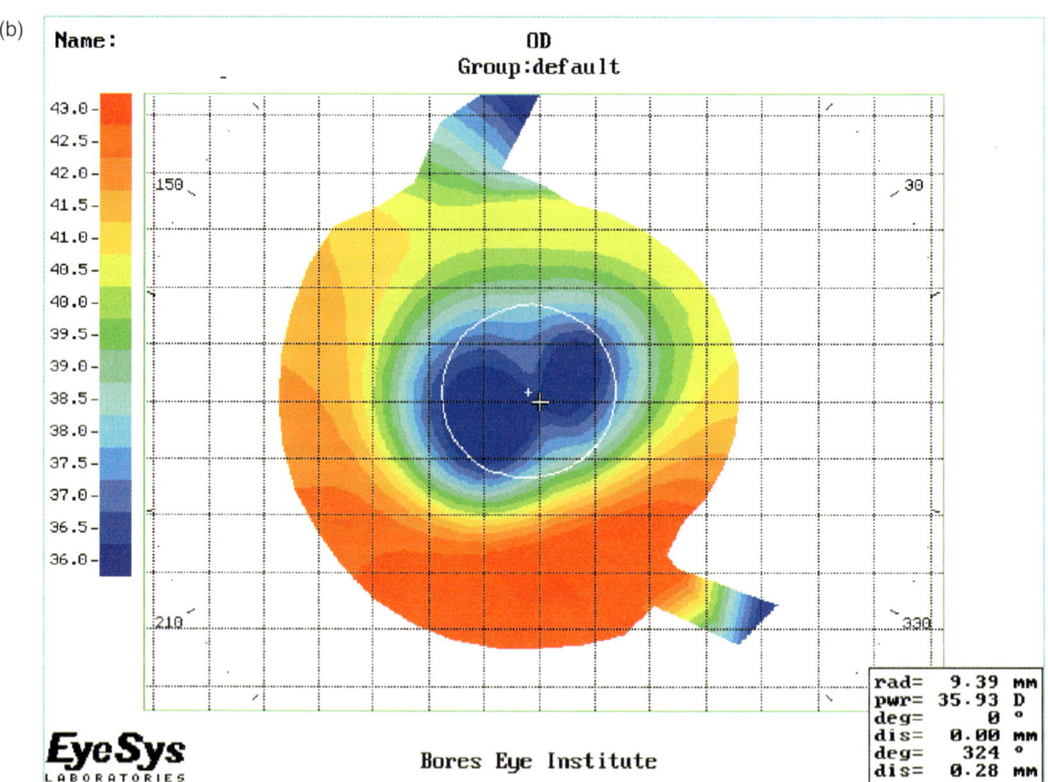

Fig. 6.40 (a) Photokeratoscopic view of an eye that demonstrates frank astigmatism. (b) This sphere-based map nicely shows this astigmatism as well as the typical inferior steepening often seen in post-RK patients. The astigmatism is well defined and reasonably regular. Predicted best uncorrected visual acuity is 20/25, but actual best-corrected visual acuity is 20/40⁻. (c) A contrast sensitivity (modulation transfer test) plot shows her visual efficiency to be 20/100⁻. She has difficulty driving at night. (d) The wavefront contour map shows why this patient cannot see. The patient has a deep furrow right along the axis of cylinder; not only that, but the true cylinder is against-the-rule—90° away from its representation on the sphere-based map, a common problem with such devices. (e) Higher-resolution map of the same surface in 0.5-D steps. By selecting the curvature (Z-height) view. (f) An elevation map or curvature map. Not only is the generalized elevation of the midperiphery easily seen, but so are some of the incisions. (g) An isometric of the same eye demonstrates the severe distortion. This patient's surgical OZ was 1.0 mm in diameter.

(c)

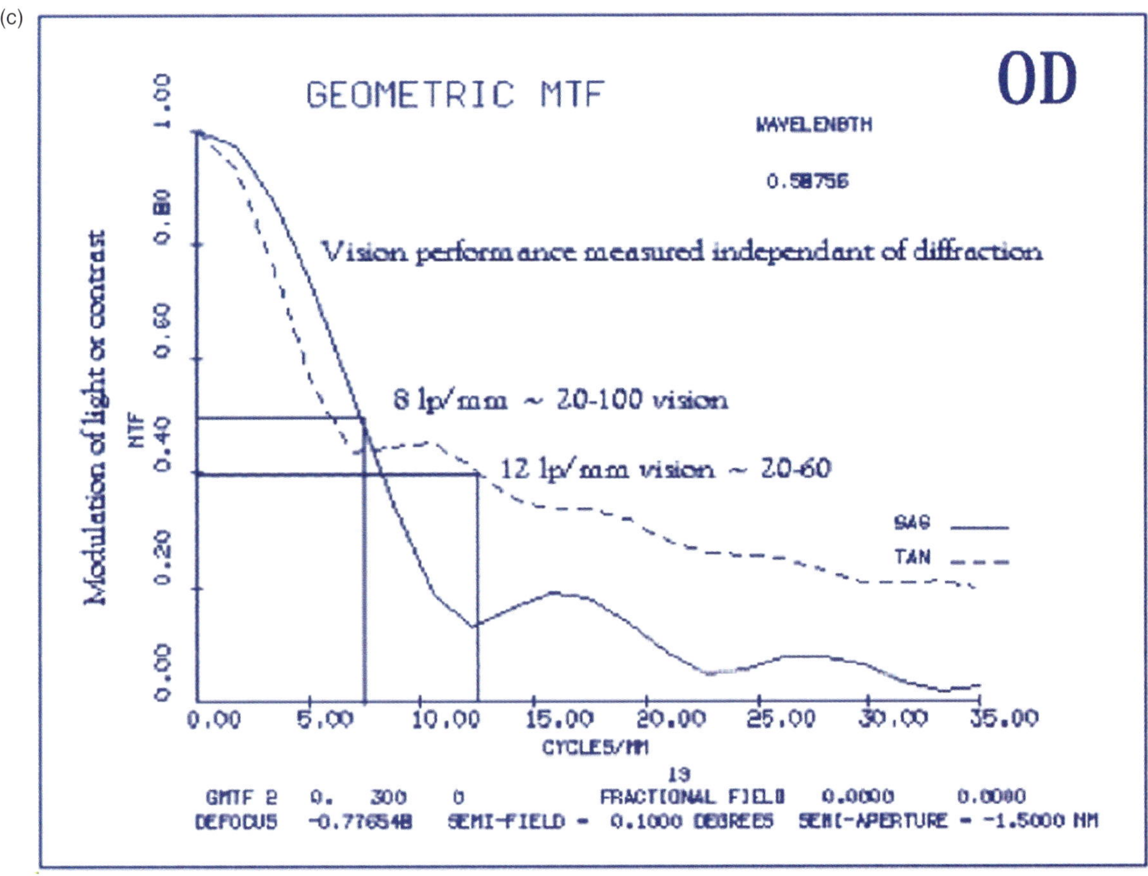

(d)

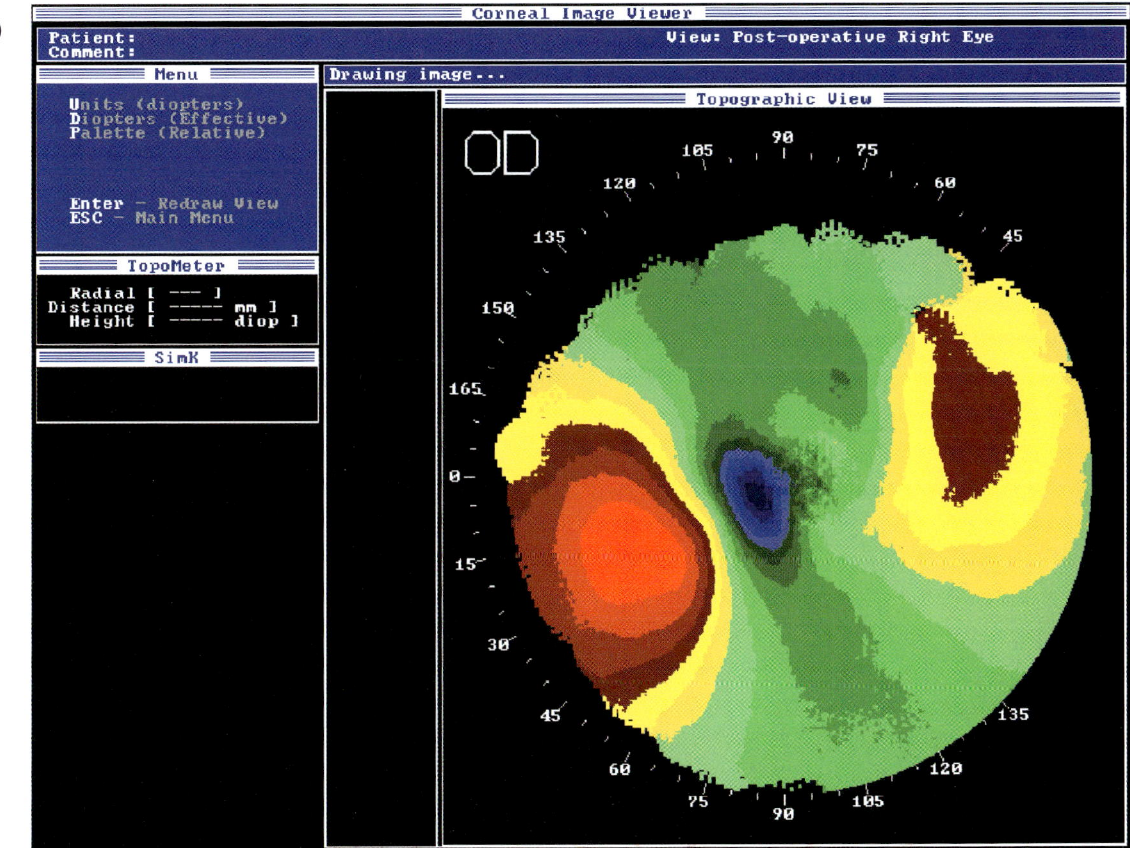

Fig. 6.40 *(Continued)*

(e)

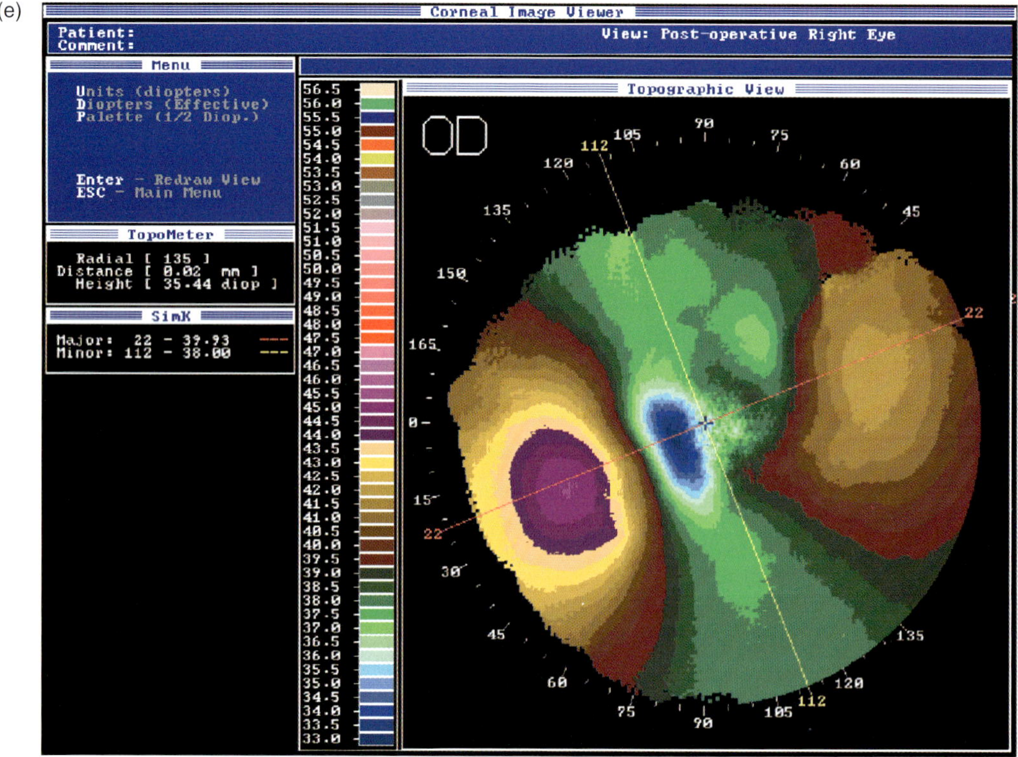

(f)

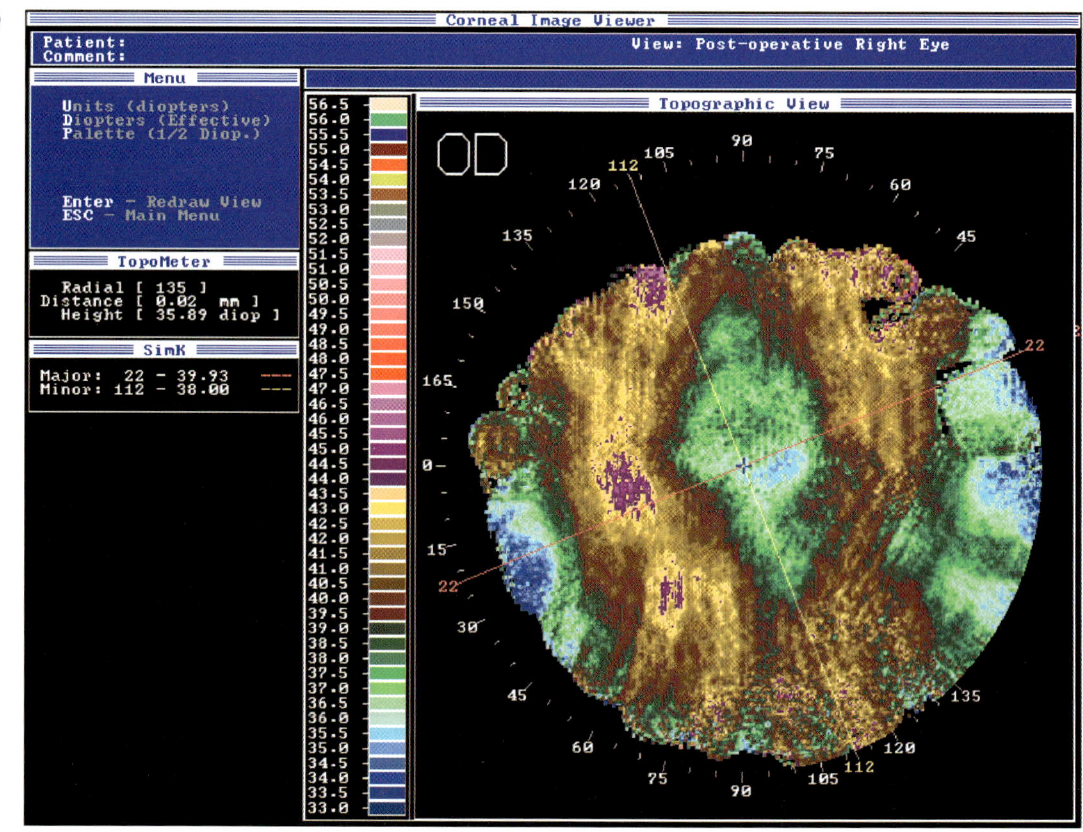

Fig. 6.40 *(Continued)*

(g)

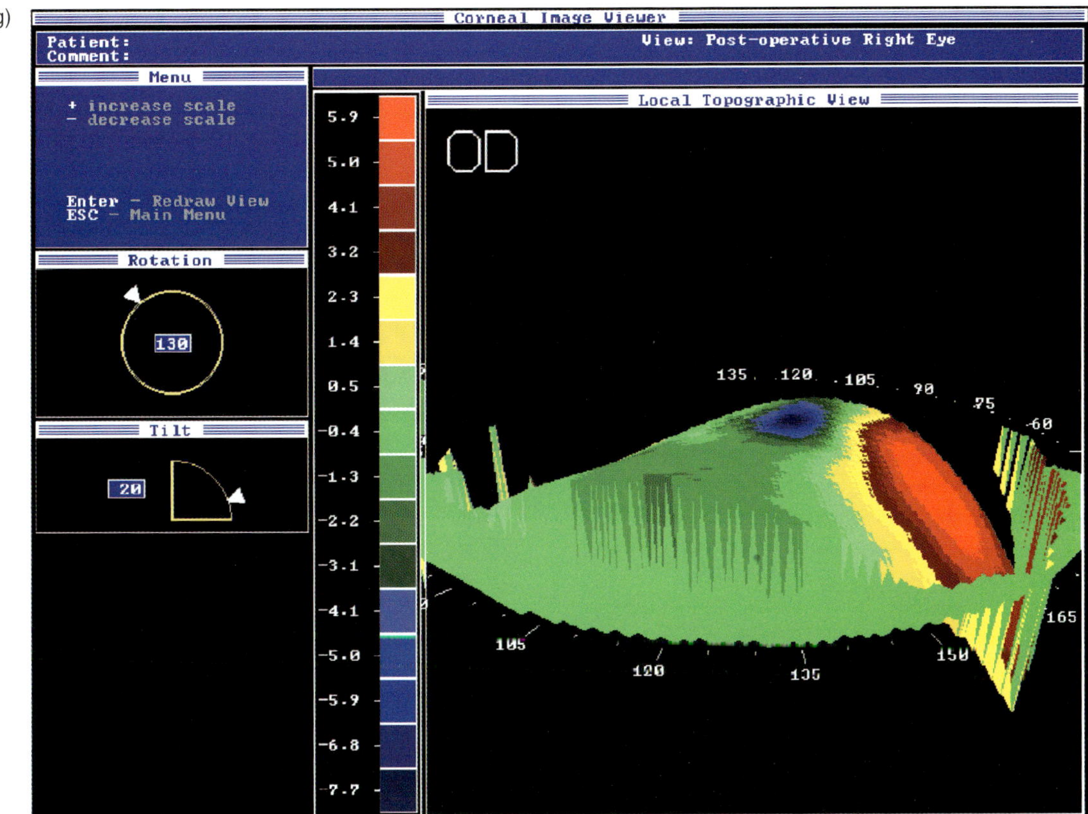

Fig. 6.40 *(Continued)*

gins of the ablation can play the very devil with vision in decentered small zones, and even a small decentration can become evident as glare and flare under darkened conditions.

These maps, representative of only a small percentage of patients examined, clearly demonstrate the value and utility of devices capable of rendering highly aberrated surfaces with precision.

What's on the horizon?

While it is obvious that the corneal surface shape is important in evaluating the outcome of keratorefractive procedures, it does not stand alone as the sole determinant of the refractive power of the eye. This salient fact seems to be overlooked in the overweening rush to climb aboard the topography bandwagon.

When I first began to speak about RK in the late 1970s, I stressed the importance of considering the eye as a refractive unit. That is, any operation performed on the cornea to convert ametropia to emetropia should be based on the ametropia existing within the ocular system as a whole and not just a part—the corneal surface.

This consideration should be obvious even to the most casual practitioner. After all, the term *residual astigmatism* is not new in our lexicon. Something less obvious, but equally important, is revealed when considering keratometry readings. Many forget that the dioptric values returned by these instruments are approximations only and reflect an arbitrary *effective dioptric power* of the cornea. This curious condition comes about because of the nature of the cornea. It is not, after all, an infinitely thin meniscus lens. It is a transparent body of measurable thickness whose back-surface curvature does not correspond to that of its front. What this posterior curvature may be in life is not known. The only data extant are taken from cadaver eyes, which, I submit, are not the best model for a living, breathing eye.

Another factor clouding the issue of the refractive power of the cornea is its refractive index—a factor whose value varies somewhat depending on which authority is cited. Hence the refractive index used in the B&L Keratometer differs from that in the Gambs device, etc. The usual formula assigns a value of –5.85 D for the back-surface power of the cornea, with 0.10 D thrown in to account for the corneal thickness. This thickness is, of course, nowhere constant across the cornea. In any event, the front-surface power is combined with the back-surface power plus the thickness power to arrive at an effective corneal refractive power. These factors are

(a)

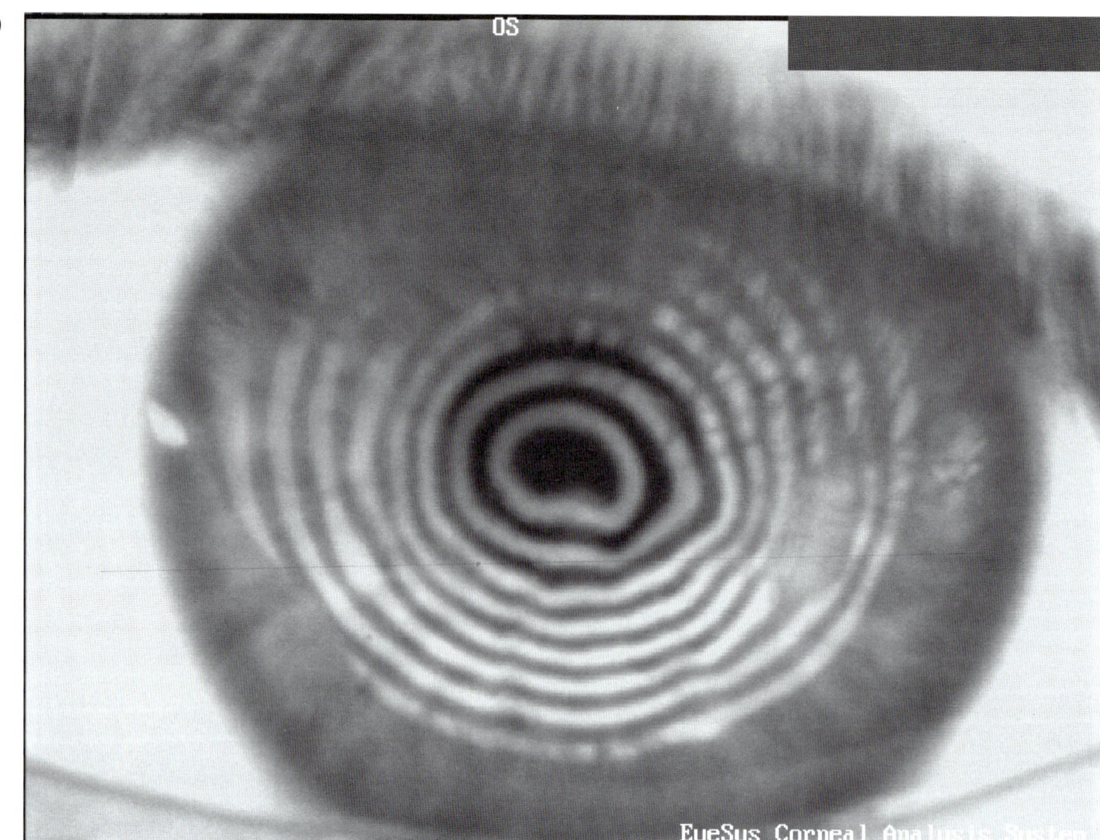

(b)

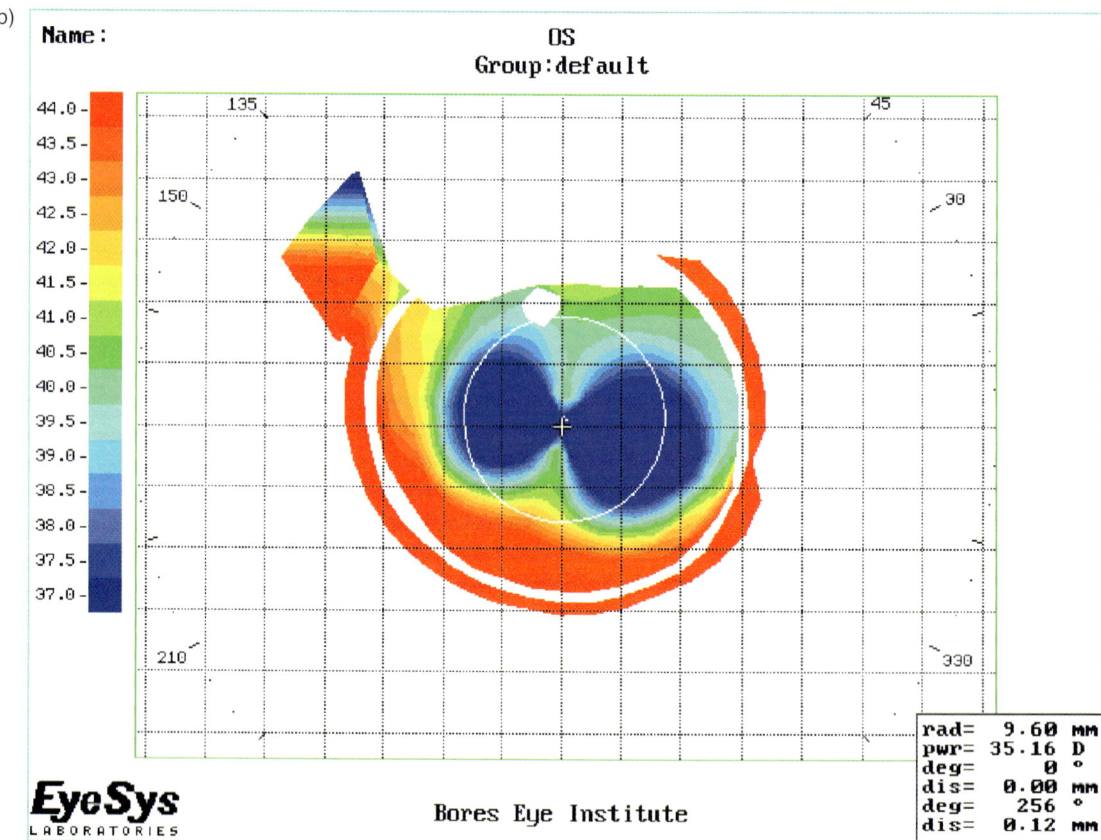

Fig. 6.41 (a) The distortion on the surface is plainly seen on this keratoscope photo. (b) However, the map of this surface shows a well-defined residual astigmatism and again predicts good vision. (c) Interferometric map is much more representative of the actual surface conditions existing on this cornea. Not only is there a large tilt, but the slope cuts through the visual axis. This does not explain her monocular diplopia however. (d) The isometric demonstrates the tilt much more graphically but does not explain the diplopia either. (e) The Zernike-generated wavefront aberration map clearly shows the two well-defined apices. Another subnominal OZ (1.0 mm) post-RK patient. This patient required a penetrating keratoplasty to recover useful vision.

(c)

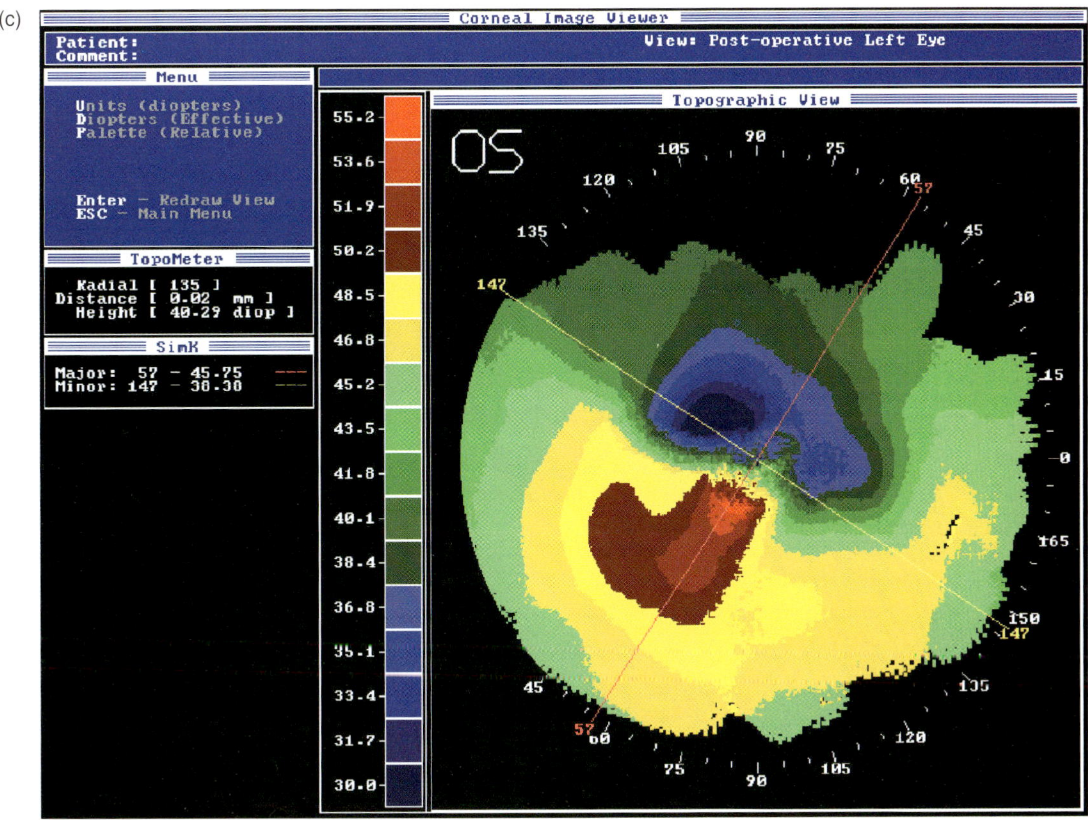

(d)

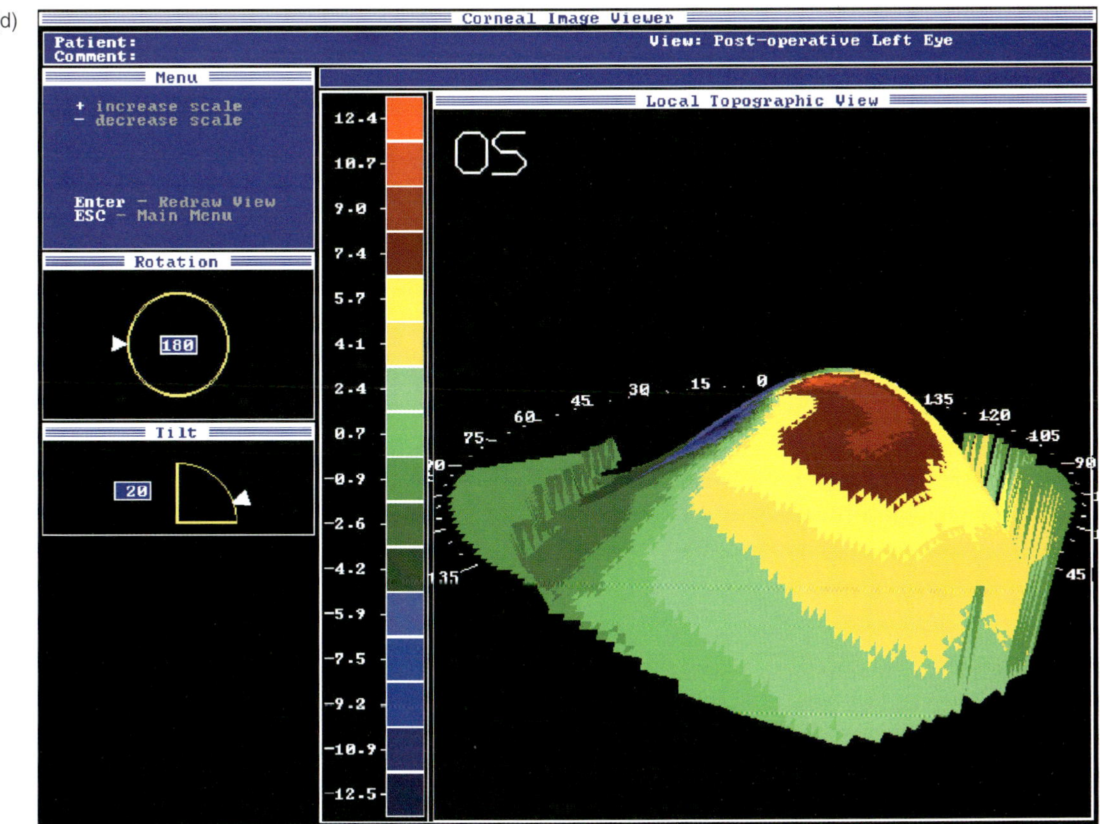

Fig. 6.41 (*Continued*)

(e)

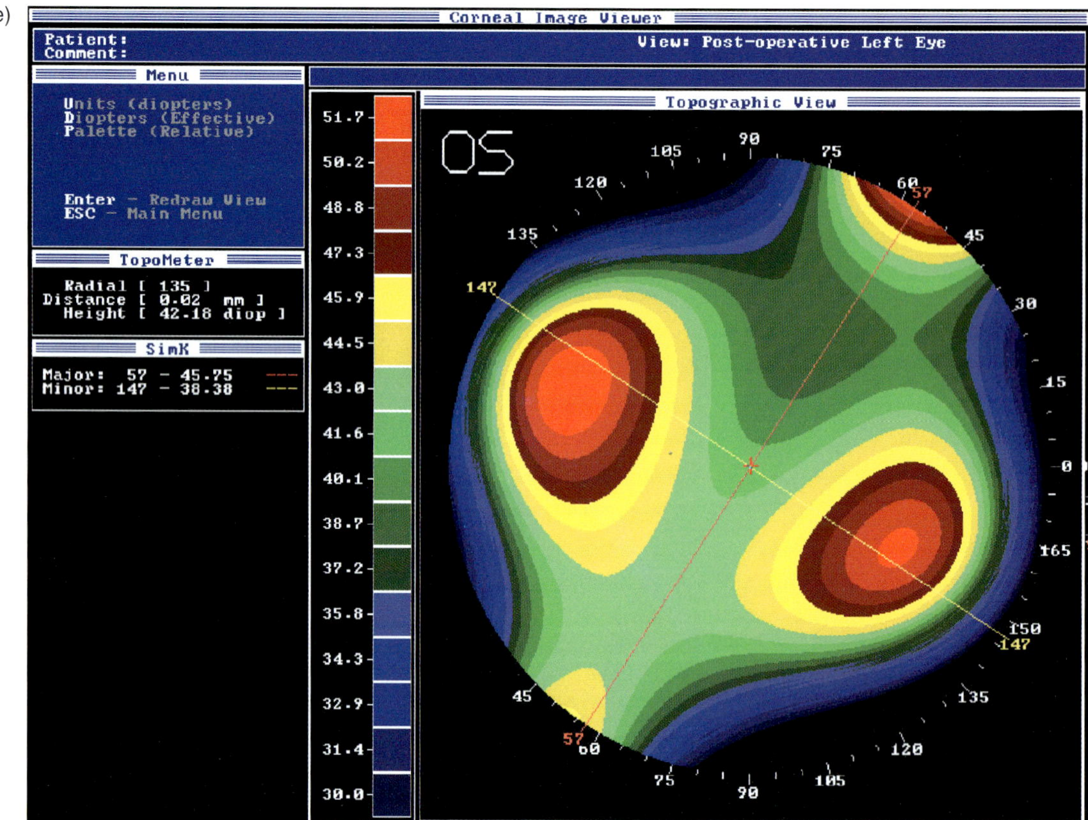

Fig. 6.41 (*Continued*)

accounted for in the usual ophthalmometer (Keratometer is a trade name) by assuming an artificially low value—1.3375—for the refractive index of the cornea.

Let me, for the moment, set aside this conundrum and consider some other facts about the cornea. In the human at least, the external vertical arc or meridian of the cornea is somewhat steeper than its compatriot meridian at 180°. Because this is usually the case, and following the penchant for codifying everything, the vertical steepness is called *with the rule*. Since, by definition, a difference in curvature of the meridians of a surface is called *astigmatism*, this type of astigmatism of the cornea is called *with-the-rule astigmatism*. The internal corneal curvature, on the other hand, tends to have the reverse trend. That is, its horizontal meridian is typically steeper than the vertical. Hence with-the-rule astigmatism for the inside of the cornea seems to be at 180°.

I have used the term *seems to be* because existing work points in that direction, and circumstantial evidence supports this premise. However, a premise is not a fact; we are not really sure. However, it should be obvious that since we can cancel a patient's astigmatism by fitting a spectacle whose astigmatic power is equal and opposite, the same is true for the eye itself. That is, the astigmatism of the internal surface modifies the effect of astigmatism of the external surface. Therefore, the true astigmatism of the cornea is a combination of both surfaces. Consequently, it is not entirely reasonable to attempt to correct astigmatism by considering the external corneal astigmatism alone. It would be hazardous enough to do so if only the cornea contributed to the astigmatism. Since, however, the lens sits astride the visual pathway in a somewhat skewed manner (not to mention the different curves of the front and back surfaces of the lens) and the retina is not axisymmetrical to the visual axis, it is trebly so.

Total ocular aberration rendering

Measuring the total optical aberration of an eye that is a potential candidate for refractive surgery *may* be the answer to the less than totally satisfactory results with current surgical methods. By adapting our surgical modifications in such a way as to compensate for such aberrations, visual acuities in excess of 20/20 (6/6) *may* be possible.

The operative word here is *may*. Newly developed devices using adaptive optics measure the total aberration of the optical system of the eye. The problem here is that *all* the aberrations are measured, including those caused by

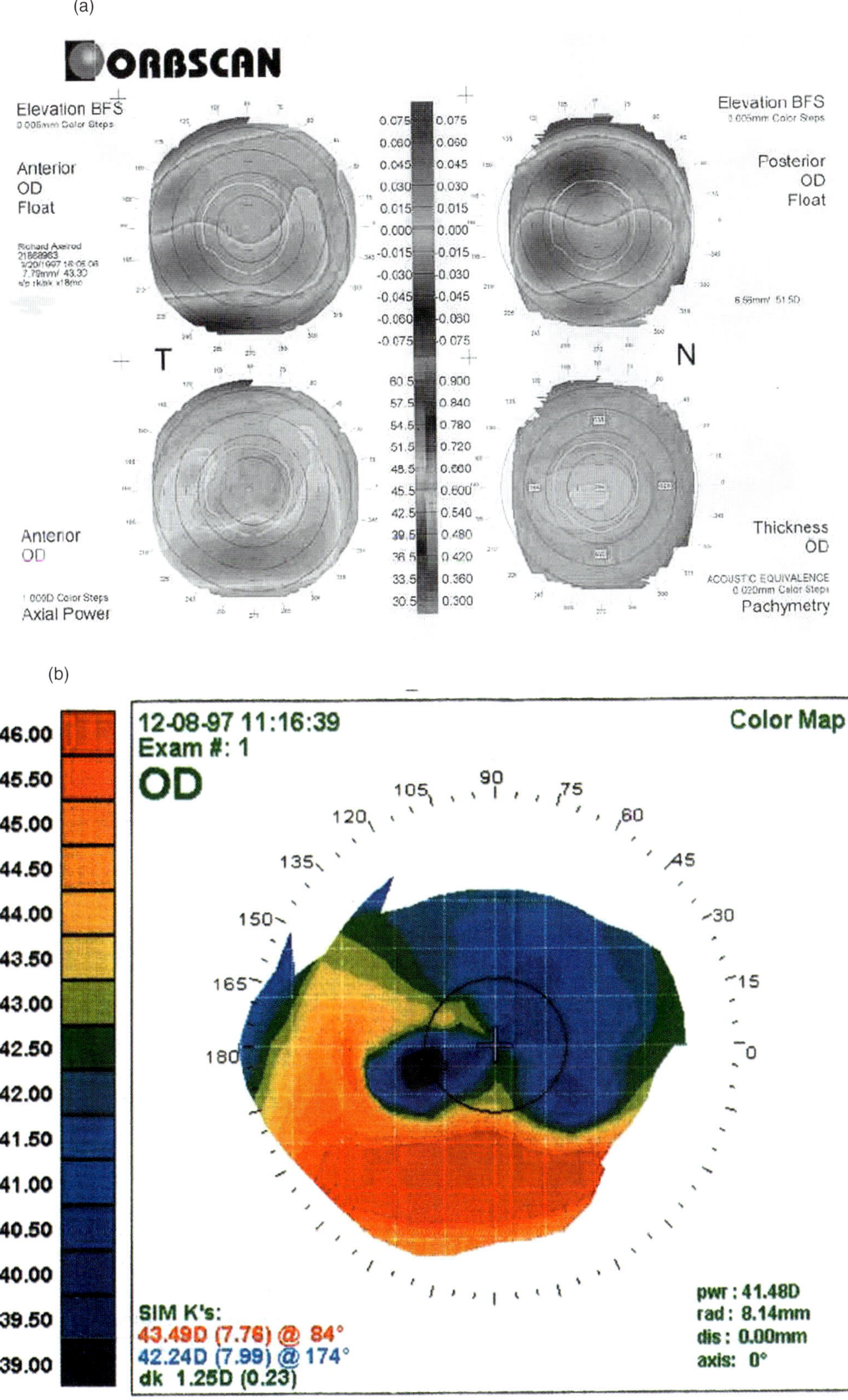

Fig. 6.42 (a) Sphere-based systems are all prone to misinterpreting surface profile. The next three images should clearly demonstrate the point. Neither the slit-scanning device, nor the Placido system (b), nor the Placido system with a step-walking algorithm (c) agree with the actual surface topography. (d) The curvature map of this post-Ruiz case in which both the radial and transverse incisions (T-cuts) can be seen. (e) The wavefront map shows the iatrogenic kerectasia (*keratoconus*). This patient required a PKP to restore useful vision.

(c)

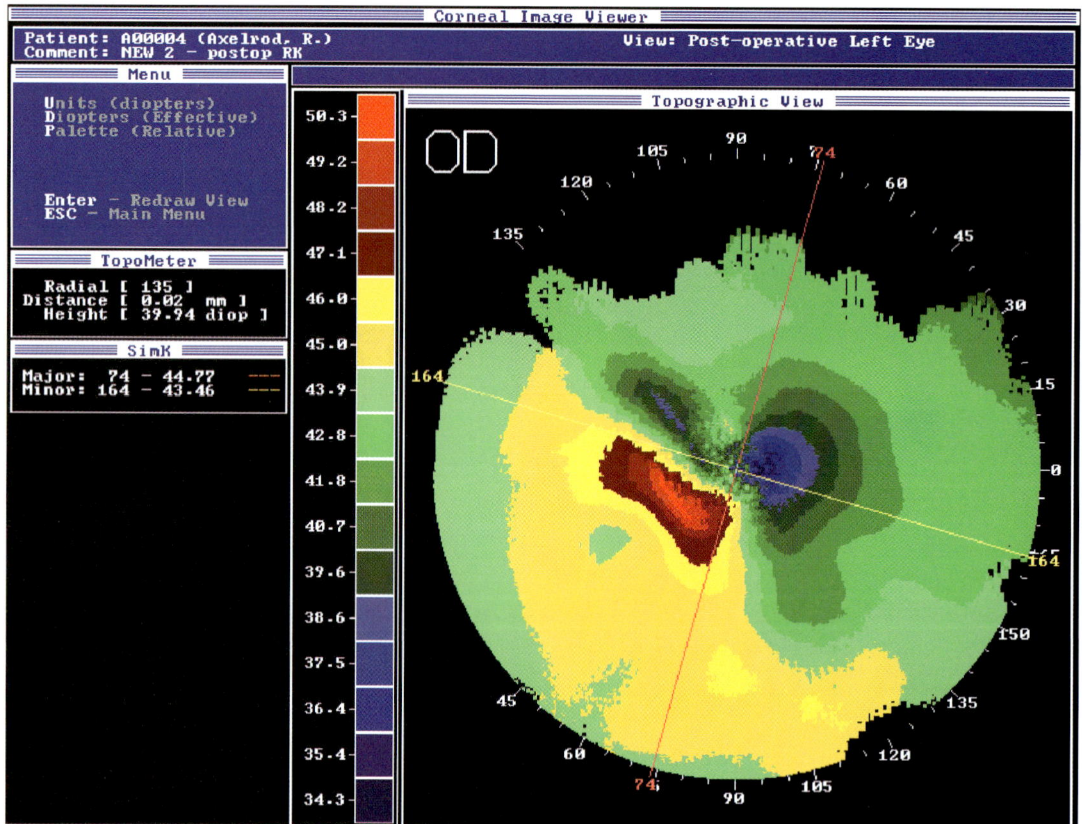

(d)

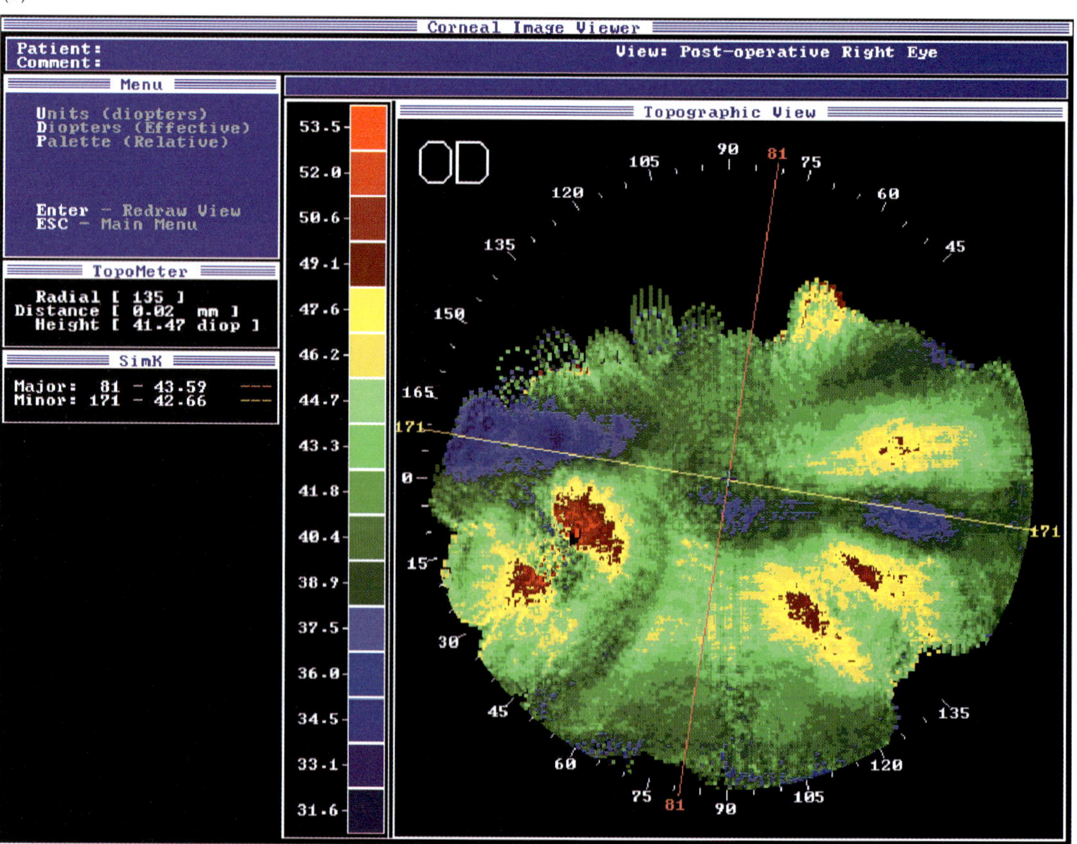

Fig. 6.42 *(Continued)*

(e)

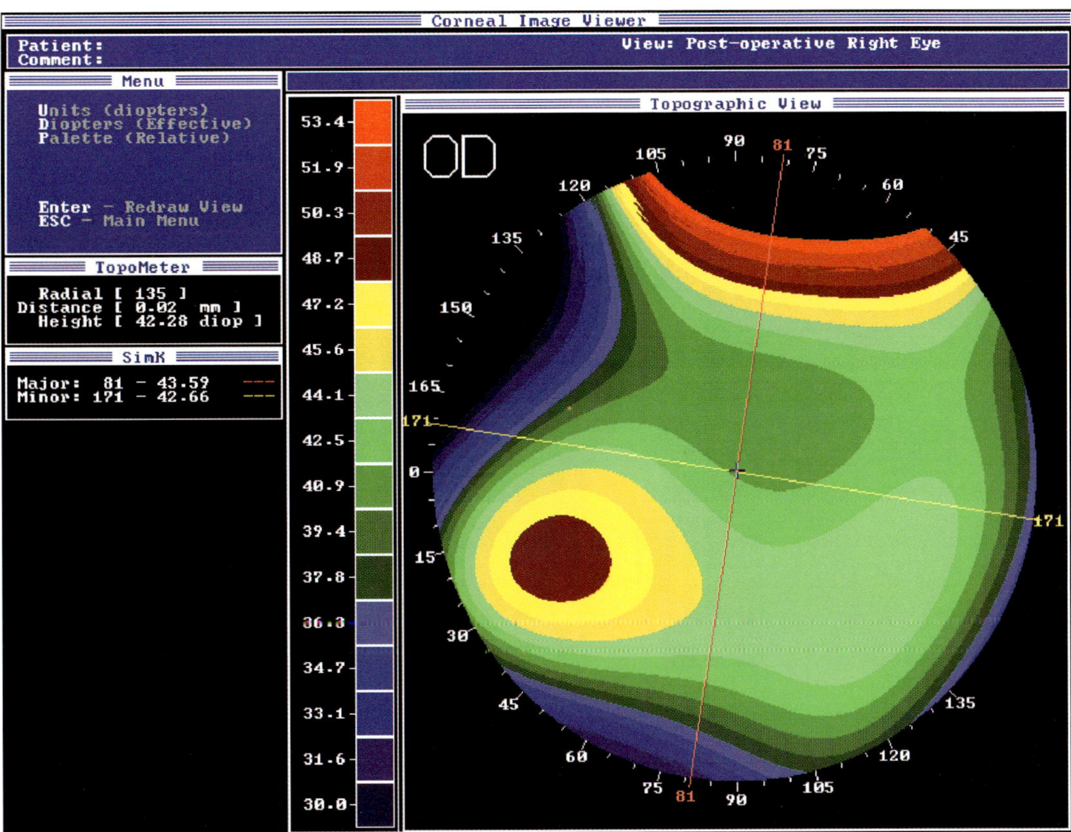

Fig. 6.42 (*Continued*)

internal lens opacities/cataract changes. Such aberrations will be dynamic—changing over time. Winnowing these out may prove to be a larger task than anticipated. It is still unclear whether the wavefront map will pick up a keratoconus suspect. And there are other aspects to be considered as well, such as structural factors—constitutive properties.

An adaptive optics system automatically corrects for light distortions in the medium of transmission. For example, if you look far down a road on a very hot and sunny day, you often will see what is usually called a *mirage*. What you are seeing is the rapidly changing temperature in the air causing it to act like a thick, constantly bending lens. An adaptive optics system measures the characteristics of this distortion and corrects for it by means of a deformable mirror controlled by a computer. The device that measures the distortions in the incoming wavefront of light is called a *wavefront sensor*.

In 1898, Marius Tscherning published his initial work on the aberroscope, a principle on which J. Hartmann expanded in the early 1900s [74]. Adaptive optics got its start in the 1970s, when Howland and Howland applied both principles to adaptive optics [75]. By 1976, the principle of adaptive optics was being applied to the field of astrophysics. The turbulence of the atmosphere blurs images to such an extent that even digital enhancement cannot improve them (Figure 6.45a, b). When the U.S. military was looking for ways to obtain clear photographs of Soviet satellites, adaptive optics provided the needed resolution. Later, as part of the Strategic Defense Initiative, popularly known as the Star Wars program, the military studied adaptive optics as a way to compensate for atmospheric distortions when focusing a ground-based laser weapon on an incoming missile.

Wavefront technology is now positioned as the hottest new thing in refractive surgery. Burned by "hot new things" in the past, however, ophthalmologists are hesitant and concerned about the hype surrounding it. They need not be; the technique is real, and its application in the profession promises to be of value. Whether "supernormal" or "super" vision will be possible is still something that only time will reveal. What *should* concern most ophthalmologists is why they were surprised by this new technology, and they should ask themselves why they have not been paying attention. Wavefront technology is not new. Holographic and interferometric technology has been used in lens design for years—on to a century.

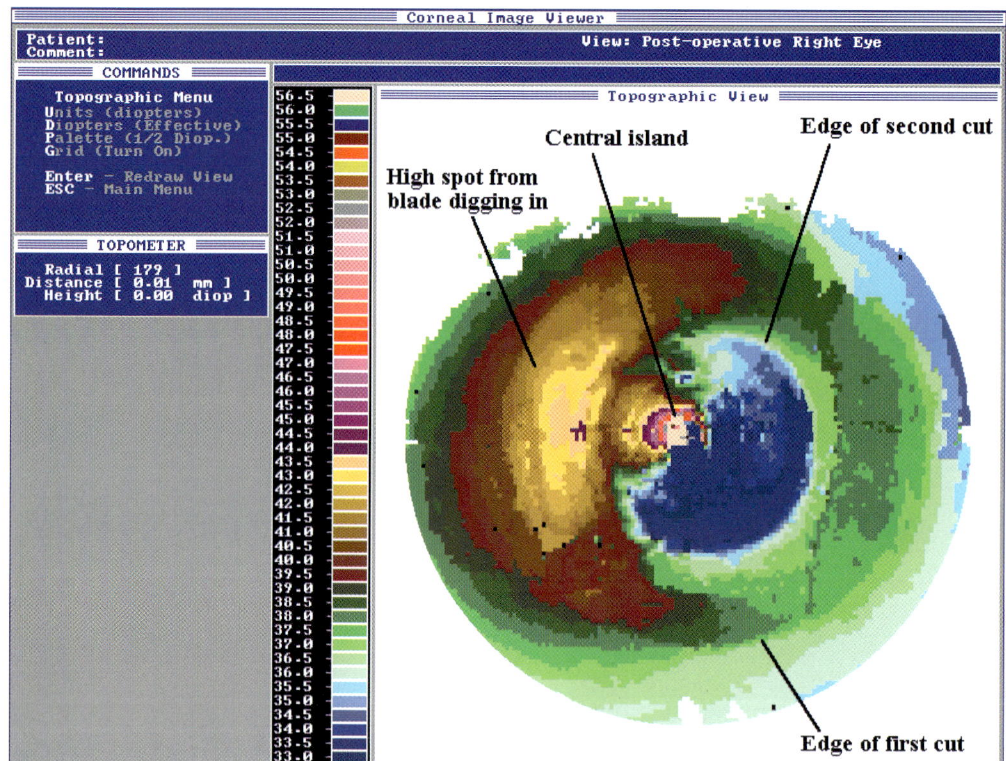

Fig. 6.43 One of the reasons ALK was abandoned. The sharp break at the margins of the second stromal cut, especially in higher myopes, produced a considerable decrease in visual efficiency. The visual aberration was exacerbated by any misalignment of the first and second cuts and by the abrupt transition at the margin of the second cut.

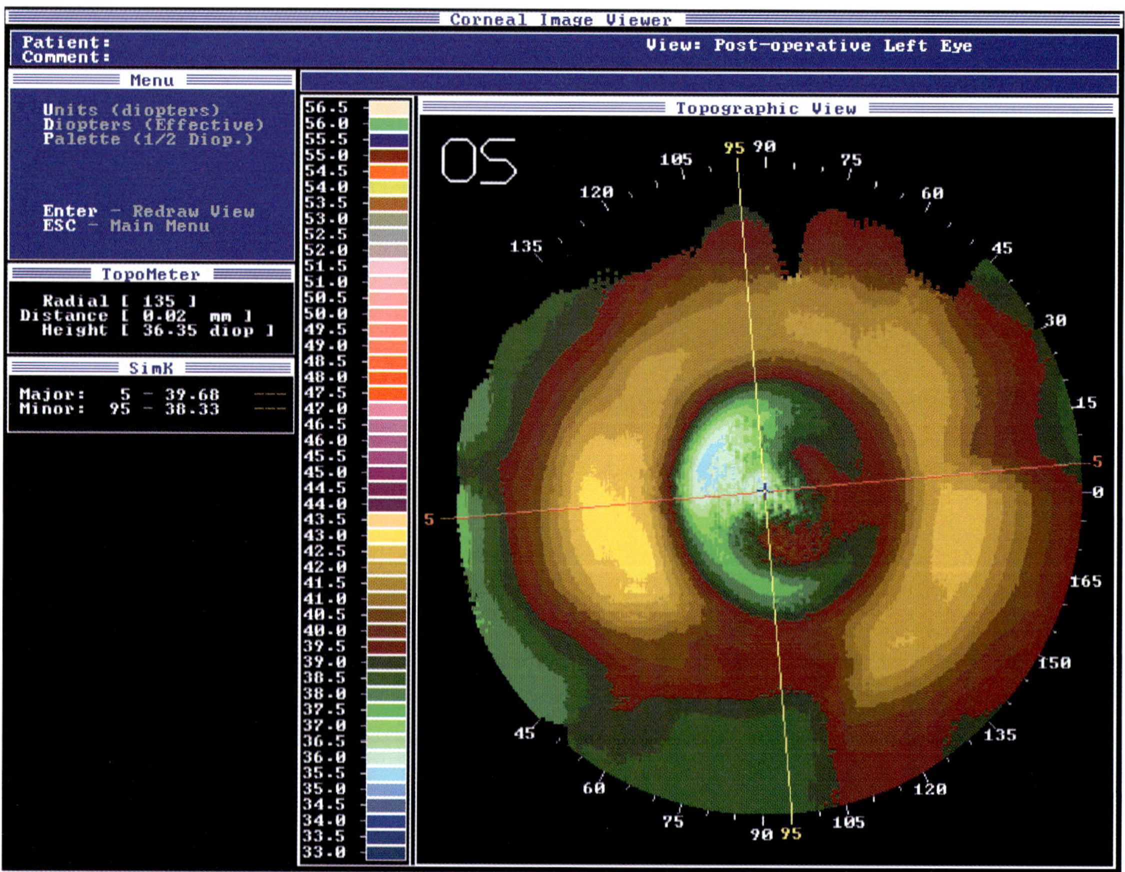

Fig. 6.44 A high-resolution rendering of a 20-week post-LASIK patient done with a Summit excimer laser. If nothing else, this map should demonstrate why precise centration of the ablation is so important.

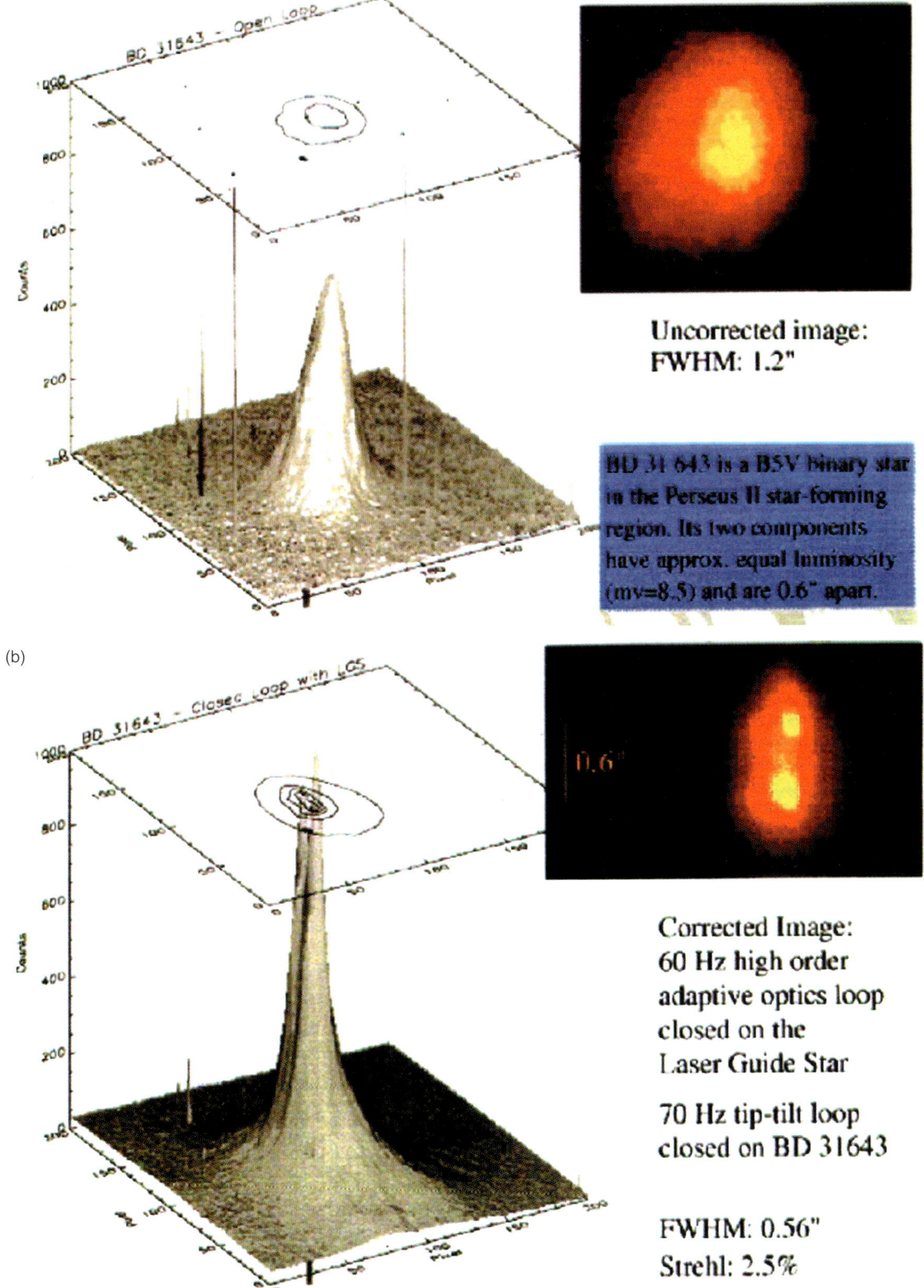

Fig. 6.45 (a) K-band photograph of BD 31,643—a binary star system whose members are of equal luminosity and 0.6 min apart. The individual stars making up this binary pair cannot be seen. (b) With adaptive optics, both stars are seen clearly separated.

How it works

Light from a nominal point source above the atmosphere enters the primary aperture and is split between a camera and a wavefront sensor. The basic strategy in adaptive optics is to collect light waves with a deformable mirror whose shape can be adjusted to compensate for distortions in an image (Figure 6.46a).

The most commonly used approach is the Shack-Hartmann method. As shown in Figure 6.46b, this approach is completely geometric in nature and so has no dependence on the coherence of the sensed optical beam. The incoming wavefront is broken into an array of spatial samples, called *subapertures* of the primary aperture, by a two-dimensional array of lenslets. The subaperture sampled by each lenslet is brought to a focus at a known distance *F* behind each array. The lateral position of the focal spot depends on the local tilt of the incoming wavefront; a measurement of all the subaperture spot positions is therefore a measure of the gradient of the incoming wavefront. A two-dimensional integration process called *reconstruction* then can be used to estimate the shape of the original wavefront and from there to derive the correction signals for the deformable mirror.

The incoming wavefront sample is analyzed into spatial subapertures by a miniature lens array that creates a pattern of spots on a two-dimensional array. The deviation of each spot from its nominal center is proportional to the input tilt at the corresponding subaperture.

The transformation from spot array to wavefront output is illustrated in Figure 6.47. The processing steps are shown clockwise from upper left: digitized spot pattern, vector representation of the spot deviations from nominal, reconstructed mirror profile, and Zernike decomposition. At center is the simple optical arrangement that makes the measurement possible.

In 1978, Professor Josef Bille, director of the Institute for Applied Physics at the University of Heidelberg, developed a system to measure wavefront distortions that occurred when light traveling through the atmosphere entered a telescopic lens. He was awarded a U.S. patent in 1986 and founded 20/10 Perfect Vision in 1999 [76]. The device produces an objective map of the ocular aberrations. Subjective information comes from real-time patient feedback. As the device shines light into the patient's eye and the mirrors correct for aberrations in the returning rays, the patient reads off the lines he or she is able to see, just as with an eye chart. The surgeon then knows if the patient's sphere, cylinder, and any aberrations are potentially correctable with surgery. Theoretically, this could help create the perfect ablation, especially for the patient with an irregular cornea.

The aberroscope

Theo Seiler and colleagues developed the Dresden wavefront analyzer based on Tscherning's aberroscope [77,78]. The system uses a frequency-doubled Nd:YAG laser emitting at a wavelength of 532 nm and a mask system for creating 128 equidistant and parallel light rays, which are projected through the cornea (Figure 6.48a). Via optical imaging, the system focuses these rays onto the retina. A computerized low-light CCD camera then uses indirect ophthalmoscopy to measure the deviation of the spots as they appear on the retina (Figure 6.48b-e). The system reconstructs the wavefront using Zernike polynomials (Figure 6.49).

Why wavefront?

The correction of higher-order aberrations can increase our ability to see "out," thereby offering the possibility of increased visual acuity, perhaps beyond the typical limit of 20/15. In theory, diffraction-limited optical cutoffs for 3- and 8-mm pupils would be high enough to yield retinal images of letter targets as small as 20/6.7 and 20/2.5, respectively. To illustrate what the retinal image would be like with supernormal optics, imagine yourself viewing the Statue of Liberty at a distance of 3 km from a boat in the New York Harbor. At this distance, the statue subtends almost 0.9°, which is equivalent to that of a U.S. quarter at 5 ft away. Under optimal viewing conditions and 20/15 vision (i.e., a normal 3-mm pupil), your retinal image of the statue would look like Figure 6.50a. If you view the statue through adaptive optics, programmed to fully correct all ocular aberrations across your 3-mm pupil, then the retinal image of the statue would look like Figure 6.50b. Notice the finer detail and higher contrast in the retinal image when the eye's aberrations are corrected. This illustrates that retinal image quality can be noticeably increased even for pupil sizes as small as 3 mm. Maximum retinal image quality can be obtained with the largest physiologic pupil diameter (8 mm) and full correction of all ocular aberrations. This situation is depicted in Figure 6.50c, which shows that the theoretical maximum optical bandwidth that can be achieved with the human eye is six times greater than the optical cutoff of a normal eye with a 3-mm pupil (i.e., 20/2.5 versus 20/15).

Improving the quality of the retinal image is an important first step toward achieving supernormal visual acuity, but it may not be sufficient. This is so because when optical limitations have been removed, visual performance now becomes constrained by neural factors. Specifically, the spacing between retinal photoreceptors represents a neural limitation to visual resolution that is only slightly higher than the normal optical limit. Consequently, increasing the quality of the retinal image probably will not yield a major increase in resolution acuity, although it could have a large impact on detection acuity.

Improving vision in one way may degrade it in others, however. In fact, the system improves resolution so well that the retina's mosaic arrangement of photoreceptors ultimately gets in the way. Given a dramatic increase in

(a)

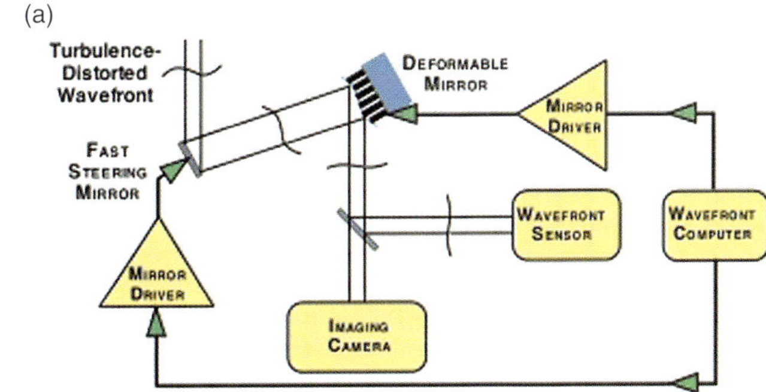

(b)

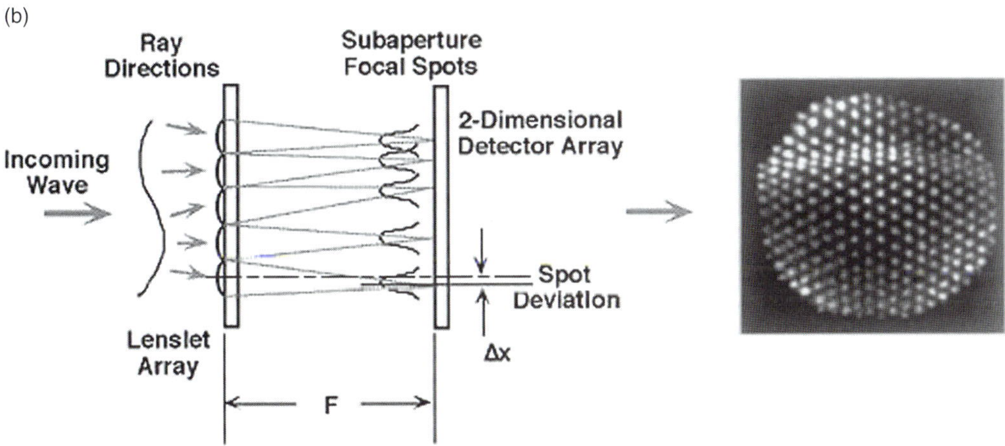

Fig. 6.46 (a) Schema of an adaptive optics system. (b) Schema of a Shack-Hartmann system.

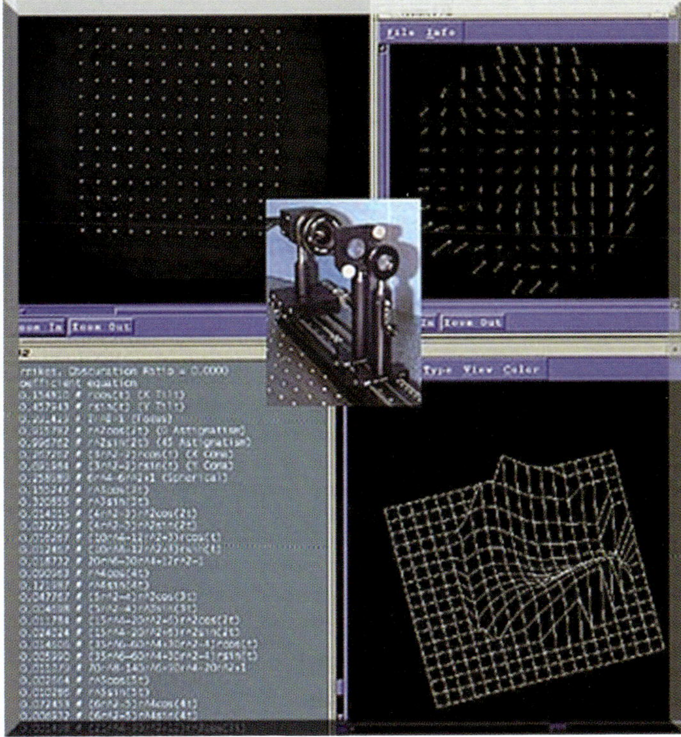

Fig. 6.47 The transformation from spot array to wavefront output processing steps are shown clockwise from upper left: digitized spot pattern, vector representation of the spot deviations from nominal, reconstructed mirror profile, and Zernike decomposition. At center is the simple optical arrangement that makes the measurement possible.

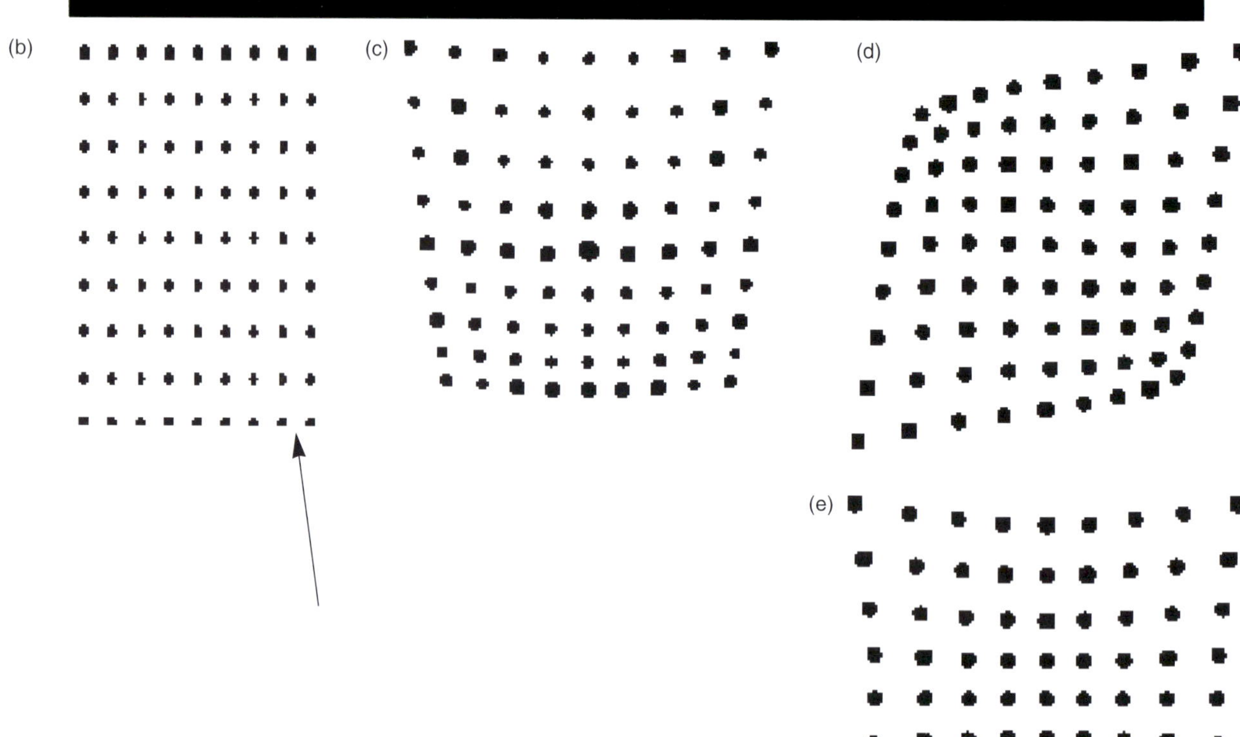

Fig. 6.48 (a) Schema of an aberroscope using a frequency-doubled Nd:YAG laser and a mask system for creating 128 equidistant and parallel light rays, which are projected through the cornea. (b) Astigmatism in a singly aberrated system. (c) Coma in a singly aberrated system. (d) Tilt in a singly aberrated system. (e) Higher-order astigmatism sometimes called *pincushion distortion*.

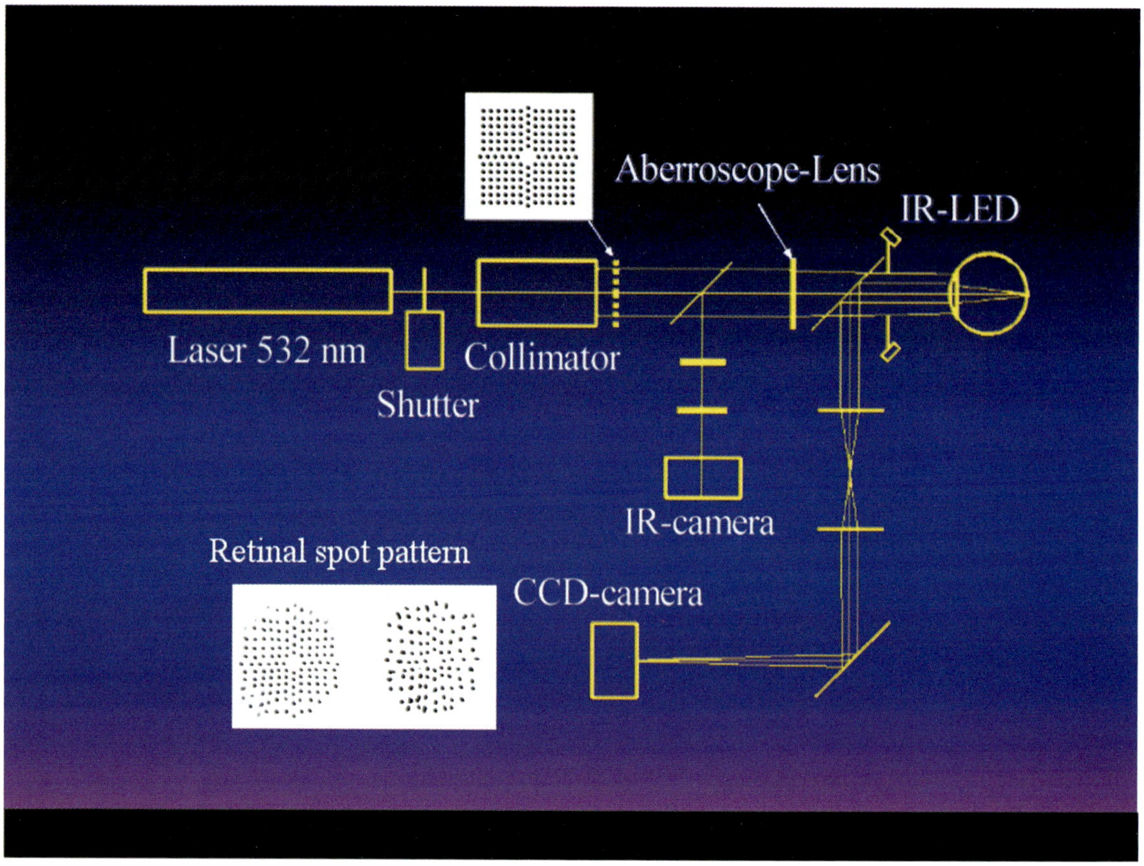

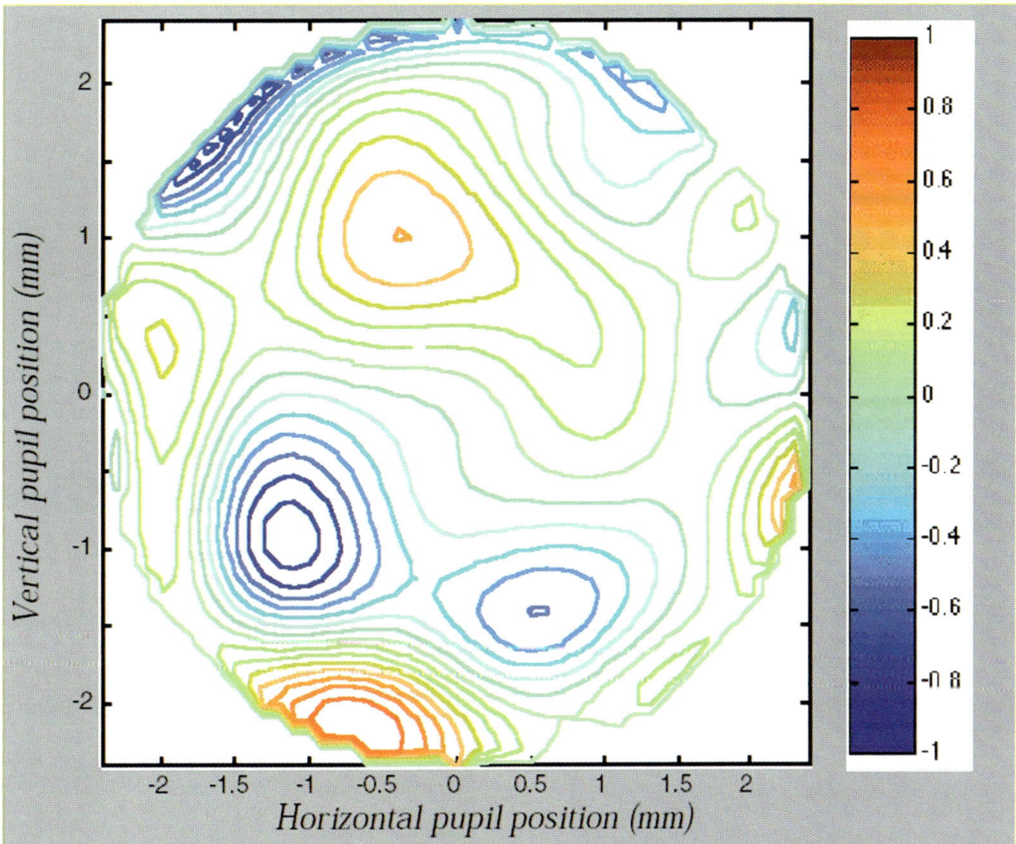

Fig. 6.49 Wavefront using Zernike polynomials derived from aberroscope data.

optical quality of the retinal image, the photoreceptor mosaic will appear relatively coarse by comparison, as shown in Figure 6.51. As a result of this mismatch, very fine spatial details in the retinal image will be smaller than the distance between neighboring cones and therefore will not be registered properly in the neural image. This misrepresentation of the image due to neural undersampling by a relatively coarse array of photoreceptors is called *aliasing*. For example, when volunteers looked at tiny points of red light that had a wavelength of 633 nm, the color sometimes appeared green—depending on which type of cone cell the beam happened to hit. The perceived color of an object normally arises from the stimulation of a large patch of cone cells, but in the experiment, the point of light seemed to fluctuate between colors [79].

However, for everyday vision, the penalty of aliasing is likely outweighed by the reward of higher contrast sensitivity and higher detection acuity. Therefore, one anticipates that correcting the eye's optical aberrations will yield a net increase in the quality of the patient's visual experience and therefore is worth pursuing. Indeed, preliminary observations indicate that stimuli seen through adaptive optics have a strikingly crisp appearance expected of an eye with supernormal optical quality, which is consistent with the sixfold increase in contrast sensitivity the author has measured experimentally.

Beyond wavefront

Wavefront technology can determine exactly what final corneal shape would produce an eye with 20/10 vision. Yet there is much yet to be learned about the basic biological mechanisms of LASIK surgery and its effect on the cornea before we can accurately achieve this change in the shape of the cornea.

Surface topography only provides a graphic depiction of the presence and location of corneal irregularities, not their underlying anatomic basis. Corneal thickness measurement by conventional pachymetric methods before and after refractive surgery correlates poorly with the intended amount of tissue removal because changes occur in the epithelial and stromal layers during healing. The variability and relative imprecision of microkeratome cuts make truly precise prediction of flap thickness impossible and produce an unpredictable final depth of keratectomy (and of residual stromal thickness) that may affect biomechanics.

The epithelium appears to possess the ability to remodel itself to compensate for stromal surface abnormalities caused by either flap irregularity or irregular stromal resection. This was one of the contributing factors in regressions seen after PRK [80]. A cornea with asymmetrical astigmatism thus possesses an irregular epithe-

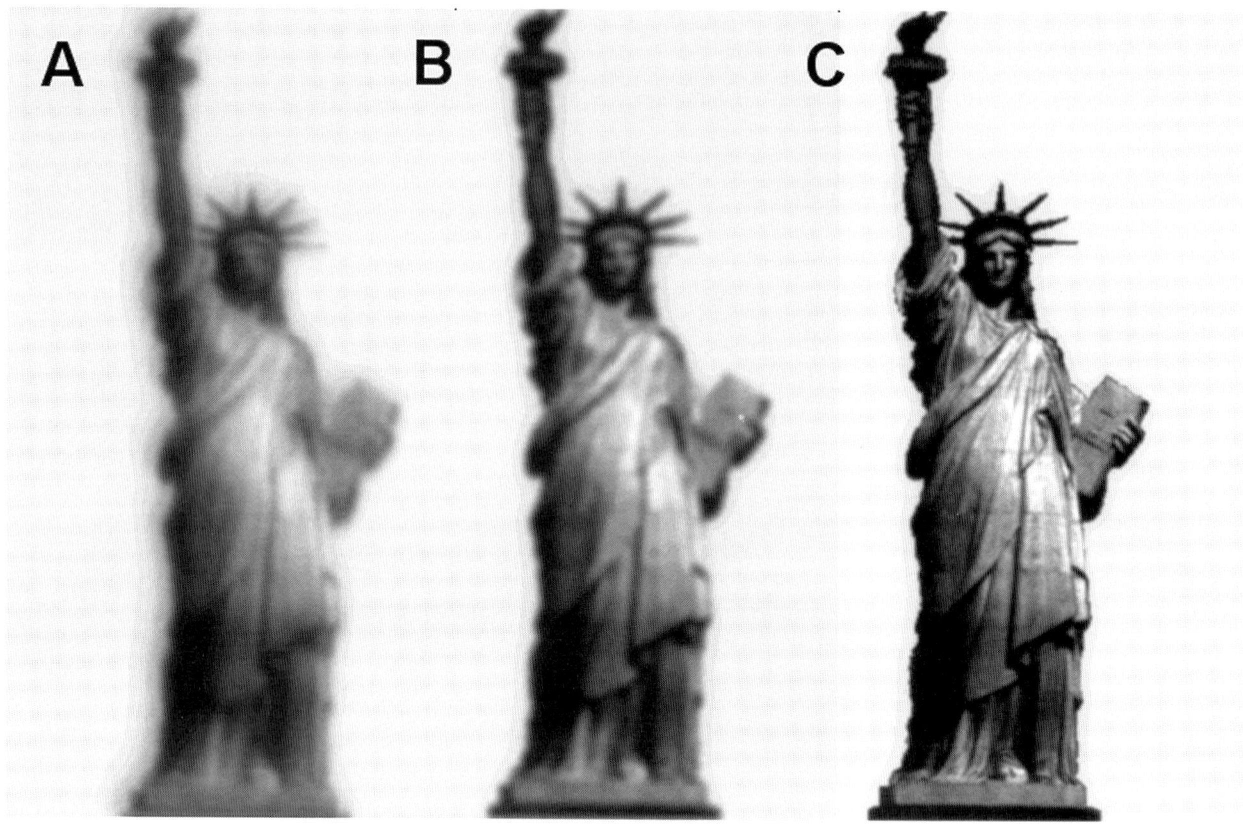

Fig. 6.50 The Statue of Liberty at a distance of 3 km from a boat in New York Harbor. At this distance the statue subtends almost 0.9°, which is equivalent to that of a U.S. quarter at 5 ft away. An individual with 20/15 best-corrected visual acuity would see the statue as in (a); correcting the aberrations across a 3-mm pupil theoretically results in a best-corrected visual acuity as in (b); and fully correcting across an 8-mm pupil results in (c).

lial thickness profile. Some compensation will mask the anatomic irregularities and cause miscalculation from topographic and wavefront measurements currently used to plan customized surgery.

Wavefront measurement may address none of these. It is still unclear whether the wavefront map will pick up a keratoconus suspect, for example.

Reinstein has been working with a digital very high frequency ultrasound system. By using digital signal processing, he is able to clearly resolve the epithelial layer from the stroma and the LASIK flap from the residual stromal bed in three dimensions [81,82]. Epithelial and biomechanical factors together could help to explain the inaccuracy of current LASIK [83].

Quoting Reinstein, professor of ophthalmology at the University of Paris:

> Wavefront gives us an enormous amount of information about the optical aberrations in the eye but no information about the corneal anatomy. . . . We're unable to accurately put the lower-order aberrations—known as sphere and cylinder—on the finish line, and that's only two numbers. How could we expect that adding another 10 Zernike coefficients would help? Only 60% to 70% of low myopes are 20/20, not because of extraneous ocular aberrations, but because there are epithelial and biomechanical changes in LASIK that we are not measuring and, therefore,

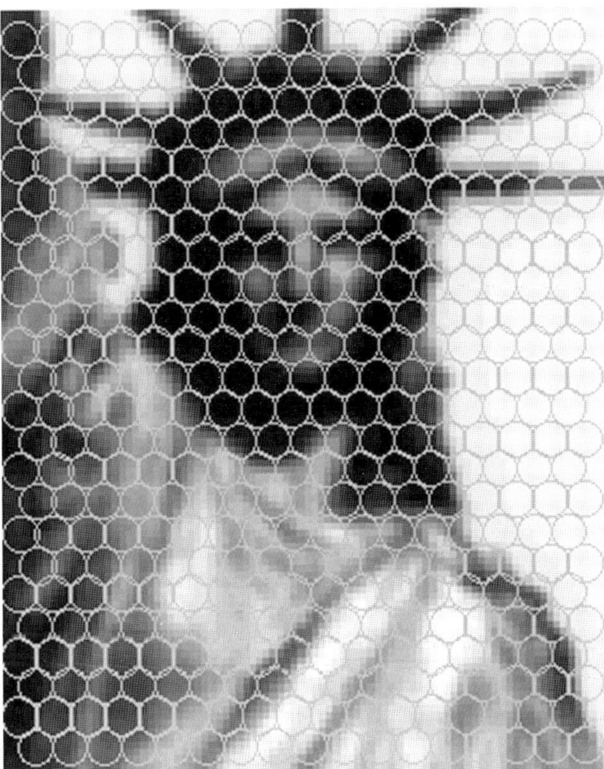

Fig. 6.51 With a dramatic increase in optical quality of the retinal image, the photoreceptor mosaic will appear relatively coarse by comparison. As a result of this mismatch, very fine spatial details in the retinal image will be smaller than the distance between neighboring cones and therefore will not be registered properly in the neural image. This misrepresentation of the image due to neural undersampling by a relatively coarse array of photoreceptors is called *aliasing*.

not controlling for. We have failed to ask some fundamental questions about the stability of refraction in an eye. About 15% of the refractive-cutting effect of the laser can be lost by this bulging after LASIK [84].

Biomechanical properties of the eye

Still less is known about the internal structural, *constitutive properties* of the cornea than is understood of its surface. The ultrastructure of the cornea has been detailed in many publications [85–87] (see also above). However, the mechanical role of these elements has not been established conclusively. Moreover, morphologic examination of corneal wound healing has not included extensive quantitation of this process and has shed little light on constituent properties [88–92]. The tools for measuring these processes are available, however, and have been used in other medical specialties, such as, in orthopedics to evaluate the requirements for prosthetic devices [93,94]. While some of the methods employed in this work are not suited for use with soft tissue, such as the cornea, the underlying process certainly can be applied in ophthalmology [95]. These methods, relying as they do on proven techniques of hypothesis, experimentation, and comparison of data to hypothetical models, yield quantitative data in distinction to the morphologic, qualitative measurements more commonly employed in ophthalmology today.

Whether any one of us means to or not, as ophthalmologists, we are taking into account biomechanical properties of the eye on a daily basis. Historically, tonometry is an example that first comes to mind [96–100]. As a matter of fact, Friedenwald dealt with the "rigidity" of the cornea when he established his coefficients [101]. Constitutive properties have been linked, albeit loosely, to parameters of age, sex, and medical health. Fyodorov and Bores, in their earlier work, have emphasized the importance of a rigidity factor in predicting the outcome of RK [102–104]. Others have attempted to account for the same elements by factoring in age, intraocular pressure, and/or sex in various ways [105,106].

In a system as complex as the human cornea, it is not surprising that although a number of closed mathematical models have been proposed for the prediction of various procedures on the cornea, their reliability has been limited by the complexity of the corneal structure, especially the limbus [96,107–109]. A different approach is the so-called iterative or open solution, in which a complex structure is broken into many small simpler components or *finite elements*. Here, the cornea is assumed to be a structure that conforms in a predictable way to accepted laws of physics in response to applied forces. Such a model, however, requires foreknowledge of the geometry of the cornea and supporting tissue along with the material properties of the constituent soft tissues making up the eye. An analogy would be a wall constructed of bricks—said bricks being the small bits or elements constituting the wall. We can say something about the wall by knowing something about the bricks. Besides, it is easier to handle and test one brick than the entire wall. As can be seen, the number of such elements could be quite large. In a typical corneal model, for example, there will be as few as 300 elements, although there are usually many times that number. Each of the elements (bricks) has nodes at each corner and at each midpoint (Figure 6.52a, b). It is at these nodes that each brick is attached to another. In the model, each of these nodes is conceived as being perfectly joined, forming a continuum—each element deforming in synchrony to every other element. Within each separate element, a simple displacement field is assumed, and the continuity of these fields is enforced rigorously within the polynomial interpolation.

Interest in refractive corneal surgery, particularly RK, has resulted in several published mechanical models of

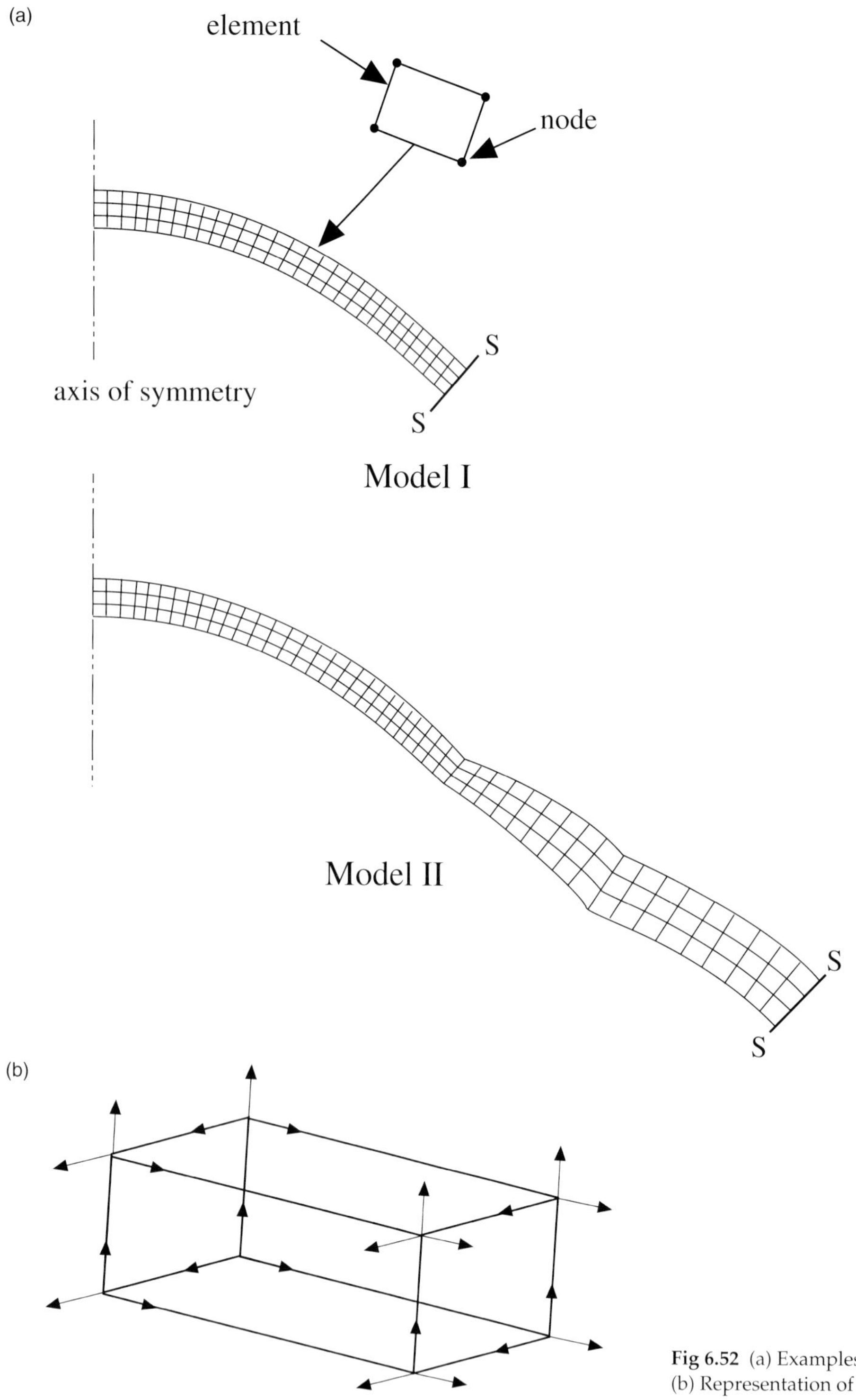

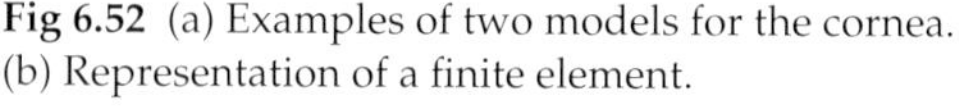

Fig 6.52 (a) Examples of two models for the cornea. (b) Representation of a finite element.

the cornea that attempt to simulate the effects of this surgery [110–112]. Many of these use the finite-element method primarily because this approach holds promise for systematically dealing with the complexities of modeling corneal surgery [113]. The predictions of even relatively simple finite-element models are in qualitative agreement with certain observations on patients when surgical parameters, such as incision length and depth, are varied [114,115]. Unfortunately, the assumptions inherent in biomechanical modeling of the cornea have not been tied rigorously to experimental observation—clearly, the key to the use of such models by refractive surgeons for quantitative rather than qualitative purposes. There are, nonetheless, caveats in a too-rigorous acceptance of such data because of certain shortcomings of method.

Constitutive properties

Structural engineering often concerns itself with "mob action." That is, it is more concerned with "macro" than with "micro" elements, even though it may deal with finite elements of minute order—hence the oft-repeated concept of a *continuum*. Thus a steel beam is a continuum of iron atoms admixed with a few carbon, cobalt, and boron atoms for flavor. This continuum will exhibit certain characteristics apart from the fundamental properties of the constituent atoms. So too the cornea. While its fundamental microstructure is important, the individual collagen fibrils and their matrix are lost within the crowd, and their individuality is lost as well. Consequently, the characteristics of the collagen molecules per se need not be considered to obtain useful information about the structure—as any mob psychologist can attest.

The characteristics of the continuum in question will be modified to some extent by the *homogeneity* of that continuum. Steel and aluminum—even concrete—are homogeneous materials, and it is relatively easy to predict their behavior. Nonhomogeneous materials, on the other hand, are not. For example, when studying the universe, astrophysicists note certain aberrations in their calculations when matter is present in greater density in one spot than elsewhere. It is still possible, nonetheless, to make some generalizations about the universe that can explain some observed phenomena. Since the universe is distinctly inhomogeneous, so too is most biologic tissue.

Biologic tissue may be homogeneous in certain areas, however. The scleral coat of the eye is relatively so, but the cornea is not. The cornea is really a composite layered material made up of collagen fibrils and ground substance. Each of these distinct layers (Bowman's, anterior and posterior stroma, and Descemet's) is homogeneous in its own venue, but taken together, they are not. This, of course, complicates the study of corneal biomechanics because all the methods employed to model structures assume homogeneity of that structure in order to produce meaningful results. Thus some average microstructure is assumed.

In general, measurement of gross material properties in substances such as the cornea, with significant internal structure, results in some error. A better approach involves measurement of the more homogeneous subcomponents of the material—in the cornea, the properties of collagen and ground material. Ideally, the material properties of collagen would be measured on a single collagen fibril, and likewise, the ground substance would be measured in a small, well-defined shape. Measurement of noncorneal collagen material properties (e.g., in rat tail tendon) will give approximate values for collagen, but these may be contaminated by differences in tertiary collagen structure and in ground substance [116]. Nevertheless, it is a place to start.

Making sense of biomechanical modeling

While it is possible to model aspects of corneal behavior based on our knowledge of certain corneal properties, some observations and cautions regarding these computer models are in order:

- *Do not generalize from the results of modeling*. Unfortunately, many authors do just this. They assume that since their modeling matches *some* clinical observations—*ergo sum*—their modeling must be correct. This is a dangerous assumption to make. It leads to the equally erroneous conclusion that since certain clinical observations are not supported by the model, such observations are wrong. I would like to point out the only "universal truth" of refractive surgery: Eye—12; Theory—0. This is to say that the eye has defied and confounded theorists successfully for years. This has been evident from the outset, especially as regards refractive surgery. Hence the second observation is
- *Credit clinical observations before theoretical notions*. One of the assumptions made in modeling is that shear effects are minimal in the cornea. This is patently not the case, as evidenced by the internal corneal folds described by Bores, Fyodorov, and Seiler, as well as others [117,118].

With all the new technologies being brought to bear on the subject, it looks like the dawn of a new day in refractive surgery to me.

Validation of corneal topography devices

After all the preceding discussion regarding the methods for the computerized reconstruction of the corneal surface from various automated approaches, it is essential to mention the importance of validating instruments. Validation of corneal topography analysis systems is slow in appearing primarily because the best data are gathered by independent research laboratories, and the publication process is lengthy by nature. Such a demonstration must include not only precision spherical surfaces but also aspherical surfaces such as done by Wang [119,120].

Assessing and describing the accuracy of corneal topographers present a set of problems not previously encountered in keratometry. One of the major difficulties encountered is that current corneal topography analysis instruments have the potential to be more accurate than traditional methods used for the production of accurately defined aspherical surfaces—particularly holographic systems. This has the potential to confound certification studies. In the past, irregularities of these surfaces have not been a problem because the instruments that they were intended to calibrate lacked the sensitivity to detect many imperfections or alert one to inaccuracies. Where the concern was for an approximate average, as is the case in keratometry, relatively small irregularities of the calibrating balls were of little importance.

Clinicians tend to compare a new instrument with an old one with which they are familiar, but in the case of corneal topographers, such a comparison might be like checking the measurements of a micrometer with those of a common wooden yardstick. Perhaps the validation of corneal topography instruments for the purposes of Food and Drug Administration acceptance, as with clinician acceptance, should be judged on the basis of accuracy in permitting diagnosis of clinical shape anomalies.

"Keratospeak"—The vocabulary of corneal topography

Confronted with shapes and colors reminiscent of Cézanne or Kandinsky, the refractive surgeon is also forced to cope with a new vocabulary—a "technobabble" unique to this emerging field or, as Waring phrased it, "keratospeak" [121,122]. It is confusing enough to try to equate data gathered on different devices or even to try to understand what each one does—if anything—without compounding the problem by having terms employed of which no two are used the same way nor whose meaning can always be agreed upon. This form of technical obscurantism serves no useful purpose. In an effort to shed some light into this dark medical corner, the author presents this section on the vocabulary of the corneal surface. Some of these definitions are covered in greater detail in Chapter 3.

Curvature

Curvature is an expression of the rate of change of the degree a given point on a line deviates from a straight line. Actually, it is the rate of change of the rate of change. Since the second part is derived from the first, curvature is the *second derivative* of the deviation. A *perfect circle* is perfect because each point deviates the same degree, and the rate of change is constant. A solid representation of such a circle would be a *sphere*. Any curvature that deviates from a perfect circle would be an *ellipsoid*. A solid representation of such an ellipsoid would not be spherical—it would be an *asphere* (see also Chapter 3).

Aberroscope

This device measures the spatial refraction of an optical system, such as the eye, and thereby can tell the spherocylindrical refraction and optical aberrations of the system.

Adaptive optics

Wavefront systems using adaptive optics feature a flexible membrane mirror, on the back of which electrodes are mounted. When a wavefront, distorted by the patient's optical system, emerges from the eye, it hits this mirror. The electrodes move the mirror in order to adjust the wavefront back into perfect alignment.

Higher-order aberrations

When a light ray enters the eye, it can be bent and distorted by the optical system before it strikes the retina. Higher-order aberrations include irregularities of the anterior and posterior corneal surfaces, lenticular changes, and retinal imperfections.

Wavefront

A beam of light is commonly thought of as a bundle of light rays. These rays are perpendicular to the normally bowl-shaped wavefront. The concept of a wavefront can be understood easily by picturing ocean waves approaching the shore. The direction in which each part of the wave is moving is analogous to a light ray. The crest, or trough, of the wave is the wavefront. Light travels in a procession of wavefronts, or flat sheets. A wavefront is an isochronic surface, meaning it is of equal time.

After light has left a point source, the rays must converge simultaneously on the retina to form a perfect image. Wavefront sensing is a new way of mapping the spatial refraction (spherocylindrical error) and aberration profile (spherical aberrations, coma aberrations, higher-order astigmatic aberrations, and more) of the eye.

Seidel aberrations

The Seidel aberrations were developed in the mid-19th century to account for the monochromatic geometric aberrations of *centered optical systems*, that is, defects from perfect imagery in optical systems that have an optical axis. The magnitude of the aberrations is expressed in terms of an aberration polynomial.

The types of aberrations can be developed from considerations of symmetry and are given names such as *spherical aberration, coma, astigmatism, field curvature,* and *distortion* [123]. In addition to their type, aberrations usually are specified according to their order (third-order, fifth-order, etc.), although sometimes they are called *primary, secondary,* etc. Higher-order aberrations introduce new types. For example, fifth-order aberrations add the types *oblique spherical aberration* and *elliptical coma*. Seidels are rarely used to describe the corneal surface.

Zernike polynomials

The Zernike polynomials were introduced by Fritz Zernike in the early 20th century and later developed to describe the properties of an aberrated wavefront [124]. Like the Seidel aberration polynomial, Zernike polynomials describe defects from perfect imagery, but the nature of the Zernike expansion is different from the Seidel expansion. Zernike polynomials describe the properties of an aberrated wavefront *without regard to the symmetry* properties of the system that gave rise to the wavefront. Today, they have a use in representing aspheric surfaces (either refractive or diffractive), particularly in systems that produce higher-order aberrations [125].

Petzval's surface

This is the curved image plane that is formed when astigmatism is eliminated (see also Chapter 3).

Coma

Coma is a form of astigmatism caused by a displacement of an optical surface so that its center is no longer aligned on the optic axis (see Figure 6.30a, b).

Tilt

Tilt is a form of astigmatism caused by a rotation of the plane of an optical surface so that it is no longer perpendicular to the optic axis (see Figure 6.31a, b).

Keratometer (ophthalmometer)

A Keratometer should more rightly be called an *ophthalmometer,* a term coined by Helmholtz in 1852 for his device that measured the central corneal curvature [126]. Keratometer, unfortunately, is a trade name owned by the Bausch and Lomb Company, but it has, like Xerox and Kleenex, entered the common lexicon and hence is used synonymously (if incorrectly) with ophthalmometer. The act of measuring the corneal curvature can be rightly termed either *keratometry* or *ophthalmometry* without fear of trade name infringement.

Radius of curvature and refractive power of the cornea

The radius of curvature of the anterior and posterior corneal surfaces affects the cornea's refractive power. A shorter radius of curvature creates a steeper arc and greater refractive power. Conversely, a longer radius of curvature creates a flatter arc and less refractive power. The image formed by light reflected from the convex anterior corneal surface is called the *first Purkinje image,* the *corneal light reflex,* or the *corneal light reflection.* This virtual, first-order, erect image is viewed during keratometry and keratoscopy and is located approximately 4 mm posterior to the surface of the cornea at the level of the anterior lens capsule.

Keratoscope

Fortunately, no one has trademarked the term *keratoscope,* which describes an instrument that projects a series of mires, most commonly rings, onto the corneal surface; all are based on Placido's original idea [57]. Keratoscopes fitted with a still-film camera are called *photokeratoscopes;* those fitted with a video camera are called *videokeratoscopes.* The term *Corneoscope* is the trade name owned by the Kera Corporation but seems headed in the same direction as Keratometer.

Keratoscopy

Direct observation of the images of mires reflected from the surface of the cornea is termed *keratoscopy,* in the same sense that examination of the ocular fundus with an ophthalmoscope is termed *ophthalmoscopy.*

Keratography

The term *keratography* denotes a record or portrayal of the cornea in the same sense that angiography records the pattern of vessels—the Greek word γραφειν (*graphein*) means "to write." Currently, there are four methods of recording pictures (keratographs) of the mires reflected from the corneal surface:

1 With photographic film, one uses a photokeratoscope to produce a photokeratograph, a process called *photokeratography* (in the same sense that one uses a photomicroscope to take a photomicrograph).

2 With video recording, one uses a videokeratoscope to produce a videokeratograph, a process called *videokeratography.*

3 Via electronic capture using a video camera and a device called a *frame grabber.*

4 With CCD (charge-coupled device) arrays that consist of tiny photoreceptors that send signals directly into a computer.

A keratograph can be interpreted qualitatively or quantitatively. A qualitative interpretation is done by visual inspection of the shape and spacing of the mires and has considerable practical value in qualitatively diagnosing corneal disorders such as keratoconus or in adjusting sutures after penetrating keratoplasty. Quantitative keratography is attempted by assigning numerical coordinate values to points on the mires and describing mathematically the curves that the points form. Complex formulas and algorithms are required for accurate quantitation of the surface topography.

Topography

Topography is the science of accurate and detailed descriptions of surface features whether they are of the

Earth, the Moon, or even the eye. The most common representation is a topographic map on which the relative elevations of the surface are delimited by contour lines. The term *topology* is often used to describe the study of such surfaces—typically in mathematical terms. Either word is correct, but within this book, I will use the more common one—*topography*.

Topographic displays

The mires used to study corneal shape have many configurations: circles, arcs, parallel lines, interference fringes, steps, etc. Those most commonly used are circular rings, as in keratoscopes. The concentric ring mires are commonly called *Placido's rings,* but strictly speaking, this designation should describe only Placido's flat disk with the equally spaced circular white rings. Modern keratoscope rings are designed differently. By convention, the rings are numbered from innermost to outermost. This can be confusing, because a specific ring (e.g., ring 3) in different instruments may cover a different location on different corneas. Therefore, it is important to designate the diameter of a projected ring and indicate the area on the cornea that it covers. There are four basic methods of displaying corneal topographic information:

1 The keratograph

2 Representation of the radius of curvature or dioptric power at various locations on the surface of the cornea, either in a fixed pattern on a faceplate or at any location identified by a cursor in a computer-assisted videokeratoscope

3 Graphic 3D figures often with exaggerations to show changes in curvature

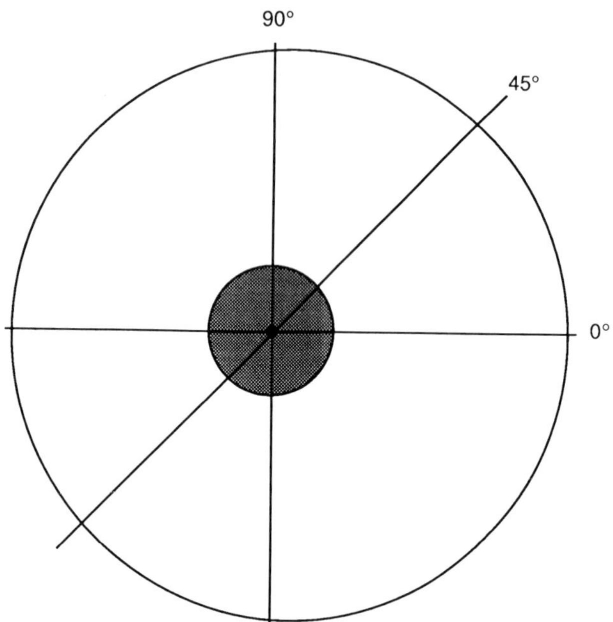

Fig 6.53 Corneal meridians.

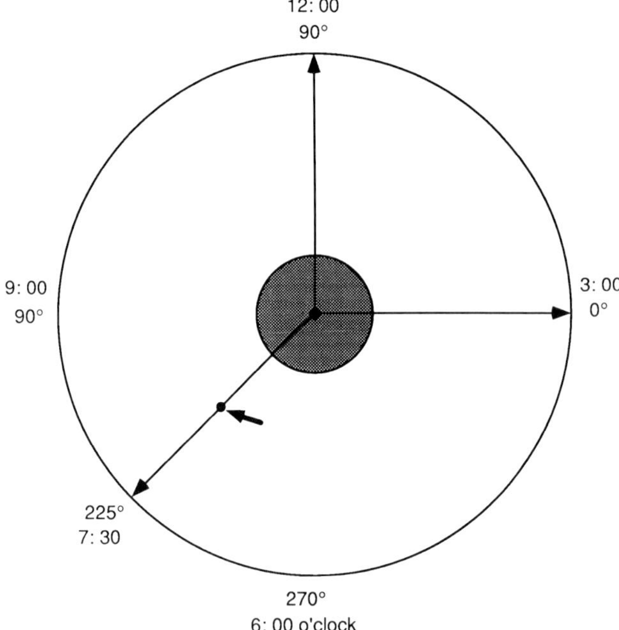

Fig 6.54 Corneal semimeridians.

4 Color-coded maps using colors to designate areas of uniform radius of curvature and refractive power

The most widely used system of color coding is reds and oranges (warm colors) to indicate steeper areas with greater refractive power and greens and blues (cool colors) to indicate flatter areas with less refractive power [67,72,127]. A quantitative scale indicates the values corresponding to each color.

Optical axis

Theoretically, this is the apex of an optical surface around which point all optical elements rotate symmetrically. I have mentioned a visual axis as if all the optical components of the eye were somehow symmetrically aligned along a common axis. Strictly speaking, such a condition does not exist. In fact, the best-derived optic axis that can be conceived—assuming such an alignment—does not strike the center of vision, the fovea, at all!

Meridians, semimeridians, and axes

Locations on the surface of the cornea are designated along *meridians*, lines that span the diameter of the cornea from one point on the limbus to the opposite point and which have a common center. Meridians are designated from 0° to 180°, proceeding counterclockwise starting at 3 o'clock for both the right and left eyes (Figure 6.53). The term *axis* designates the direction in a cylindrical lens along which there is no power. Because clinicians align the axes of cylindrical lenses with meridians on the cornea, it is common practice to substitute the term *axis* for *meridian* when referring to directions on the cornea. Thus clinicians commonly refer to the "steep axis" of a cornea when they really mean *steep meridian*, an unfortunate habit that is unlikely to ever change. Thus, when clinicians refer to the "steep axis" or the "flat axis" of the cornea, the term *axis* is used incorrectly; the term *meridian* should be used when referring to the direction of corneal refractive power and *axis* when referring to spectacle power.

Designating meridians as 0° to 180° is conventional, but unlike geographers, ophthalmologists have no north-south longitude lines to indicate a point along a meridian. Thus, if one refers to removing a tight corneal suture in the 90° meridian, it is not clear whether the activity occurs in the 12 o'clock direction or in the 6 o'clock direction. Therefore, directions from the center of the cornea are designated as *semimeridians* and are located around the 360° circumference of the cornea in degrees, such as "the 225° semimeridian" (Figure 6.54). The term *semimeridian* is preferred, since both components are derived from Latin.

A specific point on the surface of the cornea is designated by indicating its location in millimeters from the center of the cornea along a semimeridian. For example: "at 3 mm from the center (6.0-mm zone) along the 225° semimeridian, the corneal power may be 41.00 D." The location of a transverse incision could be described as follows: "It was placed 3 mm from the center (i.e., at the 6-mm zone), perpendicular to the 225° semimeridian," or better: "It was centered on the 225° semimeridian, transverse to a 6-mm zone."

References

1 Helmholtz H. *Treatise on Physiological Optics.* JPC Southall, Editor, Opt Soc Amer, New York, p. 211, 1924.
2 Maguire LJ. and Bourne WM. Corneal topography of early keratoconus [see comments]. Am J Ophthalmol 1989; 108 (2): p. 107–12.
3 McDonnell PJ, Garbus J, and Lopez PF. Topographic analysis and visual acuity after radial keratotomy [see comments]. Am J Ophthalmol 1988; 106(6): p. 692–95.
4 McDonnell PJ, McClusky DJ, and Garbus JJ. Corneal topography and fluctuating visual acuity after radial keratotomy. Ophthalmology 1989; 96(5): p. 665–70.
5 Rowsey JJ, Balyeat HD, Monlux R, *et al.* Prospective evaluation of radial keratotomy: Photokeratoscope corneal topography. Ophthalmology 1988; 95(3): p. 322–34.
6 Santos VR, Waring GO, Lynn MJ, *et al.* Relationship between refractive error and visual acuity in the Prospective Evaluation of Radial Keratotomy (PERK) Study. Arch Ophthalmol 1987; 105(1): p. 86–92.
7 Maguire LJ. and Lowry JC. Identifying progression of subclinical keratoconus by serial topography analysis. Am J Ophthalmol 1991; 112: p. 41–5.
8 Miller D. and Carter J. A proposed new division of corneal functions. In: *The Cornea. Transactions of the World Congress on the Cornea III.* Raven Press, New York, 1980.
9 Mandell RB. and Helen RS. Stability of the corneal contour. Am J Optom Arch Am Acad Optom 1968; 45(12): p. 797–806.
10 Mandell RB. *Contact Lens Practice: Corneal Topography. 3rd ed.* Charles C Thomas, Springfield, 62–3, 1984.
11 Clark B. Mean topography of normal corneas. Aust J Optom 1974; 57: p. 107–14.
12 Clark B. Topography of some individual corneas. Aust J Optom 1974; 57: p. 65–9.
13 Ludlam W. Photographic analysis of the ocular dioptric components: Part 3. Am J Optom Arch Am Acad Optom 1967; 44: p. 276–96.
14 Dingeldein SA. and Klyce SD. Imaging of the cornea. Cornea 1988; 7(3): p. 170–82.
15 Mandell RB. Everett Kinsey Lecture. The enigma of the corneal contour. Clao J 1992; 18(4): p. 267–73.
16 Snellen H. Die Richtunge des Hauptmeridiane des Astigmatishen Auges. The axis of the major meridians of the astigmatic eye. Albrecht Von Graefes Arch Klin Ophthalmol 1869; 15: p. 199–207.
17 Tomlinson A. and Scwartz C. The position of the corneal apex in the normal eye. Am J Optom Physiol Opt 1979; 56: p. 236–40.
18 Knoll H. Corneal contours in the general population as revealed by the photokeratoscope. Am J Optom Arch Am Acad Optom 1979; 33: p. 389–97.
19 Rowsey JJ. and Schanzlin DJ. *Corneal topography, in Contact Lenses. The CLAO Guide to Basic Science and Clinical Practice,* OH Dabezies, Editor. Grune & Stratton, Orlando, p. 411–6, 1984.
20 Garner LF, Owens H, Yap MK, *et al.* Radius of curvature of the posterior surface of the cornea. Optom Vis Sci 1997; 74(7): p. 496–8.
21 Smith T. Corneal topography. Doc Ophthalmol 1977; 43(2): p. 249–76.
22 Klyce S. and Beurman R. Structure and function of the cornea. In: *The Cornea,* H Kaufman, *et al.* Editors. Churchill Livingstone, New York, p. 5–55, 1988.
23 Wilson G, Bell C, and Chotai S, The effect of lifting the lids on corneal astigmatism. Am J Optom Physiol Opt 1982; 59(8): p. 670–4.
24 Vihlen F. and Wilson G. The relationship between eyelid tension, corneal toricity and age. Invest Ophthalmol Vis Sci 1983; 24: p. 1367–73.
25 Manchester PT. Hydration of the cornea. Trans Am Ophthalmol Soc 1970; 68: p. 425.
26 Kiely PM, Carney LG, and Smith G. Menstrual cycle variations of corneal topography and thickness. Am J Optom Physiol Opt 1983; 60(10): p. 822–9.
27 Kiely PM, Carney LG, and Smith G. Diurnal variations of corneal topography and thickness. Am J Optom Physiol Opt 1982; 59(12): p. 976–82.
28 Scheiner C. *Occulus Hoc est: fundamentum opticum.* Daniel Agricolam, Innsbruck, 1619.
29 Kepler J. *Ad vitellionem paraliponema.* Claudium Marnium et HJ Aubrii, Frankfurt, 1604.
30 Kepler J. *Dioptrice.* Augustii Vindelicorum et Davidis Franci, Frankfurt, 1611.
31 Newton I. *Opticks.* Smith and Walford, London, 1704.
32 Gullstrand A. *Einfuhrung in die Methoden die Dioptrik des Auges.* S Hirzel, Leipzig, 1911.
33 Young T. On the mechanism of the eye, the Bakerian lecture. Phil Trans R Soc Lond 1801; 91: p. 23–88.
34 Boerhaave H. *Prælectiones publicæ, de morbis oculorum.* A Vandenhoeck, Göttingen, 1746.
35 Javal L. and Schiøtz H. Un ophthalmometre pratique. Annales d'Oculistique 1881; 86: p. 5–21.
36 Helmholtz HLF. *Handbuch der Physiologischen Optik. Vol. 1.* Leopold Voss, Leipzig, p. 211, 1867.

37 Kohlrausch J. Uber die messung des radius der vorderflache der hornhaut am libenden menschlichen Auge. Okens Isis Jahrg 1840; 5: p. 886.

38 Coccius A. *Ophthalmometrie und Spannungsmessung am kranken Auge. Eine Monographie.* Alexander Edelman, Leipzig, 1872.

39 Landolt E. L'ophthalmometre. In: *Congres Periodique International des Sciences Medicales.* Geneva, 1878.

40 Sutcliffe J. One position ophthalmometry. Optician and Photographic Trades Review 1907; 33(suppl): p. 8.

41 Hartinger H. Über ein Neues Ophthalmometer. Z Ophthalmol Optik 1935; 23: p. 75–95.

42 Fincham EF. The changes in the form of the crystalline lens in accommodation. Trans Opt Soc London 1925; 26: p. 239–69.

43 Berg F. Vergleichende Messungen der Form der vorderen Hornhautflache mit Ophthalmometer und mit photographischer Methode. Acta Ophthalmologica 1929; 7: p. 386–423.

44 Berg F. Bemerkungen zur theorie der ophthalmmetrischen messungen von flachen-krummungen. Acta Ophthalmologica 1929; 7: p. 225–43.

45 Mandell RB. and St Helen R. Position and curvature of the corneal apex. American Journal of Optometry 1969; 46: p. 25–9.

46 Aubert H. Näher Sich die Hornhautkrummung am meisten der Ellipse. Pfluegers Arch 1885; 35: p. 597–621.

47 Tscherning MHE. *Physiological Optics,* C Weiland, Editor. Keystone, Philadelphia, 1904.

48 Gullstrand A. Photographisch-ophthalmometrische und klinische Untersuchungen über die Hornhautrefraktion. Kongl Svenska Vetenska Akad Handl 1896; new series 28(7): p. 64.

49 Reynolds A. and Kratt H. The photoelectronic keratoscope. Contacto 1959; 3(3): p. 53–9.

50 Feldman ST, Frucht-Pery J, Weinreb RN, *et al.* The effect of increased intraocular pressure on visual acuity and corneal curvature after radial keratotomy. Am J Ophthalmol 1989; 108(2): p. 126–29.

51 MacRae S, Rich L, Phillips D, *et al.* Diurnal variation in vision after radial keratotomy. Am J Ophthalmol 1989; 107(3): p. 262–67.

52 Bores L. Pseudo-accomodation following radial keratotomy. In: *Quintum Forum.* Instituto Barraquer, Bogota, 1987.

53 Bonnett R. New method of topographical ophthalmometry, its theoretical and clinical applications. Am J Opthal 1962; 39: p. 227–51.

54 Brewster D. Comments on "On a Peculiar Defect in the Eye and a Mode of Correcting It". Edinb J Sci 1827; 7: p. 326.

55 Goode H. On a peculiar defect of vision. Trans Camb Phil Soc 1847; 8: p. 493–96.

56 Placido da Costa A. *Letter.* Centralblatt für praktische Augenheilkunde, p. 157, 1882.

57 Placido da Costa A. Novo instrumento de esploracao da cornea. Periodico d'Oftalmologica Practica 1880; 5: p. 27–30.

58 Placido da Costa A. Novo instrumento par analyse immediate des irregularida des de curvatura de cornea. Periodico d'Oftalmologica Practica 1880; 6: p. 44–9.

59 Placido da Costa A. Neue instrumente. Zbl Prakt Augenheilk 1882; 6: p. 30–1.

60 Nordensen E. Reserches ophtalmométriqes sur l'astigmatisme de la cornée chez des éscoliers de 7 a 20 ans. Ann Oculist (Paris) 1883; 88: p. 110–38.

61 Rowsey J. Ten caveats in keratorefractive surgery. Ophthalmology 1983; 90(6): p. 148.

62 Roberts C. The accuracy of 'power' maps to display curvature data in corneal topography systems. Invest Ophthalmol Vis Sci 1994; 35(9): p. 3525–32.

63 Roberts C. Characterization of the inherent error in a spherically-biased corneal topography system in mapping a radially aspheric surface. J Refract Corneal Surg 1994; 10(2): p. 103–11.

64 Roberts C. Analysis of the inherent error of the TMS-1 Topographic Modeling System in mapping a radially aspheric surface. Cornea 1995; 14(3): p. 258–65.

65 Adachi I. *Real Time Analysis Corneal Keratometer.* United States Patent #4,692,003, Sept 8, 1987.

66 Gross GW, Baker P, and Bores LD. Corneal topography via two wavelength holography. In: *Soc Photo Inst Eng.* SPIE-The International Society for Optical Engineering, Los Angeles, 1990.

67 Bores LD. Corneal topography: The dark side of the moon. In: *Ophthalmic Technologies.* SPIE-The International Society for Optical Engineering, Los Angeles, 1991.

68 Seiler T. and Quurke AW. Iatrogenic keratectasia after LASIK in a case of forme fruste keratoconus. J Cataract Refract Surg 1998; 24(7): p. 1007–9.

69 Townsley G. New equipment and methods for determining the contour of the human cornea. Contacto 1967; 11: p. 72–81.

70 Edmund C. Location of the corneal apex and its influence on the stability of the central corneal curvature. Am J Optom Phys Optics 1987; 64(11): p. 846–52.

71 Dingeldein SA. Pittman SD, Wang J, *et al.* Analysis of Corneal Topographic Data. Invest Ophthalmol Vis Sci 1988; 29(Suppl): p. 389.

72 Klyce SD. Computer-assisted corneal topography. High-resolution graphic presentation and analysis of keratoscopy. Invest Ophthalmol Vis Sci 1984; 25(12): p. 1426–35.

73 Smith WJ. The modulation transfer function. In: *Modern Optical Engineering.* McGraw-Hill Book Company, New York, p. 311, 1966.

74 Tscherning MHE. *Optique physiologique; dioptrique oculaire, fonctions de la rétine, les mouvements oculaires et la vision binoculaire.* Carré et Naud, Paris, p. 335, 1898.

75 Howland B. and Howland HC. Subjective measurement of high-order aberrations of the eye. Science 1976; 193(4253): p. 580–2.

76 Liang J, Grimm B, Goelz S, *et al.* Objective measurement of wave aberrations of the human eye with the use of a Hartmann-Shack wave-front sensor. J Opt Soc Am A 1994; 11(7): p. 1949–57.

77 Mierdel P, Kaemmerer M, Krinke HE, *et al.* Effects of photorefractive keratectomy and cataract surgery on ocular optical errors of higher order. Graefes Arch Clin Exp Ophthalmol 1999; 237(9): p. 725–9.

78 Seiler T, Kaemmerer M, Mierdel P, *et al.* Ocular optical aberrations after photorefractive keratectomy for myopia and myopic astigmatism. Arch Ophthalmol 2000; 118(1): p. 17–21.

79 Liang J. and Williams DR. Aberrations and retinal image quality of the normal human eye. J Opt Soc Am A 1997; 14: p. 2873–83.

80 Spadea L, Fasciani R, Necozione S, *et al.* Role of the corneal epithelium in refractive changes following laser in situ keratomileusis for high myopia [In Process Citation]. J Refract Surg 2000; 16(2): p. 133–9.

81 Reinstein DZ, Silverman RH, and Coleman DJ. High-frequency ultrasound measurement of the thickness of the corneal epithelium. Refract Corneal Surg 1993; 9(5): p. 385–7.

82 Reinstein DZ, Silverman RH, Sutton HF, *et al.* Very high-frequency ultrasound corneal analysis identifies anatomic correlates of optical complications of lamellar refractive surgery: anatomic diagnosis in lamellar surgery. Ophthalmology 1999; 106(3): p. 474–82.

83 Holland SP, Srivannaboon S, and Reinstein DZ. Avoiding serious corneal complications of laser assisted in situ keratomileusis and photorefractive keratectomy. Ophthalmology 2000; 107(4): p. 640–52.

84 Stonecipher KG. Wavefront technology in refractive surgery. In: *EyeWorld.* p. 52–8, 2000.

85 Jakus MA. The fine structure of the human cornea. In: *The Structure of the Eye,* GK Smelser, Editor. New York Academic, New York, 1961.
86 Pratt-Johnson JA. Studies of the anatomy and pathology of the peripheral cornea. Am J Ophthalmol 1959; 47: p. 478–88.
87 Polack FM. Morphology of the cornea. I: Study with silver stains. Am J Ophthalmol 1961; 51: p. 179–84.
88 Troutman RC. and Buzard KA. *Corneal Astigmatism: Etiology, Prevention and Management.* CV Mosby, Chicago, 1991.
89 Sawusch MR, Wan WL, and McDonnell PJ. Tissue addition theory of radial keratotomy: a geometric model. J Cataract Refract Surg 1991; 17(4): p. 448–53.
90 Sawusch MR. and McDonnell PJ. Computer modeling of wound gape following radial keratotomy. Refract Corneal Surg 1992; 8(2): p. 143–5.
91 Serdarevic ON, Hanna K, Gribomont AC, *et al.* Excimer laser trephination in penetrating keratoplasty. Morphologic features and wound healing. Ophthalmology 1988; 95(4): p. 493–505.
92 Smith RS, Smith LA, Rich LF, *et al.* Effects of Growth Factors on Corneal Wound Healing. Invest Ophthal Vis Sci 1981; 20: p. 222–29.
93 Cheal EJ, Hayes WC, Chong HL, *et al.* Finite element analysis of the proximal tibia with the Miller porous–coated tibial component. In: *ASME Biomechanics Symposium.* ASME, 1984.
94 Hoeltzel DA, Simon FD, and Fernstrom KA. Computer–Aided Knee Prosthesis Design and Analysis. Automedica 1980; 10: p. 201–33.
95 Hoeltzel DA, Chang CK, Troutman RC, *et al.* A nonlinear finite element model of the whole human globe with experimental verification. Invest Ophthalmol Vis Sci 1987; 28 (suppl): p. 223.
96 Mow CC. A theoretical model of the cornea for use in studies of tonometry. Bulletin of Mathematical Biophysics 1968; 30: p. 437–53.
97 Kobayashi AS, Woo SLY, and Lawrence C. Analysis of the corneo-scleral shell by the method of direct stiffness. J Biomech 1971; 4: p. 323–30.
98 Woo SL, Kobayashi AS, and Lawrence C, *et al.* Mathematical model of the corneo-scleral shell as applied to intraocular pressure-volume relations and applanation tonometry. Ann Biomed Eng 1972; 1(1): p. 87–98.
99 Arciniegas A. and Amaya LE. Physical factors that influence measurement of intraocular pressure with a Goldmann tonometer. In: *Biomechanics: Principles and Applications.* Martinus Nijhoff, Dordrecht, p. 425–32, 1982.
100 Phillips CI. and Quick MC. Impression tonometry and the effect of eye volume variation. Br J Ophthalmol 1960; 44: p. 149–63.
101 Friedenwald JS. Contribution to the theory and practice of tonometry. Am J Ophthalmol 1937; 20: p. 985–1024.
102 Fyodorov SN. and Durnev VV. Operation of dosaged dissection of corneal circular ligament in cases of myopia of mild degree. Ann Ophthalmol 1979; 11(12): p. 1885–90.
103 Bores LD, Myers W, and Cowden J. Radial keratotomy: an analysis of the American experience. Ann Ophthalmol 1981; 13(8): p. 941–8.
104 Bores LD. Historical review and clinical results of radial keratotomy. Int Ophthalmol Clin 1983; 23(3): p. 93–118.
105 Deitz MR, Sanders DR, and Marks RG. Radial keratotomy: an overview of the Kansas City study. Ophthalmology 1984; 91(5): p. 467–78.
106 Salz JJ. A Consumer's Guide to Radial Keratotomy Predictive Software. J Refract Surg 1985; 1(2): p. 60–7.
107 Au YK. and Rowsey JJ. Bending Moment Modeling of Corneal Topography: Surgical Applications. Invest Ophthalmol Vis Sci 1986; 27(suppl)(3): p. 1–12.
108 Rand RH, Lubkin SR, and Howland HC. Analytical model of corneal surgery. J Biomech Eng 1991; 113(2): p. 239–41.
109 Schachar RA, Black TD, and Huang T. Understanding Radial Keratotomy. In: *Understanding Radial Keratotomy,* R Schachar, Editor. LAL Publishing, Dennison, p. 25–6, 1981.
110 Bryant MR, Velinsky SA, Plesha ME, *et al.* Computer-aided surgical design in refractive keratotomy. CLAO J 1987; 13: p. 238–42.
111 Bryant MR. and Velinsky SA. Design of keratorefractive surgical procedures: radial keratotomy. In: *Advances in Design Automation.* American Society of Mechanical Engineering, New York, p. 363–91, 1989.
112 Bryant MR. and McDonnell PJ. Constitutive laws for biomechanical modeling of refractive surgery. J Biomech Eng 1996; 118(4): p. 473–81.
113 Vito RP. Biomechanics: a primer for cornea surgeons. In: *Refractive Keratotomy for Myoia and Astigmatism,* GO Waring, Editor. CV Mosby Yearbook Publishers, St Louis, 1991.
114 Vito RP, Shin TJ, and McCarey BE. A mechanical model of the cornea: the effects of physiological and surgical factors on radial keratotomy surgery. Refract Corneal Surg 1989; 5(2): p. 82–8.
115 Shin TJ, Vito RP, Johnson LW, *et al.* The distribution of strain in the human cornea. J Biomech 1997; 30(5): p. 497–503.
116 Fung YC. *The Mechanics of Living Tissues.* 1985.
117 Seiler T. Biomechanics of Transverse Incisions of the Cornea. In: *Refractive Keratotomy for Myopia and Astigmatism,* GO Waring, Editor. Mosby Yearbook, St Louis, p. 1243–8, 1991.
118 Bores LD. *Refractive Eye Surgery.* Blackwell's Scientific Publications, Cambridge, p. 550, 1992.
119 Wang J, Rice DA, and Klyce SD. A new reconstruction algorithm for improvement of corneal topographical analysis. Refract Corneal Surg 1990; 6: p. 379–87.
120 Wang J, Rice DA, and Klyce SD. Analysis of the effects of astigmatism and misalignment on corneal surface reconstruction from photokeratoscopic data. Refract Corneal Surg 1991; 7: p. 129–40.
121 Waring GO. Making sense of 'keratospeak'. A classification of refractive corneal surgery. Arch Ophthalmol 1985; 103(10): p. 1472–1477.
122 Waring GO. Making Sense of Keratospeak II: Proposed Conventional Terminology for Corneal Topography. Refractive and Corneal Surgery 1989; 5(6): p. 362–367.
123 Smith WJ. *Modern Optical Engineering* (Second Edition). McGraw-Hill, New York, 1990.
124 Zernike F. Beugungstheorie des Schneidenver-Eahrens und Seiner Verbesserten Form, der Phasenkontrastmethode. Physica 1934; 1: p. 689.
125 Poularikas A. *Handbook of Formulas and Tables for Signal Processing.* CRC Press, Boca Raton, 1998.
126 Helmholtz HLF. Üeber die Accomodation des Auges. Graefes Arch Ophthalmol 1855; 1(2): p. 1–74.
127 Maguire LJ, Singer DE, and Klyce SD. Graphic presentation of computer-analyzed keratoscope photographs. Arch Ophthalmol 1987; 105(2): p. 223–30.

7 The Beginning and the Evolution of Radial Keratotomy

There is nothing more difficult to take in hand, more perilous to conduct, or more uncertain in its success, than to take the lead in the introduction of a new order of things.
[Machiavelli]

I will begin this discussion of the surgical treatment of refractive disorders with *radial keratotomy* (RK)—which is only fitting. Because, with all due respect to the late Jose Barraquer, my mentor and friend and the man who carried the banner for all those who went before, the modern era of *refractive surgery* began on November 28, 1978. It was on that date that the first RK was performed in the Western world. Thus was inaugurated a period that in 20 short years has seen more advancement in this field than has occurred in all the centuries preceding. Prior to that date, the flame was kept alive only by a select few stalwarts who worked in relative and unappreciated obscurity. The year 1978 saw refractive surgery thrust into the hands of the work-a-day ophthalmologist. More important, this surgery became available to the mainstream patient, who now—and for the first time—had a viable, low-risk alternative to ocular appliances.

This story is very much a personal one, inasmuch as I am the surgeon who performed that first operation in 1978 (Table 7.1). Because I am also responsible for not a little of the early development of RK, as well as the training of most of its practitioners, I hope that you will forgive the use of the personal pronoun (Figures 7.1 through 7.3a, b). It is, additionally, a story of deep-felt personal responsibility and anguish.

RK is an elegant solution to a serious ocular deficit—myopia. By simply making partial-thickness, *ab externo*, corneal incisions, which radiate from a common center and whose length and depth are variable, the refractive surgeon can alter not only the shape of the cornea but the life of the patient as well. Having said this, what must be added is this: What looks simple—isn't. It is not enough just to make the incisions—anyone can do that. Rather, it is the understanding of how, when, and where to make them that spells the difference between success and failure in this surgery. Thus RK can be likened to genius, which has been described as "1% inspiration and 99% perspiration." In RK—as well as in refractive surgery generally—it is 10% *incision* and 90% *decision*, that is, thinking before doing. To this end, it will serve us well to discuss how it is that this surgery works and how it was that the surgery evolved into what it is today.

Early history and development of RK

Much has been made of the failure of Sato's work (Figure 7.4). In fact, RK was—at first—deliberately confused with the Sato procedure. I say *deliberately* because no one familiar with both techniques could possibly have confused one with the other—unless, of course, the criticism was irrational and based on ignorance of either or both procedures. I suppose that this is understandable—a wagon *does* resemble a truck in a general sort of way; both have a wheel in each corner. It was this tendency for generalization that was to produce so much difficulty—not to say anguish—for myself, my family, and my colleagues as we struggled to get RK a fair hearing on its

Table 7.1 The results of the first radial keratotomies performed by Bores in the Soviet Union in 1976

	Preoperative				Post-operative			
	Refraction (D)		Uncorrected vision		Refraction (D)		Uncorrected vision	
Patients	OD	OS	OD	OS	OD	OS	OD	OS
1	3.00	3.25	20/160	20/200	Plano	–0.25	20/20	20/25
2	4.50	4.50	20/200	20/200	Plano	Plano	20/25	20/25
3	3.75	3.25	20/200	20/160	Plano	–0.37	20/20	20/30
4	3.00	3.00	20/160	20/160	Plano	–0.25	20/20	20/25
5	7.00	7.25	20/400	20/400	–1.50	–1.25*	20/60	20/60
6	10.50	4.50	20/400	20/300	–4.00	Plano	20/200	20/20

* Reverted to –3.25 D OU (incisions too shallow). Remainder stable at 3 years.

merits. It was with extreme difficulty that the results of my and Fyodorov's work, as well as that of those other stalwarts who had joined us—Myers, Schachar, Jensen, Deitz, Katzen, Hoffer, Sawelson, and some others—were given a hearing (Figure 7.5). In fact, such was the snubbing of RK papers that two organizations sprang up almost simultaneously for the purpose of providing a forum: The Kerato-Refractive Society and The International Society for Refractive Keratoplasty (ISRK, now ISRS). By that time (early 1979), I had long since given up hope of acceptance personally, so I just went on "sailing my own race"—as a sailing companion once advised. It was not until early 1995 that the American Academy of Ophthalmology formed an ad hoc study group for this surgery and only later gave this and other refractive surgical techniques a "voice."

The Sato operation

Tutomu Sato, M.D., late of Juntendo Medical College and a brilliant and gifted surgeon, called the operation "posterior half-incision of cornea. . . ." It was conceived originally as a solution to the problem of keratoconus and was first reported by Sato in 1939, in which paper he described the results of such incisions in 10 eyes of 8 patients [1]. The technique was later applied to patients with regular astigmatism [2] and still later to patients with spherical myopia itself. This method was not without precedent; Sato was familiar with the work of Lans, who stated that he had gotten the idea from something Snellen had proposed it in 1869 [3]. However, whereas Lans confined his experiments to rabbits, Sato extended the method to humans.

While studying the subject of keratoconus under the guidance of Professor Shinobu Ishihara in 1936, inventor of the Ishihara color plates and professor at Tokyo University, Sato noted a marked improvement in vision of a 20-year-old girl following spontaneous rupture of Descemet's membrane (Figure 7.5). Counting fingers vision, recorded 4 days after the rupture, improved to approximately 20/30 after 5 weeks of patching and medication. The corneal apex not only had flattened, but it also had become more regular, as evidenced by its appear-

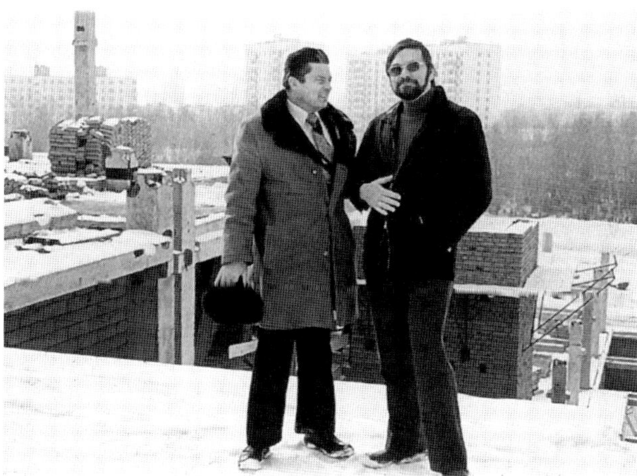

Fig. 7.1 Svatyslav N. Fyodorov and Leo D. Bores standing on the third floor of Fyodorov's unfinished institute in February 1976, the year RK was introduced to the Western world (the first RK was performed in the West in November 1978). Only 135 cases had been performed up to that time.

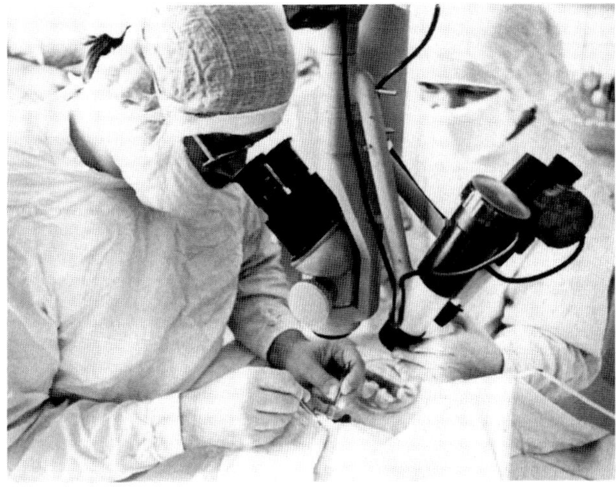

Fig. 7.2 The author performing his first RK in Moscow in 1976.

(a)

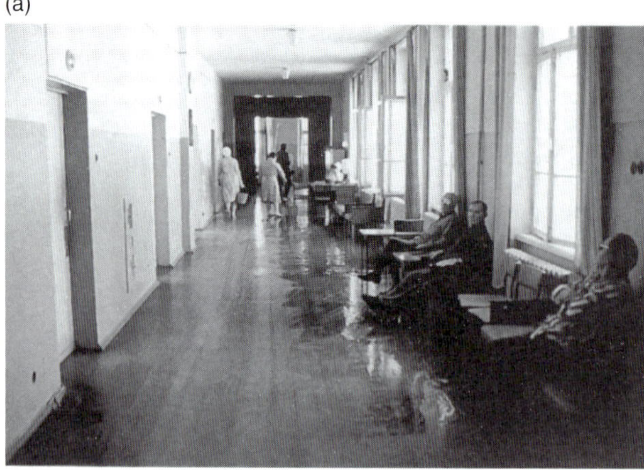

(b)

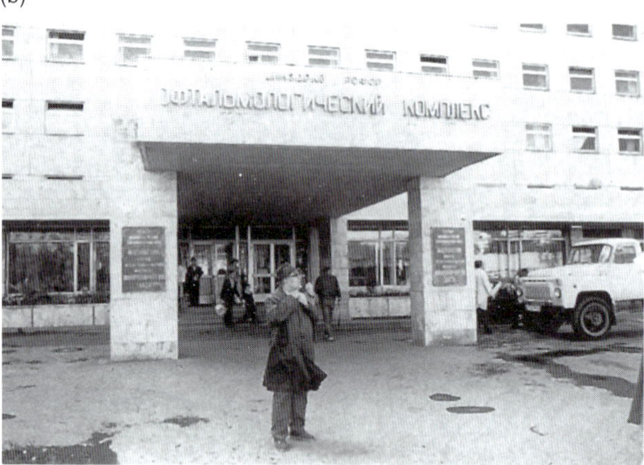

Fig. 7.3 (a) The main corridor of the original clinic—Hospital # 81, 10 Lobninskaya Street, Moscow. (b) The entrance to the Moscow Scientific Institute for Eye Microsurgery, 59a Beskudnikovsky Blvd.

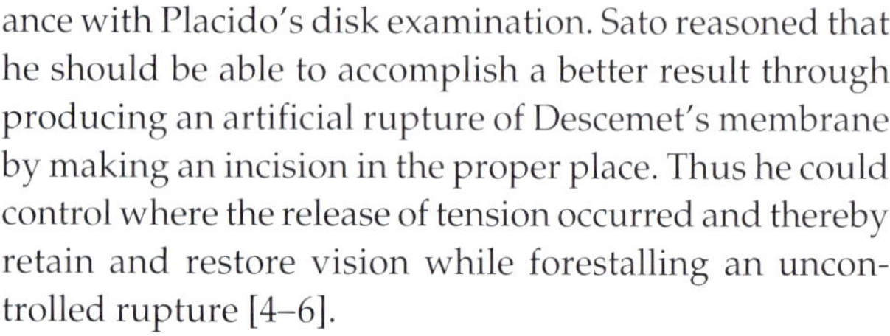

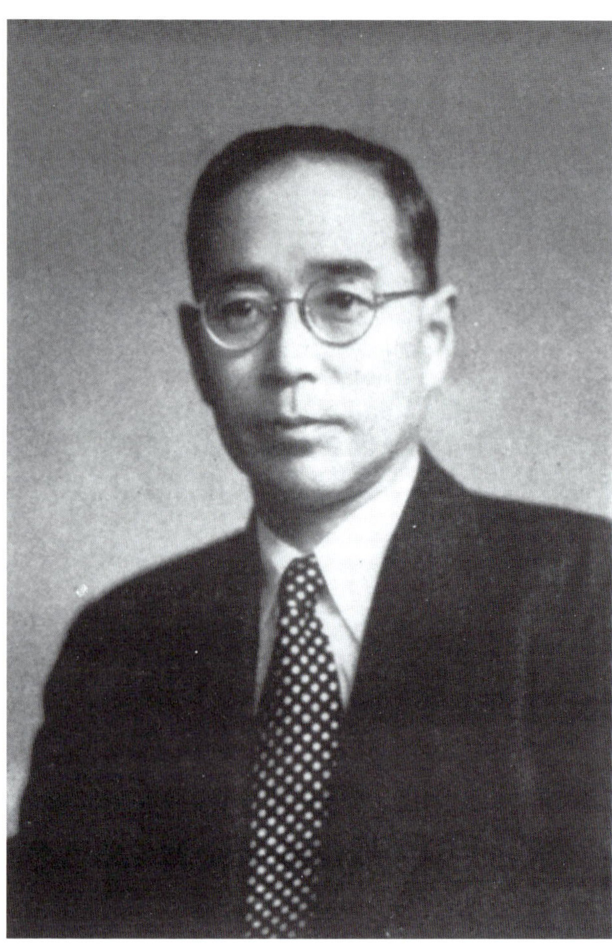

Fig. 7.4 Tutomu Sato, M.D. (Courtesy of A. Momose.)

ance with Placido's disk examination. Sato reasoned that he should be able to accomplish a better result through producing an artificial rupture of Descemet's membrane by making an incision in the proper place. Thus he could control where the release of tension occurred and thereby retain and restore vision while forestalling an uncontrolled rupture [4–6].

Sato's operation for keratoconus was straightforward, effective, and considering the alternative, appropriate. The alternative, at least for most, was poor vision, since corneal transplantation was proscribed by the religious beliefs of the Japanese. For others, it meant a long and expensive trip to either Germany or the United States. Sato himself performed 200 of these operations between 1938 and 1943. The approach was used widely by Japanese ophthalmic surgeons and was taught to medical students after the war. Nevertheless, it was a technically difficult operation to perform. It required great skill on the part of the surgeon, necessitating incisions being made *ab interno*, through half the corneal thickness, and in a straight line—close to the optic center. The method by which Sato performed these incisions is detailed in Chapter 9. For now, I will confine the discussion to the extension of this technique to spherical myopia.

Sato found that anterior and posterior incisions made in the extrapupillary portion of the cornea resulted in a

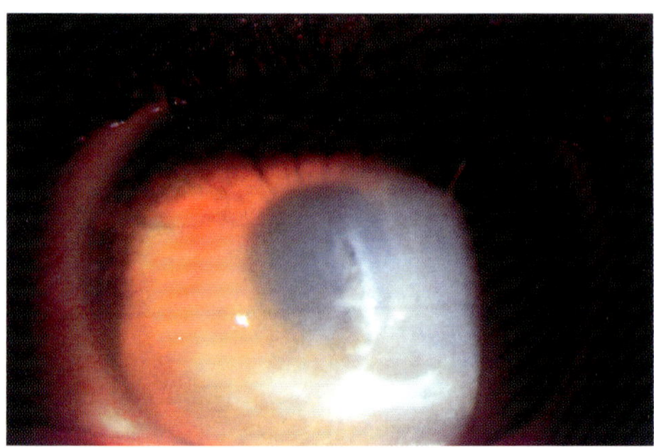

Fig. 7.5 A case of spontaneous rupture of Descemet's membrane in keratoconus.

lengthening of the radius (and the chord) of the corneal curvature overlying the pupil. This, of course, reduced the corneal refractive power—making it relatively more hyperopic. In the rabbit eye, anterior incisions produced minimal central corneal flattening, whereas posterior incisions produced a maximum flattening of 2 D [7]. Hence Sato was induced to employ incisions of this latter type when he extended this work into human eyes for mild myopia (which illustrates that preceding animal work does not always lead in the right direction—besides, I have yet to find a rabbit that can read or talk). For higher degrees of myopia, both anterior and posterior half-incisions were used.

Figures 7.6 through 7.8 show the method of performing this operation. Topical application as well as retrobulbar injection of anesthetic was used—raising the specter of possible posterior bulbar perforation (see also Chapter 15). The latter anesthesia was to ensure complete immobilization of the eye, as well as to create slight proptosis of the globe, a method still advocated today by some [8].

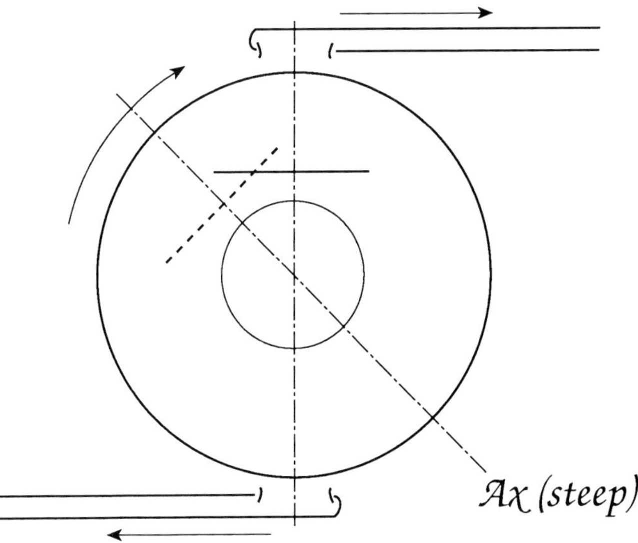

Fig. 7.6 Bridle sutures enabled the surgeon to rotate the eye as necessary.

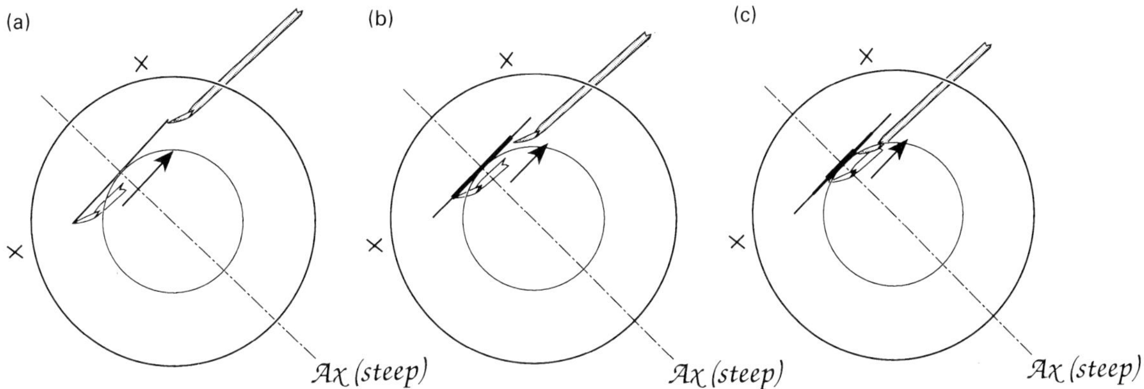

Fig. 7.7 (a) Internal transverse incisions were made tangential to the pupil. (b, c) Repeated passes were made as necessary.

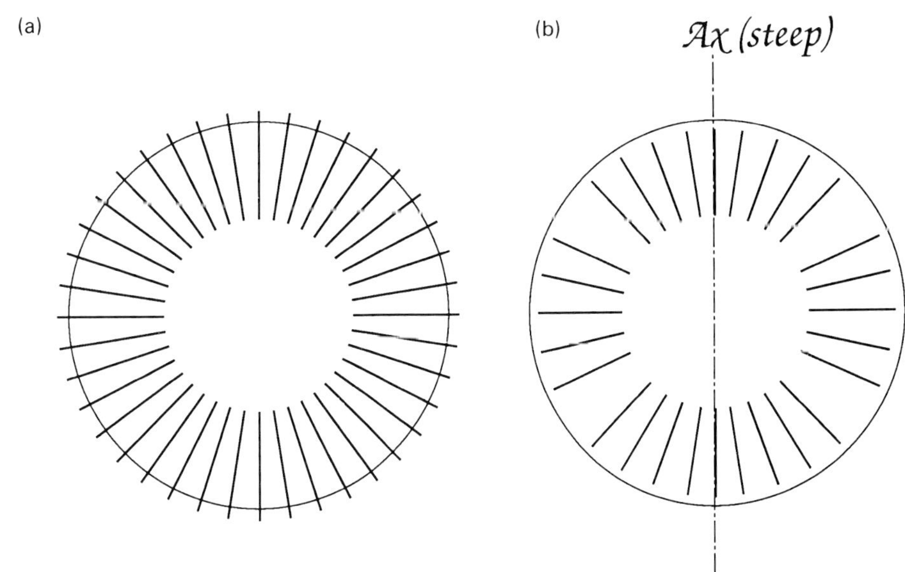

Fig. 7.8 (a) For spherical myopia, internal radiating incisions were followed by external radials. (b) In some cases of astigmatism, incisions were grouped.

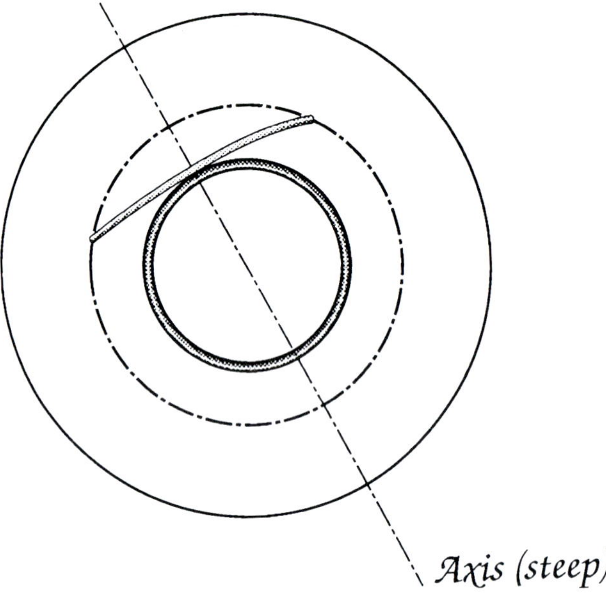

Fig. 7.9 A loop or length of human hair was used to delineate the optic clear zone and/or the extent of the T-cut.

Bridle sutures were placed around the tendons of both vertical recti so as to allow the globe to rotate freely. The optic clear zone, approximately 6 mm in diameter, was delineated by making a loop of sterile gray human hair or fine white fish gut (this was later changed to a mark made with gentian violet) and placing it onto the cornea—centered on the miotic pupil (Figure 7.9). If astigmatism also was to be treated, four additional straight pieces of hair or gut (or dye marks) were laid in place on the major and minor meridians.

A specially designed knife (Figure 7.10) was then inserted into the anterior chamber at the superior limbus through a 2-mm scleral tunnel. This tunnel was important to minimize flattening of the anterior chamber—this type of incision is self-closing. Usually five to nine incisions were made in the inferoposterior cornea—theoretically to 66% of its thickness (Figure 7.11). The operative word here is *theoretically*. I have examined several of these patients and estimate the depth of the incisions as ranging from 20% to 95% of the corneal thickness. The center of the incision was used to make the estimate, since there is a tendency in the Sato operation for both the beginnings and ends of the incisions to be shallower than the center. After each incision was made, from the limbus toward center, the knife was disengaged by turning it to the side to prevent damage to the central clear zone. These incisions were followed by the same number made in the superior cornea by entering the anterior chamber at the inferior limbus. Finally, nasal and then temporal incisions were added. Thus some 20 to 36 incisions were made, *ab interno*, with as many as six entries made into the anterior chamber.

Posterior incisions alone were found to only correct an average of –1.2 D, with a maximum of –4.5 D in the 35 patients reported in 1952 [9]. Therefore, in cases of myopia exceeding 2.0 D, an additional 40 incisions were made in a radial fashion through the anterior cornea from optical zone to limbal sclera. In this instance, a guarded knife similar to a Lancaster sclerotome (Okamura's knife) was used with the guard set to prevent perforation (Figure 7.12). How Sato determined the exact setting of this knife is not mentioned in any of his papers—however, it was set to a uniform 0.6 mm. Perhaps he used the same method described by a prominent physician (who shall remain nameless) who reported disappointing results with RK. When asked how he determined the depth of his incisions, he answered, "By intuition." How one can intuit 70% of a cornea that measures 0.5 mm in thickness in the

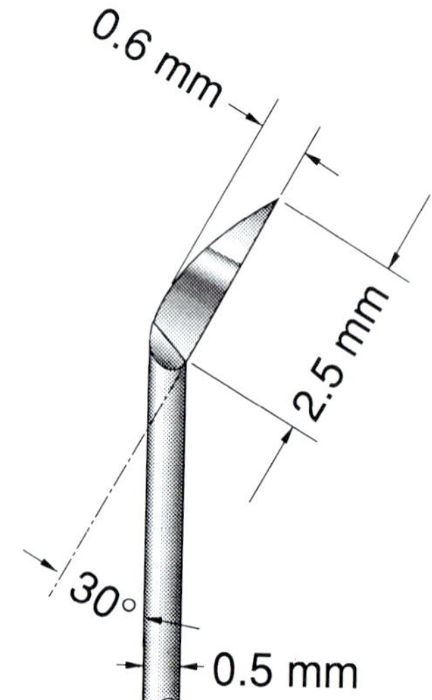

Fig. 7.10 Sketch of the blade of Sato's knife.

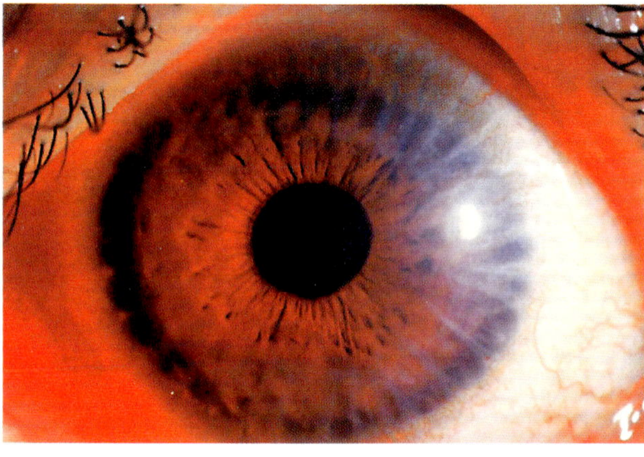

Fig. 7.11 The left eye of a 47-year-old female who had undergone the procedure of Sato 30 years previously. The other eye is similar. Distance visual acuity is 6/9, uncorrected. (Courtesy of A. Momose.)

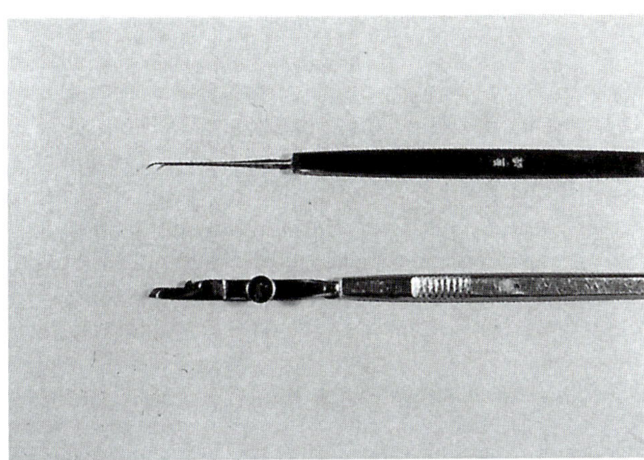

Fig. 7.12 Sato's knife (above); Okamura's knife (below). (Courtesy of A. Momose.)

(a)

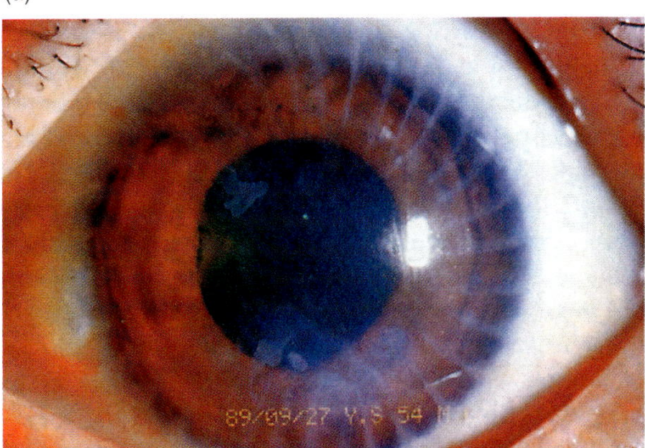

(b)

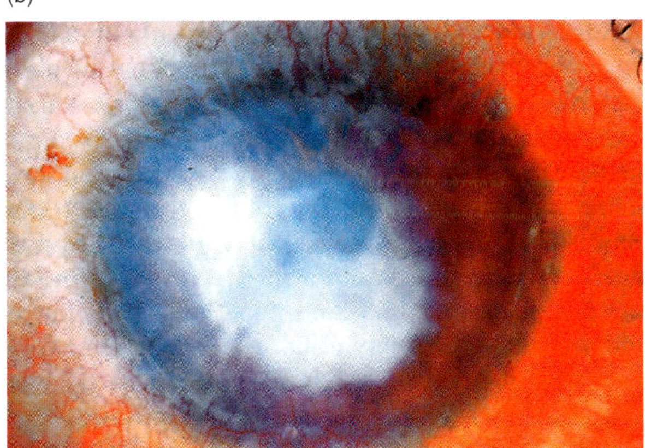

(c)

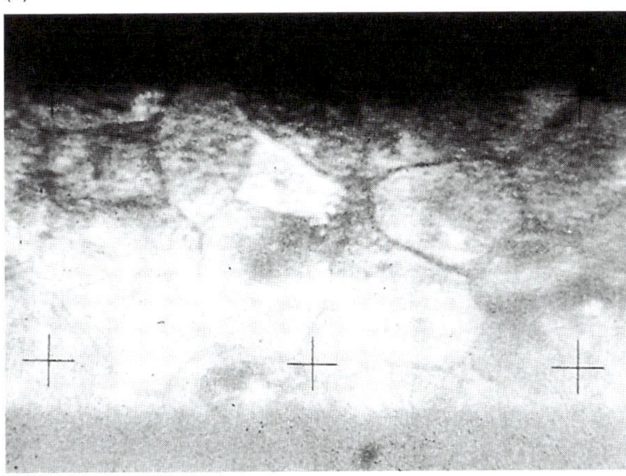

Fig. 7.13 (a) Moderate corneal decompensation following Sato's operation. (b) A more severe case with fibrous proliferation. (c) Peripheral endothelial cells in (b). (Courtesy of A. Momose.)

center was not revealed. The average corneal thickness in the human at 6.0 mm is 640 μm; thus Sato was not far off, but he was, in any case, too shallow. Nonetheless, Sato and his associates obtained a mean correction of –3.0 D in a range from –1.12 to –7.0 D for the next 32 eyes [6]. On the basis of this work, he drew two conclusions:

> We consider that this procedure, if properly performed, will safely cure myopia up to four diopters, and will produce marked improvement in myopia of from five to six diopters. This treatment, therefore, is efficacious for 95% of the myopic cases in Japan. . . . no detrimental effects from this procedure have been observed, and none of the cases demonstrated any . . . loss of visual acuity.

His follow-up was only 5 months when he made this statement; both claims proved to be premature.

Akiyama reported on the postoperative changes in two groups of eyes operated by the Sato method. In the first group of 172 eyes, operated from 1948 to 1953, the average change was –3.2 D, with a range from –0.5 to –11.5 D, 70% of the eyes achieving an effect of –1.5 to –4.0 D.

In the second group of 177 eyes, the average overall correction was –2.8 D, with a maximum of –10.5 D. In the group over –4.0 D, the mean correction was –3.9 D. Akiyama concluded, as had Sato, that more than 35 posterior and more than 40 anterior incisions should be performed. He emphasized that posterior incisions should reach as deep as possible without perforation [10,11]. From 1948 through 1959 (when contact lenses were introduced in Japan), Sato and/or his associates performed 681 similar cases, reporting similar results.

Unfortunately, the damage done to the corneal endothelium by posterior incisions frequently produced corneal opacification that only appeared 10 to 24 years later (Figures 7.13 and 7.14). In addition, certain technical deficiencies resulted in many low corrections that did not warrant the risk of the surgery. Consequently, the surgery was abandoned. It was discovered subsequently that the reason for the corneal decompensation was destruction of the corneal endothelial pump caused by the internal incisions—something never considered by the technique's author.

This should come as no surprise, since the role of the corneal endothelium in maintaining corneal deturges-

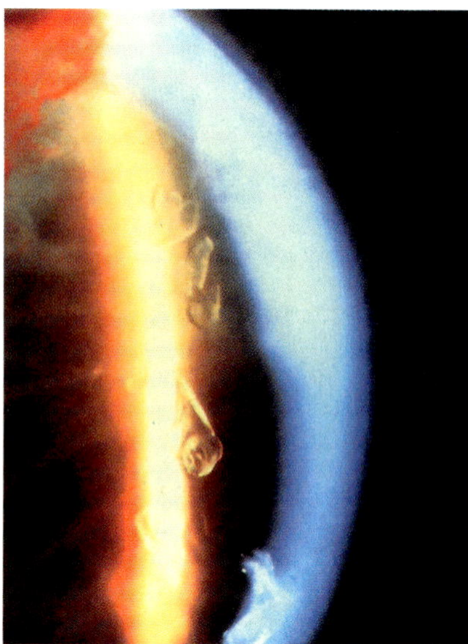

Fig. 7.14 The endothelial "tubes" and thickened cornea illustrate the cause of corneal decompensation in these cases.

cence was almost completely unknown at the time. And neither were operating microscopes available. A film of Sato operating shows him wearing loupes. These provide only limited magnification and typically a small field of view. Operating in this fashion, it made sense to make the incisions from the posterior surface because presumably the knife tip could be seen more clearly as it approached the surface. Considering the fact that the corneal reaction must have been intense (see the description of Fyodorov's early efforts below) and the availability of Okamura's guarded knife, to persist in this approach was brave—at the very least. It is obvious that the incisional depth must have varied tremendously, as evidenced by my own examination of some of these patients. Additionally, Akiyama reported a range of corrections from 0 to −10.5 D. This effect and variability are, respectively, much less and much greater than that of present-day RK, even with variable clear zones.

Kanai, working at Juntendo University in Tokyo—the school where Sato was a professor—followed 80 of the eyes of 50 patients (of 281 myopic eyes on which Dr. Sato performed the operation after 1951) from 1971 through 1980. Sixty of the 80 eyes (75%) developed bullous keratopathy. It is assumed (without any evidence) that the remaining 581 eyes shared the same fate. Interestingly, in some patients in whom identical bilateral surgery was performed, only one eye developed bullous changes with a resulting decrease in vision [12].

When Kanai and his coworkers examined the ultrastucture of several corneal buttons removed from these patients at the time of keratoplasty, they found intercellular and intracellular epithelial edema, disrupted epithelial basement membrane and Bowman's layer, increased interfibrillar distance in the stroma, and abnormal collagenous material posterior to the normal portion of Descemet's membrane. The endothelium was absent in these patients.

That this problem occurred in a sizable number of patients is not due to either the nature of Japanese corneas or the fact of incisions. That this was due solely to damaged endothelium can be seen in Figure 7.15a and b, which show Japanese corneas operated on with current RK techniques and no endothelial involvement. In fact, despite the large number of RK surgeries that have been performed in the last 12 years, endothelial cell loss and consequent corneal decompensation are not a factor (see also Chapter 15).

There has been considerable discussion of the Sato technique over the years, especially its failure to produce good results, coupled with its high complication rate in the form of corneal decompensation [13]. It has been flatly stated that 80% to 85% of Professor Sato's patients ultimately suffered some degree of corneal decompensation. This is a high percentage and, on the face of it, remarkable. How is it that a competent physician would persist in performing a surgical procedure that blinded 85% of his patients? But is this really true? Sato was not an incompetent; those who knew him have even called

(a)

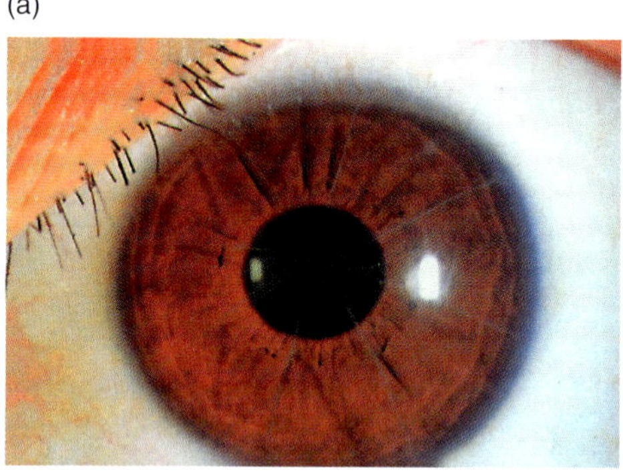

(b)

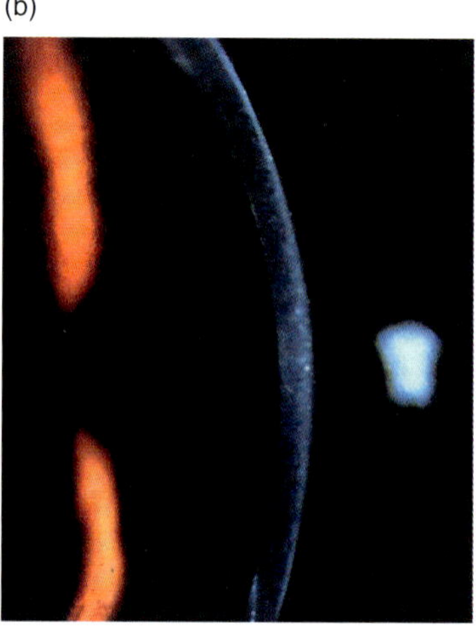

Fig. 7.15 RK in a Japanese patient. Note the total absence of endothelial involvement. (Courtesy of A. Momose.)

him a genius. It is not generally appreciated that not all of his cases were failures and that not all of the corneas became cloudy. I am struck by the lack of completed follow-up in these patients. Only 281 of 681 (40%) of the entire group of eyes—recall that Sato had performed 681 cases of this kind between 1951 and 1960—were studied to any degree. The papers dealing with decompensation all came from one group, and the total number of patients studied completely was 172 (61%) [12,13]. In this group, 129 (75%) of the eyes developed bullous keratopathy. In short, 45% of the patients retained in follow–up developed this complication. It is assumed (without any evidence) that the remaining, unfollowed, eyes shared the same fate. The question has to be asked, namely: *What happened to the rest of the patients*? Interestingly, in some patients in whom identical bilateral surgery was performed, only one eye developed bullous changes with a resulting decrease in vision. We have been painted a picture of long lines of people requiring corneal transplantation as a result of this surgery. If there is truth in the observation that only problem patients can be counted on to return for follow-up, then the picture changes dramatically. For example, 129 of 681 eyes is only 19%. High to be sure—but not the unmitigated disaster that has been described by so many (even if we were to double this number). These facts notwithstanding, the procedure was stopped because the risks outweighed the benefits. Professor Momose, however, is of the opinion that the surgery fell into disuse for two other reasons: 1) the untimely death of Professor Sato on June 9, 1960, at the age of 58 and 2) the availability of contact lenses [14].

Such a poor beginning has created considerable opposition to the adoption of a more modern and advanced technique, namely, RK. This is particularly true among Japanese ophthalmologists, who are loathe to perform RK—only 10 of whom were doing it at the initial writing of this book. Many of these physicians are still confused between modern RK surgery and the Sato procedure. Interestingly, the surgery is paid for by the Japanese national health plan but at a rate that hardly pays for the cost of doing the surgery. Professor Momose is of the opinion that this is the real reason that the surgery is not being performed in large numbers. Our better appreciation of the role of the endothelium in maintaining corneal clarity, coupled with advances such as the operating microscope, ultrasonic pachymeter, and more refined methods of corneal curvature measurement, has changed not only the performance of the surgery but also its potential

It was evident from Sato's work that incisions made in the underside of the cornea were counterproductive. Not only did they ultimately compromise the health of the cornea, they also produced little or no flattening of the center. Recall that the mean myopic reduction in Sato's series was only −1.75 D. Therefore, incisions should only be made on the outside of the cornea, and they should not penetrate into the anterior chamber. Otherwise, such an approach would be the same as making them from the underside. Hence a first principle is established: *Incisions are to be ab externo only*. A corollary to this is that they should not be made so deep as to penetrate. It was not certain at that time whether or not external incisions affected the endothelium. However, endothelial cell counts were made by myself and Fyodorov on all patients because of the concern that even incising the cornea from the outside might somehow act to produce cell damage. It was soon evident, however, from these examinations that no significant cell loss was occurring and that the cell loss described in Sato's patients was a consequence of direct trauma to the endothelium itself.

Early history and development of RK

It has been suggested by individuals with a vested interest in their own point of view that a chap named Yenaliev beat Fyodorov to the wire by claiming to have been performing something akin to RK some years before the work of Fyodorov and Durnev [15]. If this is so, it is curious that he did not publish his work until 1979—years after Fyodorov had published in 1976 and after RK had received favorable publicity throughout the world. There is a saying to the effect that "*defeat is an orphan, while success has many fathers*." Some take this to mean that it requires more than one hand to create success. I take the meaning to be the more ironic one intended by its utterer, namely, that many people wish to be identified with success—even though not earned. I certainly experienced a certain loneliness during the early days of RK while bearing the burden virtually alone. I was surprised much later to find that many others "suffered" as well—though where they were at the time escapes me. This phenomenon will be familiar to experienced students of history, but younger readers may be astonished to learn of the existence of a group known as the "sunshine patriots" of ophthalmic innovation, namely, *those who are invincible in peace (acceptance) and invisible in war (controversy)*. Many today claim to have been involved in the origins of RK who were conspicuously absent when it was "hitting the fan" back in the bad old "good old days." Twas ever thus in the annals of medicine and was well described by William Halstead at the turn of the last century:

> Surgeons are a strange breed. When something new comes on the scene—they'll say it's not true. When they find that it's true—they'll say it's no good. When they find that it's good—they'll say it's not new. Then when they've completed all three steps, they convince themselves that they started it all.

RK as we know it today had its beginning in 1973 after a chance observation of corneal flattening following ocular trauma in a child. Petrov was talking when he should have been listening it seems—some school mate punched him in the eye, breaking the glasses he was wearing at the time. Svyataslav N. Fyodorov, M.D., who at that time was director of the Hospital for Experimental Eye Surgery in Moscow, was stopped in the hallway by the patient, who proudly informed Fyodorov that he now could see clearly without glasses in his injured eye. Professor Fyodorov examined the boy and found that he had a small curvilinear incision in the paracenter of his left cornea—sparing the visual axis. The patient's myopia had been reduced 3 D by this fortuitous accident. In characteristic Fyodorov fashion, the professor mused, "*Chort vohz me*! If a fist can do this, so can I. After all, I am an eye surgeon." Accordingly, he began investigating the possibilities of such surgical intervention, assigning a young staffer named Valerie Durnev to the task (Figure 7.16). I too was somewhat skeptical of the story at first—after all, weren't the Russians the ones who claimed to have invented everything under the sun—perhaps even the sun itself? I too would have remained skeptical had it not been for my relationship with Slava Fyodorov and also for two other salient reasons: 1) I met the boy himself, and 2) some few years later I had a patient walk into my office in Detroit after having received a welding burn to his left cornea. His myopia, once –6 D, had been reduced to –3 D by a small, temporal paracentral deep stromal corneal burn. Who says that history does not repeat itself?

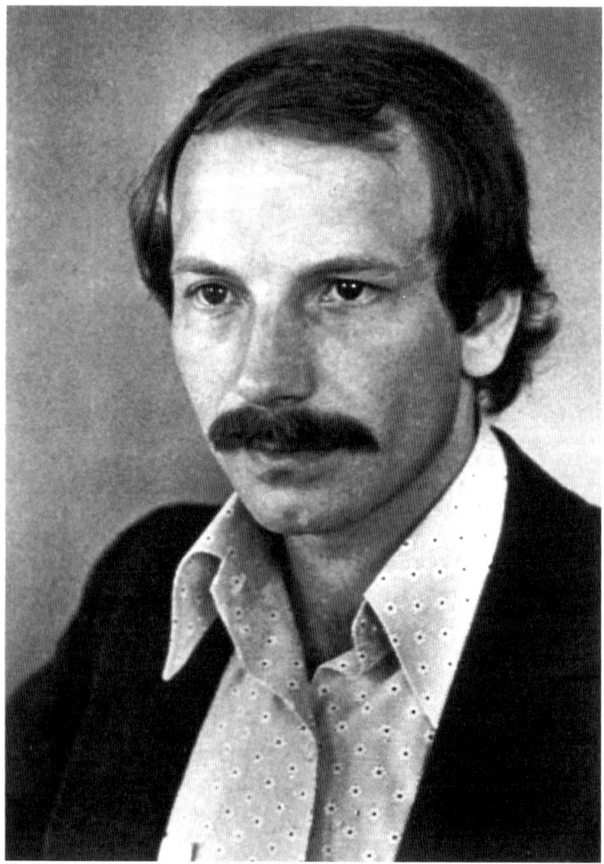

Fig. 7.16 V. V. Durnev, M.D., Fyodorov's original coworker in the development of RK.

To say that RK began in Moscow in 1973 is not to say that it sprung forth full blown and new as if from the forehead of Zeus—this is not the case. The legacy of RK is to be found in the work of Leendart Lans and Tutomo Sato and perhaps even Kokott. The latter lent his cognomen to the original name of RK: *the dosaged dissection of the circumferential ligament of Kokott*. Convinced that the surgery could not handle both controversy and a somewhat dubious name, I was struggling with renaming it when my wife, Leara, suggested (in 1979) the name by which it has since been known: *radial keratotomy*.

Kokott has a more important place in the history of RK. It was his work that certainly inspired the direction of investigations of one surgeon and may well have influenced the work of another. In three papers, Kokott detailed his extensive study of the structure of the eyeball, including the cornea [16–18]. In his 1938 paper, he described the circumferential arrangement of the deep peripheral keratocytes into the structure that bears his name. Others have described this same ligamentum in later work, whereas some others have decried it. However, the more recent studies of Meek with x-ray diffraction imaging seem to have corroborated Kokott's original thesis [19].

Fyodorov and coworkers also considered the ligamentum to be a real structure, and it was their belief that the weakening of this structure was material to the success of what came to be known as RK. This bodes ill for the so-called mini-RK and perhaps explains the less than stellar results reported from this technique. Schachar was the first to attempt shortened radial incisions and at first reported favorably on them in 1980 [20–22].

It is likely that Sato was familiar with Kokott's work and that his incisions were placed from the endothelial surface of the cornea and in the periphery in order to transect the circumferential fibers there. Hence it would not be necessary, in his view, to use a smaller optical zone—though he did say that the reason this was done was to reduce glare.

A search of the literature turned up not only the work of Sato but also that of some Soviets as well, including Pureskin [23–26], who had duplicated Sato's work. Durnev and Fyodorov also repeated some of Sato's work in rabbits and at least once in a human subject, verifying most of Sato's findings, including a tremendous corneal reaction not reported by the Japanese surgeon (Figure 7.17). Consequently, posterior incisions were rejected out of hand. Continued study showed that combining deep anterior incisions with a smaller optical clear zone resulted in a more profound reduction in corneal curvature than had been reported by Sato [27,28].

By October 1973, Fyodorov and Durnev had made several important changes in the surgery, to whit:

1 Varying the size of the optical zone from 2.0 mm (later enlarged to 3.0 mm) to 6.0 mm—depending on the degree of myopia (Figure 7.18).

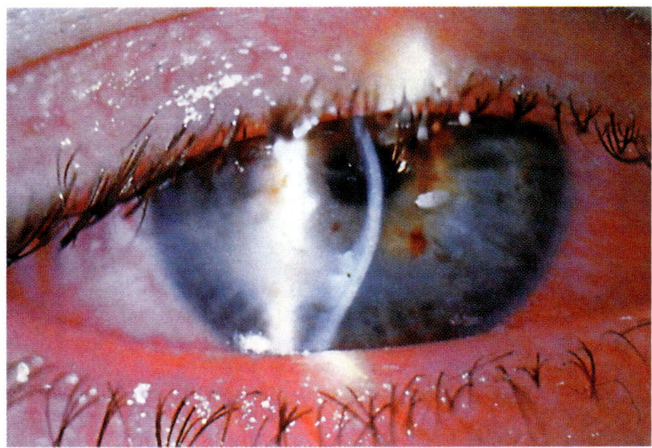

Fig. 7.17 One of Fyodorov's pre-RK patients with an internal T-cut. Note the extreme corneal reaction. Compare with Figure 7.5.

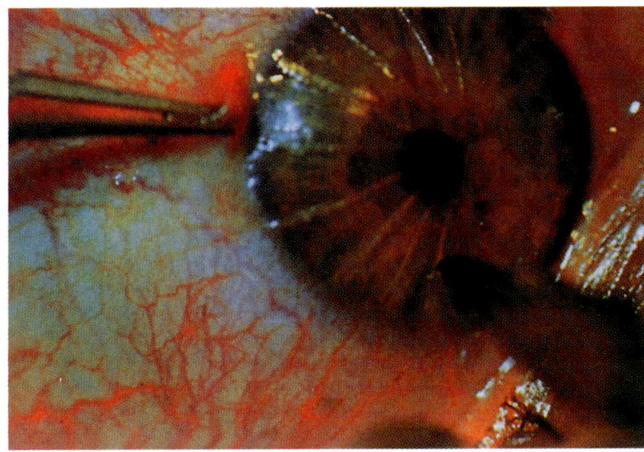

Fig. 7.19 Dosaged dissection of the circumferential ligament of Kokott, circa 1973.

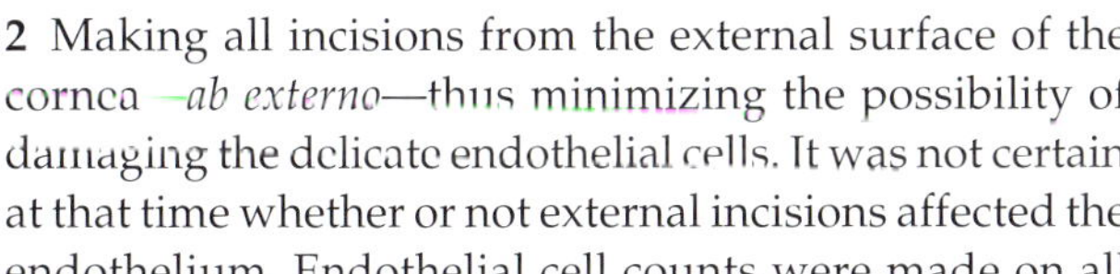

2 Making all incisions from the external surface of the cornea—*ab externo*—thus minimizing the possibility of damaging the delicate endothelial cells. It was not certain at that time whether or not external incisions affected the endothelium. Endothelial cell counts were made on all patients in the very beginning of RK because of the concern that incising the cornea might somehow act to produce cell damage. It was evident, however, from these examinations that no significant cell loss was occurring and that the cell loss described in Sato's patients was a consequence of direct trauma to the endothelium itself. (Figure 7.19).

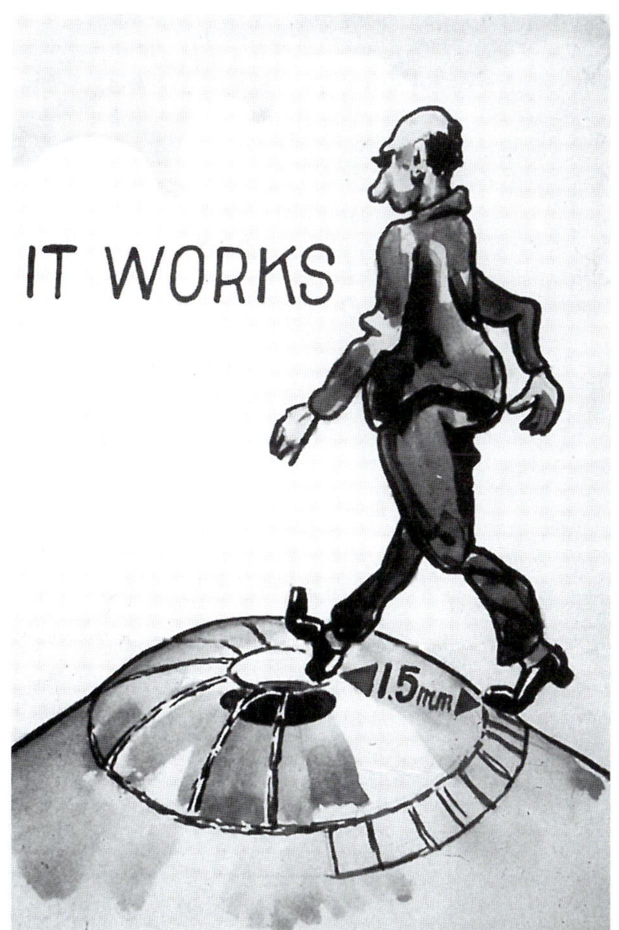

Fig. 7.18 Making the zone smaller than 6.0 mm works.

3 Basing incision depth on actual measurements of corneal thickness using optical pachymetry—verifying the depth of the incisions with specially constructed gauges or "dipsticks" (Figure 7.21).

4 Using ultrasharp disposable razor fragments to make the incisions. At first, these incisions were made free-hand with an unguarded blade using special gauges called *corneal dipsticks* to check progress.

5 Limiting incisions to 32 made from the limbus that converge on a premarked optical zone using a microscope with all its advantages to do the surgery.

It was apparent from the beginning that the use of an unguarded blade would produce an incision of uneven

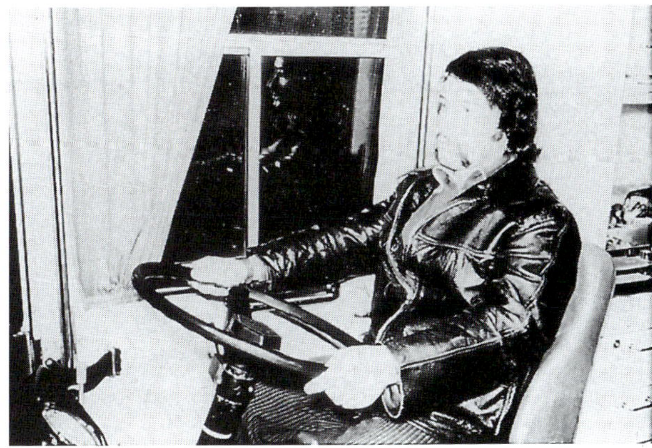

Fig. 7.20 The first RK patient—Mischa, the author's driver.

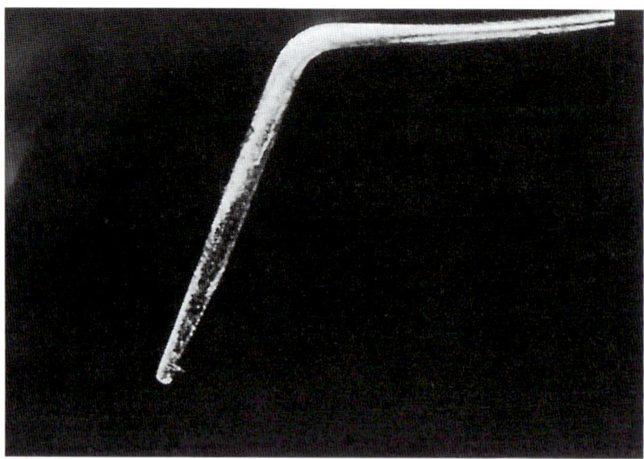

Fig. 7.21 Original Fyodorov dipstick.

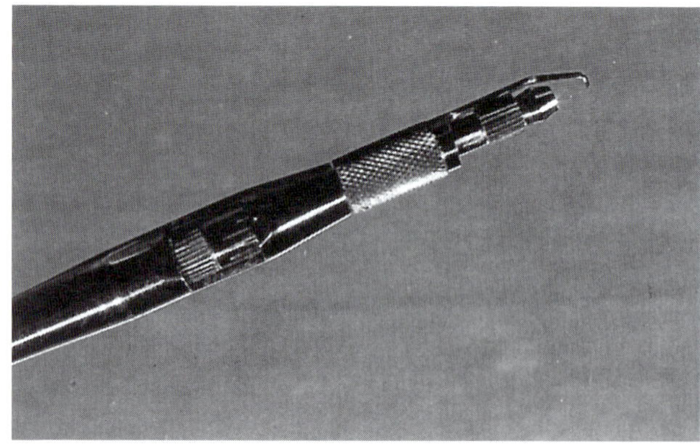

Fig. 7.22 Second-generation Fyodorov micrometer knife.

depth that could be responsible for the variation in effect from patient to patient and the consequent difficulty in predicting the outcome. In addition, the smaller optical zones (2.0 to 2.5 mm) were difficult to center. Some of these patients complained of glare at night, and some of the incisions tended to join up at the edge of the optical zone—especially in patients in whom 32 corneal incisions had been made. The first step in solving these problems was the fabrication of a micrometrically adjustable knife handle that allowed precise control of incision depth (Figure 7.22). At the same time, a marking device (originally called a *pizza-cutter*, an unfortunate choice of name because many people believed, without first checking, that this was the device that produced the incisions) was developed to make lines or marks on the corneal surface along which the surgeon could guide his knife (Figure 7.23). This was necessary in the Soviet method because incisions made from the limbus toward the center have a tendency to approach the optical zone tangentially (like turbine blades) instead of in a perpendicular manner (Figure 7.24).

Ongoing work with rabbit eyes suggested that a reduction in the number of incisions would not be accompanied by any significant lessening of effect until the number of incisions fell below 16 (Figure 7.25). This was good news because one of the difficulties experienced in the early patients was that of keeping the ends of the incisions from joining up centrally (Figure 7.26). Patients with 8 incisions at that time showed not only a profound loss of effect (40% to 50%) but also showed a significant increase in surgically induced astigmatism. Reduction of the number of incisions from 32 to 16, however, solved the problem not only of incisional joining but also, to a great extent, of glare. Comparing the results of 16 and 32 incisions of equal depth and length showed no significant difference in effect [29]. Additionally, it was found through actual application that increasing the number of incisions beyond 32 *decreased* the effect of the surgery (see Figure 7.25). It is interesting to note that the effect of 40 incisions was almost identical to that of 8 incisions. This phenomenon is undoubtedly one of the reasons for the poor overall results in Sato's patients. It should be recalled that in Sato's patients, 40 or more incisions were made routinely in each cornea, resulting in an average reduction in myopia of 3.0 D. The failure of more incisions (beyond a certain number) to produce a greater response has to do with the mechanism whereby the central corneal curvature is caused to flatten.

(a)

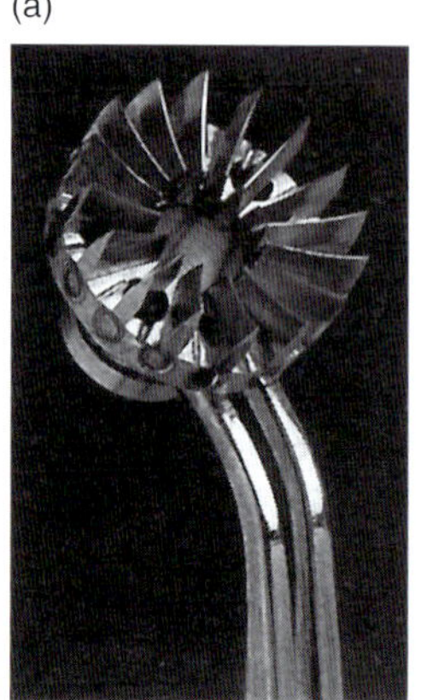

(b)

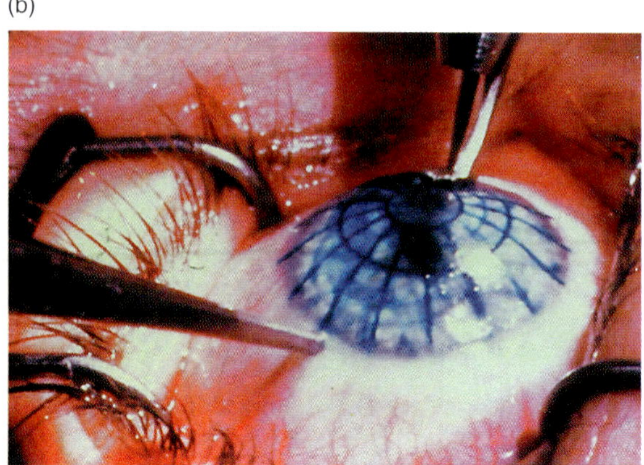

Fig. 7.23 (a) A 16-ray incision marker—the "pizza-cutter." (b) Incision guide marks are necessary in the Russian method.

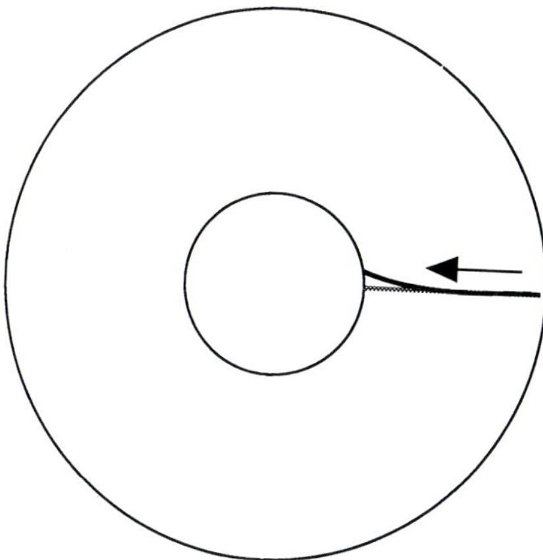

Fig. 7.24 Incisions made from the limbus tend to meet the central optical zone tangentially.

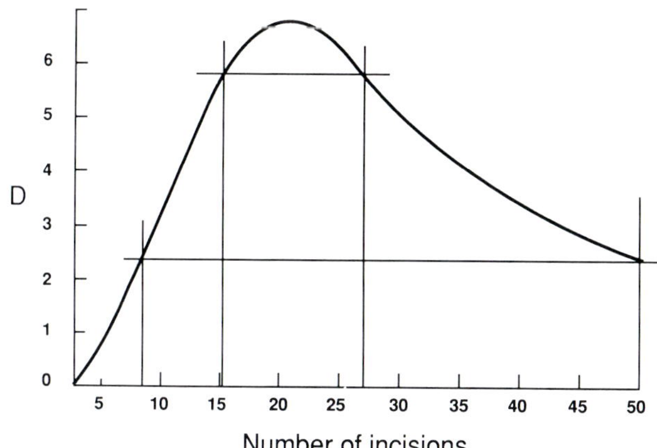

Fig. 7.25 Effect of incision number on outcome.

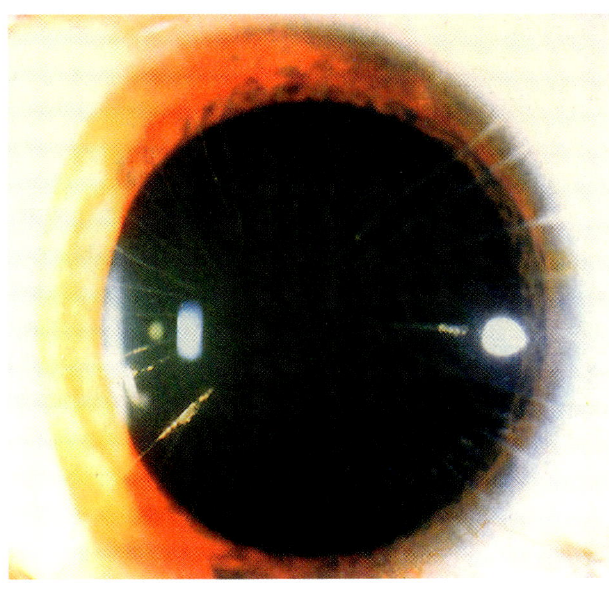

Fig. 7.26 Early 32-incision RK. Note that the central incisions join in some cases.

Mechanism of RK

The effects of the procedure depend on the temporary structural weakening of the corneal periphery, thus allowing internal ocular pressure to move this area outward (Figure 7.27). This small movement of the periphery produces tension both on the scleral ring and on the unincised central clear zone. The scleral ring resists distortion, and therefore, most of the resulting force acts on the central cornea. The effect of this force is to produce an increase in the chord length of the central arc with a concomitant reduction in its sagittal height (Figure 7.28). In short, the corneal curvature becomes more flattened (Figure 7.29).

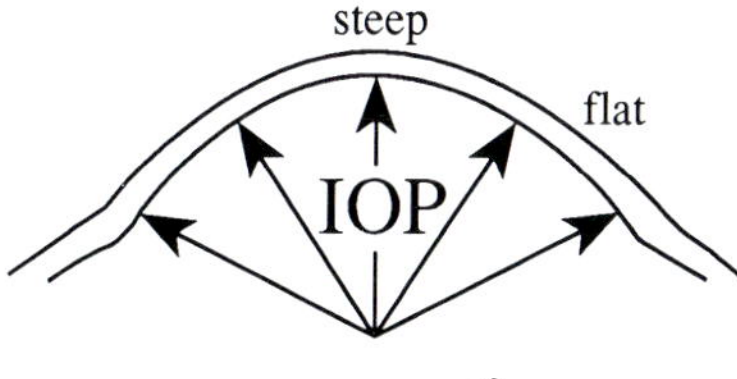

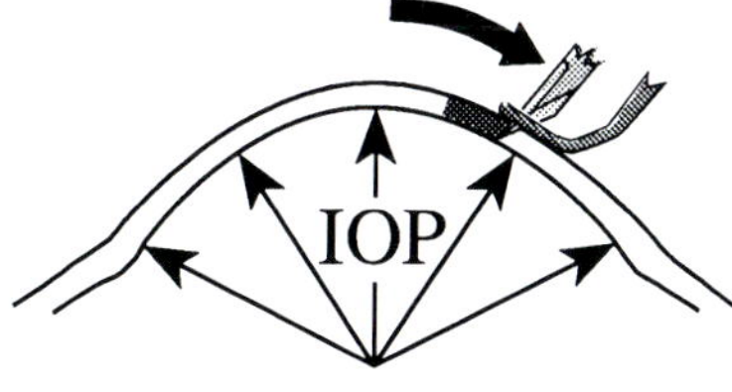

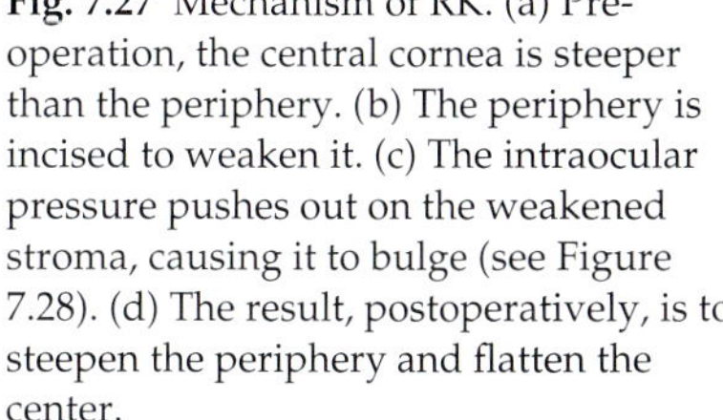

Fig. 7.27 Mechanism of RK. (a) Pre-operation, the central cornea is steeper than the periphery. (b) The periphery is incised to weaken it. (c) The intraocular pressure pushes out on the weakened stroma, causing it to bulge (see Figure 7.28). (d) The result, postoperatively, is to steepen the periphery and flatten the center.

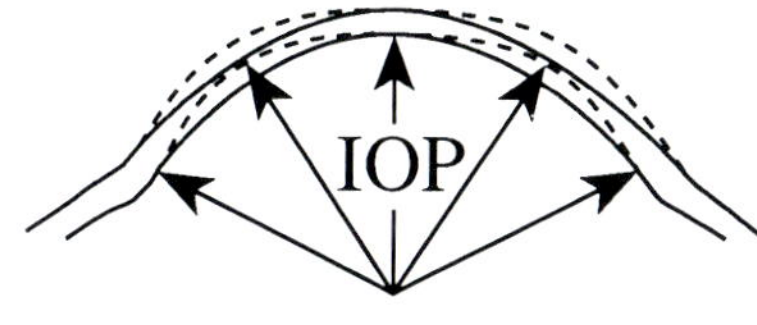

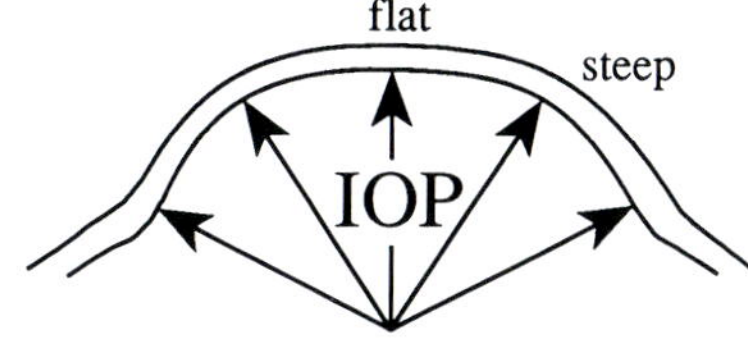

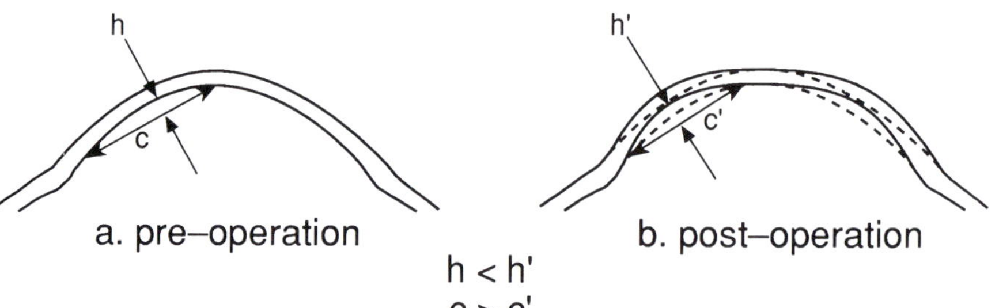

Fig. 7.28 After surgery the bulging of the cornea shortens the chord length in the periphery and lengthens the chord in the center, flattening it.

This flattening effect depends on pressure acting on the tissue bands that lie between incisions and which connect the more flexible central clear zone with the relatively inflexible limbus. In materials science, it is sometimes seen that the modulus of elasticity of a material changes when its cross-sectional dimension also changes. As the section becomes thinner, the material will distort more before fracture occurs than will a thicker section—the material has become more "stretchy" or malleable. Thus, as the pressure acts on these thinner corneal tissue bands, much of the tension is lost through stretching—the periphery bulges more—rather than acting on the clear zone to induce flattening. Therefore, incisions in excess of 16 are superfluous and not only serve to reduce the ultimate effect of the surgery but also may introduce additional problems such as glare or even irregular astigmatism (see also Chapter 15).

In the literature there are two models related to an estimation of curvature change due to RK in which the cornea is considered as a uniform sphere. The model in the current discussion is based on the concept of effective thickness associated with cutting of fibrils by the incisions and is based on the analysis promulgated by Huang [30]. These types of analyses are important in

(a)

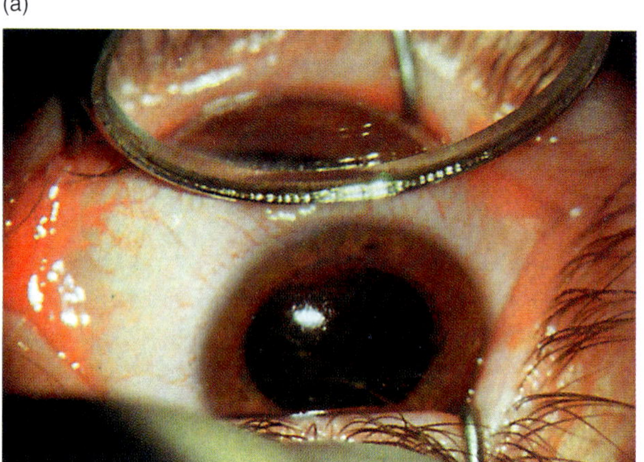

(b)

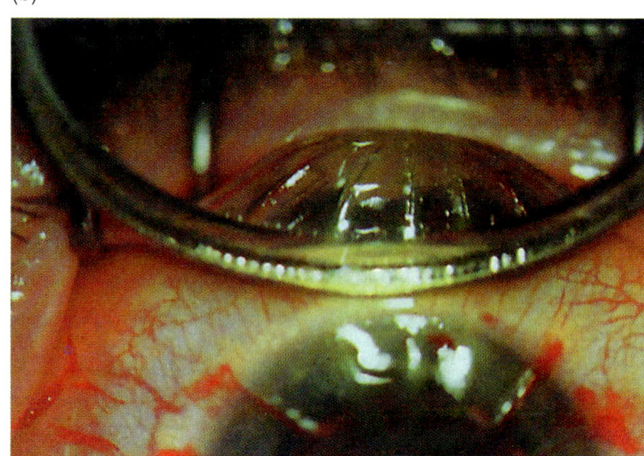

(c)

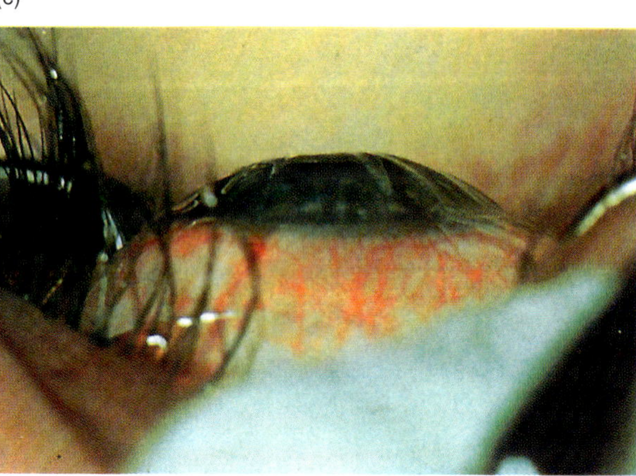

Fig. 7.29 (a) Preoperative cornea—note the prolate shape. (b) Postoperative cornea—note the oblate shape. (c) Side view shows the flattening better.

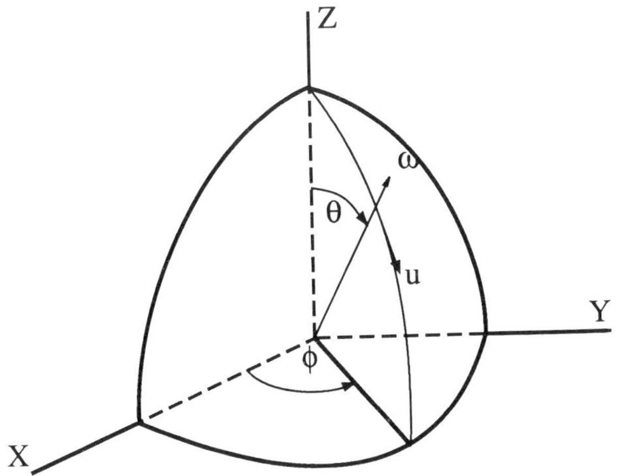

Fig. 7.30 General (simple) tensor diagram.

elastic modulus ratios are very low. The cornea is an example of such a shell. These deformations become obvious in the vicinity of some locations, such as partial-thickness incisions (Figure 7.32). Under certain circumstances, this local severe transverse shear deformation may rise sharply and influence the entire structural response. The mathematics of the analysis of such a shell are complex but are well detailed by Reissner and Whitney for those so inclined [32–34].

There are many factors that, acting together, determine the extent to which the cornea will respond to this stromal weakening. Some of these are physical properties—such as modulus of elasticity—that are poorly understood or whose elucidation is lacking in the human. However, some assumptions can be made about these factors that appear to have a bearing on the actual mechanism of RK.

deriving algorithms that can precisely predict the outcome of this surgery.

Figures 7.30 and 7.31 are tensor diagrams outlining the effect of incisions on this theoretical thin corneal shell. Figure 7.30 is a generalized tensor, whereas Figure 7.31 is specific for a cornea undergoing RK. However, Kirchoff-Love assumptions, typically used to describe thin elastic plates, are inadequate for this purpose when dealing with impaired shells such as found in the human cornea undergoing incisional weakening. Therefore, another method needs to be applied—transverse shear deformation analysis [31]. Moderate to severe transverse shear deformations appear in certain types of composite plates and shells in which the transverse shear modulus to in-plane

Early attempts at predicting outcome

The problem of predictability was tackled by an extensive retrospective analysis of the patients in whom surgery had already been performed. From this analysis it was found that certain factors seemed to control the outcome of the surgery, namely:

Optical zone. Since the size of the optical zone decreased, the amount of correction increased (Figure 7.33).

Keratometry. Since the corneal refractive power increased, the amount of correction also increased (Figure 7.34).

Corneal diameter. Since the corneal diameter increased, there was a corresponding increase in the amount of the correction (Figure 7.35).

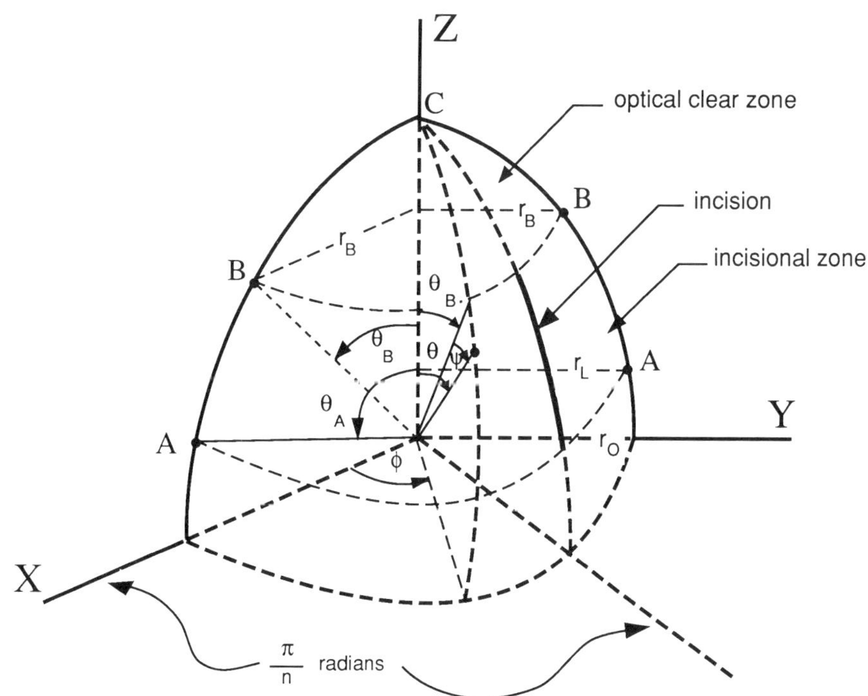

Fig. 7.31 Complex tensor diagram.

(a)

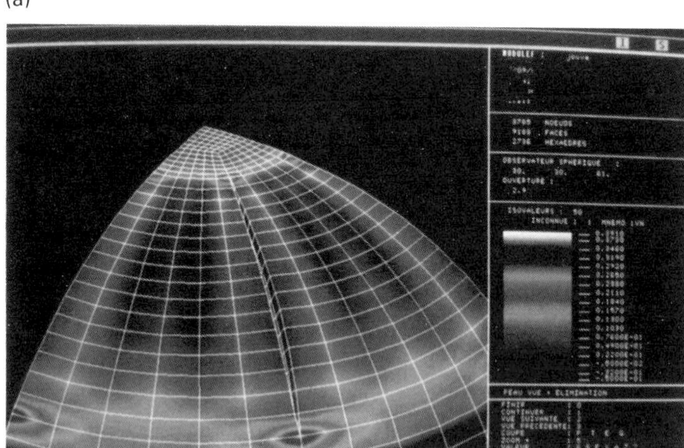

(b)

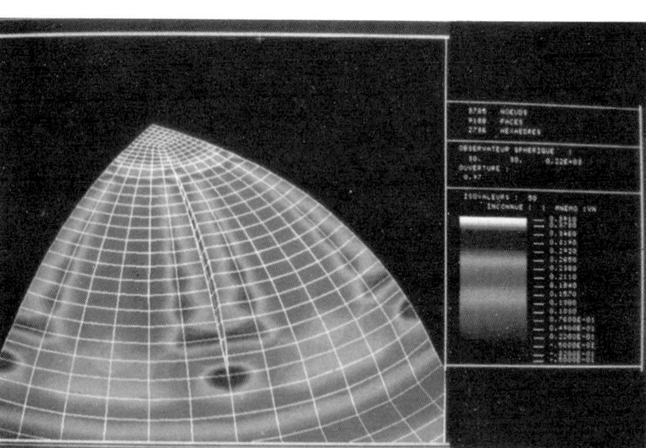

(c)

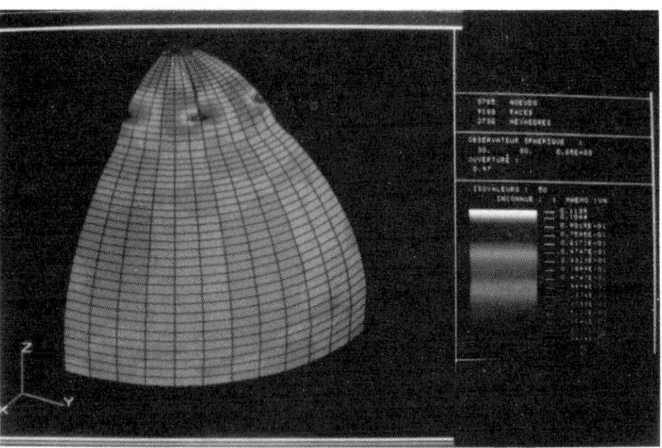

Fig. 7.32 Finite analysis of stress pattern in incised cornea. (a) Hoop stress; (b) meridianal stress; (c) combination of hoop and meridianal stress. Note the compound curvature, which could account for the multifocal effect seen in some post-RK eyes.

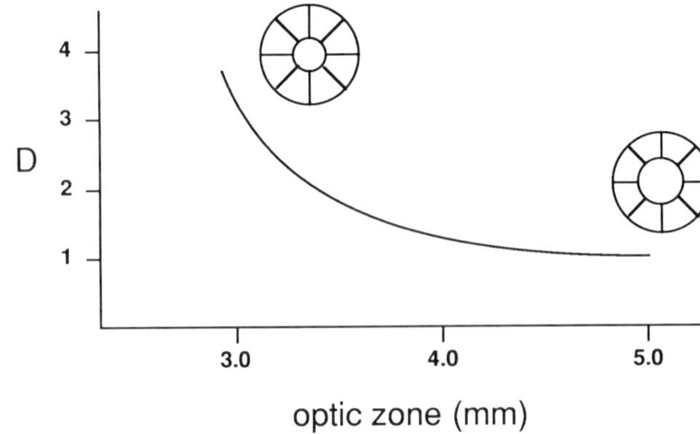

Fig. 7.33 Effect of changing optical zone size.

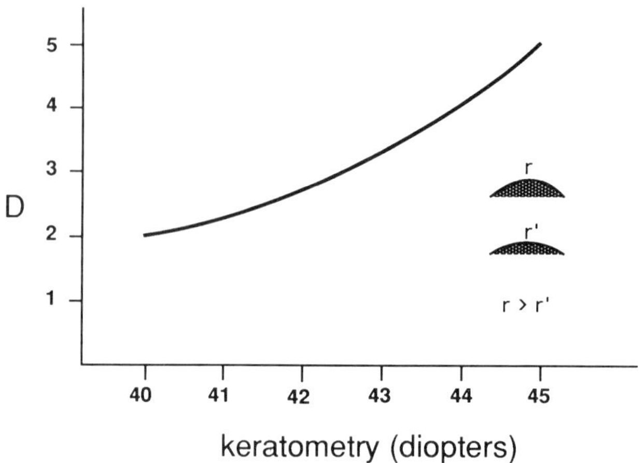

Fig. 7.34 Effect of corneal curvature.

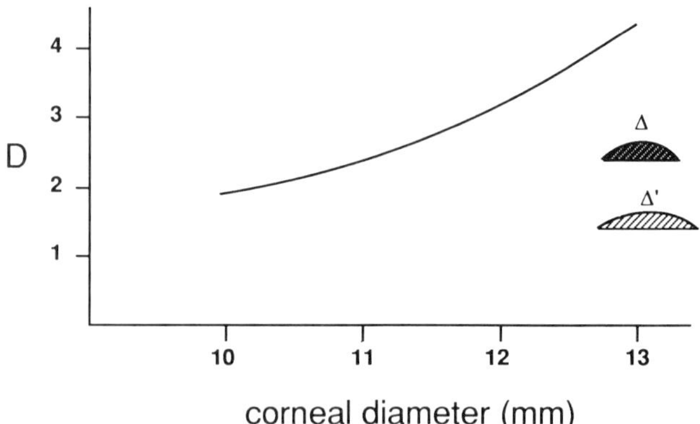

Fig. 7.35 Effect of corneal diameter.

Corneal rigidity. Since the cornea became stiffer, the amount of correction increased (Figure 7.36). This may seem illogical, but it is, nevertheless, true.

Practical coefficient of the surgeon (see below). This latter factor, which eventually became known as the *incisional depth coefficient*, was an attempt to account for individual variations in the technique of the surgeon and was designed to be optimized as experience increased. It became quickly apparent that what was really being described was the effective depth of the incisions, which increased as the surgeon became more skilled at making them and less timid in setting his or her blade (see the section on blades, below).

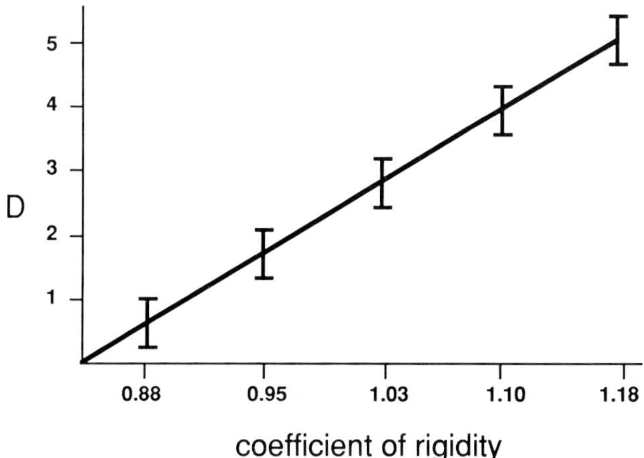

Fig. 7.36 Effect of corneal rigidity.

From these observations, a formula was constructed:

$$P = \frac{\sqrt{D^2 + \frac{16}{3}\left(R \quad \sqrt{R^2 - \frac{D^2}{4}}\right)^2 - \sqrt{d^2 + \frac{16}{3}\left(R - \sqrt{R^2 - \frac{d^2}{4}}\right)^2}}}{\sqrt{d^2 + \frac{16}{3}\left(R - \sqrt{R^2 - \frac{d^2}{4}}\right)^2}} \cdot K \cdot \alpha$$

This calculates the effect of surgery P given that D is the diameter of cornea in millimeters, R is the radius of cornea in millimeters, K is the coefficient of corneal rigidity, and α is the incisional depth coefficient. This allowed the surgeon to predict (within ±1.00 D) the outcome of the surgery in most cases—*at 1 year*. The latter is important. Many physicians ignored that bit and ended up with overcorrections through ill-advised "adjusting" of their surgery because of perceived undercorrections. Other factors eventually were found to play a role and will be discussed later in this chapter.

Early changes in technique

I made some fundamental changes in the technique with my first patient (described in the "Introduction to the First Edition") that had some far-reaching effects and which forced a different perspective to be focused on the subject of RK.

It was disturbing to me that the incisions were being made from the limbus toward the center. This methodology was then, as now, technically difficult and had the very real potential for causing a disaster should the patient move at the wrong instant—thus possibly causing an invasion of the optical zone and/or the optical axis. Even if the patient did not move, making the incisions from limbus to center requires that pressure on the blade be released at just the proper instant to prevent its stopping before the edge of the optical zone is reached. Attempts to "restart" the blade in such an event require that excessive pressure be placed on the knife to start it moving again. This is true even with ultrasharp crystalline blades—especially if the eye is soft. This excess pressure inevitably produces a sudden jumping forward of the blade as tissue resistance is overcome, almost always resulting in an invasion of the optical clear zone. Additionally, the incisions have a very real tendency to wander off-course and, unless each one is premarked, connect with the central zone mark in a tangential manner.

Therefore, beginning with my first solo patient in 1978, all the incisions were made from the central clear zone to the limbus, and all were made across from one another in pairs (i.e., 6 and 12 and 3 and 9 o'clock, etc.) and not "around the clock," as Fyodorov was doing. Doing it this way eliminated the danger of invading the optical zone. The incisions also invariably were very straight and perpendicular to the edge of the surgical clear zone, and there was an even number of them. Another benefit of making the incisions in this manner was that they spread around the effect of any incisional depth irregularity—a major concern given the quality of the blades used at that time. Because there is an ongoing change in corneal thickness during the surgery—something that begins to happen the moment Bowman's layer is incised—the order in which the incisions are made is of primary importance. In addition, the intraocular pressure of the eye decreases as each incision is made because the ciliary body is unable to keep pace with the increase in ocular volume that occurs as the incised tissue expands outward. It is reasonable, therefore, to expect that some variation in actual incisional depth will occur with each additional incision as the resistance to cutting also decreases (see the section on blades, below). While these changes may be small by themselves, they have a cumulative effect and, being grouped or adjacent, will induce more or less flattening in a localized area—thereby producing irregular astigmatism. This is not just a theoretical concern.

Some of my early patients, who had been done in the Soviet manner, did indeed show just such astigmatism—especially the "wet" cases. It therefore made considerable sense to make incisions in horizontally opposed pairs—each incision in the pair being made 180° to the other (Figure 7.37). Making the incisions in this way also tends to reduce the opportunity to "drop" an incision—something very likely to happen with premarking of the incision tracks, as in the Fyodorov (out-to-in) or even in the Bores (in-to-out) technique (see Table 7.2). This is

Table 7.2 The first nomogram used in radial keratotomy

Optical zone diameter (mm)	Effect (D)
4.5	0.75–1.25
4.0	1.50–2.00
3.5	2.25–2.50
3.0	>2.75

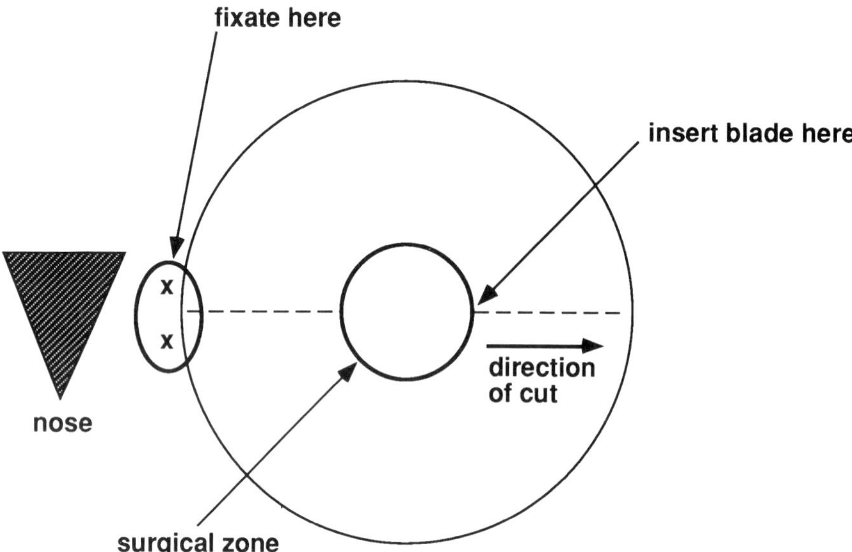

even more likely to occur with the neophyte keratotomist and is *one* of the reasons that I recommend against such marking with my method. The marking material tends to obscure the incision track and may make it seem that an incision has been made when in fact it has not. Careful attention must be paid to this potential problem when making incisions in the Russian manner, where such pre-marking is essential.

Blades and pachymetry

The evolution of blades used for this surgery is inextricably meshed with that of pachymetry—the measurement of corneal thickness. However, at first, for a given blade setting—all else being as equal as possible—the results obtained were different from what the Russians were reporting, and so were the incisions. While I and my coworker (William Myers, M.D.) were obtaining a good surgical effect initially, we were losing far more of it (56%) than Fyodorov had been reporting (20%). Our patients also were complaining of more glare at night. We also noted that our incisions were not as deep as the blade settings, and furthermore, the shallower incisions were mainly to be found in the last eight incisions. It was obvious that the blade we were using at that time (Beaver No. 76a), either because of its thickness, finish, or sharpness (or all three), was not cutting to its set depth. Also, the incisions were somewhat "ragged," and the resulting scars were slightly wider than with our current blades. This, coupled with the fact that the eye became softer as more and more incisions were made (offering less resistance and therefore causing the tissue to "flow" away from the blade), resulted in shallow incisions from the outset that became even shallower as the surgery went on. These findings necessitated a careful reconsideration of the then-current methodology.

It turned out that this incision shallowing was due in part to the direction in which the incisions were being made [35,36]. If you are one of those "logical" types used to "dry-labbing" (resorting to theory without benefit of practical experience), this statement may not make sense. Why would the direction of cut make any difference in the incision depth? Well, as I have said many times before, where this surgery is concerned, the scoreboard shows Eye 20; Theory 0. The direction of the cut does make a difference and must be considered; this observation has been corroborated by others [37]. Binder also has suggested that centrifugal incision scars (in-to-out) tend to be thinner than centripetal incision scars (out-to-in) [38]. While I have not noted this change in particular, it could be that this is related to depth of the incision, with a greater tendency of the incision to gape. It should be said that greater incision depth and subsequent wider scarring may be operational in producing the progressive corneal flattening reported in some patients (see also Chapter 15) [39–41].

The human cornea, as a rule, is thinner centrally than in the periphery—although there are exceptions to this rule. This fact introduces certain variables that affect the outcome of RK—in fact, they affect *all* refractive surgical procedures. Whereas it may be true (as taught by Barraquer) that one cannot really change the shape of the cornea without involving Bowman's layer, it is equally true that the amount of ultimate curvature change depends on distortion of the entire cornea—and this relates to tissue thickness.

The first factor to be considered is that the inner curvature of the cornea is less than the outer. Consequently, this surface is more myopic than the front and is arbitrarily given a value of –5.85 D. When this power is subtracted from the front surface curvature (in diopters), the so-called effective power of the cornea is obtained (see the discussion in Chapter 5 and "The Importance of Keratometry," below). The difficulty is that we have found that not all corneas behave the same way with respect to the gradient or delta of their thickness increase (or to put it another way, the decreasing radius of curvature toward the periphery). Naturally, this leads to errors in obtaining the true refractive power of the cornea itself. However, until recently, there has not existed—nor has there really been a need for—methods to measure the inner curvature (see also Chapter 6).

The second factor is that this variability in corneal thickness assures the surgeon that his or her incision is nowhere of uniform effect along its length—except in rare instances. It was this latter factor that led to the use of stepped incisions to overcome this handicap. This stepped-incision technique, of course, led to the introduction of other variables into the equation and, while solving some problems, created other problems in its wake.

It was evident—after examining the outcome of the early patients—that depth of incision was a major factor in the surgical result, as well as in the variability of results seen in otherwise similar patients. Several attempts were made to solve this problem, and ultimately, it required an inversion in thinking to obtain the final "solution." The first part of the solution was in recognizing that the practice of setting the blade based on a percentage of the corneal thickness was not valid. While it is true that the relationship of incision depth to initial corneal thickness is constant with this method—the effectiveness of a given incision is not. I had been taking paracentral pachymetry measurements and setting the blade to 75% of that—a method I considered more accurate and reliable than that used by the Soviets. Up to that time, they had been measuring the central corneal thickness and taking 75% of that for their blade setting. Later, they modified the method by adding 40 μm to the central corneal thickness and setting the blade to that measurement.

I at first reasoned that it would be a better idea to set the blade depth based on the pachymetry *minus* a certain amount (Figure 7.38). When I reflected on the fact that the amount of curvature change depended on stromal weakening and that the degree of that weakening, in turn, was affected by incision depth, I quickly recognized that the ultimate factor in the amount of weakening was not the depth per se but the amount of tissue left uncut at the bottom of the incision! It therefore made sense to concentrate on keeping that value as near constant as possible from patient to patient. Hence it was logical to establish a given blade length by *subtracting*, from the pachymetry, a given amount and then using the result as the blade setting. In this manner, a specific amount of tissue would be left uncut at the bottom of each incision in each patient (i.e., the amount of tissue from the bottom of the incision to Descemet's membrane)—at least at the beginning of the incision.

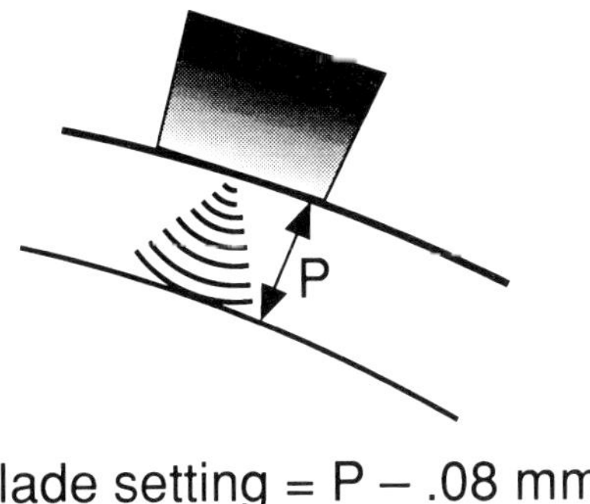

Fig. 7.38 Early method of blade setting.

The reason for this change was that I had observed that while the paracentral readings varied markedly from patient to patient (within limits) and bore no predictable relationship to the central readings, the central readings were remarkably consistent among patients. Since the surgery works by exerting a pulling force on the uncut central cornea, causing primarily flexion instead of stretch—and thereby flattening the central curvature—it seemed logical that by making the uncut corneal lamella the same thickness for each patient, the variability from patient to patient would be reduced. To test this thesis, I operated on a series of patients in whom one eye was done with the older method and the other with the new technique. I found not only more consistent results but, more important, also greater corneal flattening overall (Figure 7.39). This change did not, however, solve the need for maximizing the effect of the incision because the incision—for the most part—still became relatively shallower toward the periphery.

To compensate for the additional shallowing still occurring in the last eight incisions, I began to extend the blade even further for those incisions. That is, I extended the blade an additional 25 μm before making the last eight incisions in the pattern (see also "Wet versus dry," below). It was a natural extension of the previous thinking to take the further step of peripheral incision deepening in all patients. It was logical to assume that since deeper incisions worked with a single-depth incision, deepening the peripheral portion of that same incision—thereby keeping as constant a lamellar thickness as possible throughout its length—should make the surgical results still better. No effective way, at that time (nor yet), has been devised to adjust the blade length dynamically or continuously while incising, so a more practical method of altering incision depth was employed.

By examining a series of pachymetric measurements, it was determined that a significant change in corneal thickness occurred at approximately 6 mm from the optical center. This occurred again between 8 and 9 mm. Therefore, it was decided to make the incisions deeper in a stepwise manner. That is, each incision would be of one depth from the primary optical zone to 6.0 mm and

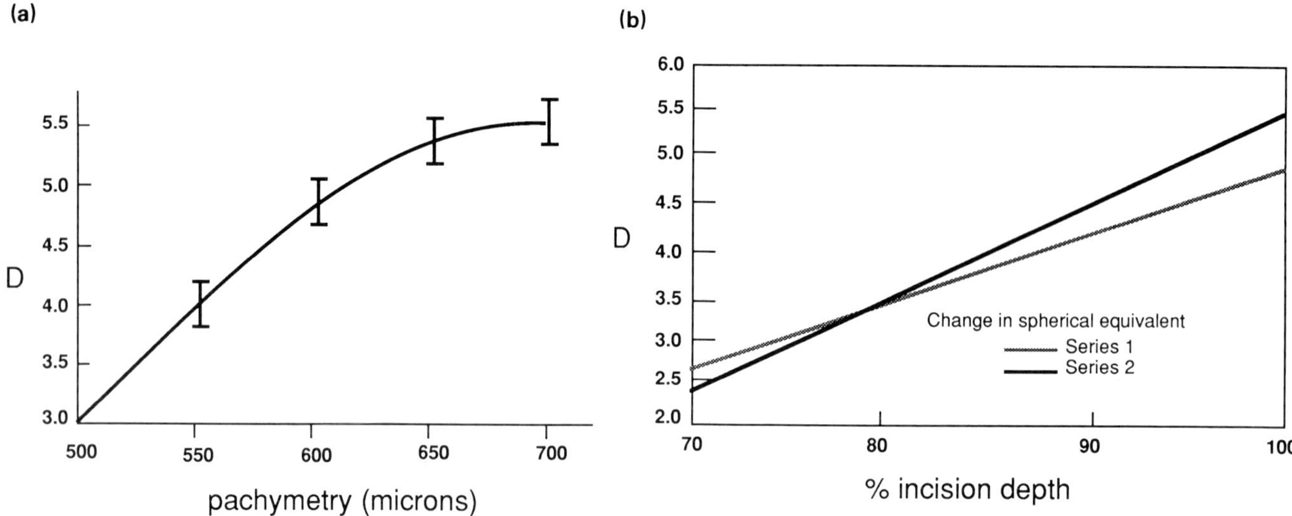

Fig. 7.39 (a, b) Effect of deeper blade settings on outcome. ((b) Courtesy of M. Deitz.)

another from there to the limbus (Figure 7.40). In some patients, an intermediate step was made from 6 to 8 mm and from there a deeper pass to the limbus. This technique resulted in considerably greater initial effect coupled with less surgical rebound [42]. This method was first applied in a series of patients in August of 1979, and the results were communicated to Fyodorov in November of that year. He began to use this technique as well and corroborated my initial findings in December 1979. With certain modifications of this principle, permanent corrections of up to 14 D of myopia have been obtained with RK (see also Chapter 8).

At first this stepping of the incisions was done by making the entire incision of one depth from the primary optical zone to the limbus. The blade would then be

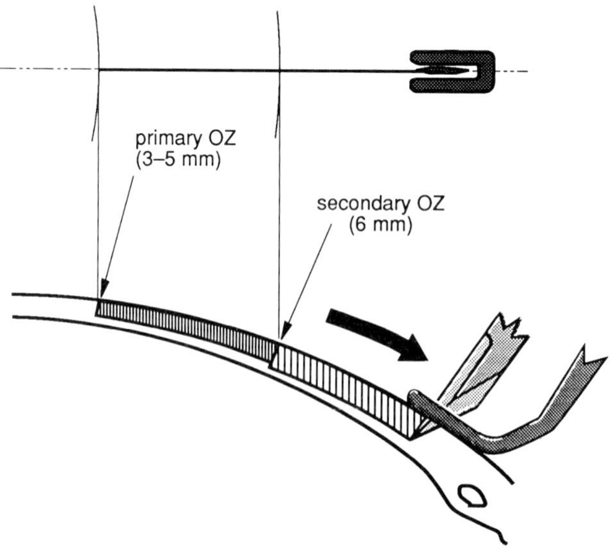

Fig. 7.40 Basic principle of the stepped incision.

advanced the required length and reinserted into the incision at 6.0 mm, and the incision would be retraced to the limbus—deepening it. This method was relatively straightforward. It was, however, not without potential problems. If the redeepening procedure was not done carefully, it was possible (at least theoretically) to produce an incision with a double bottom in the shape of an inverted Y (Figure 7.41). This could occur if too much pressure was applied to the knife handle both downward and tangentially and also if fixation was not applied exactly at 180°. This does not occur with free-hand deepening using a wound spreader and also did not occur with a guarded blade if the blade was inserted carefully into the incision and the knife blade stroked gently to the limbus, allowing the sides of the incision to guide the blade. It is only when excess pressure is applied that the blade will wander. This is true even in making primary incisions. Sufficient pressure should be exerted so as to maintain firm but gentle contact between the knife jaw and the corneal surface. In so doing, the incisions will be straight and perpendicular, and in the case of redeepening, the knife will not fall into the incision. Myers labeled this the Bores "feather touch" technique. Incisional *flaying* was never shown to be a real occurrence, except in one or two instances in which the surgeon forced the effect to prove a point (see also Chapter 8). The relatively dull edges of steel razor fragments used at that time made such a technique viable, yet it eventually was abandoned for a different and more effective approach. Interestingly, despite evidence that such incision stepping is effective in increasing the reduction of myopia, this technique is not employed by all RK surgeons—perhaps it seems too difficult.

With the advent of sharper blades, particularly those of crystalline materials such as sapphire or diamond, the danger of incision flaying became real. This reason, plus

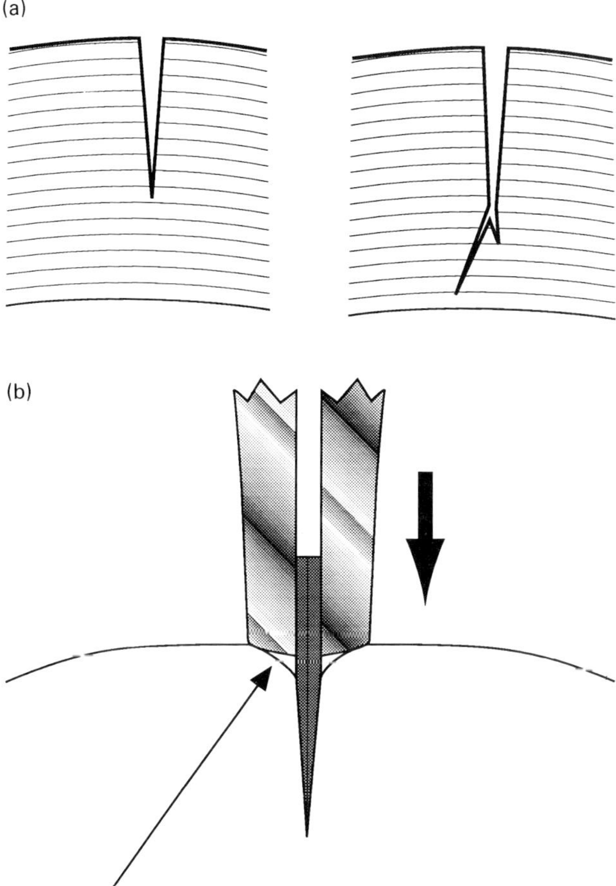

Fig. 7.41 (a) Y-shaped incision bottom. (b) The wound tends to open and spread.

another, caused me to begin to make some of the incisions in a truly stepwise manner. To avoid this potential flaying problem, a modification of technique has been made. The first part of the incision is made from the edge of the optical zone to just past the edge of the premarked midperipheral zone (usually 6 mm) (Figure 7.42). The blade is then reset and reinserted into the previous incision just before the edge of the midperipheral zone (see Figure 7.40). It is then carried to the periphery through uncut corneal tissue (see Figure 7.41). This has the advantage of producing deep peripheral incisions even with a very soft eye such as when a microperforation has occurred.

As my understanding of the dynamics of incision making grew, it became evident that the steel blades did not cut, at least initially, to the set depth. This was suggested by the fact that incisions made from the limbus (the so-called Fyodorov or Russian method) were deeper centrally than those made from the center (the so-called Bores or American method) with the same setting. The reason for this phenomenon was soon apparent.

An examination shows the corneal stroma to be made up of an interlacing network of keratocytes arranged in layers (lamella) akin to French pastry (see Figure 7.42). Each of these keratocytes has a diameter of approximately 300 Å. The edge radius of a typical steel razor blade, however, is in the neighborhood of 15,000 Å. Within and between the cells there is fluid that is kept under very precise control by the endothelium to maintain corneal transparency. The presence of this fluid makes the tissue spongelike—not in the real sense that it is compressible, because it is not, only in that it resembles a sponge in which fluid is interspersed between substance.

The cornea is also a very thin, domelike structure that receives its support primarily from the limbus. When a blade is pressed against its surface, tissue resistance is finally overcome, and the blade passes downward through the epithelium and Bowman's layer into the stroma. This resistance is not easily overcome because the tissue tends to bend over the relatively large blade edge radius (Figures 7.43 and 7.44). As the blade passes downward, it pushes tissue ahead of it until the tissue cannot move anymore, whereupon the blade cuts through it. The resistance to tissue movement becomes less the deeper the blade penetrates until, rather than cut, the blade merely pushes the tissue ahead (Figure 7.45). With further movement downward, resistance to stretch occurs, and the tissue will be cut. If, however, the blade reaches its maximum depth before this point, the tissue will remain draped over the edge (or tented up over the blade tip) and will not be cut (Figure 7.46).

Contrariwise, by introducing the blade into the thicker limbal tissue and moving it toward the center, the incision has reached its maximum effective depth well in advance of its reaching its inner extremity at the primary optical clear zone [37]. While this condition may have merit, cutting from the limbus carries with it some heavy penalties, both real and potential, emphasizing once again the old expression *"You can't get somethin' for nuthin!"*

This also means that a blade of given length inserted into the cornea and drawn toward the periphery will penetrate less far initially than the same blade inserted at the limbus, where there is more resistance. In the process of moving the blade, eventually it will cut its way down almost to its set length. Therefore, when cutting from limbus to center (out-to-in), the maximum incision depth will be in the vicinity of the optical zone, whereas in the opposite direction (in-to-out), it will be somewhat shallower there (Figures 7.47 and 7.48). In order to get maximal depth with the American method, the surgeon has to set the blade longer. In addition, I have found that while the length of the entire incision is important, the part of the incision closer to the optical zone seems to be most important. This area, which I have chosen to call the *critical zone*, extends from 3 to 6 mm (Figure 7.49). It is in this area that the maximum change in corneal curvature occurs [43]. In this transition zone, deep incisions permit a smoother curvature change without formation of the so-called knee described in the earlier patients [44].

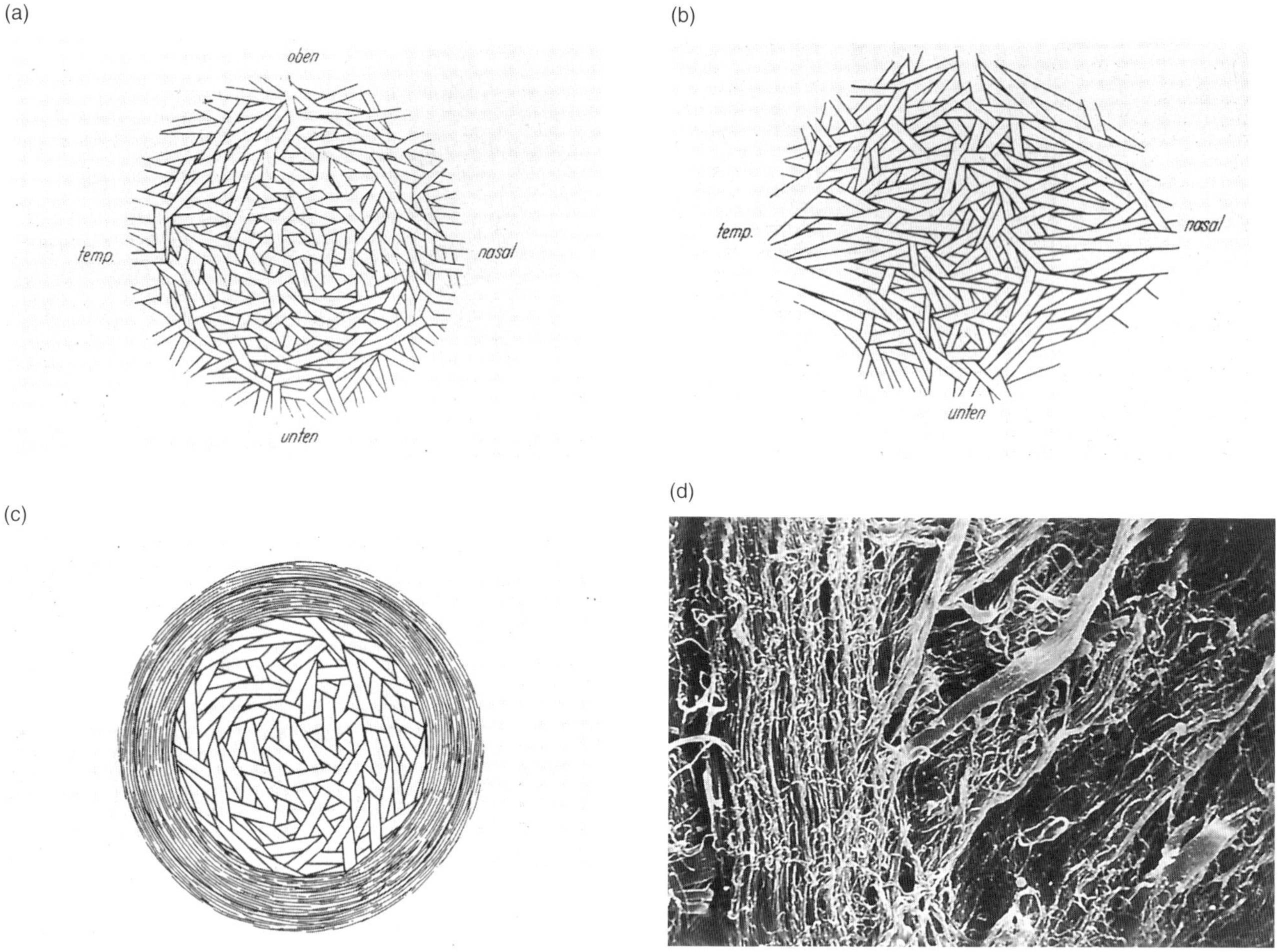

(a)

oben

temp.

nasal

unten

(b)

temp.

nasal

unten

(c)

(d)

Fig. 7.42 (a, b) Kokott's dissection of the cornea revealing the interlaced arrangement of the keratocytes. (c) The deepest layers with the peripheral cells arranged in a circular manner—the so-called circumferential ligament of Kokott. (d) SEM of corneal stroma showing the same circular arrangement.

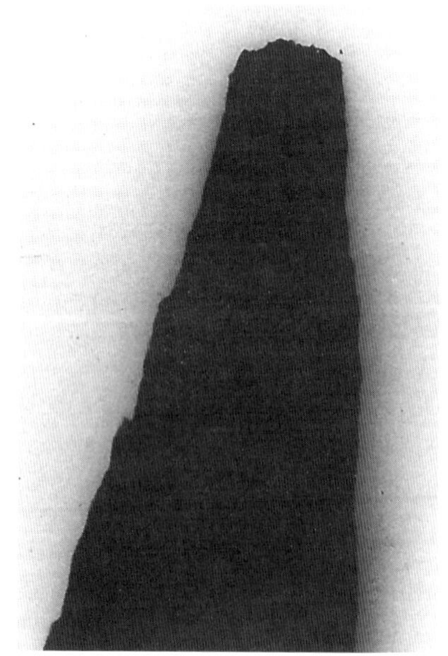

Fig. 7.43 SEM of typical razor blade.

It seemed that a practical expedient to solve the problem of the blade's not cutting deep enough would be to add a factor or bias to the corneal thickness to arrive at a specific blade setting. To test this theory, I began adding small amounts to the blade setting for each patient [36,42]. I continued to advance the blade length to attain maximal incision depth until I was setting blades up to 115% of the paracentral pachymetry (with steel blades). This additional blade length has been named *blade bias* and is blade-dependent—that is, each blade regardless of material, requires that its own unique bias be determined. Laboratory studies have corroborated my early teaching that setting to 100% of the pachymetry yields an incision depth of 80% to 85% [45].

The advent of ultrasonic pachymetry

Initially, optical pachymetry was used to obtain the corneal thickness (Figure 7.50). This method of corneal thickness measurement is fraught with difficulties. It is not the least of its problems that it is not accurate, nor can it be

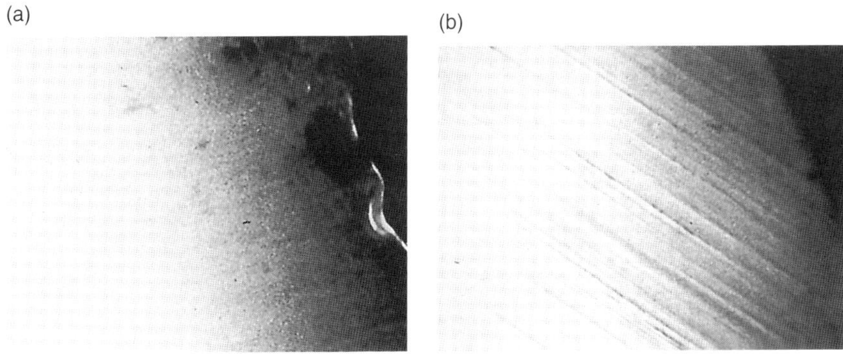

Fig. 7.44 (a) The edge of a typical razor blade fragment. (b) Honed steel blade designed for RK.

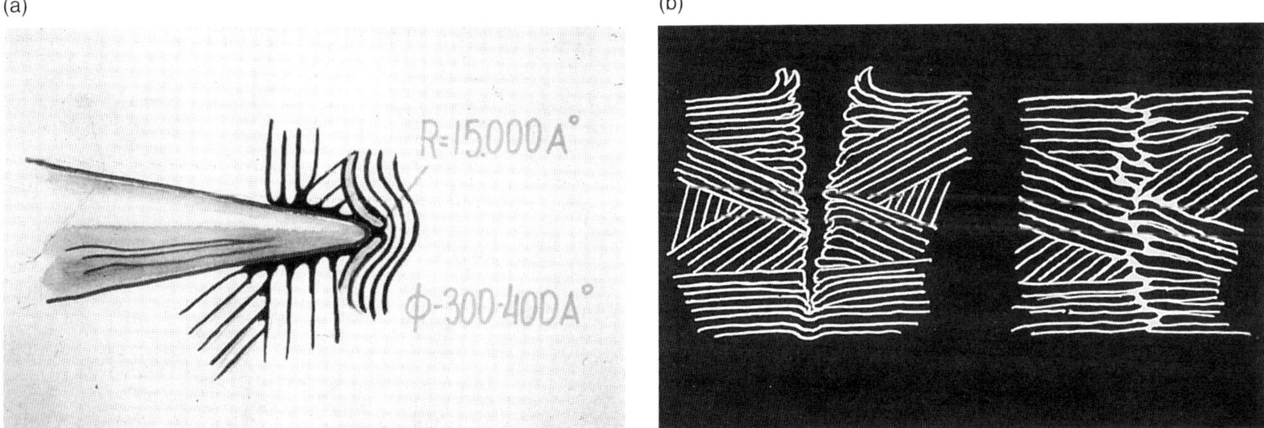

Fig. 7.45 (a) A dull steel blade pushes tissue ahead of it, tearing instead of cutting. (b) This results in wide, ragged scars.

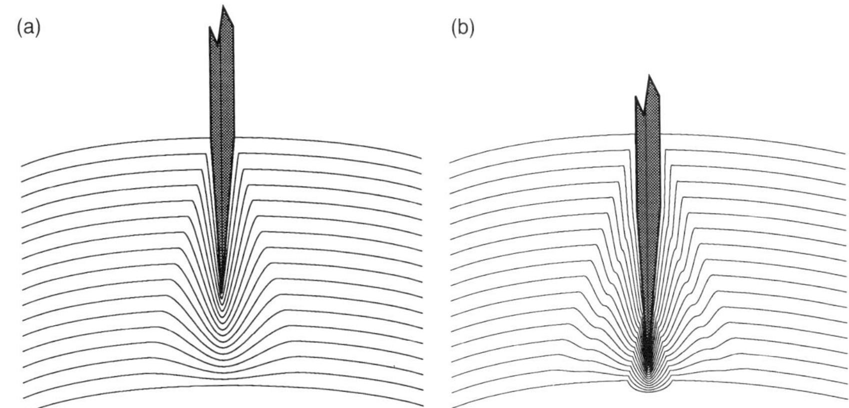

Fig. 7.46 (a) Stress lines as the blade pushes through tissue. (b) When the blade bottoms out, thinner layers remain uncut.

used with unvarnished confidence off the visual axis, even with the Mishima-Hedbys pin light attachment [46]. This method can only measure in the horizontal meridian, and Fyodorov and I were making incisions in all meridians. While we were able to get the optical pachymeter to function as a comparator and with it did hundreds of patients with reasonable success, the method still was not exact enough for our purposes. Fortunately, the problem was solved with the appearance of the ultrasonic corneal pachymeter, as conceived by Kremer (Figure 7.51a, b) Originally a modification of an existing A-scan ocular biometer (Xenotech), it soon evolved into a stand-alone unit. The original Corneometer had a hollow, open-ended tip tapering to 1.5 mm, making it easy to place the probe accurately on the cornea (see Figure 7.51c). For the first time, precise measurements of corneal thickness could be made with confidence anywhere on the surface. A corneal thickness profile also could be generated by

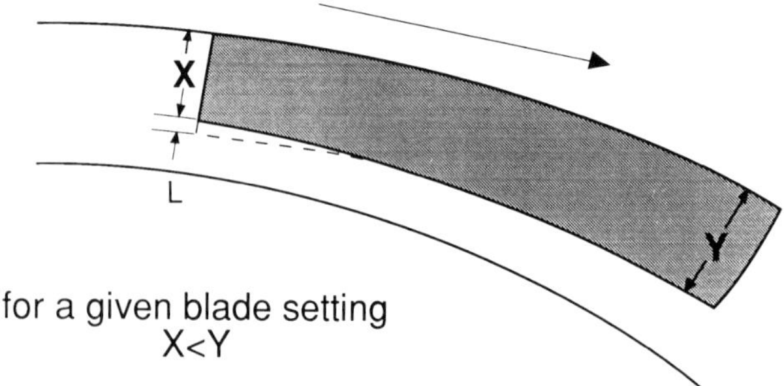

Fig. 7.47 Incision depth in American in-to-out technique.

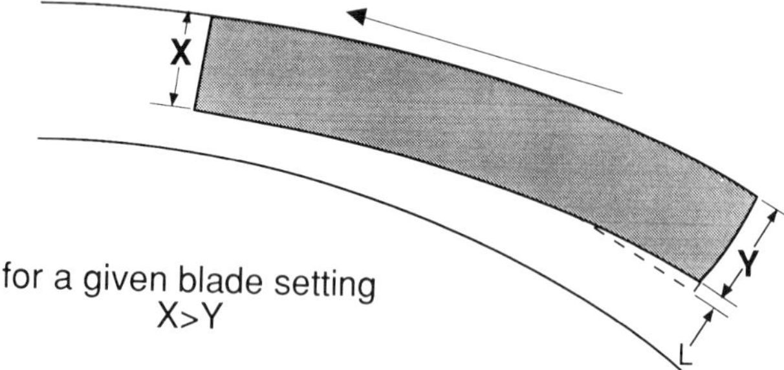

Fig. 7.48 Incision depth in Russian out-to-in technique.

taking successive measurements (mapping) in any meridian (Figure 7.52).

It was by doing these mappings that a small piece of the puzzle fell into place. Because we now "understood" the cornea by virtue of our discovery of its spongelike qualities, we expected the microperforation rate to decrease. And so it did—for a time. However, as we kept increasing the blade length, we began to experience microperforations in unlikely places. For example, most were occurring in the corneal midperiphery and not always

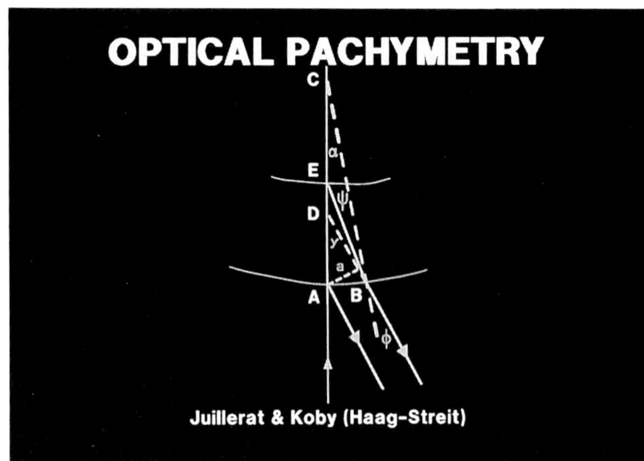

Fig. 7.50 The principle of optical pachymetry.

with the first deepening pass. Some occurred at around 9 mm and seemed to be mainly in the inferotemporal quadrant.

It was not enough to say that this was happening because continued corneal desiccation had caught up with us. While this might explain such penetrations at the midperiphery, it did not explain those in the far periphery. Some of these also might be explained through technical error such as too much blade pressure while making a stepped incision using the old method, but it was also occurring in patients in whom the newer technique was being used.

For years I had been taught that the cornea has a smooth thickness transition from center to limbus—in the absence of corneal disease. However, ultrasonic corneal thickness mapping has shown that while this may be true in some eyes, for about 11% it is not. In older patients there is a tendency for the cornea to become

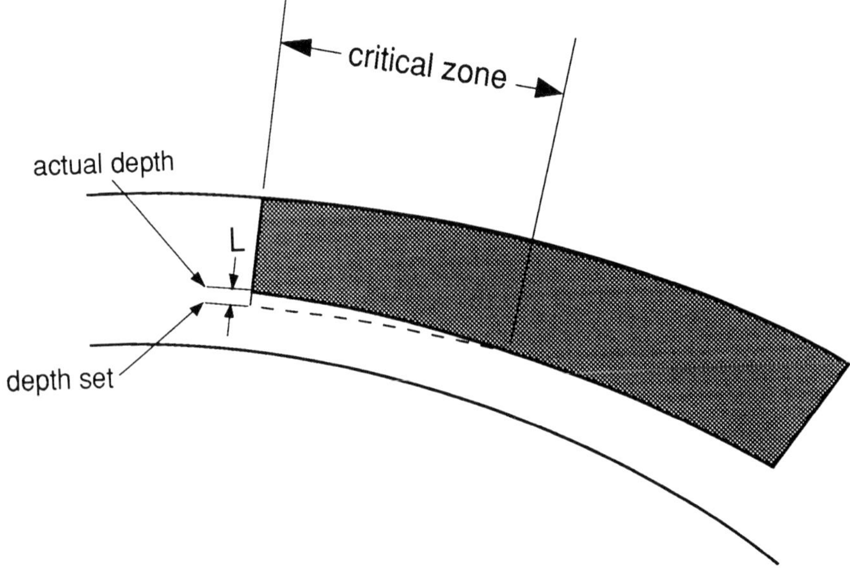

Fig. 7.49 The critical zone (3–6 mm annulus).

(a)

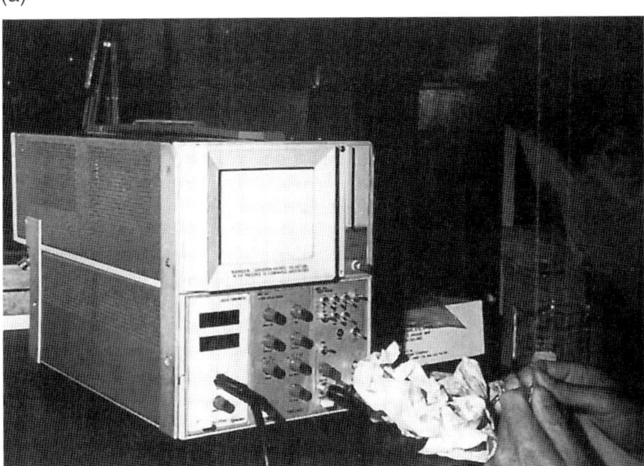

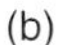

(b)

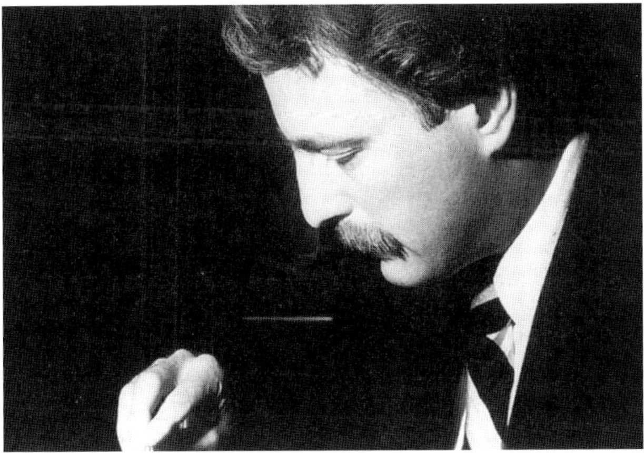

(c)

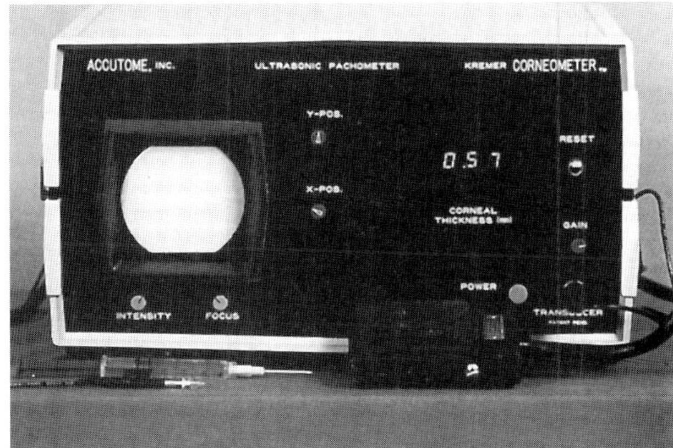

Fig. 7.51 (a) Modified Xenotech A-scan biometer used to make the first ultrasonic cornea thickness measurements. (b) Fred Kremer, M.D., originator of ultrasonic pachymetry. (c) First commercial ultrasonic pachymeter.

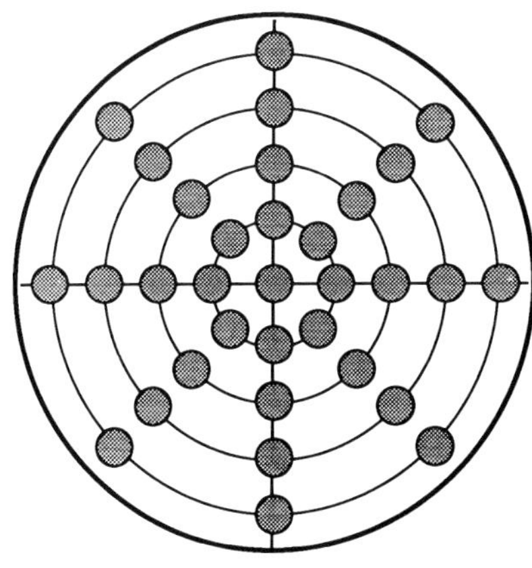

Fig. 7.52 Typical ultrasonic pachymeter mapping pattern.

thinner toward the periphery. In others, the thickness remains uniform until just before the limbus, where it thickens rapidly. Still others have been found to have small, abrupt areas of corneal thinning—which I have called *corneal dimples*. These dimples seem to occur at random and, when first encountered, were thought to be errors in measurement. An analysis of the distribution of these dimples showed a tendency to group in the midperiphery in the inferotemporal quadrant (Figure 7.53). It was in this quadrant as well that most of the instances of peripheral thinning could be found. In some cases, discovery of these areas before surgery—through mapping—allowed me to rotate my incisional pattern, thereby avoiding microperforations.

The search for the ideal blade

With the increased confidence that came with accurate pachymeter readings, I again focused my attention on the incisions. I soon abandoned the No. 76a Beaver blade in favor of razor fragments, particularly those of high carbon content, but the search for the "ideal" blade continued. A brief "love affair" with the early diamond blades promised much at first. However, until recently, I have been uniformly disappointed with the performance of the guarded diamond knife. It does not seem to cut as well as steel razor fragments after it has been used on many patients. A trifacet diamond blade remains, nonetheless, my favorite for the free-hand deepening procedure.

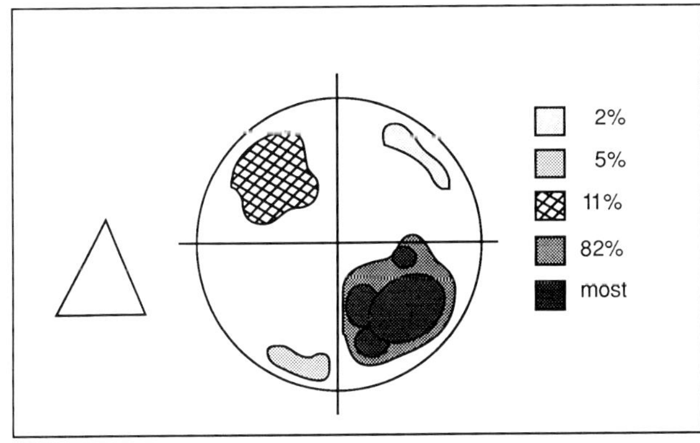

Fig. 7.53 Distribution of thin corneal areas (dimples).

This need to overset the blade was due, primarily, to the way the blades cut and in part to the pachymeter itself. The speed of sound through the cornea is not exactly known—estimates have ranged from 1540 m/s (the average speed through the human eye) to 1630 m/s [47,48]. The Corneometer had been preset to 1540 m/s at the beginning of the investigation. When I gradually advanced the speed setting (which requires more than just "twiddling" a knob), I began to get more "sensible" readings—that is, the corneal thickness measurements began to relate to the blade settings. This was so universal an experience that all instruments were recalled and readjusted to the faster speed.

This did not solve the problem entirely, however. Blades still had to be overset because of the characteristics of the corneal tissue and of the continued inadequacy of the blades being used. When I speak of inadequacy, I am speaking in relative terms, and I am talking about consistency. Certainly any blade will make an incision in the cornea. In RK surgery, however, I am talking about microns—microsurgery in a very real sense—and any blade that does not cut exactly to where it is set is bound to be a disappointment.

As crystalline blades made their appearance, the blade bias changed to 5% to 10% for diamond blades and approximately 2% for sapphire blades. The sapphire bias is usually expressed in microns rather than as a percentage, being typically 10 μm initially and up to 70 μm as the blade becomes worn (this translates to a percentage bias of 1.5% to 15%). These crystalline blades cut deeper and smoother because their edge radius is typically 450 Å for diamond and 190 Å for sapphire (Figure 7.54 a, b). Except for some very fragile experimental sapphire blades, no blade has yet reached the ideal sharpness whereby it can be *underset* to obtain a 90% to 95% incisional depth. Eventually, a new-design diamond blade made especially for me achieved a blade bias of 0%. This is the so-called LeCut double-edged thin diamond blade now marketed by KOI, a division of DGH Corporation.

It is the importance of "small" details such as this that sets refractive surgical techniques apart from others, and it is the attention to such details that sets the successful radial keratotomist apart from his or her fellows (Figure 7.55a, b). To overset a blade to maximize the incisional depth while still not cutting through the cornea may seem illogical. Nevertheless, it works. Arriving at the actual settings to use was much easier than convincing colleagues to follow suit, however. It took demonstrations of the method during actual surgery to clinch the point. In my hands, such technique actually has reduced the mean perforation rate from 12% to 7%. Microperforation of any degree during this surgery is seen by some as undesirable. Hence the suggestion has been made to make the incisions shallow. Since the data from various authors have shown that deeper incisions produce a more profound and lasting effect, I will leave it to the reader to weigh the merit of this suggestion to prevent microperforations.

(a)

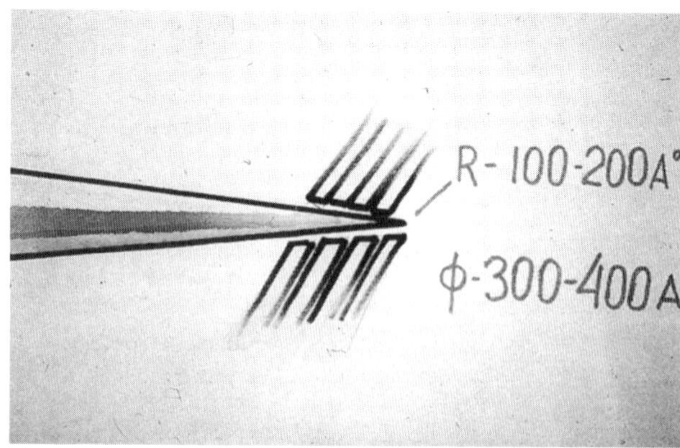

(b)

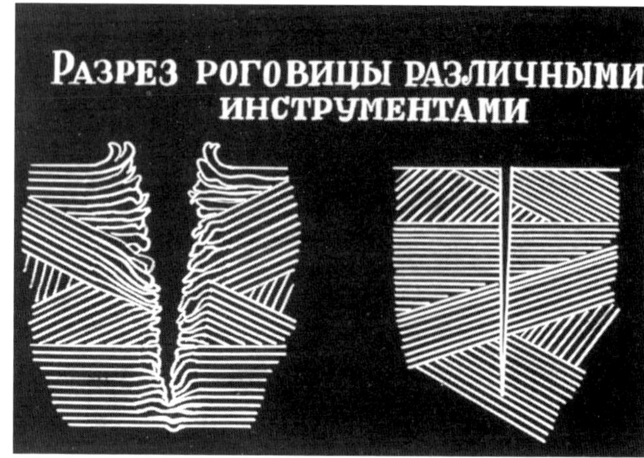

Fig. 7.54 (a) The cutting radius of the blade edge must be less than the diameter of tissue fiber to be cut. (b) A Russian slide showing the differences between incisions made with steel (left) and diamond (right).

Progressive corneal flattening

This is one caveat that should be considered whenever the question arises, "Is deeper really better?" While it has been stated, as well as shown, that deeper incisions produce an increase in ultimate effect, there may be a price to be paid for that depth increase—progressive hyperopia [39,40,49].

There is some evidence that deeper incisions may be associated with progression of effect. While progressive hyperopia will be covered in more detail in Chapter 15, it is appropriate to mention some aspects of the phenomenon at this juncture. Fyodorov and I advocated, early in the history of RK, free-hand dissection of incisions to Descemet's membrane in patients with high myopia. As the quality of blades improved—particularly their tip geometry, which allows the blade to penetrate more deeply at the beginning of an incision—and the accuracy of

(a)

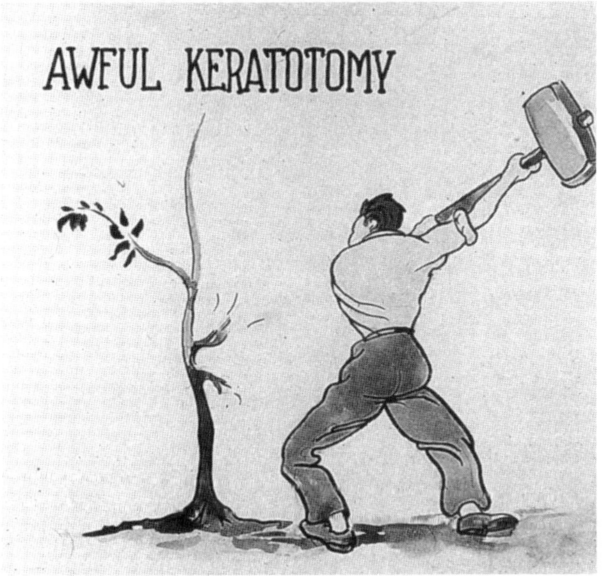

(b)

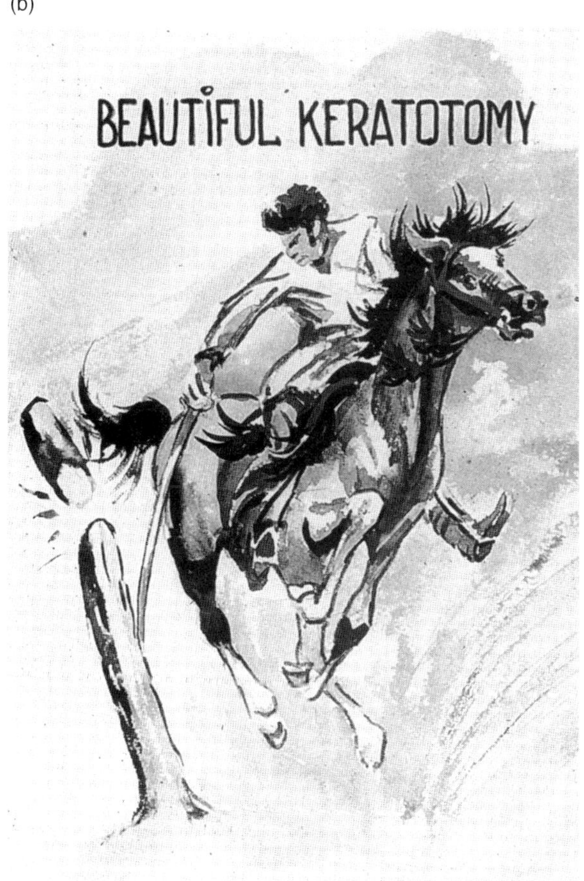

Fig. 7.55 (a) Awful keratotomy; (b) beautiful keratotomy. (Courtesy of S.N. Fyodorov.)

blade setting also increased, the number of patients in whom free-hand deepening was mandated decreased. Adding to this was the recognition that there was, as in all things, a ceiling or limit to the degree of myopia that reasonably could be expected to be eliminated by RK. The trend to "cap off" the level of myopia amenable to RK incisions also was propelled by the advent of improvements in alternative refractive surgical techniques—such as keratomileusis in situ (KMIS).

While the jury is still out on the question, it is reasonable to be alert to the possibility that incisions that approach closely or intersect with Descemet's membrane actually may induce progression in the effect of RK. It is my contention that incisions penetrating no greater than 95% of the corneal thickness will be shown to be safe with regard to progression of effect. However, the reader should carefully study the paragraphs on progressive hyperopia in Chapter 15 and consider that other factors are in play here producing this complication of the surgery (see also below).

Number of incisions

As stated earlier, 8 incisions were abandoned early on; they were revived as incisions got deeper. All accounts from individuals reporting "first experience" cases have stated that they have found little, or at the most 10%, difference between 8 and 16 incisions. However, that has not been my experience. I have, for example, a group of 48 patients in whom 8 incisions were done on one eye and 16 on the fellow eye using the same technique. I found the range of difference to be 5% to 50%, with the mean 24.6%. This finding has been corroborated by Fyodorov [50]. Eight or fewer incisions are used for all patients whose myopia is –4 D or less, for some whose myopia is –5 D, and very rarely for those whose myopia is greater (usually in astigmatic patients). Sixteen incisions are used for the remainder, although 4, 6, and 12 incisions sometimes also are used. Since it is more difficult to place the 6- and 12-ray patterns symmetrically, I use a specially designed marker to ensure equal spacing of the incisions (see also Chapter 8). The 6-incision patients have shown a mean difference in effect of 50% and the 12-incision patients, 16% of that produced by 16 incisions.

Because of the physiologic changes that occur within the cornea after this surgery that seem to affect the outcome in second-stage surgery, I cannot recommend "sneaking up" on the myopia by staging the surgery. This method has been advocated by some as a preventative for overcorrection [51]—that is, doing 3 or 4 incisions, waiting, and then doing another 3 or 4 incisions. For some reason, staging never seems to produce the same amount of ultimate correction as does using 6, 8, or 16 primary incisions. While an occasional patient may be spared postoperative hyperopia by staging the incisions in this manner, still more will be subjected to additional surgery whose outcome will be even less predictable than the first go-around. Overcorrections are rare in my hands, and Fyodorov has not reported this phenomenon to any significant degree. Properly planned surgery assisted by computer prediction programs that take into account age, sex, keratometry, corneal diameter, depth of incision, and corneal rigidity is the best defense against over- and undercorrection.

Incisional depth coefficients

Because of the greater changes in corneal curvature that were accompanying the newer methods of incision making, the formulas began to fail in their ability to predict the outcome of surgery. It therefore was necessary to generate three additional surgical coefficients (since known as *incisional depth coefficients*). These factors are 1.6, 2.0, and 2.5. These coefficients relate not only to the depth but also to the manner in which the incisions are made. In January 1980, I began (as did Fyodorov) to use these factors as follows:

1.3—Used when 16 single-depth incisions were made to a depth of approximately 70% of the corneal thickness at the paracentral (primary) optical zone. (The operative word here is *approximately*. Recall that with the advent of the subtraction/stepping technique, I and my coworkers were not using percentages to set blade depth.)

1.6—The same number and type of incisions were made with a blade set to produce an incision to approximately 90% of the corneal thickness at the primary optic zone.

2.0—Used for 16 incisions with a deepening cut made in each incision from 6 mm to the periphery.

2.5—Used for a patient in whom a stepped incision was made but also 4 or more incisions were deepened to Descemet's membrane.

This latter free-hand deepening was performed with a trifacet diamond knife. With a sharp blade, very little pressure is needed to deepen a corneal wound, allowing the surgeon to maintain complete control of his or her incision. In addition, the blade is transparent, allowing light into the bottom of the wound, which makes it easier to see Descemet's membrane.

Wet versus dry

I found, almost serendipitously, that in patients in whom the cornea had not been kept wet during the surgery, the last eight incisions were much deeper than those in whom it had been kept wet. In some cases, perforations occurred at the midperiphery even when the blade was not extended. I therefore performed surgery on a number of consecutive patients in whom extended and nonextended blade settings were used with and without corneal wetting. Except to add anesthetic, which was blotted from the surface with microsponges almost immediately, no fluids were applied to the corneal surface in the "nonwetted" patients. In all patients undergoing the "dry" technique without blade extension, the incisions were found to be deeper and more uniform throughout than incisions made in the "old" manner. In the wetted patients, there was considerable variation in the incision depths—especially the last eight incisions (all corneal thickness measurements were made using the optical pachymeter). In those cases in which the blade was extended for the last eight incisions, there was an improvement with respect to depth in the wetted patients, whereas in the nonwetted patients there was a tendency to perforate at incision 9 or 10. Therefore, I concluded that corneal wetting during the surgery would result in shallower incisions from swelling of the stroma due to tissue imbibition (Figure 7.56). Villasenor, in a series of experiments, showed that the incised corneas in monkey and human cadaver eyes thinned up to 25% of their original thickness within 25 minutes if not kept wet—almost 1% per minute [52]. One other advantage of the dry technique was that the rate of operative epithelial stripping fell almost to zero.

There were, however, two other difficulties that required solution and which remain only partially solved today. The first is keratometry, and the second is the so-called corneal rigidity.

The importance of central corneal curvature

There is still some discussion about the effect of the preoperative corneal curvature on the outcome of RK. Early work by Fyodorov and his colleagues had indicated that it did affect the outcome [53,54]. I have compensated for changes in corneal curvature from the beginning of my involvement with this surgical technique—I am convinced that preoperative K-readings relate to the end result. When preoperative keratometry results were plotted against postoperative keratometry results in a group

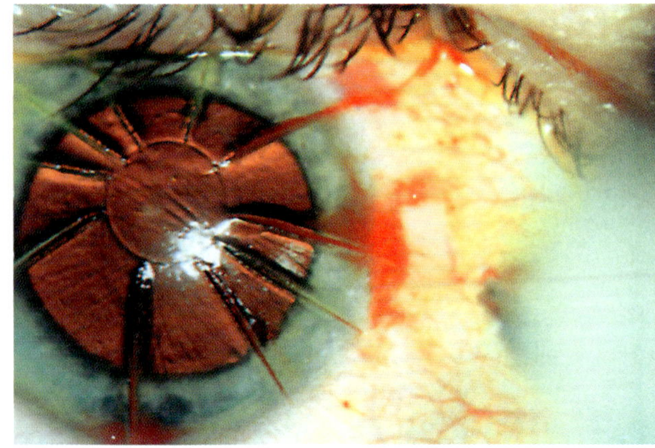

Fig. 7.56 Note the elevation of the incision edges in a wetted RK case.

of similar patients, an almost straight line resulted (Figure 7.57). If the preoperative corneal curvature was *not* an influencing factor, there should have been less effect shown for higher curvatures—however, there wasn't. There was, instead, more effect shown—thus indicating that more compensation should have been made for steeper corneas—up to a point—since if corneas are *too steep*, the effect gets less (see Figure 7.57b). Therefore, I am forced to conclude that preoperative curvature is a factor in surgical outcome, and I continue to compensate for it.

Corneal rigidity

The other factor—that of corneal rigidity—is still somewhat of a puzzler. All of us remember Freidenwald's constant when rigidity is mentioned. In fact, it was this association that produced some difficulty for me in the beginning. Freidenwald's "constant" seems to vary with the extent of the myopia and generally ranges between 0.018 and 0.025. Fyodorov kept describing factors of 1.5, 0.96, 0.88, etc. What kind of "constant" was he talking about, and where did he get it? He was really talking about the same thing that Freidenwald was, except that he measured it differently. It was found that the integration of this factor into the original formulas more accurately predicted the outcome of a specific case. As the rigidity increased, so did the effect of the surgery. In general, the rigidity increased with age and was somewhat less at a given age for a woman than for a man. The difference is convergent, however, and beginning at age 45 to 46, the corneal rigidity is essentially the same for a man or a woman. That this variable is significant can be seen by examining the evidence described in Chapter 5. Scleral rigidity is always factored into my case planning.

(a)

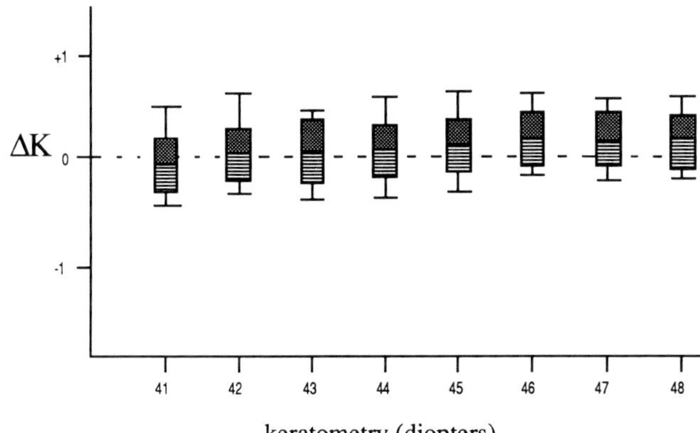

(b)

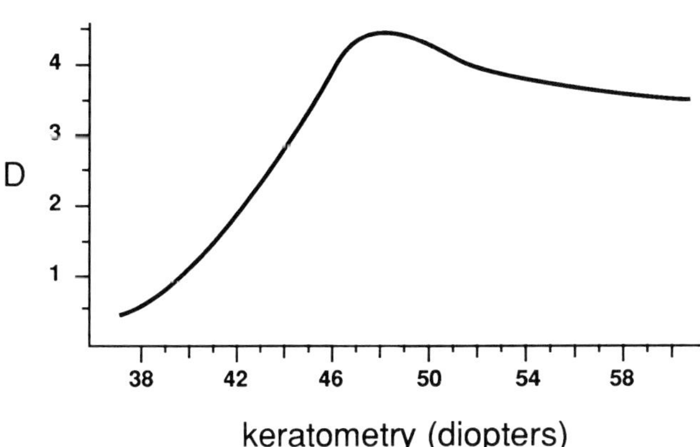

Fig. 7.57 (a) Effect of K-reading on outcome. (b) Steep corneal curvatures can decrease the effect.

Corneal diameter

Corneal diameter is a different matter. I have not found that there is much deviation in corneal diameter between patients. In addition, it is difficult (if not impossible) to take this measurement with confidence. Incisions that stop just before the limbus produce excellent results, and there is no indication to show that making them longer would make a difference (unless they extended onto the limbus, in which case they would cause a loss of effect). There is no justification for making incisions much shorter than they are now—in my view. There is no advantage in so doing, and one runs the real risk of increasing the incidence of postoperative astigmatism. The cornea must be weakened sufficiently that the overall corneal curvature has a smooth transition; it must have "room" to flex. Moreover, as Fyodorov and coworkers indicated in an earlier work, as the incisions get shorter, the effect gets less [27].

Intraocular pressure

It remains to be seen whether intraocular pressure (IOP) per se has any real effect on the procedure. There have been some patients in whom the results were not as predicted and in whom the preoperative IOP was below 12 mm Hg. Some of these patients did not have rigidity measurements taken, so I do not know what part low rigidity may have played. The possible influence of IOP in this surgery is still under investigation. Nonetheless, I recommend that surgery be avoided in patients in whom the IOP is less than 12 mmHg.

Other factors in the surgery were dealt with as they surfaced. The first patients were done with incisions that extended across the limbus. As the need for deeper incisions became apparent, concern grew for the angle structures. In addition, such incisions tended to promote fibrous ingrowth at their most peripheral portions, producing conjunctival "peaks" at the limbus. Surprisingly, these peaks were not accompanied by neovascularization, except in some patients, in whom soft contact lenses were fitted early (to stabilize the cornea) and only in those patients who wore extended-wear lenses [55]. This problem vanished when the lenses were stopped or changed to daily wear and thus seemed more related to oxygen deprivation in healing tissue than to the type of incision. The major factor in shortening these incisions was the theoretical, experimental, and clinical evidence that showed that perhaps this type of incision actually reduced the effectiveness of the surgery. I therefore began to make the incisions just to the capillary plexus and not beyond. I found that not only were the eyes quieter, but the effect also was not reduced and may well have been enhanced.

This experience prompted some workers to theorize that perhaps even shorter incisions would be just as effective, whereupon some wag observed that if shorter incisions was the answer, why not just make punctures at the edge of the optical zone? Mendez has advocated the use of deliberate punctures through the cornea and has claimed 1 D of correction per puncture. Despite the reported success with such punctures, this methodology is *not* recommended. Some patients have been done with short (3-mm) incisions, and the results were reported to be satisfactory [20] (Figure 7.58). However, no one, to my knowledge, is currently using this method.

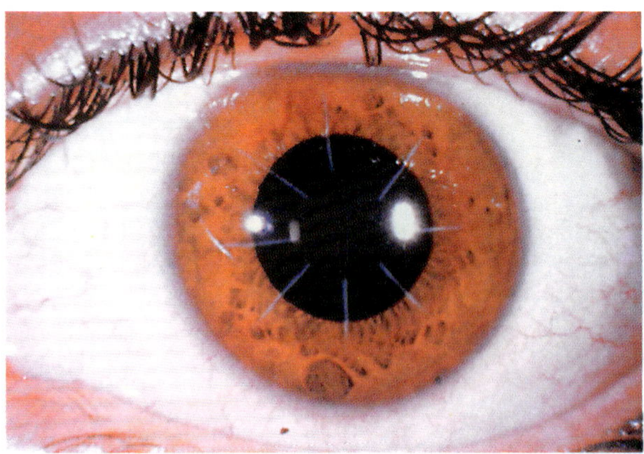

Fig. 7.58 Short (3 mm) incisions advocated by one surgeon to correct myopia on the grounds that computer simulations show that most of the effect of the incisions occurs in this area.

Circular keratotomy

Another "innovation" did not produce such happy results. It has been observed that transverse incisions across a radial incision made in the meridian of myopic astigmatism produce a profound change in corneal curvature (see also Chapter 9). Why not then extend this concept and make the transverse incisions concentric? Such an idea is not new; in fact, it was discussed by Sato in an answer to a letter from an interested surgeon [56]. Sato stated that he had tried it and it did not work. Nonetheless, a sizable number of these cases were performed, and while there was tremendous flattening of the cornea almost immediately, this disappeared along with the edema, leaving the patients with the same myopia as they started with [57]. Some had the added problem of increased glare and profound corneal instability, whereas in others the myopia had increased considerably [58]. By transecting the columns of tissue that connected the central cornea to the limbus, all means of placing stress on the center were removed; therefore, the effect was lost, and the central cornea was bowed forward. Its chord length became shorter, and its sagittal height became greater—all characteristics of myopic corneas. These concentric incisions also tended to gape because of tissue relaxation, and many were found to have "marsupialized"—therefore, they never healed (see also Chapter 15).

Final thoughts

The technique of RK is quick and relatively painless, making it ideally suited for outpatient surgical facilities (see Table 7.3). In addition, the recovery period is relatively short, and most patients return to normal activity within hours—something not always true of PRK and sometimes following LASIK. While seemingly easy to perform, the technique requires careful attention to preoperative details and nuances of surgical technique. It is truly "microsurgery" in its strictest sense, since a few microns of incision depth can affect the outcome. The seeming simplicity of the technique has led to variations

Table 7.3 Results of a study on postoperative use of steroid drops. From J. Hayes

	No steroids			Steroids		
	All	Males	Females	All	Males	Females
Number	25	13	12	33	21	12
Age (years)	33.6	34.6	32.5	36.5	36.3	36.7
Range of ages (years)	22–57	25–52	22–57	21–56	21–56	27–49
Preoperative intraocular pressure	17.2	18.1	16.3	16.3	15.9	17.2
Preoperative K(SE)	–5.66	–5.65	–5.68	–5.78	–5.11	–6.16
Range of corneal refraction	–3.62 to –8.00	–3.62 to –8.00	–3.75 to –7.62	–4.00 to –7.75	–4.00 to –7.75	–4.25 to –7.00
Delta corneal refraction	+3.99	+4.63	+3.29	+5.36	+5.44	+5.23
Range of the delta	+1.75 to +8.00	+1.75 to +8.00	+2.13 to +5.25	+3.12 to +10.12	+3.12 to +10.12	+3.25 to +8.00

or "improvements" in the method bolstered neither by experimental evidence nor by clinical experience. While "good" results have been reported with these variations, they are not optimal, as further study has revealed.

A surgical procedure is difficult to study in the classic sense—it is always on the move, like a positron. The uncertainty principle therefore enters into this type of examination. If we stop the evolution of the surgery to examine it in a so-called controlled study, we end up by becoming paleoophthalmologists studying "ancient" eye surgery. If we try to study it on the fly, we cannot apply the scientific method because each case is slightly different. Therefore, we can only get a feel of the efficacy of the surgery—some uncertainty remains. If a number of the investigators insist on an attempt to study the surgery by adopting strict guidelines while the remainder continue to alter and improve the technique, then the first investigative group is faced with a dilemma: Can they morally deny the latest treatment to their patients on the grounds that the study must be kept pure? The second group has an equally important dilemma: Are they exposing their patients to needless risk?

There is no absolute answer that is fitting because there are no absolutes in biologic processes—there are only approximations. The science of biostatistics is really a stochastic art form full of assumptions and definite maybes. As the amount of data increases, an idea of the behavior of a biologic system can be obtained, and from this idea, certain guidelines can be constructed to assist individuals working with that system.

The title of this chapter is "The Beginning and the Evolution of Radial Keratotomy," as if the final word had been written on the subject. This is not the case. As more knowledge is gained, the procedure matures and transforms. It may even metamorphose into something entirely different. One thing is for sure—this is only the beginning. Sir Frances Drake said it well in his prayer before engaging the Spanish Armada:

> Give us to know that it is not the beginning but the continuing of the same until it is entirely finished which yieldeth the true glory.

References

1 Sato T. Treatment of Conical Cornea (incision of Descemet's membrane). Acta Soc Ophthalmol (Jpn) 1939; 43: p. 541.

2 Sato T. Experimental study on surgical correction of astigmatism. Juntendo Kenkyukai Zasshi 1943; 589: p. 37.

3 Lans LJ. Experimentelle untersuchungen uber die entstehung von astigmatismus durch nicht Perforirende corneawunden. (Experimental studies of the treatment of astigmatism with non-perforating corneal incisions). Albrecht von Graefes Arch Klin Exp Ophthalmol 1898; 45: p. 117–52.

4 Sato T. Experimental study of posterior half-corneal incisions for myopia. Acta Soc Ophthalmol Jpn 1951; 55: p. 219.

5 Sato T. Experimental study of anterior and posterior half-corneal incisions for myopia. Rinsho Ganka 1952; 6: p. 209.

6 Sato T, Akiyama K, and Shibata H. Posterior half-incision of the cornea for astigmatism; operative procedures and results of the improved tangent method. Am J Ophthalmol 1953; 36: p. 462–6.

7 Akiyama K. A new surgical approach to myopia. Acta Soc Ophthalmol Jpn 1952; 56: p. 1142.

8 Shepard D. Personal communication. 1988.

9 Akiyama K. Study of the Surgical Treatment for Myopia. I. Posterior Corneal Incisions. Acta Soc Ophthalmol (Jpn) 1955; 56: p. 1142–50.

10 Akiyama K. Study of the surgical treatment for myopia. II. Animal experiments. Acta Soc Ophthalmol (Jpn) 1955; 59: p. 294–312.

11 Akiyama K. Study of the surgical treatment for myopia. III. Anterior and Posterior Incisions. Acta Soc Ophthalmol (Jpn) 1955; 59: p. 797–853.

12 Kanai A, *et al*. The fine structure of bullous keratopathy after antero-posterior incisions of the cornea for myopia. Folia Ophthalmol (Jpn) 1979; 30: p. 841–9.

13 Yamaguchi T, *et al*. Bullous keratopathy after anterior-posterior radial keratotomy for myopia. Am J Ophthalmol 1982; 93: p. 600.

14 Momose A. Personal communication.

15 Yenaliev FS. Experience in the surgical treatment of myopia. Vestn Oftalmol 1979; 3: p. 52–5.

16 Kokott W. Das Spaltlinienbild der Sklera. I. Beschreibung. Klin Monatstbl Augenheilkd 1934; 92: p. 177–85.

17 Kokott W. Das Spaltlinienbild der Sklera. II. Der Nachweis der funktionellen Struktur der Sklera. Klin Monatstbl Augenheilkd 1935; 94: p. 33–45.

18 Kokott W. Uber mechanisch-funktionelle Strukturen des Auges. Graefes Arch Ophthalmol 1938; 138: p. 424–85.

19 Meek KM, *et al*. Interpretation of the meridional x-ray diffraction pattern from collagen fibrils in corneal stroma. J Mol Biol 1981; 149(3): p. 477–88.

20 Schachar R, Black T, and Huang T. Surgical implications of the theory of radial keratotomy. In: *Radial Keratotomy*, R Schacher, *et al*, Editor. LAL, Dennison, p. 269–82, 1980.

21 Schachar R, Black T, and Huang T. A Physicist's View of Radial Keratotomy with Practical Surgical Implications. In: *Keratorefraction*, R Schacher, *et al*, Editor. LAL, Dennison, p. 195–219, 1980.

22 Schachar RA, Black TD, and Huang T. Understanding Radial Keratotomy. In: *Understanding Radial Keratotomy*, R Schacher, *et al*, Editor. LAL, Dennison, p. 25–6, 1980.

23 Pureskin N. [The surgical treatment of myopia and astigmatism (review)] <Original> Khirurgicheskoe lechenie blizorukosti i astigmatizma (obzor). Vestn Oftalmol 1966; 79(5): p. 81–5.

24 Pureskin NP. [Weakening ocular refraction by means of partial stromectomy of cornea under experimental conditions] <Original> Oslablenie refraktsii glaza putem chastichnoi stromektomii rogovitsy v eksperimente. Vestn Oftalmol 1967; 80(1): p. 19–24.

25 Pureskin NP, and Boguslavskaia ES. [Changing corneal curvature through anterior and posterior nonpenetrating incisions] <Original> Izmenenie krivizny rogovitsy putem ee perednikh i zadnikh neperforiruiushchikh nadrezov. Vestn Oftalmol 1967; 80 (6): p. 16–22.

26 Pureskin NP. *Experimental investigation of possibilities of surgical treatment of myopia and astigmatism*, Moscow; 1968.

27 Durnev VV, and Ermoshin AS. Determination of dependence between the length of anterior radial non-perforating incisions of the cornea and their effectiveness. In: *IV All Union Conference of Inventors and Rationalizers in the Field of Ophthalmology*. Minister of Health, U.S.S.R., Moscow, 1976.

28 Durnev V. Decrease of corneal refraction by anterior keratotomy method with the purpose of surgical correction of myopia of mild and moderate degree. In: *Tenth Meeting of Transcaucasian Ophthalmologists*. Tbilisi, 1976.

29 Durnev V. Characteristic of the results of myopic surgical correction after performing 16 and 32 primary anterior radial non-perforating incisions. In: *Surgery of Refractive Anomalies of the Eye*, A Ivashina and S Kolmanovskii, Editors. Moscow Scientific Research Institute for Eye Microsurgery, Moscow, p. 148, 1981.
30 Huang T, Bisarnsin T, Schachar RA, *et al.* Corneal curvature change due to structural alternation by radial keratotomy. J Biomech Eng 1988; 110(3): p. 249–53.
31 Chen Y. *Transverse Shear Deformation in an Impaired Thin Shell.* University of Texas, 1990.
32 Reissner E. The Effect of Transverse–Shear Deformation on the Bending of Elastic Plates. J App Mech 1945; 12(2): p. 69–77.
33 Reissner E. Stress–Strain Relations in the Theory of Thin Elastic Shells. J Math and Physics 1952; 31: p. 109–19.
34 Whitney J. The Effect of Transverse Shear Deformation on the Bending of Laminated Plates. J Comp Materials 1969; 3: p. 534–47.
35 Bores LD, Myers W, and Cowden J. Radial keratotomy: an analysis of the American experience. Ann Ophthalmol 1981; 13(8): p. 941–8.
36 Bores LD. Historical review and clinical results of radial keratotomy. Int Ophthalmol Clin 1983; 23(3): p. 93–118.
37 Melles GR, and Binder PS. Effect of radial keratotomy incision direction on wound depth. Refract Corneal Surg 1990; 6(6): p. 394–403; 1990.
38 Binder PS. What We Have Learned About Corneal Wound Healing From Refractive Surgery (Barraquer Lecture). Refractive and Corneal Surgery 1989; 5(2): p. 98–120.
39 Deitz M, and Sanders D. Progressive hyperopia with long-term follow-up of radial keratotomy. Arch Ophthalmol, 103(6): p. 782–4; 1985.
40 Deitz M, Sanders D, and Raanan M. Progressive hyperopia in radial keratotomy. Long-term follow-up of diamond-knife and metal-blade series. Ophthalmology 1986; 93(10): p. 1284–9.
41 Bores LD. Unpublished data.
42 Bores LD. Results of radial keratotomy after two years. In: *Keratorefractive Society*. LAL Publishing, Chicago, 1981.
43 Cowden JW, and Bores LD. A clinical investigation of the surgical correction of myopia by the method of Fyodorov. Ophthalmology 1981; 88(8): p. 737–41.
44 Rowsey JJ, and Balyeat HD. Radial keratotomy: Preliminary report of complications. Ophthalmic Surg 1982; 13: p. 27.
45 Hernandez-Meijide R, and Croxatto JO. Experimental radial keratotomy. Journal of Refractive Surgery 1988; 3: p. 224–6.
46 Mishima S, and Hedbys B. Measurement of corneal thickness with the Haag–Streit pachymeter. Arch Ophthalmol 1968; 80: p. 710–3.
47 Oksala A. Use of the echogram in the location and diagnosis of intraocular foreign bodies. Brit J Ophthalmol 1959; 43: p. 744–52.
48 Vanysek J, Preisova J, and Obraz J. *Ultrasonography in Ophthalmology*. Butterworths, London, p. 213–8, 1969.
49 Deitz M, Sanders D, and Marks R. Radial keratotomy: an overview of the Kansas City study. Ophthalmology 1984; 91(5): p. 467–78.
50 Fyodorov SN, Ivashina AI, Fedchenko OT, *et al.* [Surgical correction of myopic anisometropia by anterior keratotomy] <Original> Khirurgicheskaia korrektsiia miopicheskoi anizometropii metodom perednei keratomii. Vestn Oftalmol 1984; (1): p. 15–9.
51 Salz J, Villasenor A, Elander R, *et al.* Four-incision radial keratotomy for low to moderate myopia. Ophthalmology 1986; 93(6): p. 727–38.
52 Villasenor RA, Salz J, Steel D, *et al.* Changes in corneal thickness during radial keratotomy. Ophthalmic Surg 1981; 12(5): p. 341–2.
53 Fyodorov SN, and Durnev VV. The use of anterior keratotomy method with the purpose of surgical correction of myopia. In: *Practical Problems in Ophthalmic Surgery*, AI Ivashina, Editor. Minister of Health, U.S.S.R., Moscow, p. 47–8, 1977.
54 Fyodorov SN, and Durnev VV. Operation of dosaged dissection of corneal circular ligament in cases of myopia of mild degree. Ann Ophthalmol 1979; 11(12): p. 1885–90.
55 Binder PS. Physiological effects of extended wear soft contact lenses. Ophthalmol 1980; 87: p. 745–9.
56 Sato T. Correspondence, a reply on surgical correction of myopia. Am J Ophthalmol 1954; 36: p. 280–2.
57 Gills J. Trephination in combination with radial keratotomy for myopia. In: *Radial Keratotomy*, R Schacher, N Levy, and L Schacher, Editors. LAL, Dennison, TX, 1980.
58 Perry L, and Taylor L. Worsening of myopia following a circular keratotomy. Ophthalmic Surg 1982; 13(2): p. 104–7.

8

Instrumentation and Technique of Radial Keratotomy

I hear and forget.
I see and hear and I remember.
However, when I see, hear and do,
I understand and succeed.
[Anonymous]

Instrumentation

As I have stated repeatedly, radial keratotomy (RK) is true microsurgery. Not only does the outcome depend on careful consideration of numerous, seemingly unimportant factors, but it also depends on the instrumentation as well. Next to the preoperative workup, the most important consideration in this surgery is the blade. In the beginning, razor fragments were used for this surgery. Because such blades were inconsistent in their quality, the search began immediately for an improved blade. While it is true that specially processed steel blades (such as the Katena K2-5550) are available today that surpass in quality any previously available razor fragment and in some cases even the early diamond blades, it is the consensus among most experienced practitioners of this surgery that some form of crystalline blade (not necessarily diamond) will produce the smoothest and deepest incision.

I also have stated repeatedly that incision depth is a paramount factor in the outcome of RK. As was pointed out first by Fyodorov and his coworkers and amply demonstrated since by the author and others, there are three factors that affect the depth of incision [1–6]. These are:

1 Blade length
2 Blade sharpness
3 Tissue resistance

All these factors are interrelated, but only the first two can be controlled directly. The third factor can be compensated for to some degree by oversetting the blade.

Blades and blade handles

The ideal blade should have an extremely sharp point to penetrate to the maximum depth set instead of pushing the tissue ahead of it. In addition, the edge must be as sharp as possible to make an incision that is as smooth as possible. Depending on the material, there seems to be a practical limit to the sharpness of the point and the edge. Steel does not readily take an edge much sharper than 1000 Å (Figure 8.1a, b). Material such as diamond can be taken to a theoretical limit of 20 to 50 Å in edge radius. However, in practical terms, diamond is extremely difficult to cut into slabs much thinner than 0.30 mm. Getting an edge radius of less than 300 Å requires an expensive process that makes the price of such blades prohibitive. In addition, the bevel angle of the typical diamond blade is 43° (although some newer blades have been able to reduce this angle to 35°), resulting in a "snowplow" effect while cutting (Figure 8.2). In fact, the performance of the early diamond blades, in my hands, had been so disappointing that I, as well as many others, had gone back to the steel blade and was recommending that beginning RK surgeons not even consider the purchase of a crystal knife for some time. This recommendation has since changed with the advent of the sapphire (see below and Figure 8.3) and newer diamond blades.

(a)

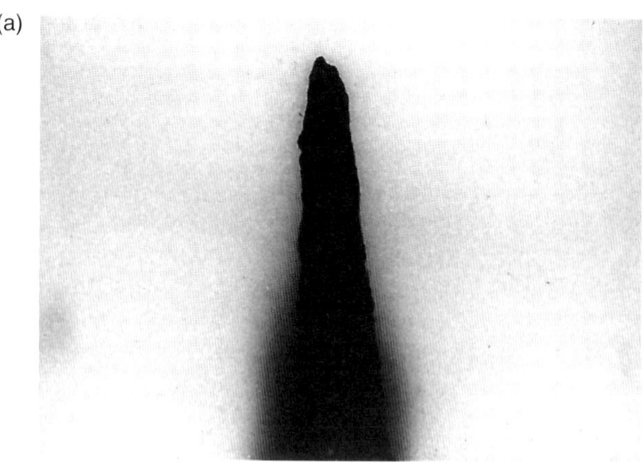

(b)

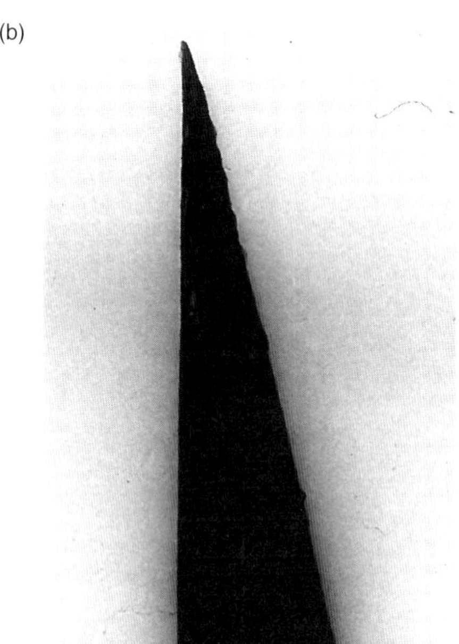

Fig. 8.1 (a) SEM of a steel blade tip ×50. (b) SEM of a sapphire blade tip ×50.

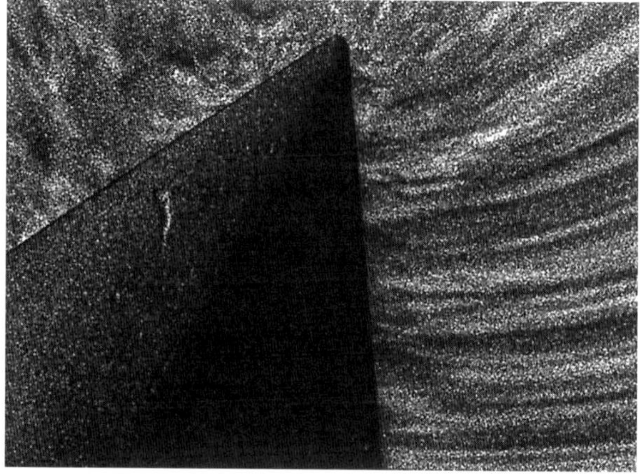

Fig. 8.2 SEM of the blade tip of a second-generation diamond blade ×400.

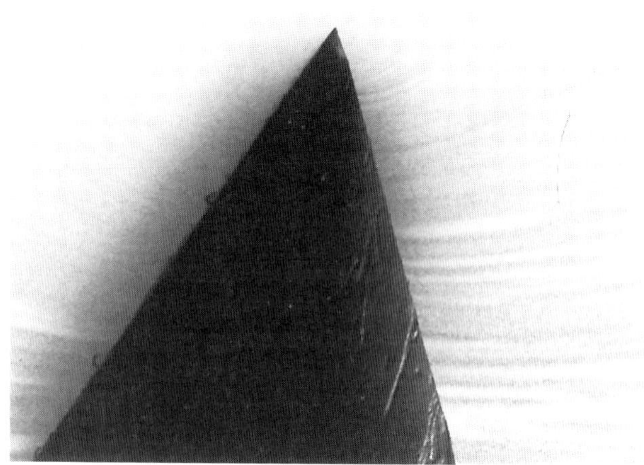

Fig. 8.3 SEM of sapphire RK blade.

Ruby is second in hardness to diamond and is somewhat easier to work, but it is difficult to get a uniform crystalline structure. I am very disappointed in its performance. Despite its hardness, it does not seem to hold an edge well. In addition, it tends to "drag" when passed through tissue.

Sapphire has the same hardness characteristics as ruby but is easier to handle. Under the right circumstances, it is possible to grow the crystal at a particular crystalline angle that, when sliced and chemically machined, produces a smooth, ultrasharp edge, in many cases surpassing diamond and in all cases surpassing steel blades. Such a blade is available commercially under the trade name XTAL and is still marketed by the Katena Corporation.

Sapphire blades, while tougher than steel, still have a finite life and eventually must be replaced. Unless broken, the tip of such a blade wears evenly and smoothly, however. If the operator possesses an optical comparator (such as the DGH-800 Bores Shadowgraphic Blade Gauge), it is possible to monitor the wear and compensate for it (see the section on optical or indirect gauges, below). Some sort of optical magnifier/comparator device is highly recommended as essential in proper performance of incision-based refractive surgical procedures. This type of monitoring extends the life of the blade some threefold. In a busy practice, this device will pay for itself very quickly in terms of blade life and successful surgery. Even in a worse-case situation, where 70 to 80 μm of bias must be used, such a blade will cut significantly more smoothly and evenly than any steel blade and many diamond blades.

Diamond has an advantage over sapphire in that it is much harder. Properly cared for, it can last considerably longer. Coupled with the use of a shadowgraph-type gauge, one blade could last for many years. The problem with diamond has been that its very hardness has placed practical limits on the quality of the blade produced.

(a)

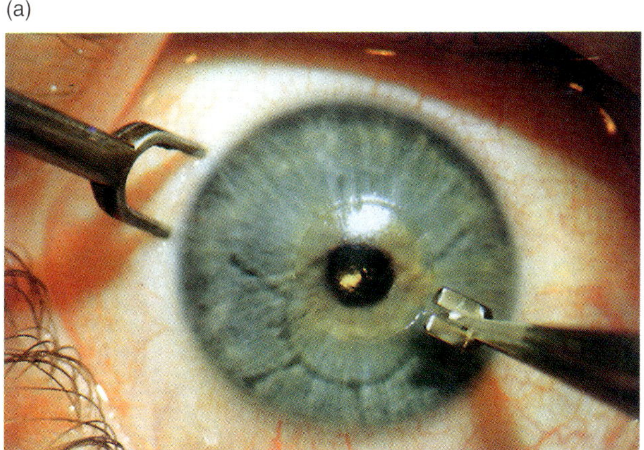

(b)

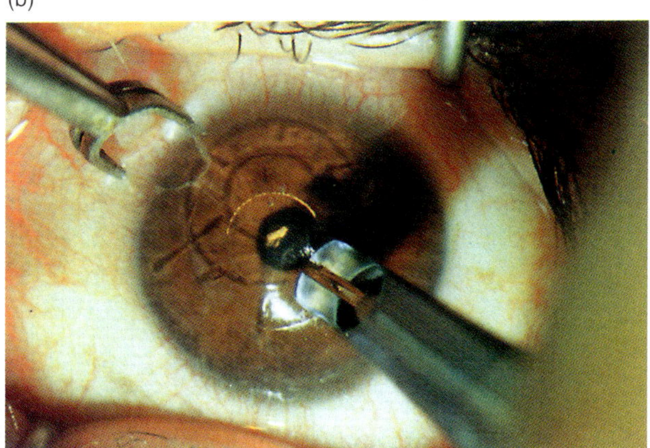

Fig. 8.4 (a) Katena footplate on cornea; (b) Micra (old style) footplate on cornea.

Recently, manufacturers have been making great strides in improving quality. The Western Medical Products WMK 200 KOI (LeCut) ultrathin diamond blade, made to the author's specifications, is a quantum improvement over previous blades. It is only 0.15 mm in thickness with an included bevel angle of 33°, giving it an edge thickness of 220 Å—very similar to sapphire, until recently the sharpest unicrystalline blade made. This double-edged blade is designed to fit into the Katena K2-6500 series handles and is completely interchangeable with the XTAL series sapphire blades.

It has been the practice, even with sapphire, to set the blade longer than the measured corneal thickness. This overset (bias) has amounted to as much as 15% of the corneal thickness (typically 60 to 70 μm) with some diamond knives—best case. With the XTAL sapphire single-edge blade, it is necessary to overset the blade only 20 to 30 μm (0.02 mm) to ensure adequate depth—again, best case. The new double-edged XTAL requires only a 10-μm overset—again, best case—whereas the WKM KOI diamond requires a bias of 0 μm. This latter bias requirement makes the WKM KOI one of the sharpest blades yet available for RK with a price comparable to that of a similar double-edged sapphire blade. The ability to make consistently deep incisions is increasing the accuracy of our predictions considerably, as well as increasing the surgical effect.

Another factor to be considered is blade interchangeability; that is, can the blade be removed from the handle and replaced with another in the case of breakage or dulling or if a different edge shape is needed? Most commercially available diamond knives presently lock the surgeon into a fixed handle/blade situation. This, coupled with unreliability and high cost, makes such knives—in my view—a second choice to an interchangeable sapphire blade or the new diamond from Western Medical KOI.

The handle should have an open L-shaped (or "sewing machine") foot with ample distance from the jaw or collet to the foot to allow an unobstructed view of the back of the blade for the Bores (American) technique or leading edge for the Fyodorov (Russian) technique (Figure 8.4). The footplate, in addition, should have the foot extend in front of the blade at least 1.0 mm (Figure 8.5). The tip should have a gentle upward curve (like a ski tip) starting ahead of the leading blade edge, and all footplate edges must be smooth and parallel with all surfaces and polished to a mirror finish. The slot for the blade should be wide enough to allow free movement of the blade during adjustment but not wide enough to trap debris or corneal tissue. Each half of the footplate should be between 0.75 and 1.00 mm in width—wide enough to provide adequate support and stability but not so wide as to obstruct the view of adjacent incisions. The spine of the blade should describe an angle of 90° to the footplate and should be set

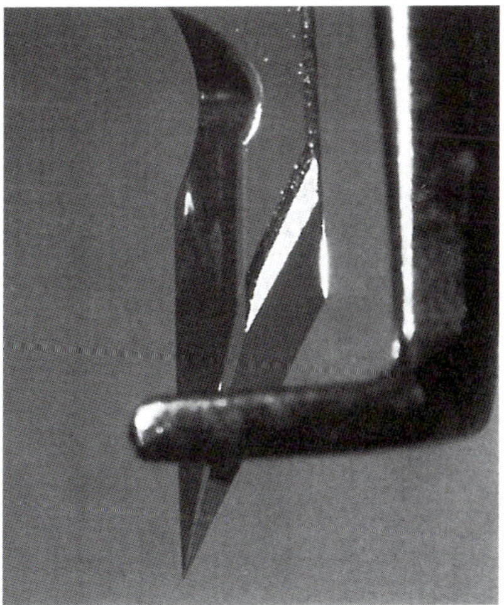

Fig. 8.5 The footplate on the Bores knife handle as supplied by Katena Instruments. Note the extension of the footplate ahead of the blade and that the curve of the footplate lies in front of the vertical cutting edge.

in sufficiently that if the handle is tipped backward or forward, a deeper cut does not occur. Some knives have the front curvature beginning at the centerline of the blade, thus materially affecting the depth of the incision depending on the direction of cut (Figure 8.6). The handle should allow smooth, continuous adjustment of blade length from a maximum of 1.0 to a minimum of –2.0 mm. Ideally, it should be equipped with a zeroing micrometer scale for fine adjustments of the blade once set (Figure 8.7).

With this type of system, the blade is advanced and checked against a gauge. After the proper length has been set, the micrometer scale is zeroed (see Figure 8.7a). Each division on the micrometer barrel should correspond to some even multiple of a millimeter, such as 0.01 or 0.0125 mm. However, no micrometer handle should be trusted to set the blade initially. The initial setting *always* should be checked against a proper gauge—preferably an optical one. There is too much play in any adjustment system to be completely accurate, particularly over a long range. However, with a zeroing micrometer barrel, small advances in the blade can be made with confidence. Because of this built-in play or looseness in the screw mechanism (backlash), always set the blade while advancing it. Never set the blade by backing up on the micrometer barrel and expect the setting to be correct—it never will be. Always check the blade setting against a gauge (Figure 8.8).

The blade should be removed easily for cleaning and replacement. If it cannot be removed, it should be able to be retracted sufficiently to clean it mechanically on all sides, as well as allow access to the foot for cleaning without damaging the blade tip. Finally, the handle should not be excessively heavy or bulky but should be able to be held easily in the fingers without fatigue. The Bores XTAL

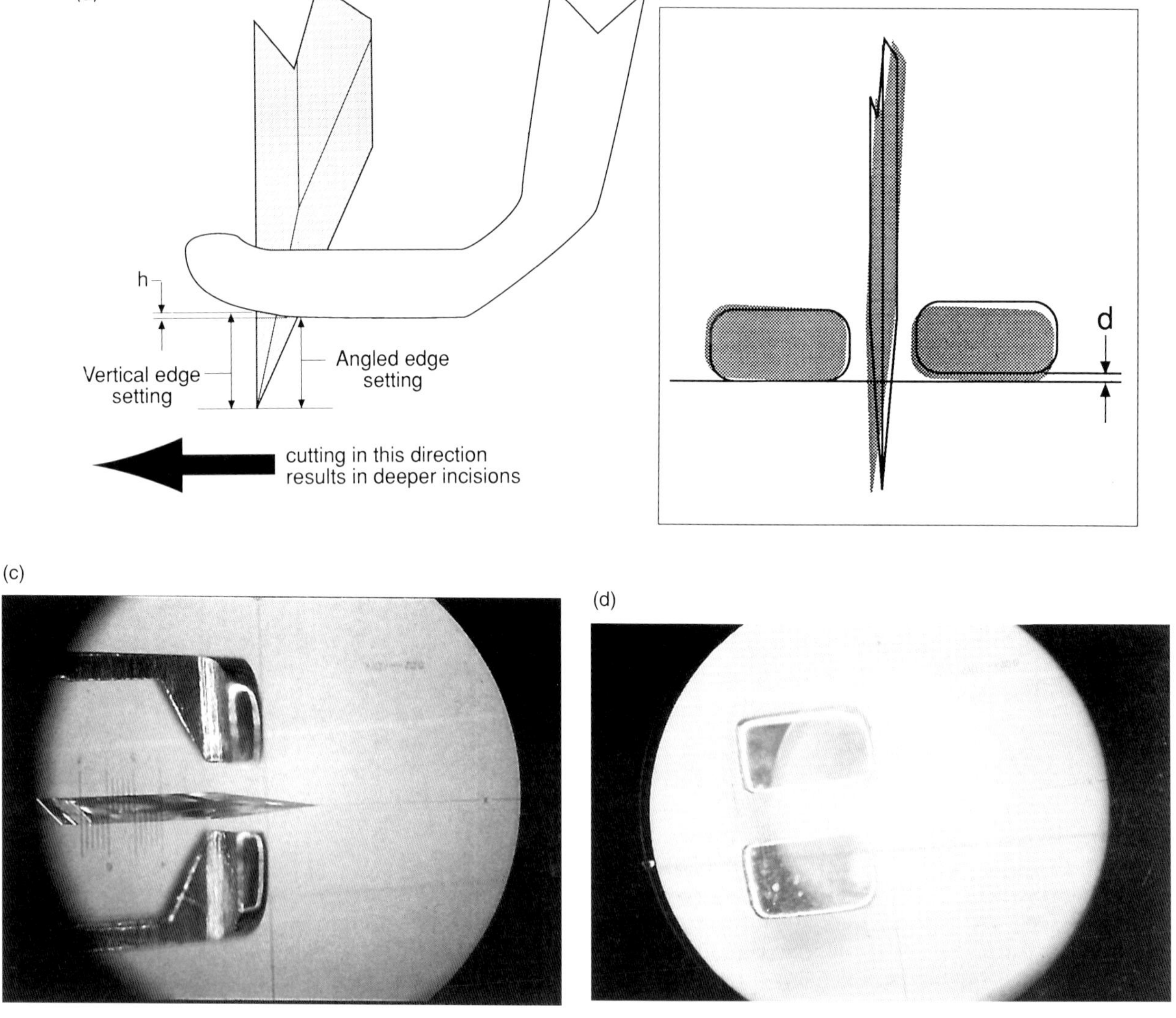

Fig. 8.6 (a) Difference between cutting with the vertical and angled blade edge. (b) Displaced footplates result in oblique incisions. (c,d) Using an optical comparator can readily detect displaced footplates.

(a)

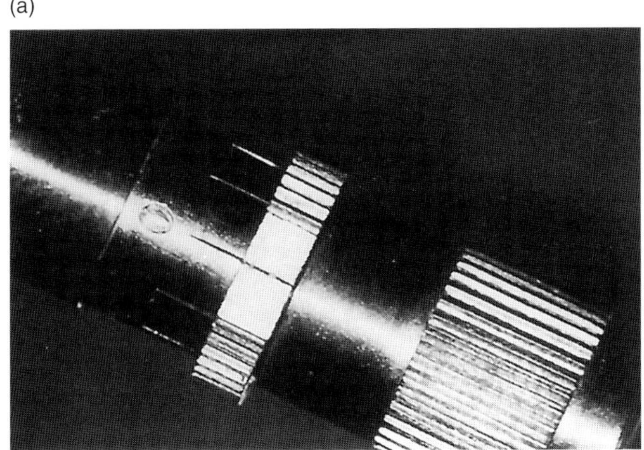

(b)

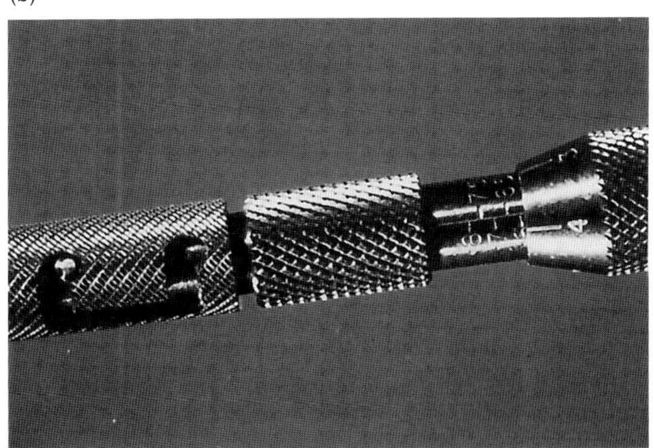

Fig. 8.7 (a) The micrometer adjustment dial on the Bores knife handle is used for fine adjustment once the blade is set with a gauge. (b) The micrometer adjustment on a typical fixed-blade diamond knife is used for all blade settings.

Micrometer Knife Handle available from Katena (K2-6505 and –07) meets all these requirements (Figure 8.9).

Handles with removable blades should be cleaned in an ultrasonic cleaner from time to time with the blade removed, rinsed with warm distilled water, and blown dry before storing in their carriers (K2-6555). Blades should be rinsed carefully in distilled water and wiped with a wet Weck-Cel or other microsponge. For stubborn residue, contact lens enzyme cleaner is useful. *Do not ultrasonically clean any crystalline blade of whatever material.* Avoid the use of potassium or sodium hydroxide as well, which tends to etch such blades. Blades can be stored in their original carriers or in the micrometer handle and may be steam or dry-gas sterilized.

Blade gauges and gauging

As the quality of blade edges has improved, there has been an ever-increasing emphasis on the accurate measurement of blade length. A precise, linearly stable gauge is a must. While many so-called coin gauges are sold with diamond and other knives, their only advantage is ease of use. Their disadvantages include measurement error due to parallax, error due to dimensional instability, and error in manufacturing. Unfortunately, many manufacturers have not gotten the message about the need for extreme accuracy in this surgery. Either that or they have let expediency guide them or, worse, are second-guessing the needs of the surgeon (a frequent occurrence). Gauges do not lend themselves to mass production; this is why so many small gauge shops thrive in industry today. Such instruments cannot be made of nylon, aluminum, glass, or combination materials. They cannot have the ticks photo-etched in (at least with commonly available methods)—such a process leads to wide lines with imprecise edges. Gauges cannot be black chromed to reduce glare—such a process will in time wear off, destroying the accuracy of the gauge. They must be made of stainless tool steel with the ticks scribed under a microscope by an expert in gauge making.

Direct-measuring gauges

One such gauge block is the Bores Corneal Gauge Block, once manufactured by Crawford Precision Grinding in Wixom, Michigan, and unfortunately no longer avail-

(a)

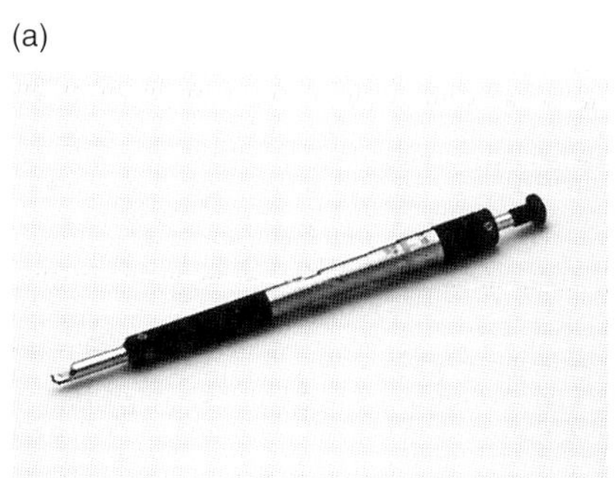

(b)

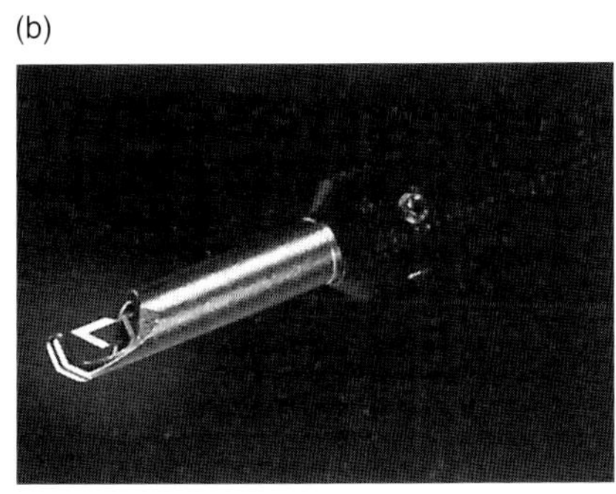

(c)

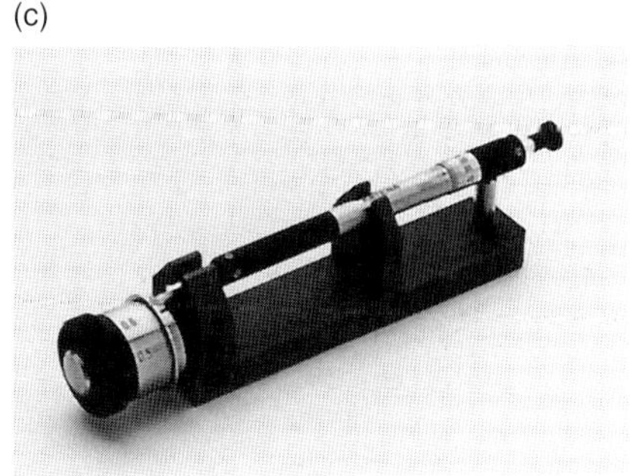

Fig. 8.8 (a) Typical micrometer diamond knife. (b) The footplate is short and does not extend sufficiently in front of the vertical blade edge. (c) Dial-type gauge and holder for this knife. This type of gauge is somewhat less prone to parallax errors when setting.

(a)

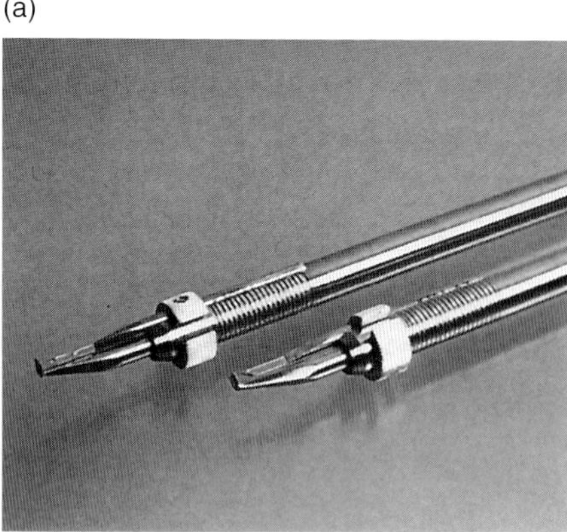

(b)

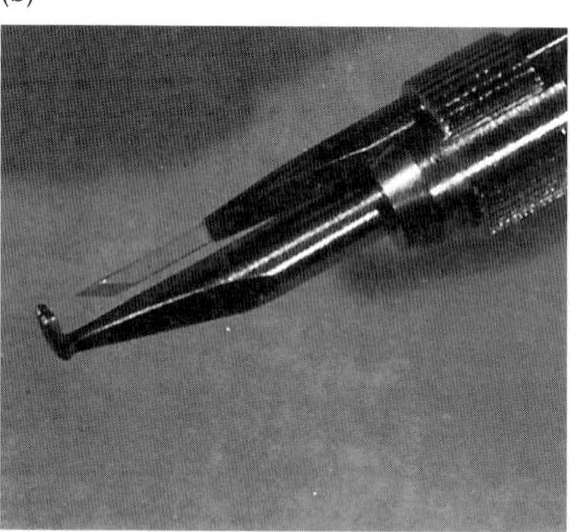

Fig. 8.9 (a) Author's knife handle design with vertical and angled blades—as manufactured by Katena. (b) Note the open construction which allows excellent visibility of the blade, which is easily changed.

able (Figure 8.10). It was the first blade gauge made for this surgery, and since 1979, this instrument has served as the standard for RK blade gauges. This gauge is made of tool steel and is certified to an accuracy of ±3 μm. Professor Fyodorov used it exclusively until recently, when he duplicated it in his own shop. Other manufacturers have used it as a "check" gauge while making their own.

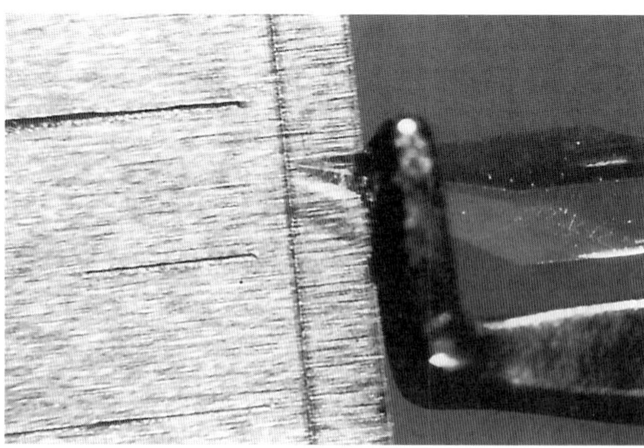

Fig. 8.11 Bores gauge in use with double-edged sapphire blade.

If this gauge is not used correctly, however, an erroneous measurement will result, as with any other gauge. The measurement must be made from the edge of the block to the *front edge* of the scribed datum line (Figure 8.11). This is so because the scribe marks were made with a flat-sided diamond scriber with the flat side held against the straight edge. This results in a half-V-shaped scribe mark whose straight edge is perpendicular to the gauge surface. Other gauges require the measurement to be made to the *bottom* of a V-shaped groove (Figure 8.12). Small changes in steel hardness can cause the scriber to wander as it moves, changing the distance of the point from the straight-edge guide. In addition, the fact that the scriber is V-shaped prevents its being held perpendicular to the edge of the guide. Both these problems result in wandering of the bottom of the V-groove with respect to the edge of the block and thus can produce errors in measurement. You should acquaint yourself with the characteristics of your gauge prior to using it in any event.

The Bores gauge has proven itself more than equal to the task of measuring blade settings but has disadvantages that make it difficult to use. First, despite efforts to make it less so, this gauge is quite reflective. The resulting glare

(a) (b)

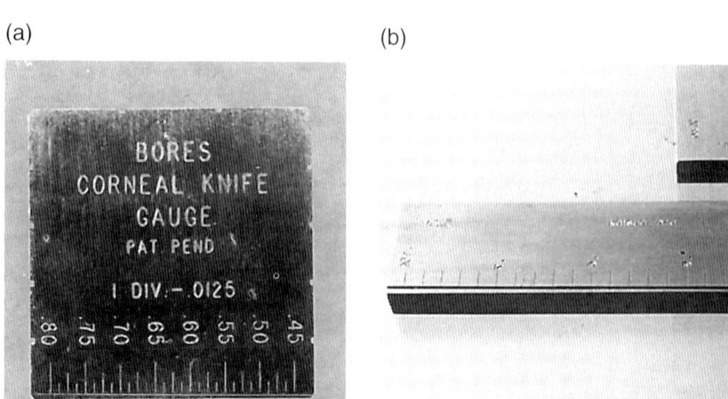

Fig. 8.10 (a) Bores corneal gauge block; (b) Kremer corneal knife gauge.

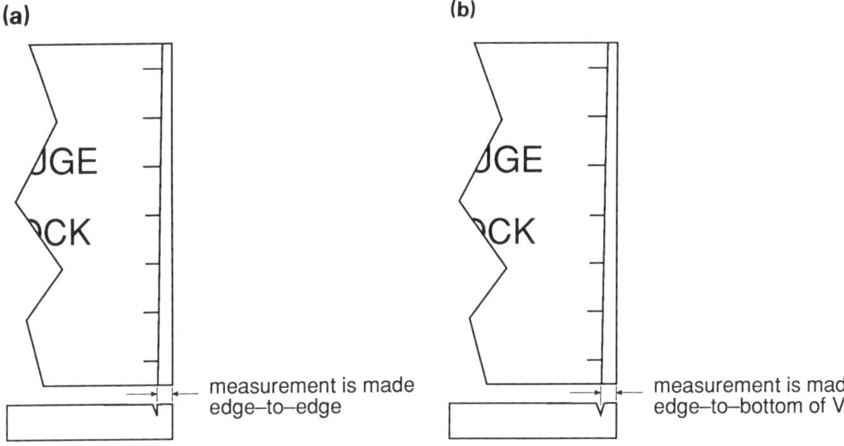

Fig. 8.12 (a) The scribe mark should be made with a flat-sided scriber. (b) A V-shaped scriber tends to wander.

makes precise measurements difficult but not impossible. This is a larger factor with the crystalline blades because of their transparency. Black chroming, while reducing the glare somewhat, will wear off in time, destroying the accuracy of the block. It is not generally appreciated that the finishing grind on the Bores block has produced the equivalent of a Ronchi ruling (see Figure 8.11). This can be verified by tilting the block slightly under the microscope and observing the color changes. It will be noted that at a certain position, the surface of the block takes on a rainbow hue. At this point, the glare falls away to almost nil. That the surface is polarizing the light reflected from its surface can be appreciated by holding a diamond blade parallel to the measuring surface (Figure 8.13). The diamond becomes black (or very nearly so) because of cross-polarization. This phenomenon extends to the XTAL blade as well, making this block suitable for any blade the surgeon might be inclined to use.

The block requires the user to steady his or her hands on some surface such as a Mayo stand, wrist rest, or even the patient's forehead to prevent "dinging" the blade edge against the steel block. As the blades have changed and their sharpness increased, the edges and tips have become thinner and more vulnerable. A mere touch of the blade against the gauge can render a crystalline blade useless for RK, be it diamond or any other material. To prevent damage to the blade (a match can burn down a house), it must be approximated carefully to the gauge surface with the blade edge rotated upward slightly along its long axis (Figure 8.14). This brings the edge up and away from the block. Care must be taken not to press the blade against the block to avoid breaking the tip or the edge. If this happens, the blade still can be used to make cataract sections but little else.

This block (and others like it) is an expensive, precision instruments and must be handled with care. It should be stored in its original container or in a specially padded plastic box and given a dip in instrument milk if the gauge is not going to be used for some time—to prevent rust. The block must not be allowed to come into contact with metallic objects.

There are limits to the resolution of the current operating microscope systems, which further adds to the prob-

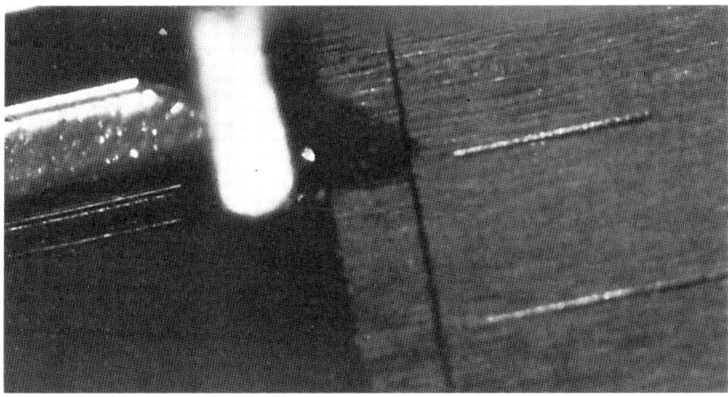

Fig. 8.13 Color change in blade caused by the cross-polarizing effect of the gauge finish and the crystal lattice of the blade.

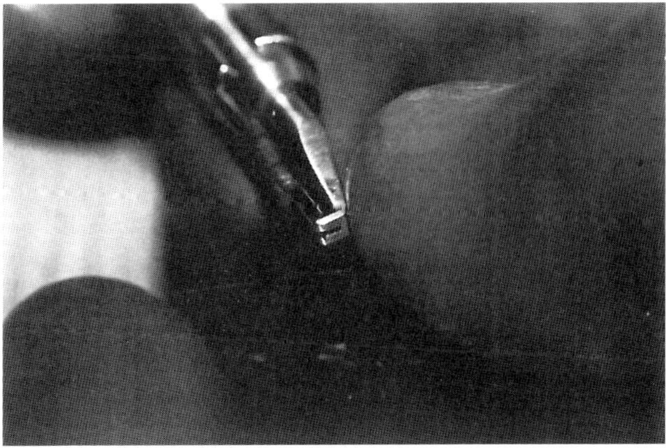

Fig. 8.14 In this single-edged sapphire the edge is rotated slightly to move the blade away from the gauge block. Measurement is taken along the back or spine of the blade.

lem of obtaining an accurate measurement. In addition, as blade tips have become finer, difficulties in judging the tip end for measurement purposes have increased. The life expectancy of a single-edged sapphire blade in experienced hands, in these circumstances, is about 80 cases. At approximately $350 per blade (single edge), this works out to a little over $4 per case. In inexperienced hands, the average life of such a blade is about 10 cases, or $35 per case, which compares with disposable steel blades at $35 per case. With the newer, sharper, thinner double-edged XTAL blades ($750), this average falls to 30 ($25 per case) and 5 ($150 per case) cases, respectively. It does not take long for this to add up; the author was changing one or more blades weekly when using the steel gauge.

Optical or indirect gauges

For years, devices called *shadowgraphs* have been used to examine and measure, under high magnification, objects made from transparent materials. These devices are usually quite large, bulky, and very expensive. They do, however, provide a highly accurate means of measurement. An early attempt to emulate, inexpensively, the features of the shadowgraph was the Magna Diamond Microscopic Blade Gauge (Figure 8.15). While the device provides an excellent view of the blade and increases accuracy of measurement, it presents the very real hazards of blade damage and contamination of a sterile knife/blade. It is awkward to use and vulnerable to dust. It is not recommended for use within the operating room but is adequate for presetting blades and examining their tips and edges for defects.

The DGH-800 Bores Shadowgraphic Blade Gauge (Figure 8.16) was designed with three goals in mind:

- Accuracy
- Ease of use
- Cost-effectiveness

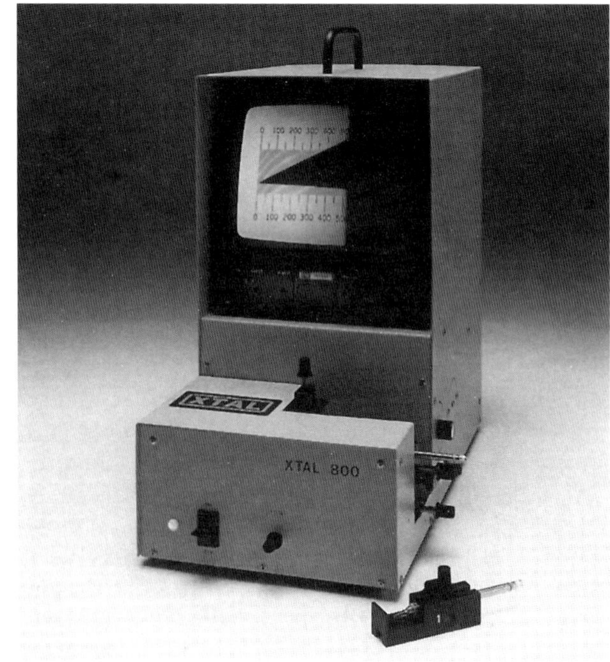

Fig. 8.16 Shadowgraph and knife carrier.

To this end, the instrument is supplied with a special sterilizable carrier into which the knife handle and blade are placed and clamped. These carriers are available for almost all makes of knife handles and blades. The entire assembly can then be transferred onto the measuring stage for final setting of the blade. The DGH-800 provides a magnification of ×190, which also allows inspection of the blade tip and edge. By using this device, it is possible to triple the useful life of the XTAL sapphire blades. This means that the instrument can pay for itself in about 2 months in the active RK practice. More important, the depth of the incisions will become more uniform, thereby

(a)

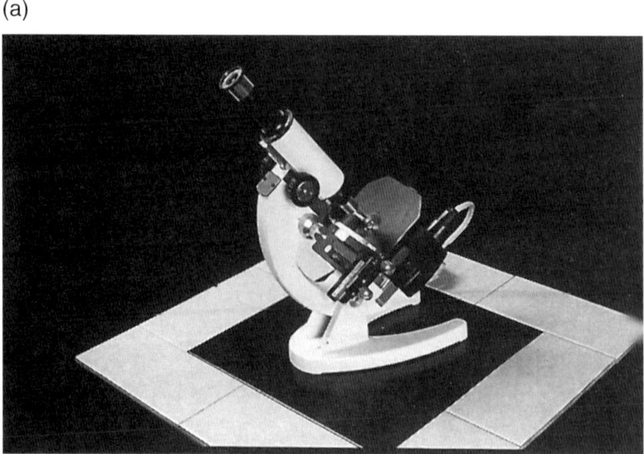

(b)

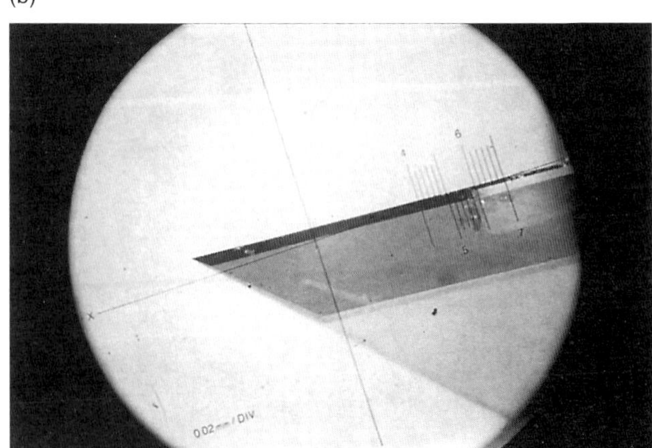

Fig. 8.15 (a,b) Magna diamond microscope and diamond blade.

increasing the confidence level of preoperative calculations. Normal rounding of the blade tip can be seen readily, and the compensating bias change can be made with ease (see below).

Fixation devices

Fixation of the eye is important to ensure that all incisions are straight and perpendicular to the corneal surface. There are many devices on the market designed for this purpose. Any such device that is used should be applied and removed easily and should not produce tissue damage. In addition, it must not interfere with the surgery.

The vacuum fixation devices based on the Barraquer fixation ring (Steinway Instruments, San Diego, CA) have not met these criteria—they always interfere with blade travel (Figure 8.17). For best results, they must be used with peribulbar anesthesia because they produce considerable pain when the vacuum comes on. In addition, the inner edge of the ring prevents the footplate of the knife from traveling its full length, requiring that the incisions be extended after the ring is removed. Expanding the inner opening to provide knife clearance requires enlarging the entire ring so as to provide an adequate suction surface. This results in a ring of such size that movement of the eye is greatly restricted, making some incisions awkward, if not impossible, to perform. It is not possible, for example, to rotate the eye downward without breaking suction and losing fixation. Considerable chemosis of the conjunctiva results from use of this device. For these reasons, the fact that it is expensive, and the fact that the job can be done better and less expensively by other means, this device is not recommended.

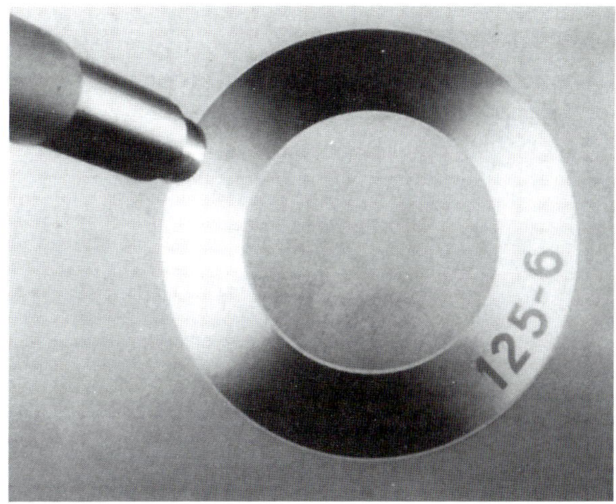

Fig. 8.17 Vacuum fixation ring.

Another ring device, this one with a number of straight teeth arranged around its rim, is available from Katena—the Thornton Fixation Ring, K3-6165 (Figure 8.18). This device is used by centering it over the front of the eye and pressing downward. This device has the advantage of pressurizing the eye, as does the vacuum ring, but it does not cause the pain—hence peribulbar injection is unnecessary. It is easy to reposition as well. It shares with the vacuum ring the problem of being awkward to use, interferes with the surgery, and in the event of a microperforation can make matters worse.

Still another ring fixation device is based on the mechanism of the "twist-pick." This device is placed onto the eye with the handle rotated to one side. Pressing down against the eye and moving the handle to the 12 o'clock position "screws" it into the sclera, thereby allowing the eye to be pulled as well as pushed. In the event of a microperforation, the device acts like a Bonnocalto ring, supporting the eye instead of allowing it to collapse. Its rim is flared outward to minimize interference with the knife jaw. It shares the disadvantages of all ring devices, however, in that it is awkward to use if kept in one position

(a)

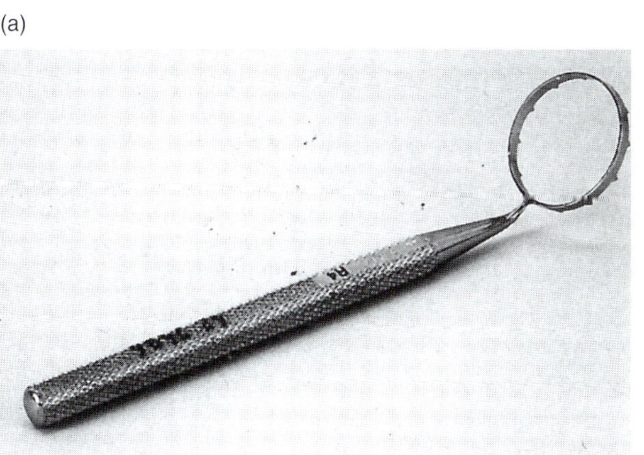

(b)

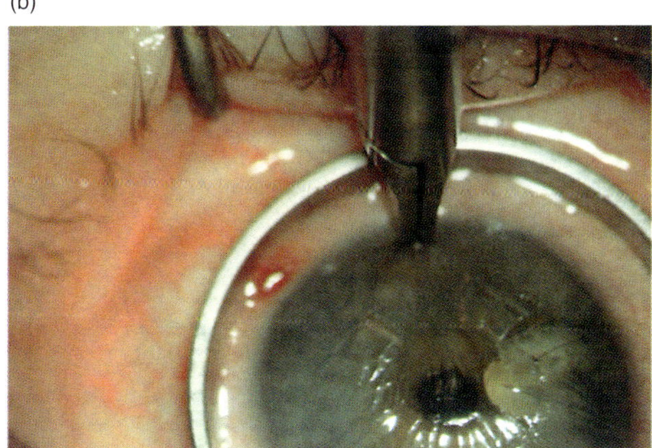

Fig. 8.18 (a) Thornton fixation ring; (b) ring in use. Note how close it is to the limbus, which interferes with knife travel. This photo shows another disadvantage of the ring, if a leak occurs.

and interferes with movement of the eye. It is available from Katena as the Bores Twist Fixation Ring (K3-6160). It has proven to be more useful in performing penetrating keratoplasties than in refractive surgery.

Fixation of the eye is obtained easily by use of a forceps applied to the limbus. Forceps that grasp the cornea or incision edge (such as the Bracken) are not recommended because of the possibility of tearing the tissue. I designed and had made for me a double-pronged fixation forceps (Katena K5-3250). This forceps has a double set of 0.12-mm corneal-scleral teeth placed 3.0 mm apart. This forceps is applied to the conjoint tendon at the limbus at 180° to the incision to be made (Figure 8.19a). The double fixation points prevent undue ocular rotation without the corneal distortion a wider jaw would produce—especially in a soft eye. Some ocular rotation will occur, allowing the track of the incision to remain straight. Forceps that totally prevent some ocular rotation usually require the surgeon to make compensating moves with the knife to keep the incisions straight.

A wide-jawed forceps such as the Bores Wide Fixation Forceps (K5-3280) provides the cross-limbus fixation essential to making straight transverse incisions—as in the Ruiz procedure (Figure 8.19b, c). Here, the eye must be prevented from rotating to prevent the natural tendency of the incision to curve. These instruments are also available with angled jaws for those who prefer it.

Compressor devices, such as the Mendez Optic Compressor—an infernal device that squeezes the eye like a grape in order "to pressurize it"—are to be avoided at all costs.

(a)

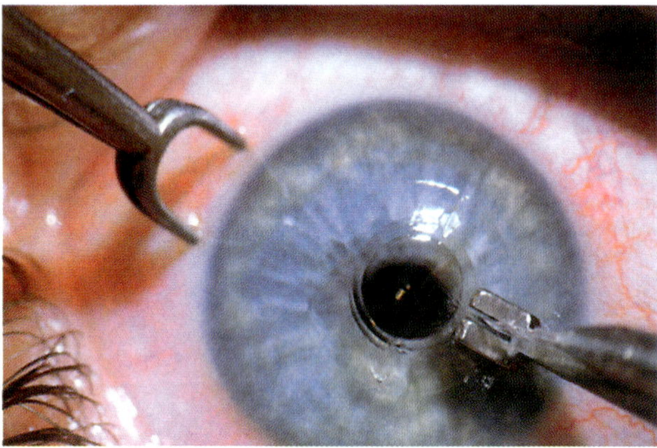

(b)

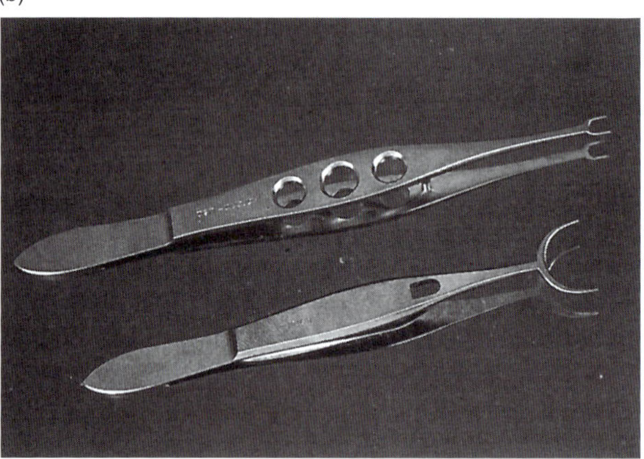

(c)

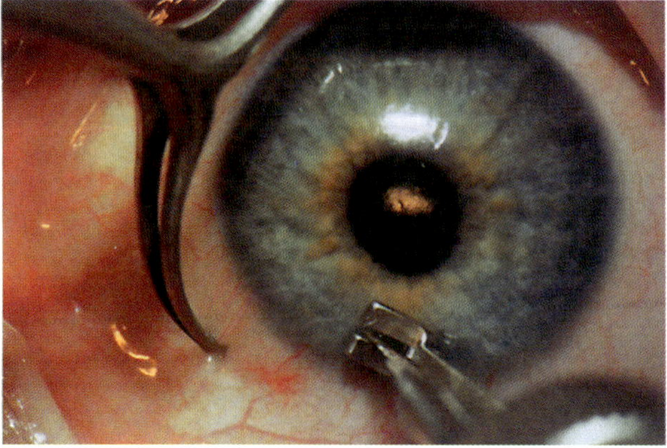

Fig. 8.19 (a) Bores fixation forceps (narrow) in use; (b) narrow and wide fixation forceps; (c) advantage of the wide forceps.

Optical zone and other markers

Corneal optical zone markers are available from various vendors. Some of these markers are not accurate (especially those for astigmatism), having been formed by stretching over a mandrel. The worst of these are the double-ended variety. Others are obviously made for people with size 2 hands. The best markers on the market today, in my opinion, are those supplied by the Katena Instrument Company (Figure 8.20).

The ideal spherical corneal marker is a perfect circle accurate to 0.05 mm and made in 0.25-mm increments from 3.0 to 5.0 mm and in 0.50-mm increments from 5.50

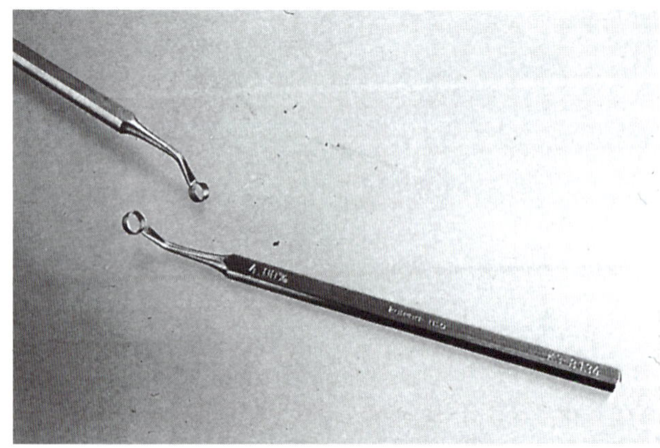

Fig. 8.20 Bores Lo-Profile optical zone marker.

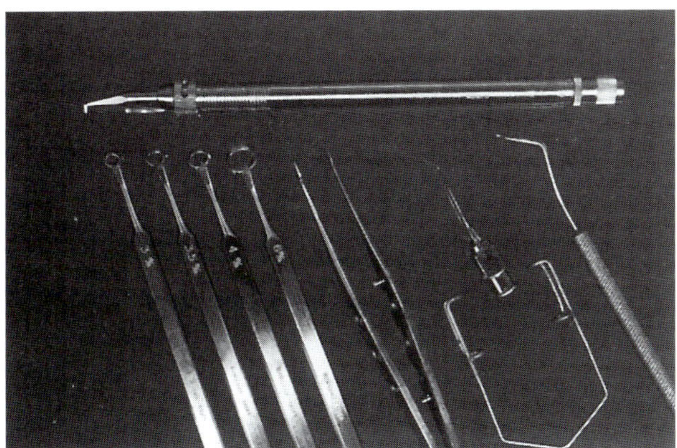

Fig. 8.21 Basic instrument set showing minimal number of markers required.

(a)

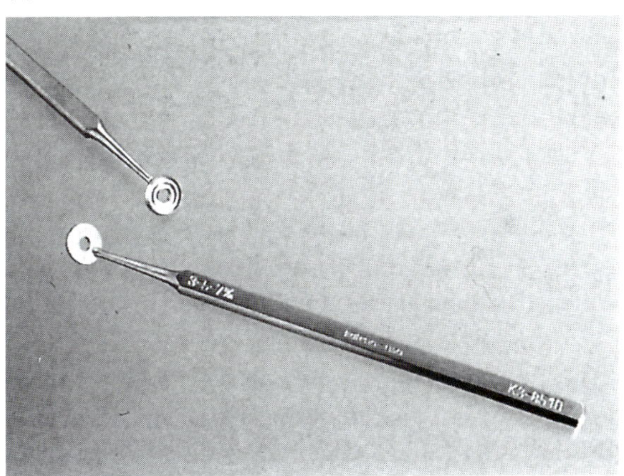

(b)

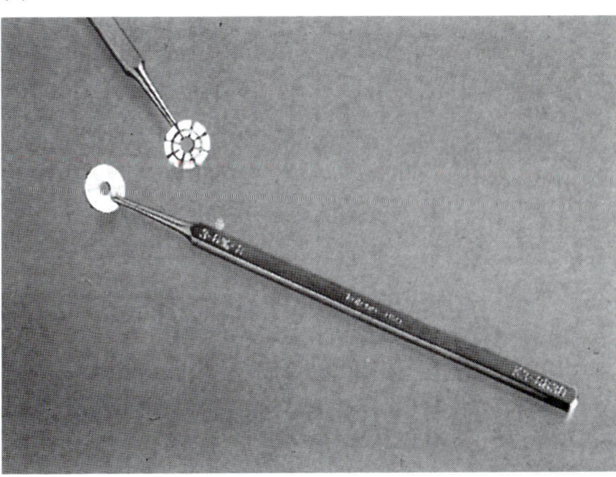

Fig. 8.23 (a) Double- and triple-ring markers; (b) double-ring/incision markers.

to 8.0 mm. Of these, the most used will be the 3.0-, 3.5-, 4.0-, 4.5-, and 6.0-mm markers (Figure 8.21). However, eventually, all the sizes will find use in a busy refractive surgical practice. These should have an outside bevel to an edge sharp enough to mark the cornea with a fine narrow mark without cutting into the corneal surface. The markers can be shallow, but if deeper than 3.0 mm, they should be wider at the top (have a conical shape) so as to provide a clear view of the entire "business end" of the marker. Deeper markers should be provided with openings in their sides to allow light to enter so as to better visualize the corneal surface. A good example is the Fyodorov series of surgical zone markers (Figure 8.22).

Cross-hairs or other centering aids are useful but not essential and frequently are aligned inaccurately. Sizes should be clearly marked on each marker, particularly astigmatism markers. All markers, especially those for astigmatism, must be handled with care to prevent damage that may distort their shapes. Double-ring markers have been produced but are not especially useful for the starting surgeon (Figure 8.23). Those of 3.0 and 6.0 and 3.5 and 6.0 mm will prove to be the most helpful. An occasional use will be found for a triple marker with rings at 3.0, 6.0, and 8.0 mm.

Special devices for marking the incision lines or spacing are available as well (Figure 8.24). However, all of these, with one exception, are optional. The one exception is the six-blade incision marker (Katena K3-8880), or the Fyodorov incision marker (Figure 8.25). While it is

(a) (b)

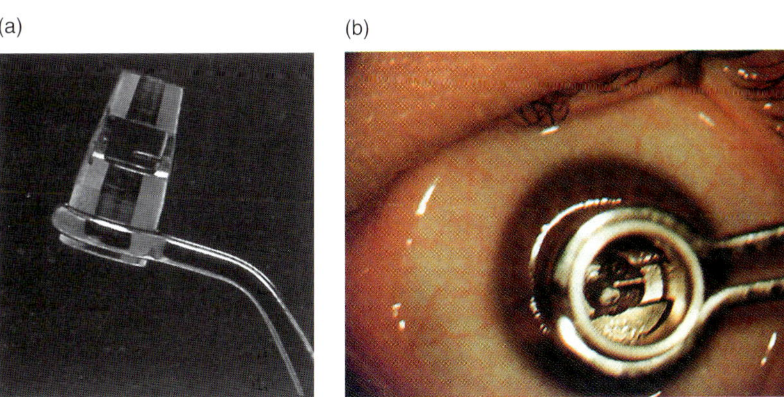

Fig. 8.22 (a) Fyodorov "bore-sight" marker; (b) the marker tapers and has an aiming stud.

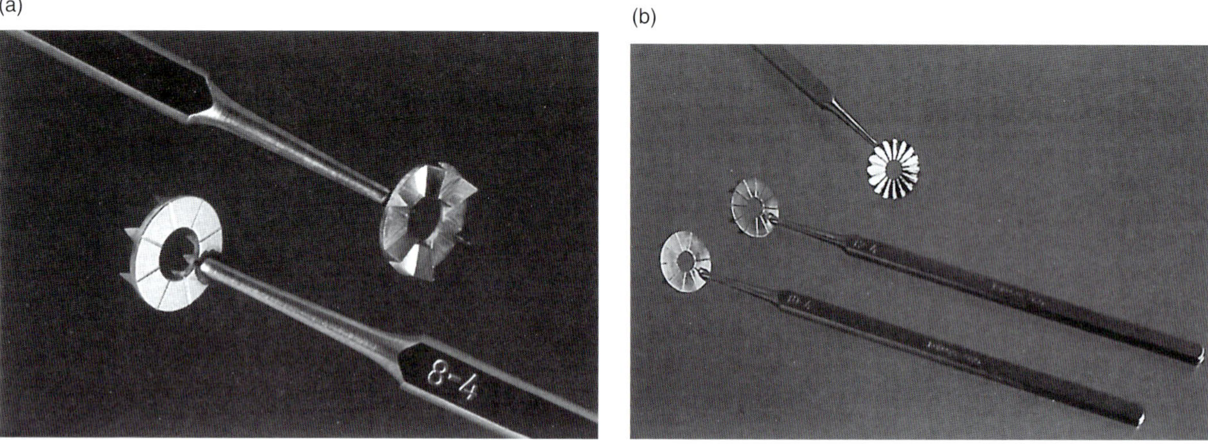

Fig. 8.24 Incision markers: (a) 6 and 8, (b) 10 and 12 incisions.

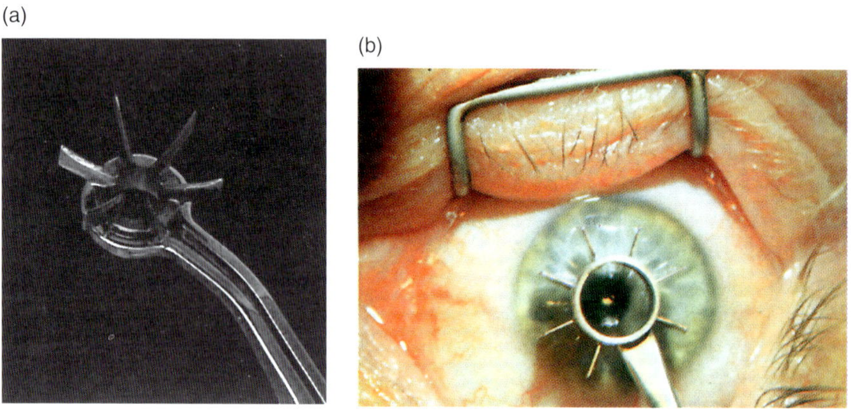

Fig. 8.25 (a) Fyodorov six-ray incision marker; (b) in use.

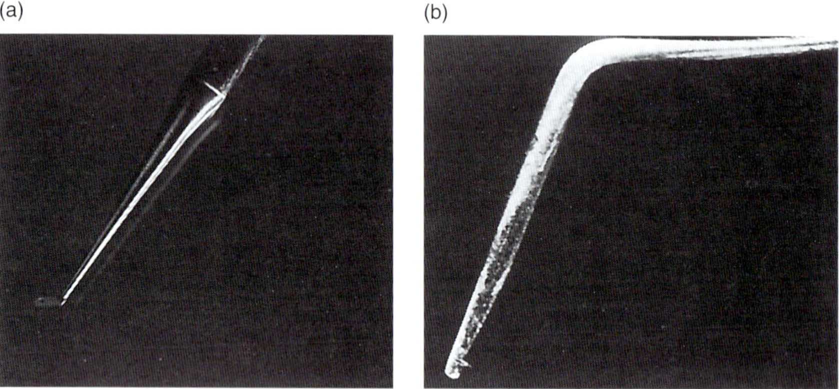

Fig. 8.26 (a) Deitz hockey stick; (b) Fyodorov dipstick.

possible to make 4, 8, or 16 incisions evenly spaced by eye, it is not quite so easy to accurately judge the 30° or 60° between incisions in 6- or 12-incision cases. Coating the bottom of this marker with brilliant green or gentian violet will enhance its usefulness—at least for the beginner or when demonstrating the surgery. More experienced surgeons will find the central ends of the marks sufficient to align their incisions.

Other useful instruments

There are some other instruments that surgeons will find of use. A thin, flexible, flat-sided probe, such as the Deitz Incision Depth Gauge (Katena K3-9600, –10, or –20) is handy (Figure 8.26). This "hockey stick" is used to measure the relative depth of incisions and check the continuity of the incision bottom, especially for "snags" from

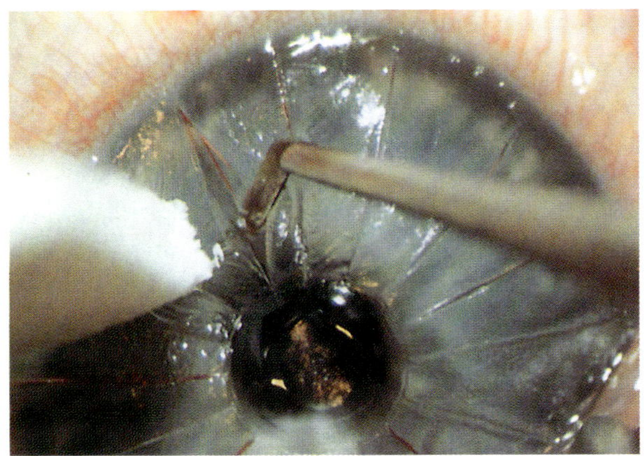

Fig. 8.27 Checking the wound with the dipstick.

improperly stepped incisions (Figure 8.27). Although available with three different blade widths, only one—K3-9620—is really needed. It is also useful for marking the optical center during optical zone marking and is recommended for this purpose over sharp needles.

Incision spreaders are used in rare patients with higher myopia to deepen previously made incisions (Katena K5-6800). These instruments should be angled to provide an unobstructed view of the bottom of the incision (Figure 8.28). They also should be provided with an adjustable stop to prevent overspreading of the wound. Those made with large teeth (inverted Colibri forceps) should not be used because of the extensive tissue damage that can result if the eye moves. A newer type of spreader with diamond (or carborundum) chips on the outer surfaces of the spreader provides greater friction against slipping without the danger of tearing tissue.

A small-bore irrigating cannula with a rounded tip and flattened bore (Rainin 27-gauge cannula, Katena K7-3580) is used to cleanse the incisions of debris postoperatively. Such an irrigation stream should be gentle and directed along the incision to flush the wound toward the limbus.

A wire lid speculum of the Barraquer type (Katena K1-5010) is recommended for supporting the lids (Figure 8.29). It should not be one with solid blades because this type will pop out with a blink. The Guyton-Park, or rigid-type, speculum is not recommended because it is too traumatizing to the lids and levator aponeurosis. Seven patients with upper lid ptosis caused by levator damage have been reported in whom this type of lid speculum was clearly implicated [7].

A suitable tray-case should be obtained that is of a size adequate to hold a basic set of surgical instruments without their being bashed together and damaged. If the lid is removable for autoclaving, so much the better. Spare instruments can be put up in sterile bags, preferably those with one clear side. Alternately, they can be placed in steel parts cabinets with padded plastic drawers such as those made by the Akro-Mills Company.

Predicting the outcome of RK

The surgery of RK is fairly straightforward. It is, however, not without its pitfalls. Careful attention to details and pre–operative planning can eliminate most problems. It is paramount for the new keratotomist to choose a single "guru" whose technique and philosophy will be followed to the letter. Do not alter or modify the technique unless and/or until your own results begin to match theirs. Only then is it safe for you to go off on your own.

The successful outcome of RK depends on the careful integration of numerous factors [8], as amply demonstrated by the mediocre and unpredictable results of the PERK study—which did not do so [9]. These factors are:

1 Degree of myopia
2 Curvature of the cornea—keratometry
3 Degree of corneal asphericity (corneal shape—the difference between the peripheral and central corneal curvatures)

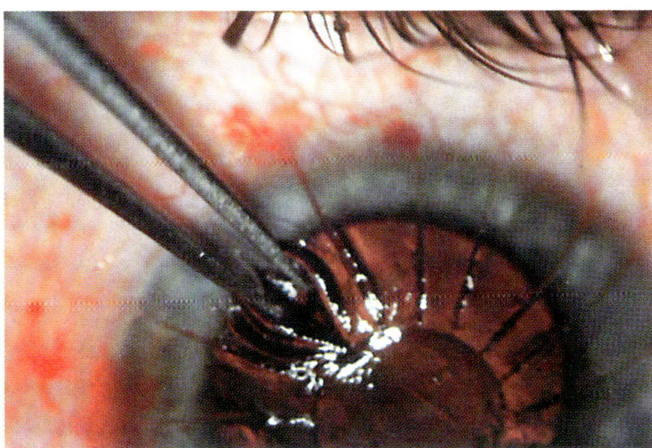

Fig. 8.28 Bores incision spreader in use.

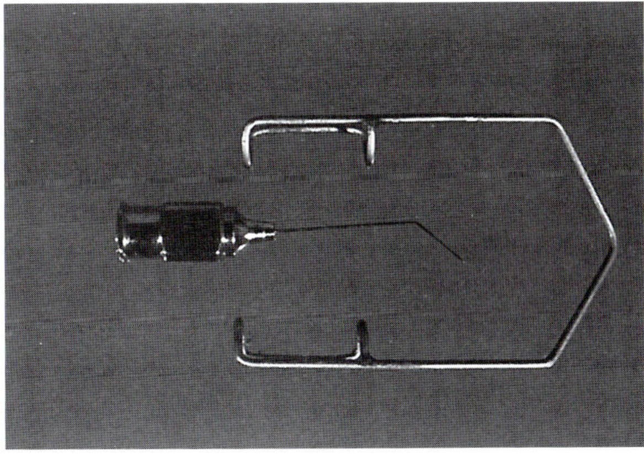

Fig. 8.29 Barraquer-type wire lid speculum; small-bore irrigating cannula.

4 Corneal rigidity (elasto-tonometric coefficient)
5 Corneal diameter
6 Age of the patient
7 Sex of the patient
8 Size of the optical zone
9 Number of incisions
10 Depth of the incisions
11 Intraocular pressure
12 Thickness of the cornea—pachymetry
13 Degree of corneal toricity (astigmatism)

It does not take much perspicacity to realize that it requires more than a crystal ball to integrate this number of variables (Figure 8.30). It also does not take too much mental energy to realize that a look-up table such as used in the early RK cases [8] or the PERK study cannot cope adequately with the problem either. Even nomograms are less than ideal because all cases will require multiple iterations, and nomograms are done manually. While all surgeons may start out using nomograms with the best of intentions, the amount of paperwork required with this method rapidly becomes onerous to the point where even a saint would look for shortcuts. This is compounded by the need for the surgeon to perform the calculations himself or herself—this is one area of ophthalmology that cannot be delegated successfully.

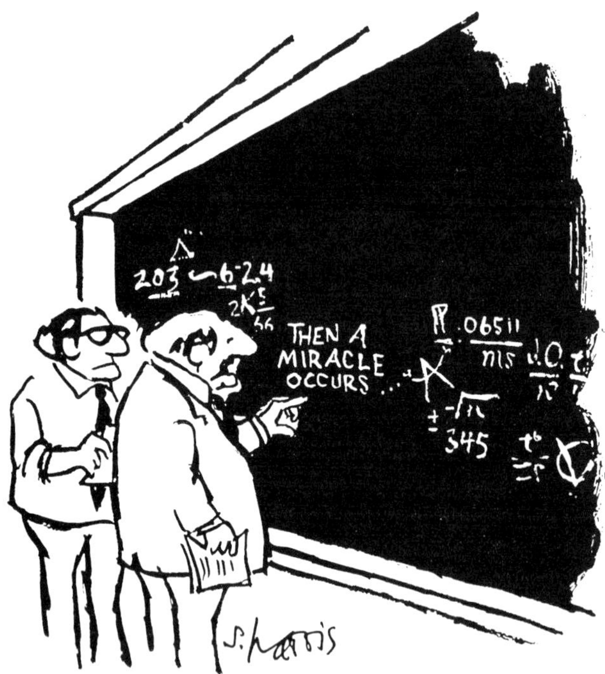

"I THINK YOU SHOULD BE MORE EXPLICIT HERE IN STEP TWO."

Fig. 8.30 More than a miracle is needed to calculate radial keratotomy parameters.

Computers and refractive surgery

A word or two are in order about establishing surgical parameters in refractive surgery. It is not possible to adequately determine how many incisions to make and/or what the optimal optical zone size should be without a computer. Look-up tables have been tried and have been found to be wanting. There is just too much data to be accounted for and correlated for two-dimensional tables, and multi-dimensional tables are too cumbersome and prone to look-up error. While it is true that "good" results have been reported by resorting to half-measures, it is well to heed an old Russian proverb: *"Better is the natural enemy of good enough."*

Data accumulate rapidly, and a paper gridlock can occur, leading to a tendency to take shortcuts with both data gathering and data processing. An effective computer program and timely data analysis can prevent error and increase the efficacy of your surgery. The computer program that you choose to use, however, should be selected with the surgical technique in mind. Each program has been tailored for a specific surgeon's approach to making relaxing incisions. If you select a particular piece of software, you are also selecting that particular surgeon's technique.

It is just not possible to "mix and match" with this surgery. You cannot be eclectic in your surgical approach and expect any prediction software to be effective under such circumstances. You must adopt the calculation and surgical method of a particular experienced surgeon and follow his or her method assiduously until such time that you have become absolutely confident in your understanding of all the nuances of this surgery. Then and only then will it be possible for you to "vary the theme" and strike off on your own.

The optical zone

Of all the factors that affect the amount of postoperative flattening of the cornea, the incisional length is one of the most important. All things being equal, the length of the incisions is controlled by the size of the surgical clear or optical zone (OZ). This is the central free zone left uncut, from which the incisions radiate toward the periphery of the cornea. These OZs are either circular (in the case of spherical myopia) or elliptical (in cases of astigmatism, under certain circumstances). It is in the selection of these OZs that the beginning keratotomist has the most difficulty.

There is a definite inverse relationship between the diameter of the OZ and the degree of myopia in the patient's optical system. Thus by varying the size of the OZ, we vary the outcome of the surgery. By keeping the incisions uniformly deep, variability in predicted result is kept to a minimum. There are, of course, other factors to consider, but the relationship of the OZ size to outcome is fundamental and a first principle.

The major problem posed for the erstwhile keratotomist is in choosing the surgical approach to be taken. I have said and have been repeatedly quoted as saying that the neophyte must choose only one guru and adhere to that person's methodology and not mix and match nor attempt modifications in technique until sufficient proficiency has been gained with the specific technique to allow such modifications to be integrated safely.

Some have chosen to interpret my admonition as meaning that one must blindly adhere to all teachings of the guru and suspend common sense. It is a sad fact that despite eons of evolution, human beings have not progressed very far in some areas. Under certain circumstances, humankind evinces all the characteristics of the lemming. I need only point to the examples of Moses, John Brown, and Jim Jones to prove my case.

The reader may say—perhaps with justification—that he or she does not fit within the group mentality associated with the aforesaid individuals and therefore is not susceptible to the lemming trap. However, if you have ever in your life followed some fashion or another, you are vulnerable; it is a funny old world, and stress can induce many types of reactive behavior. And this is the basic message of Bores' maxim: *Gurus do not exist in a vacuum*. This means that while you are adhering to the methods laid down by a particular teacher, you must stay alert for other opinions that may impinge on what it is that you are doing.

For example, it may be that your guru advocates tiny OZs for high degrees of myopia. Should you as well? You, as a beginner, have no business tackling high myopes, on the one hand. On the other, should you decide to do so, you need to ask yourself the question: *Does the application of tiny zones violate first principles*? It should be obvious that you cannot answer this question—you haven't got the experience. You know what your guru thinks. But what about the other gurus? Their opinions are equally valid. Are you a lemming after all? Most other gurus decry the use of subnominal OZs and give cogent reasons for this prohibition. Which means that should you use them, you are on your own. Under the circumstances, is applying such zones in your best interest? How about the patient's?

The answer should be: *It is not*. It does not pay to go to extremes—especially at your stage of development. If you will take my advice, you will never take on that extreme. Remember that drowning is intensely personal. Case in point: *subnominal surgical clear zones*.

Myopic regression in RK with subnominal OZs

During clinical testing of a laser interferometer designed to measure corneal surface topography, we were privileged to examine numerous patients both before and after refractive surgery. Among these was a group of post-RK patients who had been referred for excimer laser photoablation to treat residual myopia. While evaluating the results of the testing, we were struck by the appearance of a subgroup whose topographic maps showed evidence of central corneal steepening clearly isolated from the surrounding cornea by well-defined edges. Subsequent checking revealed that all these patients had subnominal surgical clear zones of 2.5 mm or less.

The advantage of using holographic techniques to map corneal surface contours is in its extreme sensitivity to minute changes in slope (see Chapter 6). Using an intermediate step—called a *phase map*—in processing of the image allows minute perturbations of a surface to be detected easily. For example, RK incisions made 10 years previously are revealed as readily as fresh ones (see Figure 6.28).

Table 8.1 lists a group of patients with preoperative and postoperative myopia measurements as well as K-readings. Figures show a typical phase map of a patient with a subnominal surgical clear zone. There is undoubtedly a consensus among refractive surgeons that the surgical clear zone in RK cases should not be less than 2.75 mm, with the vast majority preferring to go no smaller than 3.0 mm. Most, if not all, keratotomy surgeons would declare that a 2.50-mm OZ is smaller than normal. These surgeons cite difficulty in centering, increased incidence and intensity of glare, loss of best-corrected vision, induced irregular astigmatism, and loss of contrast sensitivity in subnominal OZ patients [10–12]. I concur wholeheartedly in this.

This is a troublesome issue that keeps cropping up from time to time and needs to be laid to rest. In the early days of RK, the author had occasion to do some cases wherein the OZs were 2.0 mm in diameter. Every patient in that series experienced a significant increase in glare disability. Because of this and for other reasons, Fyodorov and I decried the use of such small zones and advised against them at every meeting we attended; it soon became common knowledge, and others joined in teaching that such zones were folly.

There are limitations to the correction that can be obtained by making relaxing incisions in the cornea. Some eyes respond in much lesser degree regardless of our skill and efforts in any event. It has been said that the difference between a good surgeon and a mediocre one is that the good surgeon knows not only when not to cut but also

Table 8.1 First radial keratotomy surgical guide

Optical zone diameter (mm)	Effect (D)
4.5	0.75–1.25
4.0	1.50–2.00
3.5	2.20–2.50
3.0	>2.75

when to accept reality and quit. The practice of refractive surgery is not an Olympian struggle, wherein points are awarded for the greatest amount of diopters corrected. It is, rather, a humanistic science where the welfare of the patient is still paramount and where his or her ultimate well-being guides our behavior.

Nonetheless, from time to time, someone or other has readvocated the use of subnominal optical clear zones. They have defended their position in various ways—the most common being that newer instruments, techniques, and experience improve the outcome. This is disingenuous at the very least, arrogant in the extreme, and wishful thinking into the bargain. Some of these surgeons think that doing 10,000 cases somehow stamps their experience with academic weight. The fact that it is possible to do 10,000 cases *incorrectly* never seems to have occurred to them [13]. Neither does it seem relevant that they do so many cases that they practically never see them in follow-up. It escapes me how it is possible to learn anything from one's surgery if you do not see the results of your technique firsthand—but surely I digress?

The other point often offered in defense is that the smaller-than-normal-OZ surgeon employs an alignment device that supposedly ensures that the visual axis is located precisely. I have had the unfortunate experience of seeing many of these patients who seek improvement of a poor result subsequent to the application of tiny optical clear zones. A significant number, in fact, the majority of these cases, have misaligned OZs. In fact, the number of misaligned cases exceeds my own experience with "less sophisticated" and "imperfect" alignment methods. The crux of the matter is the patient and his or her ability to sight on the target. Unfortunately, not all patients are capable of full cooperation, and some require that the surgeon spend a little more time ensuring that they have indeed sighted the target exactly. This provision does not fit in well with the "MacDoc" approach used by too many refractive surgery specialists.

The problem is rooted in the concept of *effective OZ size*. This effective zone is controlled by tissue reaction. When an incision is made, the edges of the cut become elevated (see Figure 7.32). As the scar matures, the incision becomes depressed. These edge changes create local corneal curvature changes that distort the light striking them. These changes are relatively irreducible even in the face of steroid application—tissue reaction persists; if it did not, healing would not occur, and healing is very slow in the avascular cornea. The smaller the OZ, the more effect these edge changes have on the actual size of the clear zone. For example, the effective zone for a 2.75-mm OZ is closer to 2.5 mm (the *effective optic zone*). For a 2.5-mm OZ, it approaches 2.0 mm. For a 2.0-mm OZ, it is about 1.25 mm. Centration and radial symmetry of the incisions therefore become critical.

Irregular astigmatism and/or surface distortions therefore occur around all corneal incisions, be they performed with a knife or as a result of laser planing. This is a fact of life and has been known from the days before refractive surgery. The extent of the distortion is related to the quality of the instrument doing the incising. There is no question that thin, smooth, sharp blades produce more regularly shaped incisions and reduce distortion. But the distortion is only reduced in extent, not eliminated. There is a finite amount of distortion that persists because of the fact of the incision and the fact that healing processes are underway. These healing processes produce irreducible changes in tissue, only some of which are temporary. Thus, as the OZ gets smaller, these disturbed areas are brought closer to each other as well as to the center of vision. As the OZ gets even smaller, this clear zone gets disproportionately smaller, and the visual disturbance becomes greater even if perfectly centered.

Some individuals are nonetheless regularly performing RK surgery with zones smaller than 1.75 mm. These surgeons have defended their actions by stating that the increase in acuity offsets the loss of contrast sensitivity. However, it is not possible to suffer loss of contrast sensitivity and maintain good acuity in the real world—the two are tied together. One of the best means of determining the efficiency of an optical system is by means of the *modulation transfer function* (MTF). This is the ratio of resolution (in line pairs/mm) to contrast. The normal eye has an MTF that equates to 20 line pairs (20/20) (see Figure 6.36). If the contrast is lowered, the MTF (and therefore acuity) becomes worse (see Figure 6.40c). In the high-contrast black-and-white environment that is the Snellen chart, acuity may *appear* to be normal. However, despite its widespread use as a standard, Snellen visual acuity is not related to visual function in the real world in any quantifiable way and hence must be viewed with some skepticism [14]. The MTF ratios were uniformly subnormal in all measured cases with sub-nominal optical clear zones. Do not use OZs of less than 2.75 mm in diameter.

Selecting the proper optical zone

Selection of the size of the primary OZ is based (for the most part) on the patient's spectacle refraction, although the amount of astigmatism in the patient's optical system may not bear any direct relationship to the astigmatism on the cornea (as measured by keratometry). Remember that we are correcting the refraction of the optical system by altering the corneal surface—much like fitting a contact lens for the same purpose.

To assist in the selection of these optical clear zones, a series of tables was constructed initially (see Table 8.1). These tables soon gave way to nomograms that take into consideration as many as six separate parameters [15]

(Figure 8.31). However, the accuracy of these nomograms has been shown to be inadequate for many cases of spherical myopia and well-nigh impossible in cases with astigmatism. Continuing work on this problem produced the first of the so-called Fyodorov formulas—Formula I. Shortly thereafter, the Durnev-Fyodorov-Bores formula (Formula II) made its appearance. Both these formulas are used to predict the outcome of the surgery, the first by calculating the degree of myopia expected to be corrected and the second, the more useful Formula II, by calculating the size of the OZ to be used to affect a given amount of myopia.

The formulas

Formula I

$$P = \frac{\sqrt{D^2 + \frac{16}{3}\left(R - \sqrt{R^2 - \frac{D^2}{4}}\right)^2} - \sqrt{d^2 + \frac{16}{3}\left(R - \sqrt{R^2 - \frac{d^2}{4}}\right)^2}}{\sqrt{d^2 + \frac{16}{3}\left(R - \sqrt{R^2 - \frac{d^2}{4}}\right)^2}} \cdot K \cdot a$$

This formula calculates the effect of surgery P (after 12 months) given that D is the diameter of the cornea (in mm), R is the radius of the cornea (in mm), K is the coefficient of corneal rigidity, α is the incisional depth coefficient, and d is the prechosen OZ size. It is especially useful in cases where the minimum size OZ (2.75 mm) has to be used for a given correction. It will allow the surgeon to give the patient a reasonable expectation of the surgical outcome. It is incorporated into the RK DataMaster™ computer program (see below).

Formula II

$$d + \sqrt{-96R^2 - 3A + \sqrt{64R^2 \cdot (6(24R^2 + 2A))}}$$

where:

$$A = \left(D^2 + \frac{16}{3}\left(R - \sqrt{R^2 - \frac{D^2}{4}}\right)^2\right) \cdot \left(\frac{K\alpha}{P + K\alpha}\right)^2$$

This formula calculates the OZ size d given that P is the myopia to be corrected (in diopters), D is the diameter of the cornea (in mm), R is the radius of the cornea (in mm), K is the coefficient of corneal rigidity, and α is the incisional depth coefficient. This formula will calculate the OZ needed to fully correct a given amount of myopia in 12 months. It sometimes will result in an OZ much

(text continues on page 241)

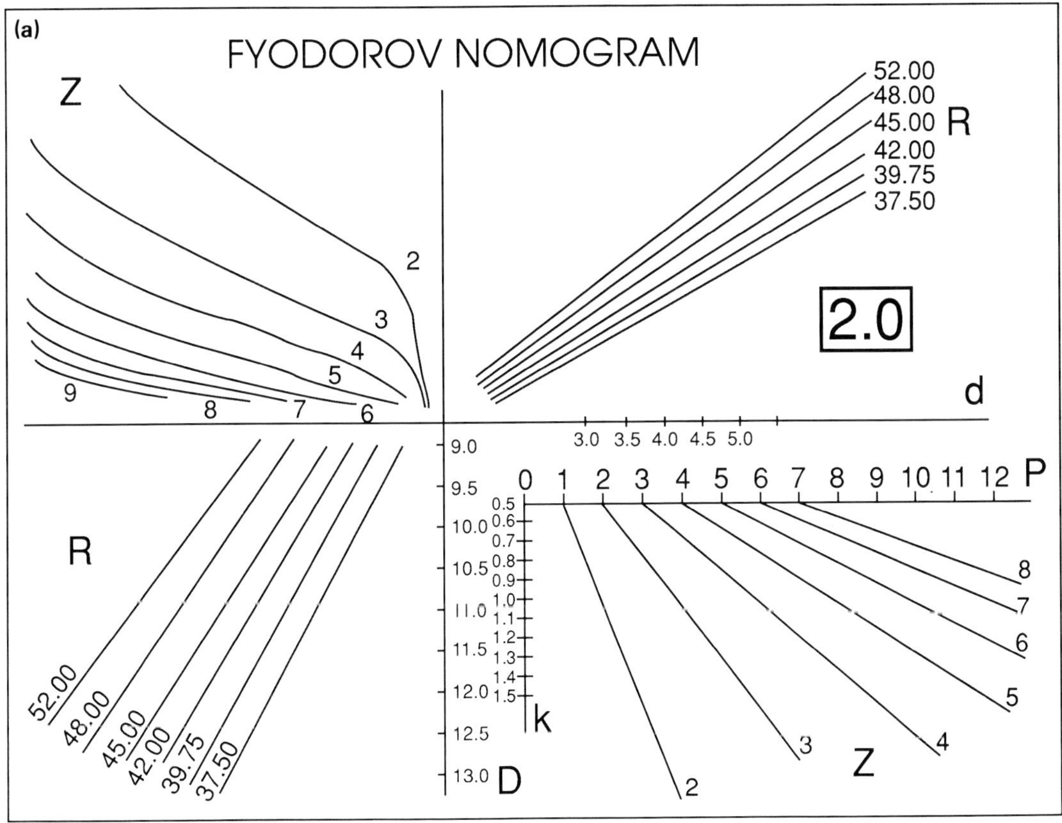

Fig. 8.31 (a) Fyodorov nomogram. (b–g) Using the Fyodorov nomogram to determine a surgical zone. (b) Select the myopia on the P line, and the rigidity on the K line. (c) Drop perpendiculars from both points. The intersection is the Z-point. (d) Draw a horizontal line to intersect the K-reading. (e) A vertical is drawn from that point to the upper Z-point. (f) A horizontal is drawn from the Z-point to intersect with the upper K-reading. (g) A vertical is dropped from that point to intersect the d line—the optical zone size.

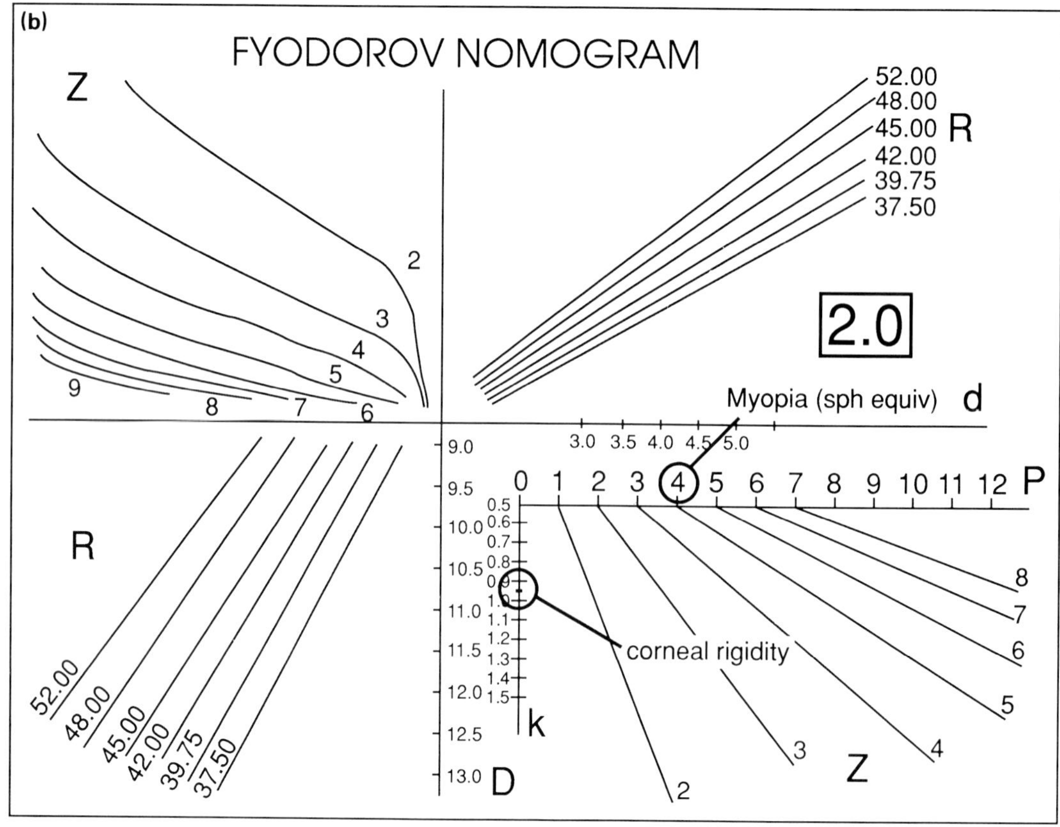

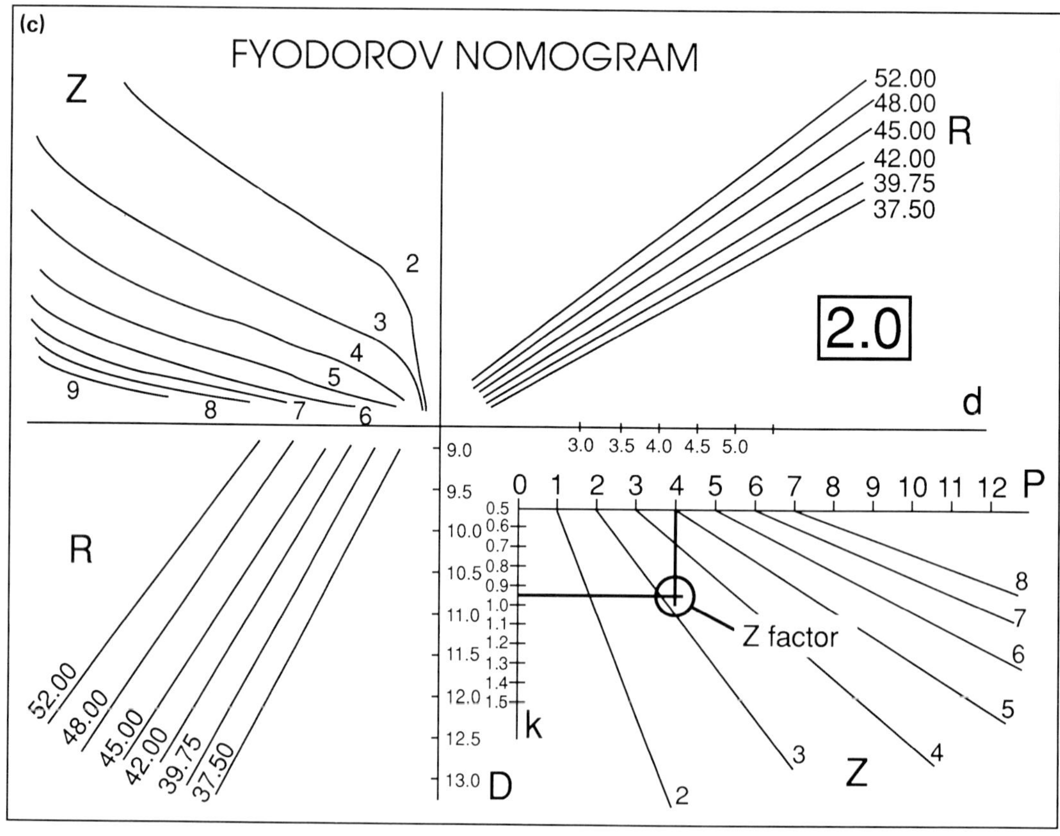

Fig. 8.31 (*Continued*)

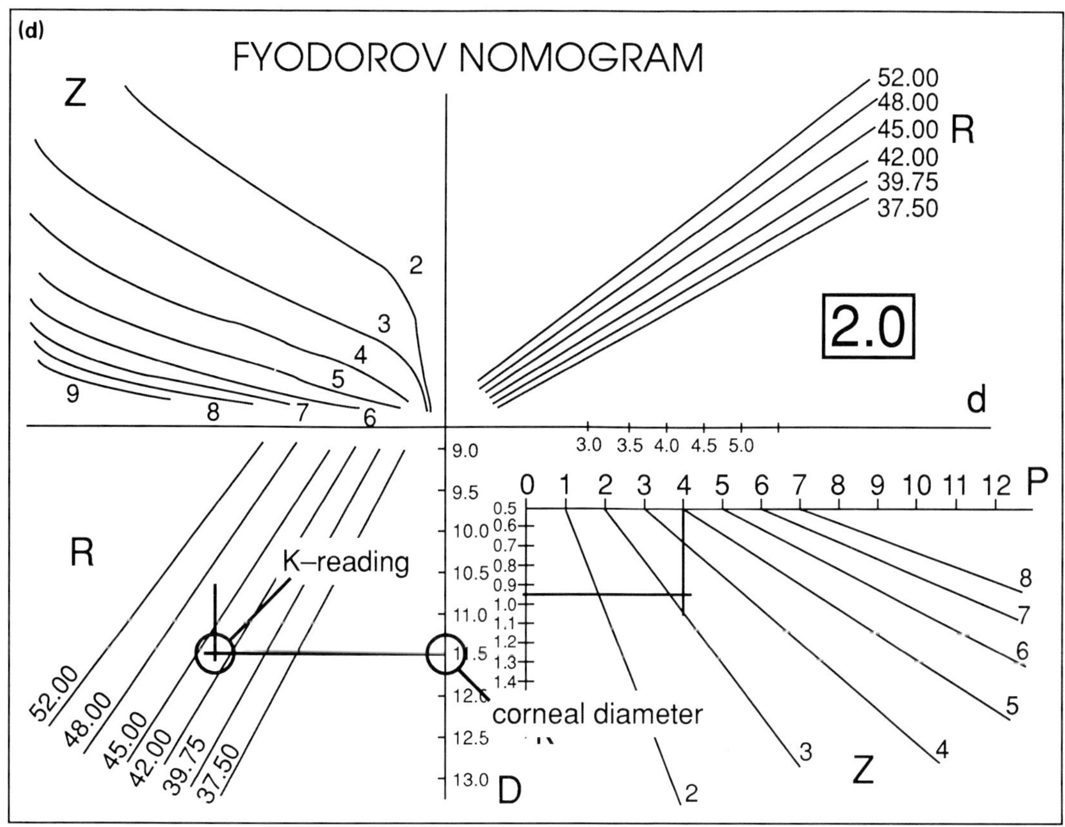

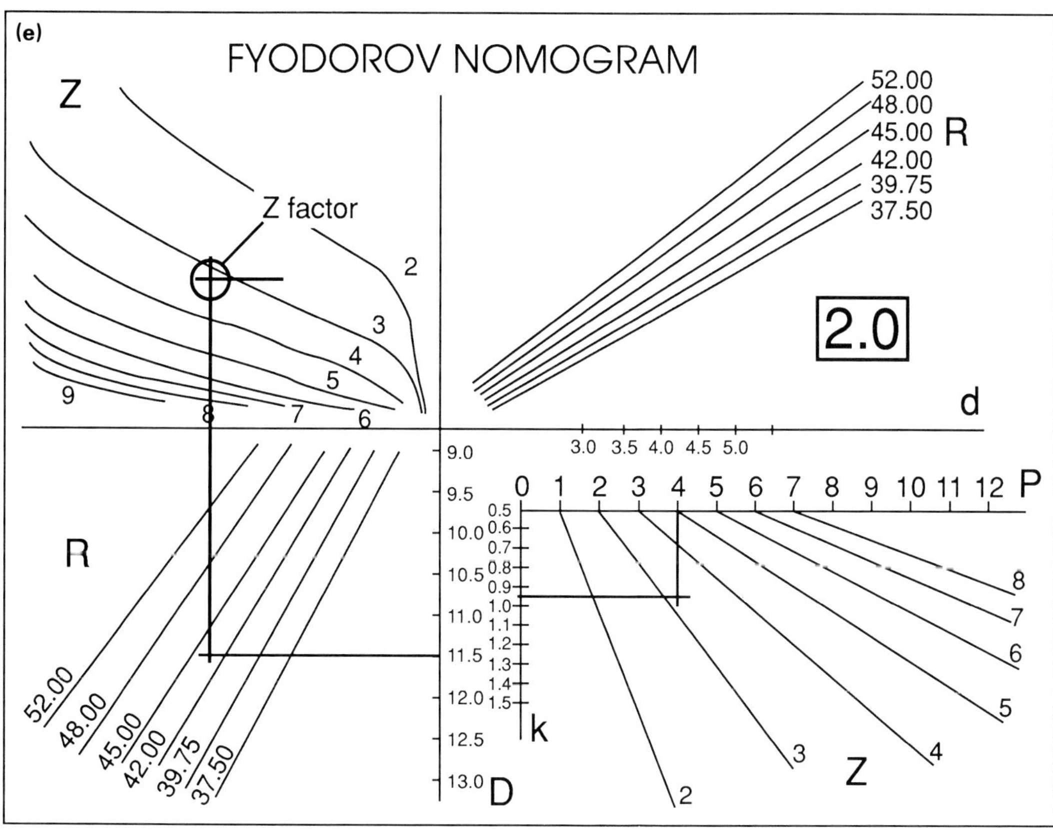

Fig. 8.31 (*Continued*)

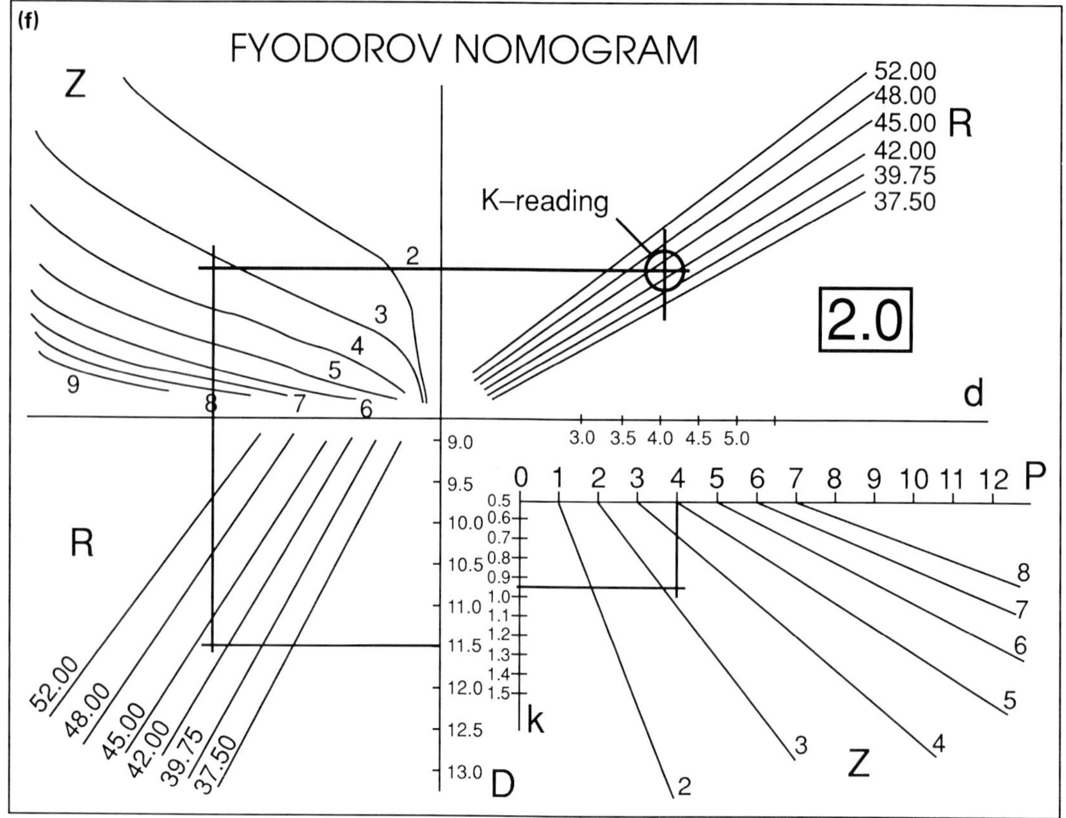

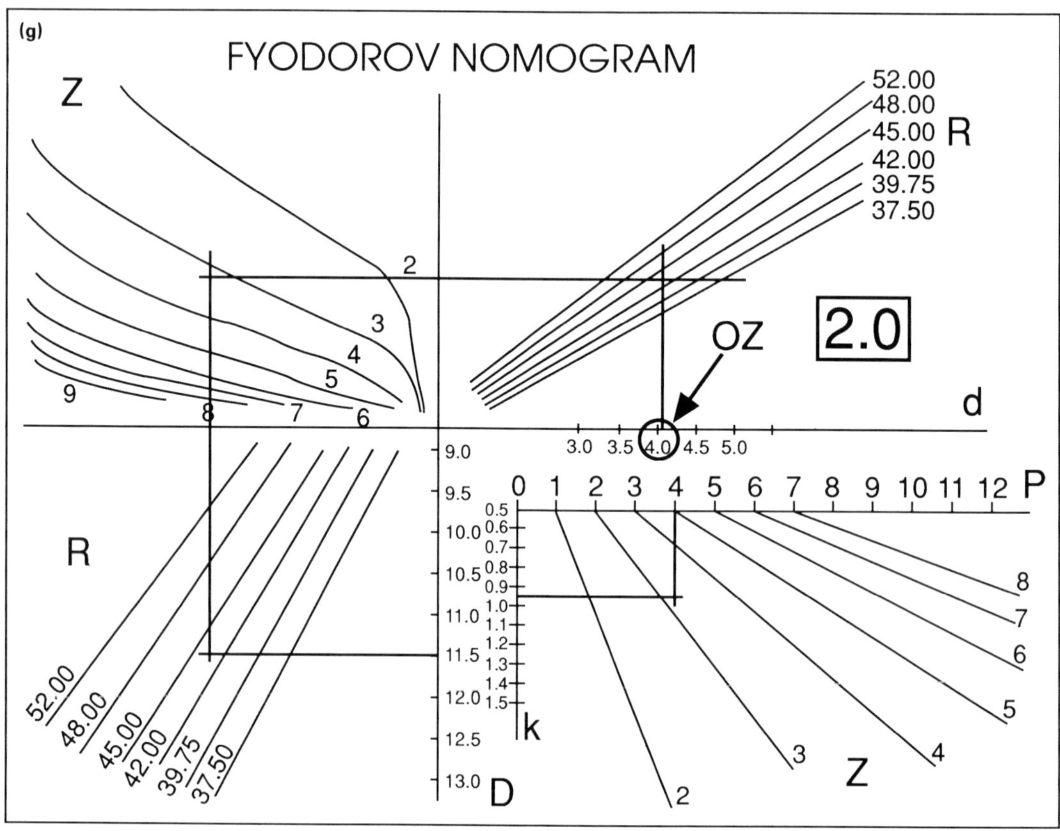

Fig. 8.31 (*Continued*)

smaller than 2.75 mm. In that case, Formula I is used with the minimal size OZ (2.75 mm) to predict how much correction can be reasonably expected. This formula is also incorporated into the RK DataMaster computer program and automatically switches to Formula I when the calculated primary OZ is less than 2.75 mm with 16 incisions (maximum surgery). Both formulas require that the surgeon input six factors:

1 The keratometry, both horizontal and vertical
2 The corneal diameter
3 The corneal rigidity
4 The number of incisions to be used
5 The incisional depth coefficient
6 The size of the surgical OZ (Formula I) or the amount of myopia (Formula II)

Using the formulas

It is necessary to make a number of measurements of each eye in order to use the formulas properly. Failure to take these factors into account leads to widely disparate results and causes confusion and disappointment not only for the patient but for the surgeon as well. Furthermore, it promotes the notion that this surgery is not predictable.

Incisional depth coefficient (IC)

This factor, originally called the *surgeon's practical coefficient of correction*, has created a great deal of confusion by virtue of its being misunderstood. Simply stated, each coefficient represents the effect on the surgical outcome by the depth of the incision. These factors are fixed in Formulas I and II. In each case, the coefficient represents the actual depth of the incision as a factor of the thickness of the cornea—at the edge of the optical free zone. The confusion arises because of the way in which these coefficients were originally expressed:

Factor 1.3 (1.29)—The earliest coefficient, this was described originally as representing an incision that was approximately 75% of the corneal thickness at the edge of the primary optical zone (PC)—which is usually 3.00 mm (minimum 2.75 mm). However, the factor was never used in this fashion. Instead, it was always used to describe any single-depth incision made by a blade set to the thickness of the cornea (measured at the edge of the OZ) that resulted in an incision whose depth was approximately 70% to 80% of the corneal thickness. This was true regardless of the size of the OZ. In short, it represented the shallowest practical incision that could be made with any hope of producing a significant—but not maximum—effect. Any incision shallower than this would produce less than 60% correction of the myopia and would be likely to regress in effect greatly over time. Typically, this depth of cut is arrived at by setting the blade at 100% of the pachymetry. This early teaching of the author has been established by laboratory studies [16]

Subsequently, three other fixed coefficients were evolved (see also Chapter 7). It is vital that the surgeon understand these factors and their relationship to each other and to the actual incisions.

Factor 1.6 (1.62)—This represents the deepest practical single-depth incision that can be made with a guarded blade. This factor describes any incision made by a blade set to the depth of the cornea at the edge of the OZ that results in an incision whose depth is approximately 90% to 95% of the corneal thickness.

Factor 2.0—This was used when making any two-stage (stepped) incision at maximal depth. That is, it describes two 1.6-factor incisions strung together, with the second blade setting determined by the depth of the cornea at the edge of a secondary optical zone (MP)—which is usually 6.0 mm in diameter. Initially this deepening was accomplished by cutting over the previously made incision with an appropriately set blade starting at 6.0 mm. However, while this technique seemed to work satisfactorily with steel blades, it often resulted in incisions whose nether regions were "flayed" and whose depth was uneven. Crystalline blades—by virtue of their sharpness, which occasioned instances of incisions wandering out of the track, and by accompanying increases in microperforations and soft eyes—caused the technique to be changed (see "Stepped incisions," below).

Factor 2.5—This originally described incisions made using a 2.0 factor in which 4, 8, or 16 incisions (or 20 in astigmatism cases) were deepened—free hand—to Descemet's membrane. This factor has since changed to represent a three-step incision in which each step is made at maximum depth, that is, 90% to 95%. It is useful to consider this incision as three 1.6-factor incisions strung together to make one. Consequently, free-hand incision deepening is no longer a requirement and actually may be undesirable.

As the technique of RK evolved, it was quickly found that the blades being used did not actually cut to the depth for which they were set. It became necessary to overset the blades in relationship to the actual ultrasonic pachymetry—that is, set them longer than the cornea was thick. Needless to say, this promoted, in many surgeons, tachycardia and hyperventilation—at least at first. This oversetting is, however, an absolute necessity and is explained in Chapter 7.

Until recently, this meant that a 1.3 factor represented an incision made by a sapphire (or similarly sharp) blade set to 100% of the corneal depth at the edge of the first OZ. A 1.6 factor was the same blade set at the pachymetry +10 μm. As can be appreciated, the amount of myopic correction was increased because of the increased depth of the incisions that resulted from this oversetting. While holding the depth of the incisions constant, compensation is made by either decreasing the number of incisions or by increasing the size of the primary OZ, or both.

Currently, the coefficients have the following meaning:

Coefficient 1.3—This requires a blade setting that produces a corneal incision of approximately 75% at the edge of the primary OZ. This is true of fresh steel and used sapphire blades. Slight undersetting of a fresh sapphire and/or diamond may be required—especially the Bores LeCut diamond.

Coefficient 1.6—This requires a blade so set as to produce an incision having a minimum depth of 90% to 95% at the edge of the primary OZ. With the Bores LeCut diamond, this would be a setting of 100% of the pachymetry. A new sapphire blade requires an overset of 10 μm, and steel and some diamond blades may need to be overset 5% to 15%.

Coefficient 2.0—This requires incisions of two steps, each step of coefficient 1.6, with the primary OZ of variable size (up to 5.0 mm) and the secondary fixed at 6.0 mm (7.0 mm if the primary is 5.0 mm).

Coefficient 2.5—This requires incisions having three steps. Each segment of the incision is to be at coefficient 1.6 and fixed zones at 6.0 and 8.0 mm (7.0 and 9.0 mm), respectively.

Figures 8.32 through 8.35 graphically illustrate the relationship of these coefficients and should clarify the situation. Regardless of the actual method of blade setting, these relationships are held constant both to the corneal thickness and to each other. It should be obvious that the actual method of blade setting used to accomplish these incision depths very much depends on blade quality as well as design and necessitates evaluation of these factors individually for each type of blade, be it steel, diamond, or sapphire. Table 8.2 summarizes the settings for commonly used blade types.

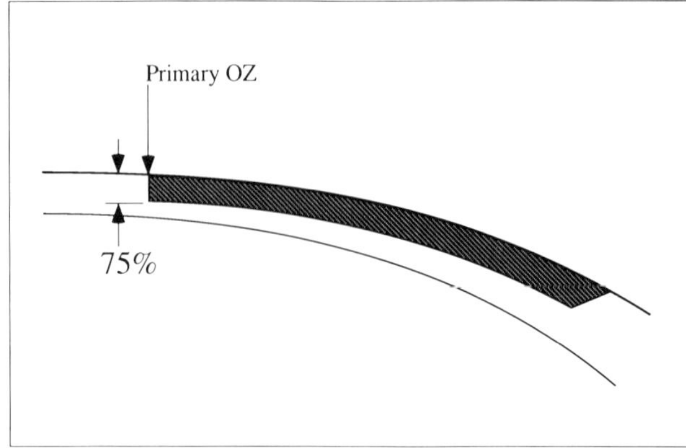

Fig. 8.32 Incisional depth (ID) factor 1.3.

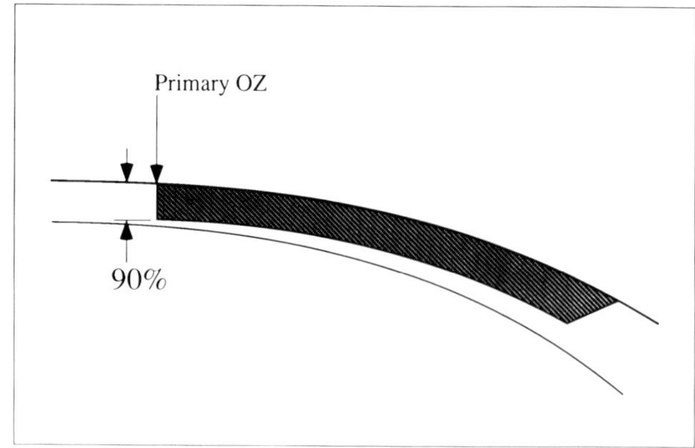

Fig. 8.33 Factor 1.6.

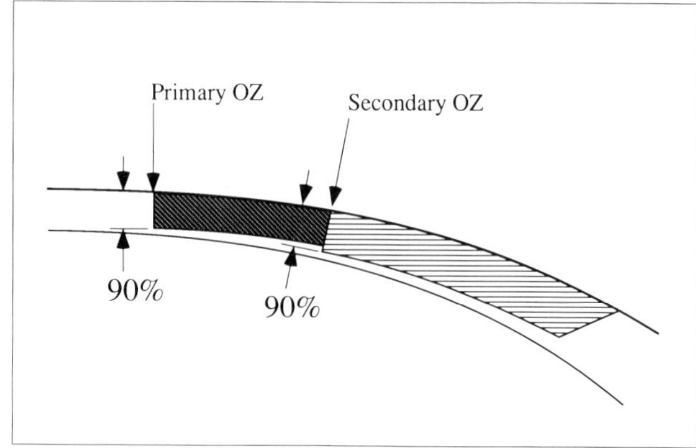

Fig. 8.34 Factor 2.0.

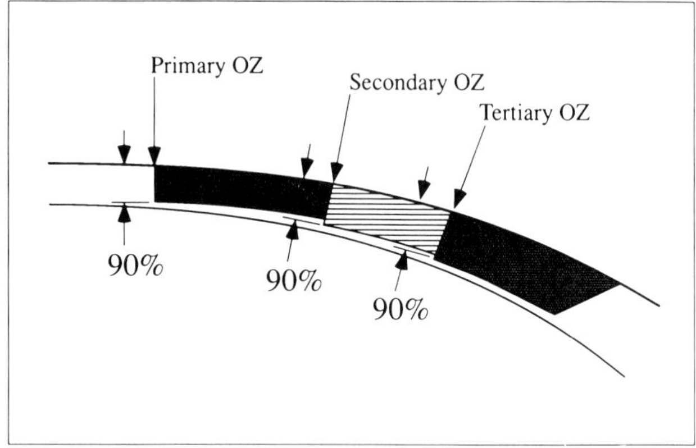

Fig. 8.35 Factor 2.5.

Corneal diameter (CD)

This is a factor that, while significant, fortunately is not a large one—yet it must be considered. Most patients will be found to have corneas that fall within the 11.5- to 12.0-mm range measured white to white. The actual measurements should be made at four points—in the vertical

Table 8.2 Initial blade bias by type

Blade type	Typical bias (% of initial pachymetry)	Typical bias* (μm)	Blade setting* (pachymetry + bias)
Steel razor fragment	15	75	575
Honed steel	7–10	35–50	535–550
Diamond— old style	10–15	50–75	550–575
LeCut	0	None	500

* Example assumes a paracentral pachymetry of 500 μm.

(6 to 12 o'clock), in the horizontal (3 to 9 o'clock), and at the 45° and 135° meridians—and then averaged. A difference of 1.0 mm in corneal diameter represents about a diopter in actual refraction effect.

Corneal rigidity (CR)

This is another factor that many surgeons have ignored either out of ignorance of its significance or because instruments to measure it have been generally hard to obtain (Table 8.3). This factor is second only to the size of the OZ in its influence on the outcome of the surgery. This parameter is related to aging—the rigidity seems to increase in older individuals and is reflected in the generally higher effect seen in these patients (the actual method of determining scleral or corneal rigidity is described in Chapter 5). The decrease in elasticity of corneal tissue, as evidenced by the cornea's resistance to deformation, causes most of the tension produced by the weakening of the peripheral cornea to be translated as a flattening of the central cornea instead of stretching—both in the center and peripherally. In addition, contraction of the healing scar meets more resistance to its tendency to produce flattening of the peripheral cornea (see also Chapter 7). This latter tendency could account for the progression of effect reported in some series [17].

Number of incisions (NI)

The number of incisions directly affects the outcome of the surgery—the fewer incisions, the less is the effect. Using 16 incisions as 100%, 12 incisions will produce 15%, 8 incisions 25%, and 6 incisions 50%—less effect. Making 32 incisions produces less than a 2% additional effect on the outcome of the surgery [18], whereas more than 32 incisions will produce an actual decrease in the effect; which helps to explain the failure of Sato's method (Figure 8.36). These ratios were arrived at by the retrospective evaluation of more than 15,000 cases over a period of several years and have been reinforced by an ongoing evaluation of patient data. Additionally, as the number of incisions decreases, the incidence of operatively induced astigmatism increases. This was especially a problem in the earlier cases and caused Fyodorov and the author to abandon 8 incisions—at least for a time.

Table 8.3 Precalculated mean corneal rigidity coefficient

Myopia (D)	Sex	Age (years) 25	35	45
1.5	Male	0.95	1.02	1.12
	Female	0.92	1.00	1.11
3.0	Male	0.90	0.95	1.04
	Female	0.88	0.90	1.03
5.0	Male	0.86	0.90	0.99
	Female	0.81	0.87	0.98
7.0	Male	0.80	0.82	0.96
	Female	0.70	0.78	0.95

Keratometry

Despite some suggestions to the contrary, corneal curvature remains one of the significant factors in determining the outcome of the surgery. Sufficient time has elapsed to bear this out (this factor is discussed in more detail in Chapter 5). Graphs plotted of cases in which compensation has been made for changes in curvature show a curve that is almost flat.

If it were true that corneal curvature has no effect, then those patients in whom the OZ was opened (widened) in compensation should show less effect—all other things being equal. However, such cases show a slight rise to the curve in the higher keratometry ranges, illustrating that there probably has been insufficient compensation for the K's (Figure 8.37). Since none of the other investigators commenting on this relationship consider age, corneal rigidity, etc., cases in their surgery, their cases are not truly representative and naturally would not show any significant effect due to corneal curvature. Recently, the work of Sanders and Marks [19], with multiple regression analyses, is beginning to corroborate our findings. It

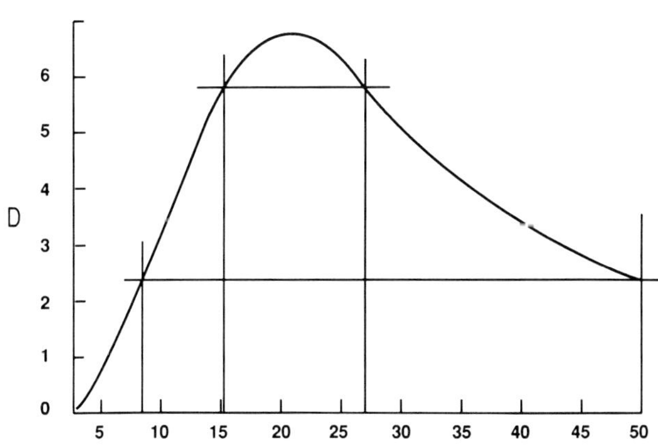

Fig. 8.36 The effect of the number of incisions on the surgical outcome.

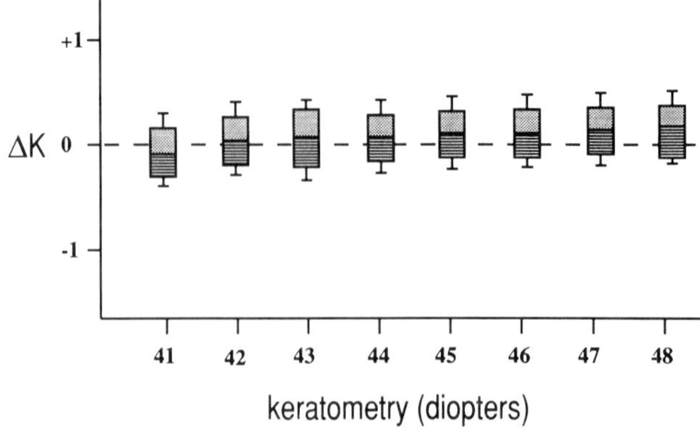

Fig. 8.37 Preoperative K-readings make a difference.

must be emphasized again that this surgery is microsurgery whose outcome depends on an integration of a number of seemingly small, outwardly insignificant, and apparently unrelated factors that, taken together, result in significant changes in corneal curvature.

Summary of patient workup

Eligible patients must be at least 18 years of age with nonprogressive myopia. They must be free of corneal or adnexal disease. They should have intraocular tensions of greater than 12 mm Hg and scleral rigidity of greater than 0.75. They must have realistic expectations of the surgery and sign an informed consent form (see also Chapter 5).

All candidates for this procedure receive the following workup in the author's clinic prior to the surgery:

1 Routine ophthalmic evaluation
2 Refraction (manifest—cycloplegic where warranted)
3 Glare testing
4 Ophthalmometry
 (a) Conventional keratometry (central and peripheral)
 (b) Photokeratoscopy (Corneoscope)
 (c) Holographic topography (CLAS II Corneal Surface Analyzer)
5 Intraocular pressure by applanation
6 A-scan ocular biometry (axial length)
7 Ultrasonic pachymetric 32-point corneal mapping
8 Determination of handedness

Calculating surgical parameters

We will review a number of typical cases of spherical myopia and detail the parameter calculation, surgical decision-making process, and actual technique of the surgery required in each case under examination. The OZ size will be calculated using the RK DataMaster program on a PC. This program will be used to select the optimal incision depth coefficient, optical zone(s), and incision number and configuration for the patient. Other computer programs are available to aid you in calculating surgical parameters. These typically call for slightly larger optical clear zones than does the RK DataMaster (Figure 8.38).

The RK DataMaster program was written by the author for this surgery and uses modified versions of Formulas I and II and the Ruiz algorithms. It will accept and process all the data, calculates the theoretical scleral rigidity, allows editing of current and previously entered records, prints out the results per eye, stores the data, and accesses compatible database files for later processing. This program is suitable for low to moderate myopia (cases recommended for the surgeon getting started in RK), as well as for complex cases with mixed astigmatism, and allows the surgeon to reasonably predict the outcome of the surgery.

These algorithms are a result of extensive collaboration between the author and the Moscow Scientific Institute of Ophthalmic Microsurgery and myself and the evaluation of over 15,000 RK cases. The calculations are accurate to within ±1.00 D in better than 85% of cases in the author's hands and are especially useful for combined myopic astigmatism and higher degrees of myopia. The Ruiz astigmatism calculations were integrated into the system so as to provide calculations for up to 8 D of associated myopic astigmatism.

The RK DataMaster program contains complex algorithms that take into account the six factors previously mentioned plus the following:

1 Age and sex of the patient
2 Intraocular pressure
3 Size of the intermediate (second and third) OZs
4 Depth of the incisions (for stepping)
 (a) Primary
 (b) Secondary
 (c) Tertiary

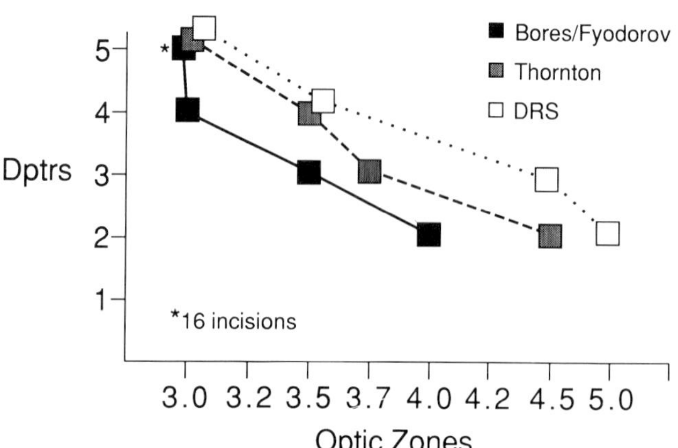

Fig. 8.38 Comparison of three popular radial keratotomy computer programs and recommended surgical zone sizes.

5 Pachymetry
(a) Central
(b) Paracentral
(c) Midperipheral
(d) Paraperipheral
(e) Limbal
6 Axial length of the eye
7 Astigmatism of the eye

The program automatically calculates the scleral rigidity by extrapolating a mean statistical rigidity—taking into account age, sex, and amount of myopia. These calculations are based on actual patient evaluations using measurements taken with the Maklakov tonometer in over 600 cases. The program also calculates the zones needed for astigmatism cases for most incisional configurations (see also Chapter 9) and suggests the particular type of incisions to use (i.e., stepped, etc.).

The current program can draw out the incisional configurations for the surgeon. Care must be taken when using this feature. Too many people assume that if the computer says a thing, it must be so. If the operator erroneously enters the wrong astigmatic axis or other value, the computer has no way of knowing that the data are in error and could draw the T or other incisions in the wrong meridian. While range checking is performed to eliminate data inconsistencies, the computer is unable to make other value judgments. Remember this adage of the computer age: *GIGO—"Garbage in, garbage out!"* It is highly recommended that the surgeon himself or herself draw out the incisional configurations personally on the surgical workup forms to avoid this potential error.

Decision making in RK

The examples considered in this section will be confined entirely to spherical patients. The specialized incisional patterns used for the treatment of astigmatism will be discussed in Chapter 9. The beginning surgeon is admonished not to attempt to correct astigmatism through any surgical means until he or she is completely familiar with the results of incisions in cases of simple myopia.

Case 1

The first case to be considered in this exercise is that of a 22-year-old male myopic patient whose preoperative workup is entered into the computer as shown in Figures 8.39. Once the operator has chosen the surgical parameters for the case, the surgical data and incisional configuration are then displayed on the surgical workup sheet (Figure 8.40). The computer will then display a summary of the case and give the operator a chance to correct or review the input data (Figure 8.41).

Case 2

In this case, we will change the amount of myopia to –5 D. The operator will choose the incisional depth (ID), number of incisions (NI), and primary optical zone (OZ) as before. In addition, a secondary OZ probably will be necessary (Figure 8.42).

Case 3

Again, only the amount of myopia has been changed—this time to –6.5 D. Take careful note, however, of the way in which the OZs and incision numbers have changed (Figure 8.43).

Case 4

Here, the myopia has been changed to 8D, an amount that exceeds that which reasonably can be expected to be corrected fully by RK. This case will require maximum surgery to even get a partial correction. This type of case is explored below under "Surgery—The technique of RK." Such cases are best avoided or corrected by other means (see Chapter 10).

Surgery—The technique of RK

The following surgical techniques are those used by the author and represent more than 20 years of experience with this surgery. These procedures have been refined considerably from the original method and should not prove too arduous for the average surgeon—provided that the proper instruments are used and the surgeon does not attempt to "wing it" or improvise. The surgery is performed under topical anesthesia in a premedicated patient. Sedation is provided by the administration of diazepam (Valium) in a dose appropriate to the patient (Figure 8.44). Generally, this will be 10 mg given orally approximately 30 to 40 minutes prior to surgery. Be advised that significant quantities of this chemical can still be found in the blood 24 hours after ingestion. The patient should be cautioned accordingly and should not drive.

The patient is placed supine on the operating table, and the eye is prepped with full-strength Betadine Solution (Figure 8.45). Betadine Prep is not recommended because it contains soap, which is extremely hard on the corneal epithelium. The microscope is then centered and adjusted, and the surgeon scrubs up. At the Bores Eye Institute we have used Septisol Skin Prep Foam successfully for this purpose for years. Draping is done using an aperture drape supplied by Alcon.

The anesthetic used is 0.5% tetracaine, followed by 1.0% non-buffered Pontocaine drops. Any additional anesthe-

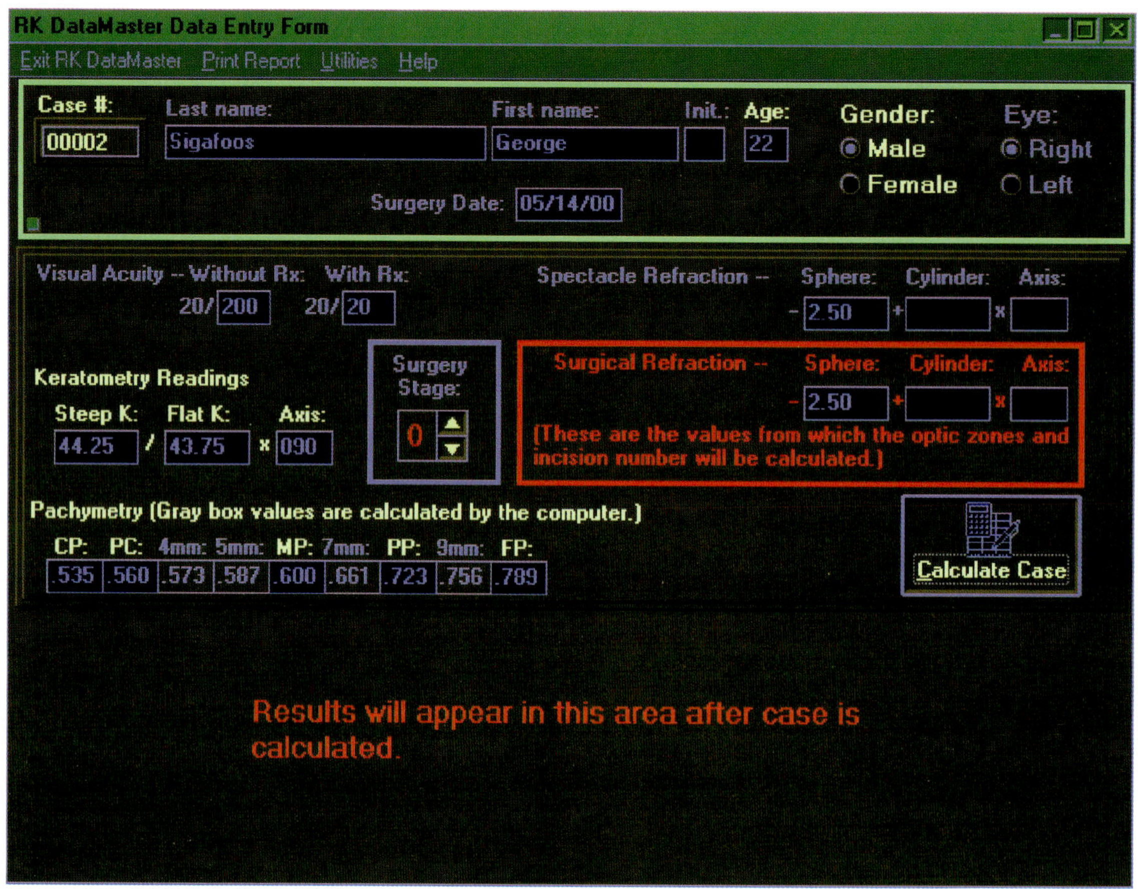

Fig. 8.39 Case 1. Data input sheet for a –2.50-D spherical myope.

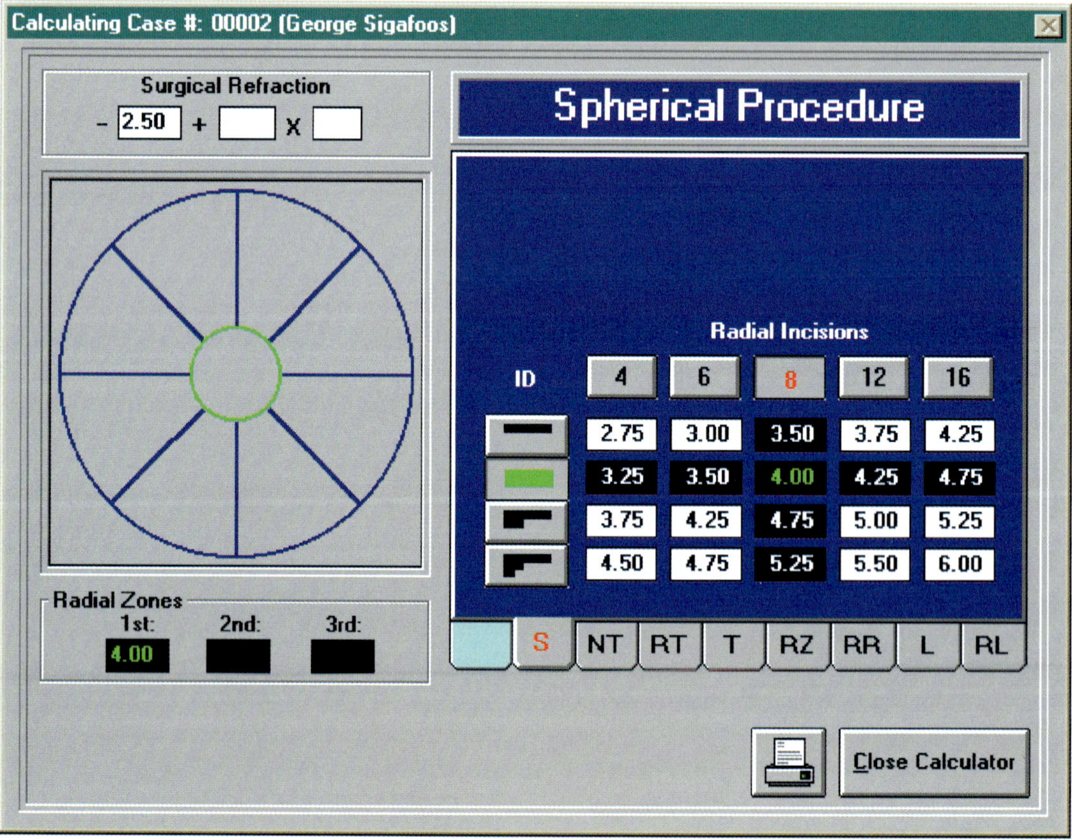

Fig. 8.40 Case 1. Surgical summary showing configuration and surgical parameters.

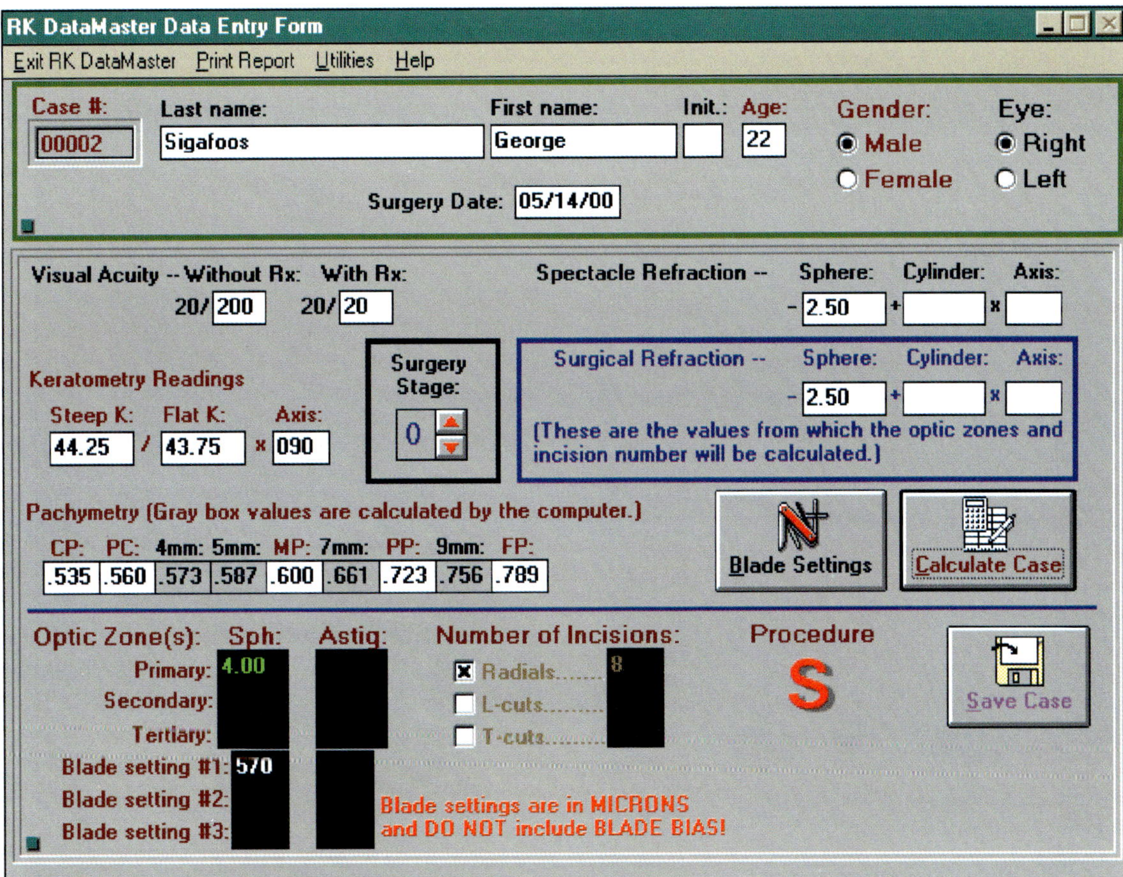

Fig. 8.41 Case 1. Summary sheet.

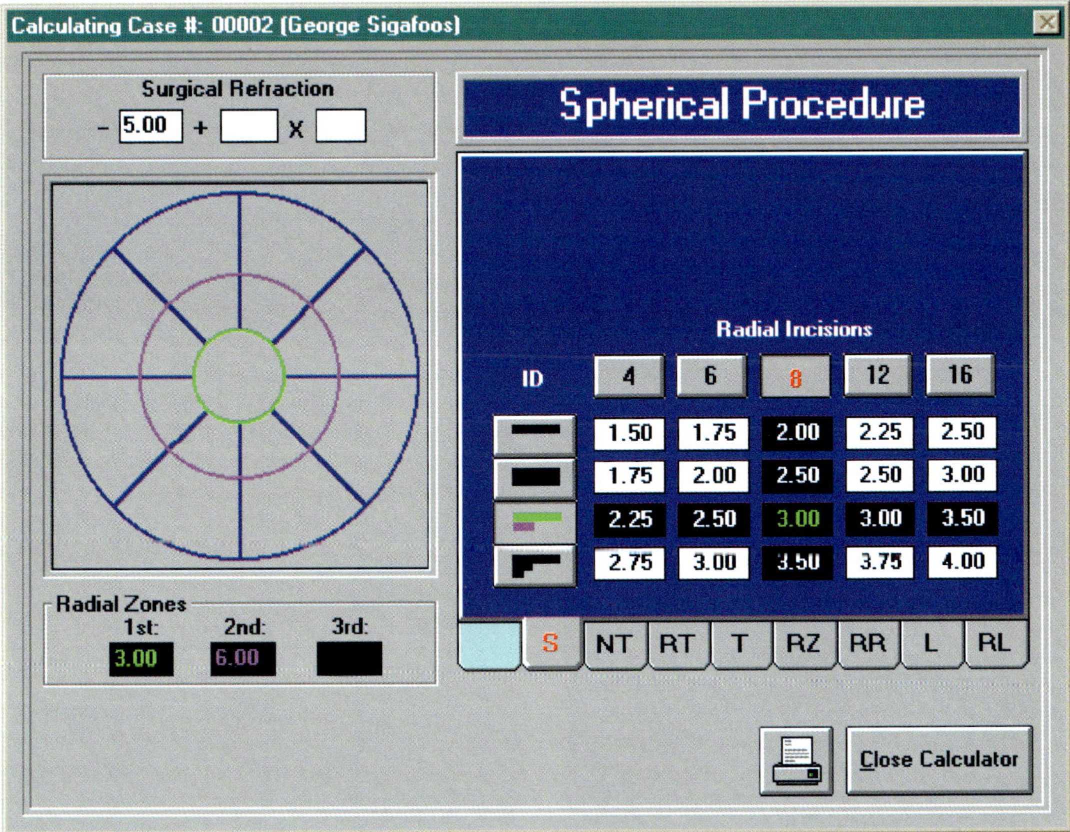

Fig. 8.42 Case 2. A –5.00-D spherical myope. Surgical summary showing configuration and surgical parameters. Note that two OZs are used here with eight incisions.

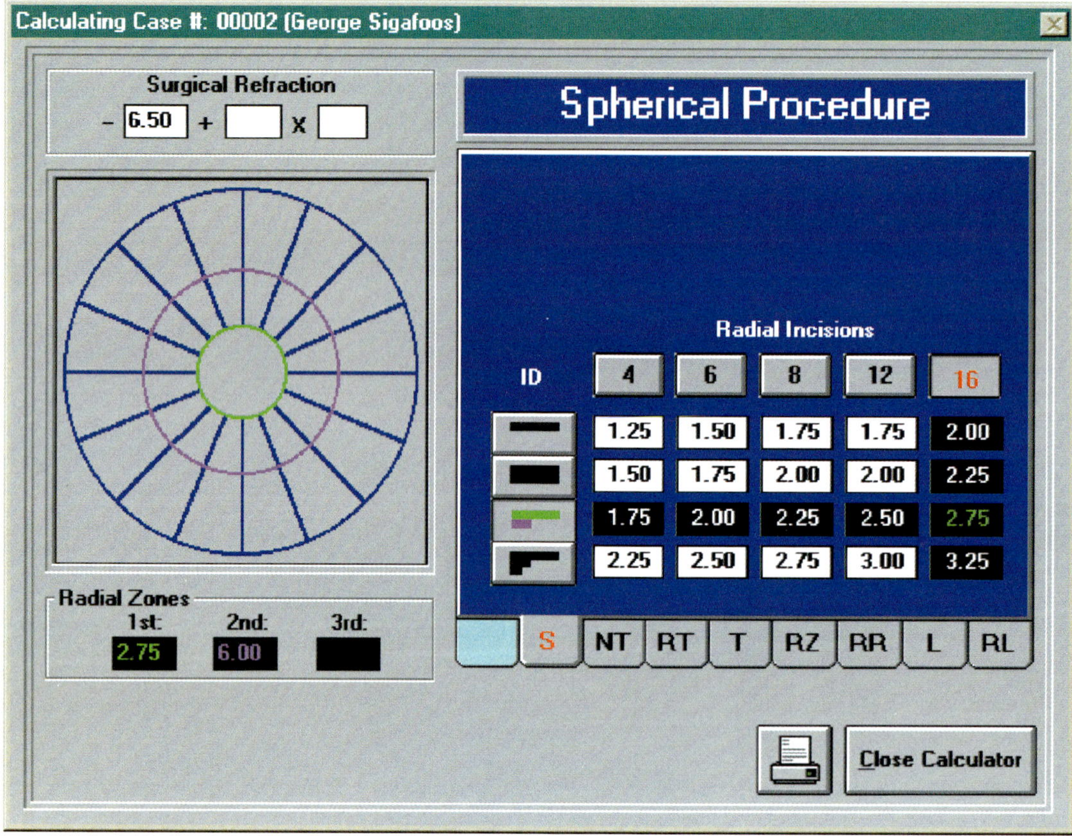

Fig. 8.43 Case 3. A −6.50-D spherical myope. Surgical summary showing configuration and surgical parameters. Note that the two OZs are indicated here along with 16 incisions. This is a "boundary" case. Some other procedure might be used instead.

sia required is provided by the application of additional 0.5% tetracaine. Occasionally, for patients complaining of discomfort from fixation (particularly in second-stage cases), 10% cocaine solution is applied to the limbus on a cotton pledget or applicator.

The instrument tray is placed on the surgeon's right side. This tray is a standard autoclave tray measuring 8 × 16 in. and supplied by the autoclave manufacturer (Castle). The bottom of this tray is lined with suitable padding. The basic instruments (supplied for every case) are a 50-mL Pyrex glass beaker, a Fyodorov dipstick (or Deitz hockey stick; Katena K3-9600), a Bores fixation forceps (Katena K2-3250), a 27-gauge Rainin irrigating cannula (Katena K7-3580), a Barraquer wire lid speculum (Katena K1-5010), a Bores adjustable handle with blade in a plastic sterilizer box, and Weck-Cel swabs. To this collection

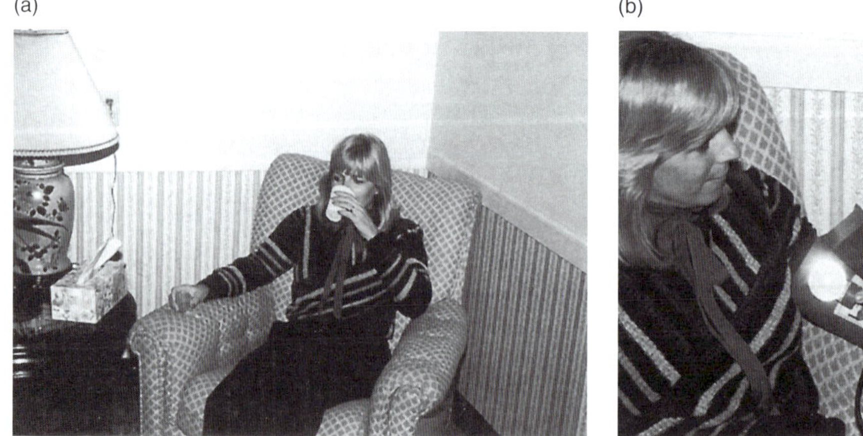

Fig. 8.44 (a) Patient taking oral sedation; (b) blood pressure is checked pre- and postoperation in all cases.

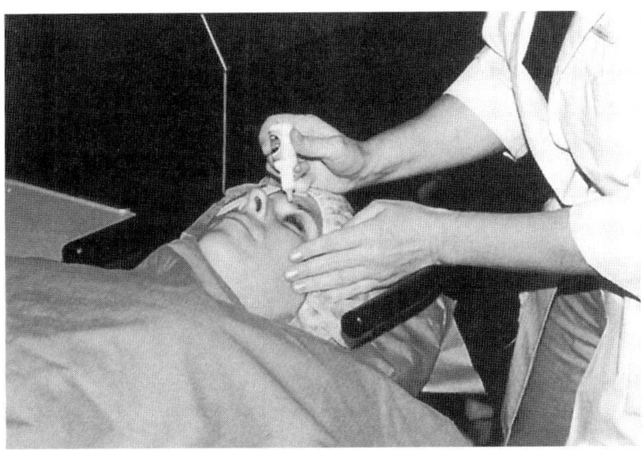

Fig. 8.45 Topical anesthetic is applied prior to prepping the eye.

are added the additional markers, forceps, etc. required in the specific case (Figure 8.46).

The blade used is the Bores LeCut™ double-edged uni-crystalline diamond blade (WMK 200) in the Bores adjustable knife handle manufactured by Katena Instruments (K2-6505). An identical blade is also available in the Bores micrometer diamond knife manufactured by KOI. The Bores sapphire blade (Katena K2-6513) mounted in the same Katena micrometer handle is also recommended. Two other blades are available from Katena for this handle. One (the K2-6501) has a single 30° angled cutting edge designed for the Bores (American) method of incising (from the OZ to the periphery). The other (the K2-6511) has a vertical cutting edge for use with the Fyodorov (Russian) technique (from the periphery toward the center), for re-incising old wounds, and for making T or transverse incisions (Figure 8.47). The single-edged blades are recommended for beginning surgeons because they are more durable.

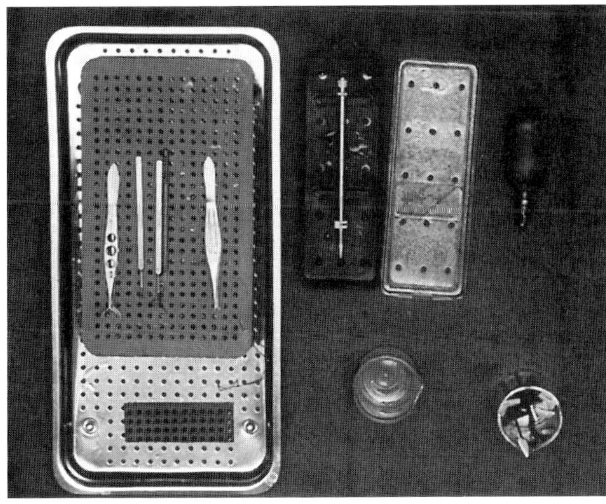

Fig. 8.46 Instrument tray set up for radial keratotomy.

The blade is set using the XTAL-800 Bores Shadowgraphic Blade Gauge, which magnifies the tip approximately 200 times. While coin or other gauges can, with care, be used, the fineness and fragility of the blade tip make such use hazardous from the standpoint of both setting accuracy and blade longevity. The blade is overset according to the desired incisional depth coefficient, as well as the blade type and style and the condition of the blade tip. This overset (bias) is typically 10 μm for new sapphire blades and zero for the LeCut diamond. After about 10 cases, the tips of sapphire blades become rounded, requiring an increase in the blade bias to maintain adequate incision depth—the diamond has not shown this same wearing pattern. This blunting is subtle and is impossible to detect under the operating microscope. Such blades, however, can continue to be used satisfactorily until the bias exceeds 70 μm or the tip breaks—in which case such a blade can still find use in cataract surgery.

Using the shadowgraph gauge

Using this instrument is quite simple. First, it must be placed in an easily accessible location. The location will depend on the volume of surgery the surgeon is currently doing on a daily basis and the number of knife handles and blades available. If less than six cases are operated on daily, the device can be placed in the instrument room

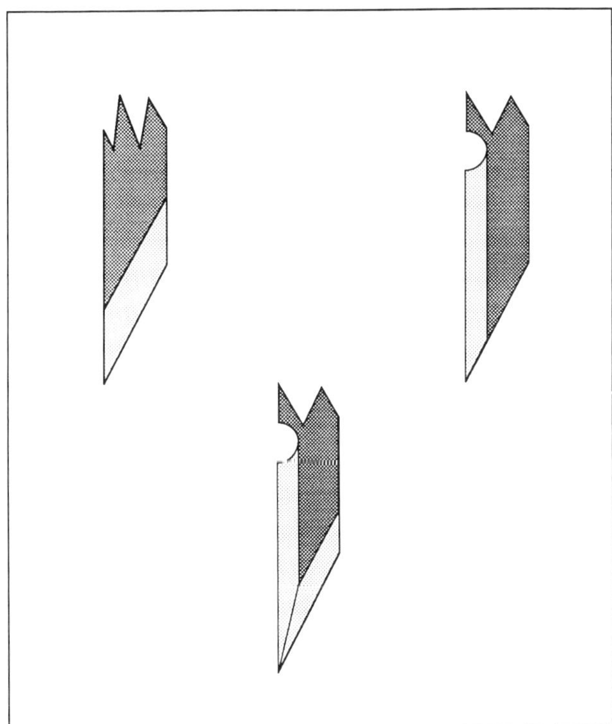

Fig. 8.47 Crystalline blade configurations.

and the blade preset before sterilization for each case. Experiments have shown that there is no measurable change in the settings after autoclaving with the XTAL-Katena handle combination. After setting, the handle is removed from the carrier and replaced into the sterilizing box, being careful not to disturb the micrometer screw. Each instrument tray is labeled with the patient's name. This system also works for higher-volume surgeons if they have a minimum of four knife handles. Care must be taken to prevent mismatching of blade and patient, however. I prefer to have the shadowgraph in the operating room, where I use it to set the blade prior to and during the surgery. The device is placed on a small glove table to my right on top of a sterile drape sheet such as a Barrier table cover. The eight autoclavable rubber knob covers are then placed over the adjustment and locking knobs.

Before initial use and from time to time, the calibration of the gauge should be checked using the special block provided with the instrument. Place the block onto the measurement stage, and lock it in place with the locking knob. Adjust the focus, brightness, and contrast controls until the reticle is crisp. The calibration bars should be superimposed over the reticle ticks. If there is no correspondence, check to see that the block is seated properly on the stage. If you are unable to align the calibration and measuring reticles, notify the company. Do not try to adjust the calibration of the instrument yourself.

To set the blade using the Katena handle, the handle is placed into the shadowgraph carrier with the back of the footplate facing up. The blade shank then fits into the groove that has been milled in the bottom of the carrier, keeping the handle from rotating. The locking plate is then slid across the handle and the knob tightened, securing the handle in the holder. The block is then transferred to the measuring stage and locked in place. This stage can be rotated while the carrier and blade are locked to it. This allows the operator to check for defects in the blade and for any misalignment either in the blade or in the footplates.

Adjust the stage up or down and in or out until the tip of the blade can be seen on the screen (Figures 8.48 and 8.49). Then retract the footplate until the blade protrudes through the footplate (Figure 8.50). Bring the blade shadow into sharp focus, and adjust the stage until the tip of the blade just touches the zero point and the back edge of the blade is in full view and superimposed on the reticle. Next, adjust the blade length by turning the adjustment screw on the blade handle. This moves the footplate and not the blade. Adjust the focus until the junction of the blade back and the footplate are well seen, and the bottom edge of the footplate is coincident with the measurement desired. Remove your hands from the controls, and ensure that the tip is still touching the zero point (you may have to refocus).

Please note in the case of double-edged blades: If you back up with your blade at this setting (i.e., cut with the vertical edge), your incision will be deeper than the actual setting because of the footplate curvature described previously (Figure 8.51). This is very important and must *never* be forgotten. Experienced surgeons can use this situation to increase the depth of the initial portion of their incisions by *gently* backing up to the edge of the OZ.

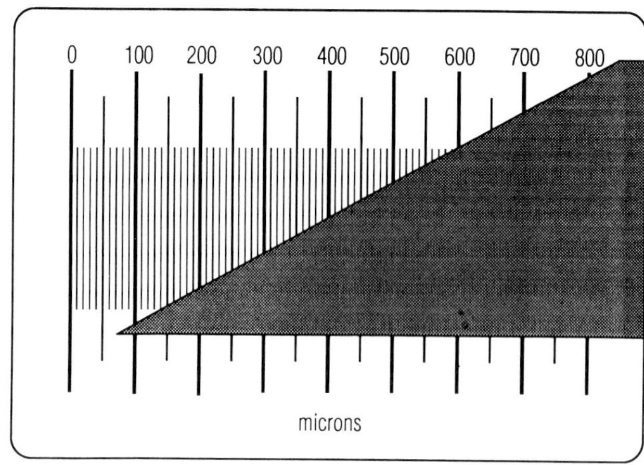

Fig. 8.48 Blade on screen in the shadowgraph.

Adjusting for direction of cut

If you are using the Russian (out-to-in) technique, then this is your initial setting. If, however, you are using the Bores (in-to-out) method, the setting may need adjusting. Using the vertical adjustment knob, lower the blade until the slanted cutting-edge–footplate junction comes into view. Adjust the focus, and note the difference, if any, in the measured setting. With current Katena handles it may be that the measured length is from 10 to 30 µm *less* at this point. This is so because the front curve of the footplate on this knife begins approximately in the middle of the blade and sweeps upward. Therefore, any measure-

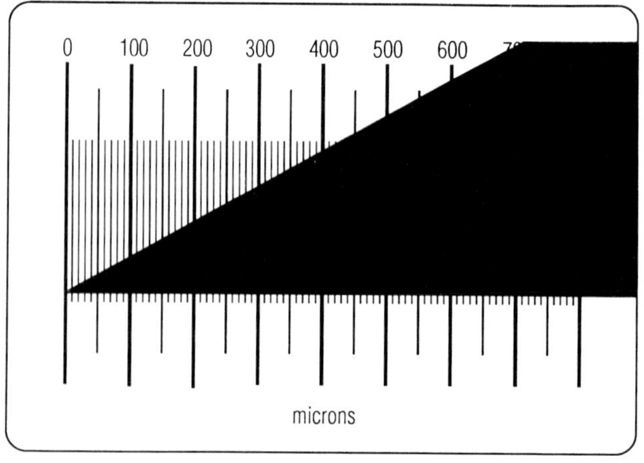

Fig. 8.49 Blade aligned with zero point on reticle.

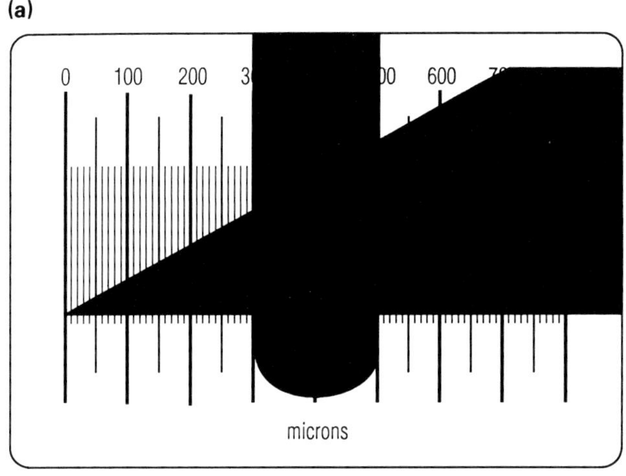

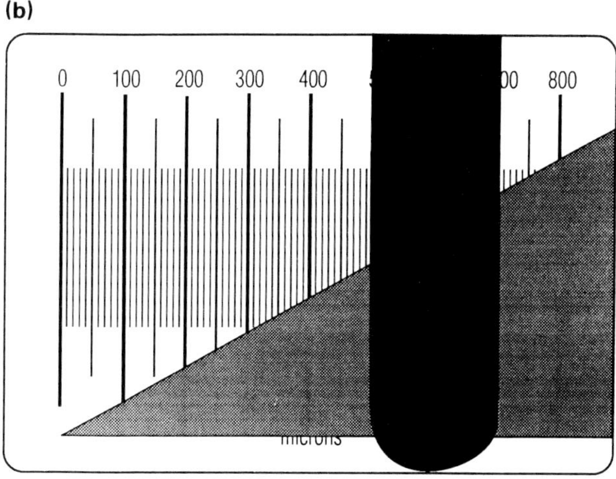

Fig. 8.50 (a) The footplate is moved into view; (b) the blade stage may have to be moved down to get the blade edge or footplate junction on screen.

ment taken there (vertical edge) will be longer than one taken at the slanted blade edge, where the footplate is flatter (and perpendicular to the midline of the blade). If you were to use the blade at this setting from in to out, the resulting incision would be shallower than that measured. Now elevate the blade until the straight edge comes into view, and adjust the focus, checking to see that the blade is still zeroed. Now *lengthen* the blade the exact amount of the difference previously noted by turning the adjustment screw on the handle. This is your blade setting.

The adjustment knob of the handle is then turned until the footplate appears on the screen; in this handle, the blade remains stationary, while the footplate moves. Keep turning the knob until the bottom of the footplate aligns with the slanted edge of the knife blade. It may be necessary to lower the stage slightly to bring the edge down to the reticle. In that case, the tip will no longer be touching the zero point. It will be necessary to move the stage up and down to check the zero point while making the final adjustment in blade setting.

You will find that while, at first, this method of setting may *seem* cumbersome, it will give the most accurate and reliable readings from setting to setting and is easily mastered. If you try to set the blade while looking at the slanted edge, you will find that the tip will be off-screen. You will then *not* know if you have introduced any lateral movement into the system sufficient to move the blade tip off zero. Remember that the stage is sprung to dampen vibrations and can be shifted if pressure is applied. The author uses this methodology on all his cases, even for the settings of each of the T's in the Ruiz procedure. The method is highly accurate, and the comparator device is recommended to refractive surgeons (Figure 8.52).

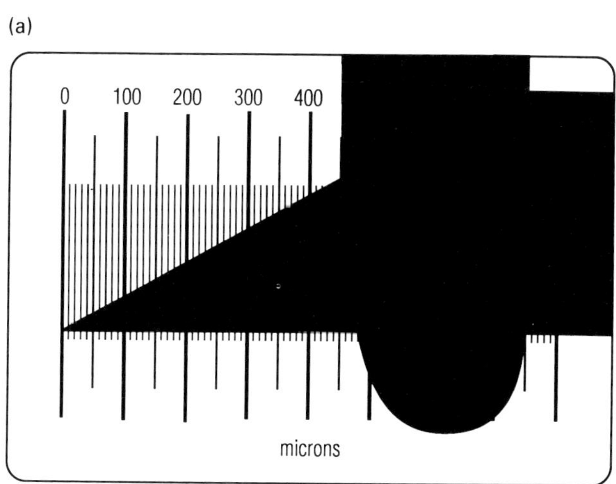

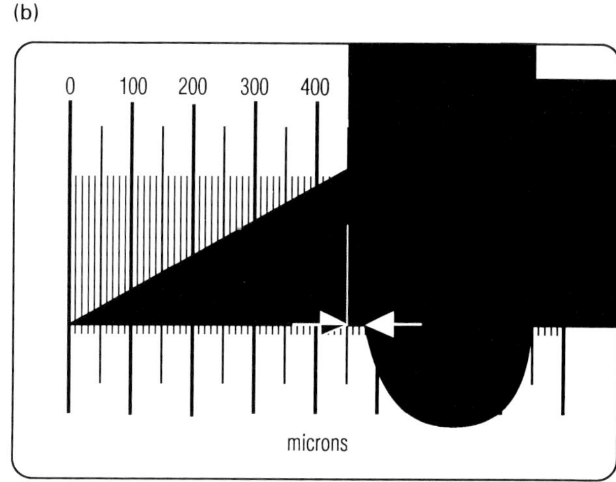

Fig. 8.51 (a) Measure along the vertical blade edge for incisions with the vertical edge and along the angled edge for incisions to be made with that edge; (b) note the difference in the two readings—this is typical for most knives.

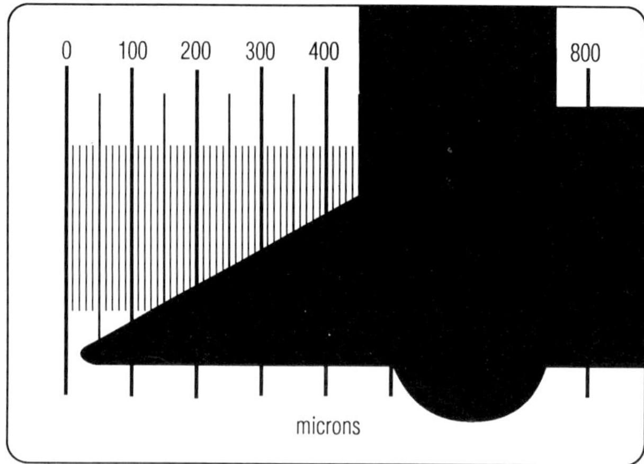

Fig. 8.52 It is very easy to see any blade defects—such as this rounded tip—with a shadowgraph. Such a defect would be missed under the microscope and would render any blade setting with a micrometer wrong.

Now unlock the carrier, and grasping it by the handle-locking knob, remove it from the stage. If the handle is sterile, sliding the carrier out will be the safest maneuver. When the carrier is free of the stage, grasp it (*not* the knife handle) and lift it to a sterile area. Since the bottom of the carrier is no longer sterile at this point, make sure to always set it down in the same place. I use a violet skin-marking pencil to outline a safe "landing" area for the stage. You could simply place the carrier onto a sterile 4 × 4 as well. Unlock the carrier and pick up the handle in such a way as to cause the head to rise first. Pushing down on the exposed end of the handle will accomplish this. Doing so will prevent damage to the blade. Remove the knife, and place it back into its sterilizing box temporarily.

Practice these maneuvers with a discarded blade until you become proficient with them. Always check the calibration before each measuring session, and be certain that the blade tip is coincident with zero when you are finished adjusting the blade. Keep the instrument covered when not in use, and take care not to bump it or drop it while moving it. Try to keep it in one place and not move it at all. This is a precision device and must be treated as such. Do not let Kathy Klutz or Fred Fumbles anywhere near it.

Establishing the optical center (fixation axis)

The patient is asked to fixate on the microscope light filament, whereupon the fixation point is marked with a blunt instrument, taking care to compensate for any parallax errors that may exist in the microscope system (Figure 8.53). This is the patient's visual axis or optical center. The light reflex seen through the Zeiss operating microscope is rectangular in shape. Because of two factors, the location of the light reflex will be displaced from the real locus of the optic axis. The position of the exit point of the light beam causes the patient to have to look down slightly in order to center the light's image (see Figure 8.53a). In addition, and because of parallax within the microscope, the reflex will be displaced laterally (in this case, *to the right*). Figure 8.53b illustrates the appearance of the reflex from the *right* ocular of the microscope. This causes the light reflex to be slightly higher than its true position. The rules of thumb for positioning the optical center mark are as follows:

1 Have the patient look at the light.
2 The surgeon fixates with one eye.
3 The mark is made in the upper corner opposite the fixating eye (see Figure 8.53b).

The Weck ophthalmic operating microscope typically produces two disks of light on the corneal surface. In this case the procedure is similar except that the surgeon alternately opens and closes his or her eyes each time,

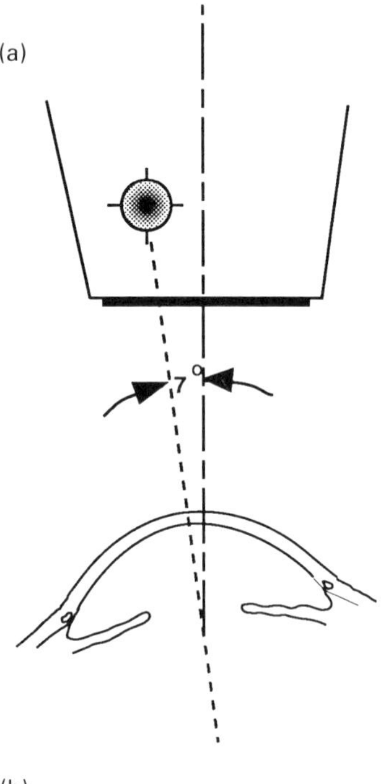

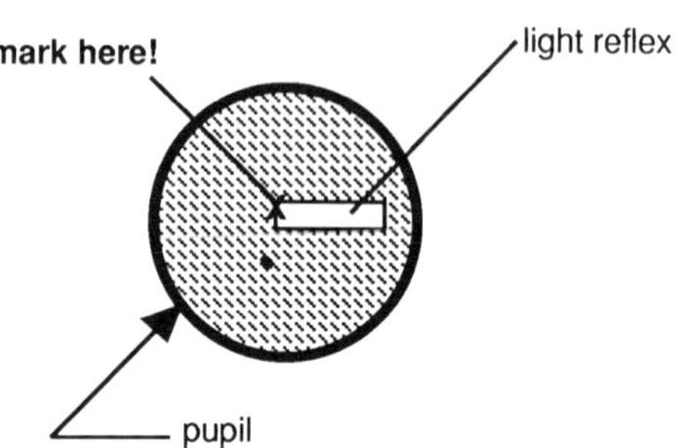

Fig. 8.53 (a) Microscope light reflex is typically higher than the visual axis; (b) the pupil is typically eccentric to the visual axis.

marking the spot *between* the light reflexes. When both eyes are fixating, two marks will be seen. The optical center lies between the two. Mastel has produced a rather nifty alignment device that clamps onto the Zeiss operating microscope (Figures 8.54a-c). This company also makes a complete line of RK instruments, including some of the most delicate and precise low-profile OZ markers (Figure 8.55).

The main OZ is then marked concentric to the optical axis-not to the pupil (Figure 8.56). This is extremely important because the pupil is not concentric with the optical axis of the eye (Figure 8.57). To verify the centration of the optical center and OZ marks, the patient is asked to look away and then back at the light. Any discrepancy is corrected. The midperipheral zone(s)—if any—is(are) then marked (Figure 8.58), and the surgery begins (Figure 8.59).

A double-pronged corneal-scleral forceps designed for this purpose (Katena K5-3250) is applied to the limbus at the 3 o'clock position with the left hand for fixation (Figure 8.60). The blade tip is then inserted into the cornea exactly at the edge of the primary OZ at the 9 o'clock position. The incision is carried to the midzone if there is one (see "Stepped incisions," below) or to the capillary plexus at the limbus. The back of the blade is your guide and should align with the midzone (if stepped) or the capillary arcade (if single depth).

The instruments are then switched to the other hand, and the second incision is made 180° to the first. The third incision is begun 90° to the first two. The surgeon continues in this manner until all incisions have been made (Figures 8.61 through 8.63).

One also must be sure that the knife footplate is perpendicular to the corneal surface and in contact with it at all times. This is especially important in the periphery, where beginning surgeons have a tendency to keep the knife handle perpendicular to the floor of the operating room and not to the corneal surface—they forget that the corneal surface is curved. This tendency is clearly evident when the incisions are examined under the slit lamp—almost all of them tend to curve up and become shallow in the periphery. Therefore, I have suggested that beginning surgeons exert extra pressure against the cornea in the periphery to ensure maximum depth of the incision there.

(a)

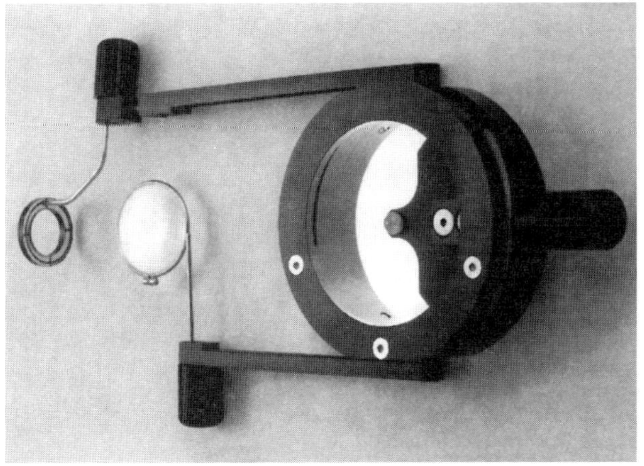

(b)

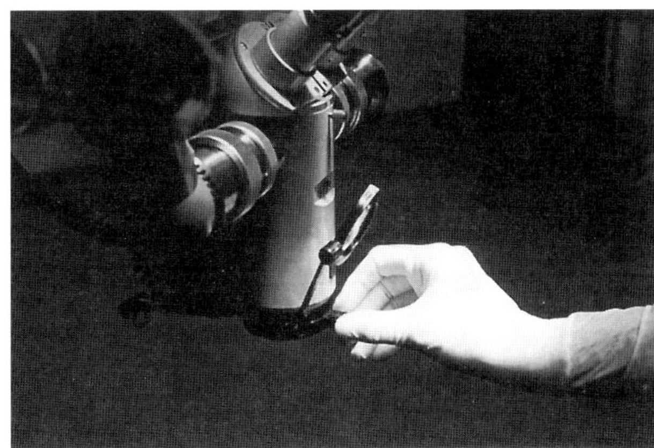

(c)

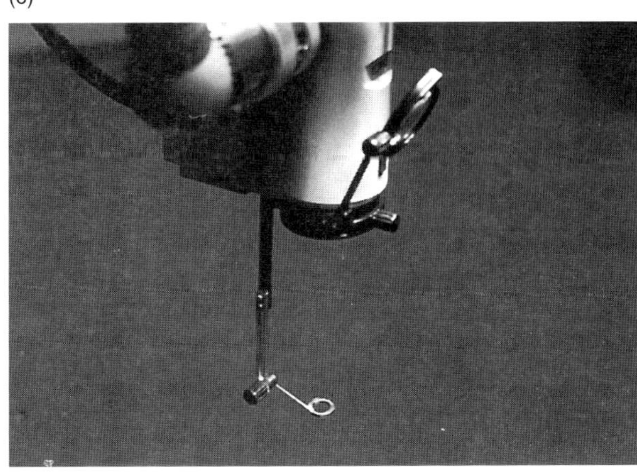

Fig. 8.54 (a) Martin aximeter from Mastel Precision Surgical Instruments. A magnifying lens and a surgical keratometer are also part of the instrument. (b,c) The apparatus attached to the microscope.

(a)

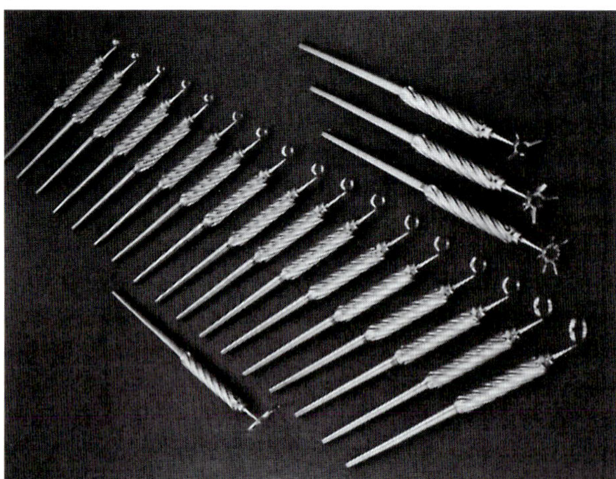

(b)

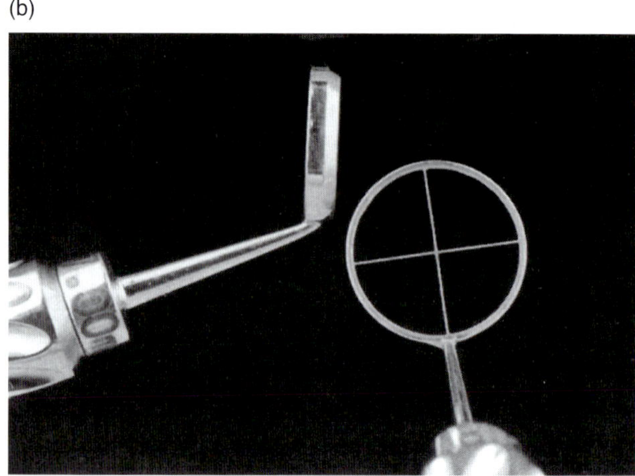

Fig. 8.55 (a) Lightweight, low-profile Mastel radial keratotomy markers. (b) Close-up of the optical zone markers.

This has prompted some "experts" to assert that the extra pressure compresses the cornea, causing the incisions to be made deeper. They carry this notion a step further and recommend that extra pressure throughout will ensure extra incision depth. While it is true that incisions will be deeper doing this, the cause is solid footplate–cornea contact, not tissue compression. I have not been able to demonstrate that normal corneal tissue is compressible to any degree, nor have I found any evidence in the literature to support the notion that it is.

Extra pressure, however, if carried to the extreme, actually may be harmful to the cornea by inducing bending/stretching of the endothelial cells. This is possibly the origin of the 22% endothelial cell loss reported by Hoffer and coworkers [20]. Videotapes of surgery being performed on the eyes included in that study show that excess pressure was exerted in these cases, causing deep furrowing of the cornea along the wound track. A similar study, reported by Smith and Cutro [21], using my technique, showed a net cell gain, demonstrating that no cell loss had occurred. It is not necessary to exert much pressure at all against the cornea using the "feather touch" technique. Simply keeping the footplate in contact with the corneal surface and arcing the knife handle to follow the curvature are sufficient to produce incisions of even depth throughout (Figure 8.64).

Stepped incisions

If a stepped incision is required, the blade is reset in the shadowgraph to the proper length, again oversetting as required. The blade is inserted into the end of the previously made incision just behind the edge of the midzone, and the incision is continued to the limbus. If the blade is

(a)

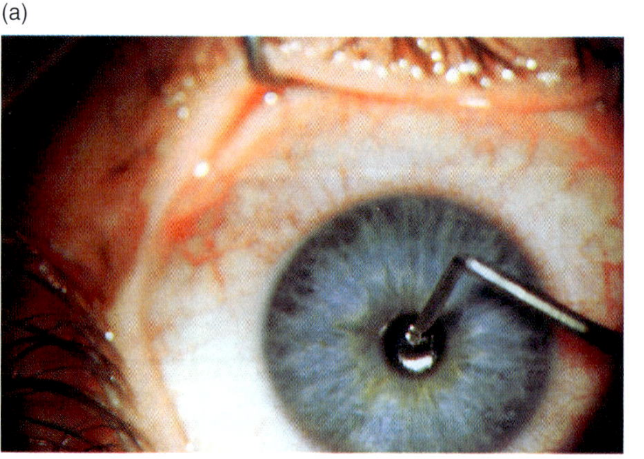

(b)

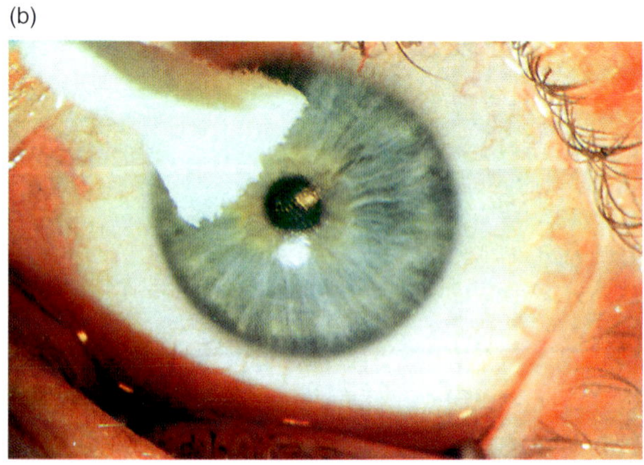

Fig. 8.56 (a) Mark the optic center with a blunt instrument—a dipstick or Deitz hockey stick is ideal; (b) wipe off the cornea with a moistened Weck-Cel sponge to reveal the mark.

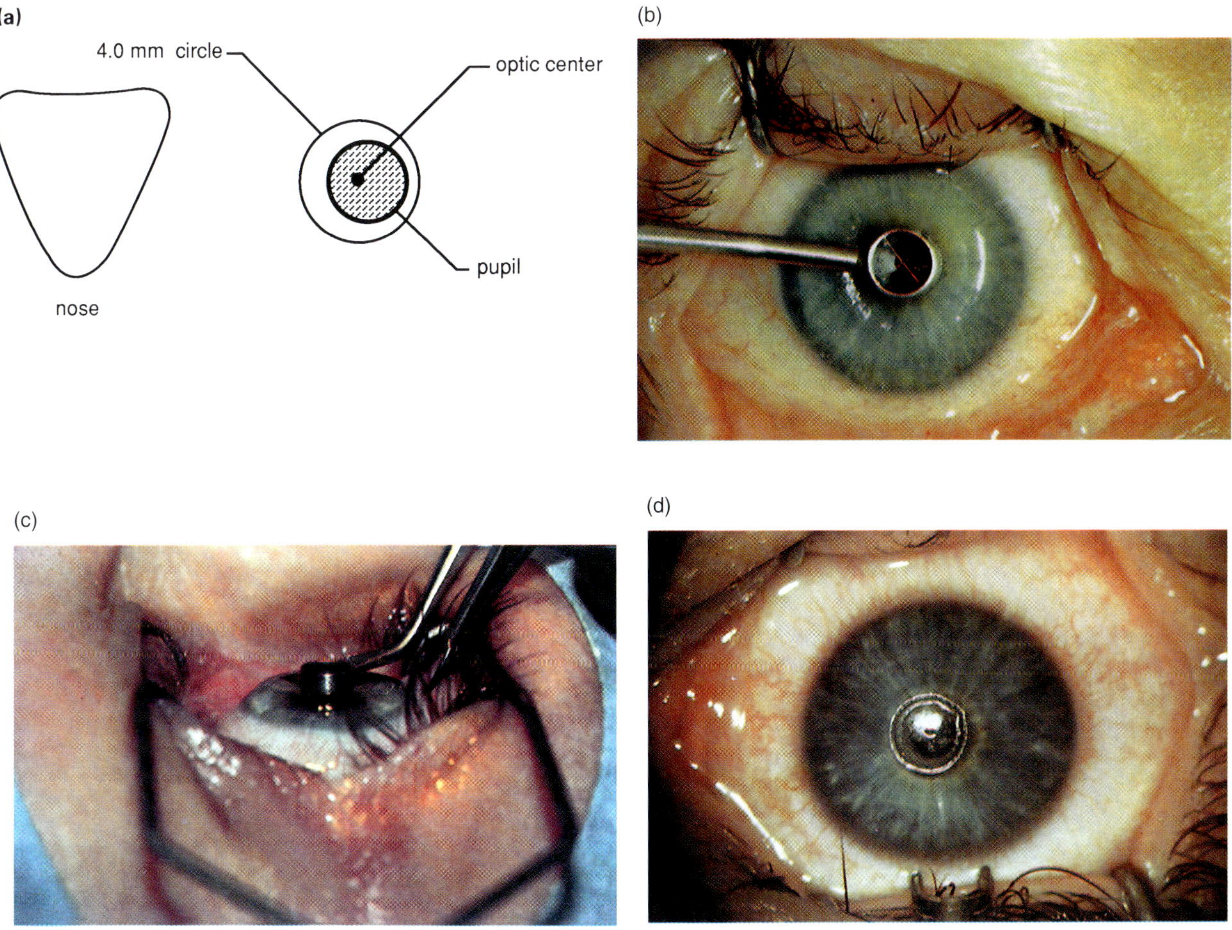

Fig. 8.57 (a) Mark the surgical zone concentric to the optic center. (b) A cross-hair is helpful. (c) Press the marker against the cornea with a slight rocking movement. Do *not* rotate the marker. (d) A dry cornea shows up the mark very clearly.

drawn up gently to the end of the preceding incision before extending it, the transition will be smooth, and no tag or "stalagmite" will be left behind (Figures 8.65 through 8.69).

After all the incisions have been made, a Fyodorov dipstick (or similar instrument) is used to ensure that no overlapping tissue tags are left behind in stepped incisions (see Figure 8.68c). If any are found, they must be incised so as not to leave a constricting band around the midzone, which would tend to reduce the effect of the surgery and/or even induce astigmatism.

The Russian way

There are times when it may be necessary or desirable to do things the Russian way—that is, make incisions from the limbus to the center. We will explain why this is necessary in our discussion about recutting over old incisions (see "Second-stage surgery—dealing with undercorrections," below). High myopia (greater than –7.0 D) is another reason (see Case 4 above). Since we have already stated that the practical upper limit of RK is somewhere around –6.0 to –6.5 D, it might be asked why we discuss cases with more myopia than that? We are discussing them because there may be times when radial incisions are warranted in high myopia. The patient, for example, may decide that part of a result is better than staying myopic, and he or she may not wish to opt for MKM or laser in situ keratomileusis (LASIK). Furthermore, despite what has been described as the practical upper limit of RK, this statement does not mean that such cases are impossible to correct—it just means that they are less likely to be fully corrected. *Less likely* does not mean "not likely" in any case. It should go without saying, though, that such a case should not be one of the first you try.

The Russian (Fyodorov) method requires a blade with a vertical cutting edge, a knife handle with an open foot (Katena/WMK), and a wide fixation forceps. It also requires that special markers be used to provide guidelines for making the incisions. There are any number of such markers on the market—I prefer those made by Katena (since most were made to my specifications). In addition, some sort of dye should be applied to the marker blades to stamp indelible marks onto the corneal

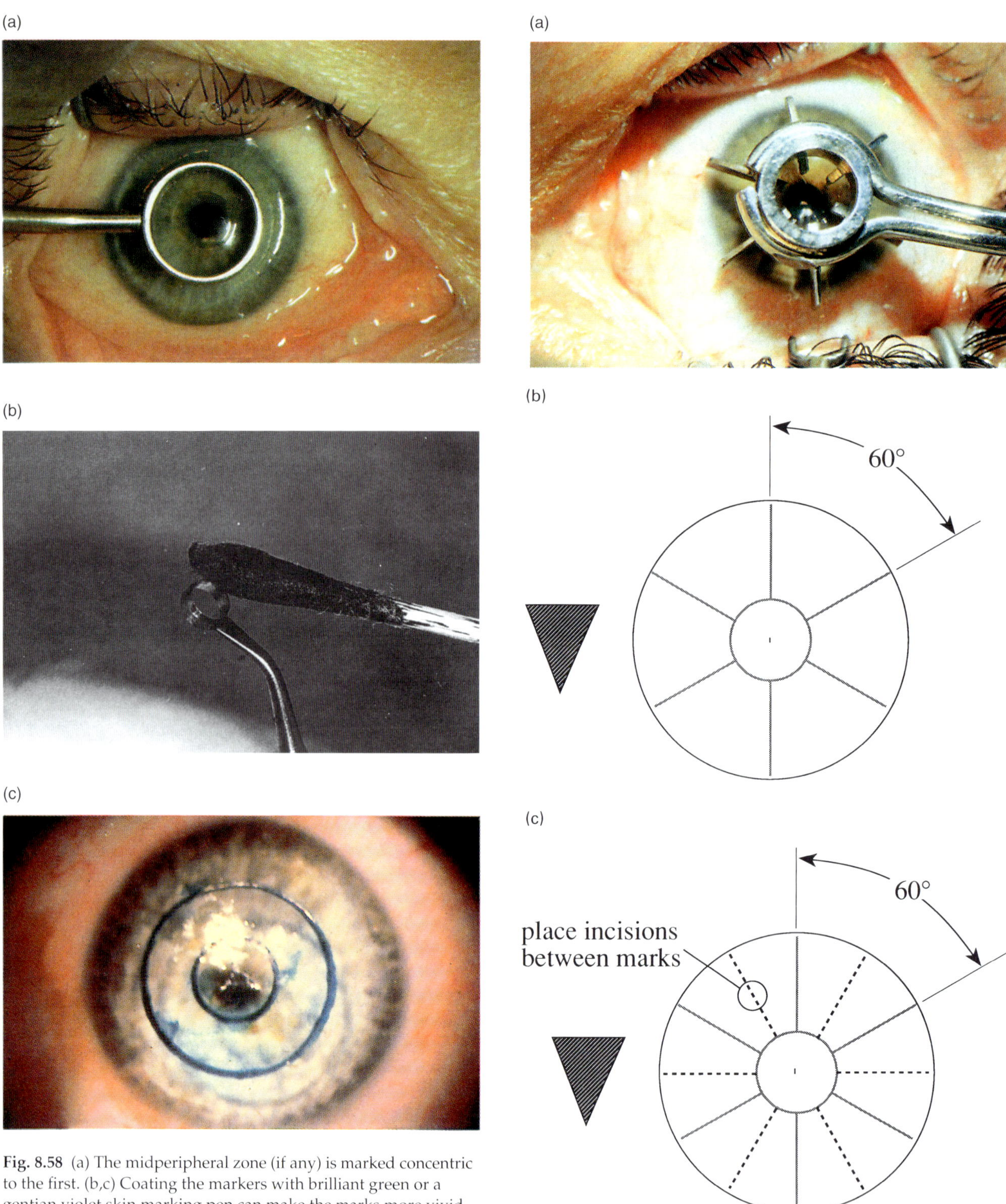

Fig. 8.58 (a) The midperipheral zone (if any) is marked concentric to the first. (b,c) Coating the markers with brilliant green or a gentian violet skin marking pen can make the marks more vivid.

Fig. 8.59 (a) Mark incisions as desired (see text). (b) A six-ray marker is useful because it is hard to line up incisions exactly at 60°. (c) For a 12-incision case, incisions are easily made between the six marks.

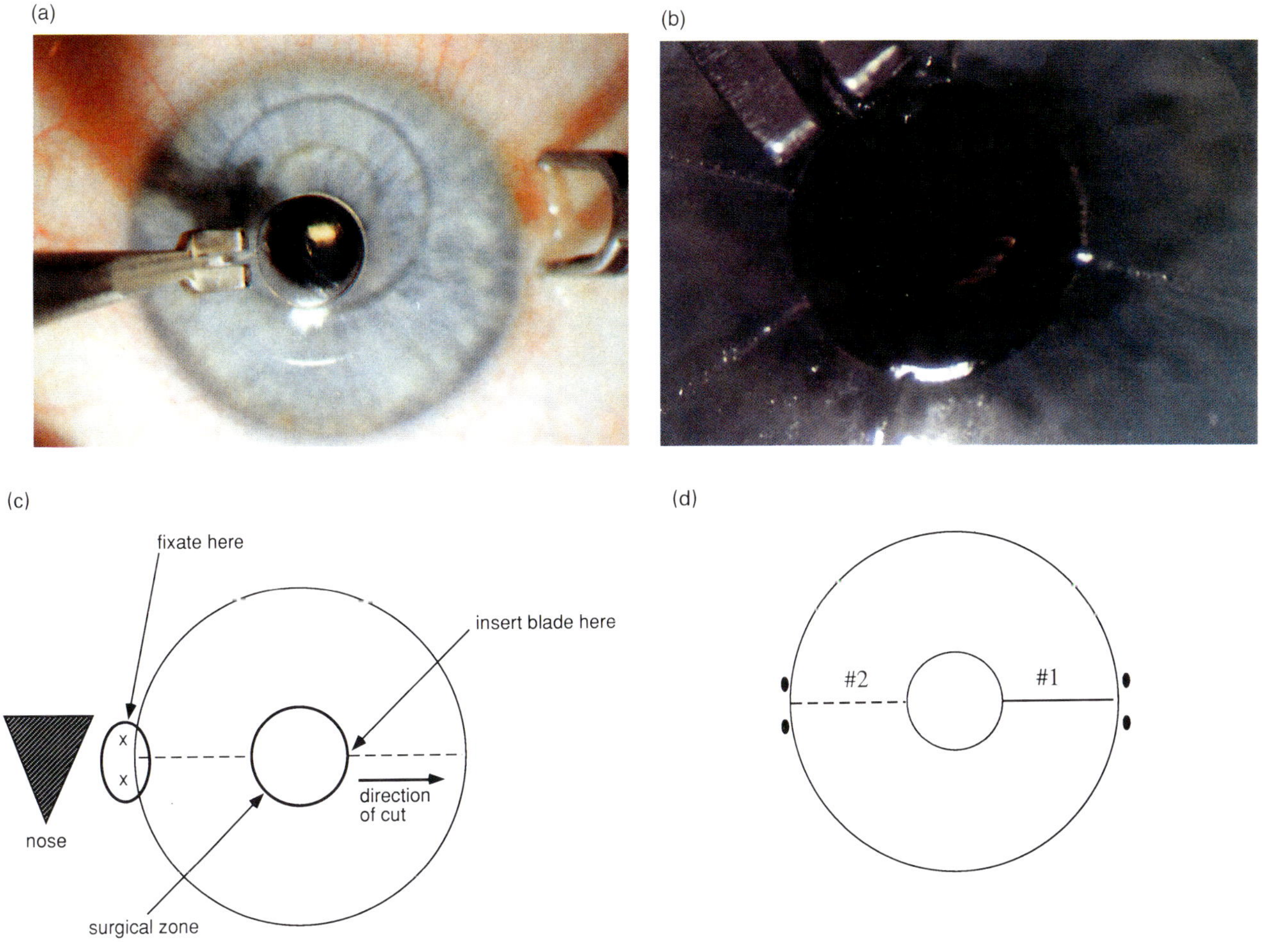

(a)

(b)

(c)

fixate here

insert blade here

nose

direction of cut

surgical zone

(d)

#2

#1

Fig. 8.60 (a) Fixation is at the limbus, 180° to the incision. (b) The blade tip is inserted exactly at the edge of the surgical clear zone. (c,d) Make the first two incisions the horizontal ones.

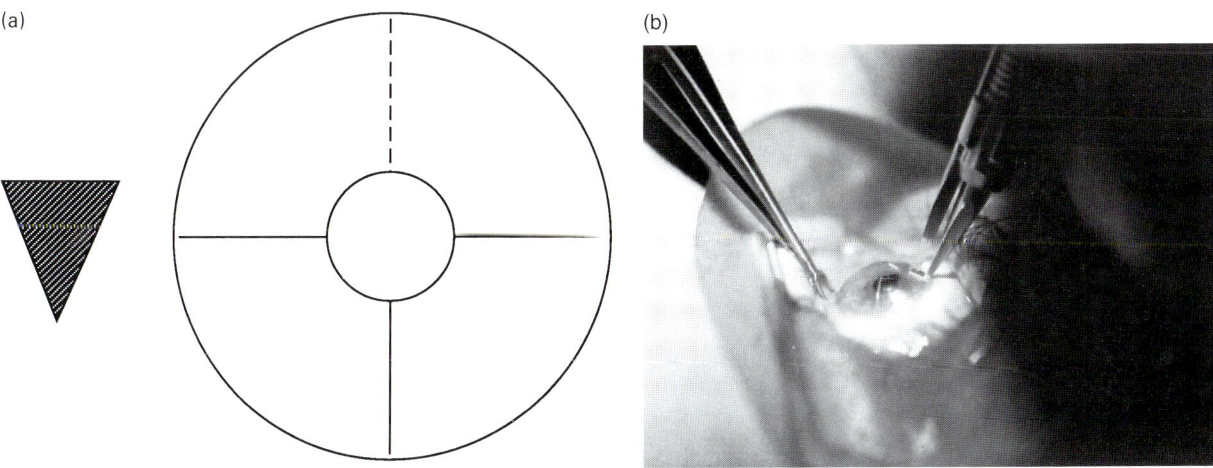

Fig. 8.61 (a,b) The 12 o'clock incision is the third to be made.

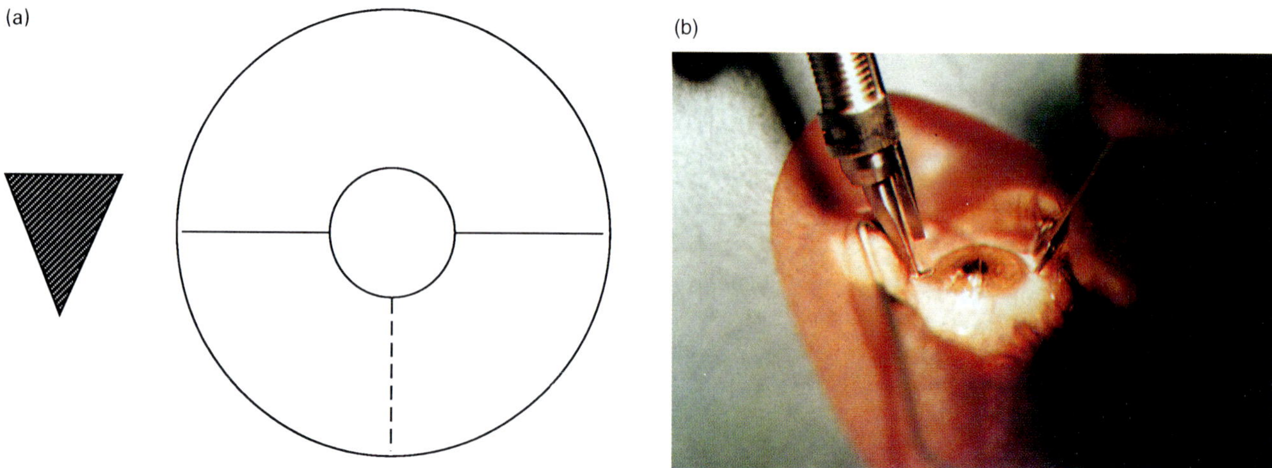

Fig. 8.62 (a,b) The fourth incision is made at 6 o'clock. Only the gentlest downward pressure is used.

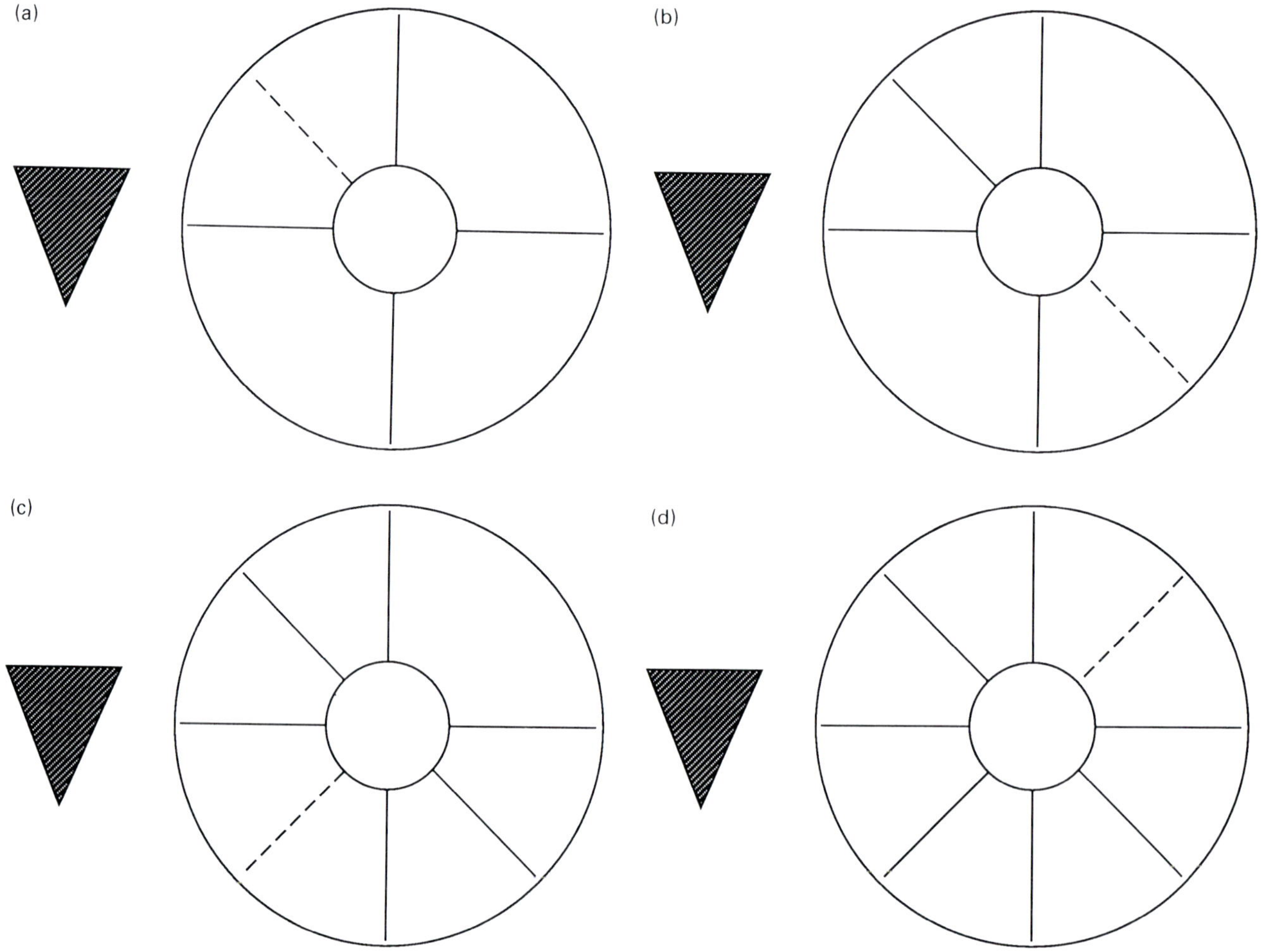

(a)

(b)

(c)

(d)

Fig. 8.63 (a) The fifth incision is made downward and nasally. (b) Incision 6 is made up and out (superotemporal). (c) The seventh incision is made in the upper nasal quadrant. (d) The inferotemporal incision is *always* last.

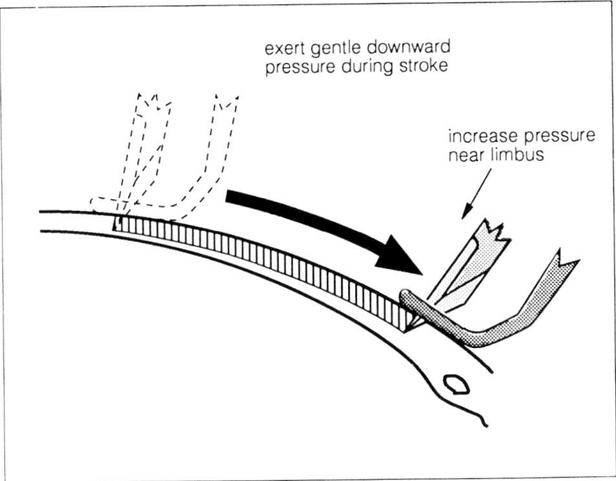

Fig. 8.64 Keep the footplate against the corneal surface.

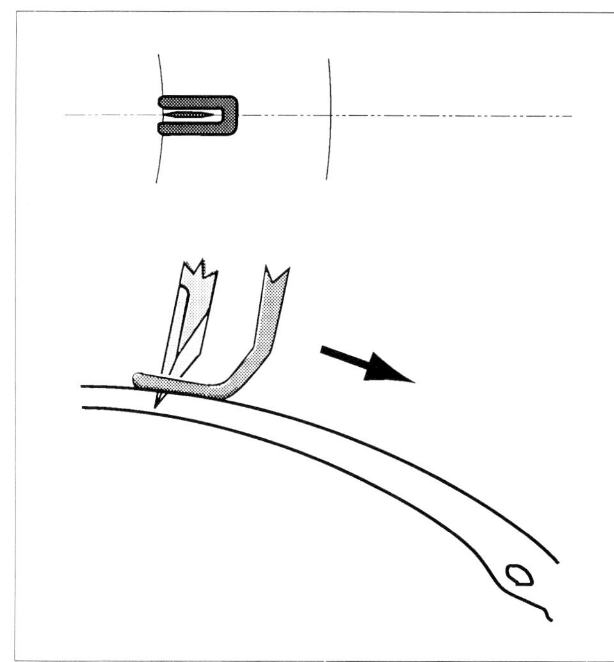

Fig. 8.65 Insert blade tip exactly at the edge of the primary optical zone as before.

surface (Figure 8.70). These are necessary because the Russian method is somewhat slower to perform, and the impressions of the marker blades alone will fade before the surgery is completed. Gentian violet from a skin-marking pen (Katena K20-4500) can be used, but I prefer a 1% tincture of brilliant green for my marks because they are more readily seen on the cornea. This is applied to the OZ and incision markers with a cotton swab and allowed to dry thoroughly. Absolute alcohol is used to make this tincture, and if any gets on the cornea, it will destroy the epithelium, so make sure it is dry.

The optical center is marked in the usual way, and the blade is set to the corneal thickness of the largest OZ to be used. Make sure, if using the shadowgraph, that the readings are taken at the juncture of the vertical blade edge and the footplate. Next, the surgical (optical) zones are marked starting with the smallest. Since the smallest zone almost always will be 2.75 or 3.00 mm (see the discussion

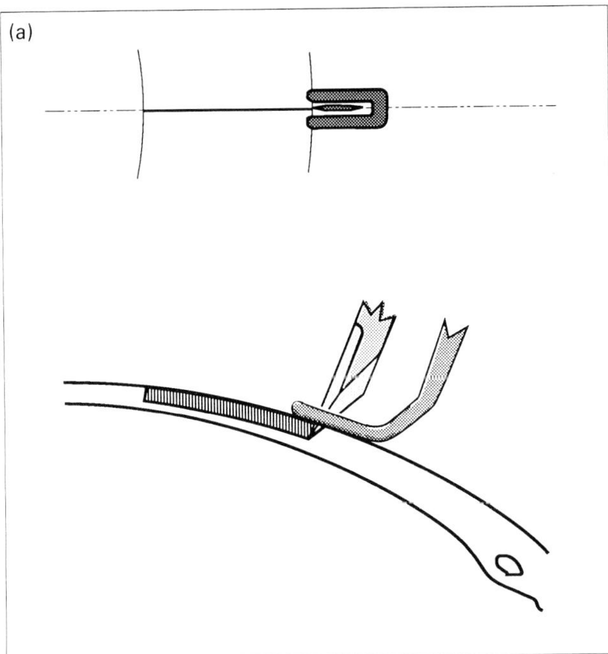

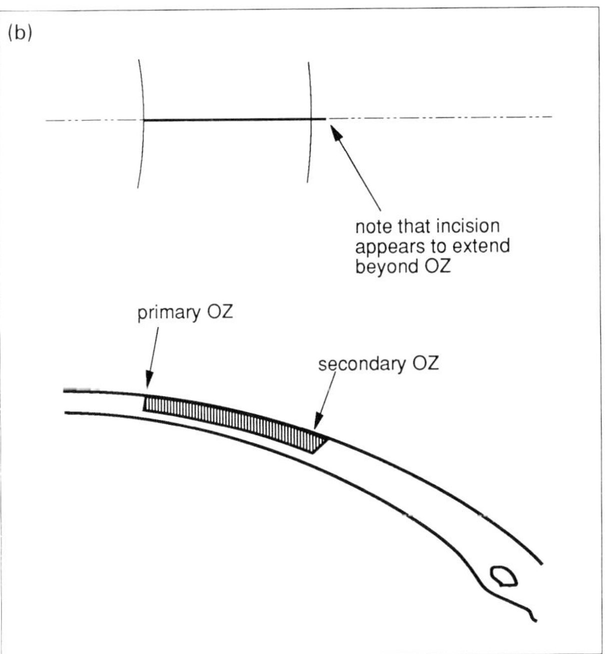

Fig. 8.66 (a) Stop at the secondary zone. (b) The incision will appear to extend beyond the secondary zone.

(a)

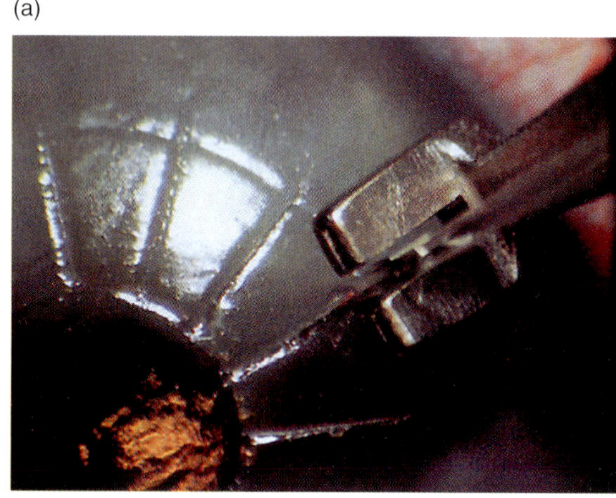

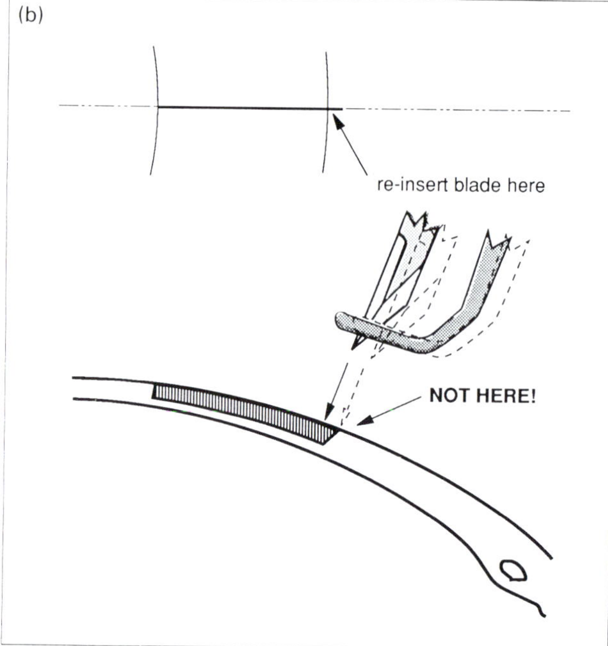

Fig. 8.67 The second step starts inside the first, not at the end.

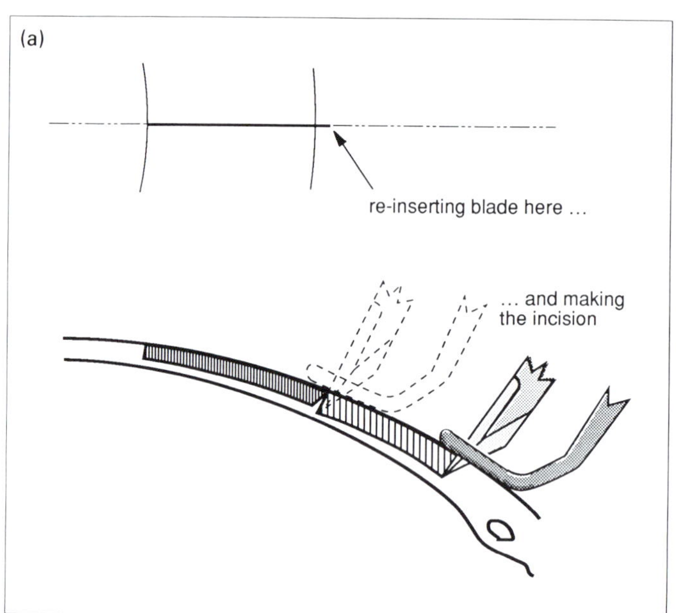

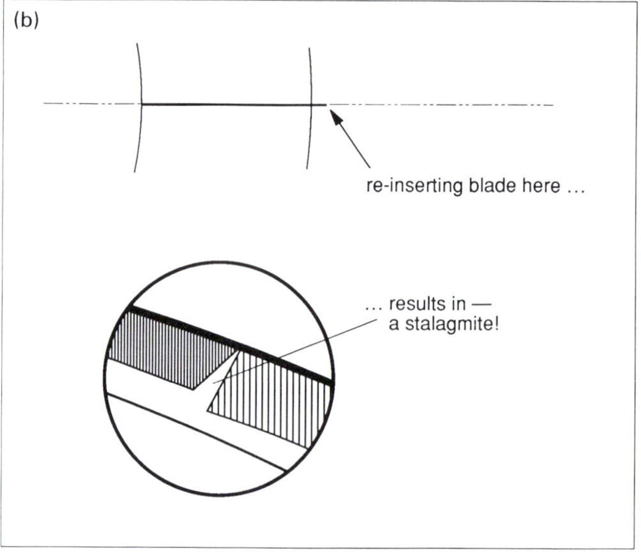

(c)

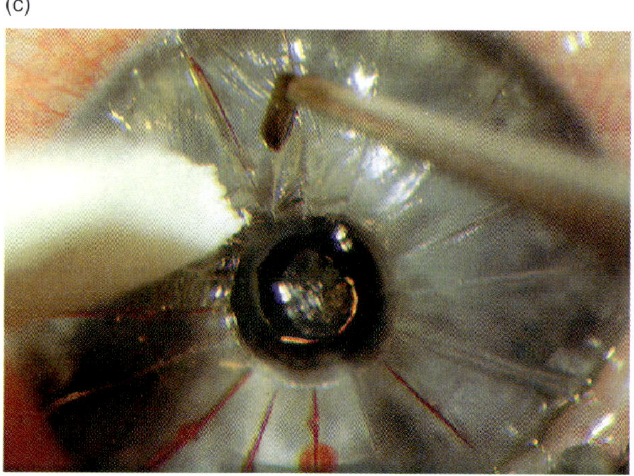

Fig. 8.68 (a) Inserting the blade at the end of the first incision results in (b,c) a stalagmite (between dipstick and swab).

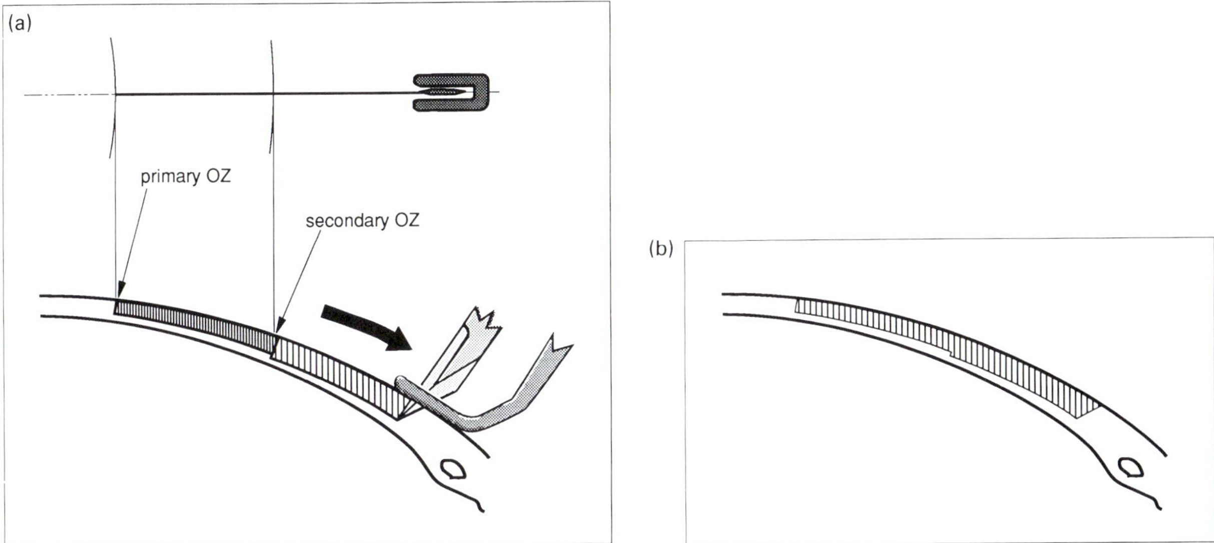

Fig. 8.69 Proper stepping technique. (a) Insert the blade just inside the previous incision. (b) Continue the incision to the limbus if the two-step procedure is being used.

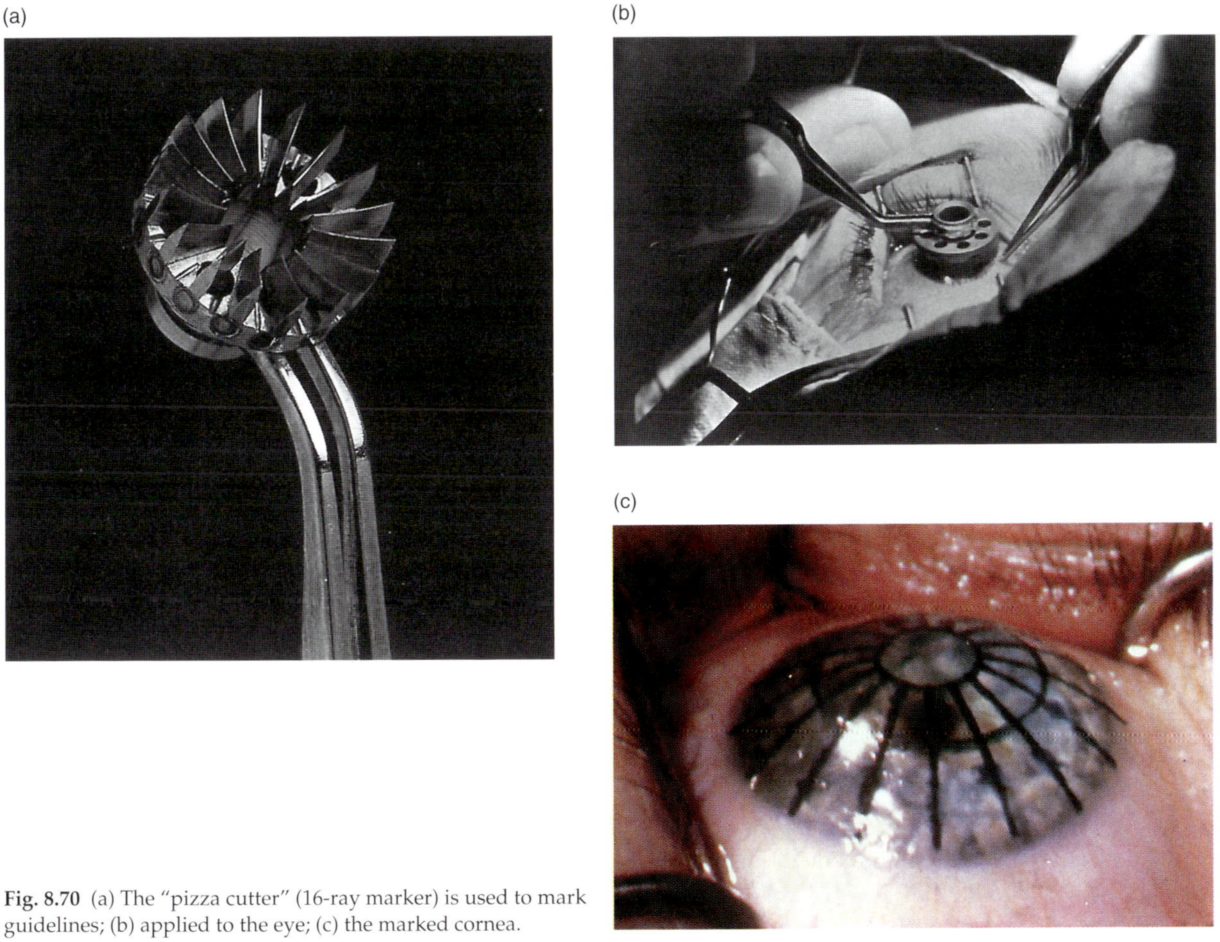

(a)

(b)

(c)

Fig. 8.70 (a) The "pizza cutter" (16-ray marker) is used to mark guidelines; (b) applied to the eye; (c) the marked cornea.

of subnominal OZs above) and the incisions will have steps at 6 and 8 mm, respectively, a triple-ring marker with these dimensions can be purchased for this purpose. Once the zones are marked, the incision guides are stamped onto the corneal surface. Fixation is made in the same manner as in the Bores technique—directly across from the incision at the limbus. If you are using a wide or limbal fixation forceps, fix the cornea at 12 and 6 o'clock. In any case, make the first incision, the horizontal one, at 9 o'clock if you are doing the left eye and at 10:30 o'clock if you are doing the right eye. It is important to do this because the central OZ is shifted slightly nasally, but the corneal thickness taper is not. Insert the blade at the limbus with the slot in the footplate straddling the incision mark (Figure 8.71).

Holding the eye steady and watching the corneal surface just in front of the blade, move the blade forward. It is futile to attempt to watch the leading edge of the diamond and sapphire blades—they are too fine to see even under the microscope. However, it is easy to see the incision being made, especially as the tissue separates and flows away from the blade edge like water being cleaved by the prow of a boat. As the blade approaches the first zone mark, pay very careful attention to the incision. Keep the blade moving until the first hint of aqueous appears; then stop immediately and remove the blade. Wait while the cornea in that area swells, sealing the wound—it should take no longer than a minute or two. You will be surprised just how far past that first mark it is possible to go. Note the point at which aqueous appeared, and make all the rest of the incisions to that point, saving the inferotemporal one to the last. You will appreciate the "feather touch" technique here because using it is very unlikely to promote leakage from the microperforation. The perforation will be very much a "micro" one, in contradistinction to what would be the case were the "ham-handed" ultraheavy-pressure technique used (Figure 8.72). Herein it is vital that all incisions be made 180° apart.

When the first step incisions are completed, reset the blade to the corneal thickness at the secondary zone. Do not forget to add any blade bias that may be necessary. Reinsert the blade just behind the end of each preceding incision—saving the one with the microperforation until last—and carry the incision toward the next zone, all the while watching for aqueous; stop and remove the blade in that event. Note that point and proceed. When all incisions have had the second step made, re-set the blade to the pachymetry at the primary optical clear zone (2.75 or 3.00 mm).

By now the eye will be much softer than it was at the beginning. Now you will likely find that fixation behind the blade, thereby pulling the cornea under the footplate, provides better control and a smoother cut (Figures 8.73 and 8.74). Carry each incision *up to* the central optical clear zone.

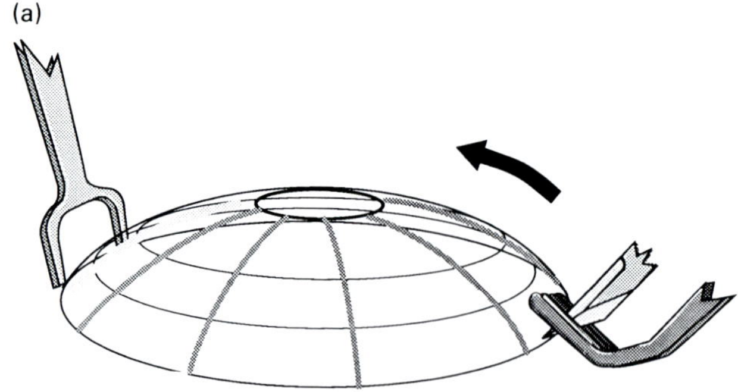

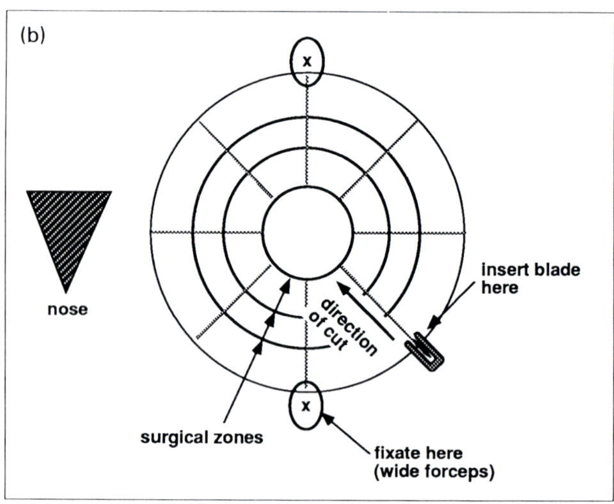

Fig. 8.71 (a) Insert the blade at the limbus. (b) Incisions are made toward the center.

CAUTION: This endpoint is not that clear-cut (no pun intended). The tissue tends to roll under the footplate, obscuring the edge of the zone. Watch the marked edge. As it passes under the tip of the footplate, begin easing the forward movement of the knife, stopping when the mark completely disappears under the footplate. Remove

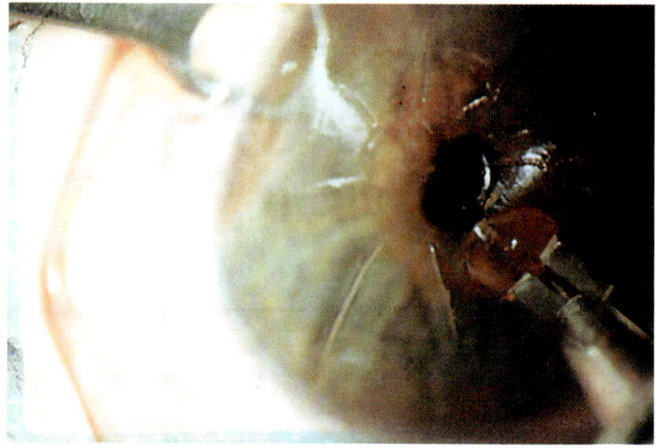

Fig. 8.72 The blade is carried forward until a microperforation occurs.

the blade, and you should find that the incision has stopped exactly on the mark.

If you find that you are consistently overshooting the endpoint, use a central marker whose diameter is 0.25 mm greater than the smallest zone you are trying to achieve. Because the eye is soft, more care will need to be taken to keep the incisions straight. Speed is a hindrance here—it only makes matters worse. Make your incisions with a slow, steady, and even pace. Do not be surprised if the terminal portions of the incisions tend to be curved or slightly irregular—while experience will minimize this effect, it is almost inevitable. Do not allow any incision to veer into and join another incision, however.

Second-stage surgery—dealing with undercorrections

The response of the eye to relaxing incisions, as in any biologic system, produces a typical Gaussian curve. That is, while most corneas flatten to a narrow range of predicted values clustering around emmetropia, there are a fair number that do not—some fall on the plus side—of emmetropia, whereas some fall on the negative side. Those which fall on the plus side—are overcorrected (or more properly, have overresponded)—and are more difficult to correct; there is no eraser on a scalpel after all. The correction of such errors is dealt with in Chapter 15. Because there is no good method to correct hyperopia as yet (although hyperopic LASIK and PRK show promise),

(a)

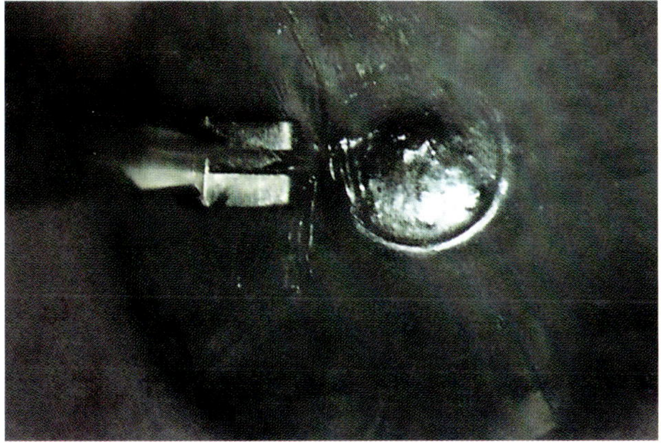

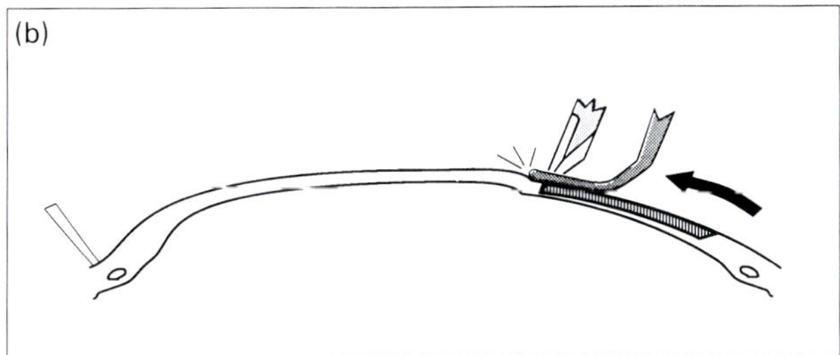

Fig. 8.73 (a,b) A "bow wake" or wrinkles will occur unless fixation is behind the blade or with limbus-to-limbus fixation.

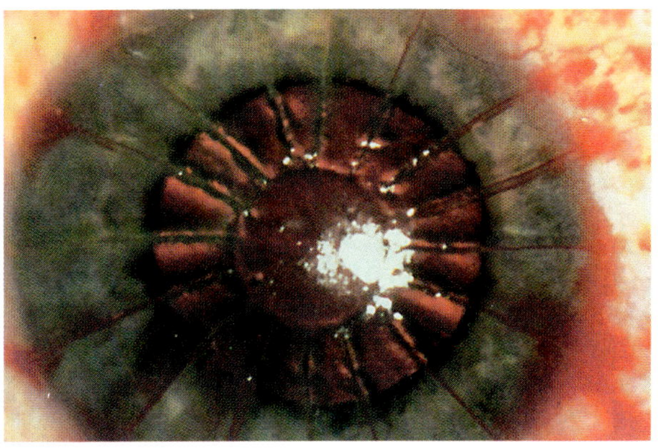

Fig. 8.74 Sharp blades, wide fixation, and a steady hand result in straight and even incisions.

the RK DataMaster algorithms have been weighted so as to skew any calculation errors to the negative or myopic side. Therefore, anyone using the author's technique will find that, on balance, they will be contending with more cases requiring a second stage of the surgery but fewer overcorrections. This, however, is better than the alternative—an overcorrection. Incisions cannot be erased in the event of overcorrection.

Some authors—with the best of intentions, no doubt—have advocated staging the surgery, at least in certain cases. By this they mean that the patient receives half the incisions (usually four), and then, after a suitable period of time has elapsed, the remainder (also usually four) of the incisions are added—if needed. This sounds like a good idea—especially if one is concerned about overcorrections—but ultimately, it is not a good idea. An impartial observer could be forgiven if he or she were to conclude that the surgeon who took this approach was either unsure of his or her technique or was less than convinced of the validity of the surgery itself. If the former, then it would seem prudent to adopt another method of parameter selection, and if the latter, perhaps it would be better if the surgeon stopped doing the surgery altogether.

There are enough variables in the equation to contend with without introducing another—which is exactly what happens once Bowman's layer is incised. No one has yet devised a formula to take into account the profound changes that occur in the cornea once this has happened—especially when days, weeks, or months have passed. All suggestions made to contend with the corneal shape after this event are purely empirical; here, the surgeon is truly flying by the "seat of his or her pants." One fact does seem irrefutable, however, and that is that the second group of incisions never results in the same effect as when all incisions are made at the same time. My advice, therefore, is to go for the whole of the myopia all at once and to do the nondominant eye first. After a suitable period of time, do the second eye, making any necessary adjustments in the technique to secure an even better result. Do it this way even if monovision is the plan. Since, as Robert Burns put it, "*The best laid plans o' mice an' men, gang aft go a-gley,*" this mind-set will keep the surgeon out of hot water most of the time. For this and other reasons, do not perform simultaneous surgery (see below).

Having said all of this, what is a person to do in the event of having "missed the mark"? The first piece of advice (and the second and the third) is not to be in a hurry. The fourth is to learn how to evaluate the depth of the incisions on which all depends. Figure 8.75 illustrates the appearance of RK incisions under the slit lamp and their approximate depths. The observer should keep in mind several points. First, early on, corneal edema can distort the appearance of incision depth, making incisions appear far deeper than they actually are. Since such edema can persist upward of a year, the task might seem impossible, except that most of the edema subsides within the first 3 to 4 weeks. Consequently, it is essential that new pachymetry readings be taken before additional surgery is performed. Usually a central reading is sufficient because the cornea swells up uniformly—add the difference to the old pachymetry measurements to get the new thicknesses. Second, the appearance of the incisions depends on whether the slit-lamp beam is coming from the nasal or temporal side of the eye. Incisions seen with the slit-lamp beam on the nasal side will seem somewhat shallower than if viewed from the temporal side.

To add incisions or to deepen them, that is the question (apologies to William Shakespeare). If the incisions are shallow, either from plan or inadvertence, it will be well to deepen them as soon as possible—that is, within the first 30 days postoperatively. To deepen incisions requires a steady hand and a sharp blade with a vertical cutting edge because the incisions have to be traced over from limbus to center. Do not even think of doing this using an angled blade and moving from center to limbus—it will not work. It does not work because the surgeon will not be able to see the incision well enough to stay within it, and it will not work because angled blades are almost impossible to keep from wandering out of the incision.

Figure 8.76 illustrates the technique of incision deepening. Note that fixation behind the blade is recommended. This is especially crucial for beginners in this technique. The surgeon will find that he or she will have much better control over both the direction and the endpoint of the incision doing it this way—corneal rippling is avoided completely.

If the surgeon has an extremely sharp blade at his or her disposal and some experience, the same thing can be accomplished using a wide limbal fixation forceps. Note, however, that the fixation points still must be behind the endpoint. Such deepening can either be single depth or in steps—just remember to set the blade according to the corneal thickness of the endpoint. One other tip (or pearl, if you will), recut alternate incisions only—do not attempt to deepen them all. This is especially important where 12 or more incisions were made primarily. The eye will become extremely soft very quickly, and attempts to recut

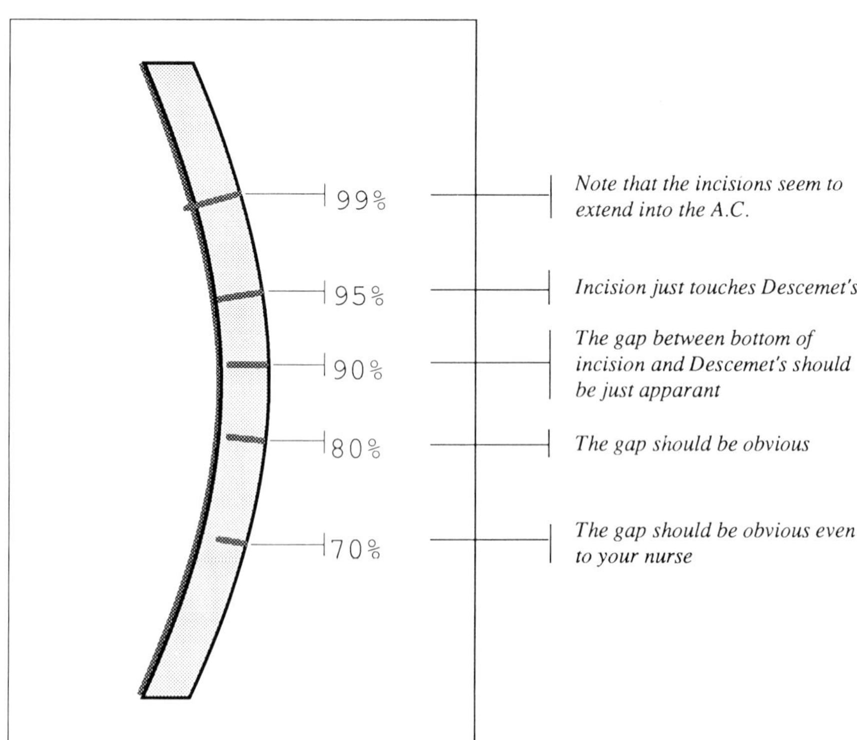

Fig. 8.75 Estimating incision depth at the slit lamp. Slit beam should be finely focused.

adjacent incisions will very likely end with one or more of them hook-shaped, where the blade has inevitably wandered out of the track or, worse, *joins* another incision.

Of course, all this could be avoided if the incisions were made deep enough in the first place. Practically every surgeon I know has had difficulty with the recommendation (nay, necessity) that blades be set longer than the corneal thickness. The entire idea seems so illogical. However, if we were letting logic alone guide us, we would *know* that RK cannot work—but of course it does; so much for logic. At any rate, most surgeons therefore will not overset the blade in their first few patients, thus obtaining less than ideal results. Some few of these will blame the procedure rather than their own timidity. Once they start oversetting the blade, however, their results start getting up to speed. It is also true, though, that some eyes will not react to the surgery as predicted—a case requiring single-depth incisions will turn out to need increased depth in the periphery. The eye will always be right, however, so take some comfort from that.

If the incisions are of an adequate depth throughout, they can still be recut to lengthen them. In this case, fixation behind the blade is essential because absolute control of the endpoint is a must. In the preceding example, the incisions are merely being deepened, not lengthened, and the blade will stop almost by itself when the inner extremity of the cut has been reached—especially if the surgeon is using what William Myers, M.D. (Dr. Myers was my former chief resident and was the second U.S. surgeon to learn RK, he assisted at most of the earlier surgeries and was the first to suggest that the cornea be kept dry when making incisions) calls the "Bores feather touch tech-

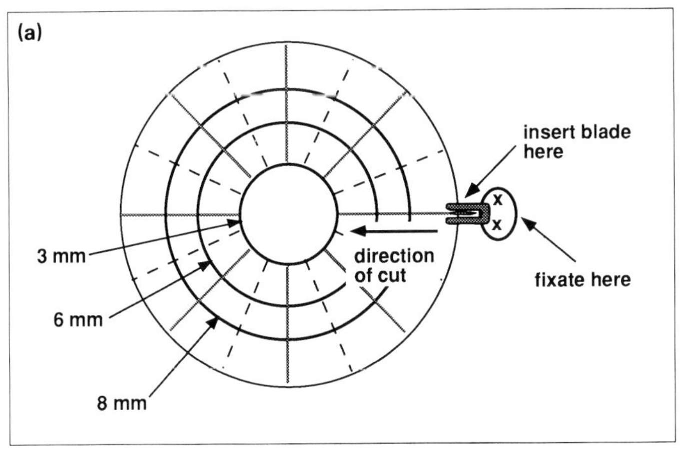

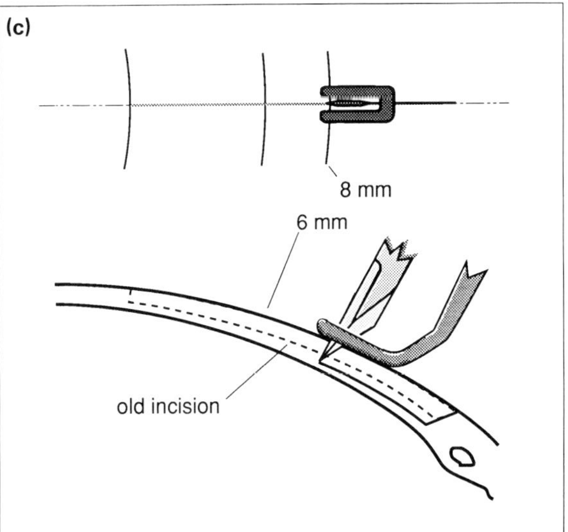

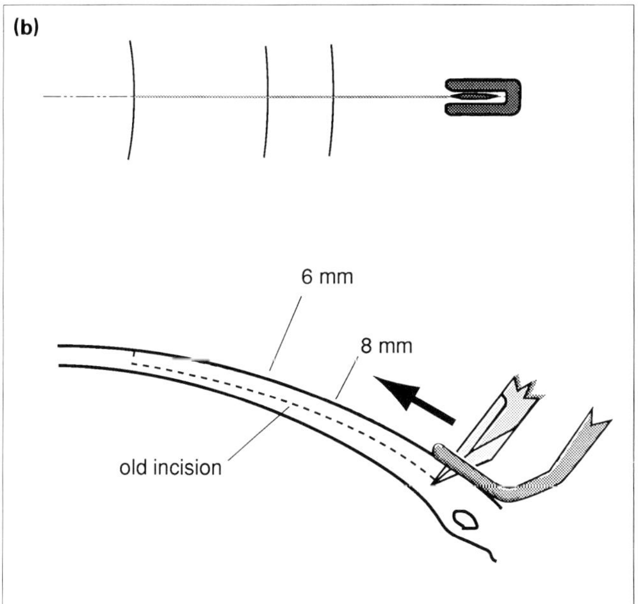

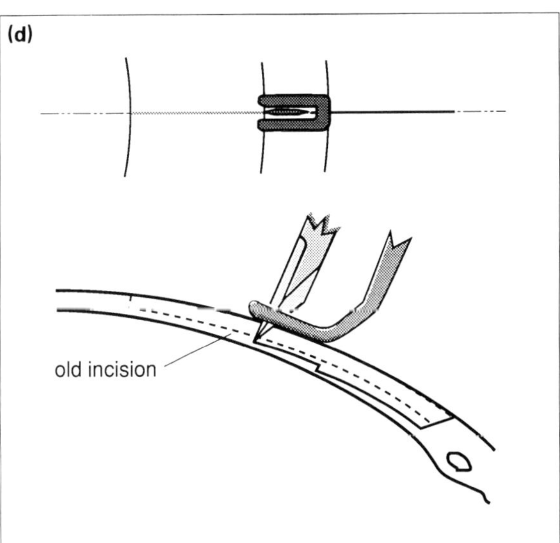

Fig. 8.76 Recutting over old incisions. (a) Straddle the old incision at the limbus. Recut alternate incisions. (b) Cut toward the tertiary optical zone. Reset the blade and (c,d) continue the incision.

nique." In this technique, only sufficient pressure is exerted against the cornea to maintain contact between the knife handle footplate and the corneal surface. This method minimizes corneal distortion, rippling, and blade wandering—our object being to incise the cornea, not bludgeon it.

All the preceding suggestions should be carried out within the first 30 days after the initial surgery or after waiting for at least 6 months. Doing additional surgery in the intervening period can result in no further effect at the very least and complete loss of effect at the most. I am not quite sure why this should be so, but both Fyodorov and I have experienced just this in some of our earlier cases. If the surgery is not redone within 30 days, the keratotomist is admonished not to do any additional surgery until at least 6 months have elapsed. There are three good reasons for this. The first is that whatever seems to be affecting the cornea after 30 days has lost that influence by 6 months. Second, and more important, some corneas will seem to lose ground between 5 to 6 months, only to gain back the effect lost. Some eyes have had additional surgery done prematurely in ignorance of this phenomenon—to the everlasting sorrow of both surgeon and patient; to act in haste is often to repent in leisure. Third, the cornea will be much more stable at this time, and the incision scars will be firmer.

Assuming that the initial incisions were of adequate depth and length and their number does not exceed eight, the only alternative left is to add more incisions. There are no hard and fast rules that apply in such a situation, but there are some guidelines that can be of help. Typically, although the additional incisions will not gain the patient as much as if all the incisions had been done together, the difference will only be 20%—if the new incisions are made in the same manner as the old. Depending on the amount of undercorrection, it may be possible to make the new cuts longer or deeper than the old. Avoid doing both in a patient over 40 years of age if the residual is less than 25% of the original myopia, though. In this case it would be best to "sneak up" on the myopia and do it in stages. This is the only situation in which I would recommend staging.

Calculate the surgical parameters using the new myopia but the old K-readings. Post-RK keratometry is notoriously inaccurate. The pachymetry must be repeated as in recutting incisions except that the central reading will reflect the additional corneal thickness. It is advisable to do a partial mapping of the corneal thickness at each of the main zones between the old incisions. The surgery can then be done as if the cornea had not been incised previously.

Postoperative management

Irrigation of the incisions with a gentle stream of BSS follows completion of the surgery (Figure 8.77). Look at each incision in turn. Some will be filled with red blood cells, whereas others will appear to be clean. These latter may be leaking and are clean looking because the flow of aqueous has washed them out. In these incisions or in those in which a microperforation is known to exist, irrigation should be very gentle indeed. It is not a good idea to either extend the perforation or cause fluid to be forced into the eye by too-vigorous irrigation.

In all cases, antibiotic drops are instilled into the cul-de-sac, followed by a cycloplegic/mydriatic such as 1% cyclopentolate or 5% homatropine. If a perforation has occurred near the limbus and blood has entered the AC, or if you have any doubts, a subconjunctival injection of 20 mg Garamycin is warranted. Usually a light patch is all that is necessary (Figure 8.78). In cases of a perforation or flat chamber, however, a pressure dressing may be warranted as well. In these cases, 1% atropine drops are advised instead of the milder cycloplegics. The patient, in such a case, is told to leave the dressing in place until morning rather than removing it in 2 hours, as is usual. If there has been a perforation, or if one is suspected, begin the patient on a regimen of Keflex (cephalosporin or some other broad-spectrum antibiotic) 500 mg b.i.d. for at least 5 days. Patients who are allergic to penicillin can be prescribed tetracycline or another antibiotic of choice.

Light analgesia, such as aspirin with codeine, should be enough to help the patients with any postoperative discomfort they may have. It has been my experience that in at least 50% of the patients who complain of postoperative pain, the pain subsides when the patch is removed. Patients with flat chambers or very soft eyes, on the other hand, will be found to be more comfortable with the patch. In such instances, it may be well to send the patient to bed with some extra diazepam (Valium). Generally speaking, all patients will benefit from 3 to 4 hours of sleep immediately following the surgery.

All patients should be examined the next day. Putting a drop of proparacaine (Ophthaine, Alcaine, etc.) in the

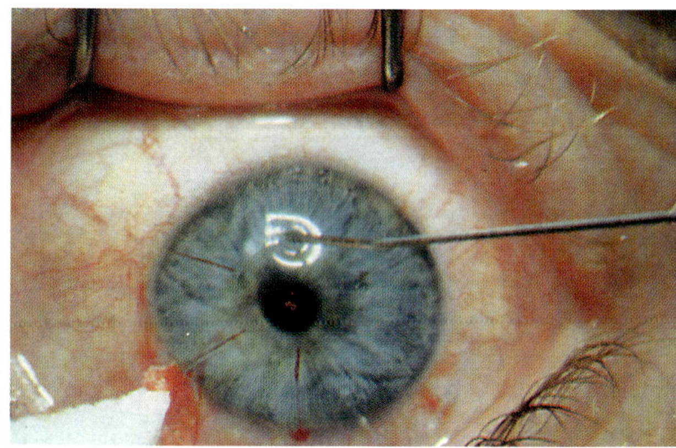

Fig. 8.77 Gently irrigate with balanced salt solution all but the incisions which have a microperforation.

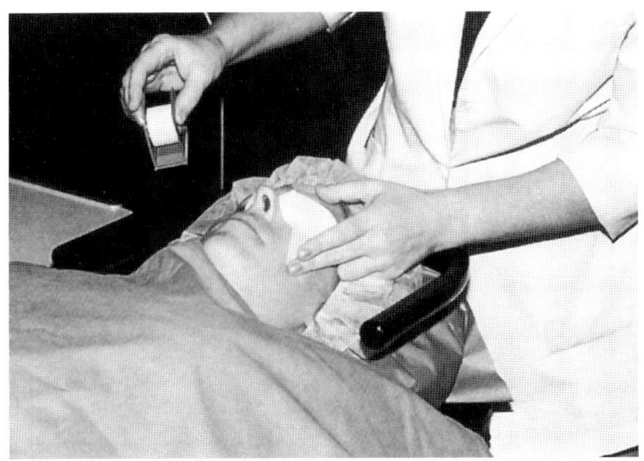

Fig. 8.78 Patch the eye for no more than 2 hours (see text).

operated eye will facilitate this examination. The visual acuity can be taken at this visit, but the result is not meaningful, except that I tend to be somewhat disappointed if the patient sees better than 20/25. This usually, but not always, is an indication that a full correction has not been obtained. The rule of thumb is: *Morning vision blurry—good news; morning vision good—bad news*. The refraction on the day following is usually spurious, ranging from highly myopic to highly hyperopic. The K-readings are a jumble as well. The patient should be encouraged, advised, and begun on an antibiotic-steroid combination (my preference is Tobradex) eye drop to be used twice daily for 2 weeks. I have used this combination (or a similar one) in all my RK patients. I have found that the addition of the steroid not only promotes patient comfort but also enhances the effect as well—even in steroid nonresponders. The only time that I have stopped this drop prematurely has been in those evidencing an allergic response and in one or two cases showing extreme overcorrection at 1 week. In no case is use beyond 14 days warranted or desired. There is some circumstantial evidence that use at 6 to 8 weeks might cause a loss of effect.

In this vein, a word of caution: Some "experts," noting that the effect of the surgery is enhanced with an increase in intraocular pressure, have advocated and have used high steroid drop dosages for upwards of a year in cases of undercorrection. In so doing they have induced glaucoma and, in some cases, cataract to increase the effect of their inadequate surgical technique. I find no medical, moral, or ethical reason to subject a patient to such increased risk of harm to gain a diopter or so of additional myopic correction. I have treated some of these unfortunates, first discontinuing the offending medication. Fortunately, in all but one case, the increased effect disappeared over time, and in the remaining case, best vision continues at a line less than preoperatively, probably due to the residual cataract, despite the almost full myopic correction.

As I have said before, there are limitations to the correction that can be obtained by making relaxing incisions in the cornea. Some eyes respond in much lesser degree regardless of our skill and efforts—so be it. The difference between a good surgeon and a mediocre one is that the good surgeon not only knows when not to cut but also when to "throw in the sponge" and accept reality and quit. The practice of refractive surgery is not an Olympic struggle wherein points are awarded for the greatest amount of diopters corrected. It is, rather, a humanistic science wherein the welfare of the patient is still paramount and the patient's ultimate well-being guides our behavior.

The second eye usually can undergo surgery at 1 week. This time should be sufficient to ascertain where the patient's cornea is going to be at 1 year. At first, it may be better to let 30 days elapse until you are more comfortable with this surgery—this is for you to decide—many of us did just that in the beginning. Except in experienced hands, it is not a good idea to do the surgery before 7 days. Likewise, I find no justification for performing the surgery on both eyes on the same day. Not only is the risk of infection not justified, but even in the best of hands, mistakes in judgment and execution can occur. Furthermore, the patient can well tolerate the delay between eyes and the temporary anisometropia that results. In the event that the patient experiences intolerable glare, he or she can still function with one eye until it subsides. Additionally, how could you explain bilateral overcorrections when it could have been avoided by delaying surgery on the fellow eye? And the presbyopic patient may decide that he or she likes monovision after all.

Further follow-up visits should be scheduled at 1, 6, and 12 months with complete evaluations—vision, K's, topography, glare testing, refraction, and symptoms recorded. Spectacles, if needed, usually can be prescribed at 1 month, but contacts, particularly soft, should wait 8 weeks or more.

Results

Like a good recipe, any good surgical procedure is subject to change. A pinch of this is added to a dollop of that—stirring, testing—making it better and better. This is what makes a surgical procedure so difficult to "study" in the classic sense—it is always on the move—like a positron. The *uncertainty principle* enters into this type of examination, as in the study of subatomic physics. If we stop the evolution of the surgery to examine it in a so-called controlled study, we end up by becoming paleoophthalmologists studying "ancient" eye surgery. If we try to study it "on the fly," we cannot apply the scientific method because each patient is slightly different. Therefore we can only get a "feel" of it—some uncertainty remains. If some of the investigators insist on an attempt to study the surgery by adopting strict guidelines and the remainder continue to alter and improve the technique, then the first investigative group is faced with a dilemma: Can they morally deny the latest treatment to their patients on the grounds that the study must be kept pure?

There is no absolute answer that is fitting because there are no absolutes in biologic processes—there are only approximations. The "science" of biostatistics is really a stochastic art form full of assumptions and "definite maybes." As the amount of data increases, an "idea" of the behavior of a biologic system can be obtained, and from this idea, certain guidelines can be constructed to assist individuals working with that system.

Therefore, I cannot give you any "truths." What I can do is present you with some data that have been gathered in what I believe to be an accurate and trustworthy way and let you decide for yourselves. In this manner I hope not to convince you that I am right, because I have long since stopped worrying about my data convincing anyone. Data are never convincing—only experience or, in its absence, prejudice will result in a judgment being made. But I do hope to give you pause, to open your eyes just a little wider, to open your mind wider still, and to make your experience a little broader.

Results of surgery using current methodologies versus older techniques have been summarized in Tables 8.4 through 8.7. Instead of subjecting you to all the whys and wherefores (you are referred to the literature for that [2,4,22]), I will just touch on some salient points and use the rest of the space to discuss some areas of "difference" and conjecture on the future.

Group I consists of patients whose eyes were among the first to have had the surgery performed outside the Soviet Union. These and the patients in group II had their surgeries done in the same way and with the same blades, except that those in group II had the blades set using the Bores method and some had peripheral incision deepening. All patients in these groups had 16 incisions. The patients in group III had surgery using "Sputnik" razor blades set at maximum using ultrasonic pachymetry and the dry technique. Approximately 20% of the patients in this group had 8 incisions only. Patients who had reoperations are not included in this series. All patients with myopia greater than 8 D had stepped incisions. Your attention is called to Table 8.8, which shows the resulting visual acuities in these groups. The results in group III are remarkably similar to the long-term Russian results and those of Nirankari [23–25].

Table 8.4 Myopia range in the first three RK groups

Preoperative myopia (D)	Group 1	Group 2	Group 3
2.00–4.00	58	136	68
4.25–6.00	18	91	47
6.25–10.00	21	76	35
	97	303	150

Table 8.5 Resultant visual acuity (VA) in cases of low (–2 to –4 D) myopia in three groups (262 patients)

Uncorrected postoperative VA	Group 1	Group 2	Group 3
20/20–20/25	41 (70)	118 (87)	83 (93)
20/30–20/40	14 (25)	14 (10)	2 (3)
20/50–20/70	3 (3)	4 (3)	3 (4)
<20/70	1 (1)	—	—
Mean uncorrected VA	0.80	0.88	0.90

Percentages in parentheses throughout tables 8.5–8.22.

Table 8.6 Resultant visual acuity (VA) in cases of moderate (–4 to –6 D) myopia in three groups (156 patients)

Uncorrected postoperative VA	Group 1	Group 2	Group 3
20/20–20/25	7 (40)	58 (64)	33 (71)
20/30–20/40	2 (11)	15 (16)	7 (14)
20/50–20/70	4 (22)	2 (2)	5 (11)
<20/70	5 (27)	16 (18)	2 (4)
Mean uncorrected VA	0.40	0.50	0.55

Table 8.7 Resultant visual acuity (VA) in cases of high (–6 to –10 D) myopia in three groups (132 patients)

Uncorrected postoperative VA	Group 1	Group 2	Group 3
20/20–20/25	2 (10)	14 (18)	8 (25)
20/30–20/40	4 (18)	15 (20)	12 (33)
20/50–20/70	3 (13)	30 (39)	11 (32)
<20/70	12 (57)	17 (22)	4 (11)
Mean uncorrected VA	0.29	0.40	0.50

Endothelial cell counts show very little change. Cell "losses" are well within the error of counting (see Table 8.8). Areas near microperforations are remarkably free of either cell loss or cellular distortion. I have not seen the cellular changes in humans that were reported by Yamaguchi and colleagues in animals [26–29].

Tables 8.9 through 8.17 show the results in a later and larger series of patients undergoing RK. In all cases, the blades were Sputnik razor fragments overset approximately 15% based on ultrasonic pachymetry.

The last series shown (Tables 8.18 to 8.23) are all cases operated on using XTAL sapphire blades overset up to 15% using a shadowgraph and ultrasonic pachymetry.

Complications of a serious or threatening nature have been rare with this surgery to date. Most can be traced to "pilot error" and/or inexperience and are not inherent to the procedure itself (see also Chapter 15). Considering that over 1 million surgeries have been performed here and abroad (at this writing), the incidence of serious trouble is very low indeed.

Table 8.8 Summary of surgical results and overall vision in all three early groups

	Group 1	Group 2	Group 3
Mean K change			
3 months	3.09 D	4.79 D	6.32 D
12 months	1.74 D	4.23 D	5.44 D
ΔK/ΔR	1.21 D	1.18 D	1.23 D
Residual refraction	3.12 D	1.18 D	0.88 D
Emmetropic eyes (± 0.50 D)	24 (25)	179 (59)	96(64)
Hyperopic eyes	3 (3)	0	1 (<1)
Myopic eyes	70 (72)	124 (41)	47 (31)
Uncorrected postoperative VA			
20/20–20/25	50 (40)	137 (45)	80 (53)
20/30–20/40	20 (21)	61 (20)	35 (23)
20/50–20/70	10 (10)	64 (21)	23 (15)
<20/70	17 (18)	41 (14)	12 (8)
Mean uncorrected VA	0.29	0.50	0.58

VA, Visual acuity.

Table 8.9 Post-operative sequelae

	Group 1	Group 2	Group 3
Subconjunctival hemorrhage	39 (41.2)	22 (7)	2 (3)
Upper lid edema	16 (16.4)	48 (15.8)	24 (16)
Epithelial defect	11 (11.3)	18 (5.9)	5 (3)
Stromal edema			
14 days	90 (92.8)	91 (30)	35 (23)
14–30 days	29 (28.9)	26 (8.8)	8 (5)
Over 30 days	0	0	0
Cells/flare			
Trace	5 (5.4)	15(4.9)	7 (5)
Significant	0	0	0
Photophobia			
14 days	14 (14.4)	297 (98)	138 (92)
14–21 days	4 (4.2)	15 (5.2)	6 (4)
Keratitis (mild)	1 (1)	6 (1.9)	3 (2)
Fibrous proliferation	1 (1)	0	0
Night glare			
<3 months	87 (89.7)	273 (90.3)	136(91)
>3 months	3 (4)	12 (4)	3 (2)
Visual fluctuation			
<3 months	90 (92.8)	271 (89.4)	141(94)
>3 months	6 (1.9)	30 (10)	18 (12)
Induced astigmatism >6 months	3 (3.2)	2 (0.6)	2(1)
Neovascularization	<4%	<6.3%	<3.1%
Endothelial cell count	14 (14.4)	297 (98)	138 (92)

Table 8.10 Patient age distribution in the second RK series

Age range (years)	*n*
18–23	215
24–40	969
41–65	259
66 and older	5

Table 8.11 Range of myopia in the second RK series

Range of myopia (D)	*n*
2–4	676
4–6	438
6–8	235
8–10	99
Total cases reviewed	1448

Table 8.12 Resultant visual acuity (VA) in cases of low (–2 to –4 D) myopia in the second series

Uncorrected postoperative VA	*n*
20/20–20/25	636 (94)
20/30–20/40	20 (3)
20/50–20/70	20 (3)
<20/70	
Mean uncorrected VA	0.90

Table 8.13 Resultant visual acuity (VA) in cases of moderate (–4 to –6 D) myopia in the second series

Uncorrected postoperative VA	*n*
20/20–20/25	324 (74)
20/30–20/40	70 (16)
20/50–20/70	26 (6)
<20/70	18 (4)
Mean uncorrected VA	0.62

Table 8.14. Resultant visual acuity (VA) in cases of high (–6 to –8 D) myopia in the second series

Uncorrected postoperative VA	*n*
20/20–20/25	63 (27)
20/30–20/40	82 (35)
20/50–20/70	78 (33)
<20/70	12 (5)
Mean uncorrected VA	0.58

Table 8.15 Resultant visual acuity (VA) in cases of very high (–8 to –10 D) myopia in the second series

Uncorrected postoperative VA	*n*
20/20–20/25	21 (21)
20/30–20/40	28 (28)
20/50–20/70	37 (37)
<20/70	13 (14)
Mean uncorrected VA	0.40

Table 8.16 Summary of surgical results in the second series

Parameter	Result
Regression of K	–17%
Mean ΔK	–6.21 D
Residual refraction	–0.75 D
Emmetropic eyes (±0.50 D)	1043 (72)
Hyperopic eyes	43 (3)
Myopic eyes	362 (25)

Table 8.17 Postoperative sequelae in the second series

	n
Epithelial defect	27 (1.9)
Stromal edema	
14 days	326 (22.5)
14–30 days	66 (4.6)
>30 days	1 (0.07)
Cells/flare	
Trace	7 (0.49)
Significant	1 (0.07)
Photophobia	
14 days	1303 (90)
14–21 days	43 (3)
Keratitis	3 (0.02)
Night glare	
<3 months	1303 (90)
>3 months	43 (3)
Visual fluctuation	
<3 months	1390 (90)
>3 months	540 (37.2)
Induced astigmatism	10 (0.69)
Neovascularization	6 (0.41)
Endothelial cell loss	(4.2)

Table 8.18 Patient age distribution in the third RK series

Age range (years)	*n*
18–23	111
24–40	396
41–65	120
66 and older	5
Total	632

Table 8.19 Resultant visual acuity (VA) in cases of low (–2 to –4 D) myopia in the third series

Uncorrected postoperative VA	*n*
20/20–20/25	232 (88)
20/30–20/40	16 (6)
20/50–20/70	16 (6)
<20/70	
Total cases	264

Table 8.20 Resultant visual acuity (VA) in cases of moderate (–4 to –6 D) myopia in the third series

Uncorrected postoperative VA	*n*
20/20–20/25	160 (79)
20/30–20/40	16 (8)
20/50–20/70	12 (6)
<20/70	10 (1)
Total cases	203

Table 8.21 Resultant visual acuity (VA) in cases of high (–6 to –8 D) myopia in the third series

Uncorrected postoperative VA	*n*
20/20–20/25	49 (33)
20/30–20/40	51 (34)
20/50–20/70	42 (28)
<20/70	8 (5)
Total cases	150

Table 8.22 Resultant visual acuity (VA) in cases of very high (–8 to –10 D) myopia in the third series

Uncorrected postoperative VA	*n*
20/20–20/25	4 (25)
20/30–20/40	4 (25)
20/50–20/70	5 (36)
<20/70	1 (14)
Total cases	15

Table 8.23 Postoperative sequelae in the third series

	n
Epithelial defects	13
Stromal edema	
14 days	142
14–30 days	17
Over 30 days	0
Cells/flare	
Trace	4
Significant	0
Photophobia	
14 days	554
14–21 days	3
Keratitis	1
Night glare	
<3 months	620
>3 months	332
Visual fluctuation	628
Neovascularization	0

The future of RK

The future for RK surgery still looks very bright to me. Despite the current popularity of the LASIK, RK remains the only titratable method of dealing with astigmatism (see also Chapter 9). We have advanced "light years" in the short time since this surgery was first introduced. Work is going forward with sophisticated instrumentation that will provide us with simultaneous surface corneal maps and thickness measurements (see Chapter 6). This will enable us, for the first time, to obtain the inside corneal curvature. There are prototypes for knives that automatically adjust themselves to the corneal thickness—which is being monitored continuously by ultrasound. New materials are being studied for knife blades that have extreme edge sharpness that will change not only this surgery but others as well. We have finally seen the day RK was pronounced "fit" and respectable for general use by whomever it is that pronounces these kinds of things. (This was realized in part in May 1989 when the American Academy of Ophthalmology issued a statement declaring RK to be a viable form of surgery.) RK has opened the door to visual freedom for countless thousands who have been forced to live behind barriers all these years.

All in all, I believe that the controversy about this procedure has been good—good for this surgery and good for ophthalmology itself. The resulting mental stimulation and the instrument spinoffs cannot but help to improve the quality of medicine being practiced today—it already has. And this is not a bad legacy for any "heretic" to leave by any standard of measurement.

References

1 Fyodorov SN, and Durnev VV. Operation of dosaged dissection of corneal circular ligament in cases of myopia of mild degree. Ann Ophthalmol 1979; 11(12): p. 1885–90.

2 Bores LD. Results of radial keratotomy after two years. In: *Keratorefractive Society*. LAL Publishing, Chicago, 1981.

3 Cowden JW, and Bores LD. A clinical investigation of the surgical correction of myopia by the method of Fyodorov. Ophthalmology 1981; 88(8): p. 737–41.

4 Bores LD. Radial Keratotomy—Clinical Results. In: *Refractive Keratoplasty*, R Schacher and L Schacher, Editors. JAL Publishing, Denison, 1983.

5 Bores LD. Historical review and clinical results of radial keratotomy. Int Ophthalmol Clin 1983; 23(3): p. 93–118.

6 Deitz MR, Sanders DR, and Marks RG. Radial keratotomy: an overview of the Kansas City study. Ophthalmology 1984; 91(5): p. 467–78.

7 Linberg JV, McDonald MB, Safir A, *et al*. Ptosis following radial keratotomy. Performed using a rigid eyelid speculum. Ophthalmology 1986; 93(12): p. 1509–12.

8 Fyodorov SN, and Agronovsky A. Long term results of anterior radial keratotomy. J Ocul Ther Surg 1982; 1: p. 217.

9 Lynn MJ, Waring G.O.d., and Sperduto RD. Factors affecting outcome and predictability of radial keratotomy in the PERK Study. Arch Ophthalmol 1987; 105(1): p. 42–51.

10 Grimmett MR, and Holland EJ. Small clear-zone radial keratotomy [letter]. Ophthalmology 1999; 106(10): p. 1857–8.

11 Nordan LT, and Maxwell WA. Avoid both radial keratotomy with small optical zones and hexagonal keratotomy [letter]. Refract Corneal Surg 1992; 8(4): p. 331.

12 Nordan LT, and Maxwell WA. Refractive surgery and informed consent. Radial keratotomy with small optical zone hexagonal keratotomy [letter]. J Cataract Refract Surg 1992; 18(4): p. 420–1.

13 Grimmett MR, and Ogawa GS. Radial keratotomy clear zone diameter errors. J Refract Surg 1998; 14(6): p. 623–30.

14 Wachler BS, Durrie DS, Assil KK, *et al*. Role of clearance and treatment zones in contrast sensitivity: significance in refractive surgery. J Cataract Refract Surg 1999; 25(1): p. 16–23.

15 Durnev VV, and Ermoshin AS. Determination of dependence between the length of anterior radial non–perforating incisions of the cornea and their effectiveness. In: *IV All Union Conference of Inventors and Rationalizers in the Field of Ophthalmology*. Minister of Health, U.S.S.R, Moscow, 1976.

16 Hernandez-Meijide R, and Croxatto JO. Experimental radial keratotomy. Journal of Refractive Surgery 1988; 3: p. 224–6.

17 Deitz M, and Sanders D. Progressive hyperopia with long-term follow-up of radial keratotomy. Arch Ophthalmol 1985; 103 (6): p. 782–4.

18 Durnev V. Characteristic of the results of myopic surgical correction after performing 16 and 32 primary anterior radial non–perforating incisions. In: *Surgery of Refractive Anomalies of the Eye*, A Ivashina and S Kolmanovskii, Editors. Moscow Scientific Research Institute for Eye Microsurgery, Moscow, p. 148, 1981.

19 Sanders DR, and Marks RG. Prospective clinical study of radial keratotomy [letter]. Ophthalmology 1982; 89(11): p. 1292–3.

20 Hoffer KJ, Darin JJ, Pettit TH, *et al*. UCLA clinical trial of radial keratotomy. Preliminary report. Ophthalmology 1981; 88(8): p. 729–36.

21 Smith RS, and Cutro J. Computer analysis of radial keratotomy. CLAO J 1984; 10 (3): p. 241–8.

22 Bores LD. Radial keratotomy. In: *The 2nd International Cataract, Implant, Microsurgical & Refractive Keratoplasty Meeting*. Japan Intraocular Lens Society, Nagoya, 1988.

23 Nirankari VS, Katzen LE, Richards RD, *et al*. Prospective clinical study of radial keratotomy. Ophthalmology 1982; 89(6): p. 677–83.

24 Nirankari VS, Katzen LE, Karesh JW, *et al*. Ongoing prospective clinical study of radial keratotomy. Ophthalmology 1983; 90(6): p. 637–41.

25 Nirankari VS, Katzen LE, Karesh JW, *et al*. Ongoing prospective clinical study of radial keratotomy. Indian J Ophthalmol 1983; 31(Suppl): p. 860–5.

26 Yamaguchi T, Asbell P, Ostrick M, *et al*. Endothelial damage in monkeys after radial keratotomy performed with a diamond blade. Arch Ophthalmol 1984; 102(5): p. 765–9.

27 Yamaguchi T, Asbell PA, Ostrick M, *et al*. Endothelial damage in monkeys after radial keratotomy performed with a diamond blade. Arch Ophthalmol 1984; 102(5): p. 765–9.

28 Yamaguchi T, Asbell PA, Ostrick M, *et al*. Corticosteroid therapy after anterior radial keratotomy in Primates. Am J Ophthalmol 1984; 97(2): p. 215–20.

29 Yamaguchi T, Tamaki K, Kaufman HE, *et al*. Histologic study of a pair of human corneas after anterior radial keratotomy. Am J Ophthalmol 1985; 100(2): p. 281–92.

9

Surgical Management of Astigmatism

The scientific reasons for preferring one testimonial to another are, no doubt, sometimes very strong. They are not, however, strong enough to prevail upon our passions, our prejudices or our interests, or to overcome that lightness which is common to all grave men. So that we always present facts in a manner that is either prejudiced or frivolous. [Anatole France, Penguin Island]

The correction of astigmatism has been a hoary problem down through the years, even when physicians knew nothing at all about its existence. The situation has not changed to any great degree other than to say that these days astigmatism is at least recognized, if not completely understood. This is evidenced particularly in those surgeons taking courses to perform laser in situ keratomileusis (LASIK) lately. Most of have had no experience with refractive surgery, and many have not considered astigmatism beyond their phoropters. Even surgeons familiar with incisional techniques for treating astigmatism run afoul of the positive-cylinder booby trap, about which the author will have more to say later in this chapter.

The history of astigmatic treatment

Thomas Young was probably the first person to describe the defect known as astigmatism (in his own eyes) in 1801, whereas the first astigmatic spectacles were made to order for the astronomer George Airy in 1825—about the same time an enterprising and observant clergyman named Goodrich had some made for himself in New York (see Chapter 2). Prior to these successes, astigmatism was compensated for by fitting spherical spectacles alone—a compromise at best [1]. The idea of performing surgery to correct this disorder came later.

It is always a good idea to examine the historical record not only to glean whatever pearls we may from the information collected but also to appreciate from afar the audacity of some of our early colleagues. This chapter will have occasion to mark, from time to time, the lessons to be learned from this early work, for all the techniques we currently use are really not new at all but stem from our predecessors' careful observations of specific corneal reactions to injury.

In this chapter the author uses the term *congenital* to describe astigmatism unassociated with disease and/or trauma (iatrogenic or not). The author is not especially enamored of the term and will have no objection if the reader chooses to discard it for his or her own pet term, but it seems to fit the situation reasonably well.

The first surgical attempts (paleoophthalmology)

Most discussions on this topic start out with references to Snellen, Lans, and Bates—giving the reader the pardonable impression that these three gentlemen were in the forefront of the surgical correction of astigmatism. And so they were, but they were not the first to attempt such surgery. Donders described astigmatism following cataract extraction in 1864—thus it seemed natural to ascribe the astigmatism to the corneal incision [1]. The wonder is that no one thought about trying to correct astigmatism surgically before 1869, since the incidence of iatrogenically induced astigmatism would have been high with the large, limbal-based incisions employed at the time.

Snellen's "suggestions"

The author is unable to substantiate that the Dutch ophthalmologist Herman Snellen, of Utrecht, ever performed surgery for astigmatism—although he defined both with- and against-the-rule astigmatism in 1869 (see also Chapter 2). He did, however, suggest that a corneal incision running perpendicular to the steepest meridian would induce an opposite astigmatism that would then neutralize the first; although he made no mention of the effect such an incision might have on the opposite meridian—a process called *coupling* [2]. Thus Snellen has the distinction of describing the principle of what we now call *T-cuts*—besides being the inventor of the Snellen optotypes [3,4].

Xavier Galezowski and half-moon corneal wedge resections

Around the time Fukala performed his first clear lens extraction for myopia in 1890, a chap named Galezowski attempted to flatten the cornea by resecting half-moon-shaped wedges out of the stroma—unsuccessfully—according to Fukala [5] (Figure 9.1). Since this was segmental surgery (with no sutures), the supposition is that this was an attempt at flattening myopic astigmatism through relaxation. If so, then Galezowski performed the first wedge resection for astigmatism; if not, it still predates any other recorded attempts at the surgical correction of myopia.

Schiøtz and limbal transverse perforating incisions

The next (or first?) case report predated that of Lans by some 13 years. In 1885, Hjalmar August Schiøtz, a Norwegian ophthalmologist, reported the case of a 33-year-old man with 19.5 D of postoperative aphakic astigmatism. Four months after the original surgery, Schiøtz made a 3.5-mm limbal penetrating Graefe knife section in the steepest corneal meridian—which gradually reduced the astigmatism to 7 D about 1 month later [6]. Schiøtz is, of course, better known for other contributions. The wonder is that he did not pursue this idea. Perhaps it was a response to a single need. Whatever the reason, Schiøtz has the distinction of being the first to carry out the previous ideas of Snellen.

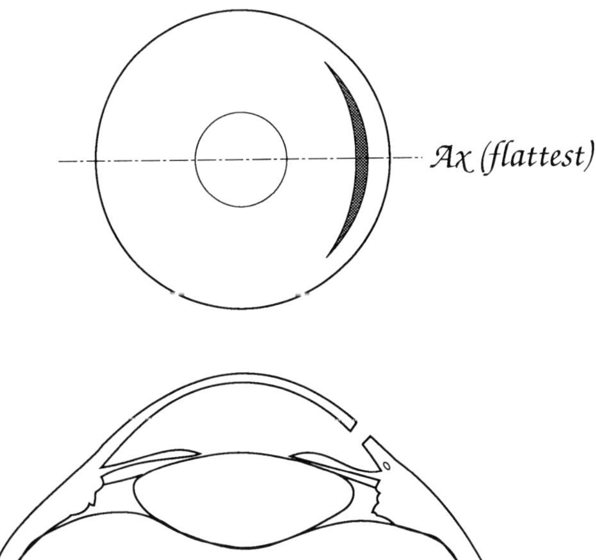

Fig. 9.1 The crescentic corneal resection of von Galezowski.

Bates and his transverse nonperforating incisions

William Horatio Bates was a physician who practiced at the New York Eye Infirmary in the late 19th century—specializing in diseases of the head. For five years (1886–1891) he taught ophthalmology at the New York Post-graduate Medical School and Hospital, leaving after a "personality conflict" with the director [7]. Actually, the dispute centered around Bates' claim that myopia could be "cured" and Roosa's insistence that it could not. In typical head-of-the-department fashion, Roosa resolved the debate by banishing Bates, thereby striking another blow for the status quo.

In 1894, Bates published a suggestion for a surgical procedure to correct astigmatism. In this paper he evaluated, succinctly, five cases of iatrogenic and one case of traumatic astigmatism. He went on to set down some basic principles or propositions of astigmatic surgery that the author has dubbed *Bates' axioms*:

1 A corneal incision lengthens the radius of curvature of that meridian which is at right angles to the line of the incision and does not flatten any other meridian. The astigmatism produced is a regular astigmatism and is corrected by a convex cylinder at an axis parallel to the line of the incision.

2 The immediate result is greater than the ultimate result.

3 The astigmatism produced is permanent after a length of time—at least a month after the cornea has healed.

4 The amount of astigmatism produced is greater near the center of the cornea.

5 The amount of correction can be regulated by the number, depth, and length of the incisions [8].

In this Bates obviously recognized the ability of relaxing incisions to produce flattening of steep curvatures—independently and before Lans. It is not likely that Bates had access to the work of Schiøtz (although it is possible).

Bates then went on to describe two cases in which such incisions actually were made. In the first, a 14-year-old girl with simple astigmatism of 2.5 D with the steep axis at 75°, he marked the 165° axis with adhesive tape and made a Graefe knife incision parallel to the tape. He noted that no aqueous escaped—hence the incision was partial-thickness. Within 5 days the patient's vision had improved, but it was not wholly satisfactory, because Bates repeated the surgery—this time making the nonperforating incision more central on the cornea. He repeated the surgery three more times—once 20 days after the second incision, once 6 weeks later, and the last time 2½ weeks after that. He did not stipulate whether these incisions were recuts or in addition to those made previously. He apparently ceased when he did because no further change by ophthalmometry was noted and the patient saw well enough. Eighteen months after the initial surgery, the patient's vision was said to still be improved, and scars were not discernible to cursory examination.

The next case was that of a 23-year-old physician with a refraction of $-1.25 - 0.75 \times 100°$ in both eyes. The astigmatism could not be measured with the ophthalmometer. Thus Bates operated for systemic or total astigmatism—not for corneal astigmatism—a concept still valid today. Bates made a shallow, transverse incision at 100° on the temporal side of the cornea in the right eye. One day later, the procedure was repeated on the left eye. Six months after that, the patient retained good, unaided visual acuity with minimal scarring. Thus Bates was the first to describe and use T-cuts—as we know them today—as well as perform repeat surgery for undercorrections.

Faber and idiopathic astigmatism

In 1895, another Dutch ophthalmologist named Faber used an anterior penetrating transverse incision in a 19-year-old patient to treat congenital astigmatism. Faber succeeded in reducing the patient's astigmatism from 1.5 to 0.75 D and improving his uncorrected vision sufficiently—from 20/60 to 20/25—to permit the patient to attend a military academy [9]. Today (at least for now), such surgery would result in quite a different outcome—in the United States, refractive surgery makes one ineligible for military service. Faber concluded that such techniques work but that the predictability would be uncertain. An interesting note is that Faber declared this procedure to be new because he had never heard of anyone performing such an operation before.

Lucciola and L-incisions

The first European surgeon to use nonperforating incisions was Lucciola, of Turin, Italy [10]. He reported 10 patients in whom he used nonperforating corneal incisions made parallel to the steeper meridian to correct astigmatism. He detailed the influence of the type and location of the incisions as well, thus establishing himself as the first to use L-cuts (which stands for longitudinal, or parallel, cuts, not Lucciolacuts).

Thus, by 1896, two concepts had been established: (1) that incisions perpendicular to the steep meridian flatten that meridian and (2) that the same thing can be accomplished with incisions parallel to the steep meridian. Additionally, these incisions need not be full-thickness.

Lans and the coupling effect

Although not the first to perform surgery for astigmatism, still another Dutch ophthalmologist, Leendert Jan Lans, was the first to perform systematic studies of refractive surgery at the University of Leiden in 1896 (Figure 9.2). He received his doctor's degree *cum laude* from the University of Leiden in 1897 by defending a thesis entitled "Experimentelle Untersuchungen uber die Entstehung von Astigmatismus durch nicht Perforirende Corneawunden" (Experimental Studies of the Treatment of Astigmatism with Nonperforating Corneal Wounds). This work was done at Snellen's clinic in Utrecht, where Lans had made a training arrangement, although his advisor was Willem Koster, chairman of the Eye Department at Leiden. Using carefully planned experimentation in rabbits, Lans evaluated patterns of keratotomy, keratectomy, and thermokeratoplasty, thereby establishing (along with Bates) the basic principles that would serve as the root of modern astigmatic surgery. He also showed that flattening in the meridian perpendicular to a transverse incision would be associated with steepening in the opposite meridian—the first description of coupling (see the section on Sato, below). Independent of Bates, Lans found that deeper and longer incisions would have a greater effect. In his paper he also admitted that he got the idea from Snellen and cited the work of Pfluger and Doganof using parallel incisions à la Lucciola [11]. However, he was unable to obtain satisfactory results with incisions, so

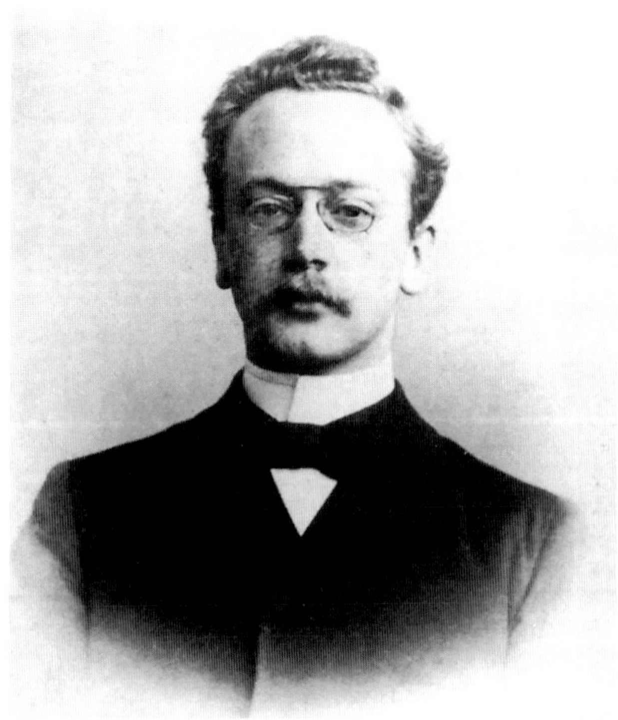

Fig. 9.2 Leendert Jan Lans, the first ophthalmologist to perform systematic studies of refractive surgery in 1896.

he turned instead to cautery. He used a fine tip to make two cauterized bands 2 by 4 to 8 mm across the selected meridian on rabbit corneas. After a 4-month follow-up, he concluded that such application could produce refractive changes of up to 6 D but that these changes were highly labile and reversible within the first 4 to 8 weeks after application. Beyond these few experiments and this paper, there is nothing further from him on the matter. He eventually settled in Arnhem, where he never again returned to the subject of refractive surgery.

Loose gears sink careers

Why is it that this idea of Bates (and later that of Lans) apparently was ignored? Lans was certainly respected. After receiving his doctorate, he went to work with Snellen. No black cloud followed him around. Bates himself appears to have been an above-average physician as well as a competent surgeon; he certainly exhibited all those qualities that Halstead wrote about. In 1886 he published a reasonable paper on the treatment of deafness [12]. Later, he conducted a study in which he demonstrated the value of sutures to close the cataract wound—an important innovation for that time [13]. Bates was a peculiar fellow, nevertheless, and probably was his own worst enemy. By 1891, he had begun his unyielding infatuation with his own ideas—and he wasn't quiet about it. He thus joined that select group of brilliant and meritorious scientists and physicians who have sometimes forsaken the orthodox and familiar scientific method for more esoteric, unorthodox, and often bizarre thinking. In short, they take counsel of their own beliefs to the exclusion of other views. In that, however, they follow in the footsteps of the great Claudius Galenus and are thereby in good, if misguided, company. Bates eventually may have become, in the vernacular, "loony-tunes"—but that looniness was singular, involving mostly the topic of myopia. He did good work in other areas and published creditable papers on other topics; hence he does not deserve to be shunted into the back alley of ophthalmology—his astigmatism axioms are still valid today.

However, surgery for astigmatism was not ignored just in the United States; it seems it was ignored everywhere else as well. With the exception of a few isolated instances, it took 42 more years—more than a generation—before reports of similar cases made their appearance in the medical literature.

Wray's reprisal of Lans' technique

In 1914, Wray used cautery à la Lans to correct a case of 6-D hyperopic astigmatism [14]. The patient was a 19-year-old whose refraction was plano +6.00 × 180° OU. A linear-type cautery was performed twice in the right eye on the hyperopic meridian inferior to the corneal apex. This was not successful, succeeding only in causing the

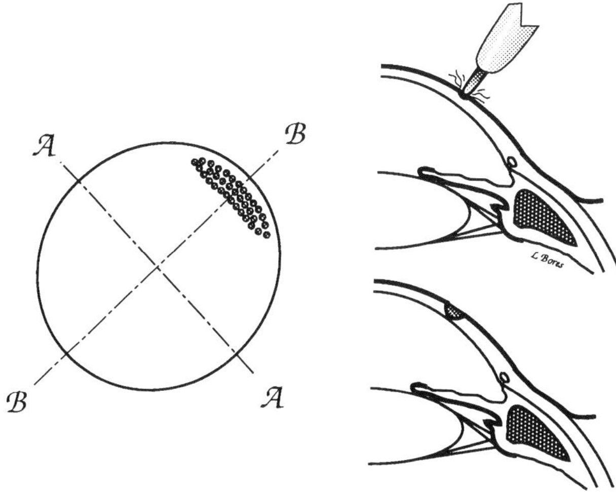

Fig. 9.3 Wray's cautery for hyperopic astigmatism.

astigmatism to rotate 30°. Somewhat better results were obtained in the left eye with four applications of what Wray called "superficial burns" (probably nonlinear) and sufficiently peripheral so as "not to interfere with reading" (Figure 9.3). The refraction improved to +0.50 + 1.00 × 180° at 1 year with a BCVA of 6/6. Wray blamed the poor result on the right to involvement of Descemet's membrane, but it is more likely that the result was due to the scars being too superficial.

Meier and the case of the peeled cornea

In 1917, Weiner reported a method of corneal peeling for keratoconus that he attributed to Meier. It consisted of resecting a two-thirds-thickness elliptical strip approximately 4 × 12 mm from the cornea [15]. Burr took this idea somewhat further by removing a full-thickness section of cornea [16]. Weiner later modified this by making a 6- to 7-mm incision about 1 mm from the limbus. A section of cornea, 1.5 mm wide at center and tapering toward each end, was removed. The wound was then sutured closed [17].

O'Connor, Bock, and corneal cautery

O'Connor was not as sanguine as Herr Doctor Lans in the use of cautery for cases of high astigmatism—only half his patients showed any improvement, and those were unstable. Patients with keratoconus fared somewhat better [18,19]. One year later (1938), Bock published his work with high-frequency cautery on the rabbit cornea (see also Chapter 14). Within a few weeks, however, the corneas had regained their preoperative curvatures [20].

Hence, by 1933, it was established that cautery does not work very well for astigmatic corrections, aside from its unpredictability. This fact did not prevent other surgeons from trying it anyway later on (see Chapter 14).

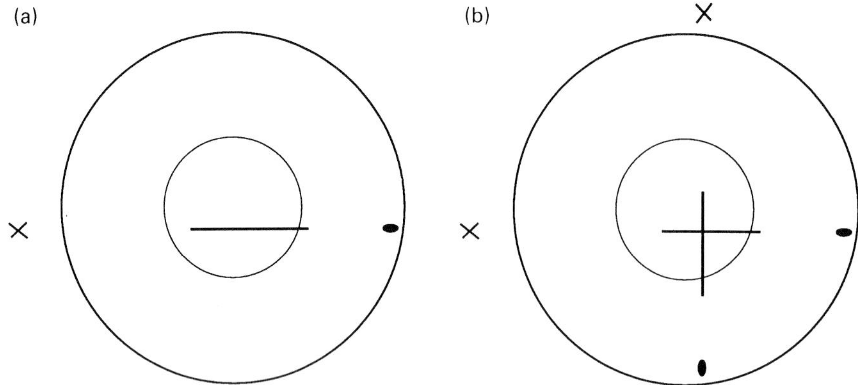

Fig. 9.4 Sato's operations for keratoconus—original pattern.

Sato and his posterior half-incisions for astigmatism

Tutomu Sato began his work with keratoconus using posterior incisions (see Chapter 7 for more details). While studying the subject of keratoconus under the guidance of Ishihara in 1936, Sato noted a marked improvement in the vision of a 20-year-old girl following spontaneous rupture of Descemet's membrane. He felt that he could do better with a knife and proceeded to demonstrate it. He reported his first 10 patients in 1939 in the Japanese literature [21]. His technique consisted in making one and sometimes two or three horizontal incisions across the corneal paracenter on the posterior corneal surface using a modification of de Lapersonne's knife—now called *Sato's knife*—introduced through the lateral limbus (Figure 9.4). While making internal incisions was original, he probably was aware of Lans work. At that time, much of the Japanese casework was being published in the German literature—Japanese surgeons studied in Germany as well. Fukala's first case reports give an address for him in Pilsen-Karlsbad. Hence Sato probably also was aware of Kokott's 1938 work on elucidating the anatomic structure of the cornea [22]. This last point is important because it may have influenced Sato's decision to use posterior incisions in the first place.

Sato's operation for keratoconus was straightforward, effective, and considering the alternative, appropriate. It became widely used in Japan [23]. Hruby and Linder also reported good results [24,25]. Gilbert introduced it in France under the name *debridement de la Descemet's* [26]. Gilbert used a Graefe knife to make the incisions, whereas Linder modified Sato's knife and also sharpened the tip of a Bowman canaliculotome—which he claimed was a safer instrument. Nevertheless, the operation was technically difficult to perform. It required great skill on the part of the surgeon, necessitating incisions being made *ab interno* through half the corneal thickness and in a straight line—close to the optical center. Nevertheless, between 1939 and 1943, Sato performed 200 such operations—successfully [27,28].

The pupil was constricted with a miotic solution presurgery. Topical application of cocaine was used at first for anesthesia. Later, retrobulbar injection of anesthetic was employed to immobilize the eye. Bridle sutures were placed around the tendons of both vertical recti so as to be able to rotate the globe freely. Straight 3- to 4-mm pieces of sterile gray human hair or catgut (later changed to a mark made with gentian violet) were laid in place on the major and minor meridians—tangential to the pupillary margin.

The specially designed knife was then inserted into the anterior chamber at the limbus through a 2-mm scleral tunnel [29]. Each incision was made from the limbus toward the center, after which the knife was disengaged by turning it to the side so as to prevent damage to the central clear zone and the underlying lens. These incisions were then followed by the same number of incisions made on the opposite side in the same manner. These internal incisions almost always were followed by external incisions made between the internals with a guarded blade.

Sato devised a crosswise technique for very advanced keratoconus that he reported in 1942 [30]. This technique was later modified and applied to the correction of congenital astigmatism using a standard incision length of 4 mm. Sato reported that in the rabbit eye, anterior incisions produced minimal central corneal flattening, whereas posterior incisions produced maximum flattening. Hence he was encouraged to use posterior incisions preferentially [31]. In this same paper he first described radial incisions made from the posterior side—a modification or extension of Lans' original idea (see above)—thus this was not the debut of radial incisions, as has been proposed.

Of his early 19 cases of congenital astigmatism, Sato achieved 0.5 to 0.75 D of flattening in 3 eyes, 1.0 D in 7 eyes, 3.0 D in 1 eye, 4.0 D in 4 eyes, 6.0 D in 1 eye, and no correction in 3 eyes [28]. These are respectable numbers to be sure, but if he counted total change (including coupling), these numbers are not quite so impressive and are, in fact, troubling (see below). The phenomenon of coupling cannot be ignored, as we shall see when we discuss tangential incisions further on, and can be disastrous (see the section on the technique of the Ruiz procedure, below).

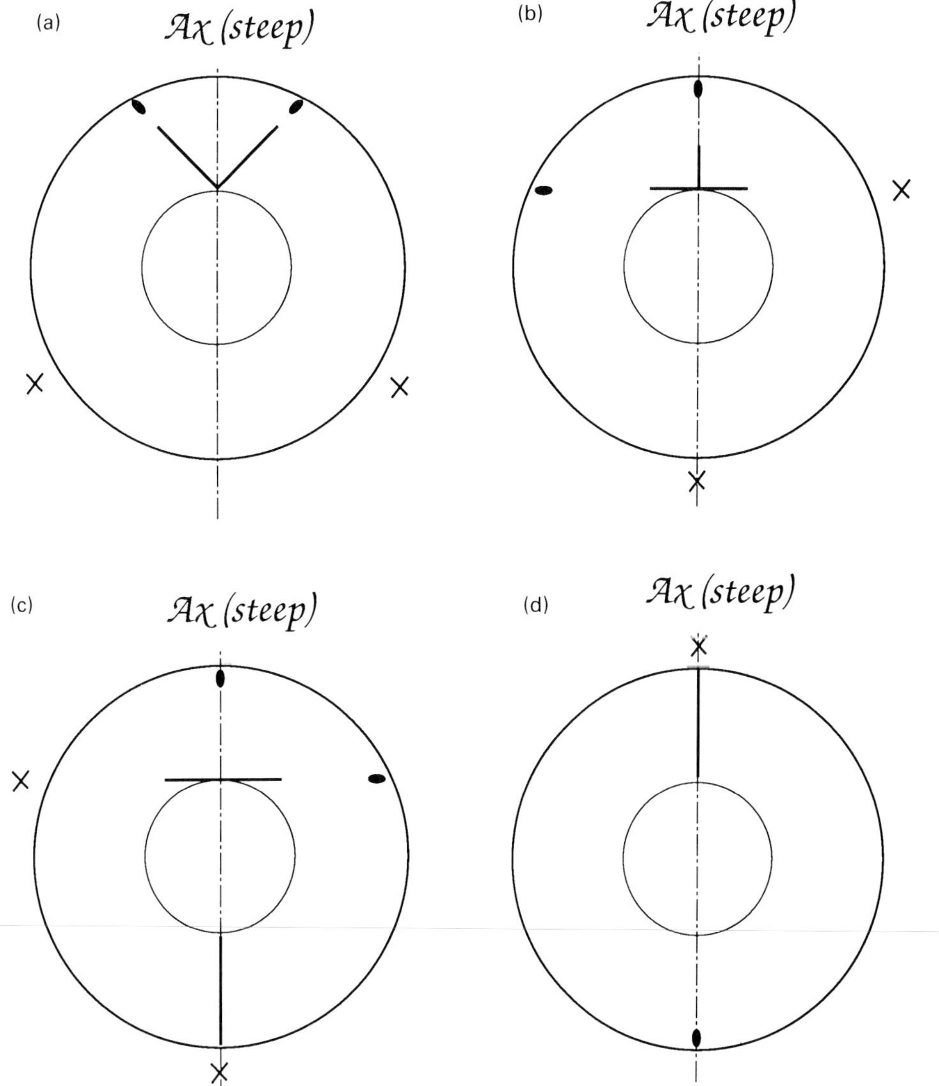

Fig. 9.5 Sato's operations for keratoconus—1950 pattern.

In 1950, Sato reported his technique in the American literature, describing at the time T- and V-incisions for astigmatism. These T-cuts were exactly that—T's (Figure 9.5). Sato declared the T- and V-shaped incisions to be unsatisfactory because of wide edge separation, thick scars, and irregular astigmatism. Later surgeons corroborated this finding (see also the section on current methods for the control of astigmatism, below).

With a radial incision in the rabbit, Sato was able to correct as much as 4 D of astigmatism, but he succeeded in eliminating only half this much in the human. With a transverse incision (T-cut), he demonstrated in the rabbit that while, in one case, he obtained a flattening of 4 D in the meridian crossed by the T-cut, 3.5 D of steepening was induced in the opposite meridian—7.5 D of corneal change had occurred in all. Thus the fact of incisional coupling was noted and described—again. He found (as did Lans before him) that deeper incisions produced more flattening in the steep meridian and that longer incisions produced more steepening in the flat meridian. He suggested that this phenomenon would be useful in compound astigmatism. The author believes that this was an error in translation and that he really meant *mixed* astigmatism, which makes more sense. Sato also made this telling statement: "There is no difference in the effect of surgical treatment between corneal and lenticular astigmatism" [28].

In another paper the same year, this time in the Japanese literature, Sato reported cases in which a lamellar dissection of the cornea was combined with a posterior incision—tangential to the steep axis [32] (Figure 9.6).

Sato's second paper in the American literature described the improved technique of tangential half-incisions (Figure 9.7). In these cases he dilated the pupils with atropine and made the incisions just inside the pupillary margin [33]. This is an interesting point. He probably did

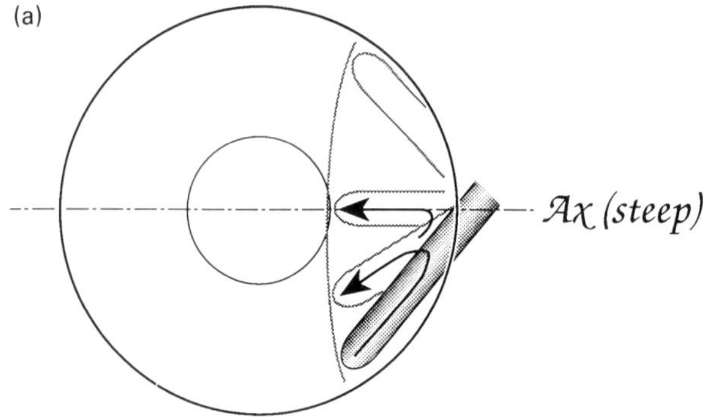

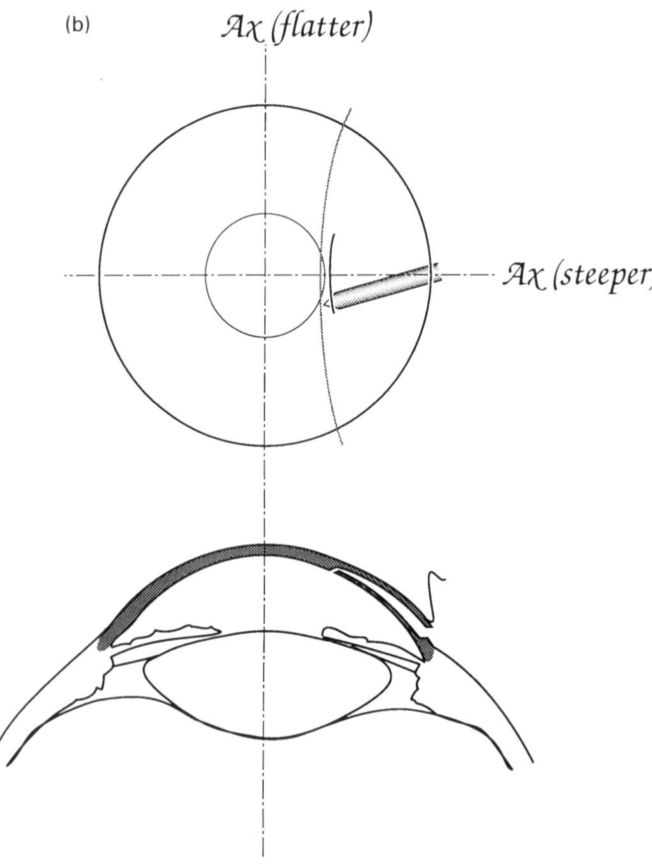

Fig. 9.6 Sato's lamellar dissection procedure.

this to reduce the incidence of glare, but he may have found—as later surgeons have—that in so doing he also reduced the incidence of iatrogenic irregular astigmatism.

Sato was enthusiastic about his "new" technique and said as much [34]. However, he reckoned without the endothelial destruction his surgery had produced (see Chapter 7 for details). Considering the fact that the corneal reaction must have been intense (see the description of Fyodorov's early efforts in Chapter 7), to persist in this approach was brave—at the very least. Sato should be given much credit, however, because many of his ideas were successful, and his work did not escape notice, even if some of the notice was unfavorable.

The evolution of surgery for astigmatism

There were, of course, others who involved themselves in this subject—for better or for worse—using various techniques and modalities.

Troutman's wedge resection for postkeratoplasty astigmatism

Troutman pioneered the technique of corneal wedge resection after keratoplasty in 1970, using a razor blade knife to excise a crescent of tissue centered on the flattest meridian adjacent to the graft–host junction [35,36]. The technique is detailed below (see the section on wedge resections for hyperopic astigmatism revisited).

Jensen introduced a double-bladed knife for more precise control of wedge resections and proposed a more quantifiable determination for the correction of large and small degrees of astigmatism [37].

Radial relaxing incisions

In 1973, Fyodorov and coworkers began using external radial relaxing incisions to correct myopia. At the same time, various arrangements of incisions were studied in an effort to correct astigmatism [38]. It was found that, as Sato had pointed out, transverse incisions, whose separation and length varied, were effective in reducing small amounts of myopic astigmatism. From this work a number of other configurations were suggested for this purpose as well. Many of these are still in use today.

Basic principles and patient workup

Astigmatism surgery is still evolving in technique, and further study is needed. Nonetheless, many patients who cannot be rehabilitated with conventional optical measures benefit significantly from surgical treatment of their astigmatism. The author considers a surgical alternative for any amount of astigmatism that exceeds 20% of the associated spherical component or, in patients with simple myopic astigmatism, when the astigmatism exceeds 0.50 D. The lower degrees are only approached if they are oblique, against-the-rule (A-T-R), and/or are symptomatic. An astigmatic refractive error in the range of 1.00 to 2.00 D may be expected to reduce uncorrected visual acuity to the 20/30 to 20/50 range, and an astigmatic refractive error of greater than 2.00 to 3.00 D could reduce uncorrected visual acuity to the 20/70 to 20/100 range [39]. However, the author has seen cases of mixed astigmatism reaching as high as 2.5 D whose unaided visual acuity has been 20/30. The refractive surgeon must be careful in these cases, particularly if this is the result of previous refractive surgery—beware not to violate Bores' first rule: *"If it ain't broke, don't try to fix it."* This is actually the first rule that a physician should learn about any treatment. It is, of course, a rule not invented

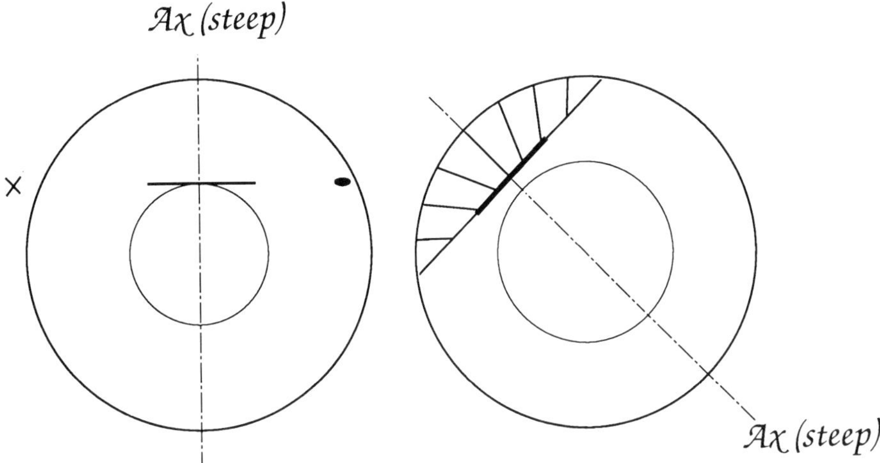

Fig. 9.7 Sato's single external T-incision alone and combined with internal radials for astigmatism.

by myself—but it is an excellent rule nonetheless. Less than careful selection of surgical parameters may well reduce the astigmatic component in, for example, a case whose refraction is −2.50 + 2.50 × 45° such that the result is −2.50 D of spherical myopia. Thus you will have reduced the cylinder along with the unaided vision. It will be difficult to convince such a patient that his or her surgery has been successful.

Astigmatism following cataract surgery is less common today with the smaller incisions being used. Still, small-incision surgery is not universal, and thus postcataract astigmatism will continue to be encountered. Astigmatism of greater than 3 D was reported by Jaffe and Clayman in 10% of a series of patients with large cataract incisions [40]. High astigmatism after keratoplasty is even more common, with astigmatism greater than 1.00 D basically being the norm [35].

Despite the attention that astigmatism has received, its treatment remains less than straightforward. To produce a lasting effect through surgery, the aspiring refractive surgeon must have a complete grasp of the fundamentals of surgical correction of spherical errors. He or she also must be experienced with this modality, having obtained good, predictable results with spherical errors, before attempting astigmatic corrections. While the cornea is somewhat forgiving in nature, there is less margin for error in astigmatism than in spherical corrections—by several orders of magnitude. You are advised *not* to tackle even the simplest case as your initiation into refractive surgery. You are also advised to read the basic rules and dicta of refractive surgery, which, if adhered to, will keep you out of "hot water."

Caveats

Astigmatism chasing

One of the biggest mistakes that can be made by refractive surgeons is committed by both the young and the old, the expert and the green. What the author is referring to specifically is the tendency to keep adding incisions in an effort to control the astigmatism. Such surgeons begin by chasing the astigmatism (violating Bores' eleventh rule: *"Chase not the astigmatism lest ye be cursed with it forever"*) and end by themselves being controlled by it.

The usual scenario is this: The patient is operated on for astigmatism—especially with T-cuts—and postoperatively, the astigmatism reappears in a different location (see Chapter 15). Sometimes it is greater, and sometimes it is the same degree. Without waiting for things to simmer down, forgetting the lessons taught them (if they ever learned them), they blithely add another T-cut or two. The astigmatism now turns up in another meridian. By now the prudent surgeon would realize that things are not in his or her control and stop—thus heeding Bores' tenth rule: *"The good surgeon knows when to quit."* But not the neophyte and certainly not the stalwart "expert" surgeon, for whom it is full speed ahead. He or she adds another T-cut or two—and so on. These surgeons are often puzzled to find—after the dust clears—a patient with unstable, sometimes irregular, often hyperopic astigmatism. The sad part in this is that it could all have been avoided in the first place. The author is unable to discover the need for haste here. The patient has had the original problem for years and now is likely to have an added one for some years to come. Please heed the moral of this tale: Wait until things have stabilized before using your knife and thereby obey Halstead's maxim: *"The biggest difference between a good surgeon and a poor one is this: A good surgeon knows when not to cut."*

There is one other error the author sees quite frequently—unpaired T-cuts. Such incisions make no sense theoretically or practically. The corneal surface is toroidal and regular in its toricity. Symmetrical surfaces demand symmetrical surgery. One unpaired T-cut, especially at 6 to 7 mm, produces an asymmetrical surface change. If the corneal thickness were even across its entire extent, such incisions might possibly produce an even curvature

(a)

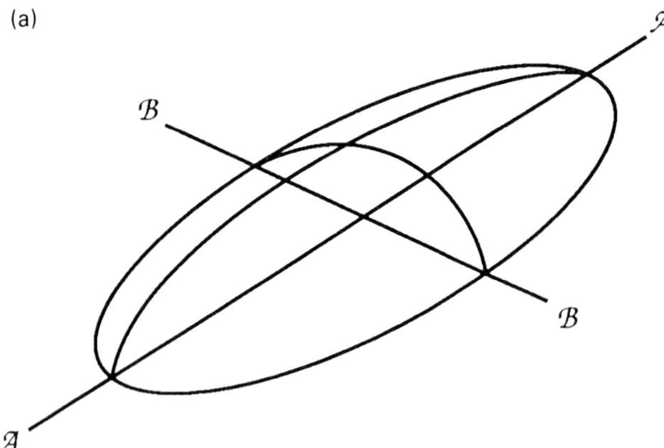

A–A ***long*** axis, ***least*** curvature, ***least*** myopic.
B–B ***short*** axis, ***most*** curvature, ***most*** myopic.

(b)

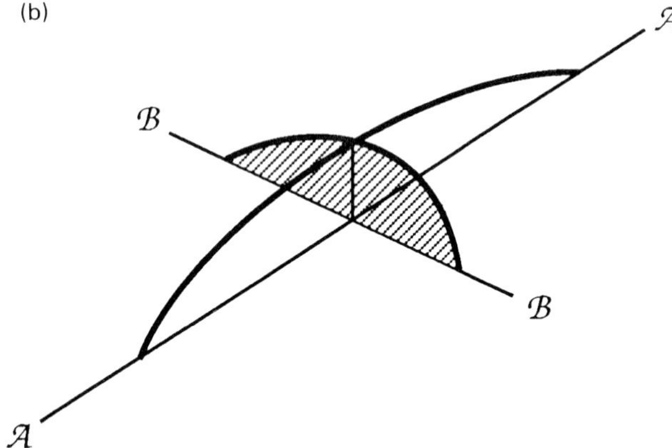

Fig. 9.8 Astigmatic meridians.

change. The normal cornea is not of even thickness; thus curvature changes from an unpaired T-cut will not be regular. The fact that the K-readings have changed in the presence of such an incision or that a patient's vision may be improved is not proof of the correctness of such application. Examination of such surfaces with sensitive holographic topography shows asymmetry of the corneal center. It is known that relaxing incisions can produce multifocal surfaces—good vision may be a happenstance related to this event [41]. K-readings are not a good criterion for the presence or absence of small areas of irregularity either—their resolution is too coarse, and they are not reliable for nonspherical surfaces; even photokeratography can miss small irregularities.

Astigmatism—By way of review

To undertake the treatment of astigmatism by the method of using relaxing incisions (or, for that matter, by any technique), the surgeon must understand that he or she is dealing with a regular toroidal surface—think of the bowl of an upside-down spoon. In a regular toroidal surface, two extremes of curvature can be identified:

- The curvature of least radius
- The curvature of greatest radius

For the sake of discussion, we will call these curvatures *major* (flatter) and *minor* (steeper). Since these curves can be represented by lines in a plan view of the surface (i.e., a head-on view), we can call these lines (curves) *major* and *minor axes* (Figure 9.8). These terms will be most helpful later on in the discussion. However, do not confuse these axes with the *axes of astigmatism*—since, in fact, they correspond to the *astigmatic meridians* (because they represent the long and short axes of an ellipse; see below).

In the case of a cylindrical refractive surface, the refractive power of the cylinder is manifest at a right angle (90°) to its axis (Figure 9.9). This *power axis* is referred to as the meridian of the cylinder. Thus in a case whose refractive error is −6.00 + 3.00 × 90°, the cylindrical axis is at 90°, whereas the meridian is at 180° (Figure 9.10). This meridian is relatively flat in its curvature (since this is the plus meridian). The minus axis is at 180°, but its meridian is at 90°. The 90° meridian therefore has the steepest curvature (it is more myopic). This is where all the action is. All the

(a)

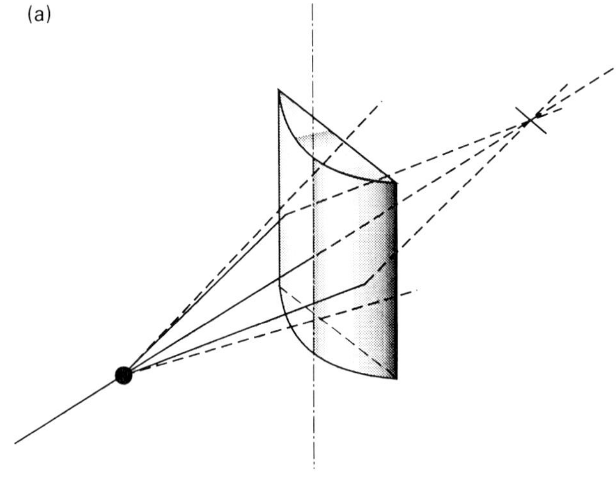

(b)

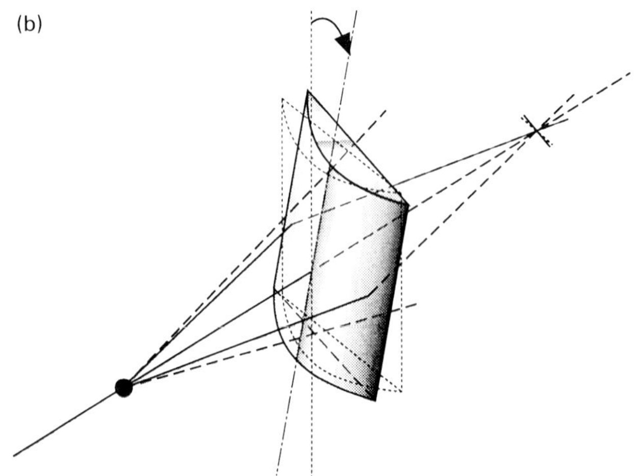

Fig. 9.9 The principle of cylinder lens.

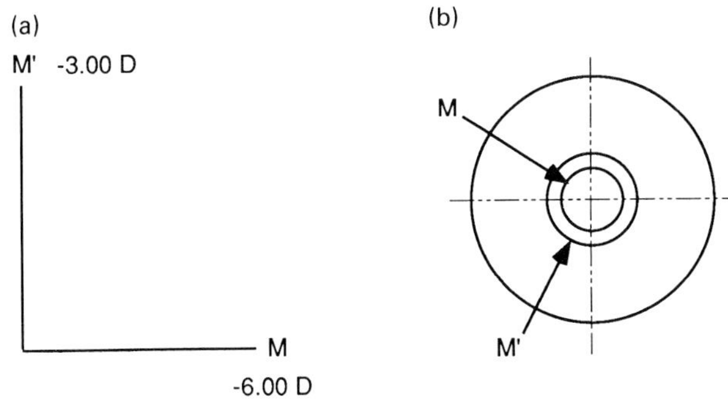

Fig. 9.10 (a) Power diagram; (b) two zones for astigmatism.

fancy configurations for myopia, incision placement, etc., are oriented on the plus-cylinder axis—hence Bores' sixth rule of refractive surgery: *"Plus-cylinder notation always must be used in planning myopic astigmatism surgery and the reverse for hyperopic astigmatism."*

Assuming a toroidal surface (with a major and a minor axis), imagine a planar section being made through this surface. In a plan view, this slice would be parallel with the floor. If we were then to turn the piece over and look at it (or trace its edge onto a piece of paper), we would find that the shape resulting would be that of an oval or, more properly, an ellipse (Figure 9.11). The short side of the ellipse would represent the minor axis and correspond to the greater (steepest, least radius) curvature on the surface; whereas the long side would represent the major axis and correspond to the lesser (flattest, most radius) surface curvature. Sections perpendicular to the surface along the major and minor axes illustrate this point. This fact explains why early attempts by Fyodorov and the author to correct astigmatism employed oval optical zone markers

Patient workup

The basic workup for astigmatism is that for spherical myopia (see Chapter 5), with some additions and special precautions. Unless you or your refractionist is particularly good at manifest refractions, cycloplegic examinations are recommended in these cases. As you become more familiar with the process of dealing with astigmatism, a return can be made to manifest refractions. This is especially important in mixed and compound astigmatism. The Jackson cross cylinder must be used to refine the cylinder axis for the same reasons of accuracy. The keratometry readings should all be done by the same person and the axes clearly defined. This is easier to do with small mire instruments such as the Haag-Streit ophthalmometer. In fact, the purchase of this instrument should be considered a priority for any keratotomist.

However, any surgery contemplated must be based on the manifest refraction because this represents the total

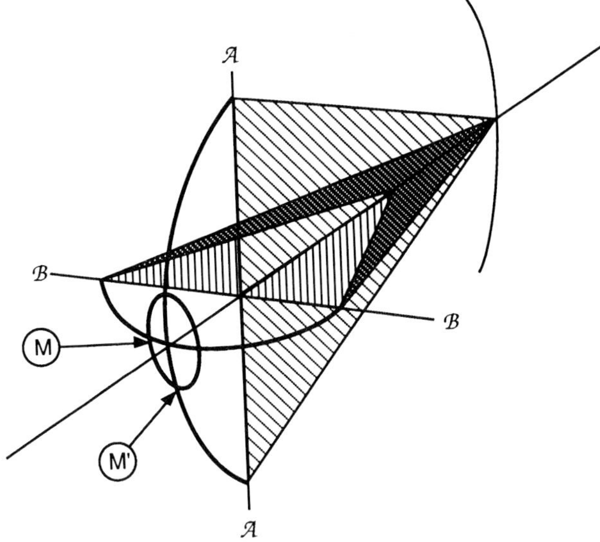

Fig. 9.11 The resulting optical zone required is elliptic in shape.

astigmatism of the eye. In such cases, the refractive cylinder axis rules—not the keratometric or topographic axis. There is a definite relationship between the diameter of the surgical optical zone and the degree of myopia of the patient's optical system; this fact is a *first principle.* Selection of the size of the primary optical zone is based (for the most part) on the patient's spectacle refraction. The amount of astigmatism in the patient's optical system may not bear any direct relationship to the astigmatism on the cornea (as measured by keratometry). Remember, we are correcting the refraction of the total optical system by altering the corneal surface—much like fitting a toroidal contact lens for the same purpose.

The problem often arises as to what should be done when the K-readings do not match the refraction. In practice, this seldom becomes a problem. Generally speaking, in higher degrees of astigmatism where the curvature and axes are more critical, the refraction will correspond quite closely to the K-readings. The K-readings always should be used when the astigmatism is high and a clear-cut refractive result is not possible. In smaller amounts of astigmatism, where the problem is less critical, the refraction should always be taken over the K-readings. In mixed astigmatism, the solution may be less clear-cut because the unaided vision is usually quite good in these patients. An incorrect assessment of the parameters could result in a loss of uncorrected vision postoperatively. The best rule-of-thumb is to always operate for total astigmatism. Trust the cross cylinder to refine the cylinder axis.

In some cases, photokeratometer may be of help because the axis of astigmatism is the critical factor here [42]. However, it takes skill to interpret the photos—although it is a skill that can be acquired in time. Be especially watchful for any indications that the limbus is less than circular. While rare, an elliptical limbus requires special techniques to deal with adequately, and each case has to be assessed individually. There are no hard and fast rules here (see the section on the Ruiz procedure, below). A photokeratometer and/or other surface-mapping device should be in the armamentarium of all keratotomists—despite the shortcomings of the photokeratometer (see Chapter 6). There are situations, unfortunately, in which nothing but experience will be of help. When in doubt, do not hesitate to seek advice, regardless how trivial the problem may seem.

In some instances, particularly those in which the patient has been wearing contact lenses, your refraction may not match that of the patient's spectacles. Here, common sense should prevail. Generally speaking, if the patient sees well and comfortably with his or her glasses, it is safe to assume that he or she will be comfortable after surgery as well using his or her old spectacle refraction in lieu of yours. Unless there is some compelling reason to alter the situation, go with the present prescription.

It is very important that the cornea be as stable as possible prior to the surgery. Therefore, contact lenses should be out as long as practical but in no case less than 1 week (Table 9.1). This goes for soft lenses as well; these are known to cause corneal warpage in as little as 20 hours [43]. If the patient has no backup spectacles, have the patient remove the contact lens from one eye for the required period. Warn the patient that he or she may experience some difficulty with depth perception and to be especially careful while driving.

Keratometry after corneal surgery

Typically, when the full thickness of the cornea has been involved—as in penetrating keratoplasty—ordinary K-readings will be as reliable as ever they were. However, after lamellar surgery, such as keratomileusis, where only the anterior curvature has been altered, K-readings are inaccurate and may underestimate the true refractive power and astigmatism by 11% or more [44] (see Chapter 6 for a more detailed explanation). This again emphasizes the author's admonition that refractive surgery demands an accurate means of evaluating the true corneal curvature.

Instrumentation

This discussion concerns itself mostly with those instruments used for astigmatism surgery and which are adjunctive to the basic tools of incisional refractive surgery. The reader is referred to Chapters 7 and 8 for a more in-depth description of basic instrumentation.

Table 9.1 Contact lens removal schedule

Lens type	Minimum time*
Hard	1 week
Soft	48 hours
Ortho-K	6 months

* See text.

Incision depth is a paramount factor in the outcome of radial keratotomy (RK) for spherical myopia—it is no less important in the control of astigmatism. As was pointed out first by Fyodorov and coworkers and amply demonstrated since by many others, there are three factors that affect the depth of incision. I reiterate:

- Blade length
- Blade sharpness
- Tissue resistance

All these factors are interrelated, but only the first two can be controlled directly. The third factor can be compensated for to some degree by oversetting the blade and by pressurizing the eye.

Blades and blade handles

As has been stated repeatedly, this surgery is true microsurgery. The outcome depends not only on careful consideration of numerous, seemingly unimportant factors but also on the instrumentation. Next to the preoperative workup, the most important consideration in this surgery is the blade. In the beginning, razor fragments were used (see also Chapter 7). Because such blades were inconsistent in their quality, most surgeons today use some form of crystalline blade.

Angled blades are not an appropriate choice for making transverse incisions. A vertical-edged crystalline blade provides the exquisite sharpness required for precise control of the length and depth of transverse incisions. An extrasharp double-edged blade, such as the XTAL sapphire blade (Katena K2-6512) or the KOI ultrathin LeCut diamond blade, is a real asset and is highly recommended. On the other hand, the author has not had a good experience with the square diamond blades advocated by Thornton [45].

A knife handle with a slightly longer than normal footplate is useful as well. Most of the current diamond blade holders do not provide a sufficiently clear and unobstructed view of the blade edge and operative area. Even if you have a favorite diamond knife, consider purchasing the Katena K2-6500 for astigmatism surgery. Keep this blade and handle sequestered, and use it for astigmatism only.

Fixation devices

Fixation of the eye is especially important in astigmatism cases to ensure that all incisions are straight and perpendicular to the corneal surface. Many devices are available for this purpose. Any such device that is used should be one that is easily applied and removed and should not produce tissue damage. In addition, it must not interfere with the surgery.

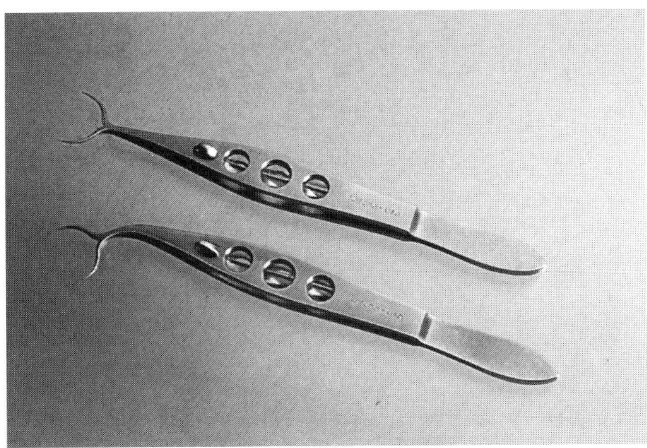

Fig. 9.12 Straight and angled wide fixation forceps.

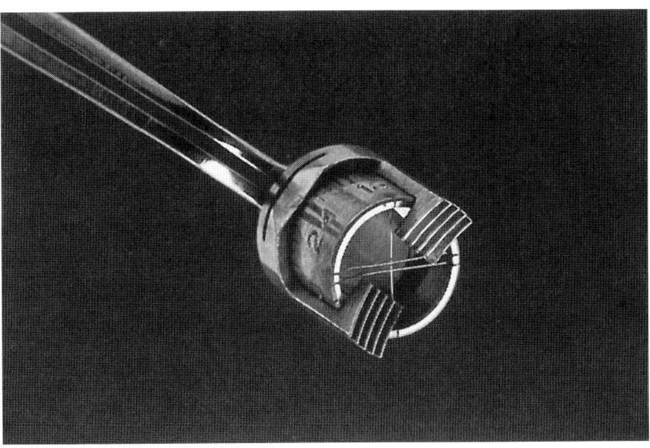

Fig. 9.13 Fyodorov L-marker.

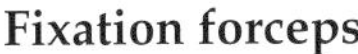

Fixation forceps

The narrow double fixation forceps prevents ocular rotation without the corneal distortion a wider jaw would produce—especially in a soft eye—for radial or parallel incisions. However, it does not provide sufficient stability for transverse incisions. For such cases, a wide-jawed forceps such as the Bores wide fixation forceps (Katena K5-3280) provides the cross-limbus fixation essential for making straight (or arcuate) transverse incisions—as in the Ruiz procedure. These instruments are also available with angled jaws for those who prefer such a configuration (Figure 9.12).

Optical zone and incision markers

Cross-hairs or other centering aids are useful but not essential and frequently are inaccurately aligned. Sizes should be marked clearly on each marker, particularly astigmatism markers. All markers, especially those for astigmatism, must be handled with care to prevent damage that may distort their shapes.

Astigmatic optical zone markers

Despite the fact that the effective optical zone in astigmatism is an ellipse, there are few occasions where an actual elliptical zone needs to be marked. Most astigmatism surgery today, which employs T-cuts, relies on circular optical zone markers.

Incision markers

Special devices for marking the incision lines or spacing are available as well. However, all these markers, with two exceptions, are optional. One exception is the six-blade incision marker (Katena K3-8880). While it is possible to make 4, 8, or 16 incisions evenly spaced by eye, it is not quite so easy to accurately judge the 30° or 60° separation between incisions in 6- or 12-incision patients. Coating the bottom of these markers with brilliant green or gentian violet will enhance their usefulness—at least for the beginner. The more experienced surgeon will find the beginning of the marks sufficient to align his or her incisions. The other exception is the Bores L-incision marker (Figure 9.13) (see the section on the RL-method, below).

Because a vertical cutting blade is used to make the transverse T-incisions, the cutting is done in reverse (toward the open end of the footplate). It is necessary to use a guideline to ensure that the incision is straight and of proper length. There are numerous guide markers available for marking individual and clustered T-incisions, with and without radials. The author recommends the Katena series of markers as being durable and accurate for this purpose (Figure 9.14).

Special markers

Special markers such as the Bores/Ruiz, Bores L-markers, and so on will be discussed under individual configurations.

Axis marker

The Bores axis marker (Katena K3-7910) is a must for astigmatism surgery (Figure 9.15). This should be used in conjunction with a Mendez protractor (Katena K3-7900) or a Zeiss eyepiece reticle to mark the axis of cylinder.

The Zeiss astigmatism reticle

The Zeiss astigmatism reticle (Figure 9.16) is supplied in a matched set of ×10 high-point oculars by Zeiss (reticle no. 30-55-83). Originally designed for use in fitting toric contact lenses, it serves admirably in the eyepiece tube of any Zeiss operating microscope. It also can be adapted to fit into a Weck scope as well.

For those of you with Zeiss operating microscopes who cannot get or do not want the expense of the first reticle,

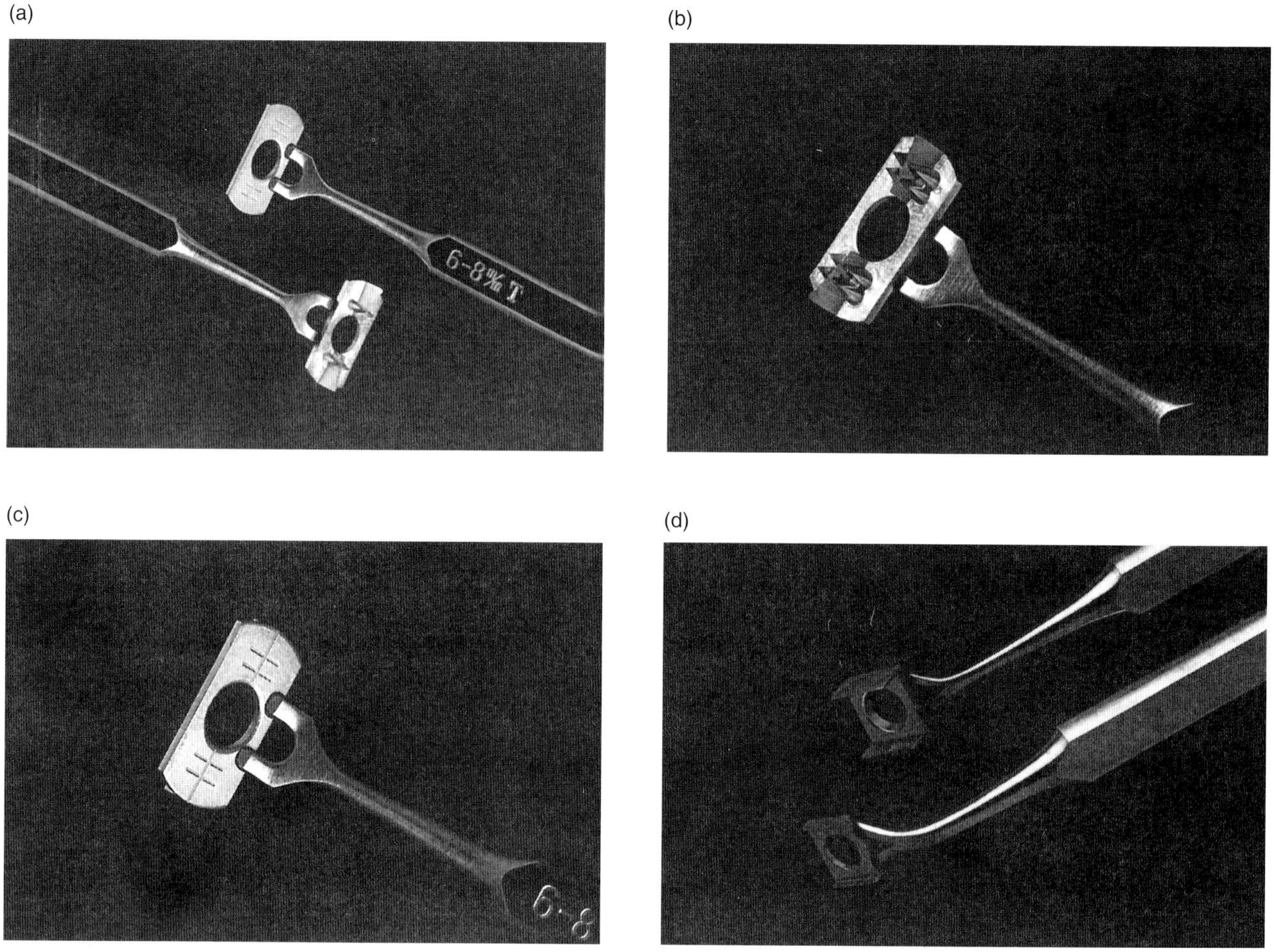

(a) (b) (c) (d)

Fig. 9.14 (a–d) Single and double T-markers (Katena).

(a) (b)

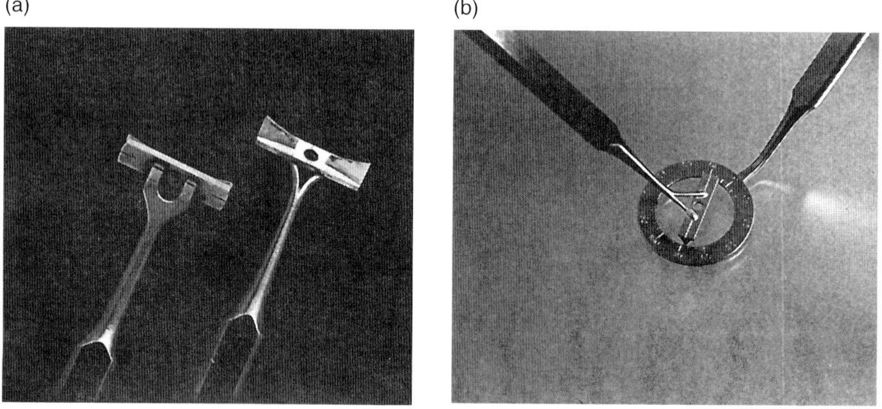

Fig. 9.15 (a) Bores axis marker; (b) used with Mendez protractor.

there are some other reticles available that can be purchased for your eyepieces. Zeiss reticle no. 30-55-98 is designed for a ×12.5 eyepiece. It has a ruler in the center and is marked off into 12 segments corresponding to 15° increments. If the eyepiece is aligned so that the 12 and 6 o'clock marks are coincident with the 12 and 6 o'clock positions of the patient's cornea, the patient's cylinder axis can be approximated closely. This reticle must be factory installed, however.

Using the Zeiss reticle

This reticle consists of a precisely engraved optical flat with a cross-hair in the center. The long arm of the cross-

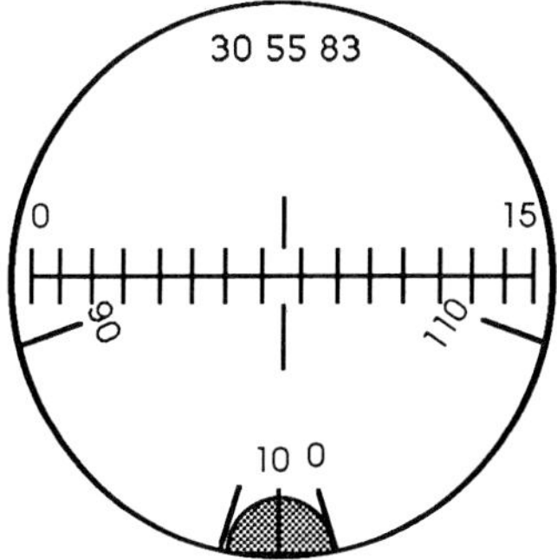

Fig. 9.16 Zeiss reticle.

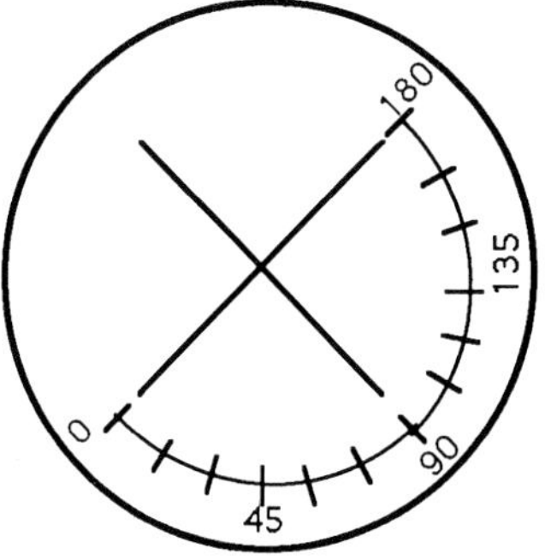

Fig. 9.18 Fenzl reticle.

hair is marked off in equal increments from 0 to 15. At the bottom edge of the reticle is engraved a 90° protractor—offset 10°. Further, the protractor is marked in major divisions of 10° and minor divisions of 2° in increments from 0° to 90° on one side and from 0° to 110° on the other. Riding in a groove under this protractor is a steel ball whose diameter is exactly 20°. When placed into the usual angled eyepiece of the Zeiss operating microscope, this ball will self-center. The reading is made off the right-hand side of the steel ball.

With the patient supine and looking at the coaxial light reflex, the eyepiece is rotated until the right edge of the ball is aligned at 90° (or 0) on the reticle. The operating microscope is then aligned sagittally with the patient's head such that the zero mark corresponds to 12 o'clock on the patient's cornea—it helps to have marked this position at the slit lamp prior to surgery. The eyepiece is then rotated to correspond to the axis of astigmatism (Figure 9.17).

The microscope is adjusted to place the cross-hair of the reticle onto the previously marked visual axis. This is done by aligning and locking the microscope head in place and then grasping the barrel of the eyepiece (below the adjustment collar) and rotating it until the cross-hair is properly aligned. It is helpful to set this eyepiece in such a way that the long arm of the cross-hair is parallel to the cylinder axis (this is not always possible). This is important—study the drawing of this reticle to understand why this is so. By aligning the reticle in this way, you have provided yourself with an additional reminder of the orientation of the steep or flat meridian—the axis you are going to be working in. Sometimes it is not possible to use the reticle in this manner—this is where the axis marker comes in.

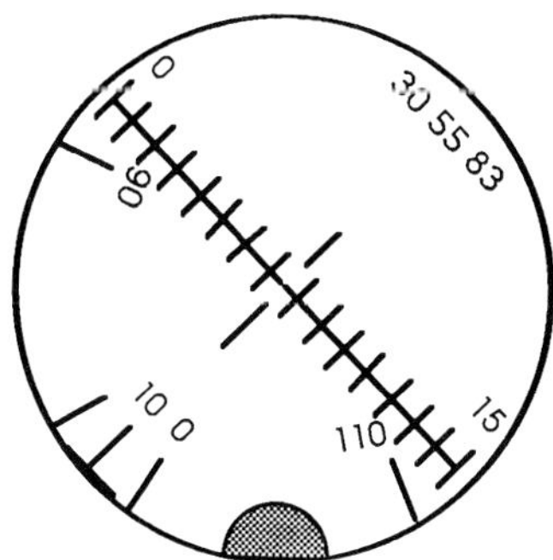

Fig. 9.17 Zeiss reticle rotated.

The Fenzl reticle

Another product is the Fenzl reticle (Figure 9.18). This is an engraved glass reticle that can be placed into any microscope eyepiece (instructions are provided). While not as elegant as the previously described Zeiss, it is serviceable and infinitely better than nothing. You will need two of these—one for the microscope and one for your slit lamp. This reticle is used in the same manner as the Zeiss product.

Mendez protractor

The Mendez degree gauge (Katena K3-7900) can be used to assist in marking the axis of the cylinder. In this case, the 12 o'clock position of the patient's cornea should be determined either at the slit lamp or under the operating microscope. The device is then placed onto the anesthetized cornea, and the 0° or 90° mark is aligned with the 12 o'clock point on the cornea. The axis marker is then rotated within the protractor ring and aligned with the proper tick mark.

Other useful things

The Thornton ruled marker (Figure 9.19) is useful as a generic marker for transverse incisions of various lengths (see also Chapter 8 for other essential instruments).

Current methods for the control of astigmatism

Wedge resections for hyperopic astigmatism revisited

This method is not the author's favorite way to control astigmatism—there are better, more predictable methods

(a)

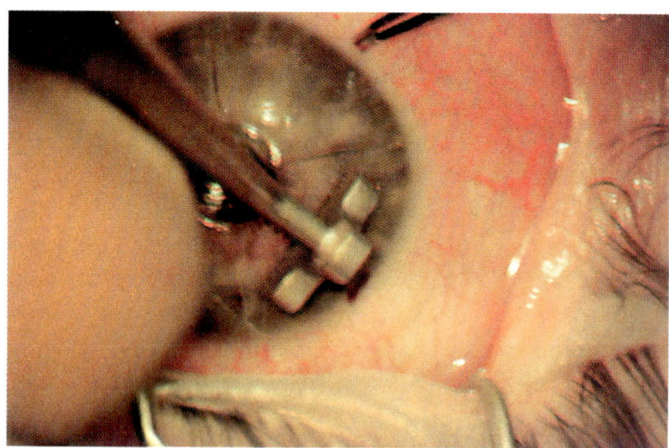

(b)

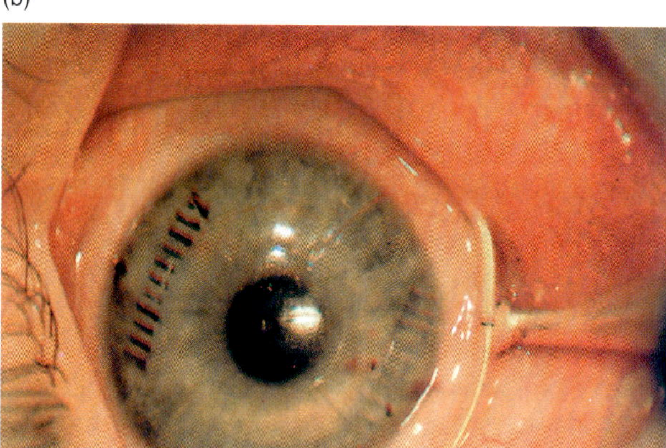

Fig. 9.19 (a,b) Thornton ruled T-marker.

(namely, relaxing incisions) to do this. Still, there are times when nothing else will do. Thus it is important that every refractive surgeon know how to perform this surgery. Troutman introduced this technique in 1970 to treat postkeratoplasty astigmatism [36]. Despite all the best efforts, postkeratoplasty astigmatism still plagues us. This is not the place to discuss the merits of double-running versus interrupted sutures, etc., however. We can leave that for textbooks on keratoplasty techniques. Suffice it to say that we do not yet have a handle on the problem—and considering what we have learned thus far from refractive surgery, we may never solve it. Nevertheless, if the problem is ever solved, the author will predict—for the record—that the answer will come from the ongoing work with refractive surgical procedures.

Before beginning a more detailed description of this technique, the student should be cautioned to *"abandon all hope for predictability, all ye who enter here."* Astigmatism surgery is a giant "can of worms" that can be dealt with successfully only by approaching it in a rational way while being prepared for occasional irrational results. It is true that some methods are more predictable than others—but wedge resections are not in this category.

This procedure steepens flat axes (even though the incision is transverse to the meridian) because it is a resection of tissue with subsequent suturing—hence the chord of the arc is shortened. The rule-of-thumb for this surgery is that for every 0.1 mm of resection, 0.67 D of cornea will be steepened—theoretically. I say theoretically because 1.0 mm of resection should gain you 10 D of correction, except that it does not—it gets you somewhat less. How much less is anyone's guess—sometimes a lot, sometimes a little. Usually, for astigmatism equal to or less than 10 D, a little more surgery is needed, whereas for more than 10 D, a little less is required. In any event, no resection width should exceed 1.5 mm—thus the procedure tops out at about 15 D—although as much as 27 D of correction has been reported [46], which is a lot of astigmatism in anyone's book. Better you should not be too exuberant with this surgery in any event—if you have undercorrected, go back and do a little more by shaving down one side of the resection—on the limbal side. The object is to reduce the astigmatism to manageable proportions. *Manageable* could mean glasses, contact lenses, or more predictable relaxing incisions (see the sections on relaxing incisions and wedge versus Ruiz, below).

Be also cognizant of Bores' axiom: *"Beware of pushing down the curvature too much over here; it might pop up over there under an assumed name."* This means that anything you do to one meridian will be reflected (in its true sense) in the opposite meridian at a ratio of about 2:1. That is, 1 D of *steepening* at 90° will be accompanied by 0.50 D of *flattening* at 180°. Thus, for every 0.67 D of steepening, there will be a corresponding 0.33 D of flattening—or 1 D of total cylinder will be induced. Better you should keep the 2:1 relationship in mind and not add up the vectors because typically you will be concentrating on one meridian and are trying to get rid of lots of cylinder. It does you no good to reduce 10 D in one meridian just to induce 5 D in the other—balance is the key here. Maybe you should only try for 7.50 D of correction. This would leave you with, for example, a residual of +2.50 D in the original meridian, and you would have induced +3.75 D in the other, opposite meridian (which is only 1.25 D difference) ultimately. Thus the final refraction would be +2.50 + 1.25 × whatever axis (I suppose you could try to figure out the exact relationship so as to end up with a plano result or even slightly minus, but you would go crazy trying to cut the exact incision width to accomplish it). For a patient who was plano +10.00 before surgery, this is an improvement anyone can live with. Be aware that some patients with mixed astigmatism, even up to 2.5 D, can record uncorrected vision as good as 20/30. An overcorrection of the astigmatism is always induced in any case with this surgery because of the compression produced by the suturing.

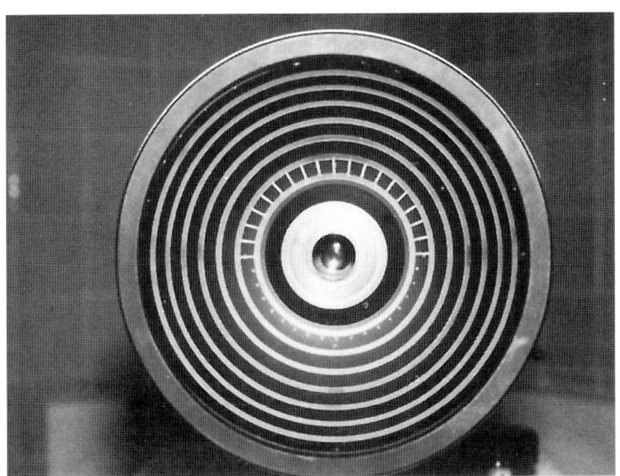

Fig. 9.20 Modified keratoscope faceplate *à la* Ruiz.

Before tackling the astigmatism, the corneal astigmatism should be stable for about 6 to 8 weeks after complete keratoplasty suture removal. Pachymetry is performed over the graft scar. Take several readings so that a thin spot will not surprise you. In performing this surgery, a surgical keratometer is almost essential to success. Retrobulbar or general anesthesia also should be employed.

To proceed, first establish the meridian of the hyperopic cylinder by photokeratoscopy and/or ophthalmometry (see Figure 9.20 for a method of modifying the faceplate of the photokeratometer); this is the one case where a Placido's disk photo can really help. Prior to surgery, seat the patient at the slit lamp and lightly mark the 12 o'clock position on the cornea—near the limbus—before administering the retrobulbar anesthesia. If the patient is already anesthetized, you will have to rely on remembered landmarks. With the patient on the operating table and anesthetized, align the microscope eyepiece reticle with the 12 o'clock mark on the cornea (see the section on using the Zeiss reticle, above). In lieu of the reticle, use the Mendez protractor for the next step.

Prep and drape the patient, and insert the wire lid speculum. Coat a Bores astigmatism axis marker with brilliant green (make sure that it dries) or gentian violet. Align the axis marker with the hyperopic (flat) meridian using the reticle or Mendez protractor, and mark the meridian (Figure 9.21). Next, coat the blades of an eight- or four-ray RK incision marker with dye. Align the marker with the flat meridian, and mark the cornea. Now you have both the axis of cylinder and the incision extent demarcated (the extent should be 90°—3 clock hours). You are now ready to take the next step.

Good fixation is a must in wedge resection. A very good method of fixation for this surgery is the vacuum suction ring of Barraquer (used for MKM/LASIK)—with or without keratome guides. If you are using the ring, the author suggests that you reverse the handle from the method described by Troutman and have it positioned at 6 o'clock. Apply the vacuum, and hold the handle with your nondominant hand.

The incisions can be made with a guarded single-blade, RK diamond knife, or the special double-blade device described by Troutman—the author uses the former for the first incision. Both methods will be described.

Single-blade method

Set the guarded blade so as not to produce a perforation. If the diamond blade is a new LeCut, underset it about 5 to 10 μm. Here's where the Bores Shadowgraph shines (see Chapter 8)—the Baribeau Micronscope also can be used. Insert the blade tip at one end of the incision, and using the vertical knife edge, incise a curvilinear incision just inside the graft–host junction using the scar as a guide.

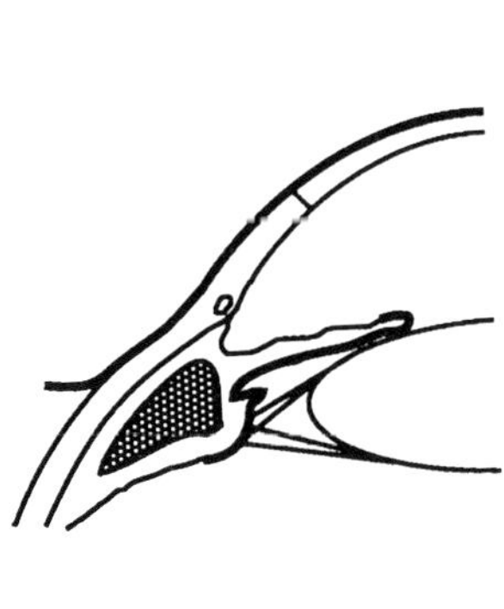

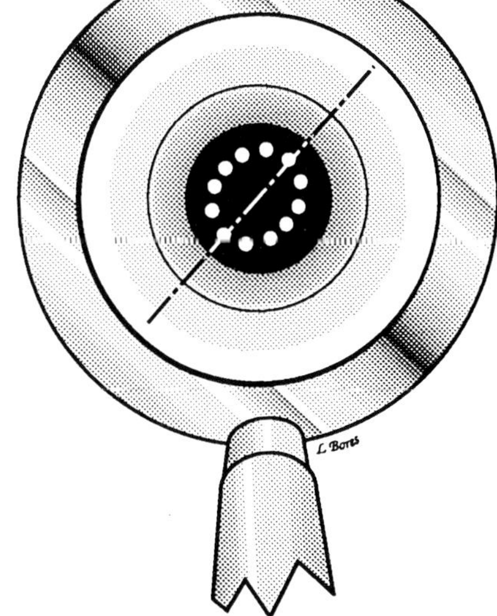

Fig. 9.21 Establishing the hyperopic meridian.

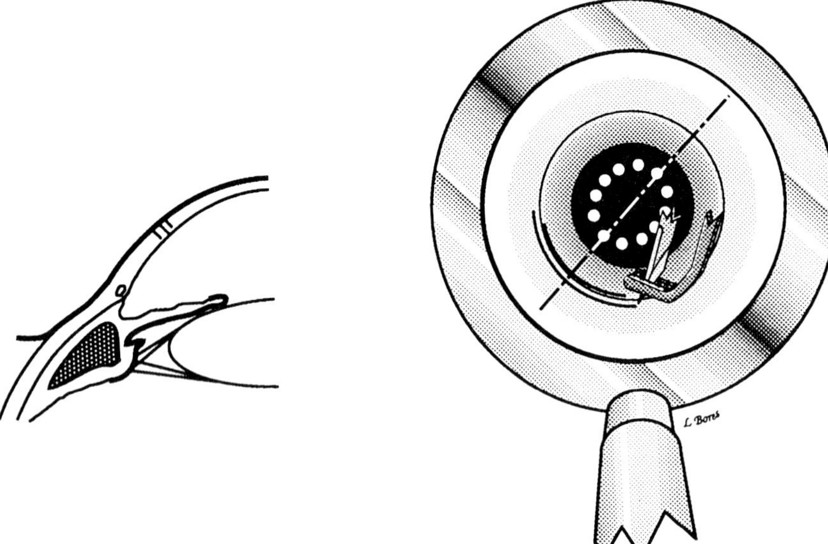

Fig. 9.22 Making the incisions.

The next part of the incision is made free-hand with a naked blade. If you have the Katena handle (K2-6700), you can remove the blade from the guarded handle and insert it into the special holder and use that. Otherwise, the author suggests the Katena K2-6705 blade in the same handle. Using a caliper, mark the widest extent of the wedge along the astigmatic meridian toward the limbus so that the incisions parallel the scar. It may help to use a fresh skin-marking pencil to trace out the incision. Trace the mark with the blade, cutting partially through the stroma. Then deepen the cut, angling toward the first incision. Avoid perforation at this juncture to ensure an even

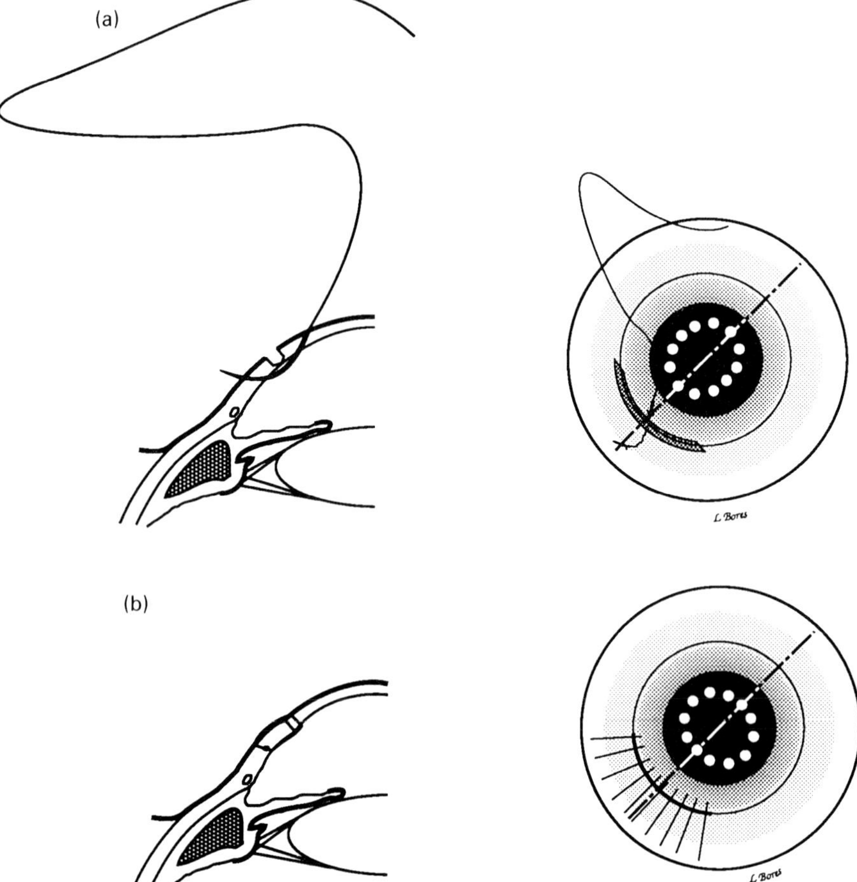

Fig. 9.23 (a) Sutures are through-and-through; (b) they are tied sufficiently tight to close the wound. Note the reversal of the astigmatism.

section. The suction ring can now be released. Finish the resection of the wedge with Vannus or other scissors.

Double-blade technique

Using the double-blade diamond knife, trace out the incision as shown (Figure 9.22). You probably will have to do this in stages to avoid entering the anterior chamber. Using the free-hand blade, extend the inner incision to join the outer. Complete the resection as described above. You probably will find that the first method yields a more even wedge than the second.

Completing the resection

A knife needle or 15° razor knife is used to make a paracentesis to reduce the intraocular pressure. This will facilitate suture closure of the wedge without tension—something that should be avoided at all costs. Care should be taken in aphakic eyes if vitreous is present in the AC. In this case, inject a small amount of air or Healon to push the vitreous away from the cornea. The wedge is closed with from eight to ten 10-0 nylon sutures placed through-and-through (Figure 9.23). Start peripherally and work toward the center. Troutman suggests tying each loop with a double slip knot, tightening them in pairs beginning in the periphery and working centrally [47]. If you have a surgical keratometer, the knots are tied so as to convert the preoperative ellipse into one with the opposite shape and extent. The extent of this overcorrection should be about 50% of the original. The sutures are then locked and the knots pulled below the limbal corneal surface.

Unfortunately, in the past, this considerable overcorrection compromised vision during the "sutures in" period—sometimes lasting up to a year. Troutman has advocated the use of compensatory compression sutures to reduce the inevitable (and necessary) astigmatic overcorrection resulting from this surgery. Two or more interrupted sutures are placed across the graft scar 60° from each end of the closed wedge. These are tightened until the reversed ellipse becomes circular (Figure 9.24). These sutures should remain until the resection sutures are removed—generally at 6 months—although, if the patient is comfortable, the sutures can remain for longer periods. Expect some reversal of effect when the sutures are completely removed. Mean residual astigmatism in the author's few patients was approximately 3 D.

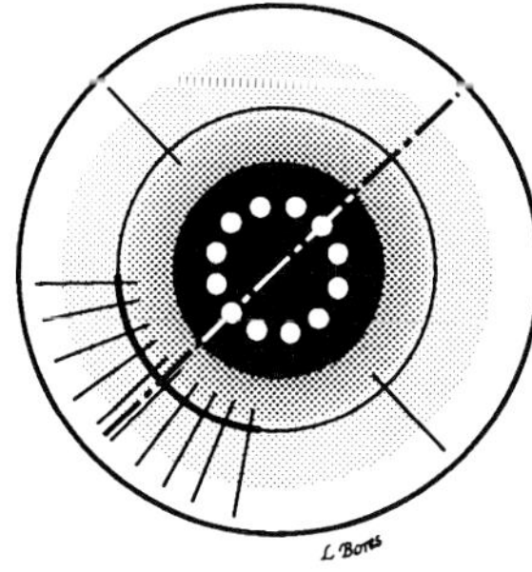

Fig. 9.24 Compression sutures are placed at 90° to the hyperopic axis to relieve the inevitable but temporary overcorrection.

Relaxing incisions for myopic astigmatism

Basic principles

Relaxing incisions have a venerable position in the hierarchy of astigmatism surgery, being among the first to be seriously applied to the problem. First used in controlling iatrogenic astigmatism, they were used eventually in congenital astigmatism as well. They have the distinct advantages of being eminently controllable through their length and depth, are easier to perform, and result in a much more rapid diminution of the astigmatic error. Typically, these procedures can be done under topical anesthesia, and since suturing is avoided, the results can be more readily anticipated.

The object of myopic astigmatism surgery is to produce corneal flattening proportional to the degree of myopia. Since the degree of the myopia is proportional to the degree of curvature of the corneal surface (all else being equal), more flattening force must be exerted in the axis of greatest corneal curvature to reduce the myopic astigmatism. Figure 9.25 illustrates a myopic astigmatic optical surface.

Note that the flattening force has to be applied to the short (steeper) side of the ellipse, with less force being applied to the long (flatter) side of the ellipse in order to bring all points to a focus on the retina. In RK, this flattening force is created by peripheral bulging (i.e., increasing peripheral corneal curvature)—in an amount proportional to the central curvature—caused by the structural weakening of the cornea by the incisions. This is the same

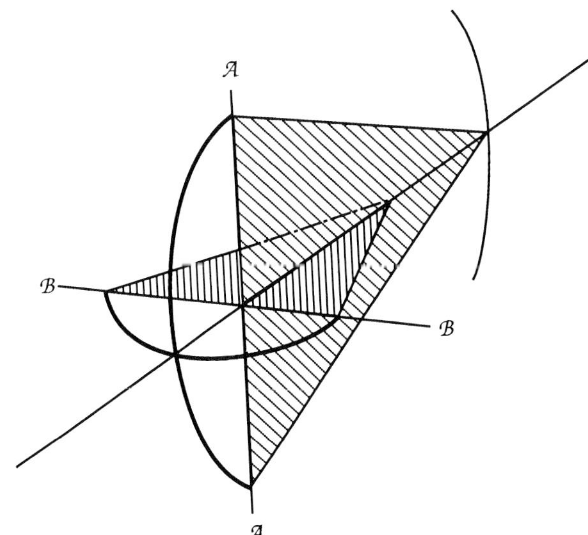

Fig. 9.25 Simple myopic astigmatism.

principle applied in quadrantic (arcuate) intracicatricial relaxing incisions used in postkeratoplasty astigmatism (see below).

The degree of peripheral bulging is directly related to the length (and depth) of the incisions. Therefore, a long incision placed parallel to the short axis will cause greater peripheral bulging and correspondingly greater central flattening along that axis. Since we are dealing with a toroidal surface, the degree of curvature diminishes as we approach the flatter axis from the steeper, and therefore, the required incision length becomes shorter.

For all practical purposes, the limbus can be considered circular (although there are exceptions). Therefore, graduating the length of the incisions produces an optical zone that has the shape of an ellipse. In classic, early RK, such elliptical optical zones were advocated in the control of corneal astigmatism [48]. However, transverse incisions and circular optical clear zones—with or without accompanying radial incisions—have since been found to be more efficient and predictable. Thus the circle is complete, and we are back to where we began in 1894.

The size of the optical zone is, of course, related to the amount of correction desired. That is, a $-6.00 + 3.00 \times 90°$ refractive error will need the clear zone diameter along the steeper axis to be of a size required to correct 6 D of myopia, whereas the diameter along the flatter axis (90° to the steeper) must be of a size to correct 3 D.

Thus, in classic RK, to correct astigmatism associated with myopia, we would need merely to make an elliptical optical zone of appropriate dimensions to obtain the correction desired. In principle, this is how it works. In practice, however, it has been found necessary to make certain modifications in the arrangement of the incisions depending on the amount of total astigmatism present. Peripheral deepening is done in the same manner as in spherical myopia (see also Chapter 8). However, for the most part, circular midzones seem to produce a better result than elliptical ones in astigmatism cases.

Decision making

The author uses his own computer program to calculate the surgical parameters for astigmatism surgery. In Chapter 8, we have pointed out the importance of not being eclectic (Bores' fourth rule). It is *not* possible to "mix and match" with this surgery and expect any prediction software to be effective under such circumstances. Thus, while I have reviewed some of the other software available for this purpose (see Chapter 8), the current discussion will be confined wholly to how the author carries out the decision-making process. Therefore, the examples the author will be using concern the output of the RK DataMaster program and no other.

The prudent keratotomist will draw out his or her incisional configuration for every astigmatic patient prior to the day of surgery. This should be done after calculating the surgical parameters. It is too easy to place the incisions off-axis otherwise. *Do not rely on a drawing made by a computer from the data that you have input.* This is so vital as to be worth repeating. It may be more convenient to have a computer do this, but there have been instances where invalid data have been used to construct a drawing, resulting in surgery being placed in the wrong axis. There also have been instances in which the input data were changed but not the drawing. It takes little imagination to follow this scenario to its end. Furthermore, by drawing out the configuration yourself, you are forced to consider the data in the light of your experience. Never, never delegate this chore—never! Comes a denouement—reliance on your technician is no defense. The author has caught errors in the data in too many instances for there to be any call to ease up on this advice—and the technicians at Bores Eye Institute are very experienced. We are all human and subject to making errors—keep this in mind.

There should be a separate surgical sheet made up for each eye, onto which all preoperative parameters are entered. Your technician can fill out the preoperative parameters—which you should check against the original workup. *Do not hesitate to question any data that seem to be at variance with experience.* Use these data to input into the computer.

The author does these calculations himself and has written RK DataMaster in a way that makes it inconvenient for a technician to do the calculations. It is not safe to let your assistant do it anyway. There are some decisions to be made while running the program that only the surgeon can make. It is possible to do as many as 20 such calculations within 30 minutes, including the data printout, so it is not an onerous task. Once you have made your decisions as to what surgical parameters you will use, enter them onto the sheet using a black or dark-blue felt-tip pen—something that will show up well. This sheet will be posted later next to your operating microscope and must be clearly legible.

The author typically employs the Nordan-T (NT) procedure for most patients with myopic astigmatism, reserving the Ruiz (RZ) procedure for those with mixed astigmatism. The Ruiz procedure is rarely used for simple or compound astigmatism because the optical zones called for are too small and prone to induce irregular astigmatism. The NT procedure uses either 6- or 7-mm-diameter optical zones that are far less likely to pronounce this nasty postoperative complication. Occasionally, the radial-longitudinal (RL) configuration will be used for some cases of postkeratoplasty astigmatism of low degree, but never employing more than three longitudinal incisions per side. The RK DataMaster application will recommend these procedures as well but is capable of calculating all the configurations.

Case examples

Case 1 This is a case of low-grade compound, myopic astigmatism (Figure 9.26). The data input sheet is dis-

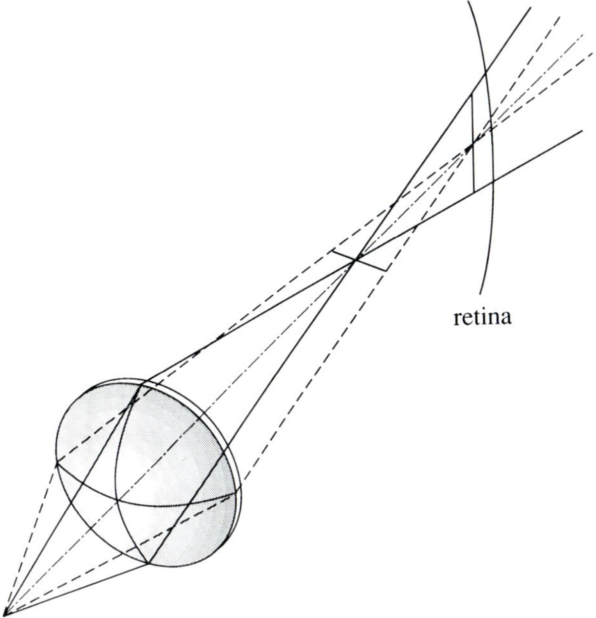

Fig. 9.26 Compound myopic astigmatism.

played in Figure 9.27. The user can choose from various procedures but either the NT (Figure 9.28) or the RT (Figure 9.29) procedure will serve here (see the section on surgical methods, below). The author prefers the NT procedure even though it results in an asymmetrical incision pattern. Figure 9.30 is the case summary sheet. A printout of this page will include the surgical configuration and should be available in the operating room. *Remember:* Double-check the computer's configuration display—garbage in, garbage out!

Case 2 This is a case of simple myopic astigmatism. There are two possible procedures to use; Figures 9.31 and 9.32 illustrate them. The RL procedure has the advantage of not producing any coupling but is difficult for the beginner to perform, whereas the NT procedure could be done here. The author would perform the T procedure.

Case 3 This case is again one of simple myopic astigmatism but higher in degree. The author chose an NT procedure (Figure 9.33) and recommends that you do the same.

(*text continues on page 305*)

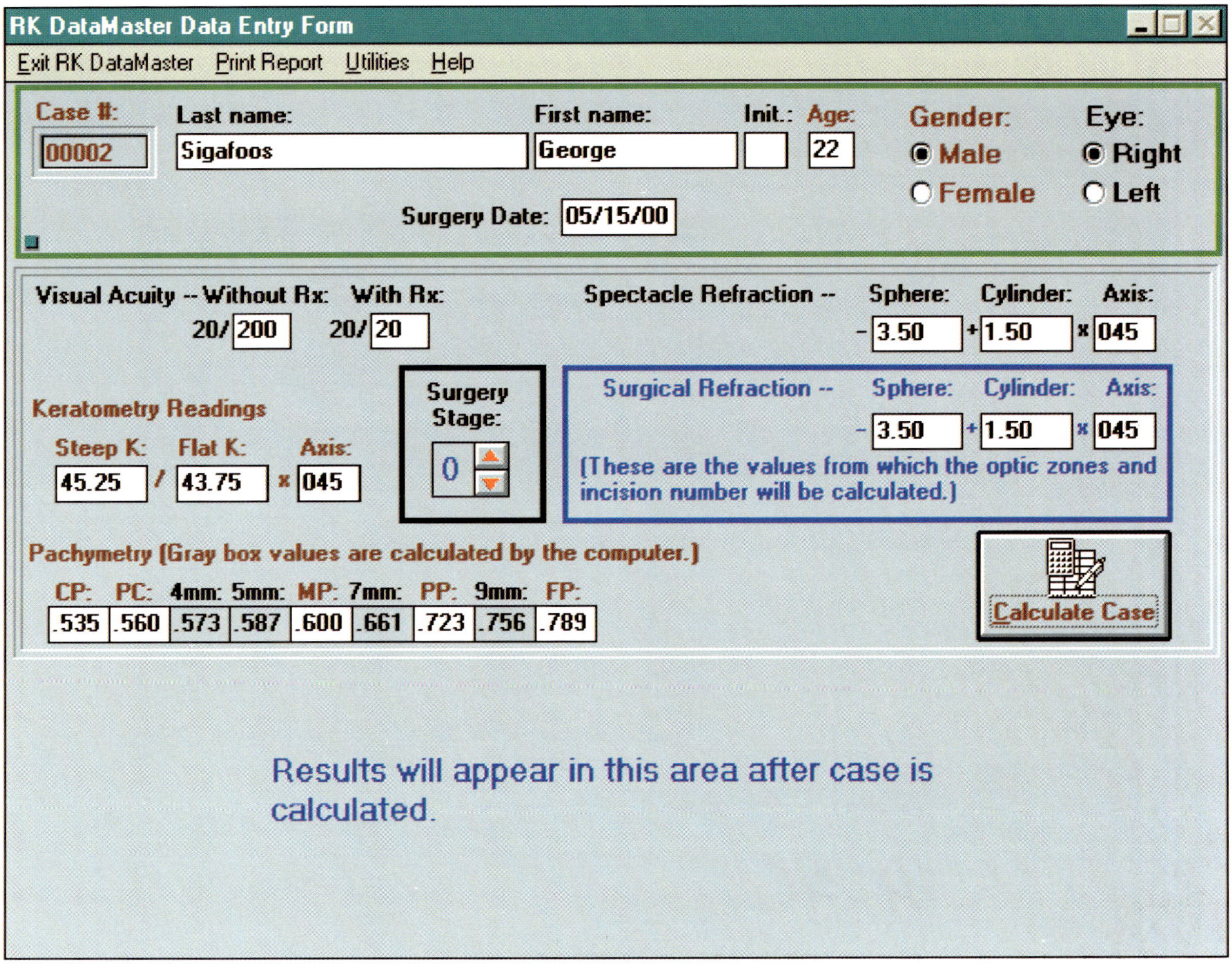

RK DataMaster Data Entry Form

Exit RK DataMaster Print Report Utilities Help

Case #: 00002 Last name: Sigafoos First name: George Init.: Age: 22 Gender: ◉ Male ○ Female Eye: ◉ Right ○ Left

Surgery Date: 05/15/00

Visual Acuity -- Without Rx: 20/200 With Rx: 20/20

Spectacle Refraction -- Sphere: -3.50 Cylinder: +1.50 Axis: ×045

Keratometry Readings
Steep K: 45.25 / Flat K: 43.75 Axis: ×045

Surgery Stage: 0

Surgical Refraction -- Sphere: -3.50 Cylinder: +1.50 Axis: ×045
(These are the values from which the optic zones and incision number will be calculated.)

Pachymetry (Gray box values are calculated by the computer.)

CP:	PC:	4mm:	5mm:	MP:	7mm:	PP:	9mm:	FP:
.535	.560	.573	.587	.600	.661	.723	.756	.789

Calculate Case

Results will appear in this area after case is calculated.

Fig. 9.27 Case 1. Data input sheet for a compound astigmatism patient, −3.50 + 1.50 × 45°.

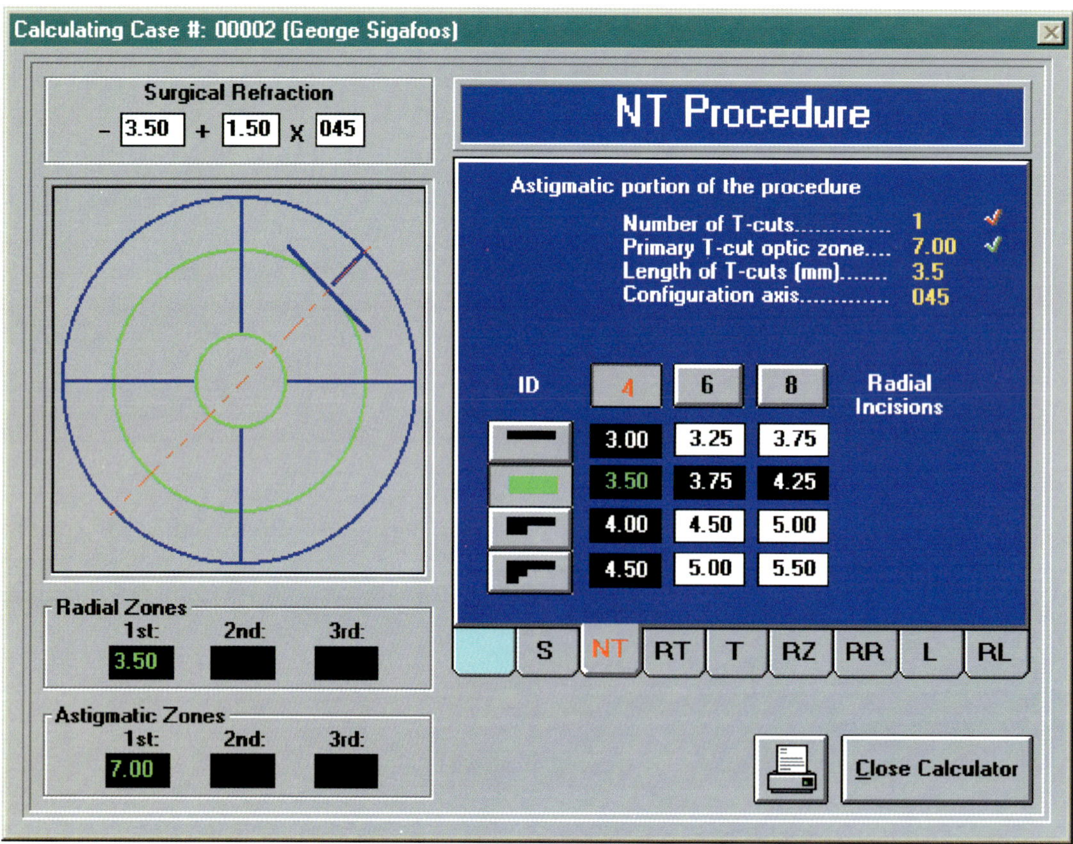

Fig. 9.28 Case 1. Surgical summary showing configuration and surgical parameters for an NT procedure.

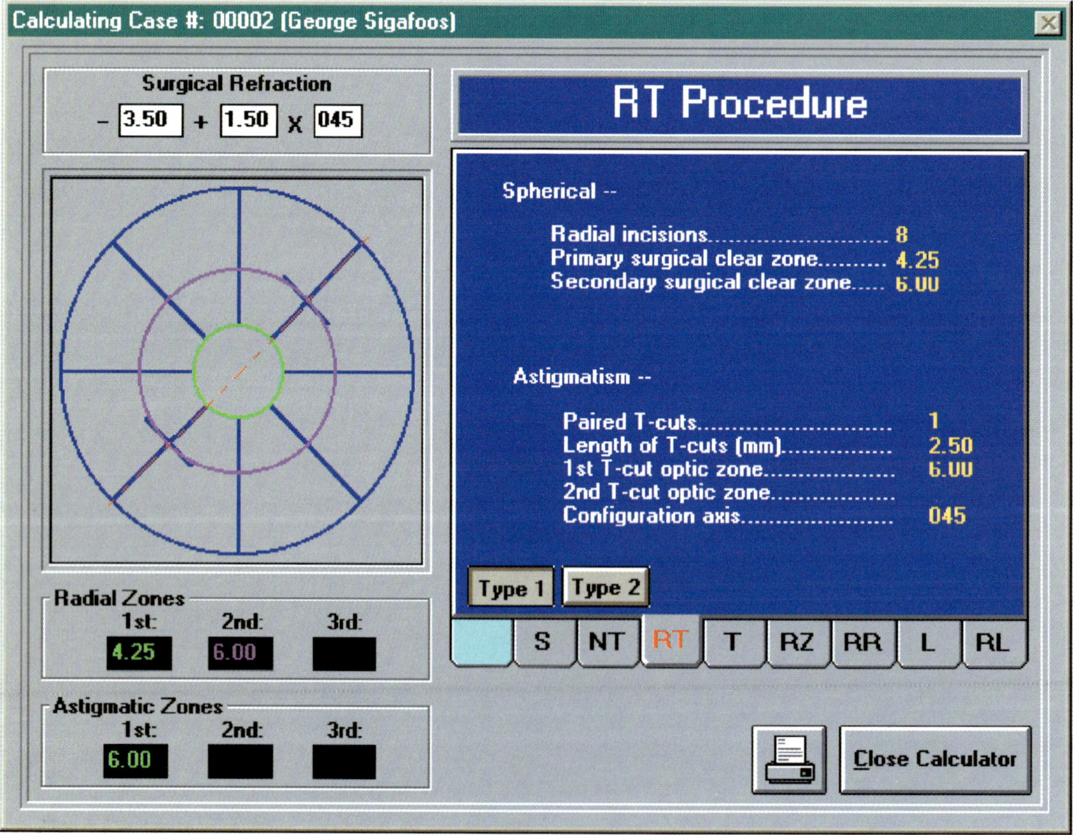

Fig. 9.29 Case 1. Surgical summary showing configuration and surgical parameters for an RT procedure.

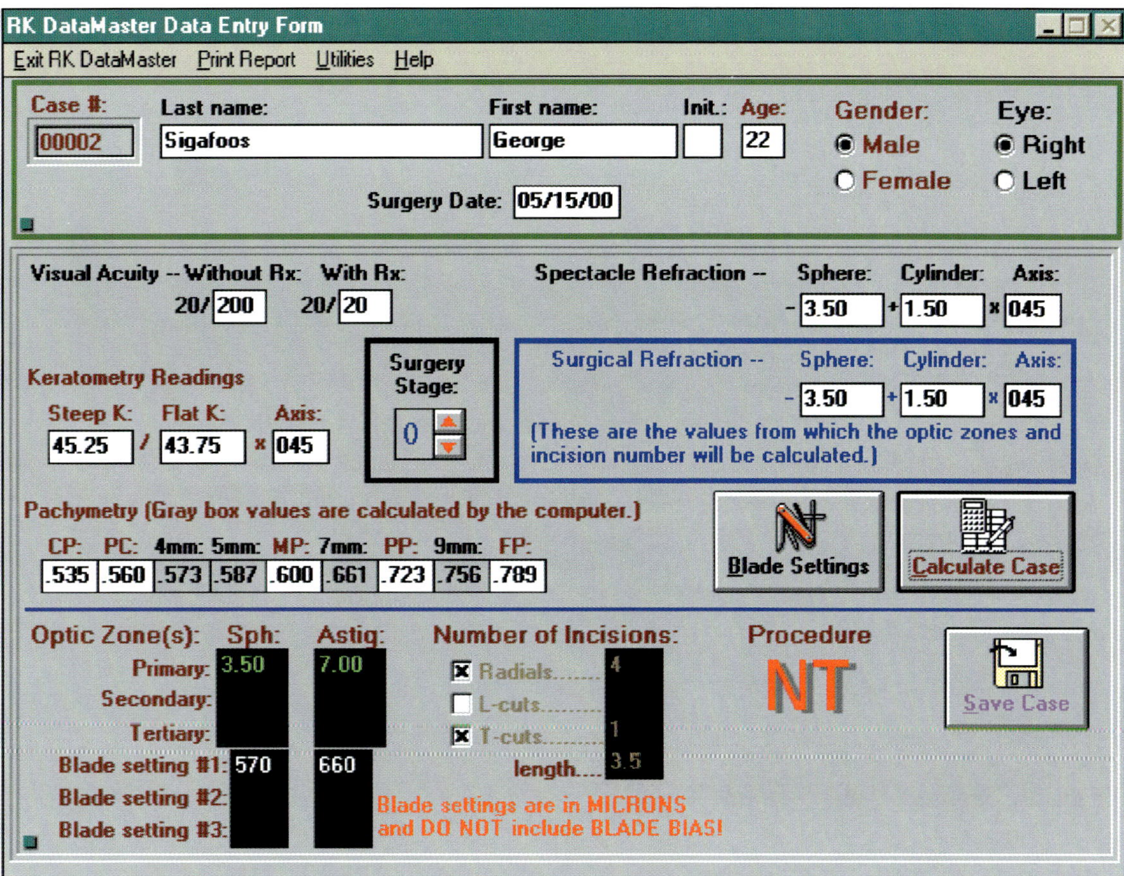

Fig. 9.30 Case 1. Case summary display.

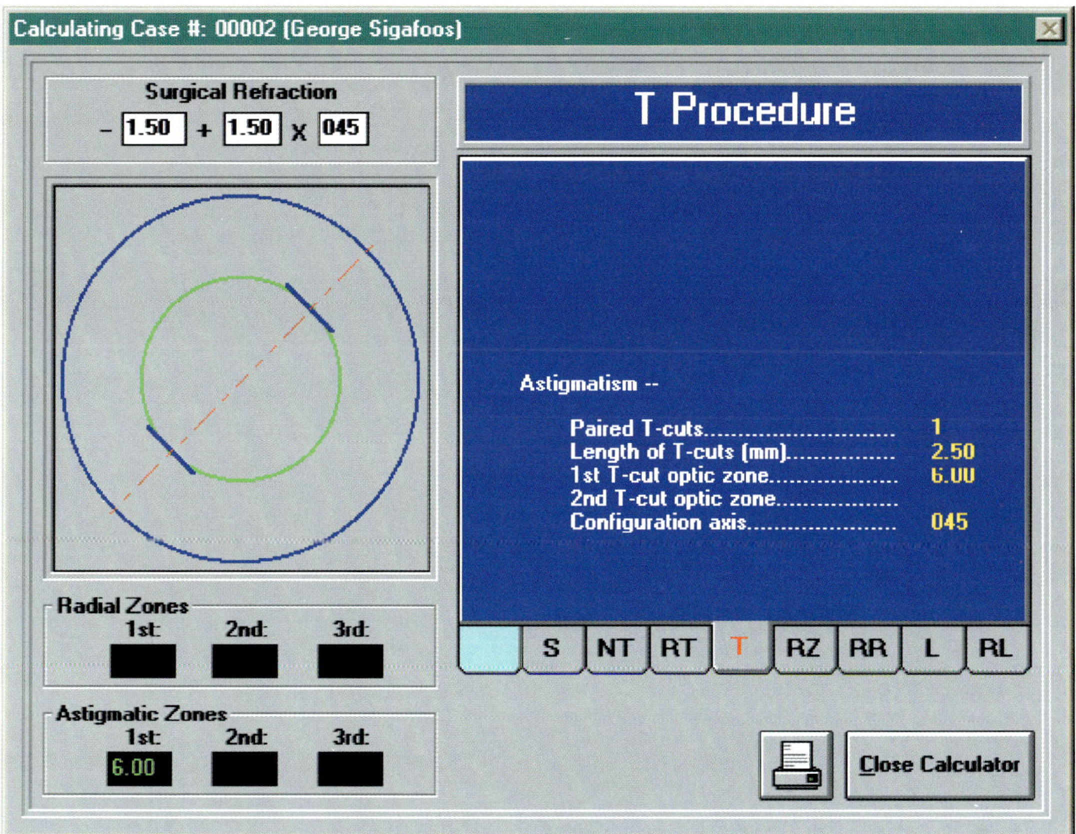

Fig. 9.31 Case 2. A case of simple myopic astigmatism, –1.50 + 1.50 × 45°, showing a T procedure.

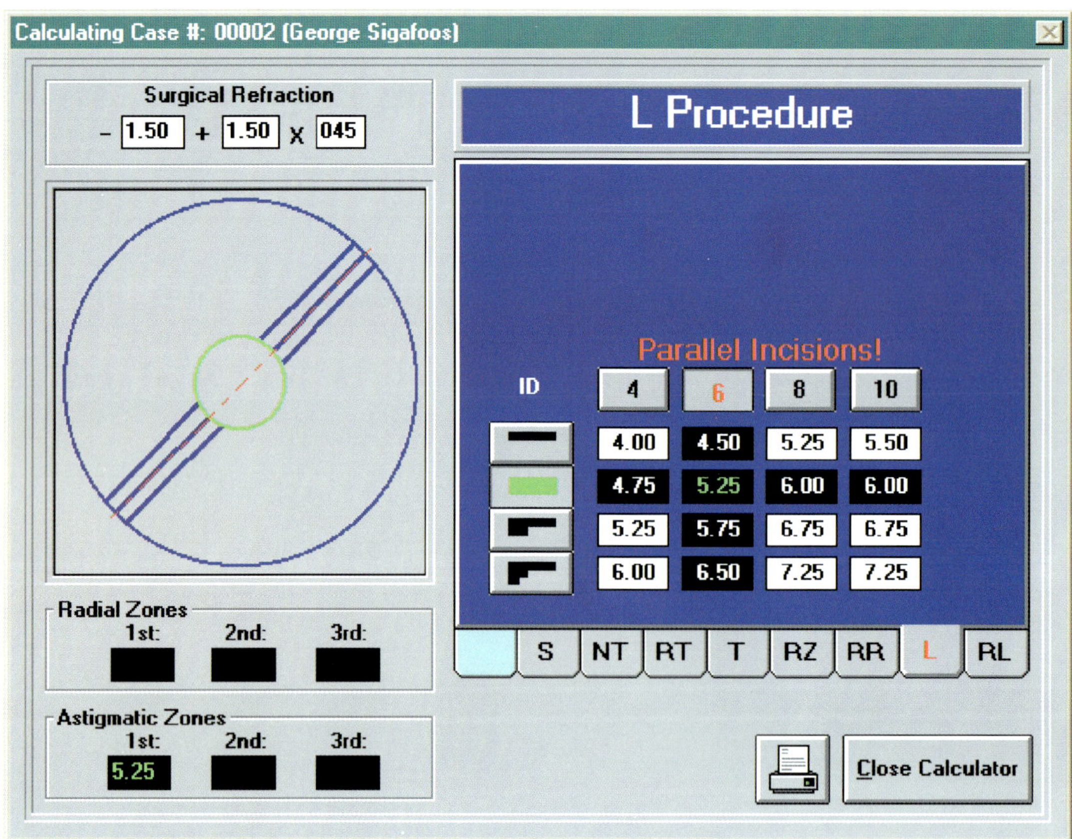

Fig. 9.32 Case 2. A case of simple myopic astigmatism, –1.50 + 1.50 × 45°, showing an RL procedure.

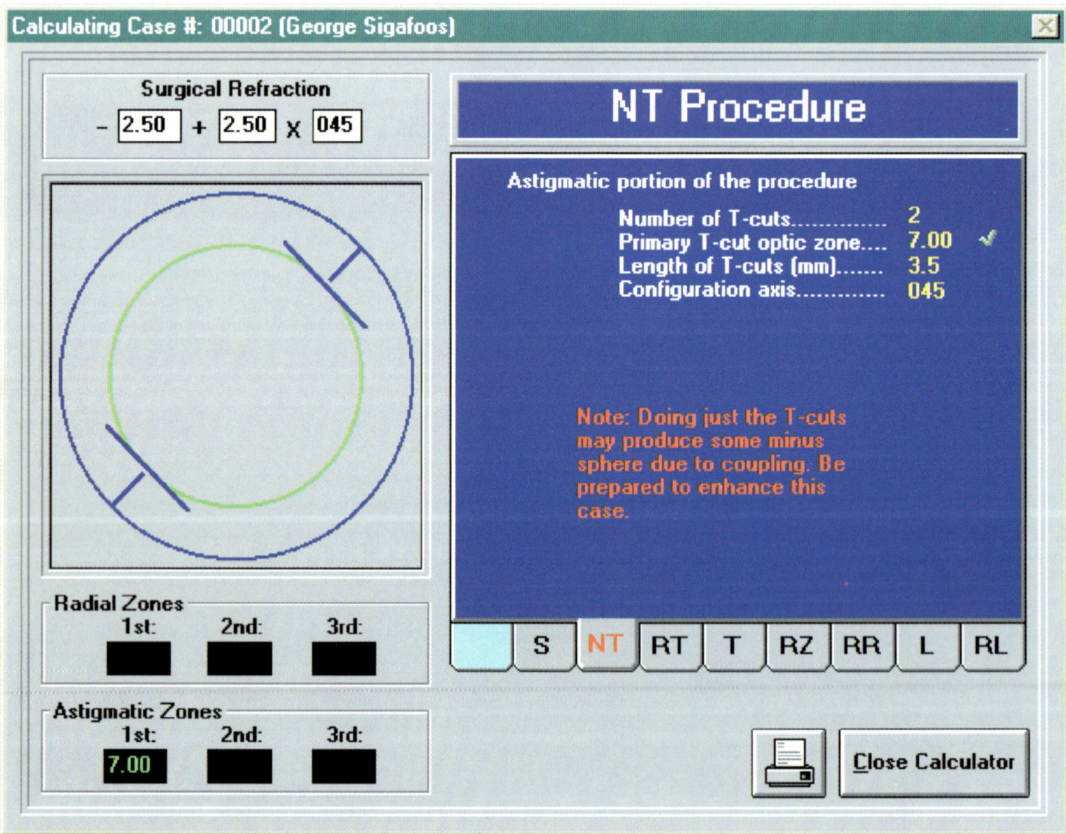

Fig. 9.33 Case 3. A case of simple myopic astigmatism, –2.50 + 2.50 × 45°, showing an NT procedure.

Case 4 This case pushes the envelope. It is a case of mixed astigmatism (Figure 9.34). The problem here is to deal with the plus cylinder. Here is where the RZ procedure shines (Figure 9.35). In this case, a modified RZ procedure is displayed using only two transverse incisions rather than the classic four on a side (see below). Using 3-mm T-cuts along with the semiradials in the steep (minus) meridian will produce sufficient coupling to steepen the flat (plus) meridian. Higher amounts of plus astigmatism (up to +4 D) can be steepened by using longer T-cuts. The computer will calculate and display the recommended lengths of these incisions.

Case 5 This is another case of compound astigmatism of higher degree. Again, the author chose the NT procedure (Figure 9.36).

Basic preparation caveats and methods

The surgery is performed under topical anesthesia in a premedicated patient. The anesthetic used is 0.5% tetracaine, followed by 1.0% nonbuffered tetracaine (Pontocaine)

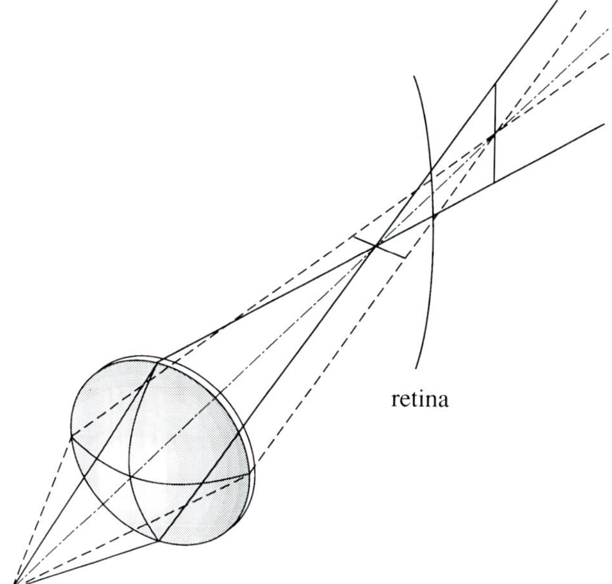

Fig. 9.34 Mixed astigmatism.

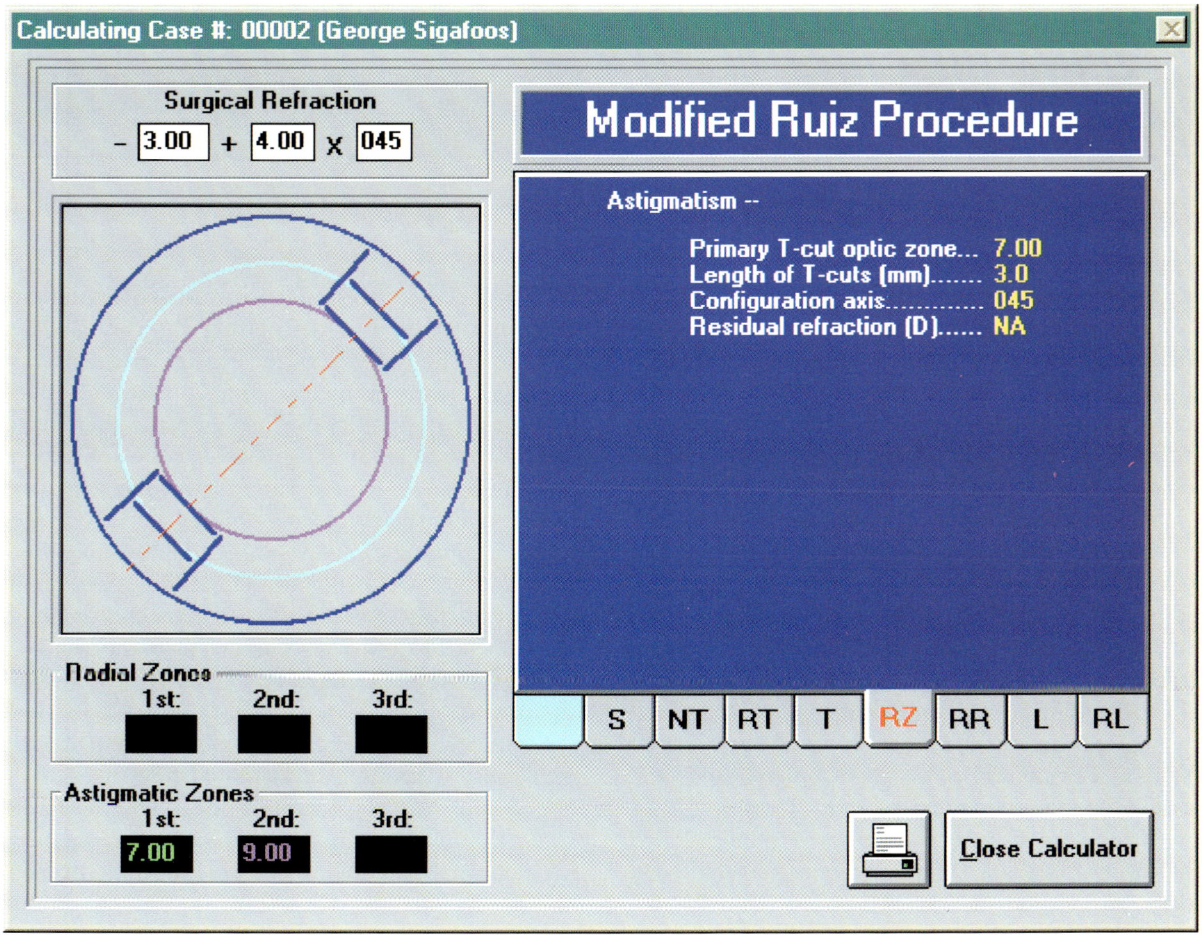

Calculating Case #: 00002 (George Sigafoos)

Surgical Refraction

– 3.00 + 4.00 x 045

Modified Ruiz Procedure

Astigmatism --

Primary T-cut optic zone... 7.00

Length of T-cuts (mm)....... 3.0

Configuration axis............. 045

Residual refraction (D)...... NA

Radial Zones

1st: 2nd: 3rd:

Astigmatic Zones

1st: 2nd: 3rd:

7.00 9.00

S NT RT T RZ RR L RL

Close Calculator

Fig. 9.35 Case 4. A case of mixed astigmatism, –3.00 + 4.00 × 45°, showing an RZ (Ruiz) procedure. This is the only configuration that can deal with this condition.

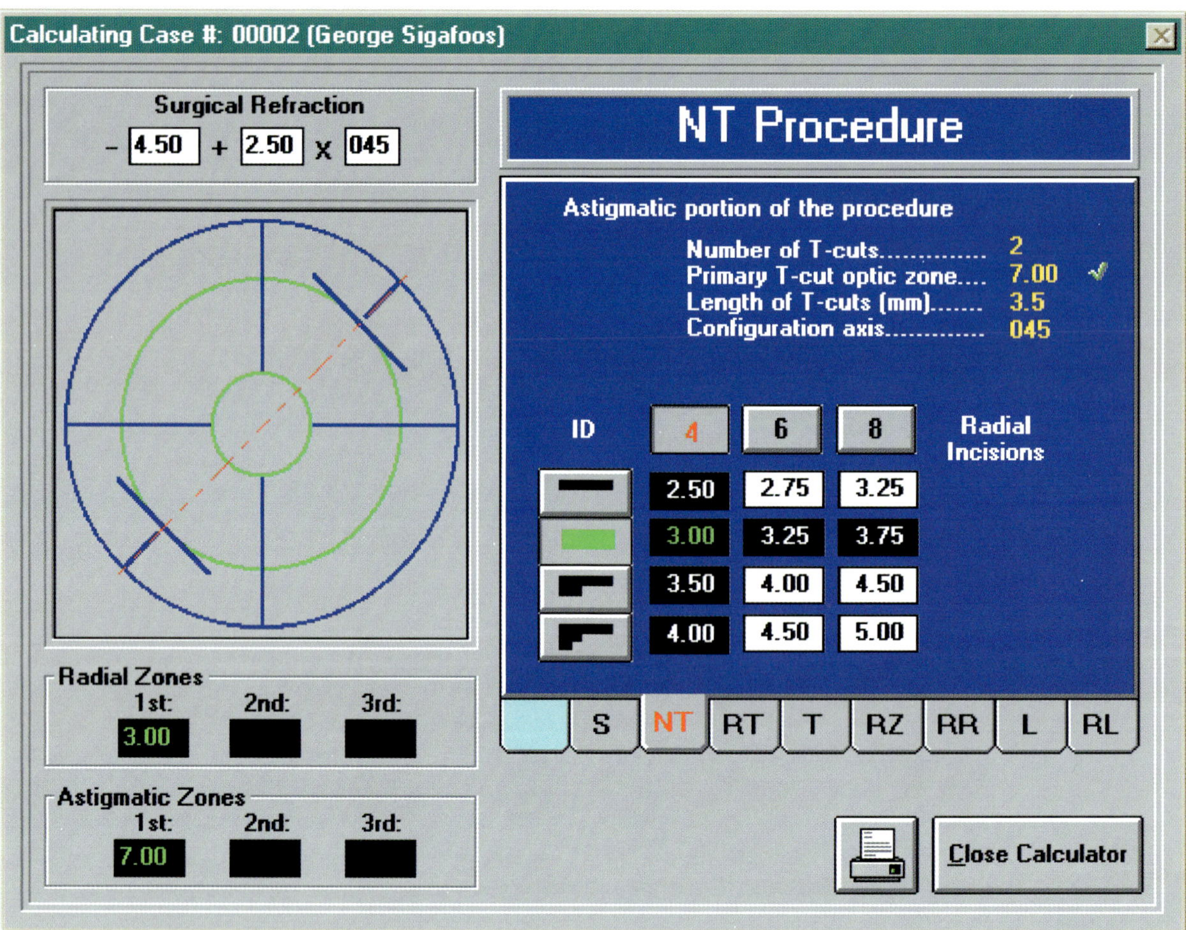

Fig. 9.36 Case 5. A case of compound myopic astigmatism, –4.50 + 2.50 × 45°, showing an NT procedure.

drops. Any additional anesthesia required during the surgery is provided with additional 0.5% tetracaine. Occasionally, for patients complaining of discomfort from fixation (particularly in second-stage cases), 4% aqueous Xylocaine solution is applied to the limbus on a cotton pledget or applicator. Sedation is provided by the administration of oral diazepam (Valium) in a dose appropriate to the patient. Generally, this will be 10 mg given approximately 30 to 40 minutes prior to surgery.

As in spherical cases, the workup is taped or otherwise placed next to the operating microscope in plain view of the surgeon. The patient is placed supine on the operating table, and the eye is prepped with full-strength Betadine Solution. (Betadine Prep is not recommended because it contains soap, which is extremely hard on the corneal epithelium.) The microscope is then centered and adjusted, and the surgeon scrubs up. At the Bores Eye Institute we have successfully used Septisol Skin Prep Foam for this purpose for years. Draping is done using the aperture drape supplied by the Alcon Company (no. 102320).

The blade used is a Bores double-edged unicrystalline sapphire or diamond blade (Katena K2-6513 or the KOI LeCut) mounted in the Katena (Bores) micrometer handle (K2-6505). Two other blades are available for this handle. One has a single 30° angled cutting edge designed for the American (Bores) method of incising from the optical zone (OZ) to the periphery—the K2-6501. The other has a vertical cutting edge for use with the Russian (Fyodorov) technique from the periphery toward the center, for reincising old wounds, and for making T-incisions—the K2-6511. The single-edge blades are recommended for the beginning surgeon because they are more durable. The blade is set using the XTAL-800 Bores Shadowgraphic blade gauge (see the section on instrumentation, above). The blade is overset according to the desired incisional depth coefficient and the blade type and style (see Chapter 8).

Establishing the optical center and marking the surgical zones are accomplished as usual. Keep in mind that it is frequently the case that the optical center is displaced somewhat nasally. This is normal. Do not position the incisions in the anatomic center of the cornea or induced oblique astigmatism will result.

Marking the steep meridian The correct *plus cylinder axis* is checked by referring to the workup sheet and speaking

(a)

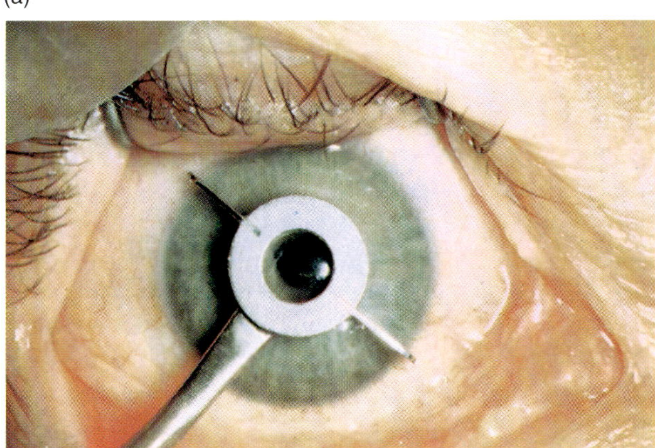

(b)

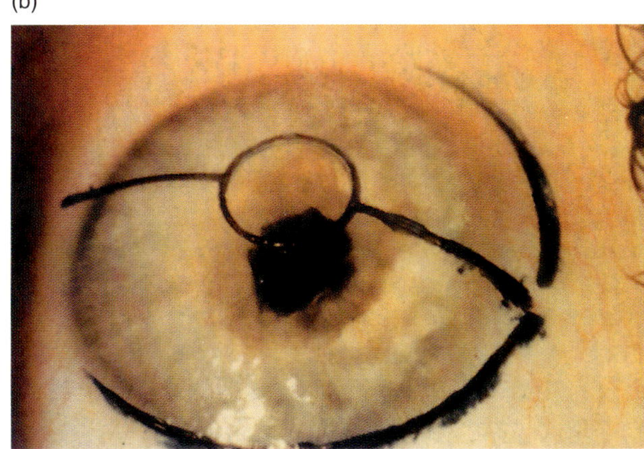

Fig. 9.37 (a) The axis is marked on the cornea after the visual axis is spotted. (b) It helps to use some dye on the marker.

the axis out loud to the circulating nurse or assistant. The axis is verified by the assistant by reference to the patient's original record. To avoid mistakes, only the specific patient's record is brought into the operating theater. Following this, the patient is again requested to fixate on the microscope light, and without holding the patient's eye, the axis of the cylinder is marked with the axis marker. To do this properly, some sort of reticle is necessary in the microscope eyepiece, or the Mendez protractor is required. Several products are available for this purpose (see the section on instrumentation, above).

Regardless of the device used, some method must be used to properly orient the surgeon with respect to the 12 and 6 o'clock positions of the patient's cornea. This is done readily by seating the patient at the slit lamp with the eye anesthetized and the head held vertical. With the patient looking straight ahead, the 12 and 6 o'clock positions are marked off on the cornea near the limbus. The occasions when recumbent cyclotorsion is sufficient to induce major error will be few, but the effort required to verify the axis is equally small. The patient is then taken into the operating theater.

The Bores axis marker is aligned with the chosen orientation device and pressed onto the corneal surface marking the plus axis (Figure 9.37). It is helpful to coat the blade of the marker with gentian violet or brilliant green first to make a more noticeable mark. This is most important in reoperations, where sometimes an old incision can be mistaken for the axis mark.

The primary OZ is then marked concentric to the fixation point—not to the pupil. This is extremely important because the pupil is not concentric with the optical axis of the eye. To verify the centration of the optic center (OC) with the OZ mark, the patient is asked to look away and then back at the light. Any discrepancy is corrected, and the midperipheral zone(s), if any, are then marked, and the surgery begins. In the absence of some sort of specialized centering device, the surgeon should close one eye when marking center, making the appropriate adjustments depending on which eye the surgeon is fixing with (see Chapter 8).

The basic surgical technique is similar to that used in marking for spherical myopia, but one additional factor has been introduced—axis of the plus cylinder. Because the OZ in astigmatism can be an ellipsoid (with a long and a short dimension), any elliptical marker must be applied to the cornea with the narrow side aligned with the plus cylinder axis (Figure 9.38).

If a third zone is to be used (i.e., the incision is to have three steps as in a patient needing a 2.5-mm incisional depth coefficient), this zone is usually marked after the first part of the incision is made. Experience has shown that marking this zone beforehand often finds the mark faded out before it is time to reference it. This is especially the case with beginning surgeons. If this happens

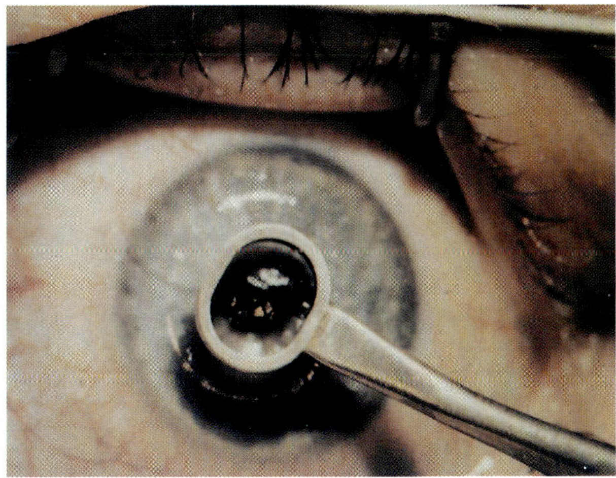

Fig. 9.38 The primary optical clear zone is then marked. Note, in the case of an elliptic zone, that the narrow portion is perpendicular to the axis.

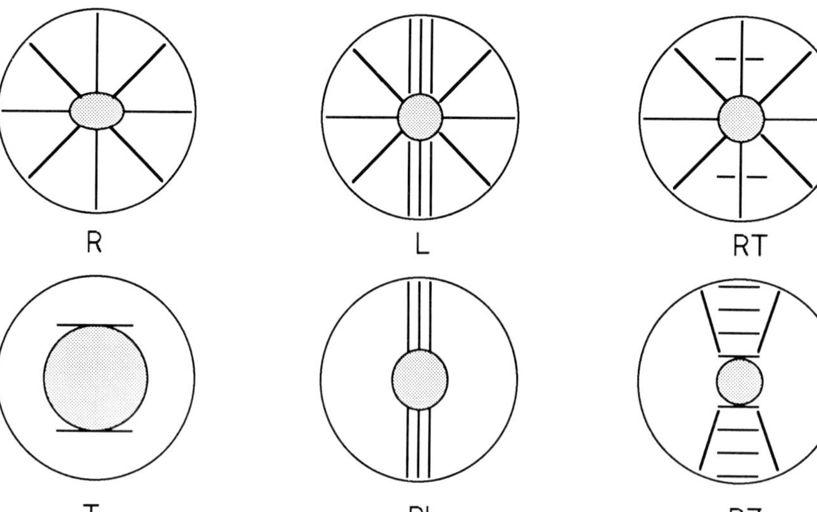

Fig. 9.39 Current incisional configurations for astigmatism.

to you and you do not choose to wait to make that last mark, use dye to make the mark last longer.

If a perforation is encountered, the surgery can be continued if extensive leakage does not occur and the eye does not get too soft; otherwise, the surgery must be abandoned. Further surgery should be postponed for at least 2 weeks. Most patients, even in the face of a severe leak (very rare), will have a deep AC the following morning. No attempt at free-hand deepening should be made in any case with a leak and a shallow or flat chamber. Suturing rarely should be necessary.

Patients receive a course of steroid antibiotic (Tobradex) drops twice daily for 2 weeks. Patients with perforations receive oral broad-spectrum antibiotics (Keflex) and mydriatics for an appropriate period of time. Patients are followed at 2, 4, 8, 12, 26, and 52 weeks when possible. Any necessary second-stage surgery is deferred for at least 6 months (see also Chapter 8).

Radial keratotomy—Surgical techniques and methods

Figure 9.39 illustrates the various incisional configurations associated with RK for correcting astigmatism. Some of these are no longer being used (see below).

Method R

Method R (for radial, formerly called method A; Figure 9.40) was the first configuration employed by Fyodorov. Its use is limited to up to 1.00 D of astigmatism. Generally speaking, however, this amount of astigmatism, especially if it is with-the-rule (W-T-R), is often eliminated by performing straightforward spherical surgery. It has been found that as much as 1.50 D of astigmatism can be lost in spherical surgery if the incisions are deep enough and there are 16 of them because of the tendency of the cornea to become spherical when incised. In this tendency the eye is obeying Pascal's law for fluid-filled spaces. It is probably this tendency of the eye that accounts for the low incidence of induced postoperative astigmatism seen in spherical surgery.

It has been the author's experience that patients tend to be a little more comfortable with a small amount of residual W-T-R astigmatism. Therefore, the need for this amount of W-T-R correction is not great, and thus the R procedure finds little application. It is useful in oblique or against-the-rule (A-T-R) astigmatism and can be employed by the neophyte to lower greater amounts of astigmatism safely (up to 2.0 D, in which case 0.5 or 1.0 D will be corrected).

This surgery is the simplest of all the configuration types to perform and is a good way for the new physician to get his or her "feet wet." The axis of the plus cylinder is marked on the cornea in the manner described previously. An elliptical OZ marker is used for the first or primary optical clear zone. If the computer calls for a secondary incision deepening or step, the OZ for that step is a standard zone marker—usually a 6-mm (sometimes a

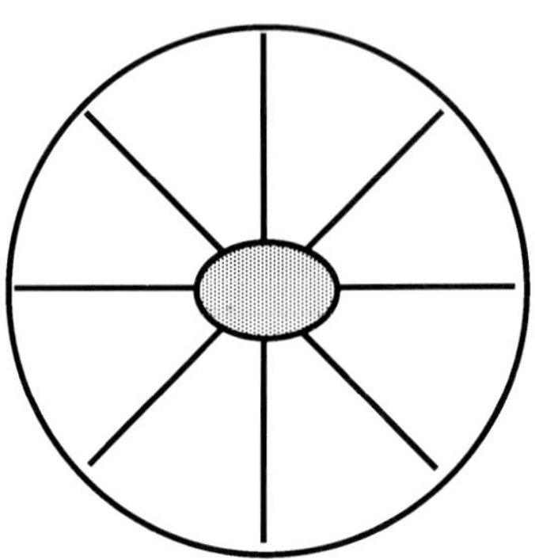

Fig. 9.40 R configuration.

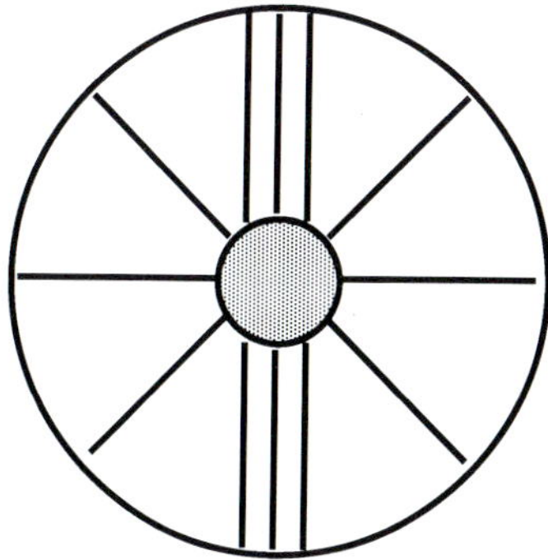

Fig. 9.41 RL configuration.

7-mm) marker. Rarely will an 8-mm marker be required. The necessary surgical zones are marked, and the incisions are made with a standard blade as if performing a simple operation for spherical myopia.

Method RL

By grouping the incisions into parallel bundles as in method RL (for radial-longitudinal, formerly method B; Figure 9.41), as much as 2.00 D can be corrected. This was the second astigmatic configuration Fyodorov tried. While technically more difficult to perform, it is more predictable and titratable than some other configurations. It also has the advantage that coupling is minimal. If you are concerned about overcorrection, this is the procedure of choice. The amount of astigmatic correction is controlled not only by the length of the incisions but also by the number of incisions made.

OZ marking resembles that of the R procedure (although it is possible to use a plain spherical marker for the primary OZ in simple myopic astigmatism). Secondary zones are also marked in the same manner. It is helpful to use some sort of parallel marker to help with the incision spacing. The special parallel markers from Katena Instrument Company (K3-8050, K3-8052) fit the bill. The use of a limbus-to-limbus fixation forceps (Katena K5-3280) can make performing this procedure much easier. Figures 9.42 through 9.48 illustrate the manner in which this surgery is performed—in this instance, in a patient with compound myopic astigmatism. Note that the parallel incisions are all made first and that all the incisions are made on one side at a time. Note also that the incisions are made from the inside of the pattern out. This is important. Do not make two incisions and then try to put one in between. This is much like trying to thin slice a piece of ham already cut from the butt—the tissue is too unstable. Your incision inevitably will run into one or the other of the preceding ones. Needless to say, a very sharp blade is mandatory for this technique to succeed. Neither the L nor the RL configuration is recommended for post-MKM/LASIK astigmatism for the reason that delamination of the lenticule could easily occur between incisions.

Methods L and T

Methods L (longitudinal) and T (transverse; Figure 9.49) produce about the same amount of astigmatic correction—1.75 D, but method T has a greater range of variance. Furthermore, T-incisions affect both the major and minor meridians, so their lengths must be controlled carefully (Figures 9.50 through 9.52). The parallel cuts are made in the manner described above. The T-incisions will be discussed below (under the RT procedure).

Method TR

Method TR (transverse-radial; Figure 9.53) was the third method employed by Fyodorov for myopic astigmatism

(text continues on page 312)

(a)

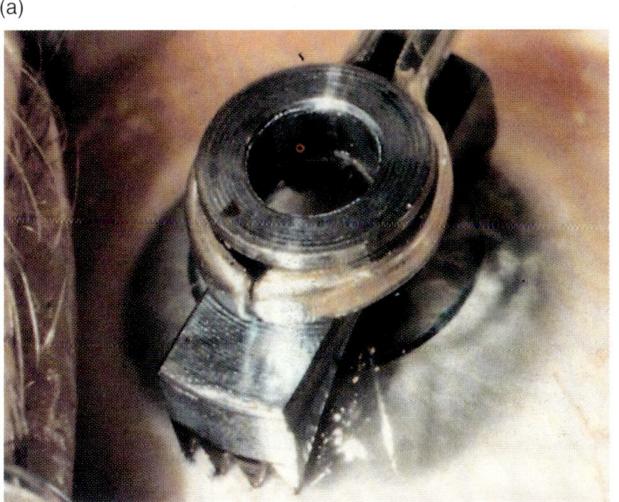

(b)

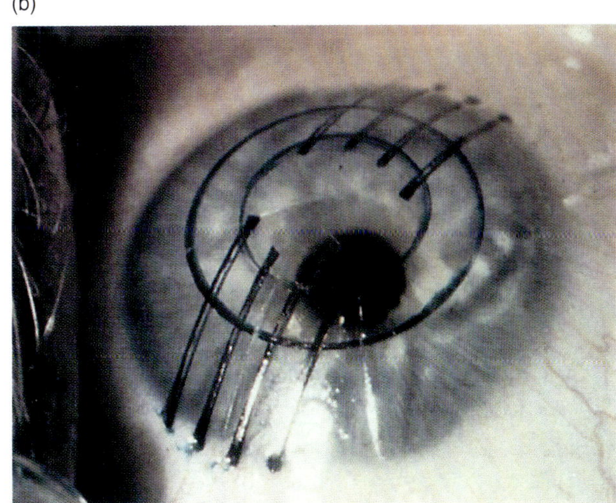

Fig. 9.42 (a) The parallel incision positions are marked with a special marker after the optical zones; (b) dye applied to the markers will help.

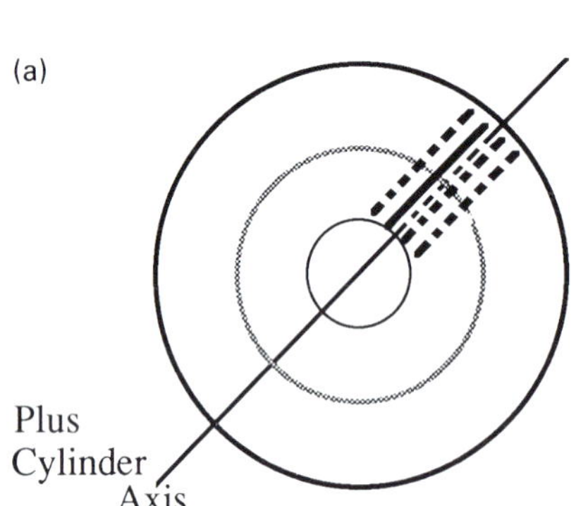

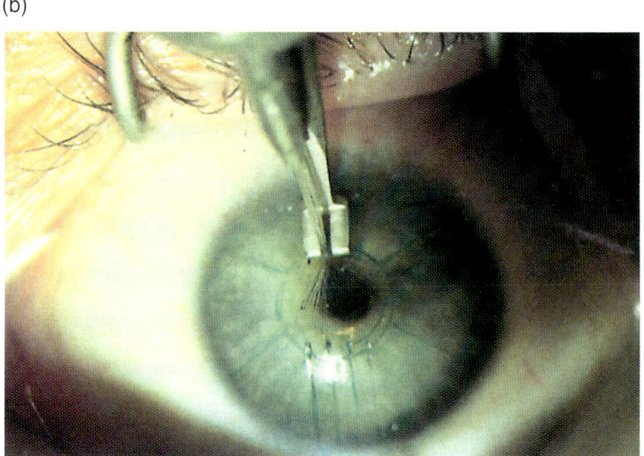

Fig. 9.43 (a,b) RL procedure—first incision.

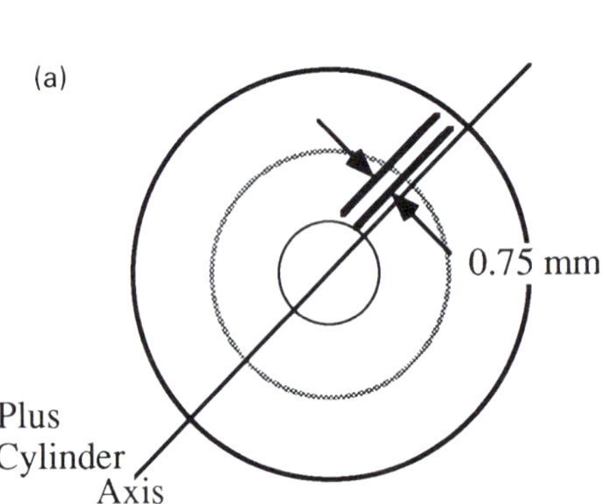

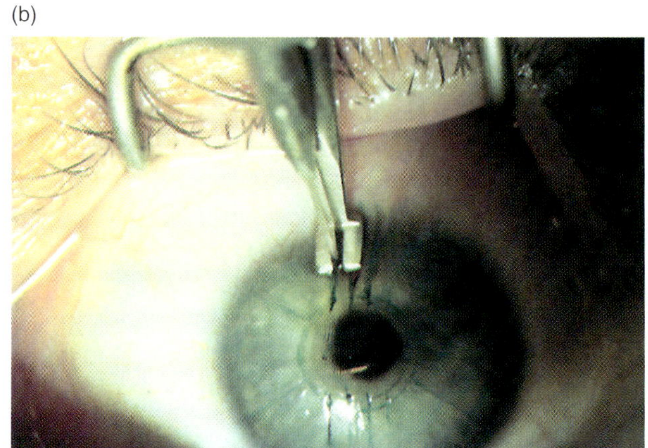

Fig. 9.44 (a,b) RL procedure—second incision.

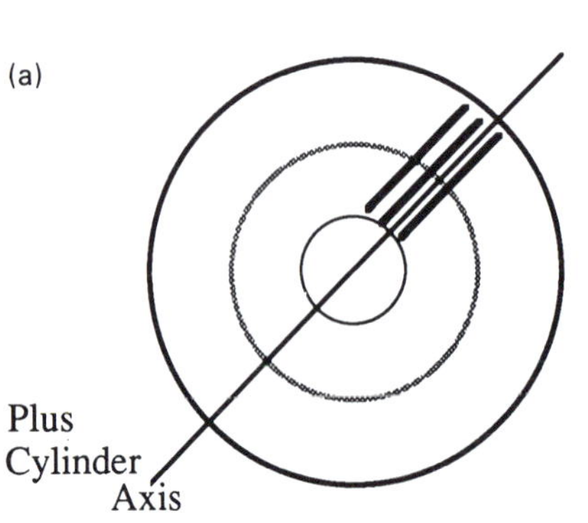

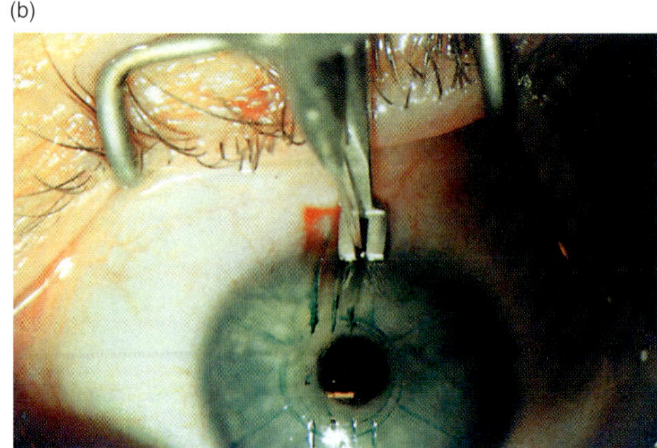

Fig. 9.45 (a,b) RL Procedure—third incision.

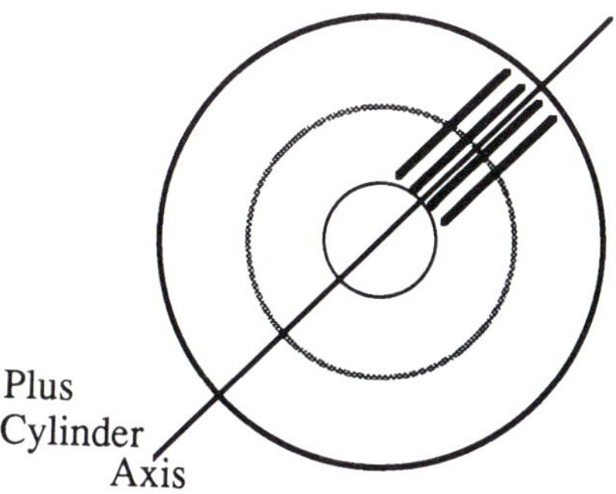

Fig. 9.46 RL procedure—fourth incision.

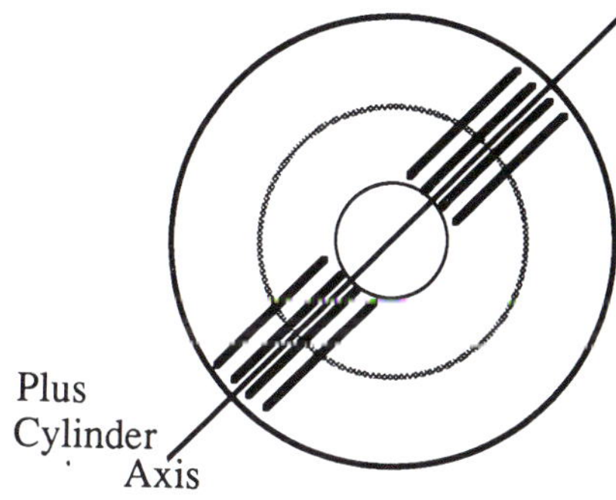

Fig. 9.47 RL procedure—parallel incisions complete.

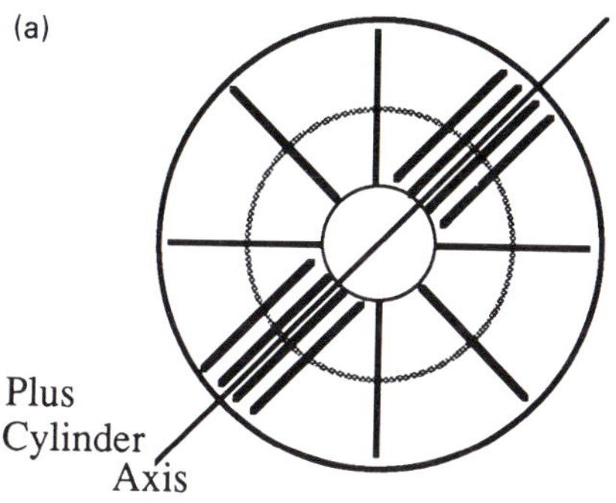

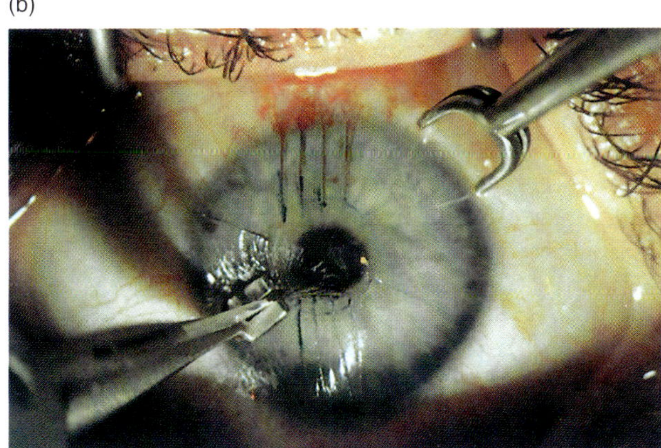

Fig. 9.48 (a, b) RL procedure—radial incisions added.

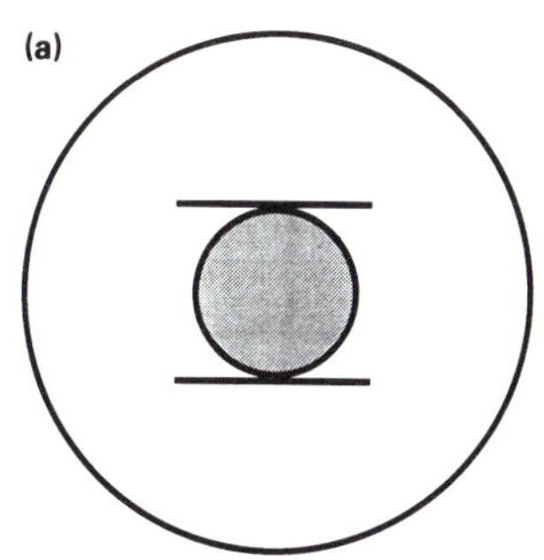

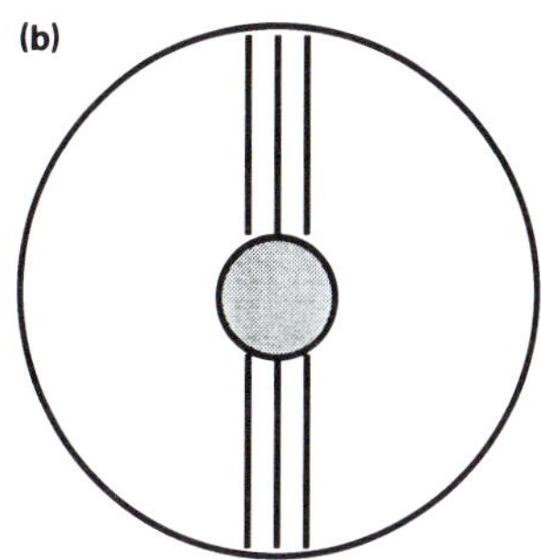

Fig. 9.49 (a) T configuration, (b) L configuration.

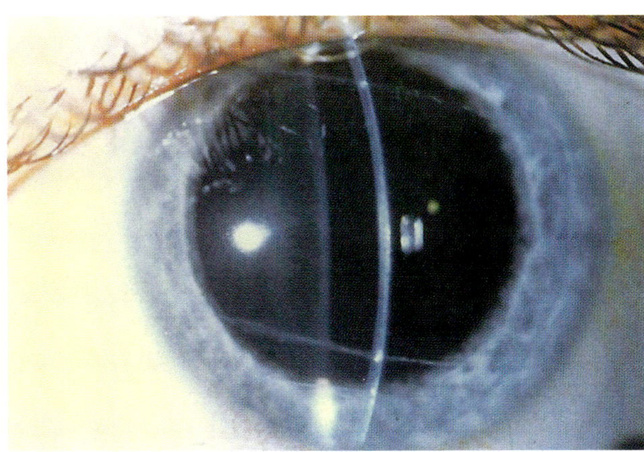

Fig. 9.50 T-incisions.

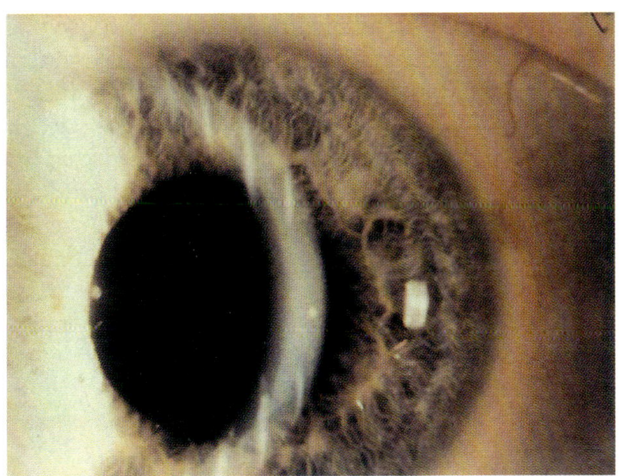

Fig. 9.51 L-incisions.

(a)

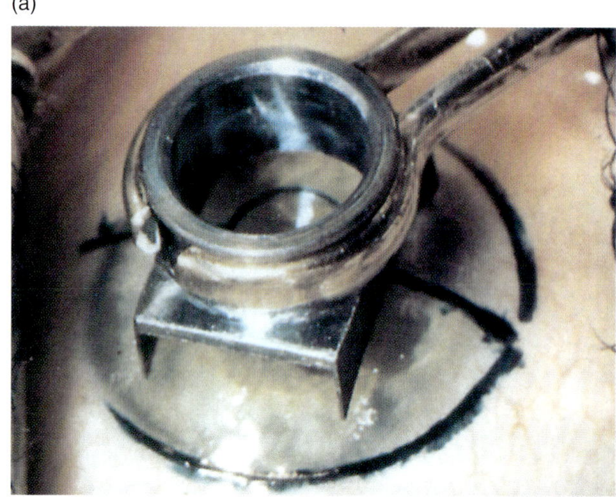

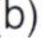

(b)

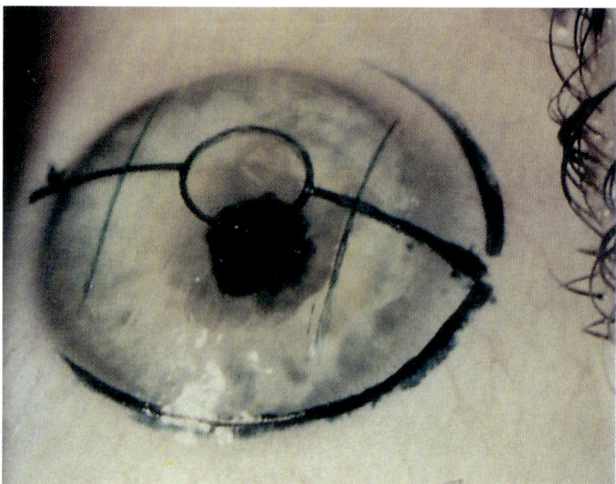

(c)

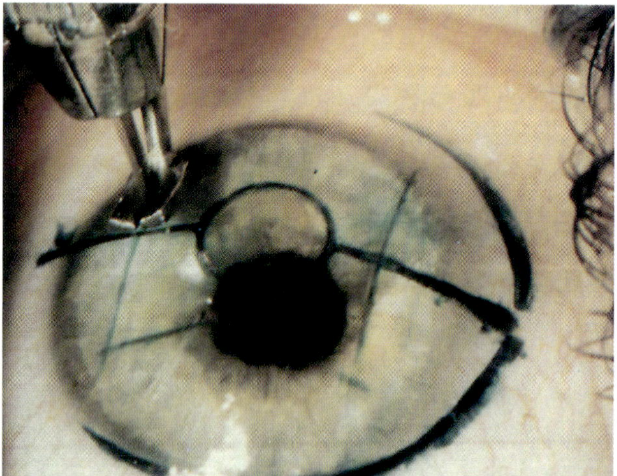

Fig. 9.52 Making T-incisions: (a) marking; (b) marks; (c) incision making.

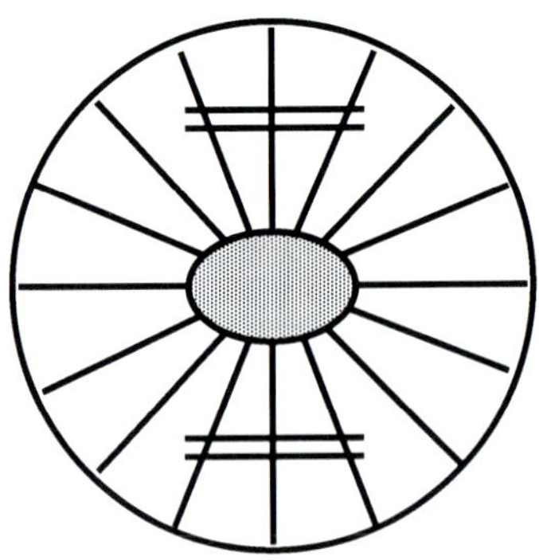

Fig. 9.53 TR configuration.

and was found to correct as much as 6.00 D. However, it is extremely difficult to perform, tends to produce isolated columns of corneal tissue that are very unstable, and thus is not recommended but is shown for historical reasons. Furthermore, it disobeys the *rule of crossing incisions.* The areas of incisional intersection are a source of difficulty, producing wide scars and longer-lasting corneal instability (Figure 9.54; see also Chapter 15). If the T portion is made secondarily (after 6 months), the intersection melting is much less (Figure 9.55). This technique and method TL have been supplanted by the RT method (see below).

Method TL

The same objection can be raised for method TL (transverse-longitudinal; Figure 9.56) as for the TR method. Crossing of incisions is to be avoided as much as possible. If incisions must be crossed, the surgery should be planned in two stages and at least 6 months allowed to elapse between stages (Figures 9.57 and 9.58). There are

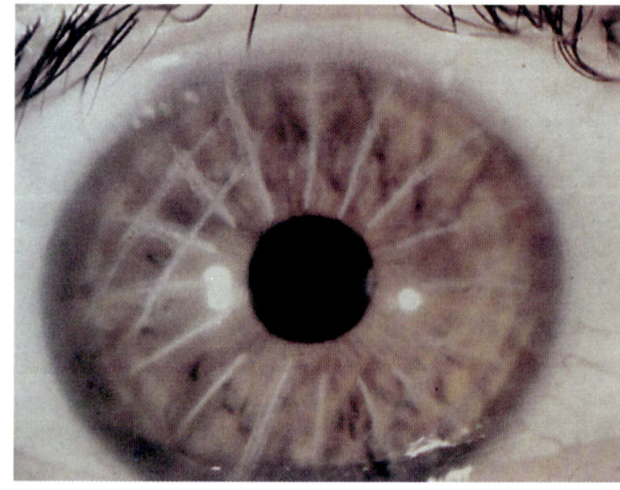

Fig. 9.54 Note wide scars at the incisional intersections.

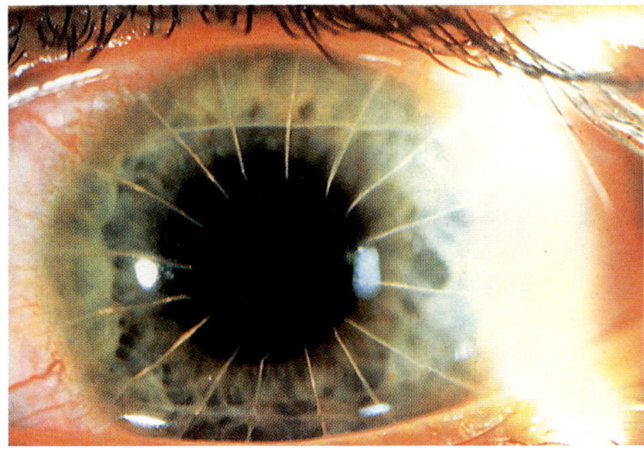

Fig. 9.55 If the T-incisions are made when the radials are partially healed, the intersection scarring is minimal.

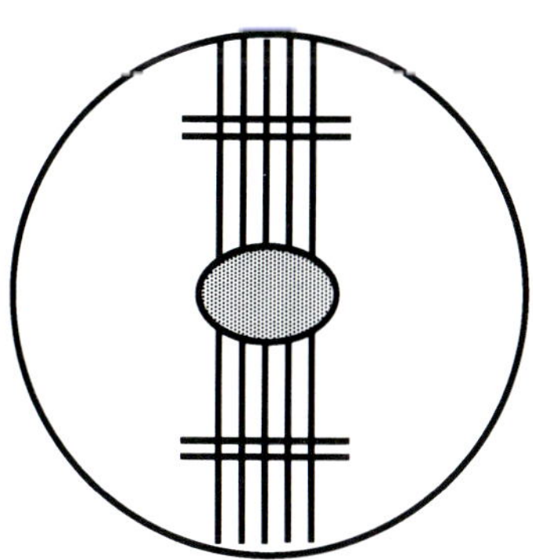

Fig. 9.56 TL configuration.

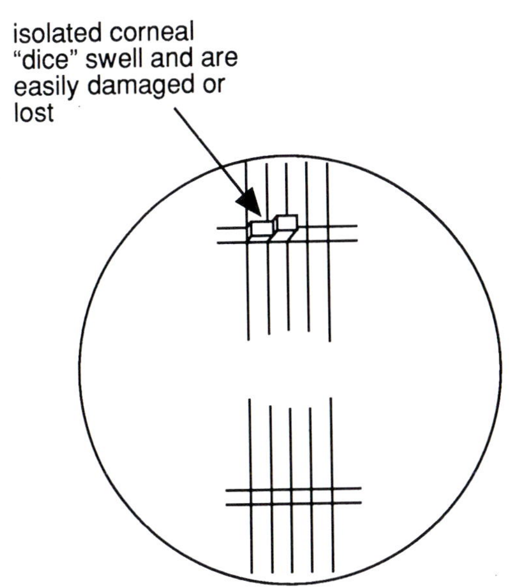

Fig. 9.57 Corneal "dice"—loose and isolated elements of stroma.

(a)

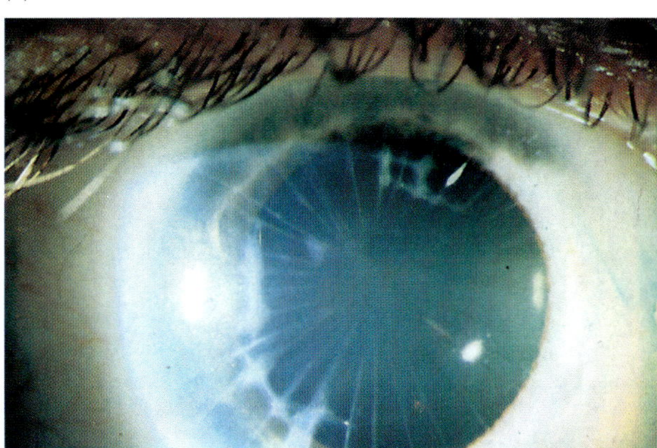

(b)

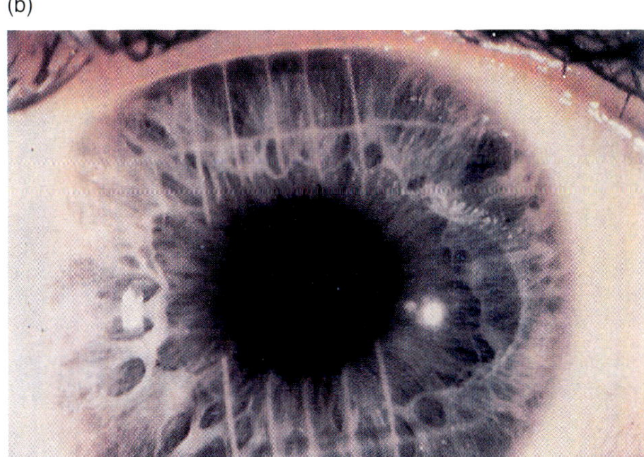

Fig. 9.58 (a) Wide intersection scars are the hallmark of T-incisions made too early. (b) Less scarring is encountered if the T's are made later.

currently much better methods to obtain the same results, so these configurations are not recommended.

Method RT

Method RT (radial-transverse; Figure 9.59), with radial incisions combined with nonjoining or interrupted T-cuts, is used widely in cases of compound myopic astigmatism and is recommended for astigmatism up to and including –2.25 D. There are numerous variations on this basic theme; however, the author uses the configuration shown, and this is the one accommodated in RK Data-Master. It is not possible to use standard look-up tables with this surgery. The computer program has to take into account the induced steepening of the flatter meridian and adjusts the spherical OZ component accordingly.

This technique is derived from the TR procedure but differs in certain important details. To avoid confusion with the earlier method, it has been designated the RT

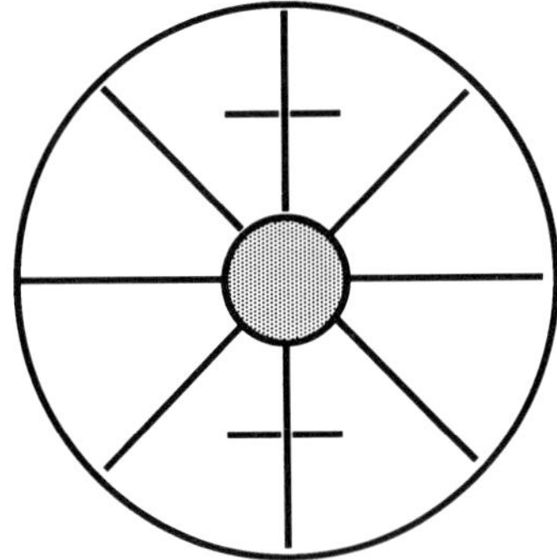

Fig. 9.59 RT configuration.

procedure (radial-transverse). The amount of associated sphere can be any amount up to the limit correctable by eight incisions.

There are certain caveats that you should be aware of with this technique. First, the depths of the T-incisions are expected to be no greater than 85% of the corneal thickness. Note that this is somewhat shallower than usually called for in RK. It has been shown convincingly that deeper transverse incisions are prone to cause progressive flattening of the meridian and some increase in curvature in the opposite axis (see the discussion under the Ruiz procedure for further details). In addition, the radial incisions are always stepped (or deepened) at 6 or 7 mm. The T-incisions are exactly 2.5 mm in length overall and do not join or cross the radials. Usually only one set of paired transverse (T) incisions is made, but in some cases there may be two. Figure 9.60 shows a typical computer display for this procedure. This procedure is definitely not for the beginner.

The procedure is basically an eight-incision spherical surgery with the addition of the T-incisions. The radial incisions should all be made *before* the T-cuts, beginning with the pair on-axis, followed by the pair at 90° to those, and then the remainder follow. The T-cut marks follow *tangential* to the T-cut OZ and centered on the axial incision. Make sure that these marks are perpendicular to the astigmatism axis. The use of brilliant green dye applied to the markers can be helpful here.

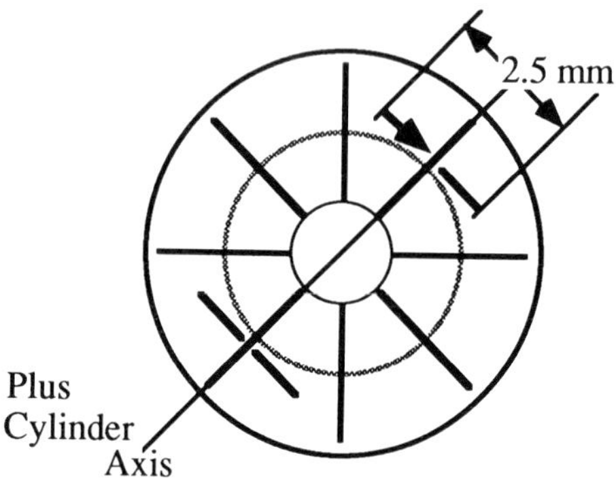

Fig. 9.60 RT procedure.

The eye is fixated employing wide forceps applied across the limbus perpendicular to the T-cuts. A vertical blade is then inserted into the cornea at the end of the T-mark, and the incision is made *toward the radial* (Figure 9.61). Making the incision away from the radial, while seemingly easier, does not work and causes the tissue to separate at the bottom of the radial. Use high magnification and stop just short of entering the radial. A small bridge of tissue should remain. It is not always possible to stop in time even with the most skilled hands. However, experience will lower the incidence of radial incision entry. The edge of the radial tends to roll under the footplate of the knife. When you see this occurring, stop. A very sharp blade does not require as much pressure to be applied, and this rolling movement is therefore minimized, making it easier to see and control the endpoint. It is for this reason that the author suggests that surgeons put aside a double-edged blade to be used *only* for T-cuts.

The radial incisions always have a step; therefore, a "dipstick" of appropriate size is inserted into each wound, and the uniformity of each incision is gauged. Any unsatisfactory incisions are recut at this time. Occasionally, the beginnings and ends of stepped incisions will override one another. This overriding connection must be separated for best effect (see Chapter 8). Each wound is then *gently* irrigated with balanced salt solution.

Method RZ (Ruiz procedure)

Method RZ (Ruiz or trapezoidal) is very useful for simple myopic or mixed astigmatism in amounts of –2.50 D and above (Figure 9.62). It can be combined with six radial incisions (method RR), to correct mixed myopic or compound astigmatism and is quite predictable and stable. Difficulties reported with this surgery are often due to the fact that the incisions either are made deeper than 85% or are too long (or both).

The RZ method of astigmatic correction combines semiradial and tangential incisions to flatten the steepest meridian of the cornea (Figure 9.63). The technique was introduced by Luis Antonio Ruiz, of the Clinica Barraquer, Bogota, Colombia, and controls different degrees of astigmatism by varying the size of the OZ and the length of the transverse corneal incisions. The OZs used vary from 2.75 to 5.00 mm, and the length of the transverse incisions varies from 1.5 to 5.00 mm. Up to 8 D of cylinder has been corrected by this method.

This surgery can induce myopic astigmatism in the opposite axis very handily. This fact makes it very useful in mixed myopic astigmatism. For example, –2.00 + 4.00 × 90° (+2.00 – 4.00 × 180°), can be converted to plano by judicious lengthening of the T-cuts (see the section on decision making, above).

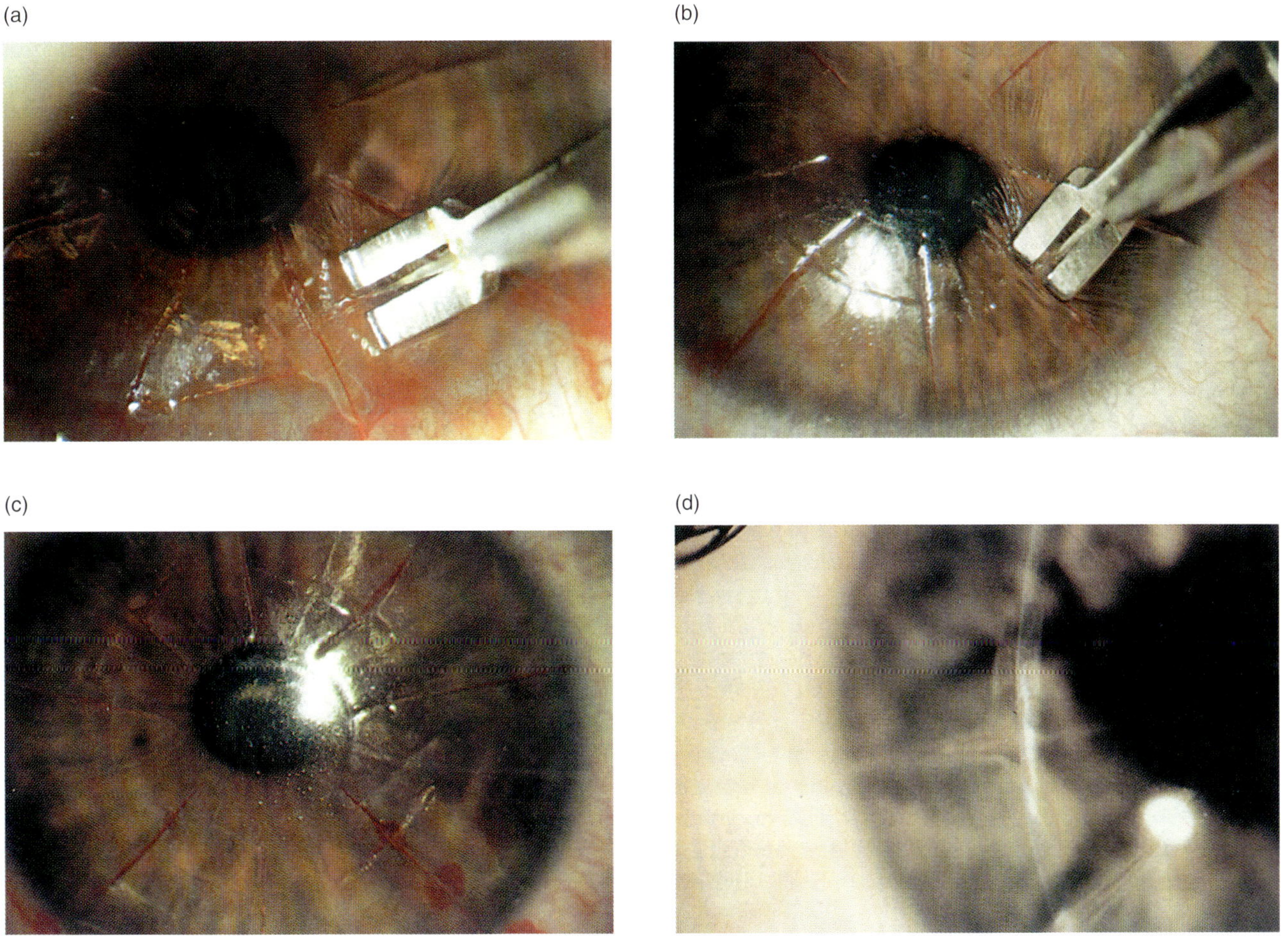

(a) (b)

(c) (d)

Fig. 9.61 (a–c) Note that the T-cuts are made *toward* the radial, stopping just short of intersection. (d) Entering the T-cut can produce wide gaping with associated wide scars and possible irregular astigmatism due to uneven healing.

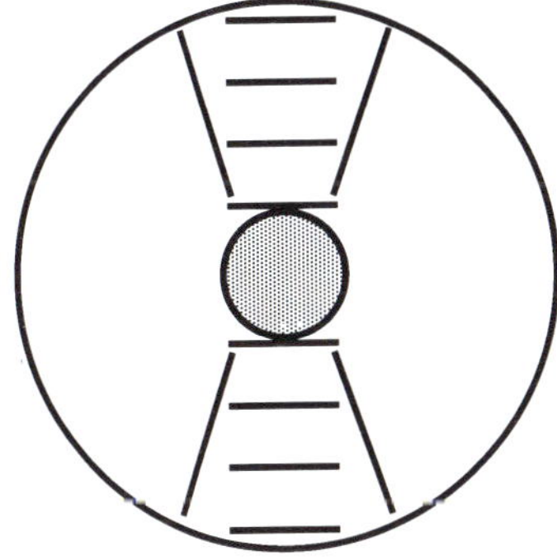

Fig. 9.62 RZ configuration.

There is an aspect to this technique that must be borne carefully in mind: The length of the incision not only affects the flattening in the steep axis, but it also affects the opposite axis by steepening its curvature (the *rule of coupling*). This can be very dangerous—it also can be very useful. If the length of the transverse component is not

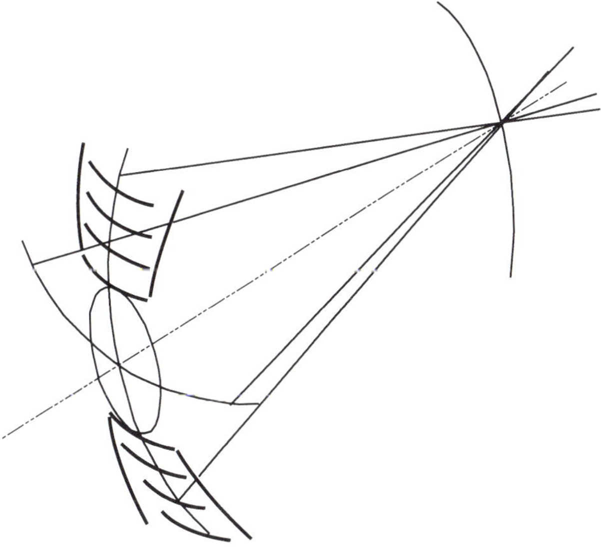

Fig. 9.63 Ruiz pattern incisions on the cornea.

carefully chosen and controlled, it is possible to actually reverse the astigmatism. By taking care and using computer analysis of the preoperative data, it is possible to completely eliminate mixed astigmatism, however. In fact, the RZ procedure is the only technique currently available that can do so in a predictable manner.

The RZ incision flattens the steeper meridian in an approximate ratio of 6:1. Troutman found that his wedge resection steepened the flatter meridian in a 2:1 ratio. That is, for every 2 D of flattening that occurred in the steeper meridian, 1 D of steepening was induced in the flatter meridian. An excellent discussion of this relationship has been detailed by Nordan and, with his permission, is abstracted below.

Wedge versus Ruiz

Consider a theoretical patient model with A-T-R astigmatism—that is, astigmatism at 180°. The vertical meridian (90°) will be flatter than the horizontal meridian (180°). If preoperative K-readings are represented by *H* and *V*, where *H* is the reading in the horizontal meridian and *V* the reading in the vertical meridian, the total amount of astigmatism *A* is represented by $H-V$.

X represents the dioptric change in the steepest meridian of a cornea undergoing either an RZ procedure or a wedge resection. If the astigmatism is fully corrected by the surgery, then $A=0$. According to Troutman, a wedge resection that increases the K-reading of the flatter meridian *V* by *X* will decrease the K-reading for the steeper meridian *H* by $X/2$ [36]. Therefore, in a wedge resection,

$$\left(H - \frac{X}{2}\right) - (V + X) = 0$$

$$\left(steep - \frac{X}{2}\right) - (flat + X) = 0$$

$$2H - X - 2V - 2X = 0$$

$$2(H - V) = 3X$$

$$X = \tfrac{2}{3}(H - V)$$

$$X = \tfrac{2}{3}A \quad (\text{because } A = H - V)$$

In this model of A-T-R astigmatism, the vertical meridian *V* is steepened by two-thirds of the amount of the original astigmatism *A*. The horizontal meridian *H* is therefore flattened by one-third of the original astigmatism. It should be noted that if performed properly, the wedge resection will steepen the meridian in which it is made—but only up to a certain point. Beyond this point, a wedge resection actually will flatten the meridian because of the effect of excessive tissue removal.

In the RZ procedure, $A=0$ if the astigmatism is totally corrected as well. According to data obtained from patients in whom the surgery has been performed, the RZ procedure decreases the K-reading of the steeper meridian *H* by *X* and increases the K-reading of the flatter meridian *V* by $X/5$. Therefore, in the RZ procedure,

$$(H - X) - \left(V + \frac{X}{5}\right) = 0$$

$$5(H - V) = 6X$$

$$X = \tfrac{5}{6}(H - V)$$

$$X = \frac{5}{6}A \quad \left(or\ \frac{5A}{6}\right)$$

Thus the steep meridian *H* is flattened by five-sixths the total astigmatism *A (H–V)*, whereas the flatter meridian *V* is steepened by one-sixth *A*.

Both the wedge resection and the RZ procedure will correct astigmatism. However, other optical considerations must be noted. Because it steepens the flatter meridian so dramatically, a wedge resection creates a significant myopic shift, increasing the myopic component of the refractive error by two-thirds of the preoperative astigmatism.

Conversely, the RZ procedure primarily flattens the steeper meridian. The myopic shift in this case will only be one-sixth the preoperative astigmatic component. There is, therefore, a fourfold difference in the amount of myopic change induced in the spherical component between the two procedures (two-thirds divided by one-sixth).

If one considers the comparative effect of the two procedures on the *spherical equivalent* (*SE*), then the wedge resection shifts the SE toward the myopic side equal to one-sixth the prewedge astigmatism. Recall that the spherical equivalent of any optical system is equal to the spherical component minus one-half the astigmatic component. The prewedge *SE* therefore would equal the sphere ($-A/2$). The postoperative *SE* would then equal sphere ($2A/3$) because the wedge resection will shift the spherical component toward myopia by two-thirds the preoperative astigmatism—assuming a perfect correction of the astigmatism. Therefore, since $SE = S - A/2$, where *S* is the sphere and *A* is the astigmatism in diopters, then if $-5.00 + 1.00 \times 9°$ (or $-4.00 - 1.00 \times 180°$), then

$$SE = -5 - \tfrac{1}{2} \quad [or\ -4 - (-\tfrac{1}{2})]$$

$$SE = -5 - 0.5 \quad [or\ -4 - (-0.5)]$$

$$SE = -4.50\text{ D} \quad [-4.50\text{ D}]$$

Thus the shift in spherical equivalent can be expressed as the difference between the pre- and postoperative spherical equivalents in this manner:

$$\Delta SE = (sphere - \tfrac{2}{3}A) - \left(sphere - \frac{A}{2}\right)$$

$$= -\frac{2A}{3} + \frac{A}{2}$$

$$= -\frac{(-4A + 3A)}{6}$$

$$= \frac{A}{6}D$$

The RZ procedure will create a hyperopic shift in the spherical equivalent equal to one-third that of the preoperative astigmatism. In this case the postoperative spherical equivalent equals *sphere* − ($A/6$) because the RZ procedure shifts the spherical component toward myopia by one-sixth the preoperative astigmatism. Thus

$$\Delta SE = (sphere - \tfrac{2}{3}A) - \left(sphere - \frac{A}{2}\right)$$

$$= -\frac{A}{6} + \frac{A}{2}$$

$$= \frac{(-2A + 6A)}{12}$$

$$= \frac{4A}{12}$$

$$= \frac{A}{3}D$$

Hence the RZ procedure creates a hyperopic shift in the spherical equivalent equal to one-third the preoperative astigmatism.

Troutman states that the corneal wedge resection produces a shift toward hyperopia due to a shortening effect on the axial length of the globe [36]. It is unclear, however, whether Troutman was referring to the spherical component or the spherical equivalent of the refraction. In either event, we can derive the amount of shortening required to produce the effect described. In Troutman's study, the amount of prewedge astigmatism averaged 11.4 D. Following the wedge resection, we have shown that the shift in spherical equivalent will equal one-sixth that of the preoperative astigmatism. Therefore, the mean shift will be almost 2 D:

$$-\frac{11.4}{6} = 1.9 \text{ D}$$

If we consider the spherical component alone, then the myopic shift will be 7.6 D:

$$-11.4 \cdot (\tfrac{2}{3}) = 7.6 \text{ D}$$

If we accept Rubin's approximation of axial myopia in a model eye, wherein 0.4 mm of axial elongation is equivalent to a dioptric change of 1.0 D, then the axial length in the first instance would be shortened 0.76 mm (0.4×1.9) and in the second 3.04 mm (0.4×7.6) [49]. This clearly does not happen.

The RZ procedure is technically easier than a wedge resection and may be performed in combination with other refractive procedures, especially RK. Furthermore, postoperative results for an RZ procedure are more predictable than for a wedge resection because sutures are not used. However, it is more variable in cases in which the corneal architecture has been altered by, for example, previous surgery. After wedge resection, there is incisional relaxation as some sutures are cut and others biodegrade. Consequently, the cornea regresses toward its prewedge astigmatism in an unpredictable manner.

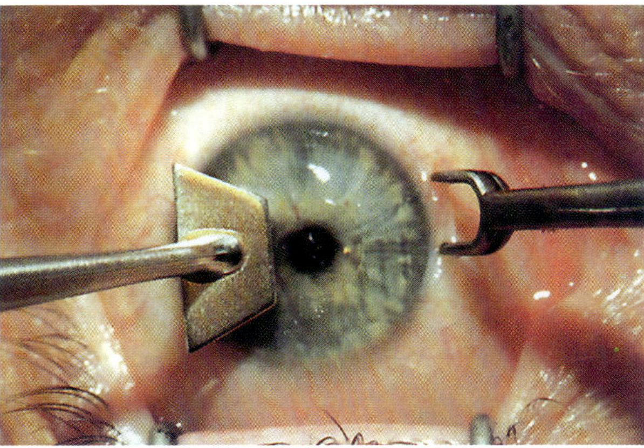

Fig. 9.64 A special marker is used for the Ruiz procedure.

The technique of the RZ procedure

Establishing the optical center is accomplished as usual, but this procedure is particularly sensitive to decentration. Mark the optical axis carefully. Next, a specially designed marker (Figure 9.64) or caliper is used to mark the positions and length of the transverse incisions. The computer would display the typical configuration for this procedure but will warn you about the suboptimal optical zone for the first T-cut. The 4.5-mm OZ is the zone at which the first transverse incision will be made. Each succeeding incision is made at equally spaced intervals to the limbus.

The transverse incisions are made first using a crystalline blade with a vertical cutting edge. The blade is set to obtain an effective depth of cut of between 80% and 90%, as determined by ultrasonic pachymetry. Deeper incisions have been shown to result in progressive flattening with this procedure, whereas shallower incisions have the opposite effect (Figure 9.65). The computer predictions assume an 85% incision depth. The eye must not

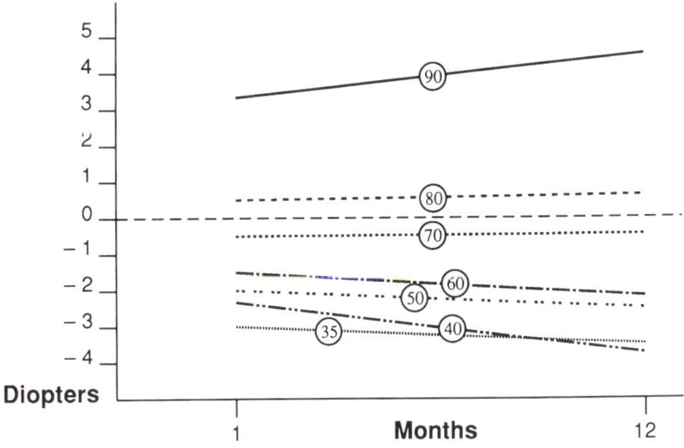

Fig. 9.65 Effect of incision depth of Ruiz "ladders" on outcome.

be allowed to rotate, so translimbal fixation using a Katena K5-3280 fixation forceps is recommended. The two central incisions are made first, the blade is advanced approximately 25 μm, and the next two incisions are made. It is here that the XTAL shadowgraphic blade gauge is most useful. The blade is advanced for each succeeding transverse incision, proportional to the corneal thickness at that point, until all eight (four on each side) "rungs" have been completed. It is important that the transverse incisions are evenly spaced and that the last one is as close to the limbus as possible. Figures 9.66 through 9.70 illustrate the various steps involved in this technique.

The blade is switched for one with an angled cutting edge and set (or reset if it is a double-edged blade) according to the corneal thickness at the primary astigmatic OZ (in the example, 4.5 mm). The semiradial incisions are then made at an angle of 20° to 22° normal to the inner tangential incision (Figure 9.71). These incisions must start *under* the outer ends of the inner ladder rung, and they must not connect with them. Making the incisions at the ends of the ladder rungs effectively increases their length. Connecting the incisions can produce wide scars and irregular healing that can lead to increased glare and irregular astigmatism (Figure 9.72). In higher degrees of astigmatism, the radial portion of the RZ pattern can be made in a stepped manner.

(a)

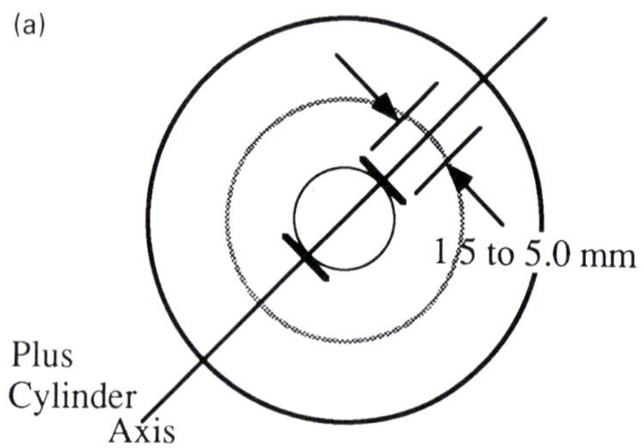

(b)

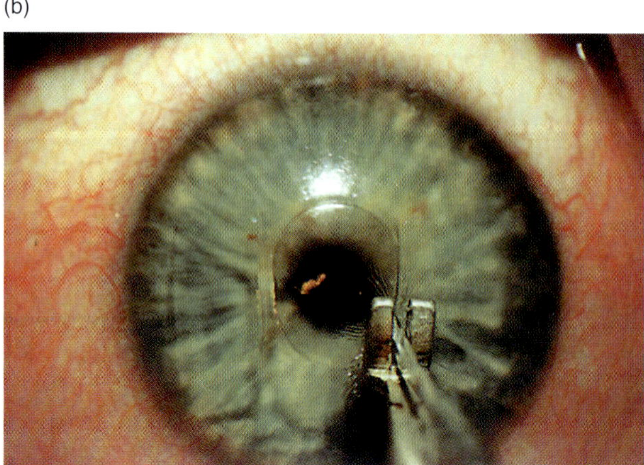

Fig. 9.66 (a,b) RZ procedure—first incision pair.

(a)

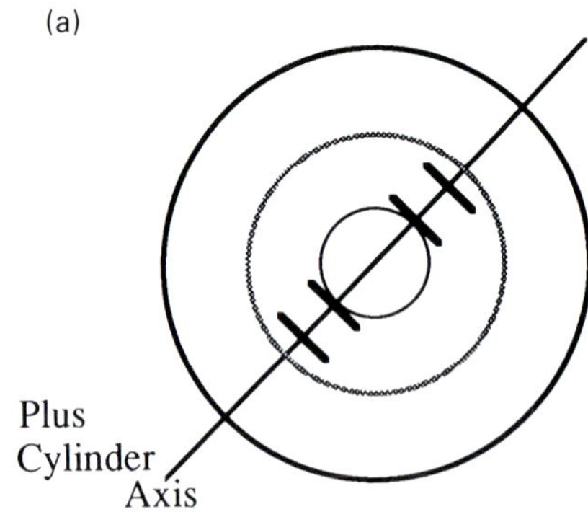

(b)

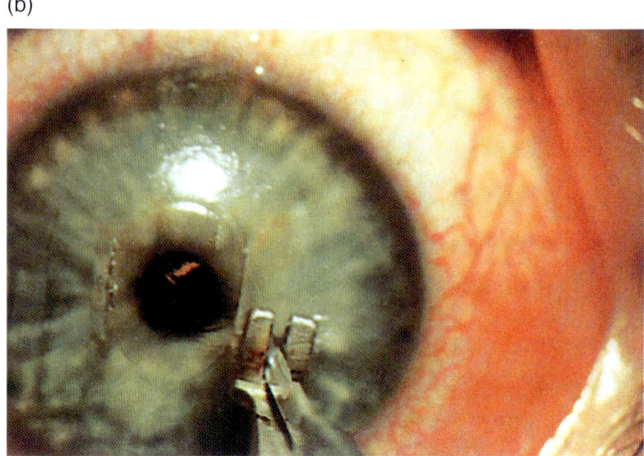

Fig. 9.67 (a,b) RZ procedure—second incision pair.

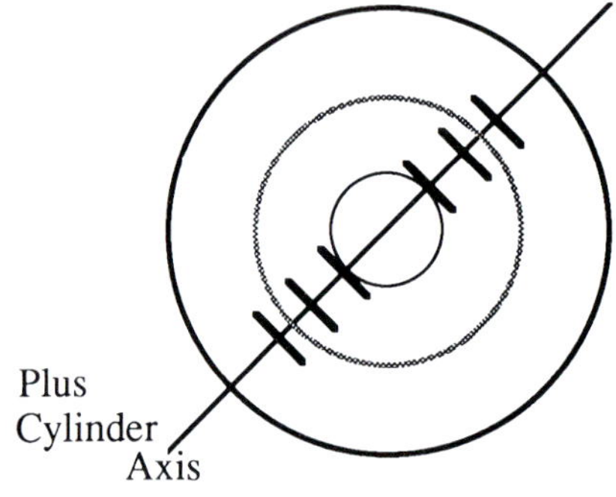

Fig. 9.68 RZ procedure—third incision pair.

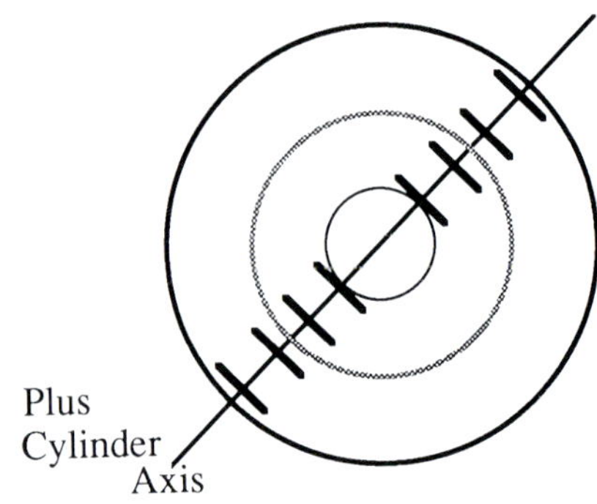

Fig. 9.69 RZ procedure—fourth incision pair.

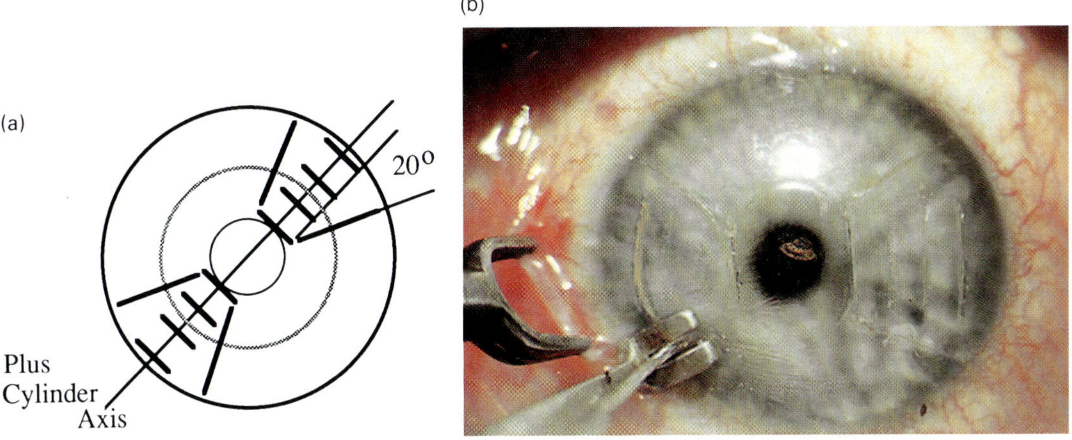

Fig. 9.70 (a,b) RZ procedure—semiradial incisions added. Note that the semiradials do not join the T-cuts.

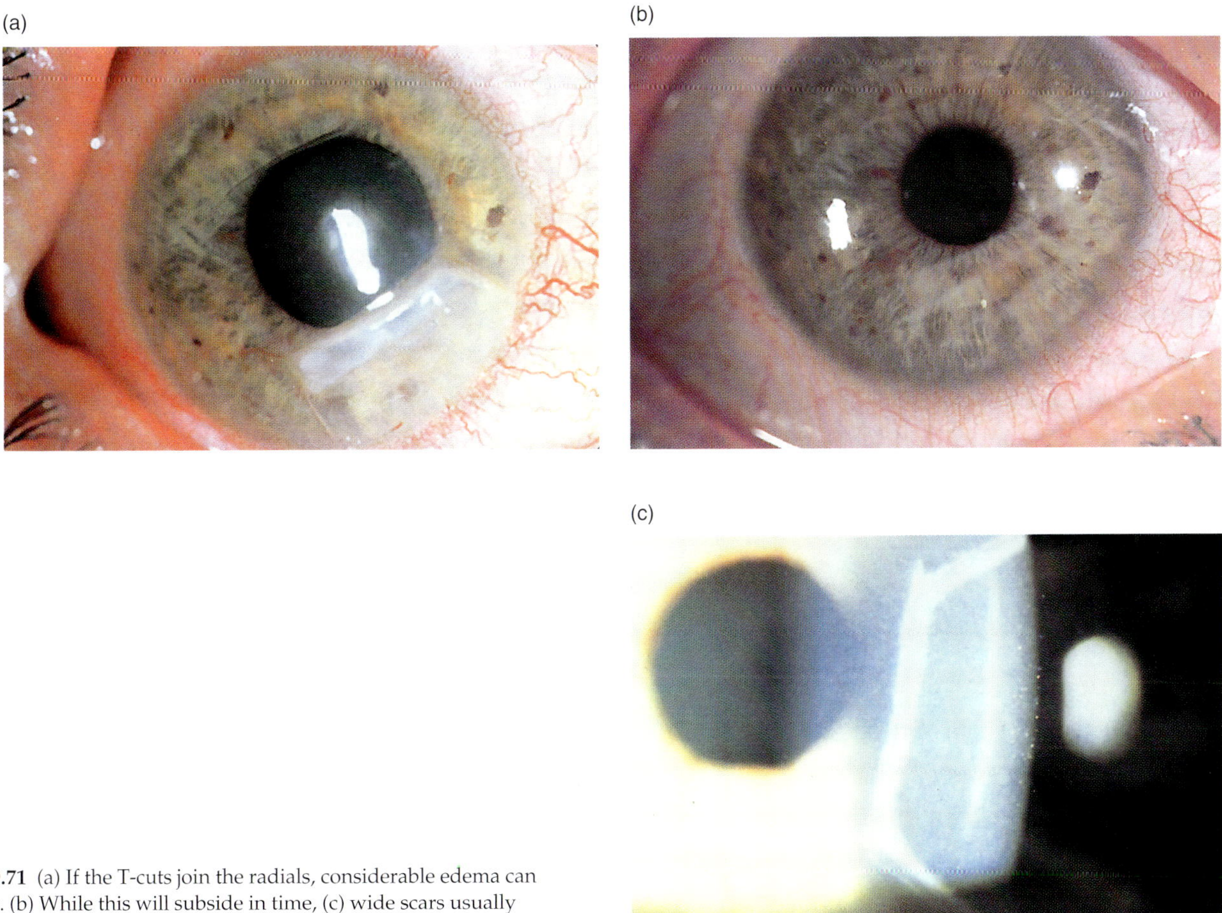

Fig. 9.71 (a) If the T-cuts join the radials, considerable edema can occur. (b) While this will subside in time, (c) wide scars usually result.

In certain instances, where the hyperopic component is effectively greater by far than the spherical component, a reversal of the pattern can be made (Figures 9.73 and 9.74). Thus in a case whose refraction is −0.50 + 5.00 × 146°, a reversed RZ resulted in the following: +1.50 + 0.50 × 180°.

RR procedure

If there is spherical myopia associated with astigmatism in excess of 2.25 D, it can be attenuated with a six-incision radial pattern added between the trapezoidal incisions and arranged around an appropriate OZ or OZs (Figures 9.75

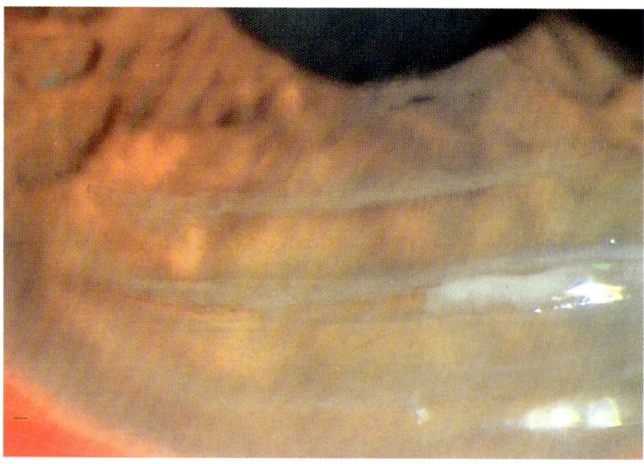

Fig. 9.72 Long T-cuts tend to gape.

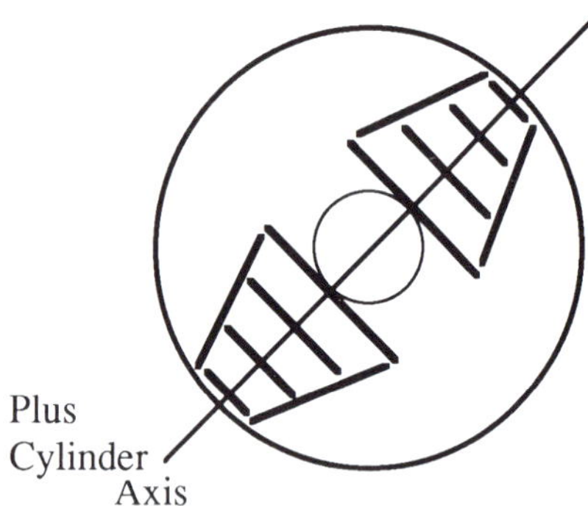

Fig. 9.73 Inverted Ruiz pattern.

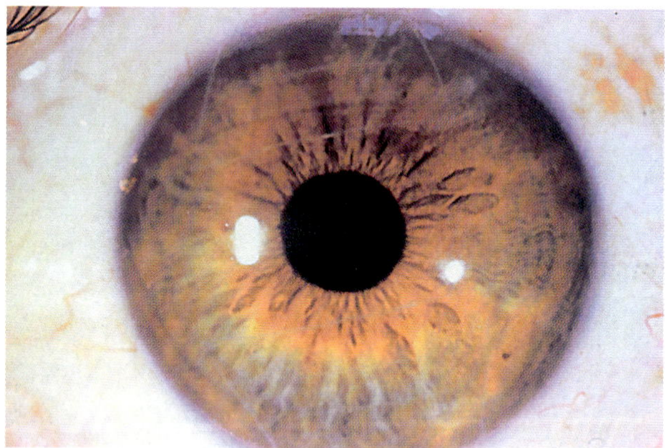

Fig. 9.74 Postoperative inverted Ruiz pattern.

and 9.76). This procedure is called method RR (radial-Ruiz). The OZ size for this part of the surgery is automatically calculated in the RK DataMaster program. A six-ray radial marker is invaluable to mark the position of the six incisions. These additional incisions have to be oriented correctly, as shown.

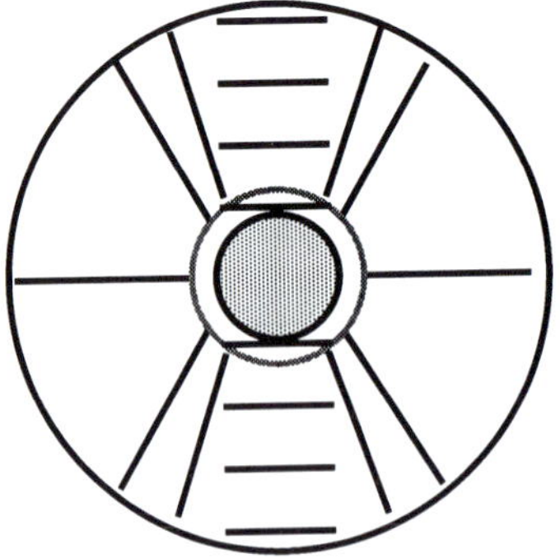

Fig. 9.75 Radial Ruiz (RR) configuration.

Do not mark the OZ for the radials or the radials themselves until *after* the astigmatic portion of the procedure is completed. There is too much danger of mistaking the (usually smaller) radial OZ for the (usually larger) astigmatic OZ if all zones are marked at the same time.

In MKM/LASIK cases, the radial incisions extend across the lenticular edge and can be stepped as in routine RR procedures. The T-incisions are arranged such that two fall within the lenticule and two fall outside (Figure 9.77). It is well to consider doing the RZ procedure in these cases only for astigmatism above 3 D. For astigmatism below this amount, use the RT or NT procedure.

In skilled hands, the RZ or trapezoidal incisions are an effective and predictable method of correcting simple myopic or mixed astigmatism over 2.25 D (up to 8.00 D) with or without associated spherical error. The use of a computer to assist in determining the surgical parameters has all but eliminated the problem of induced astigmatism. This procedure is highly recommended to skilled and experienced refractive surgeons for the purpose for which it was designed. However, take care not to find yourself in the predicament shown in Figure 9.78. Begin-

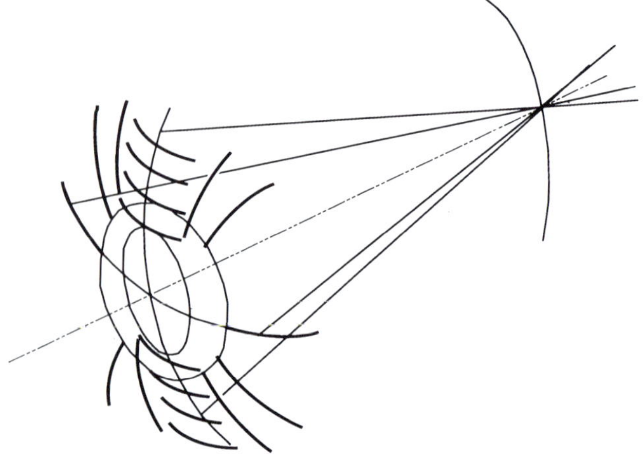

Fig. 9.76 Isometric of RR incision pattern on cornea.

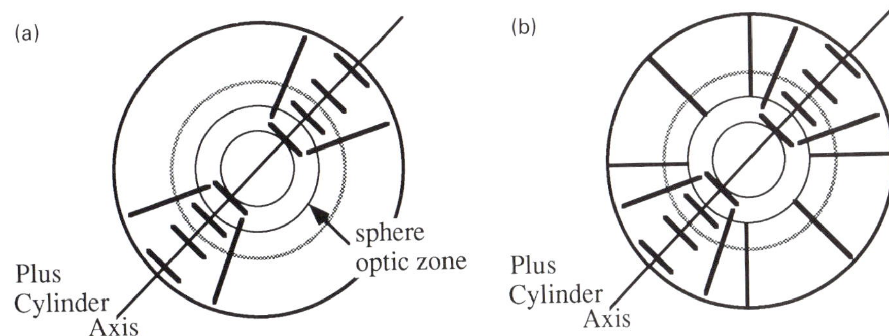

Fig. 9.77 RR procedure—showing the optical zone mark for radials to be added.

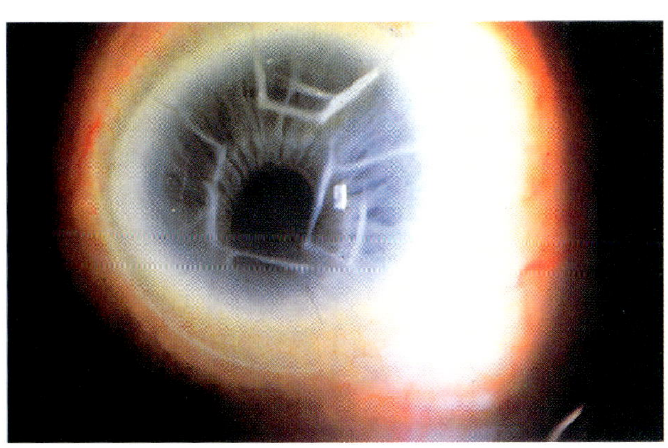

Fig. 9.78 Do not make a mistake in the axis or length of the T-cuts in the Ruiz procedure.

ning surgeons should avoid performing this or other forms of astigmatic refractive surgery until their skills and experience match their ambition.

Results with RK methods

Tables 9.2 through 9.8 summarize the author's results with the various configurations described above.

Variations of the trapezoidal procedure

Some variations of the basic incision pattern have been attempted. Figure 9.79 shows a configuration that has not proven to be sufficiently reliable in the authors hands.

Table 9.2 Early results of the application of T-cuts

Astigmatism	Preoperative	Postoperative
0.0–0.75 D		12 (21%)
1.0–1.75 D	4 (7%)	27 (47.4%)
2.0–3.0 D	26 (45.6%)	14 (24.6%)
3.25–6.75 D	27 (47.4%)	4 (7%)
Total	57 (100%)	57 (100%)

Table 9.3 Visual results of the application of T-cuts

Visual acuity	Preoperative	Postoperative
20/200–20/50	47 (82%)	21 (36.8%)
20/40–20/33	10 (17.5%)	22 (38.4%)
20/25–20/20		14 (24.6%)
Total	57 (100%)	57 (100%)

Table 9.4 Refractive results of early application of L-cuts

Astigmatism	Preoperative	Postoperative
0.0–0.75 D		22 (44%)
1.0–1.75 D	7 (14%)	21 (42%)
2.0–3.0 D	28 (56%)	6 (12%)
3.25–5.5 D	15 (30%)	1 (2%)
Total	50 (100%)	50 (100%)

Table 9.5 Visual results of early application of L-cuts

Visual acuity	Preoperative	Postoperative
20/200–20/50	32 (64%)	13 (26%)
20/40–20/33	15 (30%)	24 (48%)
20/25–20/20	3 (6%)	13 (26%)
Total	50 (100%)	50 (100%)

Table 9.6 Preoperative breakdown of patients by age and astigmatism

Parameter	*n*
Total cases	632
Age range	18–57 (31)
Dioptric range	75–8.25 D
Preoperative astigmatism breakdown	
<1.5 D	158
1.5–2.5 D	387
2.5–4.0 D	67
4.0–8.0 D	22

Table 9.7 Preoperative breakdown of astigmatism by procedure

Type	<1.5 D	1.5–2.5 D	2.5–4.0 D	4.0–8.0 D
R	126	1	—	—
L	28	73	—	—
T	4	3	—	—
RL	—	306	4	
TR	—	—	32	19
TL	—	—	11	
RZ	—	4	20	3
Total	158	387	67	22

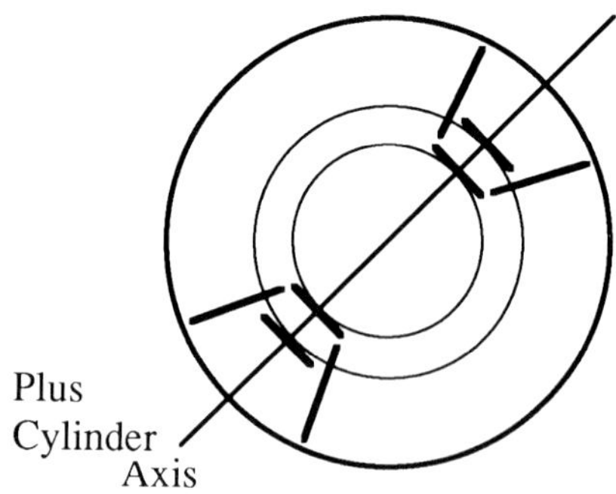

Fig. 9.79 Lindstrom's variation of the Ruiz procedure.

Table 9.8 Post-operative breakdown of astigmatism by procedure

Type	<1.5 D	1.5–2.5 D	2.5–4.0 D	4.0–8.0 D
R	127	—	—	—
L	78	23	—	—
T	4	3	3	—
RL	271	36	7	—
TR	22	21	32	—
TL	8	3	—	—
RZ	21	3	3	—
Total	531	89	13	

Lindstrom has described a technique he calls a delimited T-procedure [50]. Essentially, it is an RZ procedure with the elimination of the two outer T-cuts. Lindstrom has claimed that these outer incisions are not needed based on work with cadaver eyes that seemed to show a decreased effect when these incisions were added. The author submits for your consideration the fact that a dead eye is not a dynamic, living structure—living eyes react somewhat differently to this surgery. Furthermore, Ruiz and the author have pointed out that stability of effect is increased in the presence of these outer incisions [51–54]. Rowsey has corroborated the findings of Ruiz and the author that varying the OZ and adding the outer two incisions are effective in flattening the steep meridian [55].

Lindstrom uses a simplified method consisting of two paired incisions, either alone at 5 mm or with another pair at 7 to 9 mm (Figure 9.80). Note that Lindstrom varies the OZ for the limiting radials but keeps both the length and separation of the T-cuts constant [56]. In cases of post-keratoplasty astigmatism, he begins with a single pair of T-cuts at 5 mm. If an adequate effect is not obtained, he adds a second pair of T-cuts at 9 mm. While he states that postoperative steroids four times daily for 1 month can be used to enhance the effect, the trend of this technique is to progressive flattening—thus steroids should be used with caution. The author advises that the surgeon shoot for a slight undercorrection and use steroids twice daily for 2 weeks only (see also Chapter 8).

Intracicatricial relaxing incisions

Relaxing incisions can be placed in the host–graft interface (scar) to correct postkeratoplasty astigmatism (Figure 9.81). In some instances—such as very high astigmatism—this is a better choice than trapezoidal incisions. The author particularly favors this approach in grafts whose edges are vascularized. This procedure was first described by Troutman and Swinger for correction of high astigmatism following keratoplasty—correcting up to 15.92 D of cylinder [35]. This technique also can be used for postcataract astigmatism. The length of the incisions can vary from 70° to 90° (3 clock hours)—the author prefers the latter—with flattening/steepening ratios of 1:1 to 2:1. Stability usually occurs within 8 weeks, and

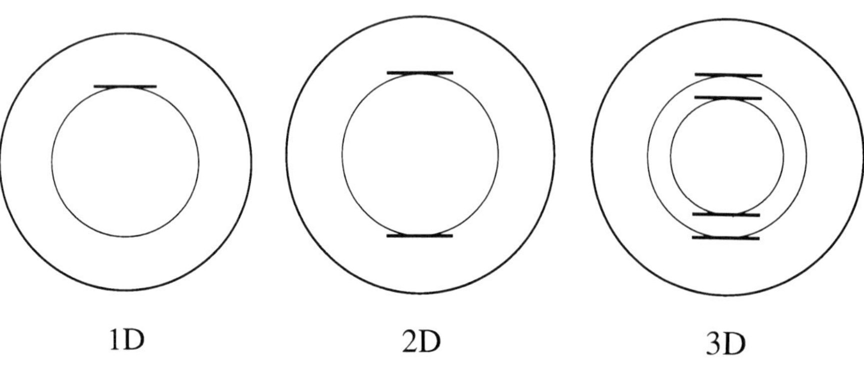

Fig. 9.80 Lindstrom's variation of the T procedure.

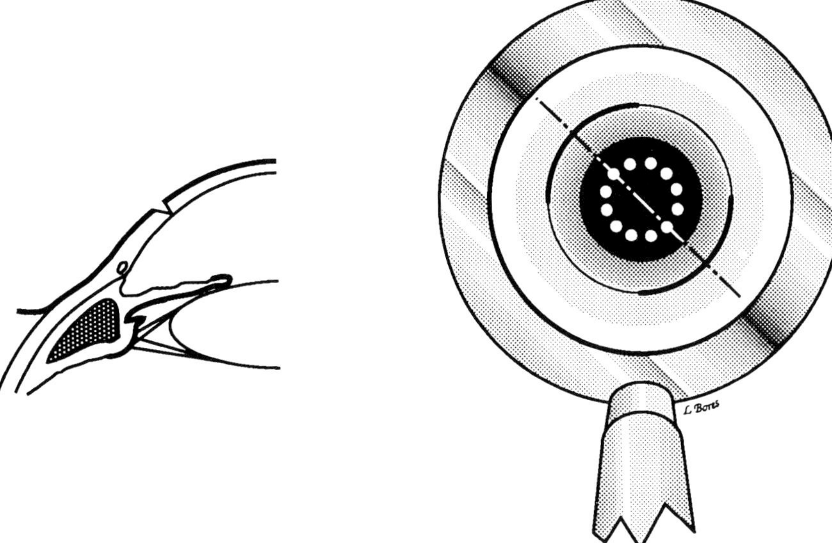

Fig. 9.81 Intracicatricial relaxing incisions.

although others have reported lessening of effect if one waits too long after removing sutures [57], the author has not found this to be the case. On the contrary, the author has found increased stability and predictability when he has waited a minimum of 4 months after suture removal to make these incisions. In any case, no surgery should be attempted after suture removal until the K-readings stabilize.

Compression sutures can be added to increase the gaping of the relaxing incisions in patients in whom insufficient flattening has occurred. This technique has the advantage of being titratable to some degree. I have combined in-the-wound relaxing incisions with wedge resections in two cases of very high second-graft post-PKP astigmatism with good results.

Arcuate keratotomy

Merlin was the first surgeon to popularize the use of arcuate keratotomy as an alternative to straight transverse keratotomy [58]. The author is using this term to describe arcuate incisions made perpendicular to the steep axis in clear cornea. We want to distinguish this procedure from the method of Troutman. Merlin based this preference on theoretical considerations, feeling that an arcuate incision would remain the same distance from the center of the cornea and would be less likely to have a distorting effect. He repeated a series of 205 eyes with arcuate keratotomies varying in length from 100° to 160° placed at OZs between 5 and 7 mm. He found increasing efficacy with increasing length of incision up to 120°. In addition, the major effect occurred at a zone of 5 mm. He found this to be a simple, reproducible procedure and noted that there were some cases of overcorrection. His results using a pair of 100° length arcuate incisions at a 7-mm OZ yielded a 2.10-D mean reduction in astigmatism. However, he only had two eyes in this group.

Lindstrom has advocated this approach for the treatment of postoperative and congenital astigmatism and uses a simplified nomogram as a planning aid for this and straight-line T-cuts. He cautions the individual trying to use his nomogram that it will have to be tailored to the individual surgeon—good advice [50]. He admits to a predictive error of ±2 D. Such a margin of error in predicting the outcome of astigmatism surgery is somewhat high in my experience. Lindstrom also has designed a special marker for this procedure (Figure 9.82), available from Katena Instruments as K3-7996 (7 mm).

Topical anesthesia as outlined above is used in all cases. The procedure is logical and straightforward. The optical center is marked in the usual manner, as is the axis. The required OZ is marked next. A six-ray marker is used to delineate the extent of a 60° arcuate incision—Lindstrom and the author do not make 120° incisions. An eight-ray RK marker can be used to mark 90° incisions, and a 16-ray marker can be used for 45° incisions (Figure 9.83). The Lindstrom marker also can be used for this purpose. The beginning surgeon is warned about the use of such a marker. It is very easy to make the incision too long when confronted with all the tick marks this marker displays. The surgeon is advised to extend the appropriate tick marks with the skin-marking pen to avoid confusion. A caliper is used to strike off the 3-mm length of the straight T-incisions, or the method of Lindstrom can be used (Figure 9.84).

The author sets the blade, as in all transverse incisions, to 100% of the mean pachymetry at 5 or 7 mm, as outlined in Chapter 8. If only astigmatism incisions are planned, mapping of the area around the planned incision site is sufficient. Arcuate incisions are always made at 7 mm. As with all astigmatism surgeries involving transverse incisions, only the very sharpest blade should be used. The eye is fixated with a limbus-to-

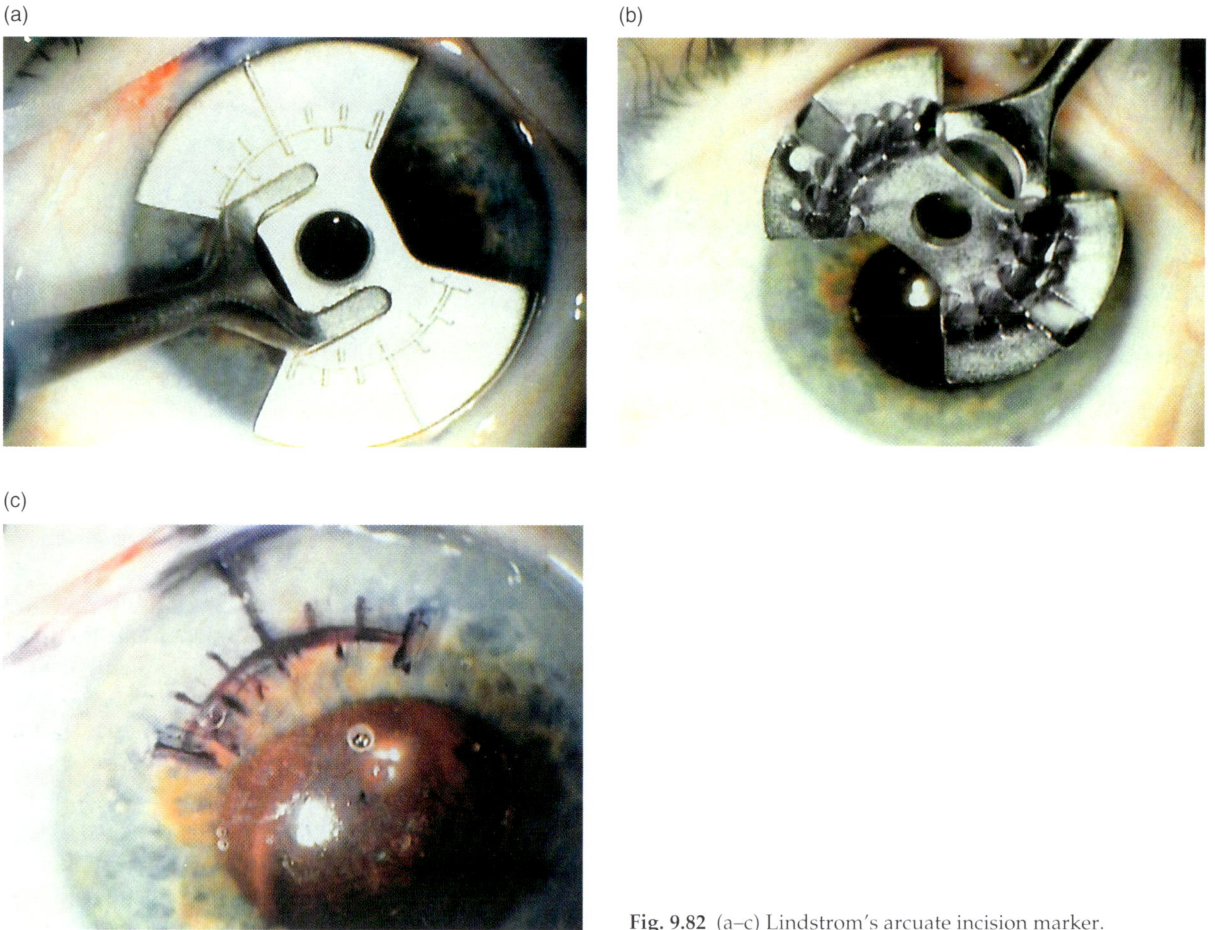

Fig. 9.82 (a–c) Lindstrom's arcuate incision marker.

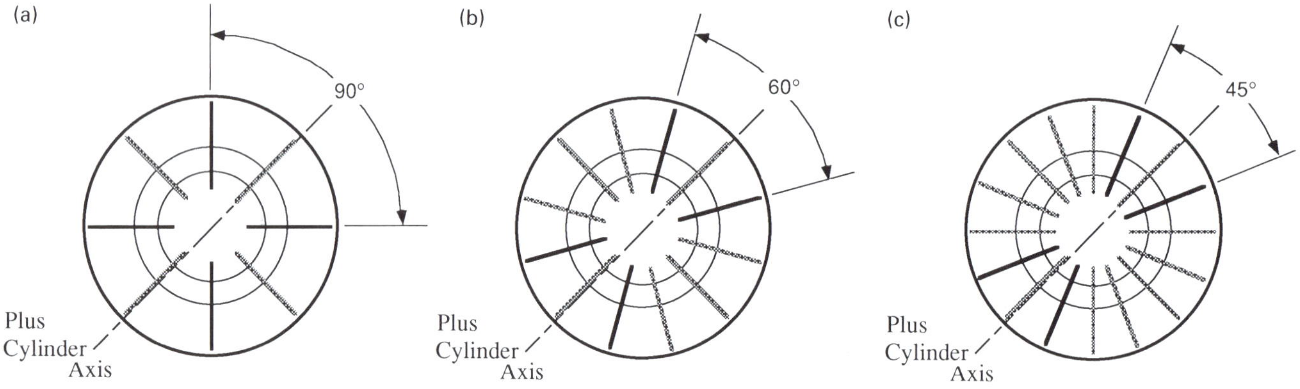

(a) 90° Plus Cylinder Axis

(b) 60° Plus Cylinder Axis

(c) 45° Plus Cylinder Axis

Fig. 9.83 (a–c) Various radial keratotomy incision markers can be used to delineate the extent of the required arcuate incision.

limbus forceps. Beginning at one end of the transverse incision, insert the blade into the cornea straddling the incision mark (Figure 9.85). Make each incision with a single smooth, even motion of the blade—stopping exactly at the end of the mark. It is not a good idea to make the incisions in halves by starting in the middle and working out to the ends. You are likely to end up with an overlapping incision this way. Furthermore, it is possible for the bottom of the incision to protrude up into the previous wound sufficiently that a penetration into the AC can occur. Transverse incisions are extremely difficult in a soft eye. The short, slanted end of the beginning of each incision is of no moment; however, the square blade of Thornton may be used to make these incisions, obviating the possible problem of a slanted endpoint (Figure 9.86). Postoperative treatment is usual (see Chapter 8). Lindstrom's nomogram is shown in Figure 9.87.

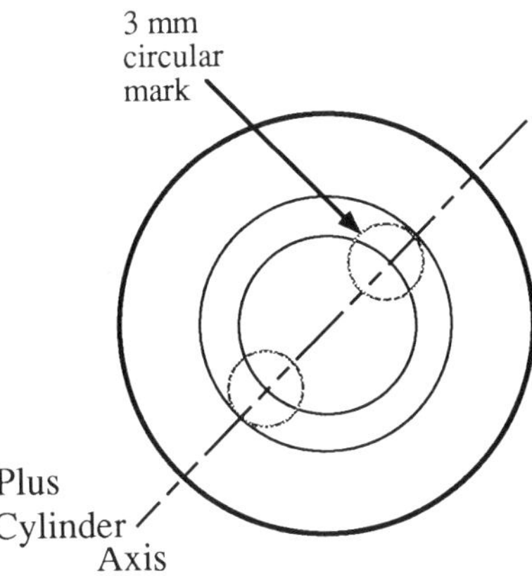

Fig. 9.84 Lindstrom's method using a 3-mm optical zone marker.

The maximum correction the author has obtained with the arcuate method is 4.5 and 5 D for the paired T-cuts. Overcorrections were seen in 6 of the 18 cases in which this procedure was used. The author has not combined arcuate incisions with radials—so far being content with the results obtained with RK methods.

Overview of relaxing incisions for astigmatism

The results obtained with these procedures confirm that straight transverse and arcuate nonperforating relaxing keratotomy incisions can be an effective tool for the reduction of naturally occurring and postcataract astigmatism with or without associated spherical error. More classical approaches to postkeratoplasty astigmatism correction through the use of intraincisional relaxing incisions with or without compression sutures may be a better alternative [35,59–64].

There is a significant range of effect with astigmatism surgery—with overcorrection and undercorrection being the rule. In addition, many patients continue to experience changes in their corneal topography and refraction

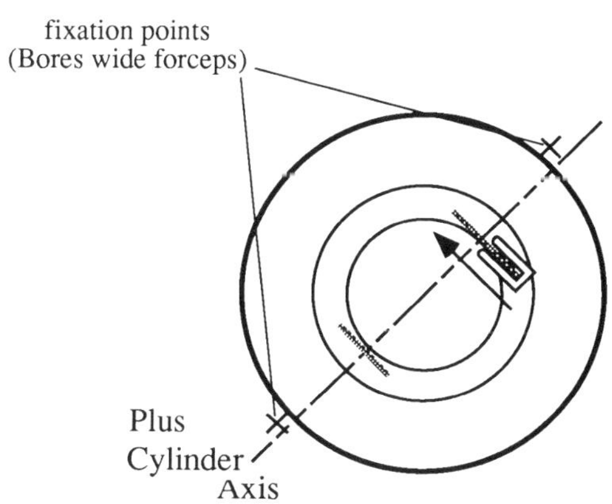

Fig. 9.85 A wide (limbus-to-limbus) fixation is necessary for precise incision control.

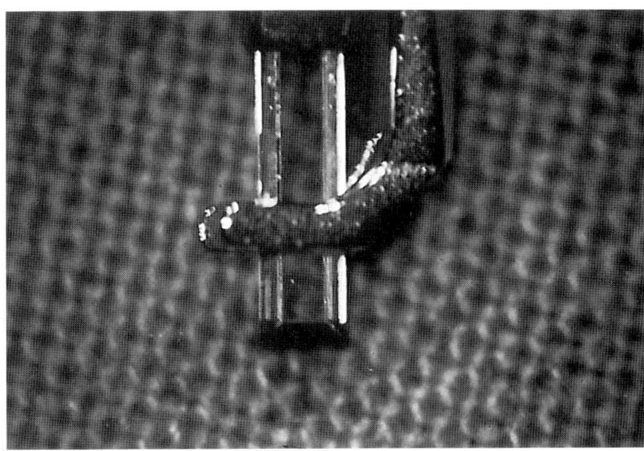

Fig. 9.86 The square diamond blade as recommended by Thornton.

beyond the expected time. This finding is especially true in patients with T-incisions.

Thornton, using his own nomogram, analyzed 60 eyes with between 1.00 and 2.25 D of preoperative astigmatism in which an eight-incision RK was combined with one to four straight transverse relaxing incisions. The transverse incision was placed between the radials. The mean preoperative astigmatism was reduced from 1.50 to 0.40 D with a short follow-up period. The astigmatism was reduced in all but two of his patients. The highest preoperative astigmatism attempted was 2.25 D in this series [62,65].

Park and Lee reported a series of 16 eyes in which a transverse incision technique intersected the radial incision. The minimum astigmatism was 5.00 D. The mean preoperative cylinder was 2.41 D, and the mean correction was 1.92 D. All but one eye achieved a decrease in preoperative astigmatism. The authors did not describe problems with intersection of the transverse incision with the radial incision. The effect decreased slightly with time, with a 23% reduction in effect at 10 months as compared with the first postoperative day [66].

Neumann also reported a series of eyes with transverse incisions placed at a 6-mm OZ. His pattern was similar to the RT procedure in that the radial incision was interrupted at the transverse—in the RT procedure, the transverse is interrupted at the radial. In 47 eyes with a mean age of 32.6 years and a mean follow-up of 3 months, he found a mean reduction in astigmatism of 1.33 D with one or two T-incisions. Four eyes had no improvement, and 9 of the 47 eyes showed an increase in astigmatism. The maximum astigmatism treated was less than 2.75 D [67].

In a series of Lindstrom-pattern patients, Agapitos evaluated 10 eyes with straight transverse relaxing keratotomy alone and 20 eyes with straight transverse relaxing keratotomy combined with RK. The mean follow-up in the transverse keratotomy alone group was 3.4 months, and in the transverse and RK group it was 7.7 months.

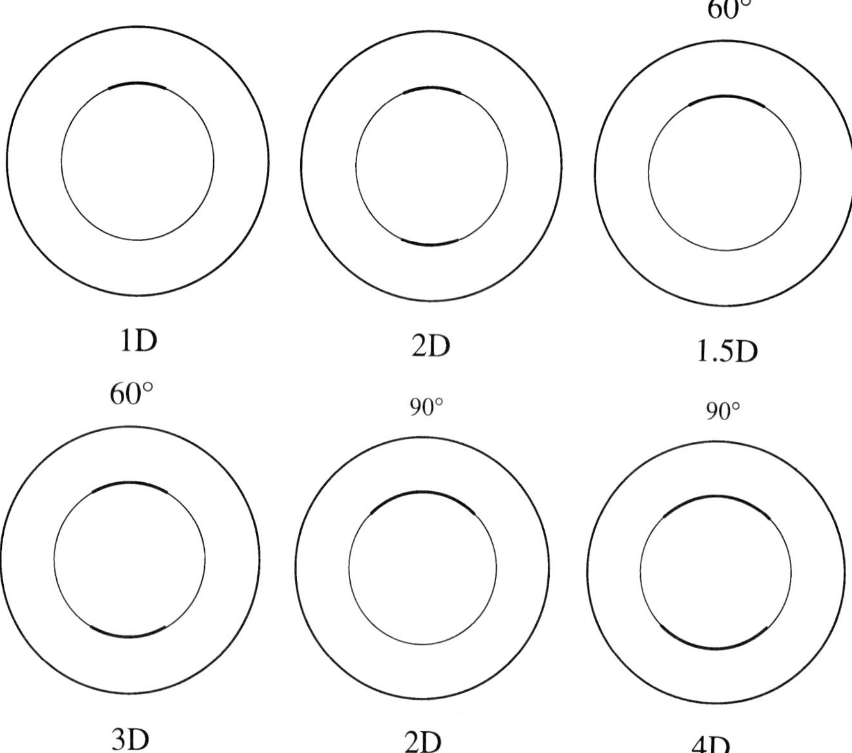

Fig. 9.87 Lindstrom nomogram for astigmatism to 4 D.

A mean preoperative cylinder of 5.30 D was reduced an average of 6.30 D in the astigmatism-only group. In the combined compound myopia series, a preoperative cylinder of 2.50 D was reduced an average of 2.90 D. The number of eyes that showed increased astigmatism was not presented. In this study, there also was a high degree of variability that has persisted in more recent series [68,69].

Currently published information, including the author's, is inadequate to determine whether straight or arcuate transverse relaxing keratotomy is superior. My results appear better with straight-T keratotomy because I find this method easier to predict with preoperative keratometry. Lindstrom has the opposite experience, preferring the arcuate T-incisions because he finds it easier to titrate with intraoperative keratometry [69]. He found that 10 of 24 patients operated on with straight transverse incisions experienced overcorrections. This can be explained by his OZ size, which he tends to keep at 5.0 mm, occasionally adding an additional pair at 7.0 mm, and also by the length, which he keeps at 3 mm. The author rarely makes T-cuts at 5.00 mm, except in cases using the RZ method, and then the T-cuts are only 1.5 mm in length.

The author was surprised to find such a low incidence (40%) of overcorrection in Lindstrom's arcuate incision cases. Astigmatism reversal could not be evaluated because the postoperative residual cylinder axis was not reported. The author also found that astigmatism tended to reverse itself in the majority of cases in which the arcuate method was applied à la Lindstrom. There is an explanation for this.

Arcuate incisions are advocated instead of straight T-incisions for the stated reason that the incision will thus be everywhere equidistant from the optical center. In the author's view, this may not be a good thing. Consider that the astigmatic surface has the shape of a regular toroid. As has been pointed out in our discussion of the nature of astigmatism (see the section on astigmatism, by way of review, above), there is a gradual lessening of corneal curvature as one progresses from the steeper meridian to the flatter. There is a direct relationship between incision length, or in the case of T-cuts, incision spacing, and the degree of the corneal curvature. That is, the steeper the curvature to be flattened, the longer is the radial incision or the closer is the spacing of the T-cut. Therefore, the primary optical clear zone is smaller. Figures 9.88 and 9.89 illustrate this principle. Note that if one were to draw the extent of the variation of this clear zone on such a surface, it would take the shape of an ellipse. It also should be obvious that the meridians that are immediately off-axis require slightly larger OZs.

This requirement is met automatically by a straight T-cut (see Figure 9.88). Note that the ends of the T-cut, regardless of length, are farther away from the center than is the central portion. This is as it should be. Note also that such an incision most closely approaches a tangent to the theoretical elliptical OZ. As the T-cut gets longer and gets closer to the flatter meridian, other factors begin to manifest themselves, and coupling occurs (see astigmatism discussion, above).

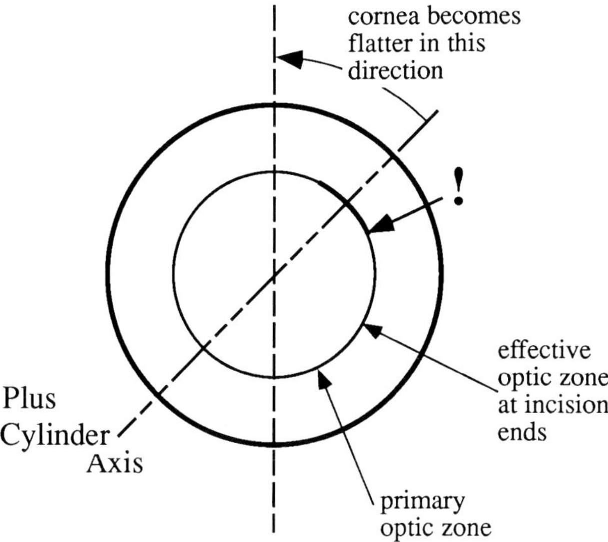

Fig. 9.88 The ends of the standard straight T-cut act at a greater distance than does the center.

In an arcuate incision, regardless of length, all parts of the incision are equidistant from the center (see Figure 9.89). This means that the ends of the incision, which are off-axis, are closer to the optical center when they really should be farther away. Thus they are exerting much more influence per increment of length than a comparable straight T-cut—they are producing excess flattening precisely where less is needed. Theoretically, for a given OZ and incision length, an arcuate cut should tend to produce more coupling effect. This is exactly what happens in the cadaver eye. This exact effect is not seen in the living eye for the reason that the OZs typically called for are larger than those used in T-cuts and also because living

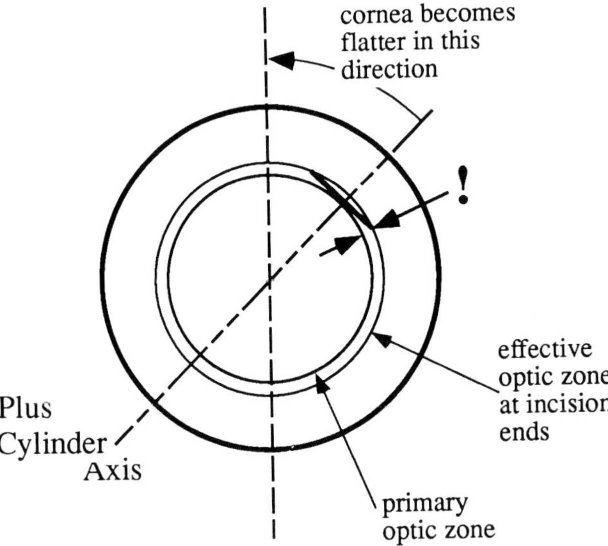

Fig. 9.89 An arcuate incision acts at the same distance throughout its length.

eyes display a different response to incisions than do cadaver eyes. Still, this aspect of arcuate cuts could help to explain the tendency the author has seen toward progression of effect (which can be explained by coupling and gradual reversal of the astigmatism). The length of these incisions undoubtedly plays a role as well. Bates and Lans established the relationship of length to effect in both meridians almost 100 years ago. Since arcuate incisions are somewhat harder to make accurately than straight T-cuts, and for the reasons outlined earlier, I urge caution in applying them.

Fortunately, in those eyes where overcorrection occurs, removal of the epithelial facet with compression suture placement can produce a good result in most cases (see Chapter 15). In undercorrection, extension or deepening of an arcuate or T-type keratotomy incision or addition of further T-cuts is possible.

Hyperopic astigmatism procedures

Cauterization techniques

These methods will be discussed in detail in Chapter 14.

Hexagonal keratotomy

The reader is referred to Chapter 14 for a discussion on failed attempts to control hyperopic astigmatism with this method.

References

1 Donders FC. *On the Anomalies of Accommodation and Refraction of the Eye,* WD Moore, Editor. The Hatton Press, London, p. 635, 1864.
2 Snellen H. Die richtunge des hauptmeridiane des astigmatishen auges. The axis of the major meridians of the astigmatic eye. Albrecht Von Graefes Arch Klin Ophthalmol 1869; 15: p. 199–207.
3 Brajkovich HL. Dr. Snellen's 20/20: the development and use of the eye chart. J Sch Health 1980; 50(8): p. 472–4.
4 den Tonkelaar I, Henkes HE, and van Leersum GK. The Utrecht Ophthalmic Hospital and the development of tonometry in the 19th century. Doc Ophthalmol 1988; 68(1–2): p. 57–63.
5 Fukala V. Surgical treatment of high degrees of myopia through aphakia [operative behandlung der hochstgradigen myopie durch aphakie]. Graefes Arch Ophth 1890; 36: p. 230–44.
6 Schiøtz HA. Ein Fall von hochgradigem Hornhautastigmatismus nach Staarextraction. Besserung auf Operativem Wege. (A case of severe corneal astigmatism after cataract extraction. Improved by surgical means). Arch für Augenheilkunde 1885, 15: p. 178–81.
7 Karatz MA. William Horatio Bates, M.D., and the Bates method of eye exercises. N Y State J Med 1975; 75(7): p. 1105–10.
8 Bates WH. A Suggestion of an Operation to correct Astigmatism. Arch Ophthal 1894; 23: p. 9–13.
9 Faber E. Operative Behandeling van Astigmatism. Operative treatment of astigmatism. Nederl Tijdschr V Geneesk 1895; 2(11): p. 495–6.
10 Lucciola J. Traitement chirugical de l'astigmie. Arch Ophtalmologie 1896; 16: p. 630–8.
11 Lans LJ. Experimentelle untersuchungen uber die entstehung von astigmatismus durch nicht Perforirende corneawunden.

(Experimental studies of the treatment of astigmatism with non–perforating corneal incisions). Albrecht von Graefes Arch Klin Exp Ophthalmol 1898; 45: p. 117–52.
12 Bates WH. Operation for relief of persistent deafness. M Record 1886; 29: p. 88.
13 Bates WH. Suture of the cornea after removal of the lens. Arch Ophthalmol 1898; 27: p. 181.
14 Wray C. Case of 6 D of hypermetropic astigmatism cured by cautery. Trans Ophth Soc (London) 1914; 34: p. 109.
15 Weiner M. Meier's method of peeling of the cornea. Ophthal Year Book 1917.
16 Burr WS. Keratoconus; results of different types of operations. Trans Ophth Soc (London) 1939; 59: p. 480.
17 Weiner M. *Ophthalmology in the war years.* The Year Book Publishers, Chicago, 1946.
18 O'Connor R. Corneal cautery for high myopic astigmatism. Am J Ophthalmol 1933; 16: p. 337.
19 O'Connor R. Corneal Cautery for conic cornea and corneal astigmatism. Trans Pacific Coast Oto-Ophth Soc 1938; 23: p. 25–31.
20 Bock J. Uber versuche, den hornhautastigmatismus durch Stichelungen mit der elecktrokoagulationsnadel zu beeinflussen. Wein Klin Wochenschr 1939; 2: p. 971–4.
21 Sato T. Treatment of conical cornea (incision of Descemet's membrane). Acta Soc Ophthalmol (Jpn) 1939; 43: p. 541.
22 Kokott W. Uber mechanisch–funktionelle Strukturen des Auges. Graefes Arch Ophthalmol 1938; 138: p. 424–85.
23 Momose A. Personal communication, 1990.
24 Hruby K. Zur Sato operation. Wein Klin Wochenschr 1949; 61: p. 653–4.
25 Linder K. Nach Sato erfolgreich operieter keratokonus. Wein Klin Wochenschr 1949; 61: p. 653–4.
26 Gilbert W. Zur behandlung des keratokonus nach Sato. Klin Monatsbl Augenheilkd 1943; 109: p. 702–4.
27 Sato T. Ueber eine Operationsmethode zur behandlung des keratoconus (Descemetspaltung). Klin Monatsbl Augenheilk 1941; 107: p. 234–8.
28 Sato T. Posterior incision of cornea; surgical treatment for conical cornea and astigmatism. Am J Ophthalmol 1950; 33: p. 943–8.
29 Akiyama K. Study of the surgical treatment for myopia. I. Posterior corneal incisions. Acta Soc Ophthalmol (Jpn) 1952; 56: p. 1142–50.
30 Sato T. Crosswise incisions of Descemet's membrane for the treatment of advanced keratoconus. Acta Soc Ophthalmol (Jap) 1942; 46: p. 469–70.
31 Sato T. Experimental study on surgical correction of astigmatism. Juntendo Kenkyukai Zasshi 1943; 589: p. 37.
32 Sato T. *Posterior half incision combined with the method of separating middle layers of cornea.* Juntendo Med Ass, 1950.
33 Sato T, Akiyama K, and Shibata H. Posterior half-incision of the cornea for astigmatism; operative procedures and results of the improved tangent method. Am J Ophthalmol 1953; 36: p. 462–6.
34 Sato T, and Komori M. Histological Findings of Posterior Corneal Incisions. Acta Soc Ophthalmol (Jpn) 1953; 57: p. 710–2.
35 Troutman RC, and Swinger C. Relaxing incision for control of postoperative astigmatism following keratoplasty. Ophthalmic Surg 1980; 11(2): p. 117–20.
36 Troutman RC. Microsurgical control of corneal astigmatism in cataract and keratoplasty. Trans Am Acad Ophthalmol Otolaryngol 1973; 77(5): p. 563–72.
37 Jensen RP, and Jensen AC. Surgical correction of astigmatism by microwedge resection of the limbus. Ophthalmology 1978; 85 (12): p. 1288–1298.
38 Fyodorov SN. Surgical correction of myopia and astigmatism. In: *Keratorefraction.* LAL Publishing, New York, 1980.
39 Duke-Elder S, and Abrams D. Ophthalmic optics and refraction. In: *System of Ophthalmology,* SS Duke-Elder, Editor. CV Mosby, St Louis, 1970.
40 Jaffe, N.S. and H.M. Clayman, The pathophysiology of corneal astigmatism after cataract surgery. Ophthalmology 1975; 79: p. 615–30.
41 Maguire LJ, and Bourne WM. A multifocal lens effect as a complication of radial keratotomy. Refract Corneal Surg 1989; 5(6): p. 394–9.
42 Ruiz LA. Personal communication, 1989.
43 Mobilia EF, and Kenyon KR. Contact lens-induced corneal warpage. Int Ophthalmol Clin 1986; 26(1): p. 43–53.
44 Swinger CA, and Barker BA. Prospective evaluation of myopic keratomileusis. Ophthalmol 1984; 91: p. 785–92.
45 Thornton SP. New diamond blade configuration for transverse incisions (instruments). Refractive and Corneal Surgery 1989; 5(1): p. 49.
46 Troutman RC. Primary astigmatism control using the Troutman surgical keratometer. In: *Current Concepts in Cataract Surgery. Selected Proceedings of Sixth Biennial Cataract Surgical Congress,* JM Emery, and AC Jacobson, Editors. CV Mosby, St Louis, p. 238–43, 1980.
47 Troutman RC. Corneal wedge resections and relaxing incisions for postkeratoplasty astigmatism. Int Ophthalmol Clin 1983; 23(4): p. 161–8.
48 Fyodorov SN, and Durnev VV. Surgical correction of complicated myopic astigmatism by means of dissection of circular ligament of cornea. Ann Ophthalmol 1981; 13: p. 1.
49 Rubin ML. The induction of refractive errors by retinal detachment surgery. Trans Am Ophthalmol Soc 1976; 73: p. 452–90.
50 Lindstrom RL. Surgical correction of postoperative astigmatism. Indian J Ophthalmol 1990; 38(3): p. 114–23.
51 Ruiz LA. Surgical treatment of astigmatism. In: *American Academy of Ophthalmology.* Atlanta, 1986.
52 Ruiz LA. Personal communication, 1991.
53 Bores LD. Radial keratotomy: current techniques. Curr Canadian Oph Practice 1986; 4(3): p. 104–7.
54 Bores LD. Mechanical modulation of the corneal surface. Int Clinics Ophth 1991; 31(1): p. 25–36.
55 Rowsey JJ. Current concepts in astigmatism surgery. J Refract Surg 1986; 2: p. 85–94.
56 Lindstrom RL. The surgical correction of astigmatism: a clinician's perspective. Refract Corneal Surg 1990; 6(6): p. 441–54.
57 Krachmer JH, and Ching SS. Relaxing corneal incisions for postkeratoplasty astigmatism. Int Ophthalmol Clin 1983; 23(4): p. 153–9.
58 Merlin D. Curved keratotomy procedure for congenital astigmatism. Journal of Refractive Surgery 1987; 3: p. 92–7.
59 Barner SS. Surgical treatment of corneal astigmatism. Ophthalmic Surg 1976; 7(1): p. 43–8.
60 Krachmer JH, and Fenzl RE. Surgical correction of high postkeratoplasty astigmatism: Relaxing incisions vs wedge resection. Arch Ophthalmol 1980; 98(8): p. 1400–2.
61 Lavery GW, Lindstrom RL, and Hofer LA, *et al*. The surgical management of corneal astigmatism after penetrating keratoplasty. Ophthalmic Surg 1985; 16(3): p. 165–9.
62 Thornton SP, and Sanders DR. Graded non-intersecting transverse incisions for correction of idiopathic astigmatism. J Cataract Refract Surg 1985; 13: p. 27–31.
63 Mandel MR, Shapiro MB, and Krachmer JH. Relaxing incisions with augmentation sutures for the correction of postkeratoplasty astigmatism. Am J Ophthalmol 1987; 103: p. 441–7.
64 Sugar J, and Kirk AK, Relaxing keratotomy for post-keratoplasty high astigmatism. Ophthalmic Surg 1983; 14(2): p. 156–8.
65 Thornton S. Thornton guide for radial keratotomy incisions and optical zone size. J Refract Surg 1985; 1(1): p. 29–33.
66 Park K, and Lee JH. Surgical correction of astigmatism using paired T-incisions. Korean J Ophthalmol 1989; 3(2): p. 61–4.
67 Neumann AC, McCarty GR, and Sanders DR, *et al*. Refractive evaluation of astigmatic keratotomy procedures. J Cataract Refract Surg 1989; 15(1): p. 25–31.
68 Agapitos PJ, Lindstrom RL, and Williams PA, *et al*. Analysis of astigmatic keratotomy. J Cataract Refract Surg 1989; 15(1): p. 13–8.
69 Lindstrom RL. Personal communication, 1991.

10
Lamellar Refractive Surgery

Discovery consists of seeing what everybody has seen and thinking what nobody has thought.
[Albert Szent-Gyorgi (The Scientist Speculates)]

Lamellar refractive surgery—MKM—has been simplified with the advent of automated, fixed-plate microkeratomes for use with the laser in situ keratomileusis (LASIK) procedure (see Chapter 11). This is both a blessing and a curse. It is a blessing because the variables of translation speed, plate thickness, and ring choice have been all but eliminated. It is a curse because most surgeons learning LASIK today have never done any refractive surgery, and very few have done any lamellar corneal surgery. The process has been so simplified as to induce many individuals to consider the process a "no brainer." However, the best admonition for any erstwhile refractive surgeon dealing with lamellar sections is this: *Make sure the brain is engaged before putting the microkeratome in gear.*

This chapter is more by way of a history lesson, since very little, if any, cryolathing is still being performed. However, a knowledge of the principles detailed herewith should come in handy when you engage your brain prior to performing LASIK. Furthermore, only grafts (epikeratophakia) are an effective alternative to a penetrating keratoplasty for keratoconus. In addition, perhaps a thorough read here will make the erstwhile refractive surgeon somewhat more respectful of the interface. The author is appalled at the condition of the interface in many of the LASIK eyes he has examined over time. Particulates in the interface, many of which appear to be detritus remaining from microsponges, are especially in evidence (see below).

Briefly, lamellar refractive surgery seeks to modify the corneal shape through mechanical means. This process can take several forms:

- Removing and reshaping the resected tissue—*keratomileusis*
- Removing tissue and reshaping the underlying stroma—*keratomileusis in situ*
- Attaching an appliqué to the corneal surface—*epikeratophakia*
- Removing tissue and sandwiching another material between—*keratophakia*
- Internal tissue ablation—*intrastromal ablation*

The latter method seeks to reshape the surface via intrastromal tissue ablation through the use of photodisruptive laser light. Hence it will be discussed in Chapter 11.

Of the remaining four methodologies, although the last—*keratophakia*—is the harbinger of the preceding three, it shall be discussed last; LASIK (a version of the second procedure on the list) will be discussed in Chapter 11.

The history of lamellar refractive surgery

The term *refractive keratoplasty* was coined in 1949 by Barraquer when he demonstrated that plastic surgery of the cornea could alter its refractive power in a predetermined way [1]. Basically the initial procedure called for double, nonpenetrating, concentric trephinations at 10 and 11 mm (Figure 10.1). The resulting annulus was resected and discarded. The central portion was then dissected to form a planar disk that was resutured to the eye, flattening the corneal curvature. The procedure was modified, in one case, to treat keratoconus, except in this instance by substituting a thicker homoplastic disk of donor cornea.

Keratomileusis and keratophakia are procedures that had their beginnings in 1961 when Barraquer reported his first eight cases of allopathic keratophakia in human eyes, followed in 1963 by keratomileusis [2]. The technique was introduced into the United States in 1977 by Richard Troutman, professor and former chairman of the Ophthalmology Department of the Manhattan Eye and Ear Infirmary. In the ensuing years, relatively few cases have been performed in the United States by relatively few surgeons.

Basic principles of lamellar refractive surgery

The premise is simple: Remove or add sufficient material within the corneal stroma to alter the external curvature of that cornea without materially affecting Bowman's layer. This precept is violated by the technique of "Bowman's blasting" with the excimer laser—which totally obliterates that structure in the visual axis (Figure 10.2; see also Chapter 11). Epithelium and Bowman's layer seem to have a special affinity—although normal-appearing hemidesmosomes are reported following laser surface ablation (see Chapter 4). Considerable variability in result has been reported (see Chapter 11).

Merely stuffing material into a pocket made intrastromally does not usually result in good effect either [3]. Typically, the resistance of Bowman's layer to distortion

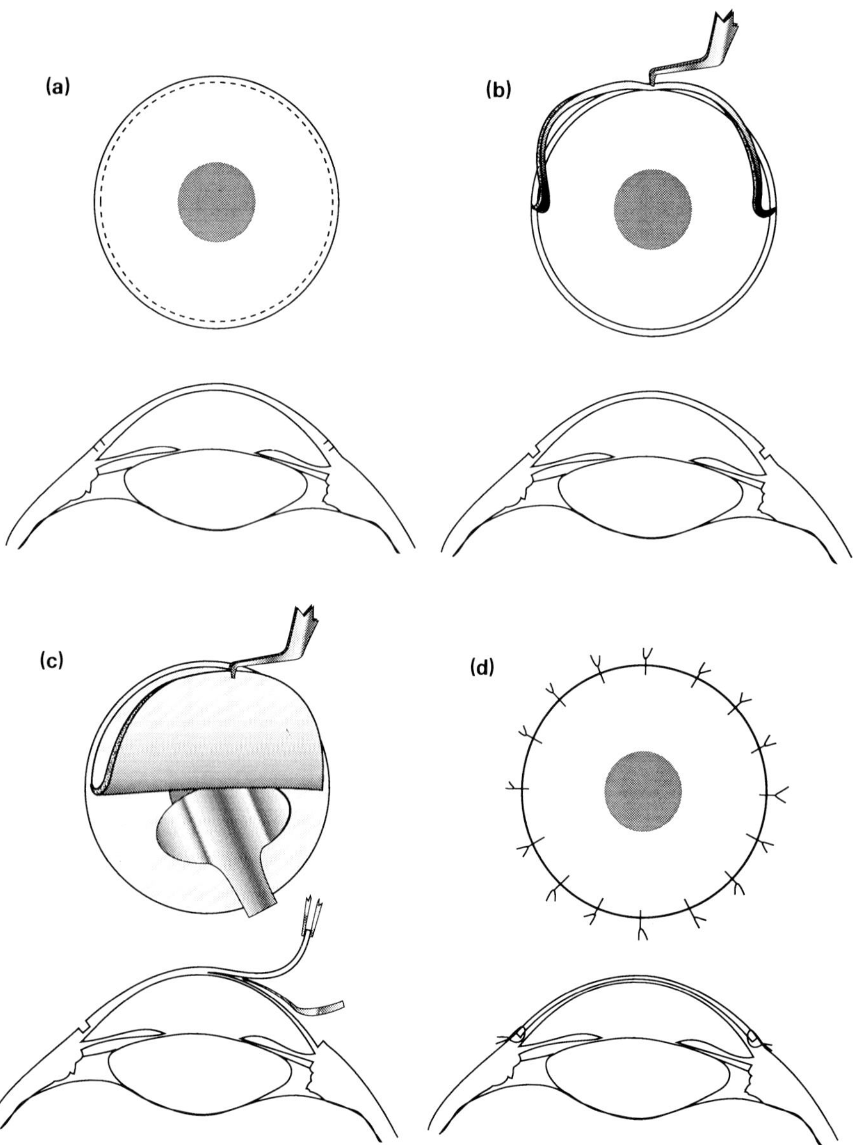

Fig. 10.1 Barraquer's lamellar stromectomy for myopia. (a) Two nonpenetrating trephinations are made—10 and 11 mm in diameter. (b) The annular ring of stroma between is dissected and removed. (c) Next the central corneal stromal disk is dissected free. (d) This freed disk is then sutured to the periphery thereby flattening the central curvature. A similar method was used to treat keratoconus. In these cases a homoplastic disk was substituted for the patient's central stroma.

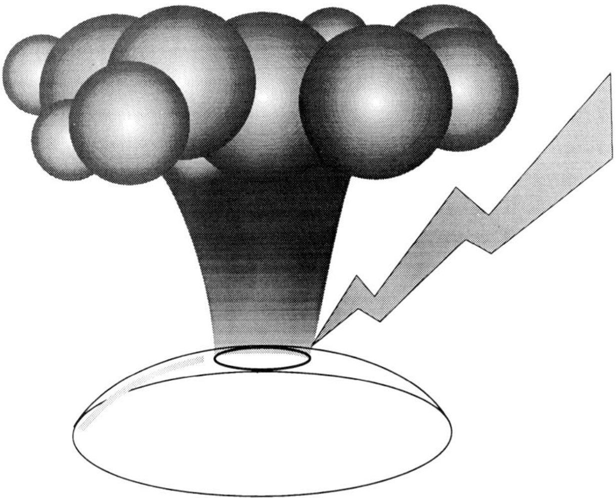

Fig. 10.2 Bowman's blasting—laser stromectomy.

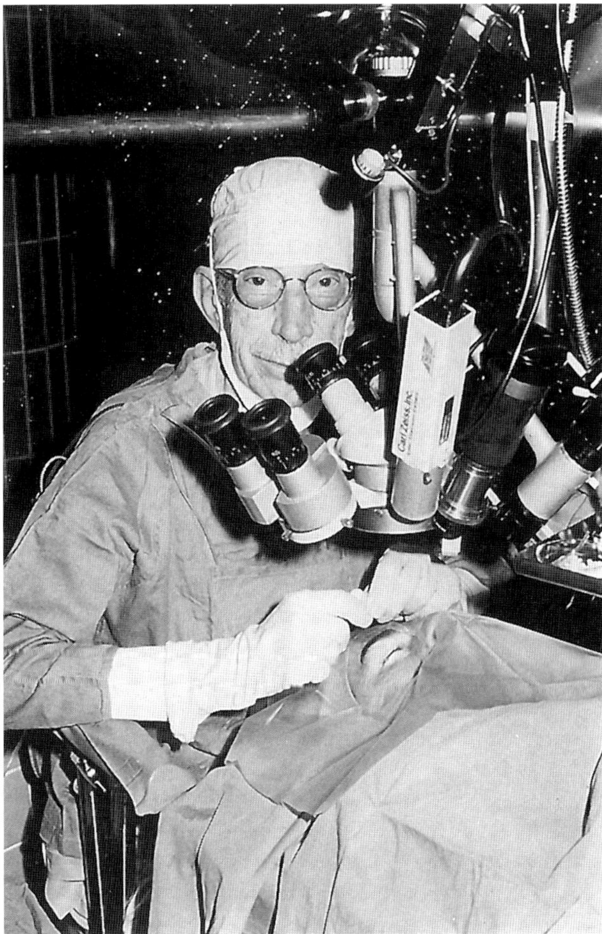

Fig. 10.3 Professor José Ignatio Barraquer—refractive surgery pioneer.

and/or stretch results in a change in the back-surface curvature of the cornea—which may (or may not) alter the total refractive power. Consequently, all successful lamellar procedures involve a complete separation of Bowman's layer from its limbal connection. This allows the front corneal layer to smoothly adjust to the induced distortion and enhances the curvature change. Various techniques have been devised to accomplish the main goal. Some have been successful, and some not. Our discussion will deal with most, if not all, such attempts.

Keratomileusis

Approximately two score years ago, a young physician began a series of experiments that culminated in a surgical technique largely unappreciated and unheralded even today. The procedure—keratomileusis; the physician—José Ignatio Barraquer (Figure 10.3). The term *keratomileusis* itself comes from the Greek words *keras* ("hornlike"—cornea) and *mileusis* ("carving")—"corneal carving." Over the years, very few ophthalmologists have taken the trouble to learn anything about this operative technique, fewer have attempted to perform it, and even fewer have mastered it. Attitudes toward practitioners of this "black art" are mixed. All are looked on as elitists or as ophthalmic buccaneers or even worse. This notion is intensified by the tendency of these "cultists" to gather together in tight little groups, to speak in tongues—"angle alpha," "base plate," "nontorque suture," etc.—and to evidence the "thousand-yard stare" of one who's *been there.*

Keratomileusis is an exhilarating, challenging, and elegant procedure whose performance is akin to flying: long moments of joy punctuated by short periods of stark terror. Having said this, we hasten to add that it is also a rewarding and satisfying procedure whose anxiety-provoking potential is in direct proportion to experience. Still—the allusion to flying pretty much sums up how many feel about this operation—terrified. It is perceived to be a technically demanding and meticulous procedure whose path to completion is studded with minefields. It *is* that and more. There is no question that the operation of keratomileusis demands levels of skill exceeding that of any other in ophthalmology. There is no question that this technique is fraught with difficulties and carries with it a high potential for disaster. There is no question that this operation is not for the "sunshine ophthalmologist" (like the sunshine patriot: *invincible in peace, invisible in war*), the occasional surgeon, or the multithumbed "instant expert." There is also no question that, properly performed, this operation provides the dedicated refractive surgeon with power over high degrees of myopia. With its encompassing ability to overcome hyperopia as well, it is a valuable tool withal, though largely supplanted by LASIK.

This section is designed to increase the reader's knowledge about this technique as well as to provide the student of refractive surgery with insight into its mechanism and performance. It is hoped that the knowledge gained will alleviate some of the understandable anxiety surrounding the procedure. Perhaps some of you will even be tempted to test the waters. This is all well but the author suggests that in that case the readers should prepare themselves for possible failure. This technique is learnable, and diligence and care will pay off.

If the reader carries away no more from reading this text than an enlightened view of this technique,—then it will be time well spent both for the reader and for the author. Regardless, a study of this approach to corneal modulation is an essential precursor to understanding and performing other techniques such as epikeratophakia, keratophakia, and laser corneal surface shaping embodied in the LASIK procedure and its ilk.

Patient selection and workup

The basic requirements that a patient must meet to be eligible for refractive surgery have been outlined in Chapter 5. However, lamellar refractive surgical candidates have additional requisites depending on the modality. For example, in autoplastic MKM (wherein the patient's own cornea will be lathed), the lower limit of refraction is –6 D, and the upper limit should be –15 D if a complete correction is expected. Furthermore, there is a limit to the degree of flattening with MKM, which has a floor of 33 D. Thus a –15-D patient should have a preoperative spherical equivalent K-reading of 48 D. If the patient has a higher myopic refraction, homoplastic MKM can be done. In such a case, corrections of up to –30 D have been obtained. However, even with homoplastic MKM, the effective optical zone (OZ) becomes quite small and centration critical. In these cases, the incidence of induced astigmatism is increased.

Corneal curvature also can affect the initial corneal disk resection. Excessively steep corneas—7.81 mm (47.54 D)—or excessively flat corneas—8.6 mm (39.24 D)—can make the resection more difficult.

The actual amount of ametropia at the cornea to be corrected (Dv in the calculations) must be the *contact lens power* or the spectacle power corrected for the vertex distance. Thus

$$D_V = \frac{D_C}{1 - (VD)(D_C)}$$

where VD is the vertex distance in meters, and Dc is the spectacle spherical equivalent. Hence, if the patient wears a –13 D spectacle whose vertex distance is 12 mm, then

$$\begin{aligned} D_V &= \frac{-13}{1 - (0.012)(-13)} \\ &= \frac{-13}{1 - (-0.156)} \\ &= \frac{-13}{1.156} \\ &= -11.25 \text{ D at the cornea} \end{aligned}$$

For a hyperopic patient wearing a +13 D spectacle at the same vertex distance, the power at the cornea would be +15.40 D.

Corneal thickness is also a factor. Generally speaking, the higher the myopia, the greater the central corneal thickness should be—as measured ultrasonically. In any case, a cornea with a central thickness of less than 0.45 mm (450 μm) should not have autoplastic keratomileusis (KM), although a homoplastic KM might be done. Such thin corneas are rare and might be cases of subclinical keratoconus—in which event the surgery should be avoided altogether.

Instrumentation for keratomileusis

In classic KM, the key instrument of the surgery is the microkeratome. In LASIK, the key instrument is still the microkeratome. While it is true, in classic KM, that the power changes in the corneal tissue are produced by the operation of lathing—still, without a proper keratectomy, the operation fails. In LASIK, the correct use of the microkeratome is paramount to the success of the operation. Shortcuts and "make do" are not appropriate approaches to the use of this instrument. Despite the difficulty of its application, however—correct usage can be learned with a modicum of diligence and practice. You are encouraged to continue such practice until you are comfortable with the instrument. Figure 10.4 shows two typical early model (manual) microkeratome instrument sets.

Microkeratome

This instrument is based on the principle of the carpenter's plane (Figures 10.5 to 10.9). The microkeratome head is divided into an anterior and posterior section in relation to the cutting blade. This blade is caused to oscillate at approximately 10,000 excursions per minute by a precision foot-switch-controlled electric or gas-turbine motor. The blade itself protrudes a fixed distance from the base of the keratome plane or head. The Steinway unit uses a fixed plate to control resection depth. In the SCMD unit, a threaded knob attached to a movable plate in the anterior portion of the head varies the relative protrusion of the blade; this in turn alters the thickness of the tissue section removed. This head will be described further below. The Draeger microkeratome operates on a slightly different principle and will be discussed, along with the Ruiz-Steinway keratome, in a separate section.

The microkeratome head has dovetail guides on either side along the bottom edge of the plane. These guides fit into corresponding guides in the pneumatic rings and position the edge of the cutting blade at a constant 0.13 mm to the plane of the pneumatic fixation ring. The position of the posterior platform of the plane is held constant to prevent any modification of the intraocular pressure during the resection. The prototype of the current

(a)

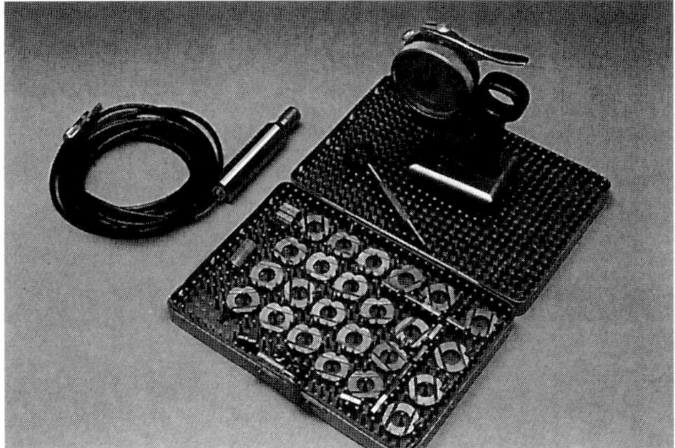

(b)

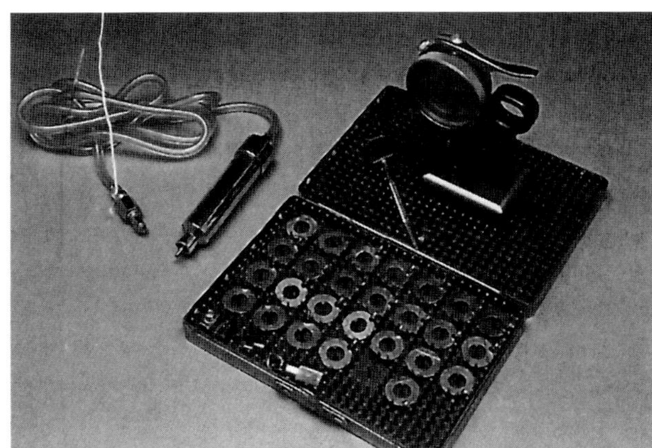

Fig. 10.4 Standard keratectomy sets. (a) Steinway *in-situ* set with electric motor handle. (b) SCMD *in-situ* set—gas-turbine handle. Both instruments can be used with the cryolathe.

keratome used an adjustable blade, had no guiding dovetails, and was passed across the surface of a flat-topped pneumatic fixation ring. The problems produced by this configuration were manifold. It was, for example, not possible to precisely gauge the thickness of the resection from case-to-case. The keratome subsequently was redesigned to provide both guides and a fixed-position blade. The resection thickness was (and still is) controlled by a variable-thickness interchangeable applanator plate.

The dimensions of the microkeratome have been selected carefully in relation to the size of the human globe and the average corneal curvature. It is a sensitive and high-precision instrument manufactured from surgical stainless steel. It is easily disassembled for cleaning and blade changing. It always should be cleaned and dried carefully after each session and should never be stored assembled or wet. The classic microkeratome is disassembled by unscrewing the knurled ring at the rear using the pronged tool provided to start—finishing with the fingers.

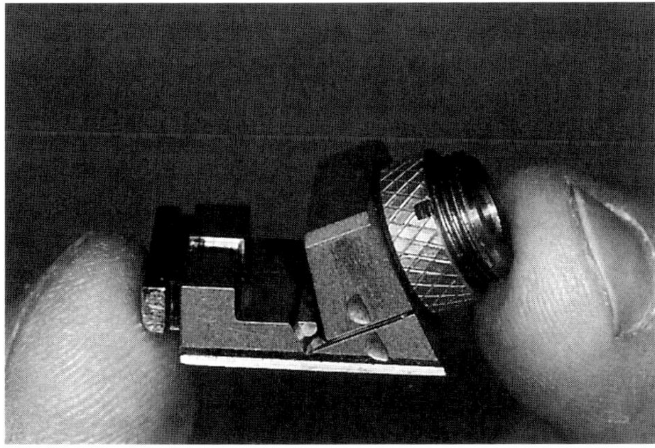

Fig. 10.5 The standard Barraquer microkeratome head.

The standard microkeratome head consists of six parts:

1 Head (posterior part) with shaft hole and blade holder slot
2 Plane (anterior part) slotted for interchangeable plate
3 Blade holder, slotted with blade boss
4 Plate
5 Blade, slotted
6 Threaded fixation collar

The head has a slot into which is fitted the blade holder. The blade holder is also slotted to engage the motor shaft, which inserts through a hole drilled in the head. There are two pins protruding from the head that engage holes in the plane to ensure complete alignment.

Head assembly To assemble the head, fit the blade onto the holder. This can best be done by placing the head, slot upwards and shaft hole toward you, onto a soft surface such as a moistened microsponge instrument wipe (Murocel—do not use a cotton 4 × 4 or a Weck-Cel because these tend to be very "linty"). Place the blade holder into the slot of the head with the holder slot facing the shaft hole and the small bosses facing up. Holding a fresh blade carefully by the side edges, place the blade onto the holder with the cutting edge facing forward. If the blade is single-edged, make sure that the bevel is facing up. Align the blade slot with the holder bosses, and press down—gently—until the blade is engaged. Next, place the plane carefully onto the head, avoiding touching the blade edges to the head, and align the pins into the holes. Holding the assembly together between thumb and forefinger, screw the knurled ring onto the threaded end of the assembly. Make sure that the keyed portion of the ring faces outward. Use the tool provided to gently tighten the ring against the head assembly. Next, insert the short shaft section into the shaft hole, engaging the blade holder. Rotate the short shaft between thumb and forefinger to

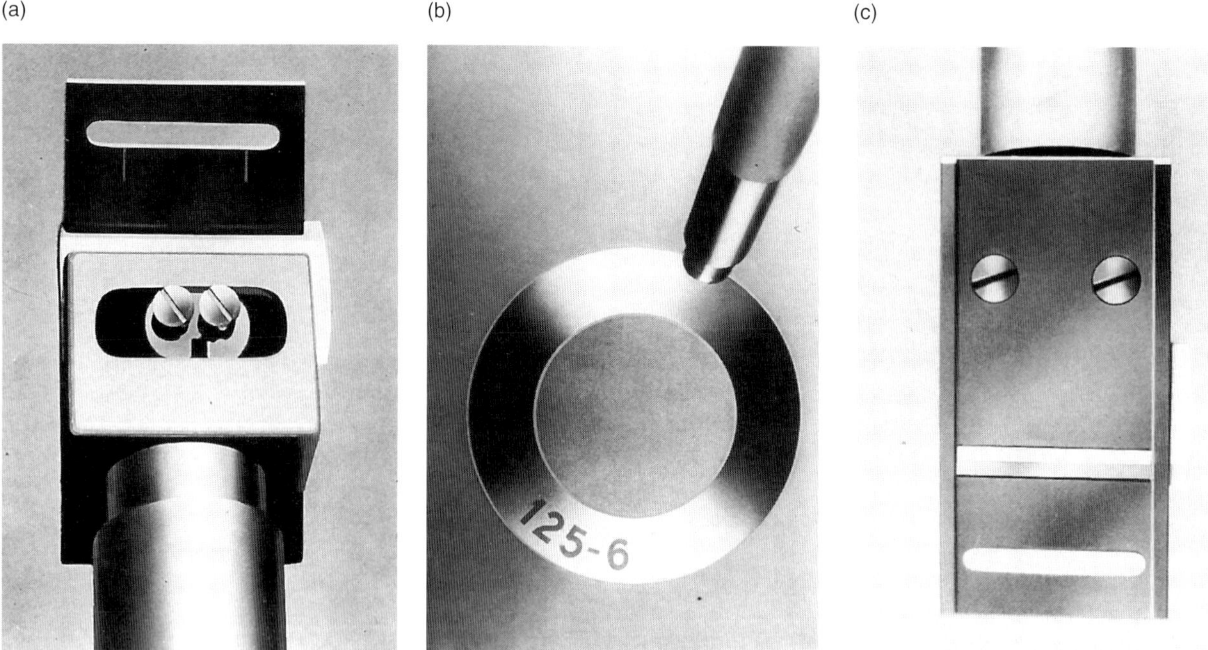

Fig. 10.6 (a,b) Top and bottom views of the prototype microkeratome. The blade is adjustable. (c) Prototype vacuum fixation ring. Note the absence of guides for the keratome (from Barraquer Jl. Historia de la cirugia refractiva de la cornea. In: *Cirugia Refractiva de la Cornea*, Instituto Barraquer de America, Bogota, Colombia, 1989).

ensure that the blade oscillates freely. Remedy any binding by disassembling the unit and carefully reassembling it. Inspect the blade edge at the microscope under high power. It will be necessary to replace the blade if it is nicked. The head for all standard design units is assembled in the same manner as the SCMD unit described above.

The microkeratome head is attached to the handle by screwing it into the handpiece. A *tiny amount* of special grease is applied to the eccentric pin at the very end of the motor shaft. The shaft is inserted into the keratome head, which is then screwed into place until seated finger tight. Apply power to the assembly by depressing the footswitch. If the head rotates, tighten the head more firmly. The microkeratome should operate freely. With practice, any problems with free movement of the shaft and blade can be detected by the sound. Pay strict attention to the sound of a properly functioning keratome while in your instruction laboratory.

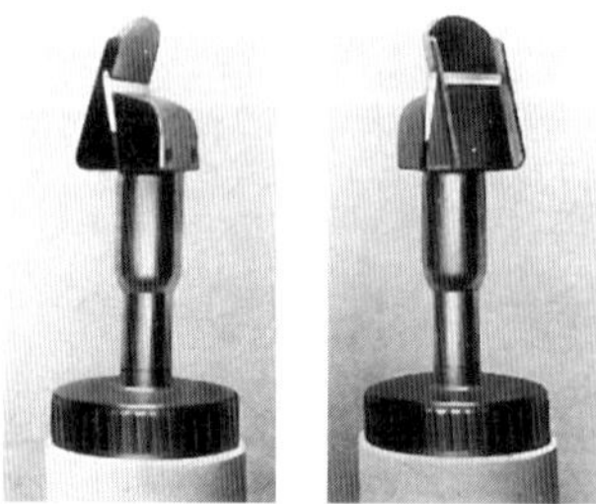

Fig. 10.7 Second-generation keratome head with dovetails, fixed blade, and provision for replaceable applanation plate (from Barraquer Jl. Historia de la cirugia refractiva de la cornea. In: *Cirugia Refractiva de la Cornea*, Instituto Barraquer de America, Bogota, Colombia, 1989).

The original microkeratome motor handle is small and must be gas-sterilized. The newer Steinway motor handle is slightly larger, operates at 12 V (instead of the 30 V of the original), is sealed, and therefore is autoclavable. It is also quieter and develops more torque by virtue of its noncogging motor. Motor speed is not adjustable on either of these model motors.

The SCMD handle assembly consists of a stainless steel handpiece with integral gas supply hose and quick release tubulature fitting. The unit is completely sealed and autoclavable and is designed to run on compressed nitrogen. Take care not to kink the supply hose. The speed of this motor is adjustable but is set at the factory to run at approximately 16,000 rpm. Its only drawbacks are its weight, size, and the fact that it is extremely noisy—sounding like a jet turbine (which in fact it is—in miniature). It also tends to vibrate at a high frequency, which actually tends to help float the head through the guides on the fixation ring.

Plate The thickness of the disk resected by the microkeratome is regulated by the plate. In the standard microkeratome head (for lathing), these plates are supplied in fixed sizes: 15, 20, 25, 30, 35, 40, and 45, corresponding to expected resections of 150 to 450 μm. Keratome sets designed for nonlathing procedures are supplied with slightly different plate sizes. There are other differences

(a)

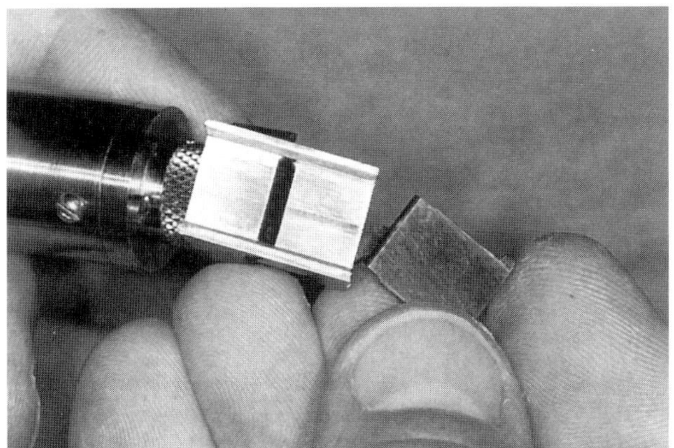

(b)

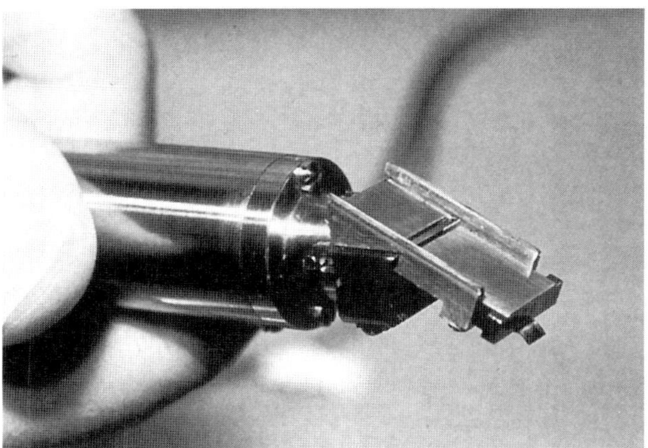

Fig. 10.8 (a) Resection depth (disk thickness) is controlled by interchangeable plates. (b) These plates snap into the anterior part of the keratome base.

(a)

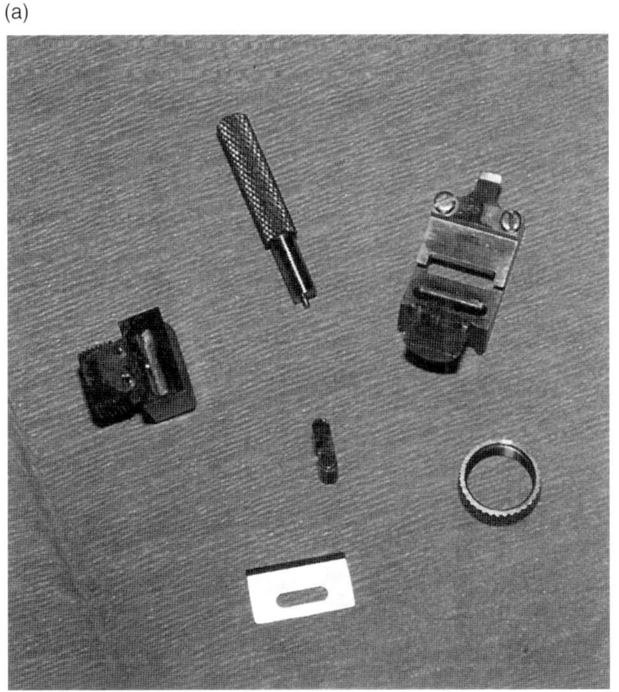

(b)

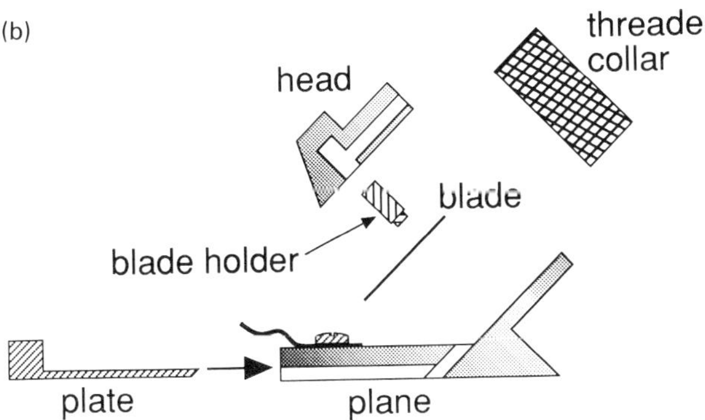

Fig. 10.9 (a) The five individual components of a standard microkeratome head. The short-shaft used to test the assembled head for binding is at the 12 o'clock position. (b) Exploded drawing of a standard keratome.

as well, which will be discussed in the section under "Non-freeze lamellar techniques."

In practice, the actual thickness of the resection will depend on two factors: speed of movement of the head across the cornea and the diameter of the disk. Typically, the instrument invariably will produce a section 20 to 30 μm thicker than the plate size. Additionally, disks cut from human eye-bank eyes can be expected to measure 20 to 40 μm more in thickness than those cut from living eyes. If the speed of the motor is less than 7000 rpm or the translation speed (speed of movement across the cornea) is too fast, the resulting sections will be thinner than expected. This has become less of a problem with the automated heads, but variability in cap thickness can still occur.

If disks of *different diameter* are cut with the same plate, it will be found that the larger disk will be somewhat thicker than the smaller one. For example, using a no. 15 plate, the operator cuts a disk of 7.25 mm diameter. Typically, such a section will measure 170 to 180 μm in thickness. A disk cut with the same setting but with a 4.25-mm diameter usually will measure 140 to 150 μm in thickness.

It should be noted that the numbers engraved on each of these plates refer to the nominal thickness of the disk expected to be resected using that specific keratome head—plus some additional amount. Despite the number engraved on the plate, a section of greater or lesser (usually greater) thickness will result. These plates are not transferable and cannot be used with other keratome heads, even those made by the same manufacturer. Each plate is custom-fitted to a specific head. This is a potential problem only if, like the author, the surgeon has more than one microkeratome in his or her operatory.

Some surgeons are concerned by apparent inconsistencies in plate thicknesses after having measured various plates with a micrometer. Some plates have different numbers but are of the same thickness! Disk thickness is, of course, related to just how much blade edge is exposed below the plate. However, remember that this unit resembles a carpenter's plane. Thickness of the section is thus also related to the aperture or space between the blade edge and back edge of the plate. Thus, if a plate is slightly shorter than another of the same thickness, the shorter plate will produce a slightly thicker section—all else being equal.

SCMD microkeratome head

In the case of the SCMD instrument, this disk thickness is determined by moving the plate up or down with the threaded adjustment knob. In actual practice this is accomplished by placing the detached head, upside down, into a special gauge ring mounted on a heavy support base. The system is zeroed by slowly lowering the Teflon anvil until it rests on the blade edge. The zero point is set and the gauge locked. The anvil is raised slightly above the blade, and the head is moved back slightly so that when the anvil is again lowered it will now rest on the surface of the movable plate—adjacent to the blade. The head is grasped firmly and the knob turned to move the plate the desired distance. Once the correct thickness has been reached, the anvil is raised and the zero point rechecked. Next the setting is regauged. It is very important that the plate blade edge spacing be measured with the anvil as close to the blade as possible. Take care to ensure that the anvil does not touch the blade. It is possible.

Rule 1: The *plate* determines disk *thickness*.

To use the microkeratome in refractive surgery, a few complementary instruments—such as pneumatic fixation rings, a preoperative tonometer, and applanation lenses—are necessary.

Pneumatic fixation rings

Regardless of the precision of the microkeratome head, accurate sections cannot be obtained in the absence of the vacuum guide, or fixation rings. These rings are designed not only to fixate the eye but also to pressurize it. In addition, they provide a precise base against which the keratome acts to produce the proper thickness of tissue section as well as its diameter.

The primary function of the rings is to ensure that the proper diameter tissue disk is cut.

Rule 2: *Rings* determine disk *diameter*.

The fixation ring is a short cylinder approximately 21 mm in diameter machined internally to fit snugly onto the eye (Figure 10.10). Those of you with lathing experience will note that the KMIS rings are slightly larger than those provided with the lathe. The central opening of the rings is 11.5 mm, through which the cornea will protrude. The upper surface is highly polished to reduce friction

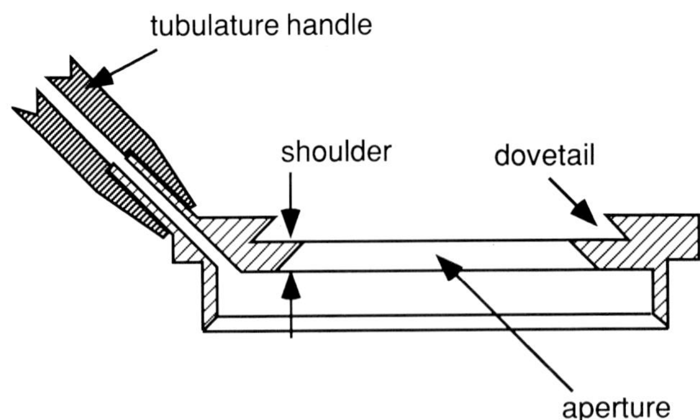

Fig. 10.10 Typical vacuum ring design. The internal shoulder varies in thickness to provide different resection diameters.

and is provided with a ridge and double-dovetail keratome guide. The author prefers the easy off-on nature of the original Barraquer rings with a single dovetail—they are easier to disengage at the end of the keratectomy. Theoretically, this feature also makes it easier to lose contact with the ring surface. If this happens, the section will be irregular in thickness. The argument in favor of the double guides is that they prevent the keratome from lifting off the ring surface. This makes it a cinch for the surgeon (especially the beginner) to maintain contact with the plate. While this is true, the double-guide rings also tend to bind, resulting in a jerky movement across the corneal surface. This also results in irregular resection thickness. That the concern surrounding the single dovetail is spurious is demonstrated by Figure 10.11. Rings can be supplied with either single or double guides.

The lower surface of the fixation ring is concave with a wide 360° groove (Figure 10.12). When applied to the globe along with a vacuum via the ring tubulature handle, the ring adjusts to the globe and holds it with suction. The diameter of the ring–eye interface (12.5 mm) and the degree of vacuum supplied by the pump (22 in. of H_2O) have been selected carefully to induce an intraocular pressure rise of 65 mm Hg. Smaller (11.0-mm-diameter) rings are used in pediatric cases and are available on special order.

There are some 10 to 25 rings, depending on the set, ranging from 0.4 (no. 4) to 1.80 (no. 18) mm. In some cases, rings as low as no. 2 or no. 3 may be needed and are available as optional equipment depending on the design and purpose of the set. It is advised that these be obtained when you take delivery of your equipment—all rings have to be matched to a specific microkeratome. The diameter of these rings is constant, but their internal and external heights vary. Inside each ring there is a small ledge or shoulder in which the aperture of the ring is cut. The thickness of this shoulder varies and increases as the ring number increases. Each ring is engraved with an identifying number that corresponds to the height of

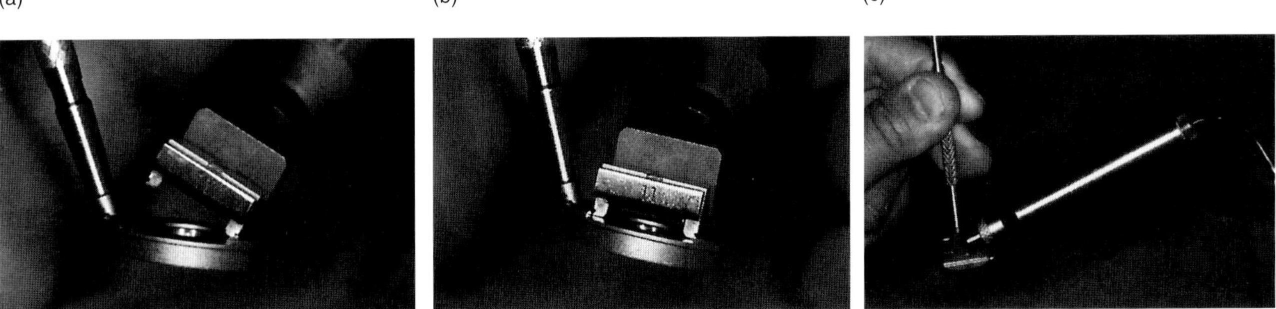

Fig. 10.11 (a,b) A single-dovetail guide allows easy engagement and disengagement of the keratome. (c) The only thing holding this assembled microkeratome securely in the fixation ring is a single-dovetail guide.

the upper ring surface as measured from the corneoscleral contact point in 0.10-mm increments. The thickness (height) of this shoulder determines just how far the cornea protrudes through the central aperture and consequently the amount of cornea flattened by the plastic applanator lens. The lower the number, the more cornea that will protrude and the larger is the diameter of the disk that will be cut. The ring size then determines the diameter of the resected corneal disk when used with the applanator lenses (see below)

The accompanying diagrams illustrate this point. In Figure 10.13, the shoulder height is low (thinner); therefore, *L* is high. In this case, the area applanated will be large. In Figure 10.14, the shoulder height is high (thicker); therefore, *L* is low. In this case, the area applanated will be small. If the applanated area is too large, less cornea must be drawn up into the ring to get a smaller-diameter disk. In that case it will be necessary to select a ring having a higher number (thicker shoulder). Conversely, if the applanated area is too small, a smaller number ring (thinner shoulder) must be selected.

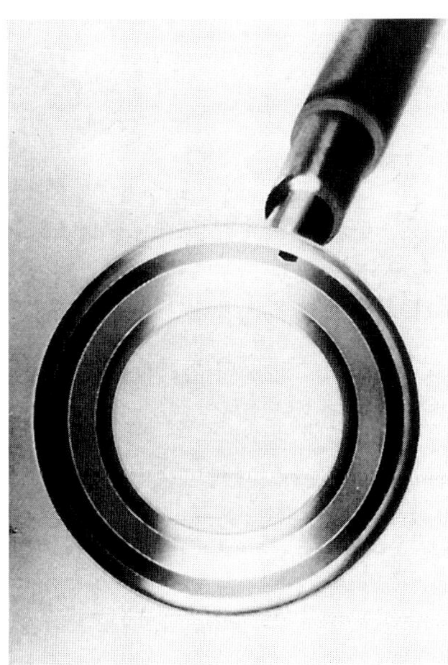

Fig. 10.12 The underside of a vacuum fixation ring (prototype) (from Barraquer JI. Historia de la cirugia refractiva de la cornea. In: *Cirugia Refractiva de la Cornea*, Instituto Barraquer de America, Bogota, Colombia, 1989).

For example, if a disk diameter of 7.25 mm is desired, that applanator is selected. In applanators having two reticle rings (Bores type), the outer, larger ring always measures 7.25 mm in diameter—therefore, the applanator will be marked with the diameter of the *small* reticle. Next, a fixation ring is selected that through experience will cause an area of cornea to be applanated (flattened) of 7.25 mm in diameter. Typically, a no. 8 (0.8-mm) ring will expose sufficient cornea to achieve this. Start the no. 8, and apply suction to the eye. Dry the cornea, and apply the applanator (Figure 10.15).

The area flattened should just fit within or be slightly smaller than the inscribed circle. If the area is too small, more cornea needs be exposed or the disk will be too small. Therefore, a ring of lower height (thinner) needs to be used to attain the diameter desired. Try a no. 5 (0.5 mm). If the area is too large, less cornea needs be exposed—therefore, select a ring of greater height (thicker). Try a no. 10 (1.0 mm).

Corollary to Rule 2: If the disk is too small, choose a lower-numbered ring, and vice versa.

Applanator lenses

These lenses are measuring instruments designed to determine that the proper fixation ring is used so as to obtain a tissue disk of the correct diameter upon sectioning. Treat them accordingly.

Some of these lenses are made from PMMA and are to be cold sterilized by soaking in CIDEX or a similar chemical disinfectant. Gas sterilization is not recommended because the carrier gas—Freon—can craze the plastic surfaces, destroying their accuracy. Recently, autoclavable clear plastic applanators have become available. Check

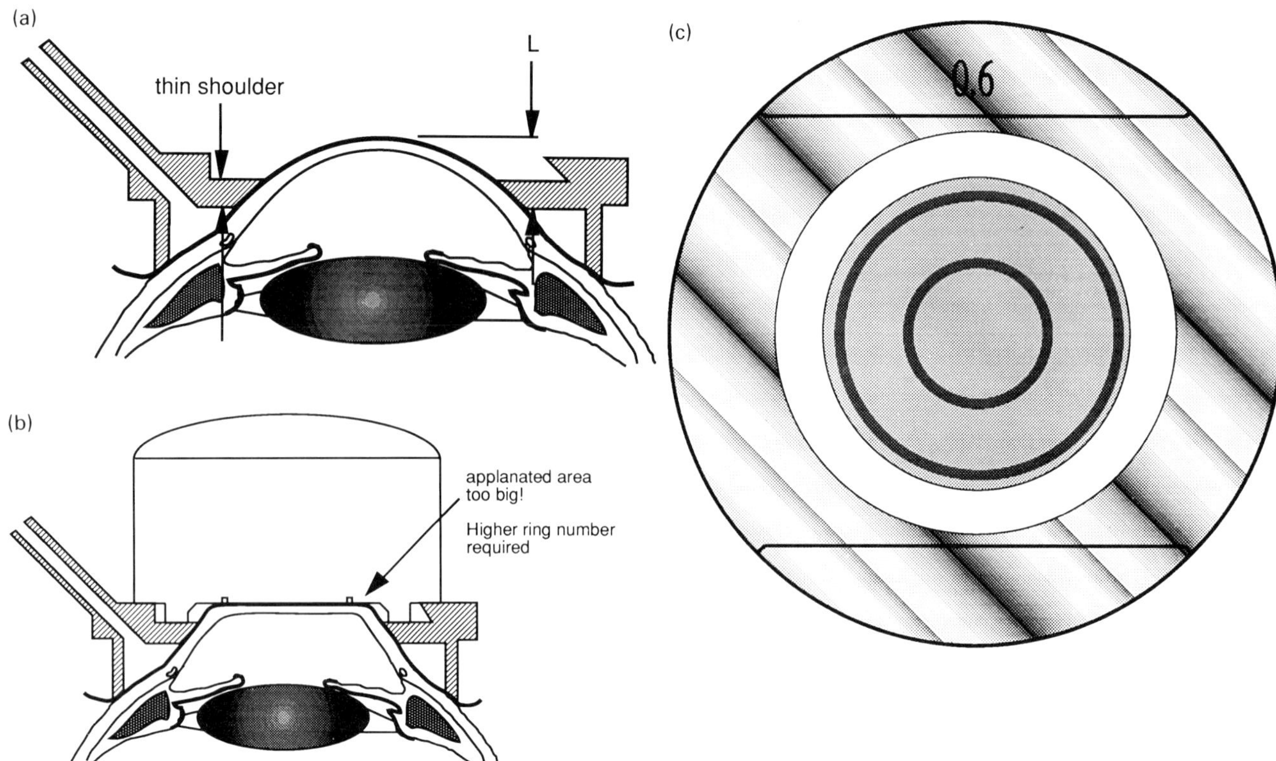

Fig. 10.13 In a low-numbered ring (thin shoulder), more cornea protrudes through the ring. (a–c) Now the applanated area is too large. Choose a slightly thicker (higher number) ring and try again.

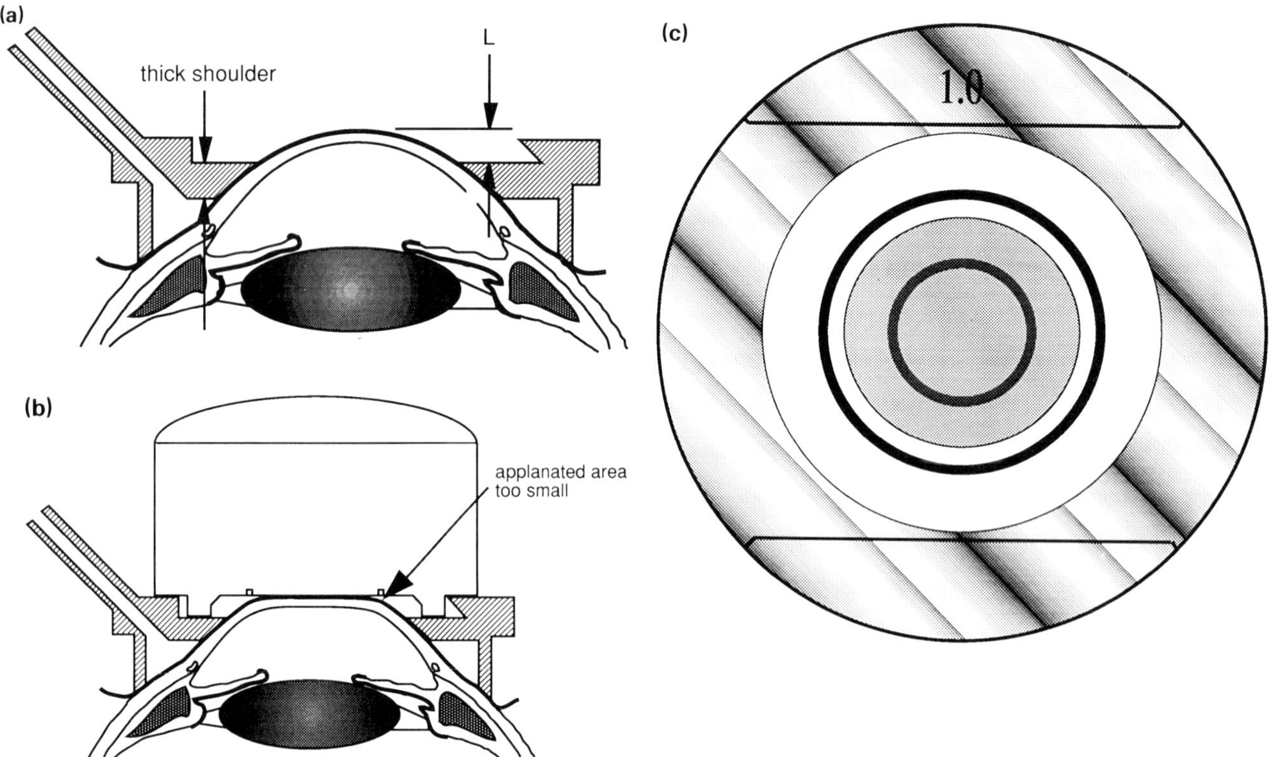

Fig. 10.14 In a high-numbered ring (thick shoulder), less cornea protrudes through the ring. (a-c) The applanated area is too small. Choose a lower number (thinner) ring and try again.

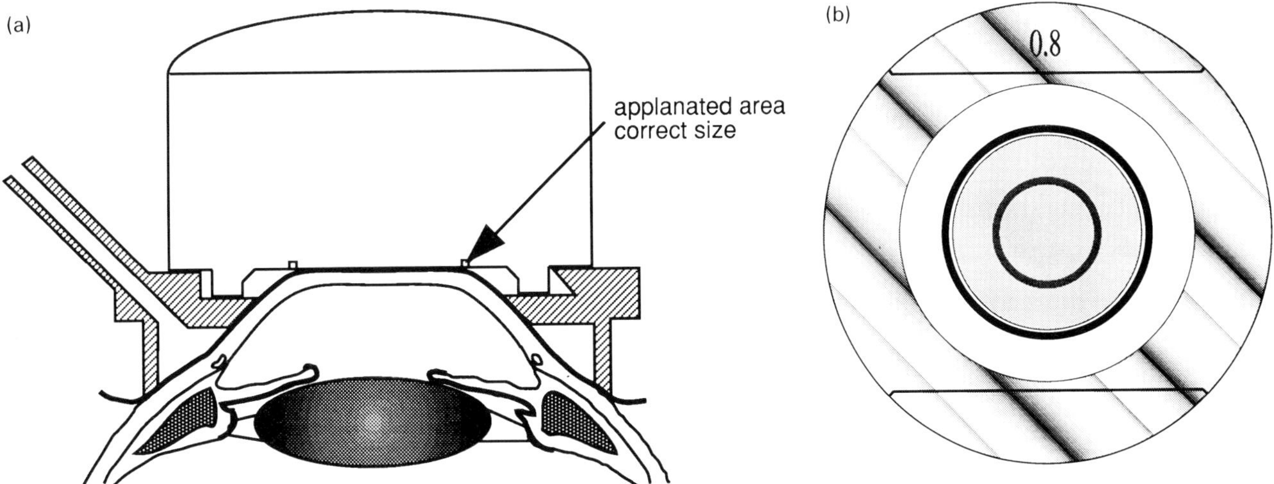

Fig. 10.15 (a,b) The no. 8 ring is the correct choice in this case. Note that the edge of the applanated area is slightly smaller than desired. This is necessary (but not critical in keratomileusis *in-situ*) because the disk will have a diameter 0.2 mm in excess of that applanated.

with your supplier to make sure which type you have do not assume.

Typically, the applanators will have an upper face made convex to serve as a magnifying loupe (Figure 10.16). The bottom surface has a matte finish and is inscribed with one or two circles (reticles). The larger of the circles in double-ring applanators is *always* 7.25 mm in diameter. These lenses are marked with the size of the smaller ring. Thus a no. 3.5 double-ring applanator has a 7.25- and 3.5-mm ring scribed on its undersurface. The smaller circles range in diameter from 3.5 to 5.0 mm in the KMIS set. The applanator set for HLK has single rings measuring from 4.8 to 6.8 mm in diameter. Standard applanators supplied for lathing typically have only one reticle, although double rings can be specified.

When these lenses are placed onto the fixation ring, the reticle is at the same height as that of the microkeratome back plane—0.13 mm. Two indentations have been made into the sides of the lenses to fit around the vacuum tubulature handle of the fixation ring (Figure 10.17). The applanator must contact the surface of the ring completely to ensure that the measurements are correct (Figure 10.18). If contact is not made, an incorrect disk diameter will result—typically larger.

The disk diameter will need to be varied somewhat depending on the amount of ametropia to be corrected—the computer will determine the disk diameter. In KMIS, for example, the diameter of the first section has been determined—optimally—to be 7.25 mm. While the ideal diameter of the first section should be 7.25 mm, there is no appreciable difference in outcome with sections varying from 6.0 to 8.0 mm in diameter. There appears to be a greater incidence of postoperative astigmatism with disks that are either larger or smaller than 7.25 mm, however. Disk diameters in classic KM should never be smaller than 7.0 mm.

To obtain a disk of the proper size, always begin with a no. 8 ring, ensuring that there is sufficient clearance between it and the lid retractor so as not to interfere with passage of the keratome through the ring. Engage the suction foot pedal, and check the intraocular pressure (IOP) with the surgical tonometer (see below). Then place the

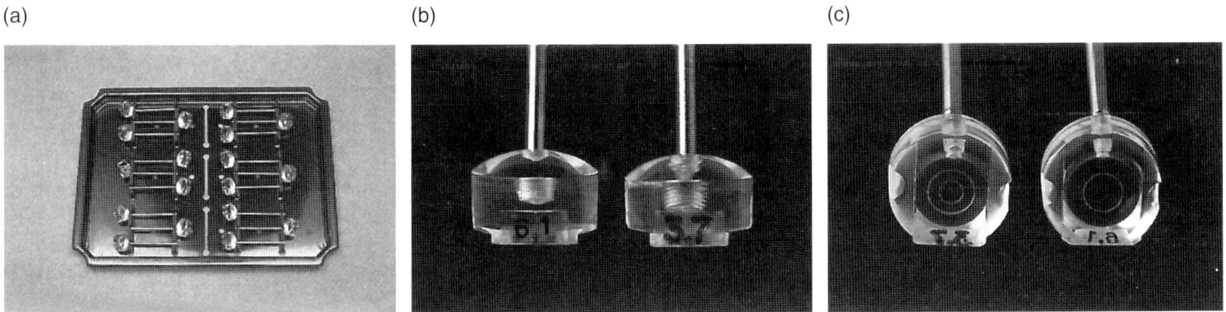

Fig. 10.16 (a) A set of plastic applanator lenses for MKM. (b,c) Double reticle applanators are marked with the size of the *smaller* reticle, the larger is always 7.25 mm.

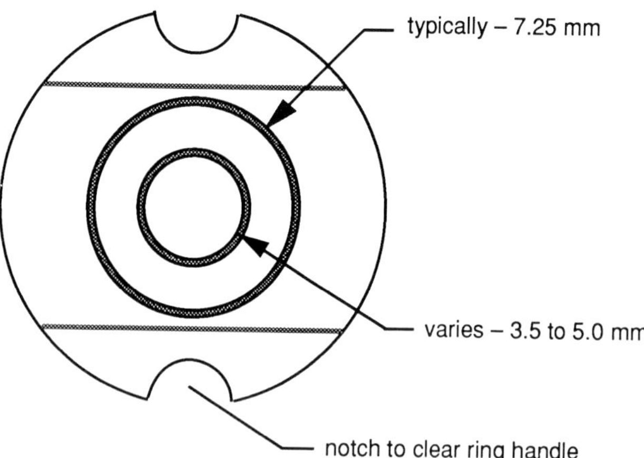

Fig. 10.17 The applanator is usually notched to clear the tubulature handle.

applanator lens onto the fixation ring. Make sure that the cornea is dry. The applanated portion of the central cornea should just touch the inside edge of the inscribed ring. Ideally, the applanated area should be approximately 0.2 mm smaller than the scribed ring because the actual diameter of the resected disk is always about 0.2 mm larger than measured. If the area is too small, then a smaller (lower-number) ring must be used. Try to select the ring size by observing the actual size of the applanated area. If it is just slightly undersize, then the next size down probably will be acceptable. If it is markedly smaller, then select a ring several sizes smaller. Details on making the keratectomy will be discussed in the following section.

Try to make the choice of ring with as few reapplications of suction as possible so as to minimize intraoperative conjunctival edema and possible subconjunctival hemorrhage. Occasionally, repeated applications of suction during surgery will result in sufficient edema of the conjunctiva to prevent adequate fixation. In such cases, a peritomy may be necessary or the surgery abandoned (see also Chapter 15). The same steps are taken for the second resection in KMIS. Remember, keep the cornea dry when measuring with the applanator lenses to avoid errors.

Remember, also, that there is a subtle relationship between disk diameter and thickness. For a given plate, a large-diameter aplanation (lower-numbered ring) will always result in a thicker disk. The flatter the corneal curvature, the smaller diameter will be the resulting corneal section. The reverse is also true. Do not forget that sections that are larger are slightly thicker as well.

Preoperative tonometer

To obtain a good resection with the microkeratome, the IOP must be raised momentarily and uniformly. Experience has shown that an IOP of approximately 65 mm Hg is required at the moment of resection to obtain an optimal disk. The pressure will not be applied for longer than 10 seconds, and thus far there have been no secondary complications because of this. The preoperative tonometer has been designed to ascertain that the correct pressure has been obtained when the suction ring has been engaged.

The device is a cone-shaped lens made of methyl methacrylate, weighing approximately 10 g (Figure 10.19). The upper face is convex to act as a magnifier to facilitate reading the reticle. The narrow or bottom face has been given a matte finish and is inscribed with a reticle 0.38 mm in diameter.

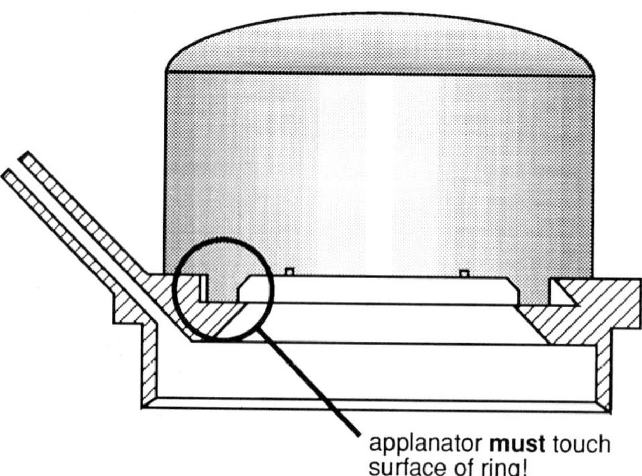

Fig. 10.18 The applanator lens has to be in contact with the ring surface to read correctly.

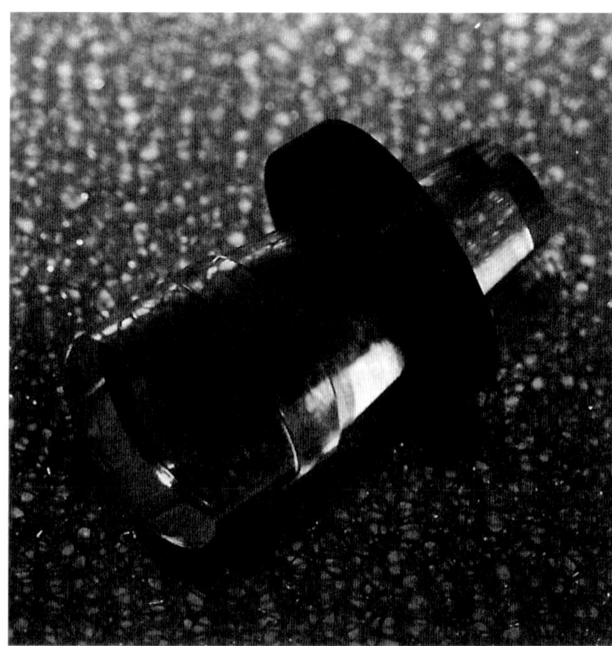

Fig. 10.19 The presurgical tonometer is in two parts: the applanator and the support ring.

Wipe the lower face with a damp microsponge to remove any trace of sterilizing solution. The instrument is then held vertically over the center of a dry cornea, being careful not to touch the ring or lid retractor. This maneuver is aided by the loose plastic ring supplied with the device. Apply the instrument to the cornea. The applanated area should just fill the inscribed circle. A wet cornea will give a false reading, so make sure that the cornea is dry.

Hand and special instrumentation

There are, in addition to the equipment described in the preceding sections, certain other hand instruments and miscellaneous equipment used with this surgery (Figure 10.20). The first of these is the Barraquer lenticule spoon (Katena K3-4250). This instrument is also available from Western Instruments in titanium. While especially designed for retrieving disks from the Kitton green preservative solution used during cryolathing, it is also extremely useful for handling the thin first disk in keratomileusis in situ. Since this tissue is only 130 to 150 μm thick, it is easily damaged by handling with the usual corneal tissue forceps such as a Colibri forceps with 0.12-mm teeth. If you must handle the disk with forceps, a Pierse-Hoskins type is recommended, and the pressure on the tissue should be very light—sufficient to hold but not crush the disk edge.

Another instrument that may be of considerable help, especially for the beginning surgeon, is the Bores-Ruiz bull's-eye marker from DGH. This marker is made of titanium and consists of an outer 10.5-mm ring joined and aligned with a smaller (4.0-mm) ring fitted with a cross-hair and off-axis reference-marker blade. This marker is used by coating it with a 1% tincture of brilliant green applied with a cotton-tipped applicator and allowed to dry. This will produce a bright green semi-indelible mark on the corneal surface. If this is done, make sure that the alcohol has completely dried on the marker before applying it to the cornea to avoid damaging the epithelium. A fresh skin-marking pen also can be used to coat the surfaces of the marker. This marker is aligned with the constricted pupil and produces two concentric marks on the cornea that serve to assist in aligning the suction ring on the eye. In addition, the off-axis blade makes the parallel reference mark simultaneously.

A 4.0-mm marker such as the Bores optical zone marker for radial keratotomy (RK; see Chapter 8) also should be included in the instrument set. This instrument is used to mark the cornea for HLK and also to circumscribe the pupil prior to making the tangential reference mark.

The Hofman-Polack forceps is an optional instrument that some find useful in this surgery to prevent the tissue disk from rotating when placing the cardinal sutures. The author uses this forceps extensively in transplant surgery but does not find it essential in MKM.

A plastic moist chamber is essential for storing the disk/lenticule while cleaning the resection bed in cases where the cap will be removed completely (Figure 10.22). A plastic corneal cap is also needed to cover the resection while cleaning and/or lathing the tissue disk in such cases. A white porcelain crucible with lid is used to hold the cryopreservative—Kitton green—if lathing is to be done. The white color makes it easier to see the disk in the solution. A stainless steel crucible with lid holds a balanced salt solution in a special heater block to thaw the lenticule after lathing.

An artificial anterior chamber completes the list of necessary equipment (Figure 10.22). This device is necessary for sectioning disks from preserved donor tissue when

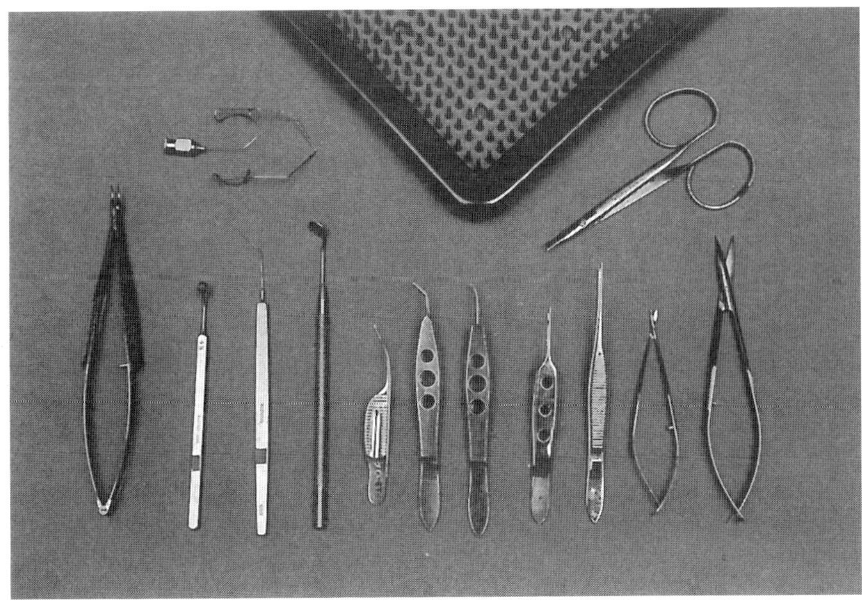

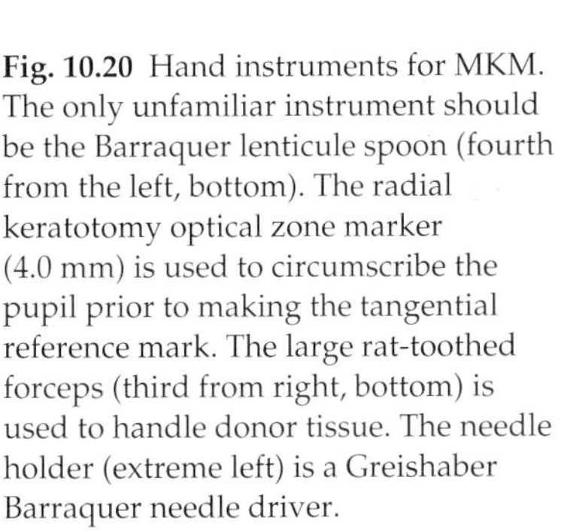

Fig. 10.20 Hand instruments for MKM. The only unfamiliar instrument should be the Barraquer lenticule spoon (fourth from the left, bottom). The radial keratotomy optical zone marker (4.0 mm) is used to circumscribe the pupil prior to making the tangential reference mark. The large rat-toothed forceps (third from right, bottom) is used to handle donor tissue. The needle holder (extreme left) is a Greishaber Barraquer needle driver.

(a)

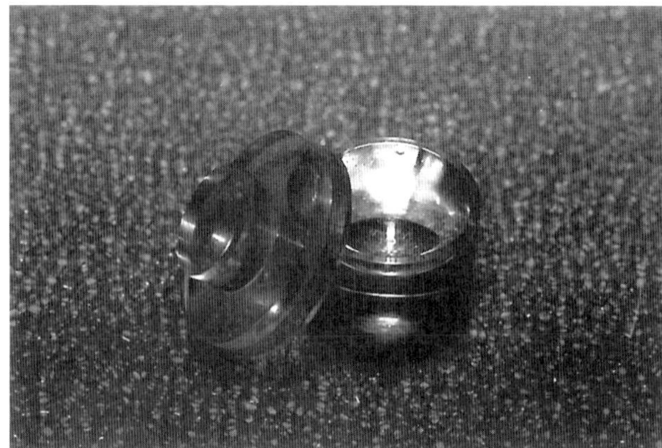

(b)

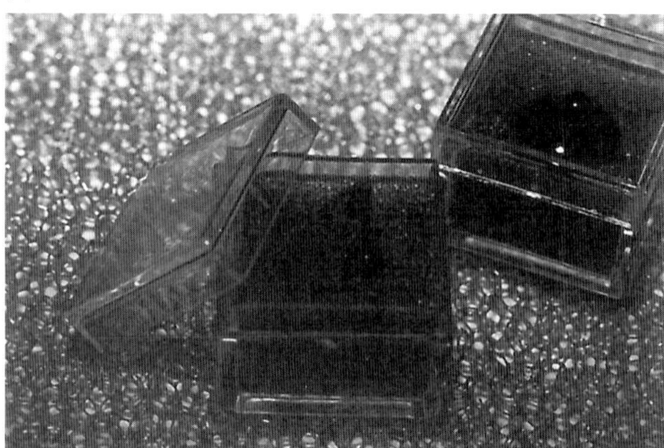

(c)

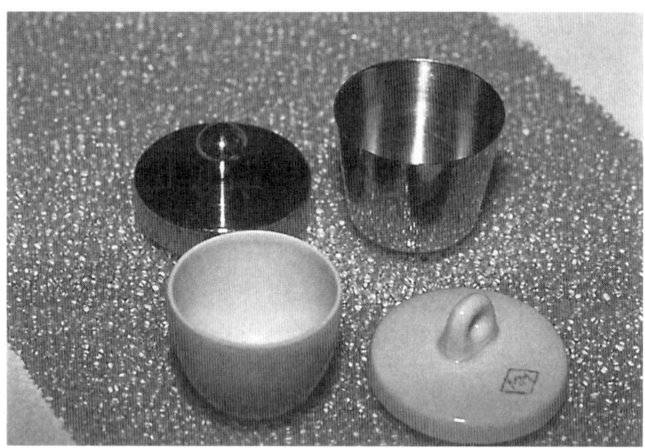

Fig. 10.21 Ancillary equipment. (a) Plastic moist storage chamber; (b) corneal dust cover; (c) the white crucible is for the cryo-preservative, the other is the tissue-thawing chamber.

whole globes are not available for backup, for homoplastic KM, or when making epikeratophakia lenticules.

Advances in microkeratome design

The keratectomy has always been the stumbling point in lamellar procedures. It is difficult to make consistently regular sections. Consequently, manufacturers have cast about in an effort to make this part of the procedure more precise and repeatable.

Draeger microkeratome

The Draeger microkeratome unit has a rotating blade powered by a geared motor (Figure 10.23). The head is driven across the cornea by a helical gear train that provides a smooth and even translation each time. The advantages of such a motor-driven translation system are, of course, the possibility of producing an even-thickness resection case after case. Disk diameter is regulated by an adjustable transparent applanator plate. Disk thickness is selectable in several discrete increments by inserting a special shim analogous to the applanator plate of the standard keratome (Figure 10.24). The unit is very quiet. Prototypes tended to produce sections of uneven thickness because of the instability of the rotating blade. Disks also tended to be slightly elliptical. The author has not found the new unit to possess these deficiencies. A special artificial anterior chamber/motor table allows the device to be used to cut disks from donor corneal buttons and produce nonlathed epikeratophakia lenticules (Figure 10.25).

Steinway-Ruiz automatic microkeratome

This unit differs from the other products of this company by being completely motor-driven (Figure 10.26). An external cogwheel system moves the microkeratome through the guide ring and across the cornea automatically (Figure 10.27). The unit depends on the pressure of the eye to force the head against the dovetail guides and keep the gear in its track. When it moves, it does so with a slightly tottering or drunken pitching movement. Theoretically, the unit should produce sections whose cut surfaces would be ridged. However, clinical experience has not shown this to be the case.

The new unit also incorporates a continuously adjustable suction ring (Figure 10.29). Theoretically, this allows the operator to retain the ring on the eye for the second

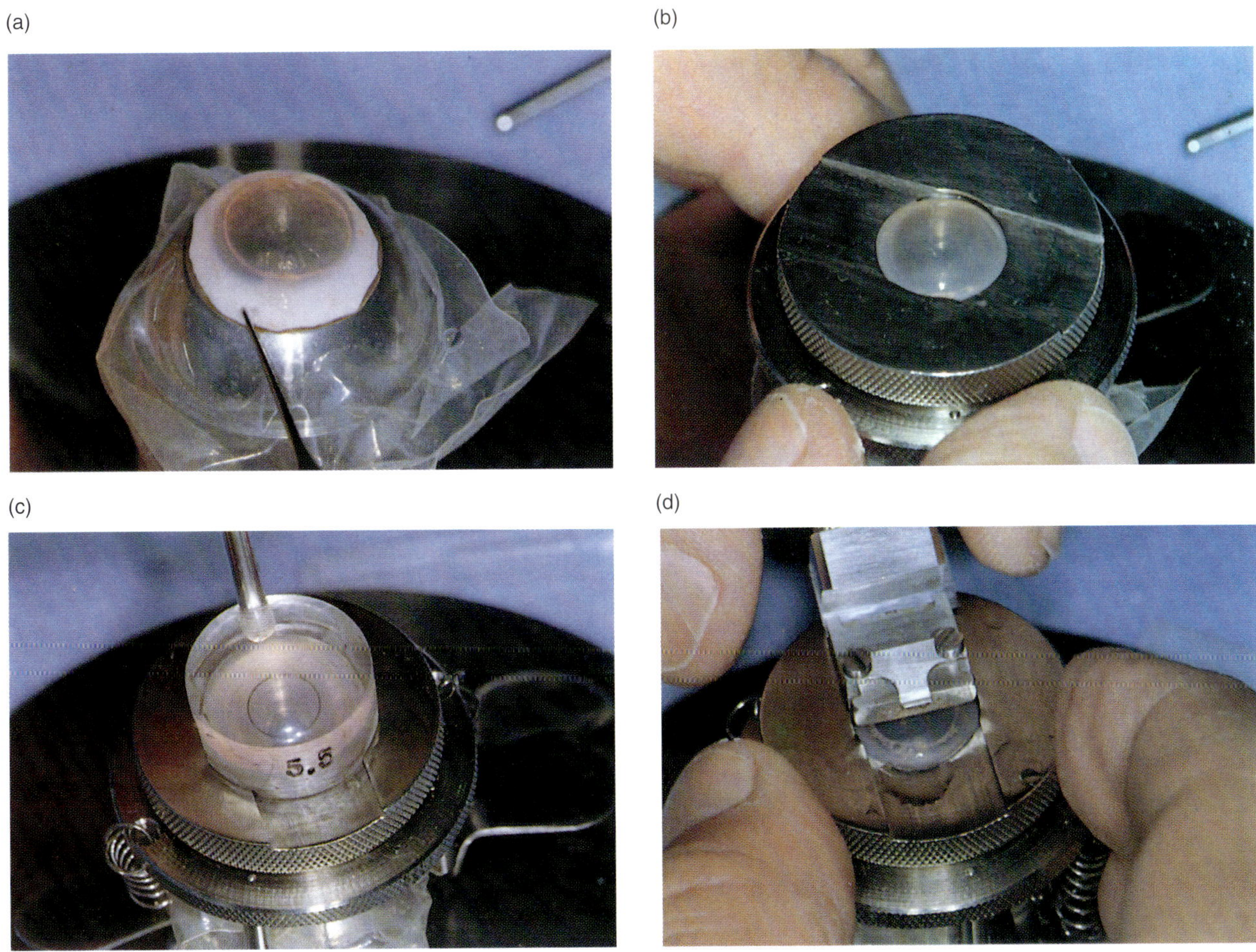

Fig. 10.22 Artificial anterior chamber. Thin rubber dam material is placed over the pressure chamber aperture and the chamber is filled with saline, expelling all air. (a) The donor cornea is centered over the chamber aperture. (b) The retainer ring is snapped over the tissue button completely covering the edges. The guide ring is then screwed onto the retainer. (c) The disk diameter is checked with the applanator. The diameter is controlled by screwing or unscrewing the guide ring. (d) Holding the guide ring firmly, the keratectomy is performed.

section in keratomileusis in situ, thereby ensuring proper centration. However, since the keratome plate has to be changed, it is not practical nor a good idea to leave the suction on the eye while this is done. It does cut down on the number of parts to keep track of, nonetheless.

The motor design incorporates a safety mechanism such that if the unit stalls in its movement, blade motion stops as well. This is an important safeguard and prevents both cutting into the anterior chamber and mangling of the resected disk. However, disengaging the unit from the tissue when this happens is not easy to accomplish without endangering the disk.

Most important is that the speed across the cornea is preset and constant from section to section. This completely eliminates the variability in sections made with the older versions of this keratome, which depended entirely on operator skill. Since the most critical part of keratomileusis is the keratectomy, this device should open the door to a more widespread application of lamellar refractive surgery.

Other manufacturers such as LaserSight with its MicroShape keratome and Solan with its FlapMaker have entered the microkeratome market with disposable cutting heads. The device chosen should deliver consistent cuts and be reliable.

Surgical technique of classic keratomileusis

The surgery should be performed at a site in which dust has been strictly controlled. This is critical to avoid interface debris that has the potential to degrade vision. The floor model laminar flow filters manufactured by Stora Filterprodukter AB of Grycksbo, Sweden, have been recommended in the past for dust control. These units are currently not available in the United States or Canada. However, Oto-Med, of Lake Havasu, Arizona, is making a low-profile, high-efficiency wall-hung unit that will serve even better. There are two units available—large and small. The larger unit can move 1600 cubic feet of air per minute. In a recent test, the device reduced a room

(a)

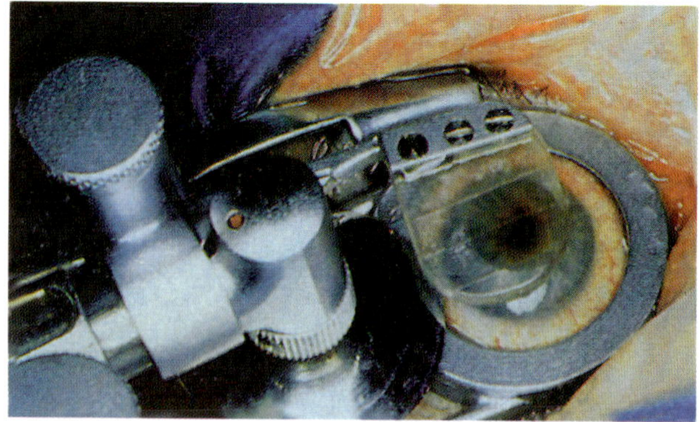

(b)

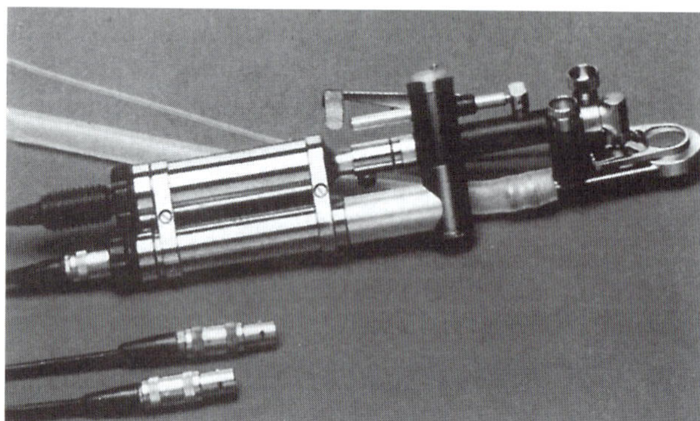

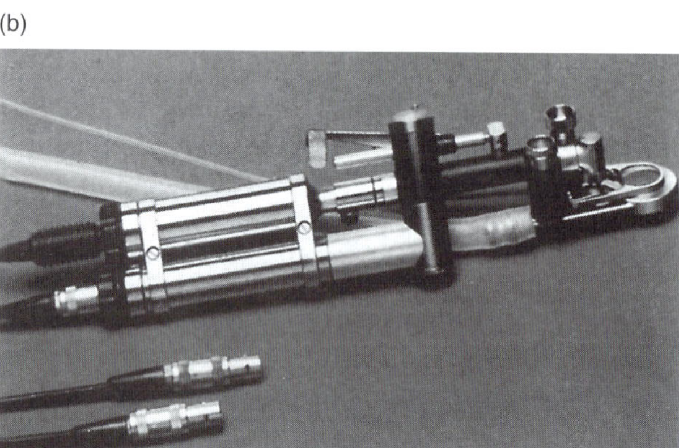

(c)

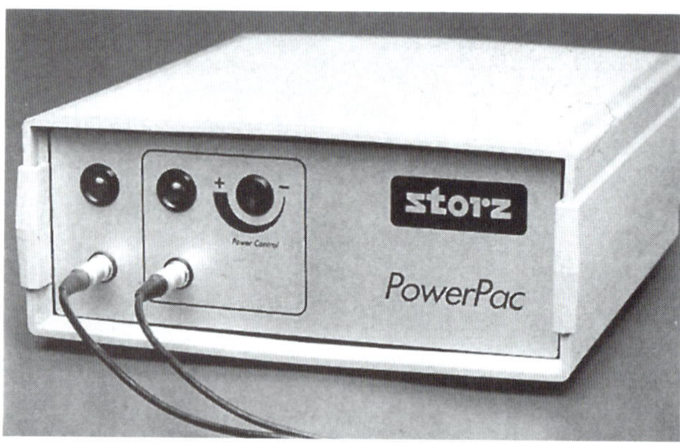

Fig. 10.23 (a, b) The Draeger microkeratome unit. It is powered by a compact power supply (c).

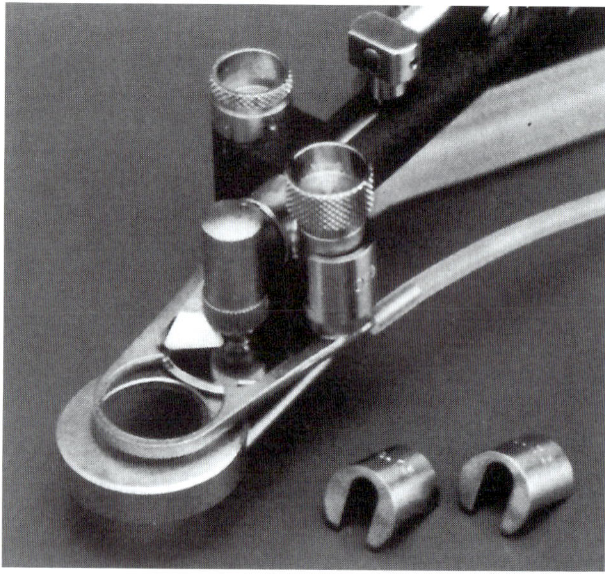

Fig. 10.24 Disk thickness is selectable by inserting special shims.

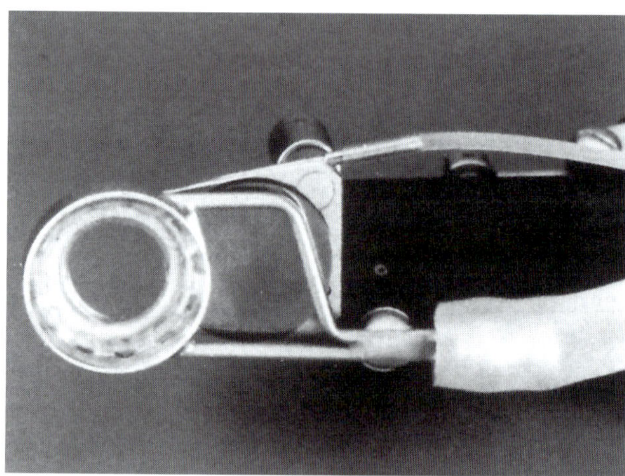

Fig. 10.25 The vacuum fixation ring is integral with the handpiece.

(a) (b)

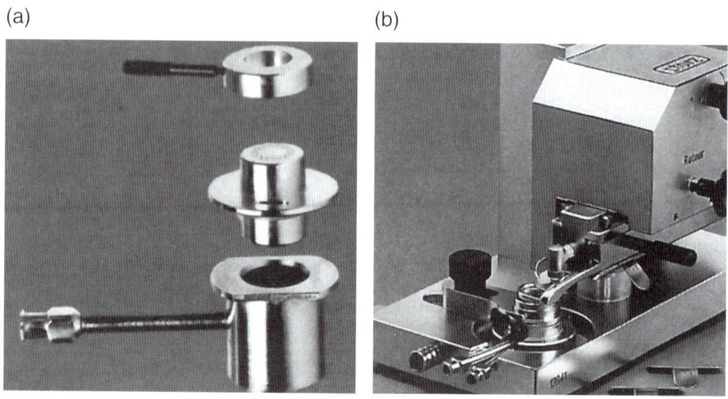

Fig. 10.26 The artificial anterior chamber (a) is inserted into the base of the motor table (b). Disk thickness is controlled by interchangeable plates. Disk cutting is automatic once the system is set up.

(a)

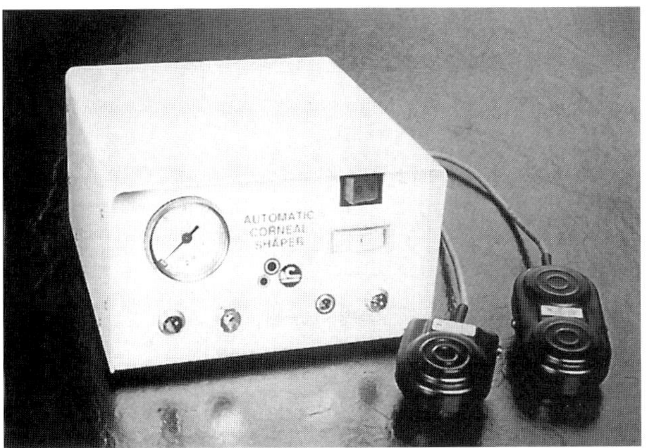

(b)

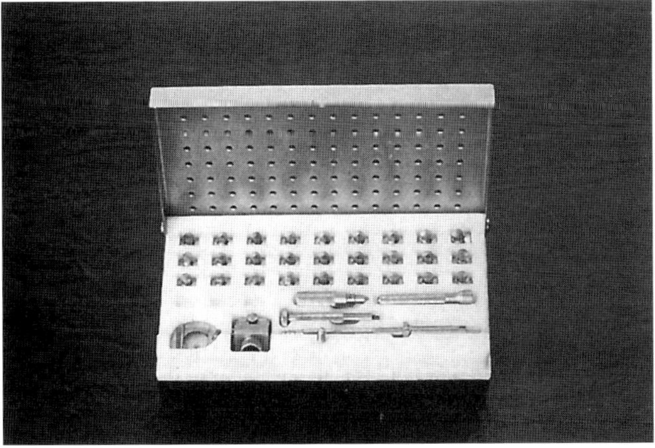

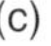

(c)

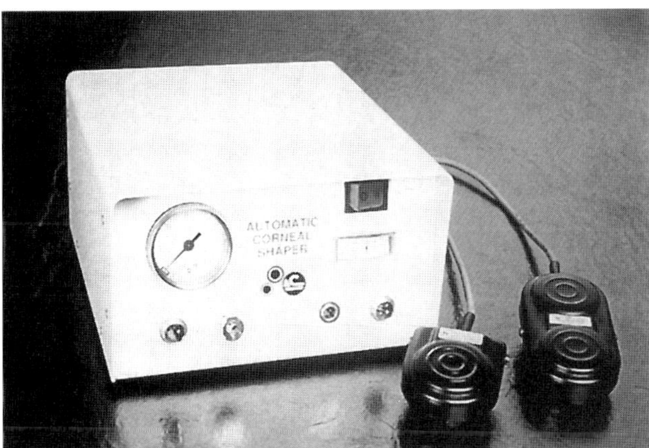

Fig. 10.27 (a–c) The Steinway–Ruiz automatic corneal shaper.

from 16,000 0.5-µm particles per cubic foot to 500 particles per cubic foot within 5 minutes. These units should be switched on a minimum of 1 to 2 hours before surgery is to take place—running full speed, although they can run at low speed overnight. At the author's clinic, the units are run for a few hours each day. If you are using

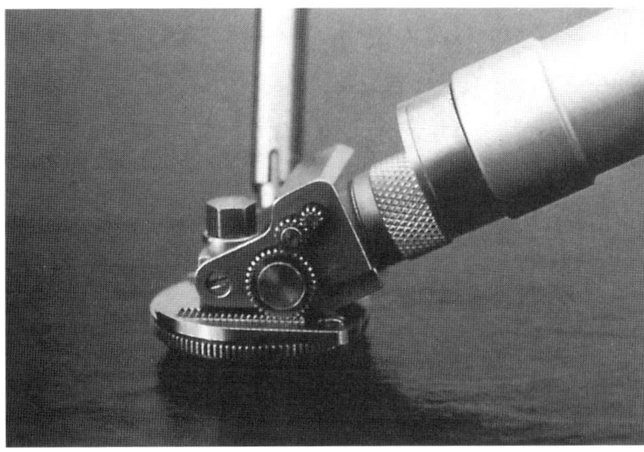

Fig. 10.28 This device is a gear-driven microkeratome.

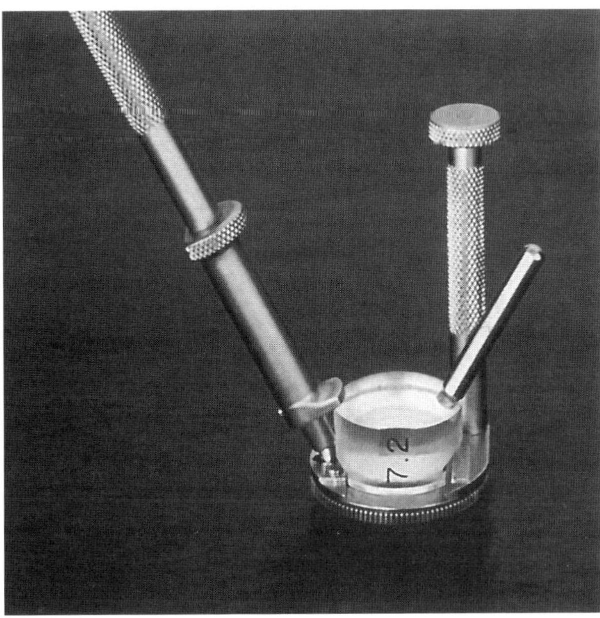

Fig. 10.29 The vacuum fixation ring is adjustable to produce the desired disk diameter.

your own facility, floor mopping and dusting should be done while the filter is running at full speed. Sterile lintless drapes are required in the surgery, and no gloves are to be worn when performing any of these procedures.

While the keratectomy may be a critical factor in the outcome of the case, the disk needs to be converted to a lenticule—this is where the lathe comes in. In classic keratomileusis, therefore, the lathe is the instrument that produces the alteration in corneal curvature that achieves the desired effect. Barraquer's experimental work was performed on a modified jeweler's lathe (Figure 10.30). The actual lathe used for the first surgical cases was a modified Levin contact lens lathe (Figure 10.31). Today's lathe is much more sophisticated, and a new device was to be more so (Figure 10.32). When the first of these cases was

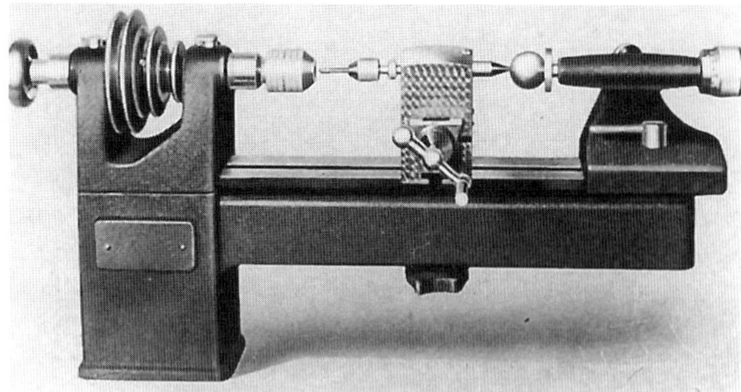

Fig. 10.30 Professor Barraquer's first lathe (from Barraquer JI. Historia de la cirugia refractiva de la cornea. In: *Cirugia Refractiva de la Cornea*, Instituto Barraquer de America, Bogota, Colombia, 1989).

done, the cryolathe was not located in the surgical suite—it was in a laboratory some 3 km distant. Thus, after the resection was done, the tissue was transported to the laboratory, where, under sterile conditions, the calculations were completed and the lathing performed. The tissue was then placed into a sterile vial to thaw and taken back to the surgical suite, where it was returned to the eye (Figure 10.33). The first lenticules were not sutured in place but were kept in place by an inverted conjunctival flap. Ultrafine suture material did not become available until almost 15 years later.

A number of calculations must be undertaken to complete the lathing. Various data are transferred into the computer, where the calculations are performed. Table 10.1 lists the most common data points and their meaning. This list is not complete, nor is the discussion below a comprehensive guide to keratomileusis—only a formal course can cover all the details and provide the hands-on experience necessary to actually perform this surgery.

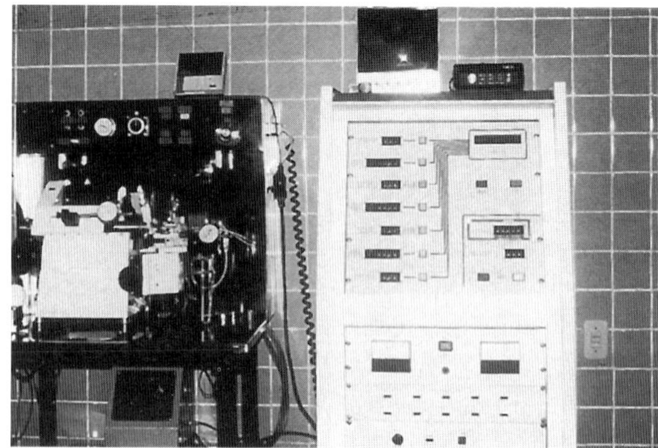

Fig. 10.32 The prototype of a completely computer-driven, automatic, cryolathe designed by Professor Barraquer (from Barraquer JI. Historia de la cirugia refractiva de la cornea. In: *Cirugia Refractiva de la Cornea*, Instituto Barraquer de America, Bogota, Colombia, 1989).

Lathe preparation

The lathe should be placed in an easily accessible location (Figure 10.34). Check the gas supply the night before, replacing any tanks whose pressure falls below the recommended levels set by the manufacturer (Figure 10.35). Make sure that the tanks are secured within their holders and that the heating collars are properly attached to the lower part of each tank. Close and latch the tank access doors—tape them closed. It is not unusual for these doors to come open through either jarring or vibration. The electrical supply of the lathe is connected via safety interlocks to the doors. When the door is open, even slightly, power is disconnected from the lathe. If this happens during the surgery—trouble. If it happens during the ultraviolet

(a)

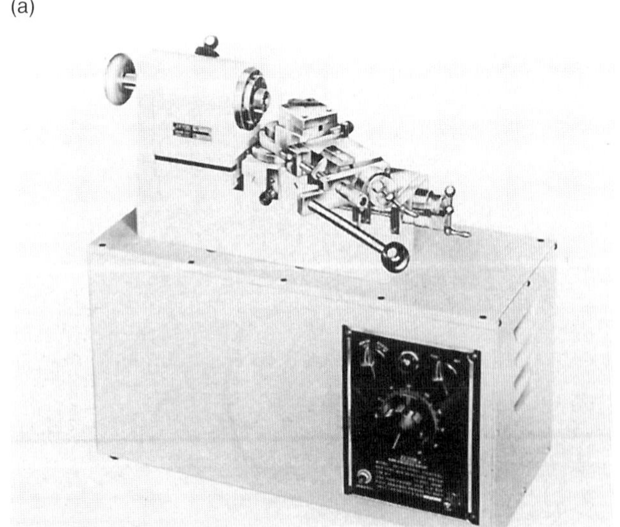

(b)

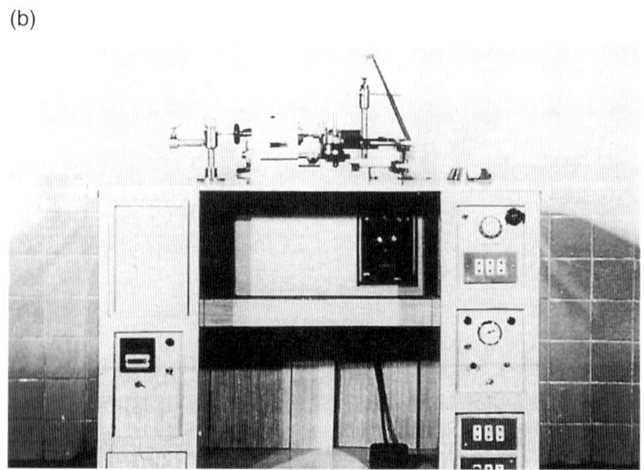

Fig. 10.31 (a) The Levin contact lens lathe. (b) The first cryolathe—a modified version of (a) with which the first human cases were performed (from Barraquer JI. Historia de la cirugia refractiva de la cornea. In: *Cirugia Refractiva de la Cornea*, Instituto Barraquer de America, Bogota, Colombia, 1989).

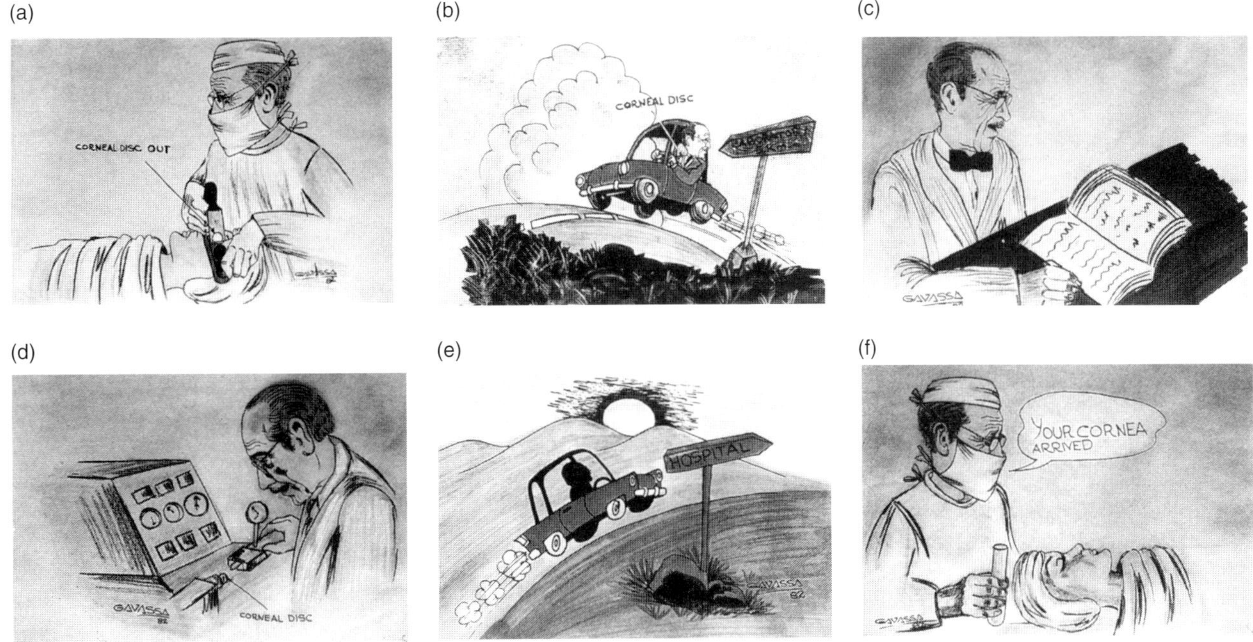

Fig. 10.33 (a–f) The first keratomileusis (from Barraquer JI. Historia de la cirugia refractiva de la cornea. In: *Cirugia Refractiva de la Cornea*, Instituto Barraquer de America, Bogota, Colombia, 1989).

Table 10.1 Abbreviations used in lamellar keratoplasty discussions and calculations

Abbreviation	Definition
Alpha	The angulation of the lathe tool in relation to the axis of rotation (determines the limit of the optic zone (Zo))
D	Diopters
Db	Diameter of the Delrin base (typically = 8.0 mm)
Dc	Diopters of spectacle correction
Dd	Disk diameter
Di	Initial anterior corneal curvature—in diopters
Dp	Displacement of the tool
Dv	Dioptric power at the corneal vertex (see text)
Ea	Thickness of the wing (in EPI and hyperopic lamellar keratotomy)
Ec	Central corneal thickness remaining after lathing
Ed	Thickness of the resected disk *before* preservation
Edp	Thickness of the resected disk *after* preservation
El	Thickness of the lenticule in hyperopia
Ezi	Thickness of the intersection zone (EPI and hyperopic lamellar keratotomy)
Rb	Radius of the base
Re	Radius of the resection base (interface)
Ri	Initial anterior corneal curvature—in millimeters (see Di)
Rt	Cutting radius
Zi	Intersection zone (EPI and hyperopic lamellar keratotomy)
Zo	Optical zone (diameter of the resection in keratomileusis and of the lenticule in keratophakia)

(UV) cycle, the lathe sterilization will be incomplete, and contamination of the patient's tissue is possible.

Remove the front cover and turn on the main power switch. Then replace the cover. If the lathe is located in an area that can be accessed by others (hospital, outpatient surgical clinic, etc.), it is a good idea to chain the cover to the lathe via the handles. Set the timer for the UV sterilizer (on the back) to the recommended time (minimum 12 hours), and turn on the UV power switch. Make sure that the UV power is off before removing the cover at the end of the cycle. On the day of surgery, untape the doors,

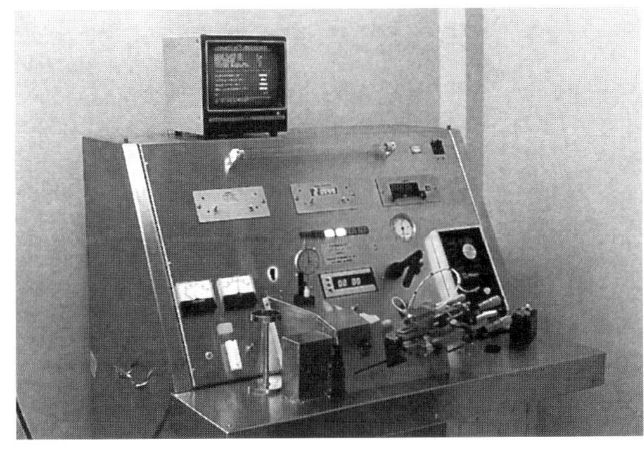

Fig. 10.34 The current model cryolathe as manufactured by Steinway Instruments, San Diego, CA. The monitor relays information from the central computer used to calculate the lathing parameters in each case.

(a)

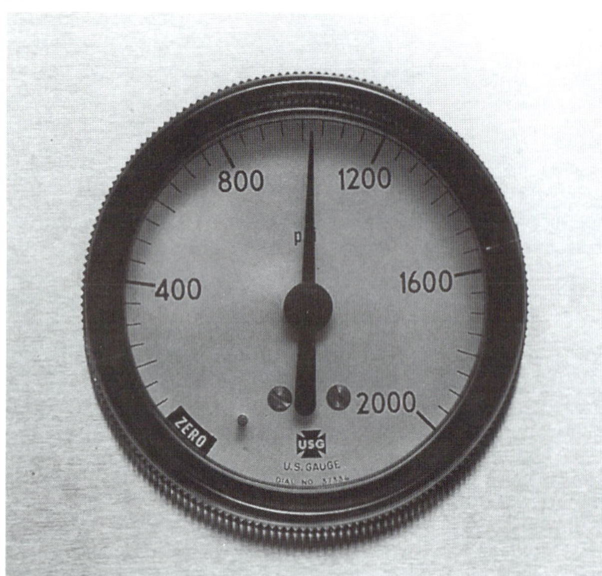

(b)

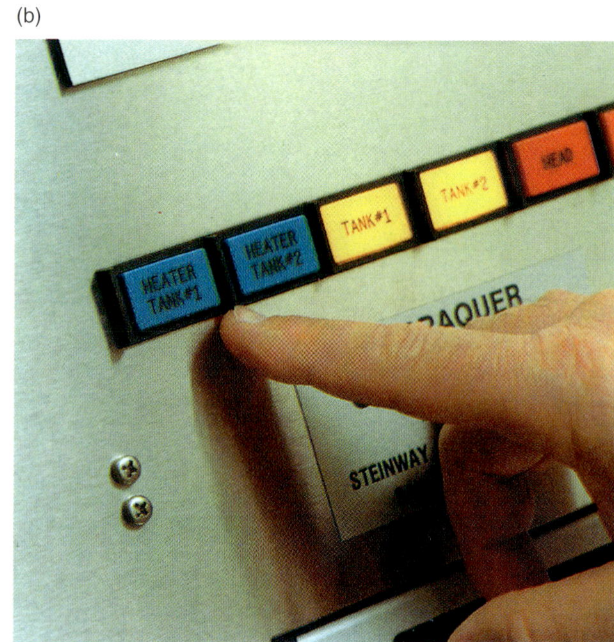

Fig. 10.35 (a) A fresh carbon dioxide tank should show a pressure of 1000 psi. (b) If the pressure falls to 800 psi, the tank heaters should be switched on.

and turn on both CO_2 tanks. Close and retape the doors. Remove the cover from the lathe, and place it outside the operating room in a safe place. Make sure that no one touches the lathe or the front panel until the surgery is completed. The author has a special shelf holding a monitor hooked up to the lathing computer. The monitor is situated directly in front of the surgeon. It is turned on at this time.

Delrin base-plate preparation

Under sterile conditions (scrubbed and gowned), turn on all console power switches and zero all digital readouts (you cannot zero the cutting-radius digital readout). Make sure that the tissue freezing timer is off and reset. Turn on the light. Put an 8.0-mm presterilized Delrin base plate into the headstock, and secure it with the threaded ring. Pull out the headstock locking knob to disengage the head, and spin it up to make sure it works. If you forget to pull out the lock, the drive belt is sure to come off the pulley. It is inside the lathe and not easy to get at.

The stop pin should be unlocked, as should the radius stop (Figure 10.36). Run the tailstock up toward the head until the tool just touches the Delrin base. Make sure that the cutting radius is set to 8.02. Turn on the lathe, and zero the displacement readout. Set the displacement micrometer readout to 20.00. Advance the tool and cut the base until the displacement readout displays –2.50. A new base has to be cut at least this much to ensure even and rapid freezing. Some surgeons forget this step and risk incomplete and/or prolonged freezing times.

Lock the stop pin. Advance the tool against the stop—the knob will be very difficult to turn, but it will move a few thousandths. Reset the displacement digital readout, and withdraw the tailstock. Bevel the edge of the Delrin base by holding a blade lightly against its edge—this removes any "flash" that may remain after the base is cut. Turn on tanks 1 and 2 from the front panel—the system is now ready for the first case.

Preoperative patient preparation

Approximately 1 hour prior to surgery, the patient should have 2 drops of 1% pilocarpine instilled in the operative eye. Repeat with 1 drop no less than 30 minutes before surgery if the pupil is not yet constricted. Using a miotic too soon before surgery presents the surgeon with congested conjunctiva, which is more likely to bleed and/or interfere with using the vacuum fixation ring. Position the patient beneath the microscope, and align the optics perpendicular to the patient's optical axis. If possible, prior to the administration of anesthesia, mark the optical center as follows: The patient is asked to fixate on the microscope light filament, whereupon the fixation point is marked with a blunt instrument, taking care to compensate for any parallax errors that may exist in the microscope system (Figure 10.37). To verify the centration of the optical center, the patient is asked to look away from and then back to the light. Any discrepancy is noted and corrected.

Anesthesia is then administered. In hyperopic eyes, retrobulbar anesthesia is safer than in myopic eyes. How-

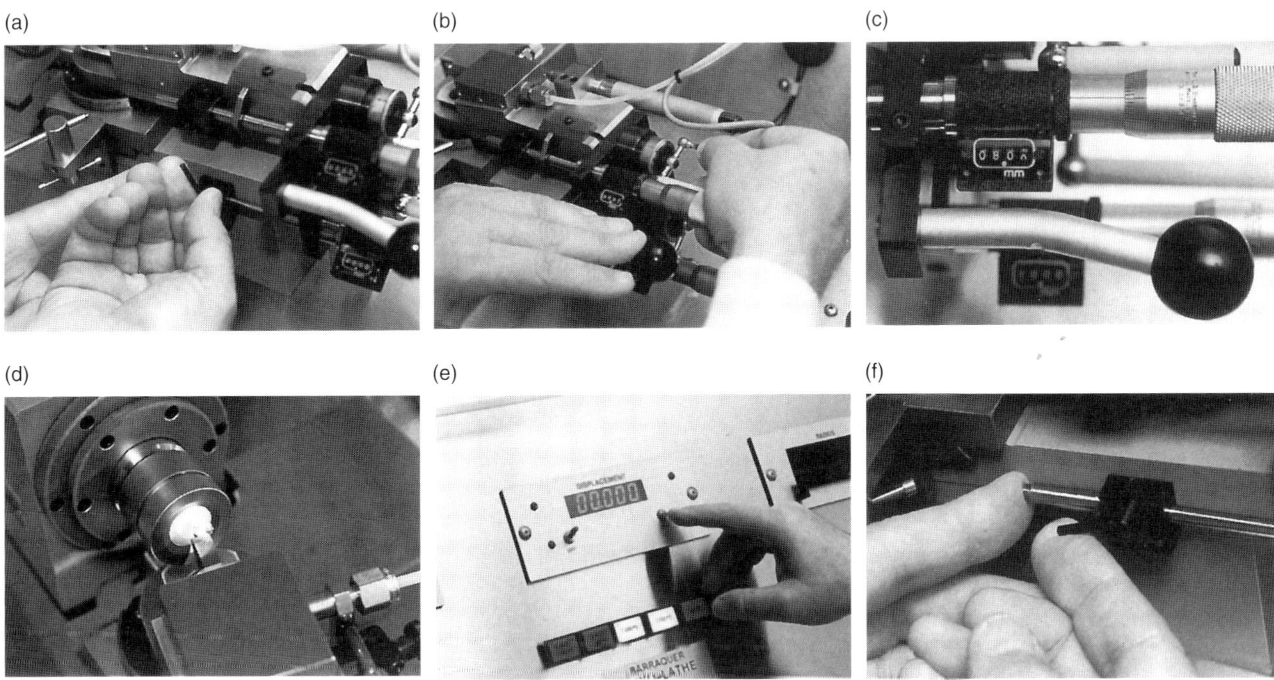

Fig. 10.36 Lathe setup. (a) Unlock the displacement stop pin. (b,c) Set the initial cutting radius. (d) After cutting the base, make sure the displacement is still set and locked at 20.00. (e) Zero the displacement readout. (f) Lock the stop pin.

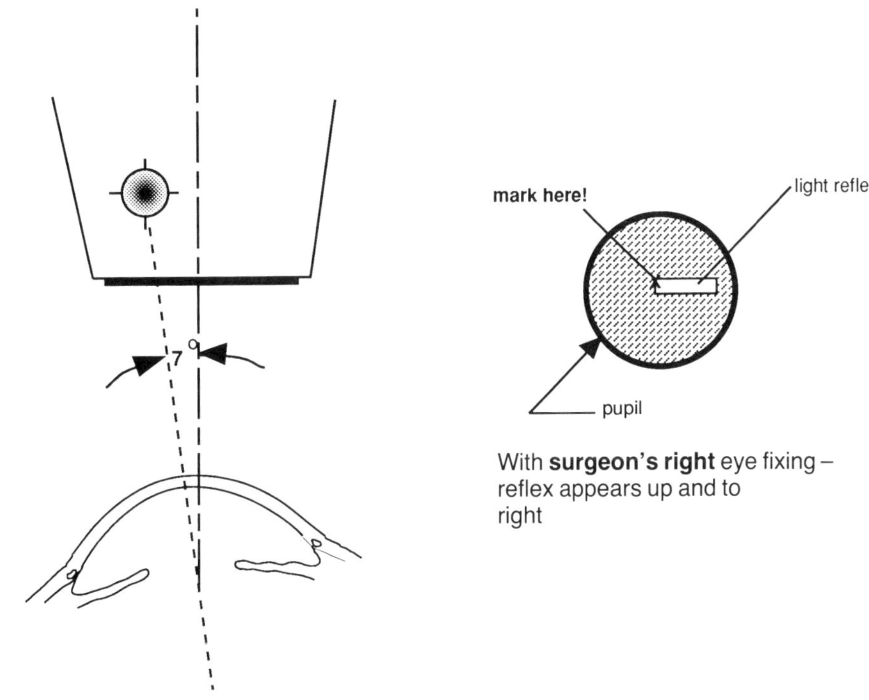

Fig. 10.37 Marking the visual axis. The light reflex is displaced downward because of the microscope design. To verify the centration of the optic center the patient is asked to look away from and then back to the light. Any discrepancy is noted and corrected. The visual axis is located as shown. The optic axis is not concentric with the pupil. Note that the visual axis is eccentric to the pupillary margin. It will be helpful to mark a 4.0 mm optical zone with an appropriate radial keratotomy marker—it helps when lining up the fixation ring.

ever, since some of these eyes will be hypercorrected myopes, it is safer to use peribulbar anesthesia coupled with a modified Van Lint (or O'Brien or Nadbath) lid block or even general anesthesia. If using local anesthesia, perform the blocks yourself unless the anesthesiologist has demonstrated his or her ability to perform such blocks without excess lid or subconjunctival infiltration.

To avoid possible injury, have the patient look down and out before inserting the needle into the orbital space. This maneuver swings the vulnerable posterior pole away from the needle tip but still allows infiltration of the cone (see Chapter 15). At the author's clinic, we use a mixture of 10.0 cc 4% plain Xylocaine, 4.0 cc bicarbonate, and 5.0 cc 0.75% Marcaine as our anesthetic medium.

The patient can now be prepped and draped for the procedure. For the prep, I recommend Betadine Solution—full or half strength. Do not use Betadine Prep. Betadine Prep contains soap, which is highly irritative to the conjunctiva and cornea—it can remove the corneal epithelium in a flash. If this happens, the surgery should be aborted. For a drape, we recommend the large 3M plastic incise adhesive drape (no. 1060). This is large enough to cover the field and to drape the Mayo stand placed over the patient's chest. More important, it is lintless. The surgeon should have prepped his or her hands in the usual manner for a full 10 minutes and be wearing no gloves. Hands should be rinsed thoroughly in sterile water and dried on low-lint or lintless towels.

The drape is opened with blunt scissors (taking care not to injure the lids or cut off any eyelashes), and a wire lid speculum is inserted between the lids. Ensure that the vacuum fixation ring fits within the space provided by the speculum with some clearance at 12 and 6 o'clock. Neither the lids nor the speculum should encroach on the ring so as to interfere with passage of the keratome. Be sure that the conjunctiva is flat and that there has been no anterior infiltration of the peribulbar anesthetic. If insufficient clearance is present, use an alternative form of lid retraction such as sutures. Take care with the placement of such sutures so as to prevent hemorrhaging.

A small canthotomy may be needed in some cases, but this will be unusual. To perform a canthotomy, first ensure that the area has been properly anesthetized. If it is found necessary to inject anesthetic, perform the injection at the posterior edge of the lateral orbit using the method of Van Lint. Next, use a straight, medium Halstead hemostat to clamp the lateral canthal area. After a brief wait, remove the clamp and perform a small canthotomy—do not involve the bulbar conjunctiva. If done properly, very little, if any, bleeding will occur. Remember to suture the canthotomy at the close of the procedure.

Assemble the microkeratome under a good light, making sure that all parts fit without forcing and that the blade moves freely. Be very careful of the blade both to protect its edge and to protect your fingers. Place the microkeratome (and handle) to the side in a secure place. Some surgeons recommend that these be placed within a special pocket of the operating gown. Do not do this! It is too easy for the blade to be damaged or lint and other particles to make their way into the microkeratome head. This goes for the rings as well. Do not put any of the rings into any gown pockets or pouches. Arrange these in a convenient place, in ascending order. Examine each one carefully for any signs of corrosion or accumulations of detritus. Clean any suspect areas, and test the fit and movement of the microkeratome in each one that you are likely to use. The microkeratome must move freely through the rings without any binding or catching.

Test the vacuum by occluding the tube and depressing the vacuum foot pedal. The gauge should read 22 in. Then attach the ring handle and test the vacuum again. Attach one of the rings and retest the vacuum by pressing the ring against your thumb with the vacuum pump on. It should hold onto your thumb as long as the vacuum pedal is depressed. Do not test the vacuum by putting the tubing into water. The system is not designed for this. Although there is a moisture trap in the system, it is a small one.

Centration of the resection

To begin the surgery, it will be necessary to mark the cornea to:

1 center and position the resection and

2 ensure that the tissue is replaced epithelial side up.

To accomplish the first goal, a 4.0-mm RK optical zone marker is applied to the cornea, concentric to a premade optical center mark. If the patient had already been anesthetized before marking the optic center, make the mark concentric and slightly nasal to the constricted pupil. This is extremely important because the pupil is not concentric with the optical axis of the eye.

Using a disposable needle (25 gauge), scribe a *tangential* reference mark on the corneal surface as shown in Figures 10.38 and 10.39a. Do not make more than one mark! This mark satisfies requirement number 2. Note that this mark is not made radially, as some of you may have been taught or read. This is so because it is easier than you might think to replace the corneal disk on the cornea—upside down! If the reference mark is made in the manner illustrated and the tissue is replaced incorrectly, the mark will appear as in Figure 10.39b. This is especially important in RK hypercorrections because of the radial scars already present. It is easy to get confused, so be careful.

Plate selection

The typical section thickness for lathing should be around 300 μm—although 350 μm is not too thick. Avoid resections that leave less than 150 μm of tissue in the resection bed. Thin posterior sections are likely to result in progressive corneal ectasia, which can reduce or eliminate the myopic correction and can even increase the myopia over time. This phenomenon is used to advantage in the hyperopic lamellar keratotomy (HLK) procedure (see "Hyperopic lamellar keratotomy," below). Conversely, do not remove such a thin disk that when lathed the center thickness is less than 120 μm. Such thin centers are often associated with irregular astigmatism due to wrinkling or actual freeze cracking of Bowman's layer. The exact plate selection will depend on the individual microkeratome as well as the experience and technique of the user. For example, some surgeons may consistently obtain sections 200 μm in thickness using a no. 25 plate, whereas others may get 280 μm with the same plate. It does not

(a)

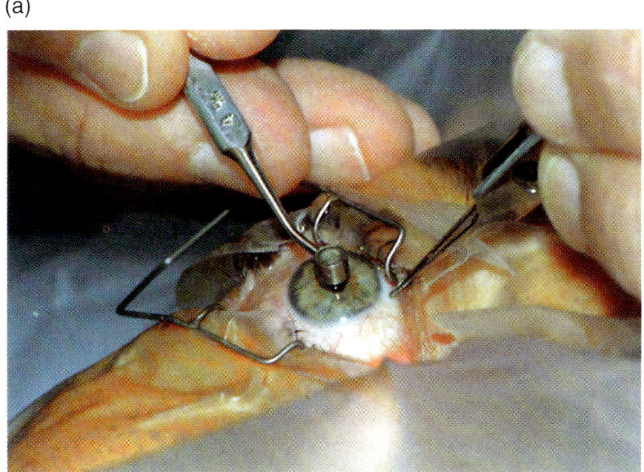

(b)

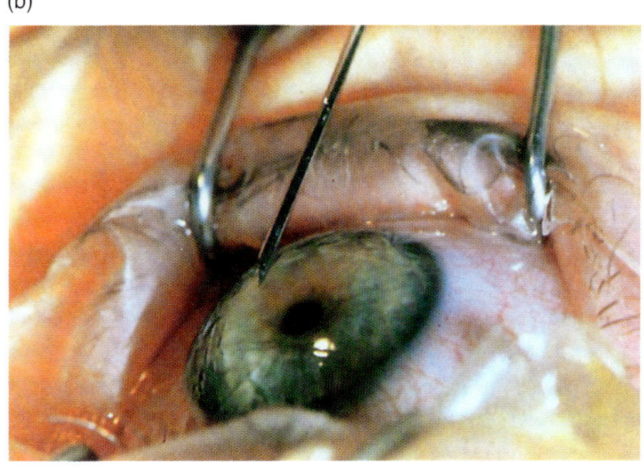

(c)

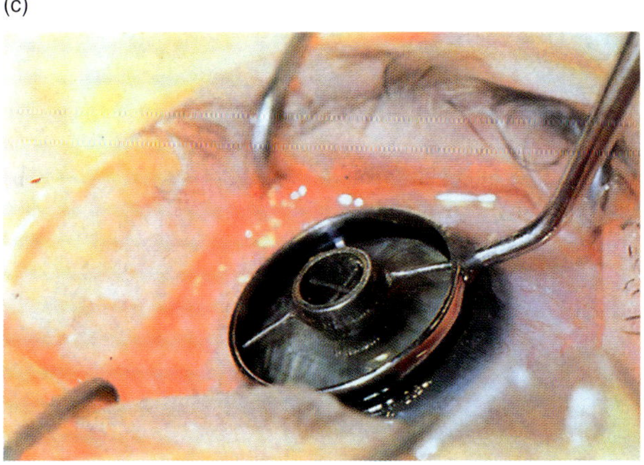

(d)

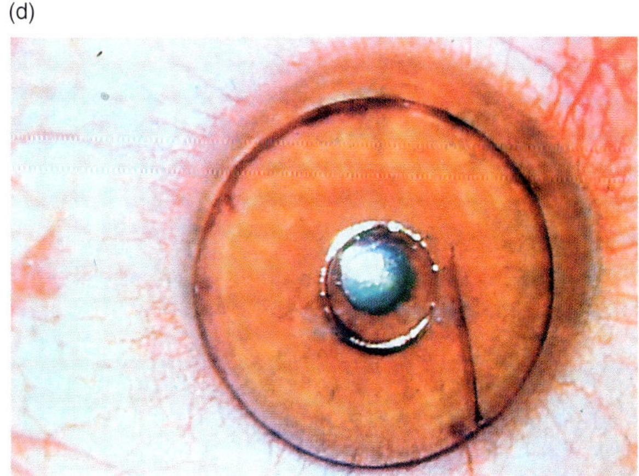

Fig. 10.38 Making the reference mark. (a) Make a 4.0-mm optical zone mark concentric to the optic center. (b) Use a fine-gauge needle held almost parallel to the corneal surface, taking care not to cut through Bowman's layer. This mark must be made tangential to the central zone—a gentian violet skin-marking pen can be used to enhance the mark. (c,d) An alternative is to use the Bores–Ruiz bull's-eye marker.

matter. The important thing is to be consistent in your technique.

Disk diameter

Always check the IOP with the tonometer before determining the resection diameter—at least for the first application of the ring (see Figure 10.40c). The disk diameter will be suggested by the computer program typically used in this surgery. The author usually uses a 7.25-mm-diameter disk for myopia and ignores the computer's suggestion. It will be necessary to try a few rings before the correct one is found. For a section having a diameter of 7.25 mm, a no. 8 ring should be tried first.

It is not enough to merely place the ring on the eye and actuate the vacuum pump—great pains must be taken when placing that first ring on the eye. Begin by making sure that the ring fits within the palpebral fissure without obstruction. Sometimes, in deep-set eyes, it will be necessary to proptose the eye somewhat by injecting more anesthetic. Be careful not to inject too much so as not to force the lids tightly against the eye. Center the ring carefully in relation to the pupil—a little exposed limbus is okay. Because the eye is not a perfect sphere, it will tend to center itself when the vacuum is applied. Unfortunately, that center of equilibrium is seldom concentric with the optical axis—hence the eye usually will shift its position. Before applying the vacuum, therefore, grasp the conjunctiva firmly with a tissue forceps (such as a Bishop-Harmon), and anchor both hands on a firm base such as the brow or arm rest. Holding the eye and ring rigidly, apply the vacuum. Resist any tendency of the eye to decenter within the ring aperture. If it gets away from you, release the footswitch immediately, reposition the ring, and try again. Once you have satisfactory centration, allow the vacuum sufficient time to seat the ring against the eye—10 to 15 seconds should do it. This maneuver will produce an indentation in the globe that will persist through the entire surgery, making centration of subsequent rings almost automatic. This is critical in keratomileusis in situ, which requires two passes of the keratome and subsequently two ring changes.

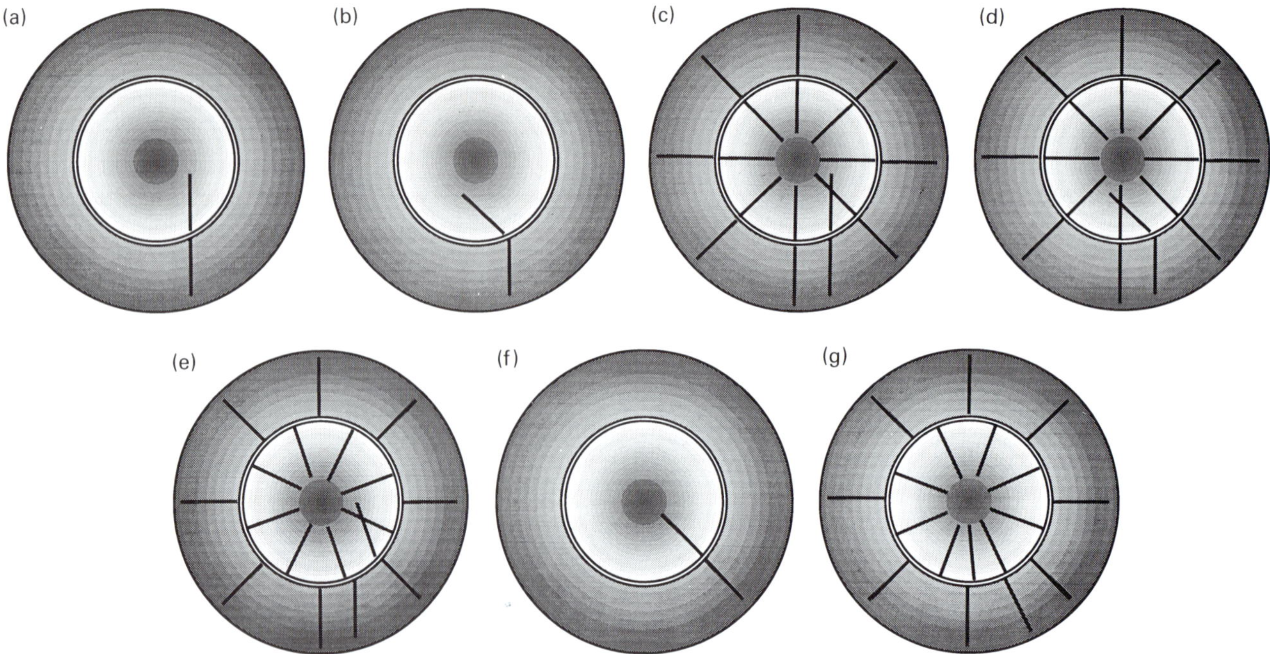

Fig. 10.39 The significance of making the reference mark tangential to the center rather than radial is illustrated in the following: (a) tangential mark; (b) if the tissue is inverted, the mark is dog-legged; (c) such a mark is especially important when operating on radial keratotomy cases; (d) tissue inverted; (e) tissue rotated; (f) there is no way to be sure this disk is inverted; (g) reference mark, reference mark, which one's the reference mark? Could the tissue be upside down? In a radial keratotomy case, a radial mark is especially confusing. With a proper mark, there's no confusion.

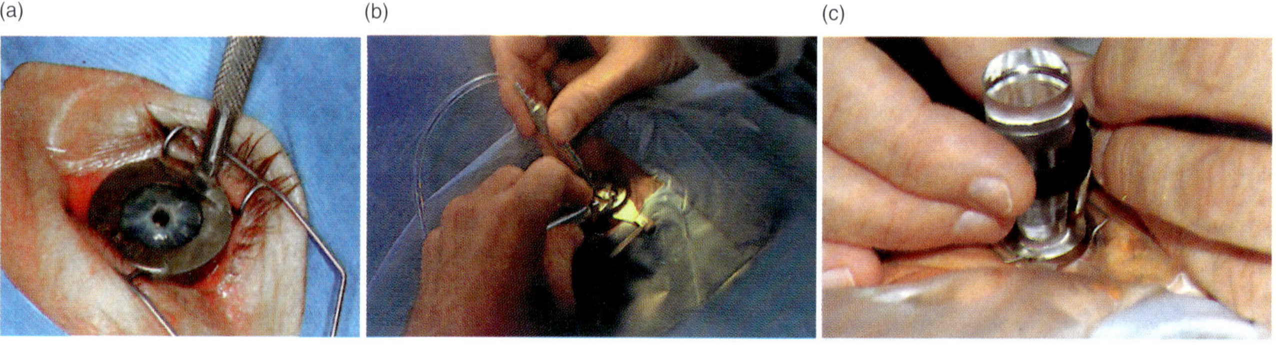

Fig. 10.40 (a) Make sure that there is plenty of clearance around the ring. The photo shows the correct position for the ring tubulature/handle. (b) The wrong ring handle position—below the eye. (c) The presurgical tonometer checks to ensure complete pressurization of the globe.

With the vacuum on, check the IOP and disk diameter (Figure 10.41). If the applanated area is too small, select a lower-numbered ring, and if it is too large, select a higher-numbered ring. Remember also to dry the cornea with a microsponge before making any measurements (Figure 10.42). If the readings seem difficult to obtain, place the lenses into sterile chilled water for a few minutes. Dry them carefully before placing them on the cornea. A slight condensation of moisture will occur outside the contact area when the applanator is placed against the patient's cornea, thereby facilitating the reading (Figure 10.43).

Note: The actual diameter of the resected disk will be about 0.2 mm larger than that applanated. This must be kept in mind to prevent a problem in HLK, where disk diameters are specified in tenths (see below).

A common mistake is not seating the applanator totally against the fixation ring. A less common mistake is mixing up applanators designed for different procedures or for different instruments. If you have a lathe or equipment from more than one manufacturer, make sure that all pieces are kept strictly isolated to avoid mix-and-match errors.

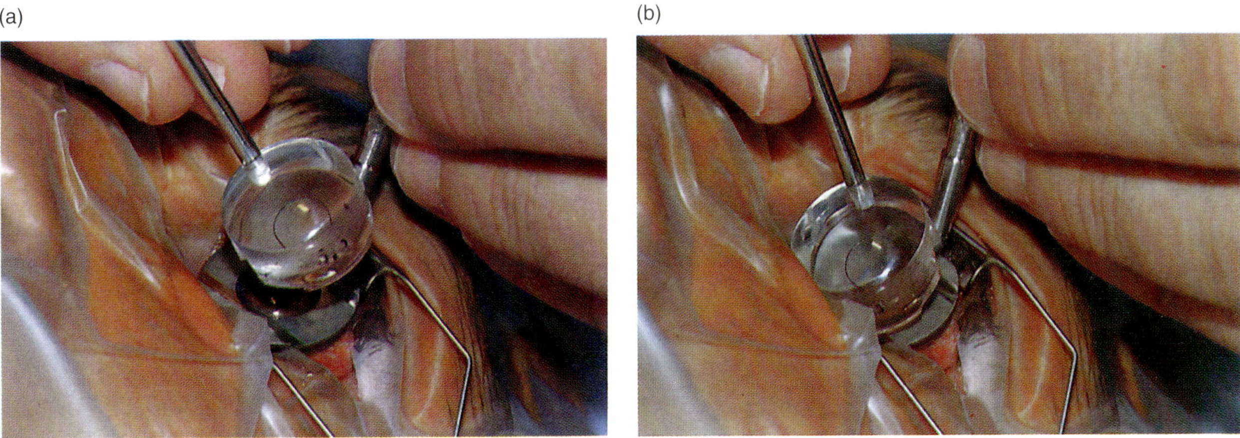

Fig. 10.41 (a) Angle the tonometer slightly and engage one edge against the lower ring guide. (b) Rotate the upper edge of the applanator down against the ring. This technique ensures proper seating of the lens. It's easier than you might think to place the applanator lens askew in the ring guides, so take pains to ensure that it is properly seated.

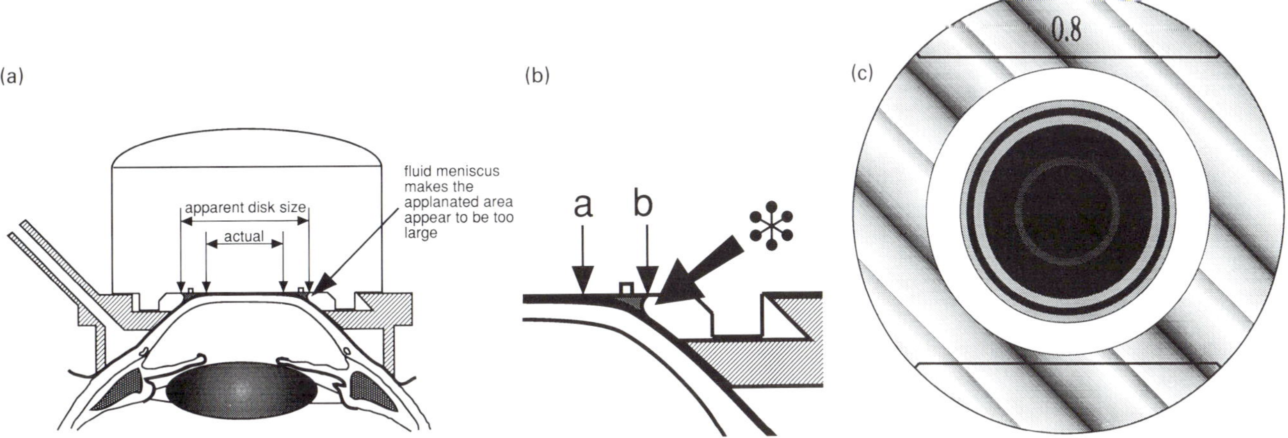

Fig. 10.42 (a-c) If the cornea is wet when the applanator is applied, the fluid meniscus will make the flattened area appear larger than it really is.

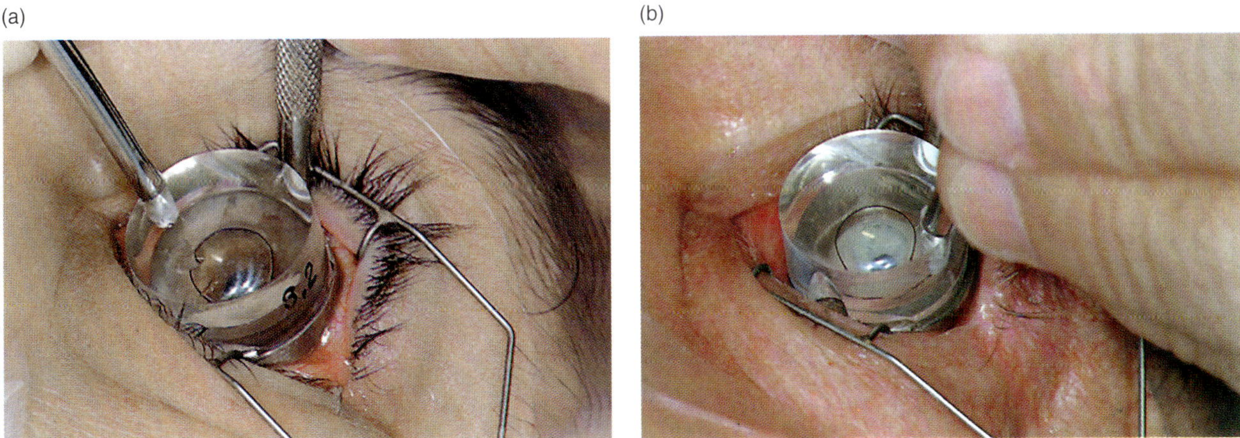

Fig. 10.43 (a) Cooling the applanators before use makes the contact zone easier to see. The applanated area lies just inside the reticle—the ring is the correct size for this case. (b) This ring is obviously too thick (high-number) for this case.

If the applanator is too large for the ring, or if it is malpositioned, the applanated area will appear much smaller than normal and will tend to be displaced. Ordinarily, such displacement can be corrected by sliding the applanator on the ring surface. If this is done and the applanation is still displaced (typically either up or down), the lens is not seating in the ring. Make certain that the applanator has not "infiltrated" from another set, and replace it on the ring. Do not accept any measurement if you are unsure of the applanator. Remember, *measure twice, cut once*. Once the correct ring has been found, you are ready to perform the keratectomy.

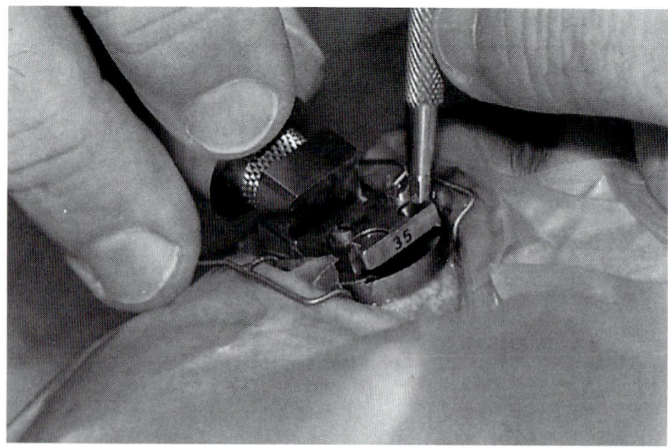

Fig. 10.44 In some patients the nose will interfere with complete excursion of the keratome head, resulting in an incomplete section. By rotating the ring temporally, the problem is avoided (see also Chapter 15).

Making the section

Check to see that the microkeratome moves freely in the ring—off the eye. If the keratome does not pass freely through the ring off the eye, it is certain not to do so on the eye. If the keratome hangs up in the ring during a resection, a disk of irregular thickness and shape is the inevitable result.

Position the ring back on the eye, making certain that it is centered in reference to the premarked central OZ, and apply vacuum to the eye—check both the IOP and the ring centration. When operating on the left eye, hold the ring with the right hand, tubulature at 12 o'clock, resting the hand on the patient's forehead—reverse hands for the right eye. Do not hold the ring with the tubulature at the 6 o'clock position—the cheek does not provide a solid base for support. Furthermore, the forearm of the holding hand will inevitably press on the patient's nose, obstructing the airway. The holding hand is also vulnerable to being hit from below—such as by the anesthesiologist's or the patient's hand trying to clear a breathing space. Rotate the ring handle temporally so that the nasal side of the ring is slightly higher than the temporal side (Figure 10.44). This will avoid the problem of the head striking the nose. Do not pull up on the ring when performing this rotation—suction can be lost if this is done, and it will always happen at the wrong moment. Neither should you press down on the ring, thereby pushing the eye back into the orbit. This maneuver is sure to decrease lid clearance, hindering passage of the head. The idea is to support or fixate the eye. Make sure that your ring hand is planted firmly against the patient's brow.

Hold the instrument as shown in Figure 10.45, and engage the microkeratome in the ring guides. Make sure that both dovetails are engaged in double-dovetailed rings. This can be accomplished more easily by angling the head slightly, as shown in Figure 10.46. Move the instrument nasally until the front blade edge is even with the temporal ring aperture (Figure 10.47). Wet the cornea with saline.

Does the blepharostat clear the ring?

Obstruction to free head passage through the ring can come from objects external to the ring itself. The end result is the same and is to be avoided at all costs. If the lid speculum is interfering, have the assistant grasp the upper and lower blades of the speculum with a hemostat to spread the lids. If this does not work, it may be necessary to do a canthotomy.

Depress the motor foot pedal, and move the instrument nasally. The keratectomy is performed in a smooth, even

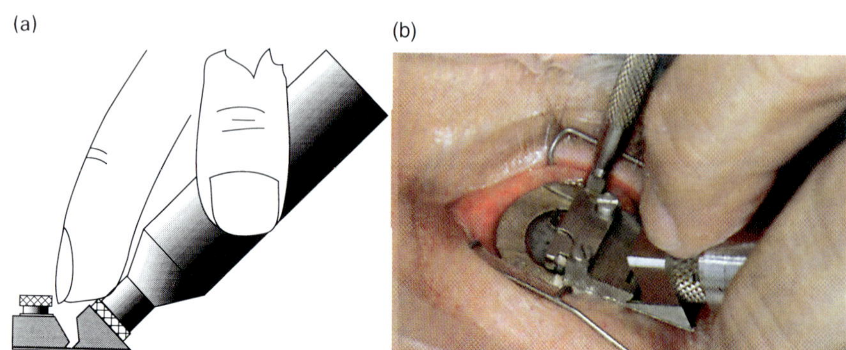

Fig. 10.45 (a,b) The correct way to hold the keratome. The instrument should be held securely but lightly. Do not force the microkeratome through the rings—let it glide through on its own. Movement of the keratome should be smooth and steady.

(a)

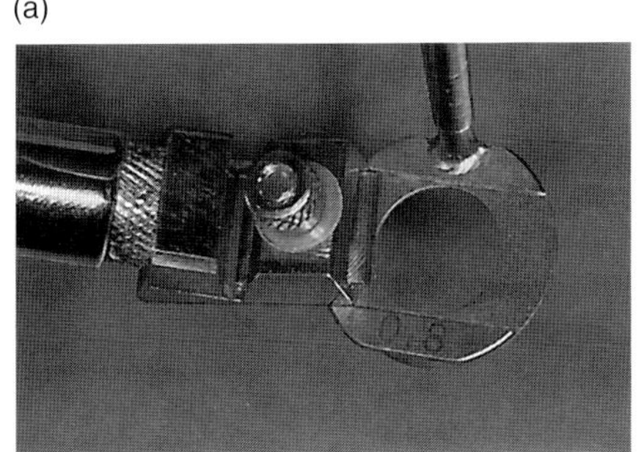

(b)

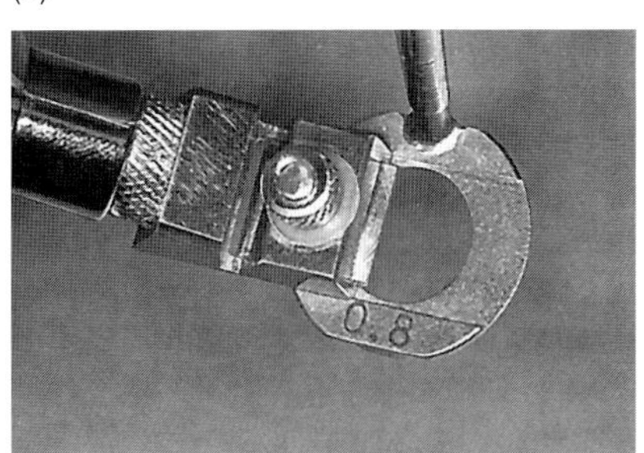

Fig. 10.46 (a,b) In double-dovetail guide rings, it helps to angle the head slightly to fit it into the guides.

manner at moderate speed. Do not stop! The translation across the ring should be smooth and even. A little BSS on the guides may help. Do not use any silicone oil or any lubricant other than water! It is vital that the movement be slow and even without any hesitation or stopping. It should take about 3 seconds (a count of one thousand one, one thousand two, one thousand three is about right). If the instrument moved freely before applying the ring to the eye, it should do so now. In the SCMD unit, the turbine sets up a high-frequency vibration which tends to assist movement through the ring—almost floating it along.

The most common error made by beginners is holding the microkeratome too rigidly. Your hand should just support the instrument and provide movement. Most right-handed people will find that left-eye keratectomies seem to go better than right-eye ones. This is so because most people are not overcontrolling the keratome with the left hand but are doing so with the right hand. Relax! Guide the instrument without any rotational force. Remember that you only have to move the head about ¼ in. to complete the cut. The author recommends that the surgeon view the microkeratome through the microscope—watching the tissue disk as it feeds through the slot (Figure 10.48). By concentrating on the movement of the tissue, you will inevitably relax. Furthermore, you can easily control the speed of the keratome by watching the feed rate—when the tissue stops moving out of the slot, the keratectomy is complete.

Do not stop the motor until the section is complete, however. When the blade edge meets the nasal side of the ring aperture, release the motor foot pedal and then the suction (Figure 10.49). *Do not release the vacuum until the motor stops at the completion of the keratectomy.* Remove both the ring and the microkeratome from the eye—together (Figure 10.50). If any resistance is met, gently disengage the microkeratome by backing it up with the motor off. If you have not stopped the motor too soon, all should be well. Disengage the microkeratome from the ring, and set the ring aside. Place the special cover over

(a)

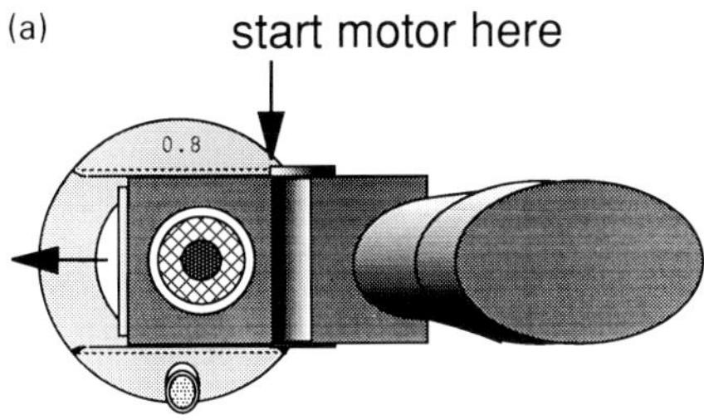
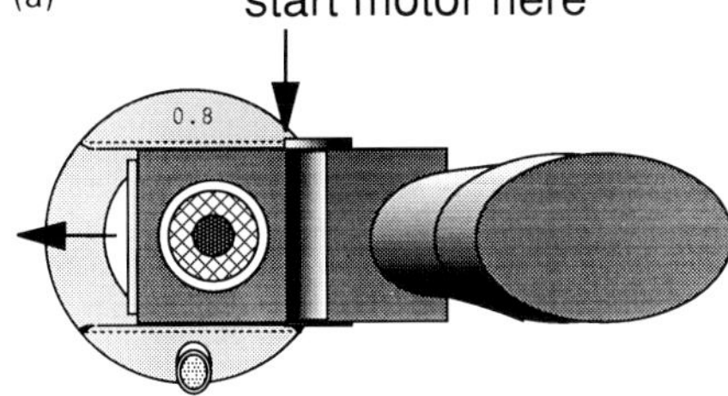

(b)

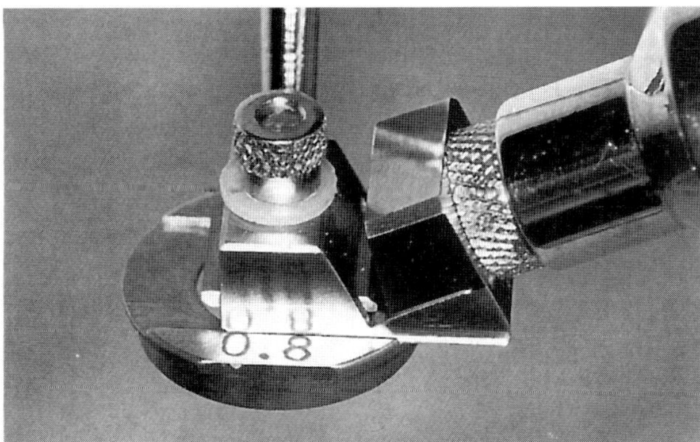

Fig. 10.47 (a,b) The keratome is advanced until the leading edge of the blade corresponds with the temporal edge of the ring aperture. Start the motor at that point. Starting the motor too late can result in a flat-sided disk with a thin edge.

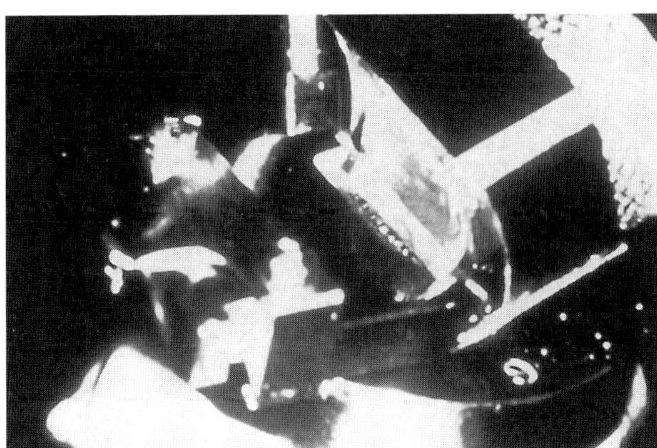

Fig. 10.48 The tissue disk issuing from the keratome feed slot. Watch the disk as it emerges from the keratome head. When it stops moving forward, the section is complete.

(a)

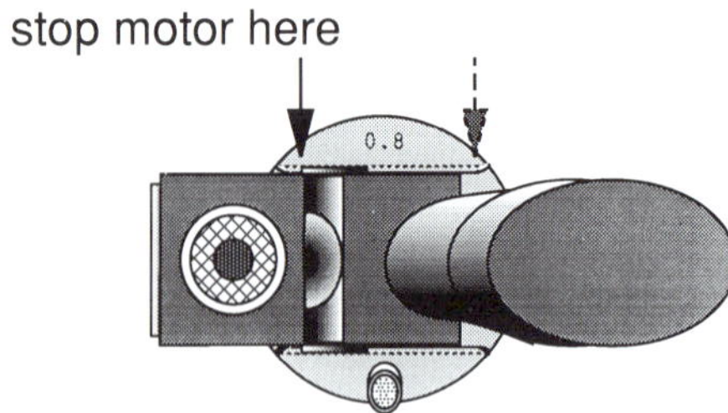

(b)

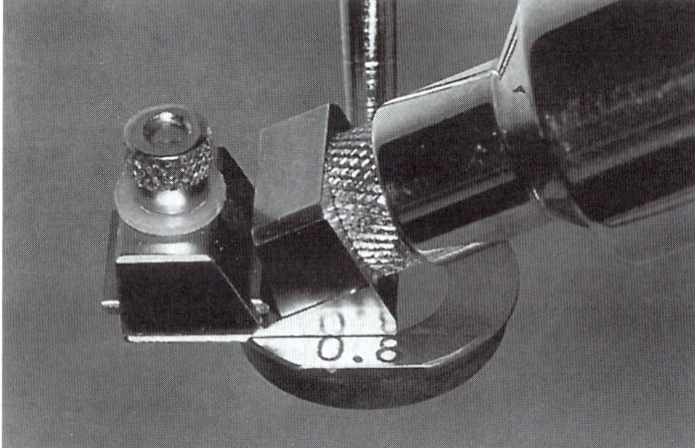

Fig. 10.49 (a,b) Stop the motor when the blade edge reaches the nasal side of the ring aperture or the tissue stops feeding through the slot.

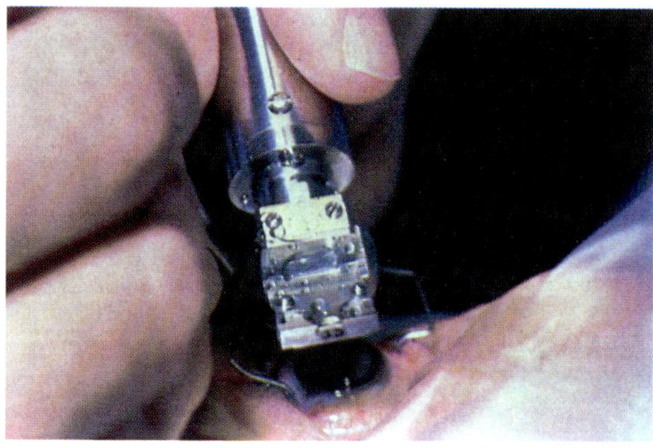

Fig. 10.50 The keratome and the ring are removed from the eye as a unit.

the cornea (Figure 10.51). Remove the resected tissue with a fine-toothed forceps by gently teasing it out of the keratome head. To do this, turn the microkeratome over and pull the exposed tissue edge out onto the plate (Figures 10.52 and 10.53). If you try to pull it in the opposite direction, it could be cut. If it is bunched up behind the head and free of the blade, move it out with a closed forceps. Place it, epithelial side down, onto the applanator

(a)

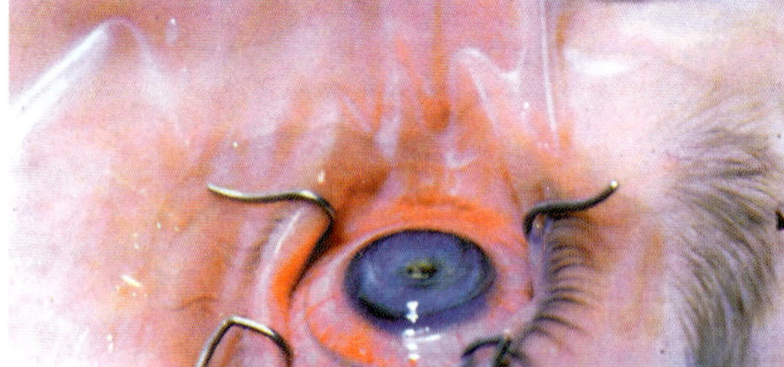

(b)

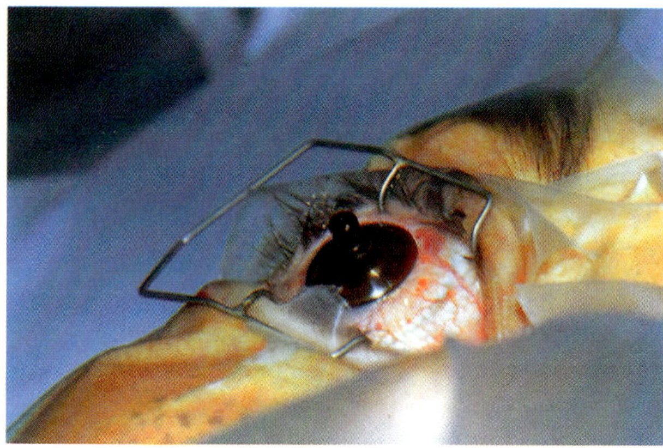

Fig. 10.51 (a) A completed keratectomy. Note the saddle depression from the ring. The appearance of this depression signals that adequate suction was obtained. Additionally, this saddle makes it easier to center the second pass in keratomileusis *in-situ*. (b) Place the cover over the cornea as soon as possible.

lens to check the diameter and the disk edge under the microscope (Figure 10.54).

Transfer the tissue to the sterile tissue gauge, and measure the thickness—record this (Figure 10.55). Since this tissue is usually quite thick, gentle handling with a fine-toothed forceps will not damage it. Moisten both plates of the gauge before putting the tissue on the bottom plate; otherwise, the tissue is going to stick to the plastic and be hard to remove. Make sure that there are no folds or wrinkles in the tissue disk. Gently lower the upper anvil onto the tissue, and take a reading. Do not tap on the knob! Did you remember to zero the gauge before use?

It may be necessary to wet the disk to remove it from the gauge—do not force it! Place the tissue, epithelial side down, into the "moist chamber," and replace the chamber cover.

Always measure the disk thickness to be sure that you are getting the depth of section that you planned on. Most beginners will find that their initial sections are somewhat thinner than expected. This occurs because the sur-

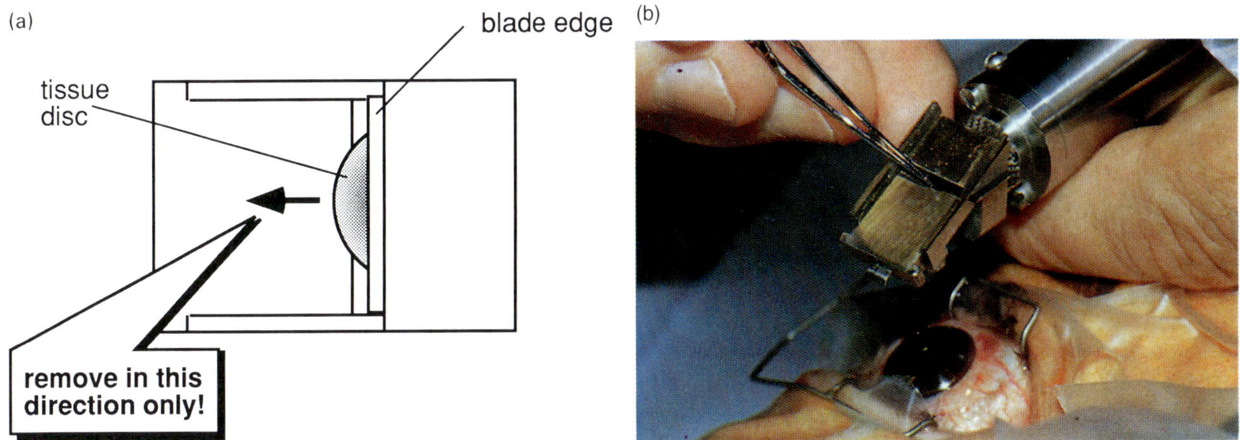

Fig. 10.52 (a,b) If an edge of tissue is protruding through the bottom of the keratome, remove the tissue by teasing it onto the blade, away from the blade edge. Do not pull it up through the feed slot.

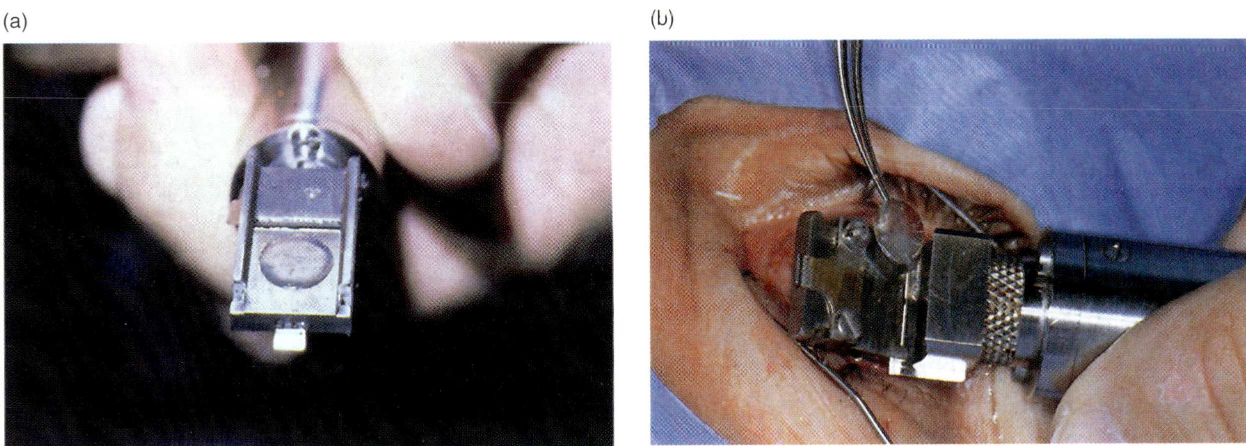

Fig. 10.53 (a) Examine the disk for defects while it is flattened out on the applanator plate. (b) A keratectomy disk on a radial keratotomy patient. Note that there is no fraying or splitting of the disk edges at the incisions.

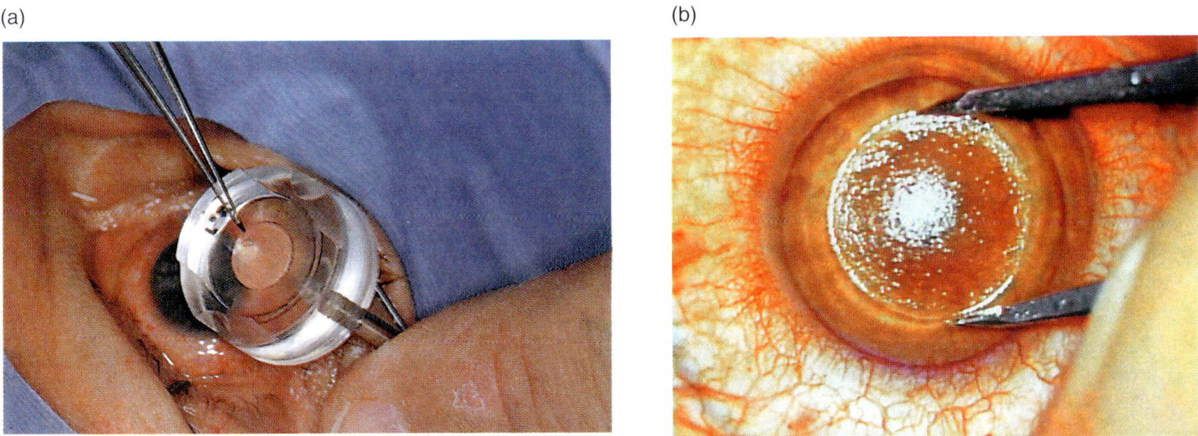

Fig. 10.54 (a) The diameter can be verified by placing the disk onto the applanator lens. This is a good way to inspect the tissue for defects under the microscope. (b) A caliper provides an alternate. Remove any lint or particles that you find.

(a)

(b)

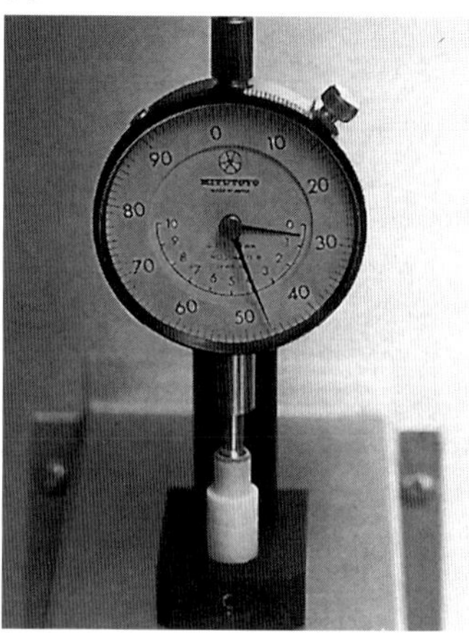

Fig. 10.55 (a,b) Transfer the disk to the tissue gauge and measure its thickness. This information is fed into the computer before and after cryo-preservation.

geon is "hurrying" the keratectomy. On the other hand, if you go too slowly, you could enter the anterior chamber. This is particularly likely to happen if you stop moving the microkeratome halfway across.

Another cause for a thinner section can be too low an IOP prior to performing the resection. If the pressure is not high enough, insufficient elevation of the cornea into the ring occurs as well. With less pressure, the tissue also tends to flow away from the blade. Experienced keratotomists can compensate for this somewhat by slowing up the rate of translation, but this is not recommended.

Too slow a movement can lead to striations or ridges in the section. This is more likely, however, to be caused by a too-slow motor speed. The motor speed is fixed in the Steinway unit. It is adjustable in the SCMD unit and has been preset at the factory. That setting should be marked or recorded before you change it. If the motor speed is too slow, not only will the cut be uneven, but it also will be too thin. Always check both the motor speed and the IOP before starting the keratectomy. If the IOP is consistently lower than 65 mm Hg. (22 in. of H_2O on the vacuum gauge) and there is no apparent problem with the rings (i.e., they seem to be holding), then the system will need adjustment. This is not something that you can do easily by yourself—it should be done by the manufacturer.

The most likely problem with vacuum will be found in the periphery and not with the pump setting. The same is true with the motor speed. The speed of the motor has been carefully adjusted to produce full rpm with the loads expected under normal circumstances. If slowing occurs, it more likely will be found as a result of binding introduced in the assembly of the microkeratome. Motor speed problems are particularly unlikely to be a problem with the gas turbine, which generates considerable torque. In fact, the motor generates sufficient torque to overcome minor binding due to misalignment of the blade during head assembly. This condition can lead to spalling and the deposition of tiny metallic particles (spalls) on the resection bed or on the undersurface of the disk (see Chapter 15). The caveat is: *Make sure that the head assembly is correct and check for binding before using the instrument.*

Checklist for keratectomy

1 Turn on power supply.
2 Attach the aspirator (suction) tube.
3 Check the vacuum by occluding the tube.
4 Release the occlusion. The vacuum should drop to zero.
5 Inspect the blade edge under the microscope.
6 Assemble the microkeratome head.
7 Ensure blade movement.
8 Set the plate.
9 Assemble the motor handle.
10 Apply grease, and attach the head to the handle.
11 Attach the gas supply tubing to the power unit.
12 Check the performance of the motor.
13 Test the microkeratome in ring(s).
14 Mark the central zone.
15 Place the reference mark.
16 Place and center the fixation ring.
17 Depress the vacuum actuator switch.
18 Check the adherence of the ring.
19 Dry the cornea.
20 Perform tonometry.
21 Check the dimensions of applanation.
22 Moisten the cornea.
23 Perform the keratectomy—slow and even movement.
24 Release the motor switch and the vacuum switch simultaneously.
25 Remove the disk from the microkeratome.

Additional steps are performed as required for the procedure at hand.

Preoperative caveats

The cutting edge of the blade must be checked under the microscope. This can be done by checking the brightness;

any irregularity in the shine of the edge means a nicked blade, which must be replaced.

Once the microkeratome has been assembled, it must be tested in the rings to make sure that it slides freely to ensure a proper cut. Finally, it must be started for a few seconds to check if the blade is moving freely and the speed is correct.

Although, as a rule, there are usually no accidents or problems during the keratectomy, failure to heed each point can lead to difficulty. If you forget to check the blade, you can be sure that it will have a nick in it. If you forget to check the vacuum, it will fail at the worst possible moment. If you neglect to check for free movement of the microkeratome in the rings, it will bind halfway across. Check every point. It is a good idea to have an assistant read off each point as you go, waiting for your response before going on. If you do this in the early cases, it will be safe to resort to a printed checklist later on.

The preceding discussion is valid for keratectomies done for lathing as well as for keratomileusis in situ, HLK, keratophakia (KP), or laser keratomileusis. I will now move on to actual lathing of the tissue disk.

Lathing

Transfer the resected disk to the crucible containing the Kitton green preservative solution (Figure 10.56). The author always places the tissue into the solution stromal (curved) side up. Make sure that the tissue is completely submerged, place the crucible in a safe place, and start the timer. The computer will ask for the preserved thickness of the tissue. The author has been advised by Ruiz to enter the same value found for the unpreserved disk thickness—this is our standard practice. While the tissue is soaking in the Kitton green, the new cutting radius, displacement, and angle alpha should be set and locked in.

After 1 minute, a Barraquer lenticule spoon is used to retrieve the disk from the preserving solution. Figure 10.57 shows how the tissue disk is transferred to the Delrin base—epithelial side against the base. A sable brush or a microsponge is used to draw off as much liquid as possible without disturbing the disk. Merely touching the bristles to the junction of the tissue and the base usually suffices.

Turn on the lathe motor to about 15 rpm or so (the disk should be turning slowly), and using the edge of the Barraquer spoon lightly touched to the disk edge, center the disk on the base (Figure 10.58). A little practice will make this an easy task. Stop the motor and reset the freezing timer (it was used to time the preservation step). Press the HEAD button to start freezing the tissue, and start the timer. Run the tool up close to, but not touching, the tissue (Figure 10.59). Start the tool freezing and the tissue slowly turning. Watch the tissue very carefully at this point. The tissue will change color as it freezes. At first it will turn a dark green and will appear granular (Figure 10.60). After about 45 seconds or so, the tissue will undergo a sudden change. It will seem to recede or shrink back against the plastic base—it does, of course, indeed shrink at this point. At the same time its color will become a light white-green. Check the tool—it should be frozen by now and look it. Increase the lathe speed. You may now proceed to carve the tissue disk into a lenticule. One caveat: Even if the tissue coloration changes early, do not begin lathing until 45 seconds, minimum, have elapsed.

Lathing continues until the displacement given by the computer program has been reached—typically the stop will prevent any advancement beyond this point. Make sure that each pass of the tool across the face of the tissue disk is smooth and even (Figure 10.61). A dry sable brush can be used to brush away shavings from the tool tip if they are obscuring your view. If this is a myopia case, this completes the lathing phase of the operation. If, however, this is a case of hyperopia, the cutting radius will have to be readjusted and the wing portion of the lenticule lathed (Figure 10.62).

When lathing is complete, turn off the gases and retract the tool to its fullest extent. Turn off the lathe motor and push in the locking knob to prevent rotation of the lathe spindle. The Delrin base, tissue and all, is removed from the lathe and plunged (tissue side up) into a bath of saline

(a)

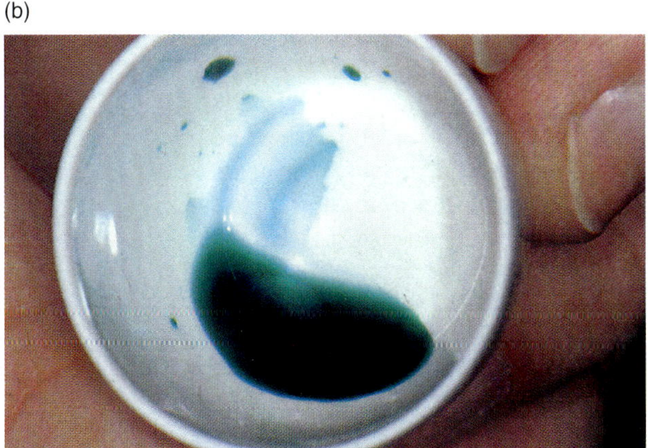

(b)

Fig. 10.56 (a) The disk is placed into a solution of kitton green for 1 min. (b) Make sure that the disk is completely submerged. It is easy to see the disk against the white background.

(a) (b)

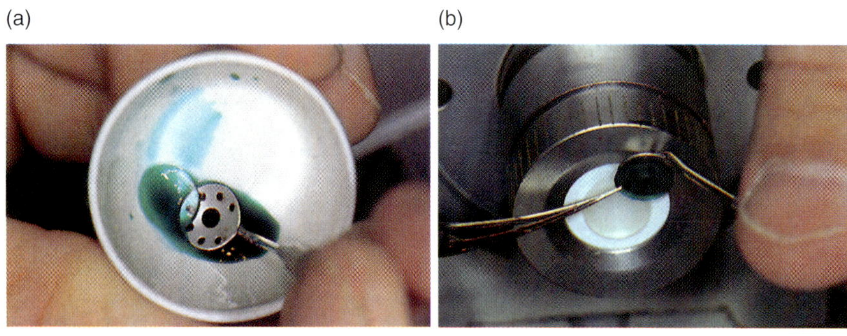

(c) (d)

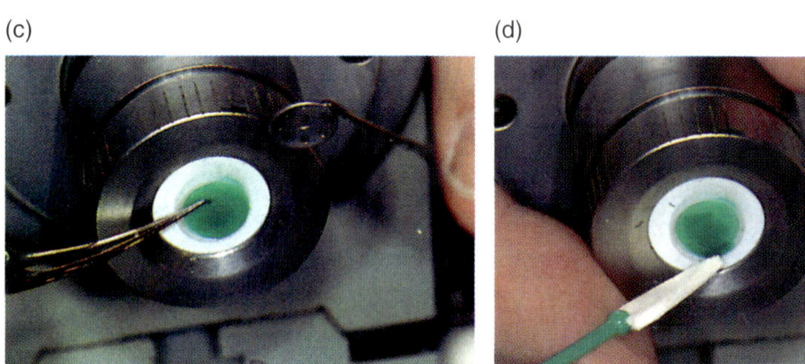

Fig. 10.57 (a) The tissue is removed from the preservative solution with a lenticule spoon. (b,c) A forceps or sable brush is used to *slide* the disk onto the Delrin base. Sliding the tissue serves to prevent air bubbles being trapped behind the disk. (d) A microsponge is gently touched to the junction of the disk edge and base. Capillary action will draw away most of the excess fluid.

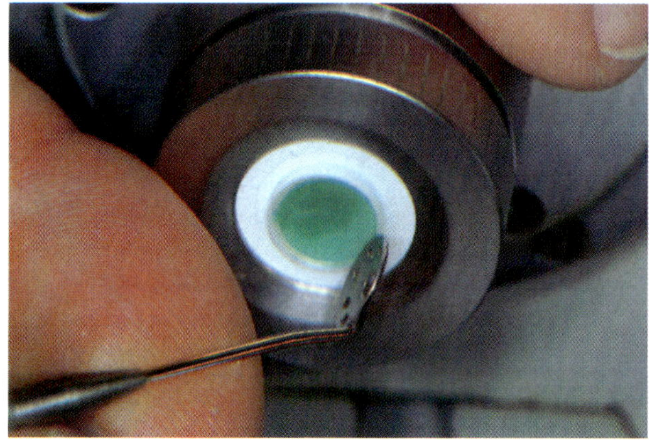

Fig. 10.58 The Barraquer spoon is used to center the disk while the lathe head is turning slowly.

heated to body temperature. The author uses a special heater block that holds a container designed for this purpose. Stop the freezing timer, and record the display.

The Barraquer spoon is now used to remove the lenticule from the thawing chamber and to transfer it to the moist chamber (Figure 10.63). Remove excess liquid from the chamber with the sable brush, cap the chamber, and place it in a secure spot. Lathing is complete. It is now time to clean the recipient bed.

Figure 10.64 shows the various lenticule configurations and the abbreviations used to label them (see Table 10.1). While not comprehensive, it is included as a guide to the topic in this and other books.

Cleanup

Remove the corneal cover, and with a sable brush and copious irrigation, "scrub" the keratectomy bed. This

(a) (b)

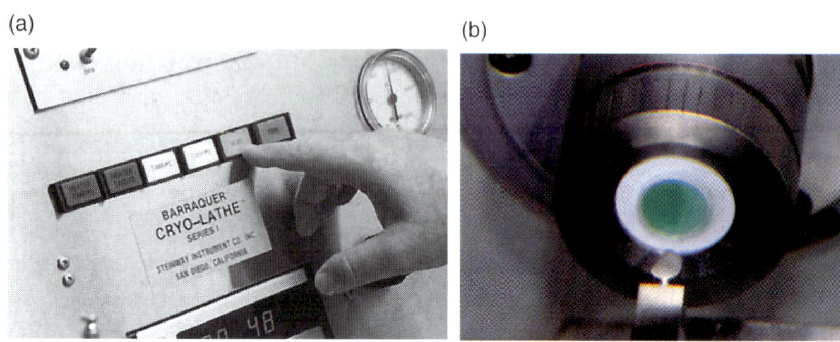

Fig. 10.59 (a) Start the head (and tissue) freezing first. The lathe head should be slowly revolving at this time. (b) Run the tool up close to, but not touching, the tissue and start the tool freezing.

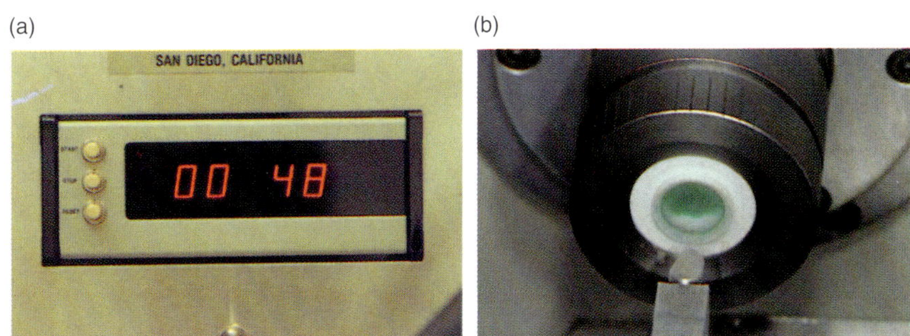

Fig. 10.60 (a) A sudden change in the appearance of the disk signals that freezing has occurred. (b) At least 45 seconds should elapse before starting the lathing process. This ensures that complete freezing/shrinkage of the tissue has occurred.

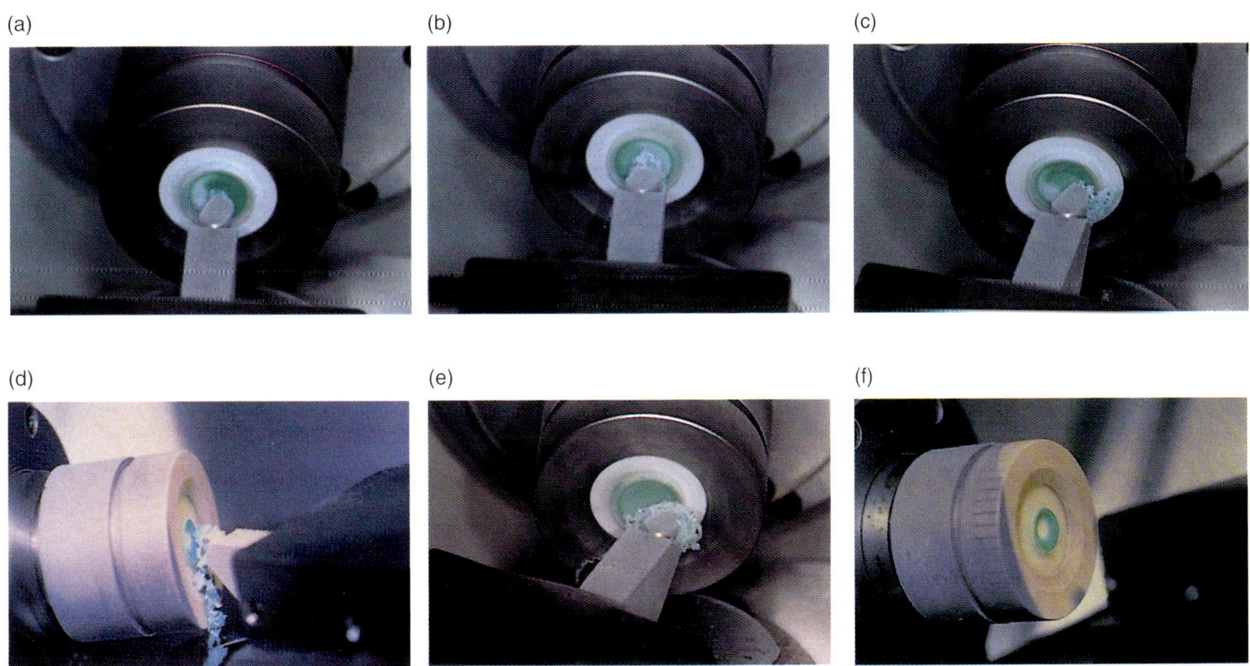

Fig. 10.61 (a–f) Lathing the disk. Advance the tool slowly, taking complete passes across the tissue surface before advancing further. Make the swing-through smooth and even. The finishing pass is made twice. Retract the head completely when lathing is complete.

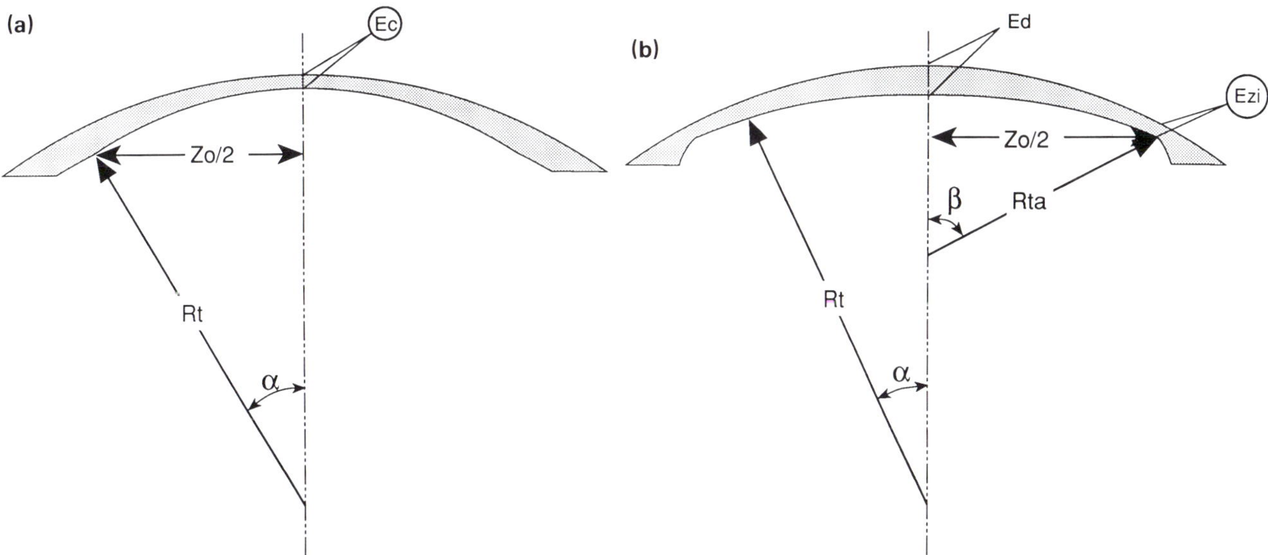

Fig. 10.62 (a) In cases of myopia, only one setting of the cutting radius and angle α is needed. The nature of the hyperopic lenticule shape is such that two separate settings of the cutting angle and radius are required (b).

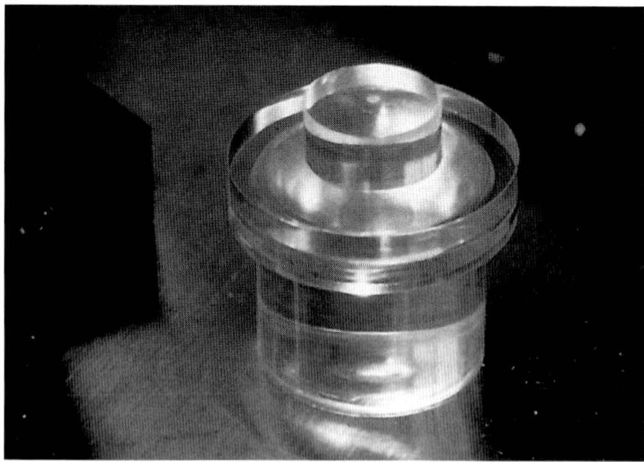

Fig. 10.63 The tissue is stored in the moist chamber while the resection bed is irrigated and debrided.

scrubbing is just vigorous brushing to ensure that any lint or epithelial cells are removed. Next, dry the bed with a moistened microsponge or, preferably, the sable brush. *Do not use the cellulose sponges* (such as Weck-Cel) for this purpose. They have a tendency to leave small particles behind. This drying step is to reveal any threads or small pieces of metal that may have come off the microkeratome and were not dislodged by the irrigation or missed by the scrubbing. Remove these with a fine forceps, and irrigate again. Use high power! Replace the cap.

Hold the moist chamber under the microscope, and remove the lid. Very gently irrigate and brush the undersurface of the resected disk (Figures 10.65 and 10.66). It may be necessary for your assistant to hold the chamber for you. If he or she does, make sure that he or she is observing through the microscope while doing so. Do not perform the cleaning by resting the tissue onto the cornea. To do so is to invite a visit from the "epithelium fairy."

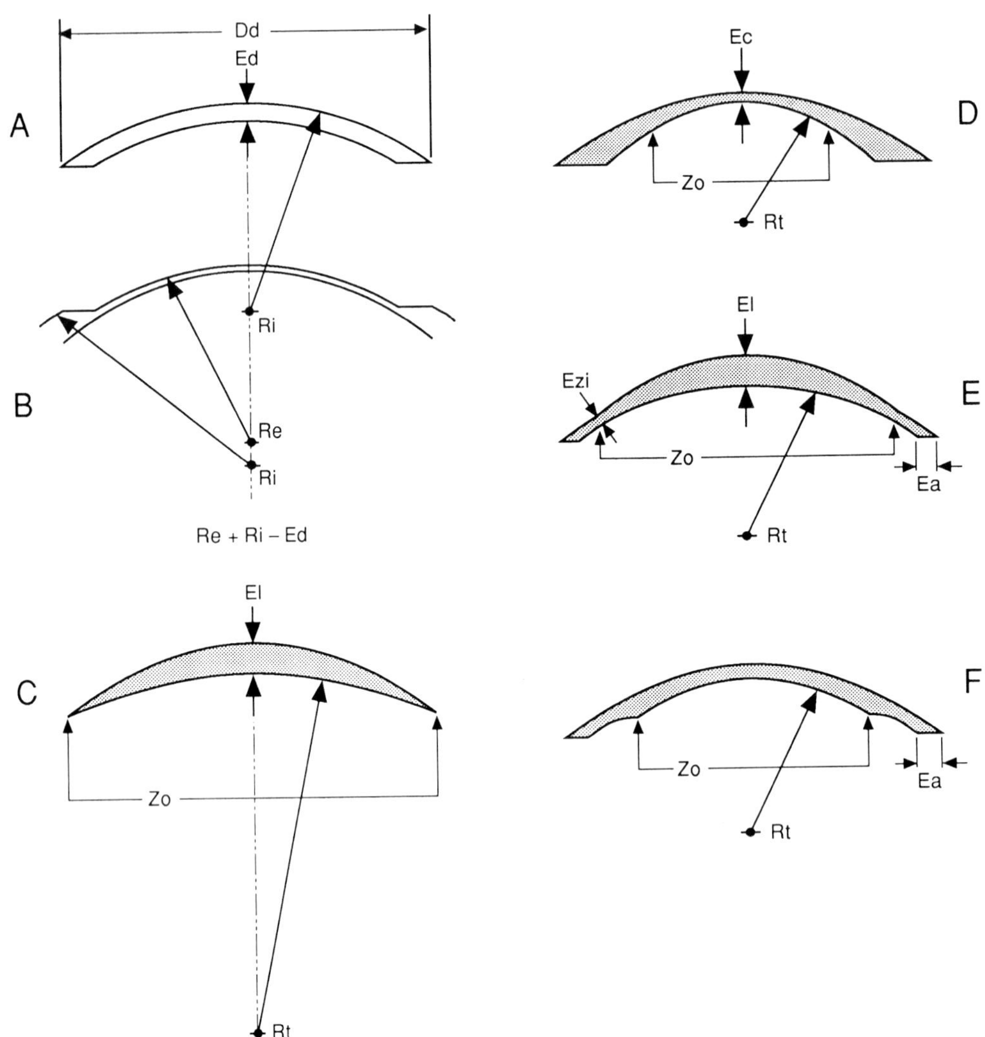

Fig. 10.64 Various lenticules and the abbreviations used in discussions of lathing (see Table 10.1). A, Resected disk; B, resection bed; C, keratophakia lenticule; D, myopia lenticule; E, hyperopia lenticule; F, epikeratophakia lenticule.

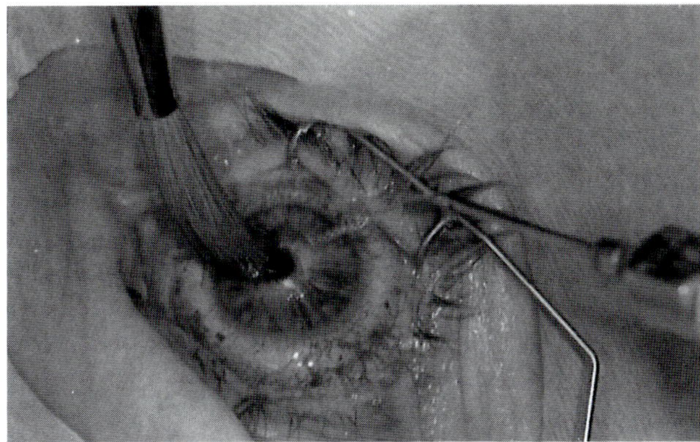

Fig. 10.65 Do not stint in the irrigation and brushing of the resection bed. Debris is easier to remove now before the lenticule is sutured in place.

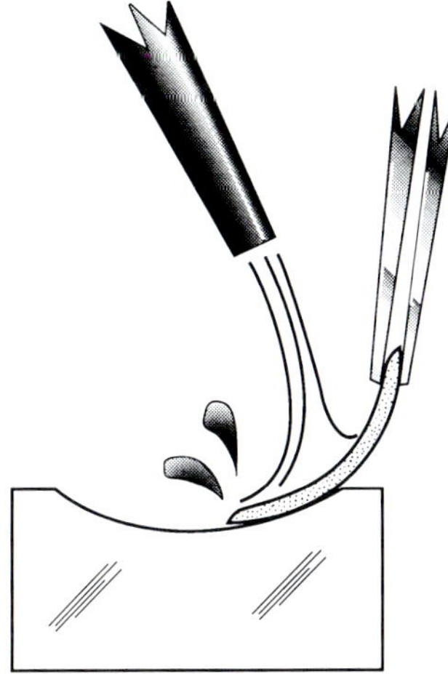

Fig. 10.66 Clean the underside of the lenticule in the moist chamber. Do not rest the tissue on the cornea to do this. That technique is sure to implant epithelial cells into the interface. Direct a gentle stream of saline downward onto the disk, using a soft brush to dislodge any particulate matter.

Now remove the tissue from the chamber using the lenticule spoon or a fine-toothed (0.12-mm) Colibri forceps. Be very gentle with the tissue at this point. Tissue for keratomileusis in situ is much thinner (135 to 150 μm in LASIK) than that encountered in HLK or in cryolathing and is easily torn—have a care. Here is where the lenticule spoon really pays for itself. Using a drop or two of BSS, float the tissue within the moist chamber so that it can be picked up easily by the spoon. If you are concerned about tearing or have a tendency to hold the tissue too firmly or do not have the spoon, try using a Pierse-Hoskins iris forceps.

Remove or have your assistant remove, the corneal cover, wet the eye, and place the tissue—epithelial side up—into the keratectomy bed (Figure 10.67). Gently, using the sable brush and/or the edge of the forceps, rotate the tissue into alignment with the previously made reference mark. It should line up exactly. If it does not and seems to join the corneal mark at an angle, you have placed the tissue onto the eye *upside down*. This is very easy to do with the thin keratomileusis in situ disk. The natural cupping seen with thicker sections, which aids in identifying the epithelial side, is absent. As mentioned in the discussion on HLK, this can be especially troublesome in RK cases with all the corneal scars (see the section on HLK, below). This is why the type of mark illustrated earlier is recommended; it is difficult to confuse it with those scars. Once the tissue is aligned, touch a microsponge or sable brush to the junction to soak up excess fluid. This also tends to "tack" the tissue down.

Suturing the corneal disk

At least three cardinal sutures of 10-0 nylon should be used (at 12, 6, and 9 o'clock) to hold the tissue in place and prevent rotation. Do not try to skimp with one or two. Even José Barraquer used three sutures. Thus, if the master did it, so should you. Alcon A-3 (or CU-11) 10-0 nylon with a spatulated (side-cutting) needle seems to work well

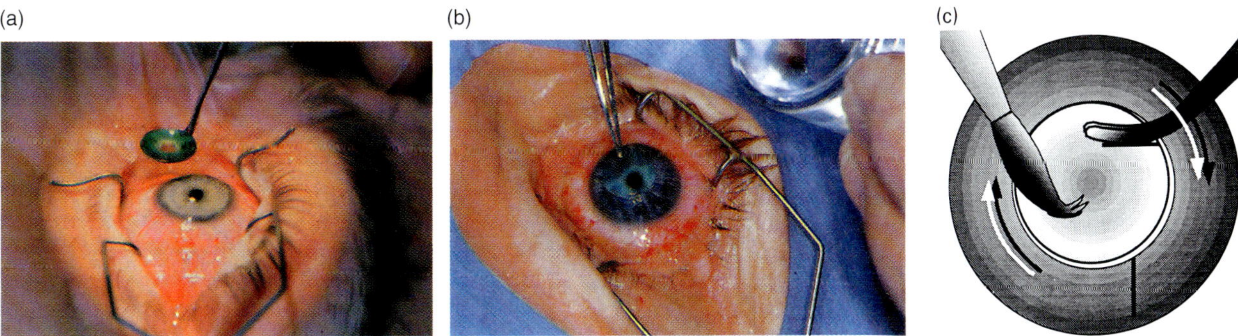

Fig. 10.67 (a) Transfer the lenticule to the eye with the tissue spoon. (b) Place it onto the resection bed. (c) Rotate the lenticule with brush and curved forceps. Align the reference mark. The disk and resection bed should be wet when performing this maneuver. Avoid sliding the disk over the edge of the resection bed to prevent seeding the interface with epithelial cells.

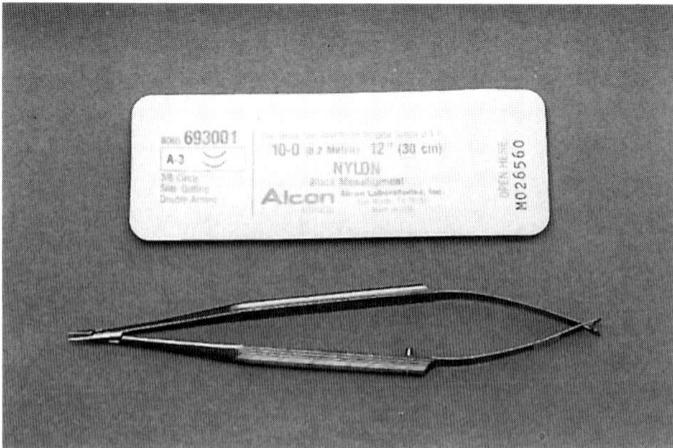

Fig. 10.68 The A-3 needle/nylon configuration by Alcon is the author's choice. A fine, straight needle holder may be easier to use by some surgeons.

in these cases (Figure 10.68). It should be cut in half, with one-half used for the cardinals.

Begin suturing with the 12 o'clock cardinal (Figure 10.69). Grasp the upper edge of the tissue disk with either 0.12-mm corneal forceps or the double-pronged Hofman-Polack forceps (Katena K5-1566) or similar, being careful not to rotate the tissue. Place the first suture through the tissue sufficiently back from the disk edge to hold without tearing out. Bring the needle through and into the cornea at the edge of the resection bed and out. Tie it so as just to coapt the edges. Pull the knot to the limbal side, and cut the ends long. The 6 o'clock suture should be placed next, again ensuring that the disk is not displaced or rotated. It is not necessary to hold the tissue with forceps, but it may be helpful for the first few cases to do so. Tie the suture so that little, if any, furrowing occurs in the disk. The last cardinal is then placed. In this case, countertraction at 3 o'clock is needed to keep from displacing or tearing the disk. Again, tie the knot only tight enough to coapt the edge.

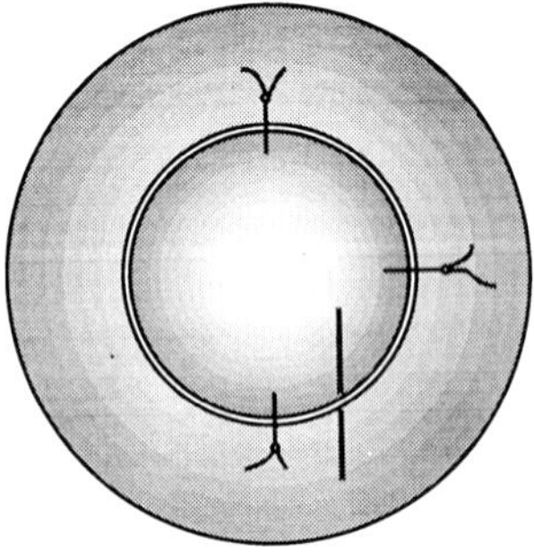

Fig. 10.69 Cardinal sutures. These sutures are for the purpose of preventing gross misalignment of the disk during placement of the running suture—do not tie them tightly. There should not be any furrows in the disk—this is not a keratoplasty! Place interrupted sutures at 12, 6, and 9 o'clock. Start at the 12 o'clock position; next do the 6 o'clock suture.

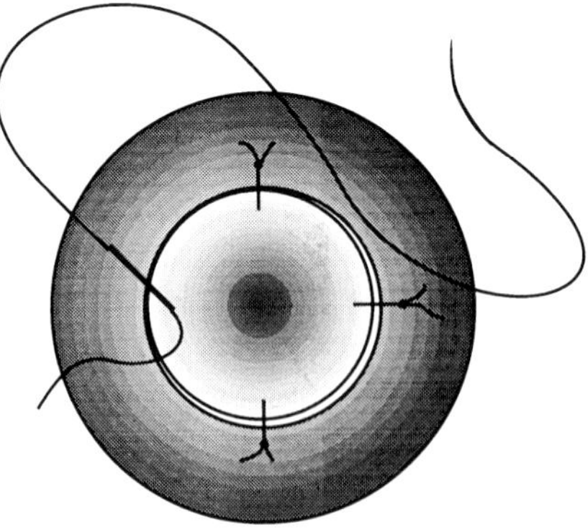

Fig. 10.70 First suture pass. Fixation at the limbus directly in line with the suture path provides good control over the procedure. The author tends to fixate behind the needle (on the opposite limbus), but some find it easier to fixate in front. When suturing the thin keratomileusis *in-situ* disk, it is best to avoid handling it with forceps of any kind. It really isn't necessary at any rate. If the needle tip is angled down slightly and pressed against the disk, the needle will easily cut its way through the tissue without undue distortion or displacement of the disk itself.

The placement of the eight-bite antitorque suture is not all that difficult if it is approached in a precise stepwise fashion. Begin suturing at the 3 o'clock position by passing the needle through the disk at 3 o'clock, approximately 1.0 mm from the edge. Angle it at 45° to the resection margin, and pass the tip between the edges of the disk and resection bed (Figures 10.70 through 10.72).

Do not run the needle through the tissue at the bottom of the bed (Figure 10.73). In keratomileusis in situ it is useful to push straight back against the eye with the slanted needle tip rather than trying to sweep it through the disk edge. In this way, the needle will penetrate the thin disk through and through without displacing it. Withdraw the tip sufficiently to make the limbal portion of the bite, entering at the bottom of the limbal edge and exiting about 1.5 mm from the edge (Figure 10.74). It helps to grasp the limbus with corneal-scleral forceps adjacent to the point where the needle will exit. Do not push the forceps toward the needle holder. This will make the cornea

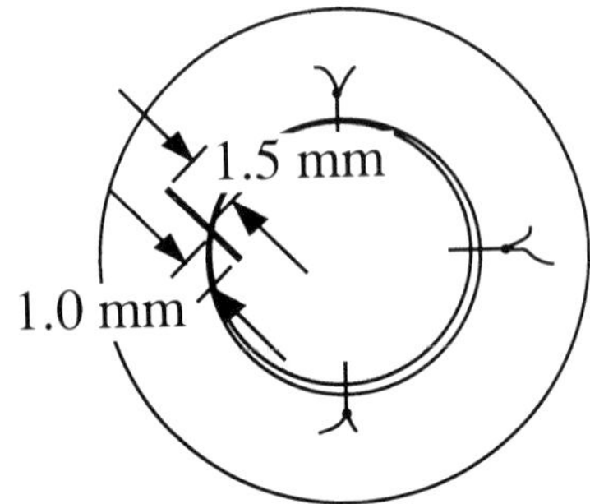

Fig. 10.71 Placement of suture bite. Try to keep the entry points on the disk as equidistant from the edge as possible. The exit points on the corneal sides are not as important.

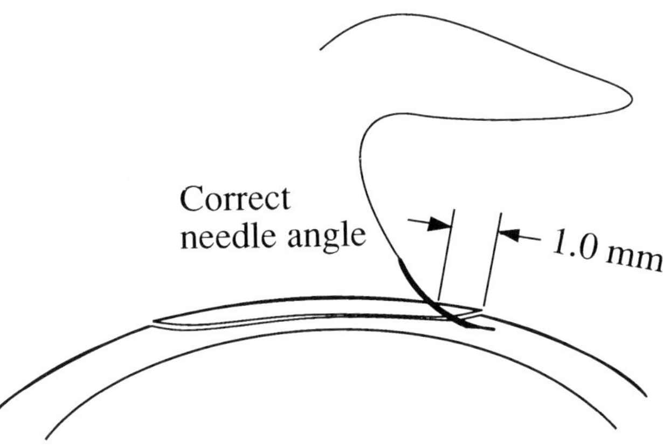

Fig. 10.72 Correct needle path. The needle should come out at the bottom edge of the disk and enter the corresponding portion of the resection edge without entering the bottom of the bed.

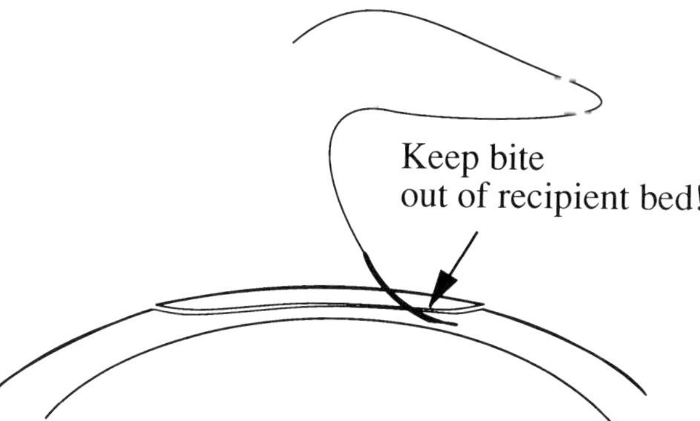

Fig. 10.73 Incorrect needle path. Avoid catching the tissue of the resection bed with your needle and suture. The tissue disk must be allowed to move and adjust itself freely over the resection surface to minimize astigmatism.

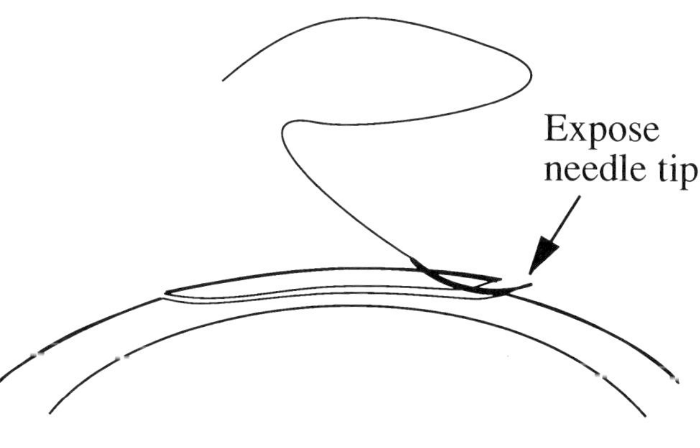

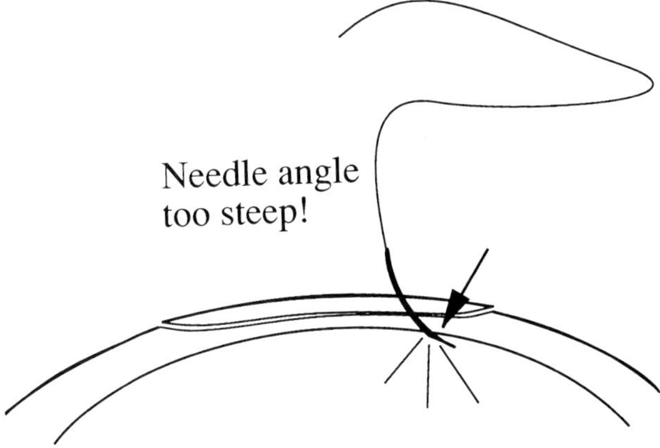

Fig. 10.75 Incorrect needle path. Shallow bites are the order of the day. Too great an angle of the suture tip practically ensures that the needle will enter the AC. If aqueous appears, withdraw the needle and place it properly—no ill effects are likely in that event.

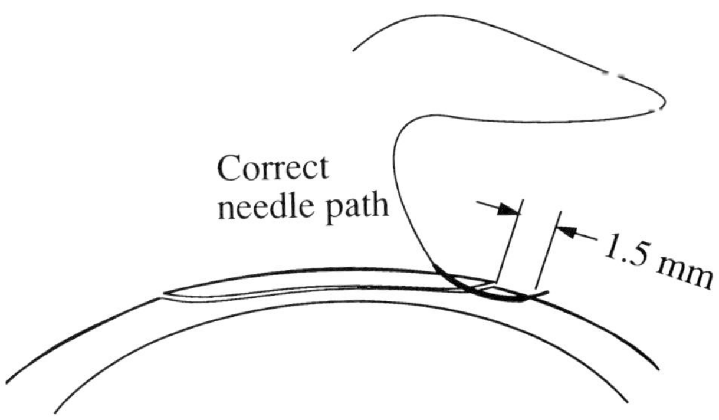

Fig. 10.76 Try to expose the needle tip. By exposing the tip of the needle each time while slightly raising up on the disk, the surgeon is assured that tissue at the bottom of the resection is not trapped.

bend upward, causing the needle to plunge deeper, possibly entering the anterior chamber (Figure 10.75). To prevent this, pick up the needle tip and expose it under the edge of the disk. Then place it flat on the recipient bed and pass it through the limbal side of the resection (Figure 10.76). Pull the excess suture through so as to leave about 1 in. (2 to 3 cm) loose. Continue with the remaining seven passes (Figures 10.77 through 10.83).

The slack in the suture is drawn up, and a three-throw or "surgeon's" knot is made, pulling the suture ends in such a way as to cause the knot to end up off the lenticule as close to the exit point on the limbus as possible (Figure 10.84). Snug up the suture sufficiently so that all limbs are straight and against the corneal surface. At this point, the disk and bed are wetted with BSS to allow the disk to slide. Cut and remove all three cardinals, taking care not to cut the continuous suture (Figure 10.85). If the cardinals are removed before tying the knot, the lenticule will be dragged or displaced toward the knot.

Some displacement of the lenticule may occur even with the cardinals in place. In this event, it must be recentered within the resection bed. By pulling up gently on the suture limbs toward the side you wish the lenticule to move, it will oblige by sliding in that direction (Figure 10.86). This maneuver may have to be done several times. Leave the lenticule slightly decentered to the side *opposite* the knot. The lenticule should end up just touching the resection

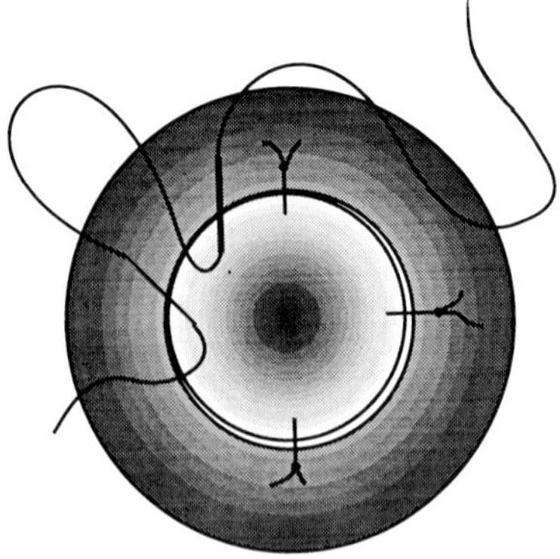

Fig. 10.77 Second suture pass. The next bite begins halfway between the 3 o'clock and 6 o'clock positions and is angled so as to produce a 90° included angle with the external limb of the previous bite. Again withdraw the needle back from the edge to ensure that none of the resection bed is included in the bite. The disk must be free to move within the resection bed.

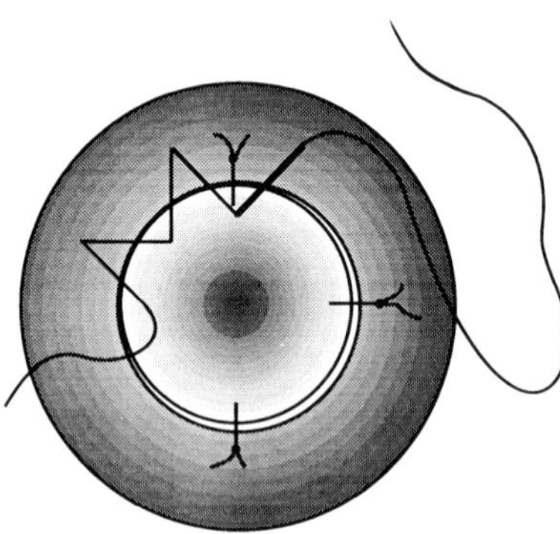

Fig. 10.78 Third suture limb. Begin the third bite at the 6 o'clock position, angling it at 45° in the same manner as the first. Draw up the slack so that the suture limbs lie flat and apposed to the corneal surface.

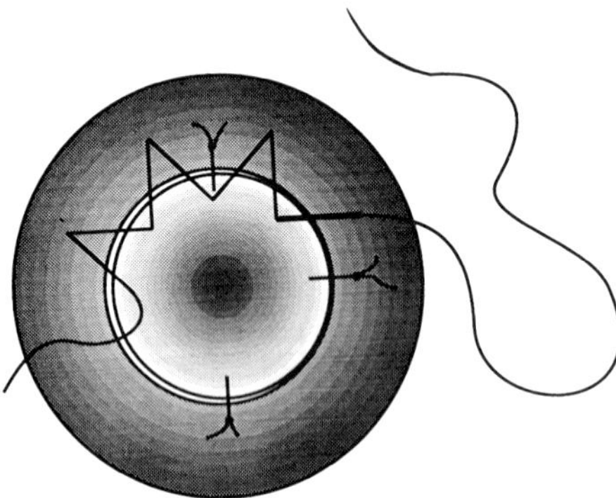

Fig. 10.79 Fourth suture pass. The fourth limb begins midway between the 6 and 9 o'clock positions and is directed at 180°. Again, take up the slack so that all the previously placed limbs are lying flat. Do not let the suture drag across the surface of the lenticule. Not only will this displace the lenticule itself, but it may tear off the epithelium. If you have displaced the lenticule, wet the area and gently, using the back of a curved forceps, move the tissue back into place. Pulling on the appropriate suture limb in the direction you wish the lenticule to move helps.

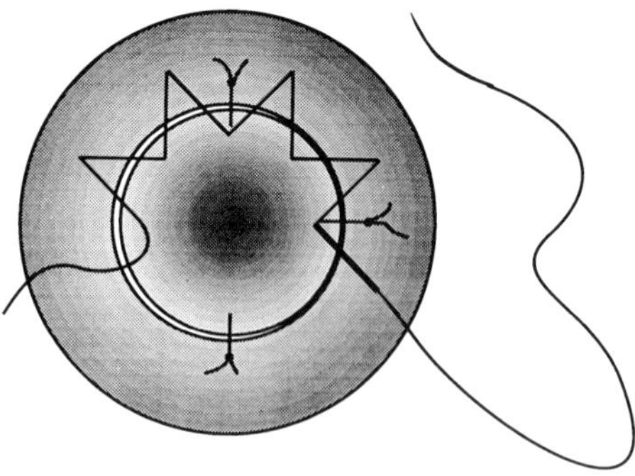

Fig. 10.80 Fifth suture pass. All of the previous limbs of the suture were placed backhand. For the next parts, reverse the needle and begin at the 9 o'clock position, positioning the needle to make the fifth bite at 45°.

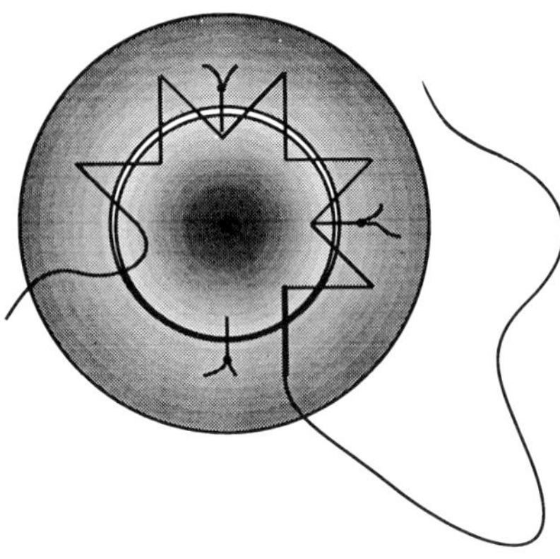

Fig. 10.81 Sixth suture pass. The sixth limb begins between the 9 and 12 o'clock positions and is directed toward the surgeon.

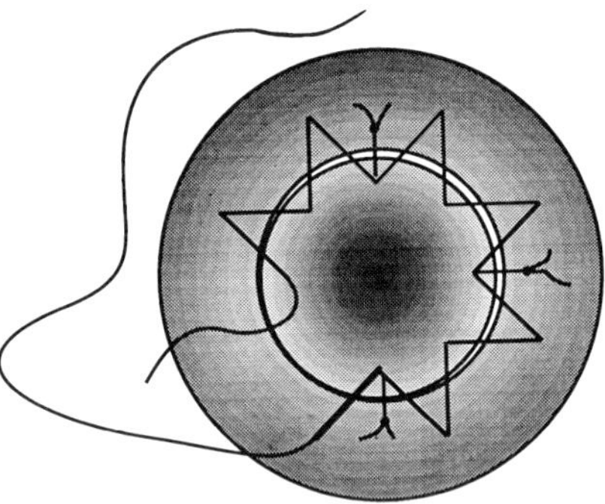

Fig. 10.82 Seventh suture pass. The seventh suture limb starts at 12 o'clock and again makes a 45° angulation to the tissue edge, making sure not to include the cardinal suture at that position.

edge at 3 o'clock, leaving a gap between the lenticule and the edge everywhere else.

The loosened suture should be snugged up and a single throw added to the previous triple. To keep the knot from "traveling," hold the standing part of the suture on tension, and pull the other limb down and away from the knot. The knot should not move and should be located at

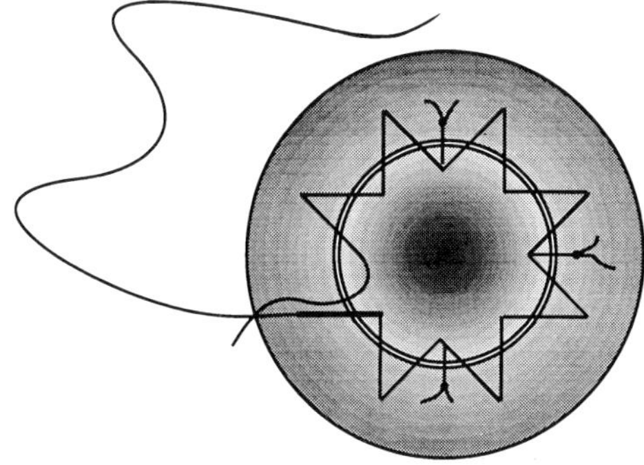

Fig. 10.83 Last suture pass. Finally the eighth bite enters the disk (lenticule) between the 12 and 3 o'clock positions and is directed horizontally. You are now ready to tie the knot.

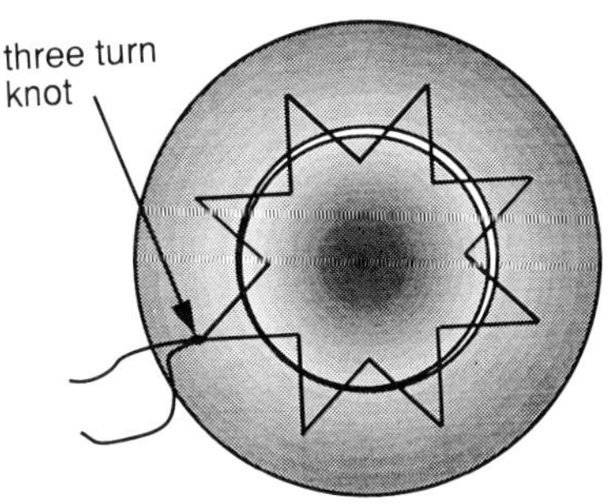

Fig. 10.84 First knot—three-turn surgeon's knot. When snugging up the first (three-throw) knot, hold the standing end on tension and aligned with the superficial limb as shown. Pull the other end of the suture down toward the limbus. This will crimp and lock the knot, keeping it from slipping.

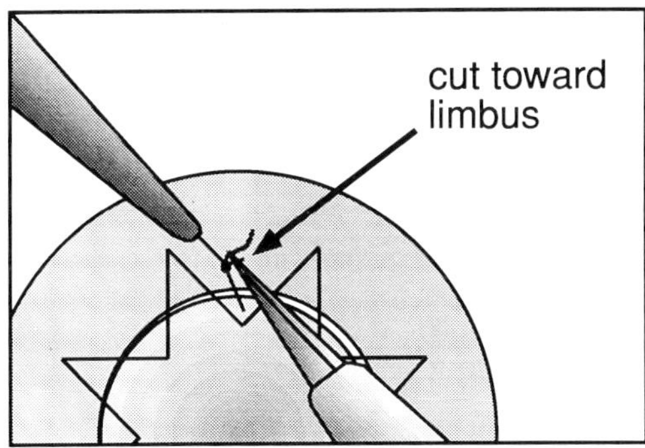

Fig. 10.85 Removing cardinal sutures. Cut and remove the cardinals carefully to avoid severing the running suture.

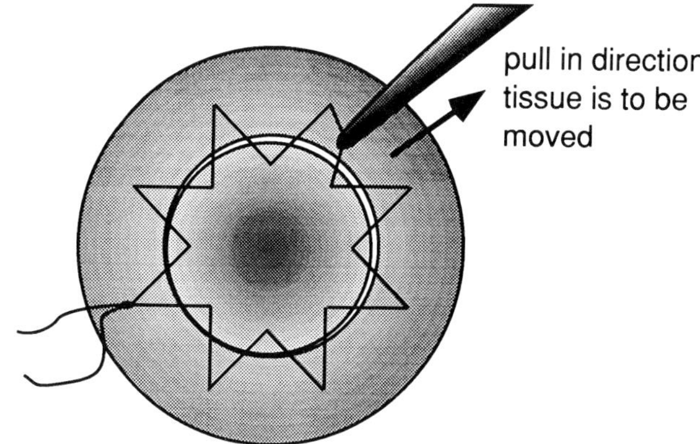

Fig. 10.86 Pull up gently on the suture limbs. Pull up all the slack in the running suture. If the disk is displaced, pulling on the suture limb in the direction you wish the tissue to move will cause it to slide over. Leave it slightly decentered directly opposite and away from the knot.

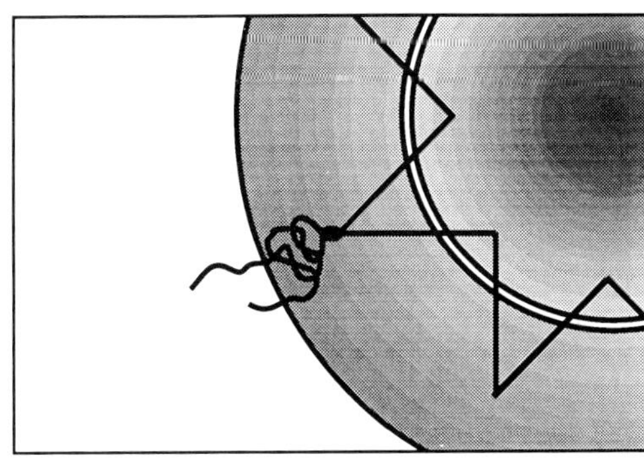

Fig. 10.87 Finish off the knot. Retighten the three-throw surgeon's knot and add a single throw. This maneuver will cause the disk to center itself. The next throw should be square to the one previous so as to lock the suture. The resulting knot should be tight and compact and will not slip.

the exit point of the last bite and on the scleral side of the keratectomy incision. Do not tie the knot so snug as to produce furrows in the disk. The ideal is to just tie the suture tight enough so that the disk lies flat against the cornea and is not loose. Add another single throw—square to finish off (Figure 10.87).

Under magnification, use a sharp razor knife to cut the suture ends on the knot. Direct the cutting edge away from the knot angled slightly up. Hold the tip against the knot with the edge extending past the knot. Hold each loose end with a forceps, and bring it up against the blade edge—bending the suture over the edge slightly. It does not take much tension to cut the suture. Repeat for the other suture end (Figure 10.88).

The next and final step is to bury the knot. This adds immeasurably to the patient's comfort but also reduces irritation and blinking, which slow epithelial healing. Using two smooth tying forceps, grasp each of the exposed suture limbs as shown. With the left hand, pull the suture toward the knot while at the same time pulling away with the right hand. The knot will disappear into the suture tract handily (Figure 10.89). Do not pull the knot into the resection bed or into the disk. If it goes in too far, ease it in the other direction. It should lie just below the corneal surface on the scleral (limbal) side of the incision (Figure 10.90). Equalize the suture limbs if necessary.

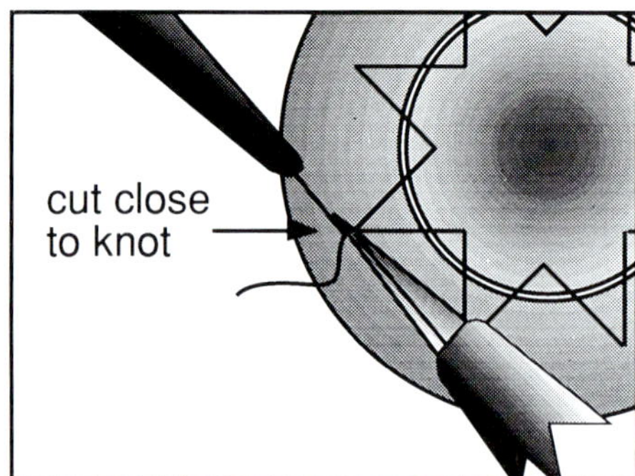

Fig. 10.88 Cut the knot flush. The suture should now be cut close to the knot, using a sharp, 15° razor knife. Lay the flat of the tip against the knot and cut the suture by pulling up on the ends, bending them over the blade edge. Do not pull too hard or the knot will also be cut.

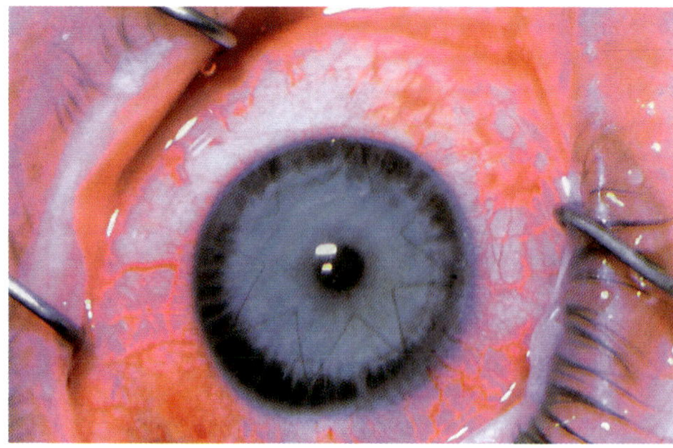

Fig. 10.90 The sutured lenticule. The suture limbs should indent the surface slightly but there should be no wrinkles in the tissue.

Perform a subconjunctival injection of Garamycin and Decadron/Depo-Medrol. Apply an antibiotic steroid drop (TobraDex) as well as a cycloplegic/mydriatic (such as 1% Cyclogyl) and a drop of anhydrous glycerin. Patch the eye with two cotton patches, a Fox eye shield, and paper or other hypoallergenic tape.

Complications and problems encountered during this surgery will be covered in Chapter 15.

Postoperative care

The patch is worn overnight, and it is recommended that it be replaced nightly (along with a shield) until the sutures are removed. The patient is placed on FML and MURO-128 drops three to four times daily until the sutures are removed—usually in 2 weeks.

Epithelialization normally will be complete within the next few days because freeze damage of the tissue has occurred (Figure 10.91). Except for the residual edema and subconjunctival hemorrhage from the fixation ring, the eyes will be essentially nonreactive. In fact, most of the postoperative discomfort will come from the latter rather than the resection. The use of cycloplegics or strong analgesics for comfort is rarely necessary. When vision in the operated eye has returned to 20/40 or better, surgery on the fellow eye can be done. This could take several months (see the section on the results of lamellar refractive surgery, below).

The sutures are left in for 2 weeks (14 days). They can be removed easily at the slit lamp with topical anesthesia. A 15° razor knife is used for this and is prepared by making a small right-angled bend in the tip, as shown

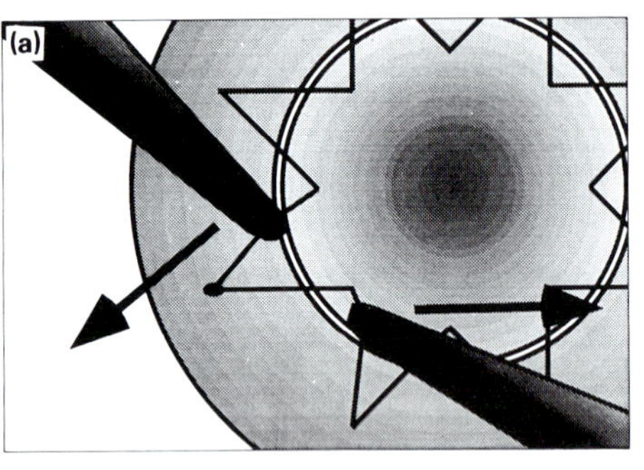

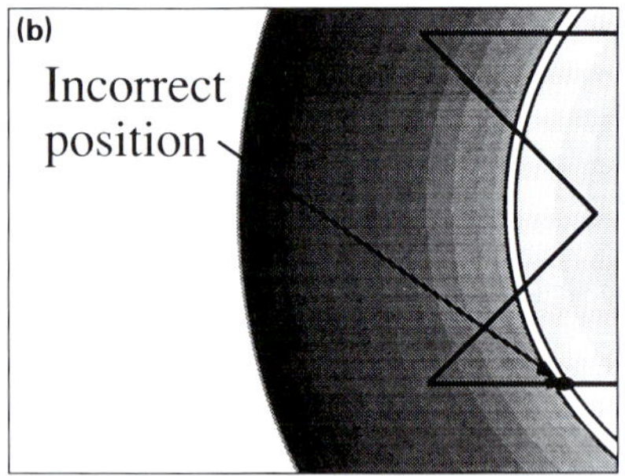

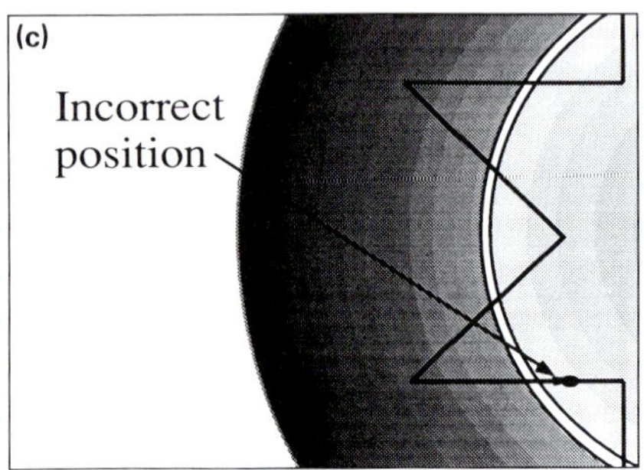

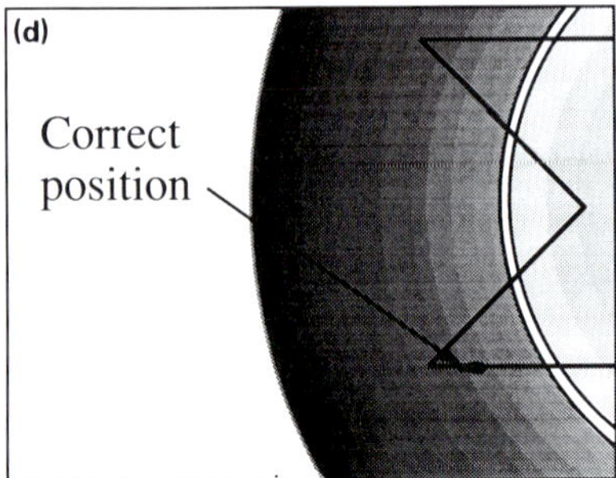

Fig. 10.89 Pull the knot below the surface. The knot must be buried to reduce patient discomfort and allow a smooth surface for re-epithelialization. Do this by pulling gently on the suture in the direction shown (a). The knot should disappear beneath the surface without difficulty. Do not neglect this step. (b) Often the knot is pulled in too far. Do not let it stay in the gap. Letting it stay in there provides a path for the epithelium to infiltrate the interface. (c) The knot cannot lie in the disk either. Leaving the knot in the disk can promote the same event as well as tissue erosion, especially through the thinner keratomileusis *in-situ* lenticule. Neither of these occurrences is a good thing and they should be avoided. (d) The correct position of the knot is just below the surface of the limbal cornea.

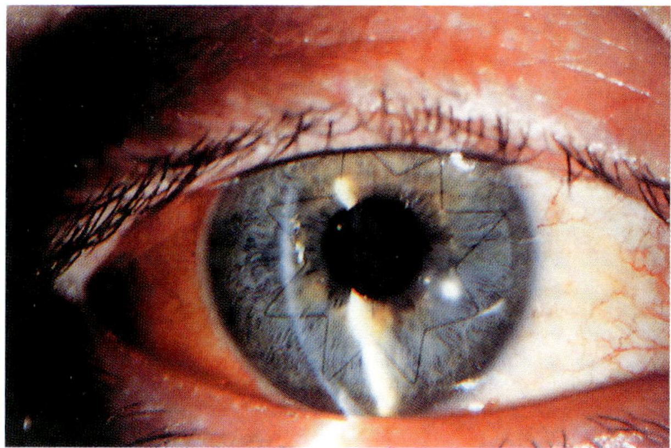

Fig. 10.91 MKM—48 hours postsurgery.

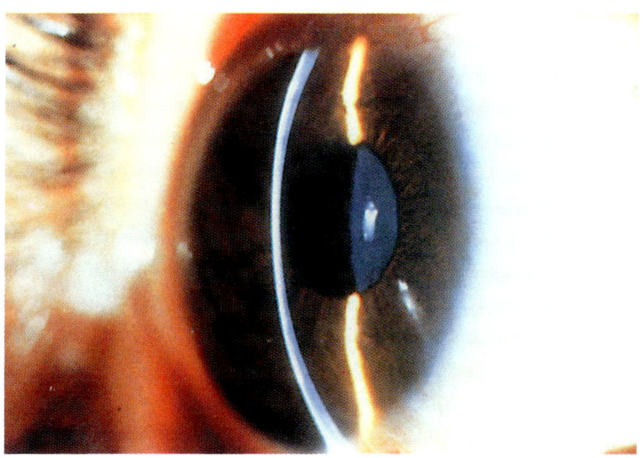

Fig. 10.93 Myopic keratomileusis. The Ec in this case was less than optimal. The correction was excellent but the transparency is poor—the patient will need a homoplastic procedure.

below. This small hook is used to pull up the exposed suture limb, and then by turning the blade 90°, the suture is cut. The running suture is cut in the middle of a limb in at least four places (Figure 10.92). The loose ends are then grasped with smooth fine-tipped forceps (Kelman-McPherson, Katena K5-5030) and the suture pulled out—*from the limbal side*. Do not pull toward the lenticule; it is very easy to pull it off the cornea at this stage. Patching after suture removal is not usually necessary, but a drop of antibiotic steroid is advised. Some patients will do much better if they are given artificial teardrops (Tears Naturale II) to use for the next few weeks as needed.

Variation in technique for homoplastic keratomileusis

In homoplastic keratomileusis, several points must be stressed to ensure success. First of all, it is important to cut the donor lenticule first. There are several reasons for this, not the least of which is possible damage to the donor lenticule. The resection has to be as thick as possible—as much as 450 to 480 μm—not especially easy to accomplish. Some cheat by removing the plate from the keratome—a technique not recommended. Second, the disk has to be at least 0.3 to 0.5 mm smaller in diameter than the recipient bed to minimize the possibility of epithelial ingrowth. Epithelialization typically is slower than in autoplastic cases, which increases the chance for this complication—a situation that is compounded if the donor tissue tends to overhang the recipient bed. Donor tissue varies in its response to the keratectomy, chiefly due to variations in water content. Preserved corneal buttons, especially those in Optisol, are less prone to variation, however. A typical disk for homoplastic KM should be cut to 7.0 mm. However, it may come off at 6.8 or 7.2 mm. It will be easier to resect the recipient disk to the required larger diameter—7.2 to 7.5 mm, respectively; thus the surgeon has a better chance at getting it right.

Time on the lathe will be longer with homoplastic and hyperopic cases. During the lathing, the thick donor disk must be converted to a thinner, parallel-sided disk. Thus the displacement is set several times—twice in myopia cases, once for the thinning and once for the optical carving, and three times for hyperopia. Figures 10.93 to 10.95 show postoperative KM eyes.

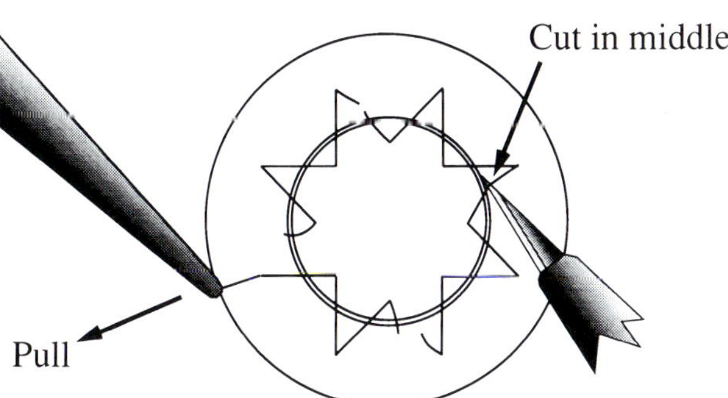

Fig. 10.92 Removing sutures. Cut the exposed limbs in at least four places using a razor knife. Lift up the severed limbs and pull the suture toward the limbus.

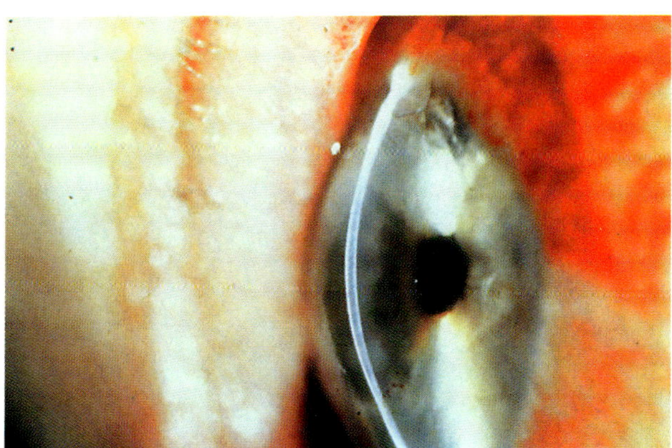

Fig. 10.94 Typical appearance of hyperopic keratomileusis.

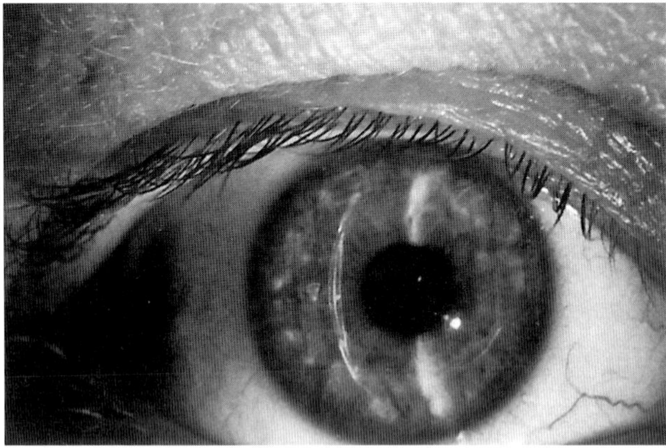

Fig. 10.95 Lathed MKM over an undercorrected radial keratotomy.

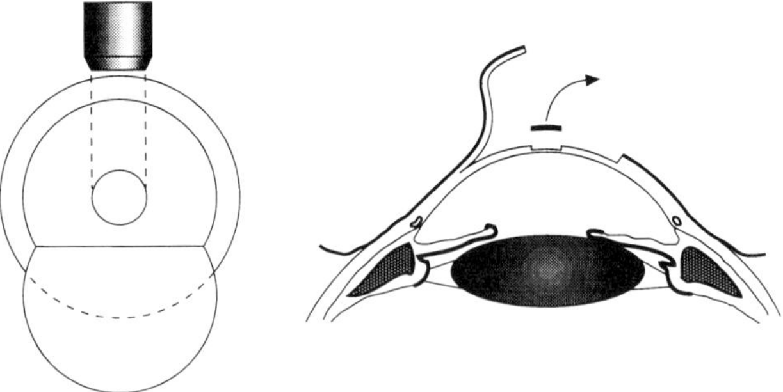

Fig. 10.97 Pureskin's modification of Krwawicz's central stromectomy.

Nonfreeze lamellar techniques

Both theoretical and experiential considerations have triggered attempts to simplify the original Barraquer procedure and possibly eliminate the need for freezing the tissue. While the process of freezing enables a precise shaping of the resected disk, it nonetheless results in death of the keratocytes and considerable edematous reaction. Both these factors contribute to a prolonged postoperative recovery period and to certain of the complications seen—such as delayed epithelialization and ingrowth (see Chapter 4).

It is not surprising that Barraquer himself conducted the first experiments with nonfreeze techniques. His most promising results came from his work with making an additional pass over the eye to remove a second thin section approximately 6.0 mm in diameter after partially removing the first resection [4] (Figure 10.96). His attempts to effect the reduction of myopia by varying the thickness of the secondary section were not wholly successful, and he eventually concluded that freeze lathing offered the best combination of accuracy and predictability.

Krwawicz followed Barraquer's work with his stromectomy cases in 1964, although he had attempted to modify the corneal curvature through other methods previously [5–7]. Pureskin modified Krwawicz's technique by using a trephine to demarcate the resection [8] (Figure 10.97). Elstein and coworkers reported their work on rabbits in 1969 [9]. In 1985, Hoffman devised a method of stromectomy using double suction rings and curvature templates called *keratokyphosis* [10] (Figure 10.98). None of these latter techniques successfully answered the challenge presented by classic KM, however.

Barraquer-Krumeich-Swinger (BKS) technique

In 1977, Swinger developed a simplified method of corneal reshaping by resecting a section of cornea and then by inverting the resected tissue over a suction die, cutting away a central portion of the disk to flatten its center [11] (Figures 10.99 through 10.102). This procedure had the advantage of not requiring freezing of the tissue but introduced a few problems of its own.

The first problem was that those who attempted the operation were misled into believing that this method somehow "simplified" the procedure. This is so because many thought that the lathing of the tissue was the toughest part of the operation, whereas, in reality, it is the keratectomy itself (the most difficult part of the operation to perform well) that is crucial to success in lamellar surgery. In addition, the technique specified a primary resec-

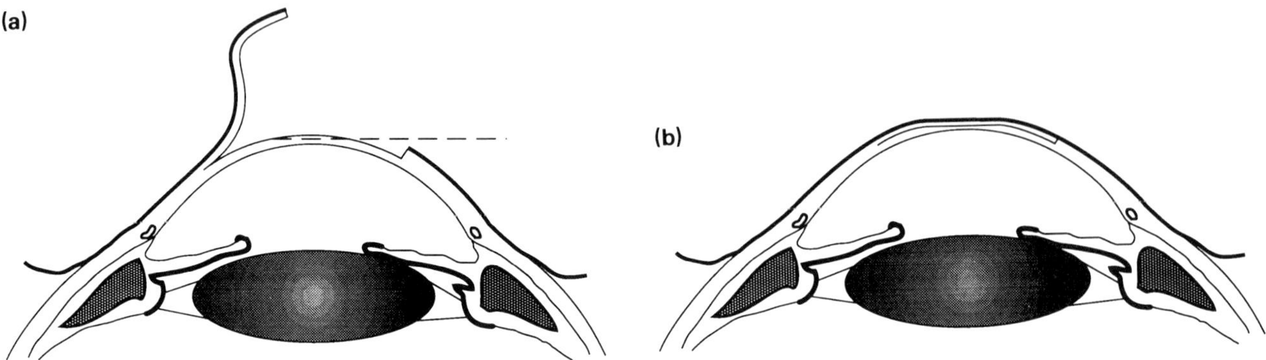

Fig. 10.96 (a,b) Barraquer's stromal resection. After dissecting the corneal cap, the keratome is used to remove the central disk.

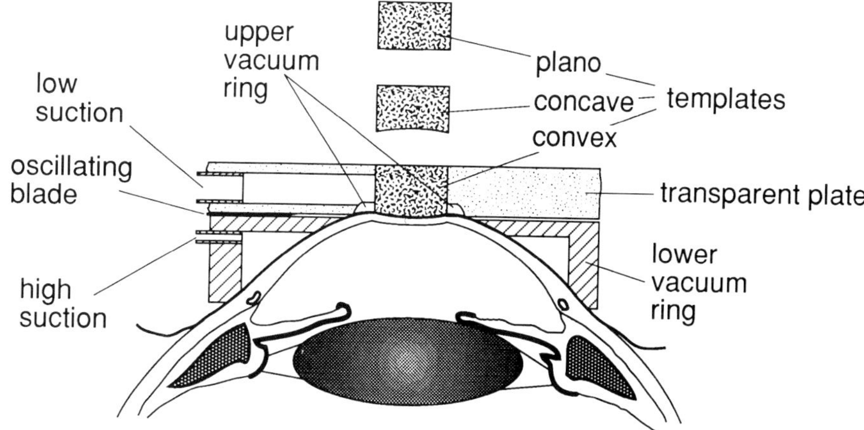

Fig. 10.98 Hoffman and Jessen's keratokyphosis.

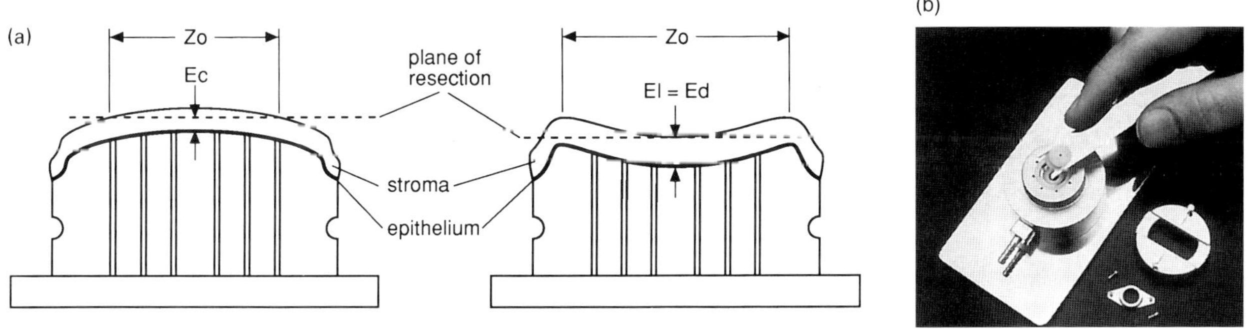

Fig. 10.99 Principle of the nonfreeze, BKS technique. (a) Plastic vacuum fixation plates in varying curvatures are employed with the BKS unit. (b) A convex plate is used for myopia and a concave plate for hyperopia.

tion whose diameter was 9.0 mm—a size difficult to cut smoothly, especially of the thickness required—300 to 350 μm. This tissue disk had next to be draped—upside down—over one of several perforated suction dies of differing curvature, precisely centered, and then secured with a serrated clamping ring that inevitably crushed the outermost portion of the disk. Vacuum was produced by a syringe that evacuated the chamber beneath the disk and a stopcock that—hopefully—held that vacuum until the surgery was complete. The thickness of the portion to be resected was controlled either by using a plate similar to the original Barraquer microkeratome or by means of an adjustable guide ring (in later models). Resection diameter was controlled by die curvature that, by being fixed, was essentially a compromise.

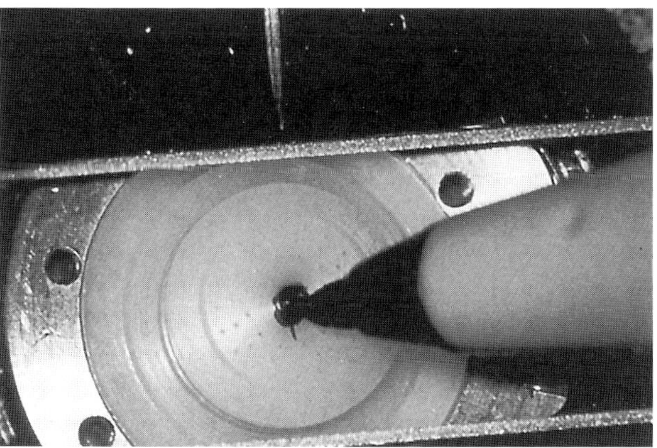

Fig. 10.100 A gentian violet pen is used to mark the center of the fixation plate.

While early success was reported in the laboratory, such success did not follow in the clinical studies [11,12]. Irregular astigmatism occurred in many cases probably due to imperfect disk centering but also undoubtedly due to poor fixation that allowed the resected disk to move during the second cut. Another factor is the character of the corneal tissue itself. Bereft of the support of Bowman's layer (which it is when inverted), the stroma takes on the consistency of jelly and tends to flow when pushed—as by the edge of a blade. This shearing of the surface introduces irregularity and elongation of the resection. Thus, what is supposed to be a circular resection actually turns out to be somewhat elliptical in shape. When such a section is laid against the cornea, it tends to match the curvature of the recipient bed. Since the major and minor meridians of the resection have different chord lengths, astigmatism results, often of the irregular variety. Further,

(a)

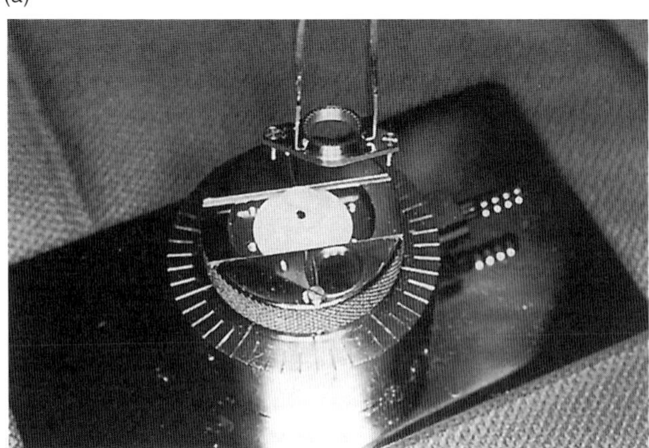

(b)

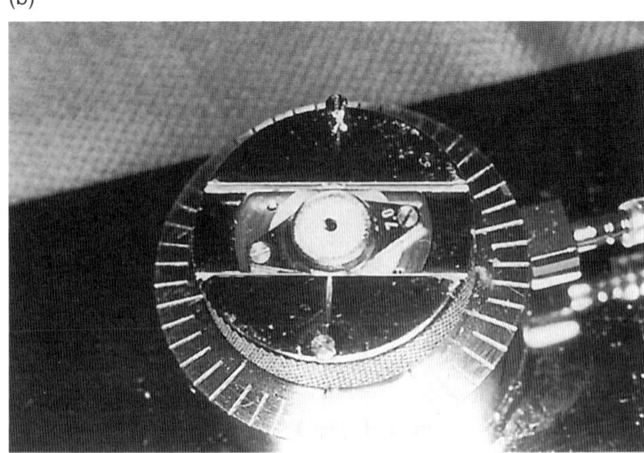

Fig. 10.101 The resected disk is centered over the fixation plate—epithelial side down (a) and clamped with the retainer plate (b).

predictability was something to aspire to but was not realized sufficiently in clinical practice. Despite some suggestions and attempts to fabricate epikeratophakia lenticules by this method, few, if any, clinical cases are being performed in this country currently [13].

Hyperopic lamellar keratotomy (HLK)

In classic myopic keratomileusis, one of the causes for loss of effect with the surgery is deep keratome sections. If the posterior corneal layers are thinner than 20% of the central corneal thickness, late low-order corneal ectasia will occur, producing a steepening of the central corneal curvature and an increase in the myopia. While reviewing cases of late loss of effect in MKM, Ruiz noted that the amount of ectasia or central steepening seemed to be related to the size of the disk removed by the keratome [14]. He experimented with rabbits and found that by making a section 80% of the central corneal thickness and varying the size of the disk removed, he could produce steepening of the cornea proportional to the disk size. No manipulation of the tissue other than the initial section was necessary. By simply replacing the tissue disk on the eye and securing it with a running antitorque suture, up to 8.5 D of corneal steepening could be obtained. He applied this technique to human corneas in December 1984. In early 1985, the author was the first to perform this procedure in the United States [15]. These first cases were in RK hypercorrections; later, cases with "pure" hyperopia were operated on.

The procedure (called a *keratotomy* because while tissue is removed, it is replaced immediately) is relatively straightforward in execution (Figure 10.103). The microkeratome head is fitted with a plate (or the plate is ad-

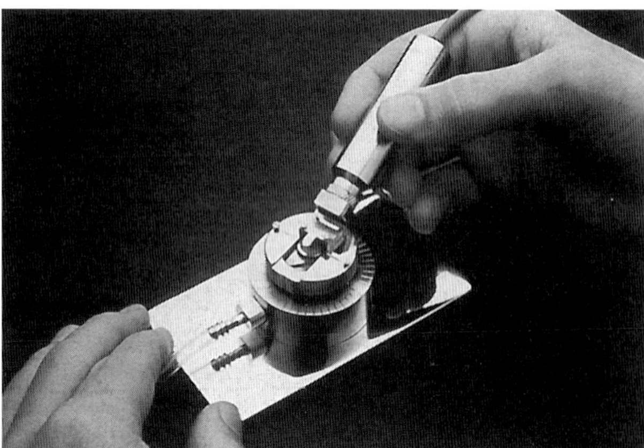

Fig. 10.102 A vacuum is drawn on the tissue via the side port. The guide ring is then adjusted by screwing it up or down, as with the Barraquer artificial anterior chamber. The keratectomy proceeds as usual.

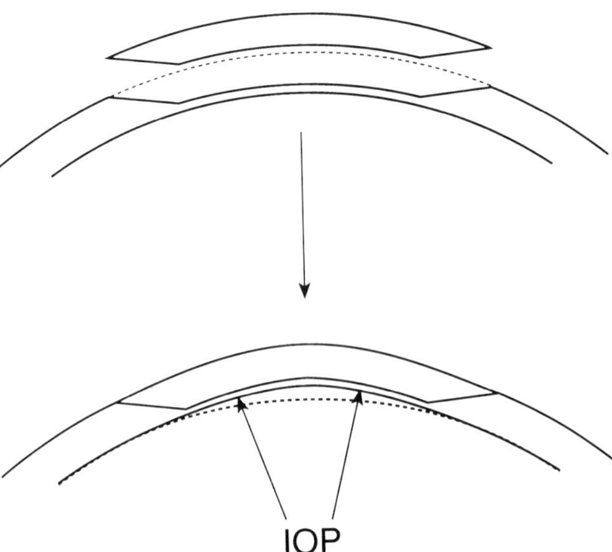

Fig. 10.103 Hyperopic lamellar keratotomy. This surgery works by allowing a controlled ectasis of the cornea to occur, therefore both disk thickness and diameter are critical. Only one section (deep) is made in this surgery.

Table 10.2 Results of epikeratophakia in aphakia

	Preoperative			Postoperative		
Cases	Spherical equivalent (D)	Mean unaided vision	Mean corrected vision	Spherical equivalent (D)	Mean unaided vision	Mean corrected vision
6	12–14	20/400	20/30	0–2	20/60	20/70
9	14–16	20/400	20/30	0–1.5	20/50	20/80
4	16–18	20/400	20/30	0–1	20/60	20/75

justed with the set screw) to obtain a resection thickness of 70% of the central ultrasonic pachymetry. The actual procedure is difficult to perform and requires great skill with the microkeratome—something only obtained through extensive practice and experience—but it can be learned. In retrospect, HLK is somewhat more difficult to perform than keratomileusis in situ because the diameter and tissue thickness are critical to success. Stabilization can be assisted by the application of 5% saline drops three times daily for up to 3 weeks to reduce tissue edema.

Disk diameter and thickness are extremely important in this surgery. Sometimes the plate that matches the disk thickness needed exactly cannot be found (in fixed-plate keratomes), and the closest size must be made to serve. Because of this limitation, the author has had made a microkeratome head that can be adjusted continuously so as to provide a closer approximation of the resection depth required. This head is driven by a gas-turbine motor that provides higher speed (rpms) and greater torque than the earlier models. This combination results in much smoother resections than before, but there are inevitable compromises that had to be made in the design.

Centration of the resection

Centration is accomplished as in classic keratomileusis (see above). Make sure that the reference scribe mark is *tangential* to the pupil or a 4.0-mm OZ mark—*not radial.*

Plate setting

In HLK, only one pass of the microkeratome across the cornea is required. Typically, the section is made to 70% of the central corneal thickness, as measured by ultrasonic pachymetry. If necessary, refer to the section on pachymetry in Chapter 5. The disk thickness is determined by the following guidelines:

1 If the central corneal thickness is 0.52 mm or less, choose the plate so as to obtain a section no thicker than 360 μm or 70% of the pachymetry.

2 If the corneal thickness is 0.53 to 0.60 mm, choose the plate so as to obtain a section of 360 to 420 μm or 70% of the pachymetry.

3 If the thickness is greater than 0.60 mm, choose the plate so as to obtain a section of no greater than 450 μm.

For example, if a patient has a central corneal thickness (CP) of 0.522 mm (522 μm), choose the plate so as to obtain a section of 360 μm. Typically, the sections taken with the SCMD adjustable keratome are some 60 to 80 μm thicker than the plate setting—but this will vary with the individual machine. Thus, in the preceding example, the actual plate setting would be 360 less 60 to 80 μm (i.e., 260 to 300 μm) depending on the characteristics of the particular head.

Disk thickness – keratome bias = plate setting

It follows, therefore, that each head must be calibrated individually. This can be done by making several sections at various settings, preferably using cadaver eyes. In doing so, be advised that the sections taken from these eyes typically will be 20 μm thicker than those from a living eye. If, then, a particular keratome is consistently cutting 70 μm more than the actual setting, the plate would be adjusted to 310 μm (70 – 20 = 50 μm). After sectioning, the disk should measure 360 μm—which is the thickness desired.

In overcorrected RK patients, the plate setting should be 10% less than that for an unoperated cornea. It has been

Table 10.3 Results of fresh epikeratophakia in keratoconus

	Preoperative			Postoperative		
Cases	Spherical equivalent (D)	Mean unaided vision	Mean corrected vision	Spherical equivalent (D)	Mean unaided vision	Mean corrected vision
17	*	<20/400	20/30	+0.50 to –3.0	20/40	20/25

* Rational refraction not possible

found that RK corneas pull up into the ring somewhat higher than do uncut corneas. This may occur because these corneas are somewhat more malleable than unincised corneas. In the example case, a disk thickness of 330 μm should be created. This would mean an actual plate setting of 280 μm—using the head described.

In no instance should the section be less than 0.30 mm (300 μm). A cornea requiring a 250-μm section would have a central thickness of 380 to 400 μm, which is approaching that seen in keratoconus. Lamellar sections probably should not be done in cases of keratoconus, except for the purpose of reinforcing the cornea—in which case a wet epikeratophakia lenticule would be a better choice.

Because of the variability in resection thicknesses required, a fixed-plate keratome is not ideal for performing this surgery. The SCMD adjustable-plate microkeratome was designed especially for this surgery and is recommended, as is the Steinway automatic corneal shaper.

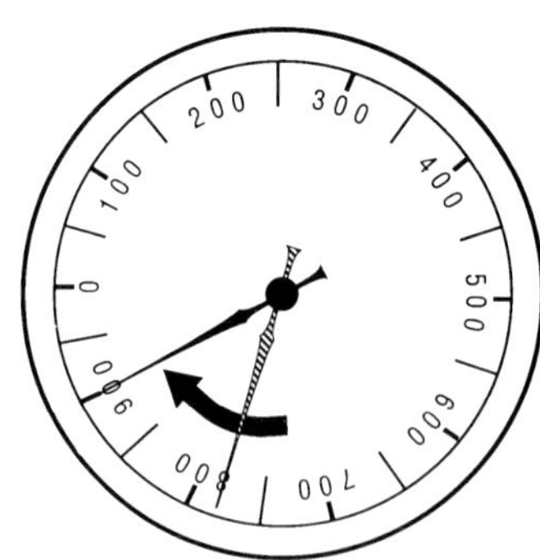

Fig. 10.105 Plate set to 100 μm disk thickness. Keep in mind that while the gauge setting indicates a plate setting of 100 μm, the resulting tissue disk is likely to measure somewhere around 170 μm. This is because the microkeratome typically cuts a thicker section than that set. The exact amount of overage (bias) that will occur is dependent on the specific instrument, requiring each one to be calibrated individually, but is usually on the order of 60–80 μm.

Plate setting with the SCMD unit

Most important, the plate setting must be done with the gauge anvil as close as possible to the blade without touching it. While steadying the keratome with one hand, turn the plate adjustment screw until the indicator stops at the desired setting (Figure 10.104). Remember that this setting is the desired tissue thickness less the keratome overage or bias. To avoid confusion and possible error, the gauge can be set to account for the bias of a particular microkeratome. To do this, set the zero point as usual, and then, while the anvil is still resting on the blade, rotate the dial face clockwise until the needle indicates the amount of bias in the system. This is your new zero point—lock the gauge ring. Now, when the plate is set at 100 μm, you will get 100 μm (Figure 10.105).

Remove your hands from the head and gauge ring for the final reading. Typically, the indicator will have moved and will now show another reading. In that case, make the corresponding adjustment to the plate until the desired setting is indicated when the microkeratome is hanging free.

Now raise the anvil again, and recheck the zero setting. If the zero point has shifted, be certain that the anvil is positioned correctly before resetting the gauge. If anything has been changed, it will be necessary to reset the plate. Once the setting is satisfactory, remove the head from the setting ring, apply a tiny amount of lubricant to the motor shaft, and reattach the keratome head to the turbine handle, making sure that it is screwed all the way in and is finger-tight.

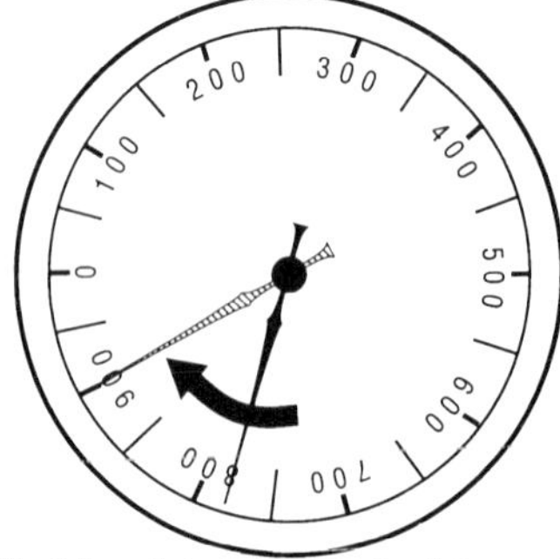

Fig. 10.104 Adjust the plate to the desired tissue thickness. Always adjust the setting so that the plate moves from thicker to thinner (i.e. open to closed), never vice versa. This prevents possible problems from the plate getting hung up. Note that the gauge is read in reverse. That is, 900 μm is really 100 μm, etc.

Resection diameter

The diameter of the resection necessary is selected from Table 10.4 or from the computer program, and the proper fixation ring is selected. It will be necessary to try a few rings before the correct one is found. Since the sections in

Table 10.4 Nomogram for HLK

Hyperopia (D)	Diameter of disk (mm)
1.5	6.5
2.0	6.4
2.5	6.3
3.0	6.2
3.5	6.1
4.0	6.0
4.5	5.8
5.0	5.6
5.5	5.4
6.0	5.2
6.5	5.0
7.0	4.8
7.5	4.6

HLK are much smaller in diameter than those for keratomileusis, it is suggested that a good size to begin with would be a no. 10—two steps higher than usually required. Always check the IOP with the tonometer before determining the resection diameter—at least for the first application of the ring. Remember also to dry the cornea with a microsponge before making any measurements.

Remember that the actual diameter of the resected disk will be about 0.2 mm *larger* than that applanated. If the table calls for a 6.2-mm disk, choose a ring that will produce an applanated area of 6.0 mm. It may not be possible to obtain an applanation this precise each time, however. You are advised in such cases to cut a disk slightly smaller than required. For example, if it is found that although the case calls for a resection diameter of 5.6 mm, one ring applanates to 5.8 to 6.0 mm and the next size up applanates to 5.2 mm, choose the ring that produces the 5.2-mm applanation. It is better for the patient to end up slightly myopic than to remain hyperopic. There are sufficient applanators within the usual instrument set that the exact size a ring applanates can be determined—so take the time to check. It does not take much time to be sure.

Making the section

Always check to see that the microkeratome moves freely in the ring before attempting to resect a disk. Put a drop or two of saline on the corneal surface and on the microkeratome head before starting. Do not, however, flood the eye. If the cornea is too wet, some unevenness of the section will result.

Make the section as described in the section on keratomileusis above, and check the thickness with the tissue gauge. Put the resected disk into the moist chamber, and clean up the resection bed. Remove the tissue from the chamber using the Barraquer lenticule spatula or a fine-toothed (0.12-mm) Colibri forceps. The tissue can be floated, epithelial side down, onto the spatula using a drop of BSS. Be very gentle with the tissue at this point. While it is less fragile than a lathe-cut lenticule, it can still be torn.

Rotate the tissue until its reference mark comes into alignment with the corneal mark. It should line up exactly. If it does not and seems to join the corneal mark at an angle, you have placed the tissue onto the eye upside down. This is a very rare occurrence with HLK because of the disk thickness, but it can happen if you have not been paying attention. It can be especially troublesome to align the tissue in some RK cases because of the radial corneal scars. This is why the tangential type of mark is recommended. It is difficult to confuse it with the RK scars. If this is a problem with RK cases, it may help to outline the reference mark by dabbing it with the skin-marking pencil, thus making the mark more prominent.

Suturing of the resected tissue back onto the cornea is the same as in KM and is covered in the section on suturing the corneal disk above. Figure 10.106 shows a postoperative HLK patient.

This technique is especially applicable to cases of RK that resulted in induced hyperopia. In these cases, resection of the corneal disk should not be attempted before 6 or, preferably, 8 months after RK. At this time, the cornea should be sufficiently stabilized and the incisions strong enough to allow a smooth resection. Sutures must be placed carefully so as not to open the incisions. Despite such care and the nature of the suturing pattern, which assists in preventing such occurrences, opening or "fraying" will occur at the extreme edges of the tissue disk in some cases. Such fraying has not produced unusual healing, nor has induced astigmatism been a hallmark in the cases of the author's experience (Figure 10.107).

Keratomileusis in situ (KMIS)

The first human cases to undergo KMIS did so in Bogota, Colombia, in May 1987. The anterior lamellar sections were secured, as in MKM, by the classic running eight-point antitorque suture. Epithelialization generally was complete within 24 hours. Useful vision was restored within days rather than the months usually seen in freeze-lathed cases. Encouraged by the results in these patients, the author performed the first KMIS surgery in the United States in November 1987 on patients whose fellow eye had received classic freeze-lathe surgery. All patients reported a more comfortable postoperative course, and all remarked on the rapidity of onset of clear vision. The results, however, were not identical to those reported initially by Ruiz [16]. The incidence of induced postoperative astigmatism was somewhat higher than that seen in classic MKM, for example, especially irregular astigmatism (see section on results, below).

KMIS differs from classic keratomileusis in that the actual change in corneal curvature is made by the microkeratome and not the lathe. In order for this to work, two passes of the microkeratome must be made. This latter requirement is easier to accomplish than one might expect—it depends, really, on correct placement of the first ring. If the first ring is centered properly before suction is applied and the eye is held until the ring is firmly seated, a saddle-shaped impression is made in the limbal sclera that makes placement of the ring for the second pass a snap.

Since both the thickness and the diameter of the first and second resections are different, two different rings and applanators must be used. An adjustable-plate keratome was designed for this surgery (see the section on the SCMD microkeratome, above).

The first pass removes the corneal "cap." This section is typically 0.13 to 0.15 mm (130 to 150 μm) in thickness and 7.25 mm in diameter. This disk is much thinner than those encountered in classic KM and requires special handling. The second pass removes a smaller-diameter disk that

Table 10.5 Ruiz KMIS nomogram

Myopia spherical equivalent (D)	Optical zone size							
	3.5	3.7	4.0	4.2	4.5	4.7	5.0	5.2
2.5	0.016	0.017	0.021	0.023	0.026	0.029	0.033	0.036
3.0	0.018	0.021	0.024	0.027	0.031	0.034	0.039	0.043
3.5	0.021	0.024	0.028	0.031	0.036	0.040	0.045	0.049
4.0	0.024	0.027	0.032	0.035	0.041	0.045	0.051	0.056
4.5	0.027	0.030	0.036	0.040	0.046	0.050	0.057	0.062
5.0	0.030	0.033	0.039	0.043	0.050	0.055	0.063	0.069
5.5	0.032	0.036	0.043	0.047	0.055	0.060	0.069	0.075
6.0	0.035	0.039	0.046	0.051	0.059	0.065	0.074	0.081
6.5	0.038	0.042	0.050	0.055	0.064	0.070	0.080	0.087
7.0	0.040	0.045	0.053	0.059	0.068	0.075	0.085	0.093
7.5	0.043	0.048	0.057	0.063	0.072	0.079	0.091	0.099
8.0	0.045	0.051	0.060	0.066	0.077	0.084	0.096	0.104
8.5	0.048	0.053	0.062	0.069	0.080	0.088	0.101	0.109
9.0	0.050	0.056	0.066	0.073	0.085	0.093	0.106	0.115
9.5	0.052	0.059	0.069	0.077	0.088	0.097	0.111	0.120
10.0	0.055	0.062	0.072	0.080	0.092	0.102	0.116	0.126
10.5	0.057	0.064	0.075	0.083	0.096	0.106	0.120	0.131
11.0	0.059	0.067	0.078	0.087	0.100	0.110	0.125	0.136
11.5	0.062	0.069	0.081	0.090	0.104	0.114	0.130	0.141
12.0	0.064	0.072	0.084	0.093	0.108	0.118	0.135	0.146
12.5	0.066	0.074	0.087	0.096	0.111	0.122	0.139	0.151
13.0	0.068	0.077	0.090	0.100	0.115	0.126	0.144	0.156
13.5	0.070	0.079	0.093	0.102	0.118	0.130	0.148	0.161
14.0	0.072	0.081	0.095	0.106	0.122	0.134	0.152	—
14.5	0.074	0.083	0.098	0.108	0.125	0.137	0.156	—
15.0	0.077	0.087	0.101	0.112	0.129	0.141	0.161	—
15.5	0.078	0.088	0.103	0.114	0.132	0.145	—	—
16.0	0.080	0.090	0.106	0.117	0.135	0.148	—	—
16.5	0.082	0.092	0.108	0.120	0.138	0.152	—	—
17.0	0.084	0.095	0.111	0.123	0.142	—	—	—
17.5	0.086	0.096	0.113	0.125	0.145	—	—	—
18.0	0.088	0.099	0.116	0.128	0.148	—	—	—
18.5	0.090	0.101	0.118	0.131	0.151	—	—	—
19.0	0.092	0.103	0.121	0.134	0.154	—	—	—
19.5	0.093	0.105	0.123	0.136	0.157	—	—	—
20.0	0.095	0.107	0.125	0.139	0.160	—	—	—
20.5	0.097	0.109	0.128	0.141	—	—	—	—
21.0	0.099	0.111	0.130	0.144	—	—	—	—
21.5	0.100	0.112	0.132	0.146	—	—	—	—
22.0	0.102	0.114	0.134	0.149	—	—	—	—
22.5	0.104	0.116	0.136	0.151	—	—	—	—
23.0	0.105	0.118	0.139	0.153	—	—	—	—
23.5	0.107	0.120	0.141	0.156	—	—	—	—
24.0	0.109	0.122	0.143	0.158	—	—	—	—
24.5	0.110	0.123	0.145	0.160	—	—	—	—
25.0	0.112	0.125	0.147	—	—	—	—	—
25.5	0.113	0.127	0.149	—	—	—	—	—
26.0	0.115	0.129	0.151	—	—	—	—	—
26.5	0.116	0.130	0.153	—	—	—	—	—
27.0	0.118	0.132	0.155	—	—	—	—	—
27.5	0.119	0.134	0.157	—	—	—	—	—
28.0	0.121	0.135	0.159	—	—	—	—	—
28.5	0.122	0.137	0.161	—	—	—	—	—
29.0	0.124	0.139	—	—	—	—	—	—
29.5	0.125	0.140	—	—	—	—	—	—
30.0	0.126	0.142	—	—	—	—	—	—
31.5	0.130	0.146	—	—	—	—	—	—
32.0	0.132	0.148	—	—	—	—	—	—

Plate setting in millimeters.

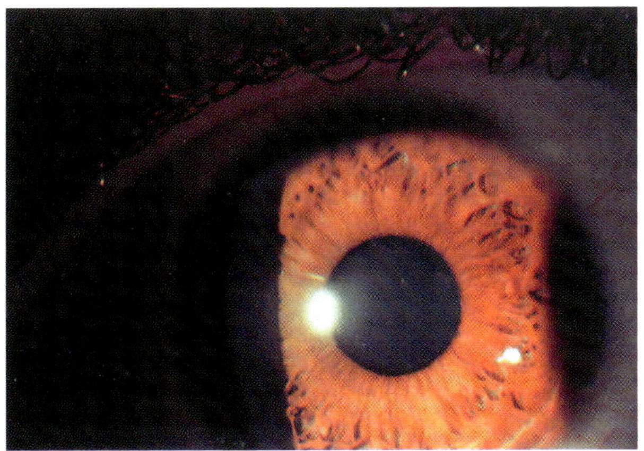

Fig. 10.106 Appearance of hyperopic lamellar keratotomy eye 6 months postsurgery.

can range from 0.05 to 0.15 mm (50 to 150 μm) in thickness and 3.5 to 5.0 mm in diameter.

Epikeratophakia (EKP)

It seems a good idea that if KM works, why not suture the lenticule to the surface of the eye—producing thereby a "living" contact lens (Figure 10.109)? Why not indeed? Building on a concept first described by Ruiz, Werblin began experimenting with the concept of corneal tissue appliqués to correct ametropia [17–31]. This work was later expanded and refined by McDonald [32]. The concept of attaching prelathed human tissue, which could be ordered up like a contact lens, to an eye to correct both near- and farsightedness was and is appealing [33,34] (Figure 10.110). In a carefully constructed prospective study that underwent three to four changes in protocol during its life, considerable useful data emerged.

Table 10.6 Side effects experienced by hyperopic lamellar keratotomy Group 1

Side effect	*n*
Glare	0
Photophobia	0
Cells and flare	0
Delayed epithelialization	0

Table 10.7 Complications experienced by hyperopic lamellar keratotomy Group 1

Complication	*n*
Thin section	1
Thick section	1
Induced astigmatism	4
Irregular	0
Epithelial ingrowth	0
Overcorrection >1 D	4
Undercorrection >1 D	6

The technique found its first application in treating aphakia. While successful, considerable discrepancy between predicted and actual final refractive error was found. Epithelialization was prolonged and in some cases resulted in failure of the lenticule. While first described as reversible, in its original form the surgery resulted in both permanent corneal curvature changes and scarring. The results in myopic cases were worse and in some cases produced as much as ±17 D of variation from that predicted. This was reduced somewhat by a redesign of both the lenticule and the incision. However, the results so far do not justify its application in myopes of any degree with the possible exception of those with keratoconus.

(a)

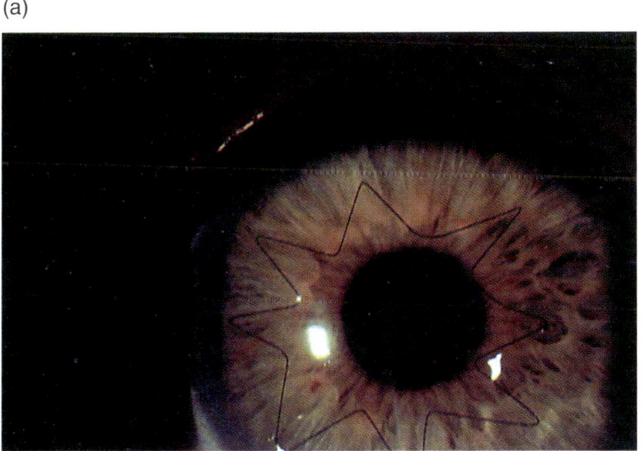

(b)

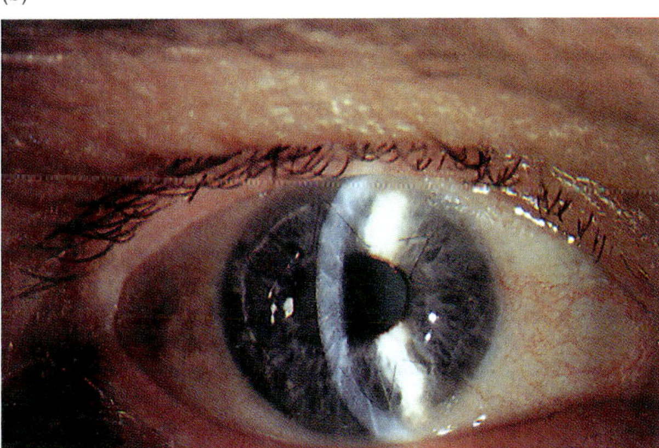

Fig. 10.107 Hyperopic lamellar keratotomy in overcorrected radial keratotomy. (a) 36 hours postsurgery in a four-incision case; (b) 7 days postsurgery. Note the smoothness of the surface.

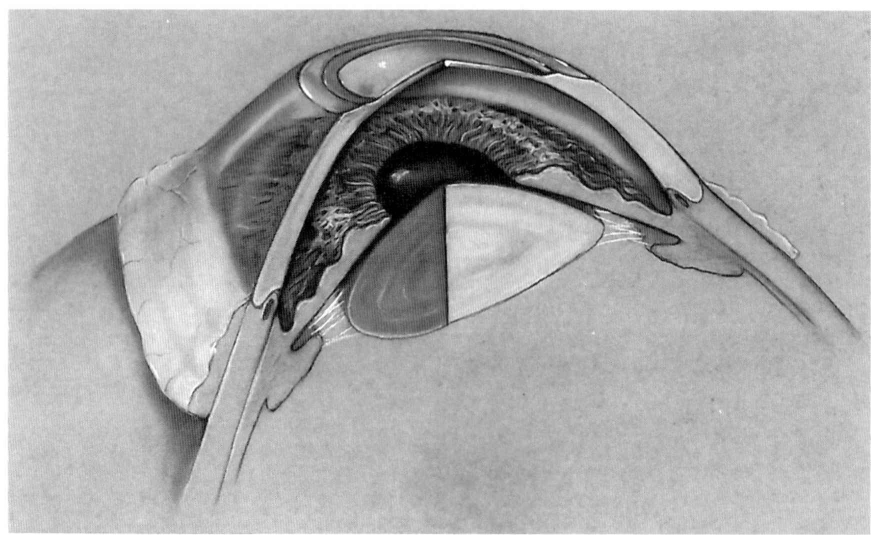

Fig. 10.108 Keratomileusis *in-situ*. Note that two keratectomies are required.

Table 10.8 Details of keratomileusis *in-situ* Group 1 cases

Parameter	Values
Age	18–47 years
Range	−6.50 to −22.00 D
Total eyes	37

Table 10.9 Side effects experienced by keratomileusis *in-situ* Group 1

Side effect	*n*
Glare	0
Photophobia	0
Cells and flare	0
Delayed epithelialization	0

Table 10.10 Complications experienced by keratomileusis *in-situ* Group 1

Complication	*n*
Induced astigmatism >0.5 D	3
Irregular	2
Epithelialization	0
Undercorrection >1 D	29
Overcorrection >1 D	3

Table 10.11 Details of hyperopic lamellar keratotomy Group 2 cases

Parameter	Values
Age	20–47 years
Range	+2.00 to +7.00 D
Total eyes	17
Iatrogenic	3
Natural	14

Table 10.12 Side effects experienced by hyperopic lamellar keratotomy Group 2

Side effect	*n*
Glare	0
Photophobia	0
Cells and flare	0
Delayed epithelialization	0

Table 10.13 Complications experienced by hyperopic lamellar keratotomy Group 2

Complication	*n*
Induced astigmatism >0.5 D	4
Irregular	0
Epithelial ingrowth	1
Overcorrection >1 D	1
Undercorrection >1 D	6

Table 10.14 Details of keratomileusis *in-situ* Group 2 cases

Parameter	Values
Age	18–47 years
Range	−6.50 to −26.00 D
Total eyes	22

Table 10.15 Side effects experienced by keratomileusis *in-situ* Group 2

Side effect	*n*
Glare	0
Photophobia	0
Cells and flare	0
Delayed epithelialization	0

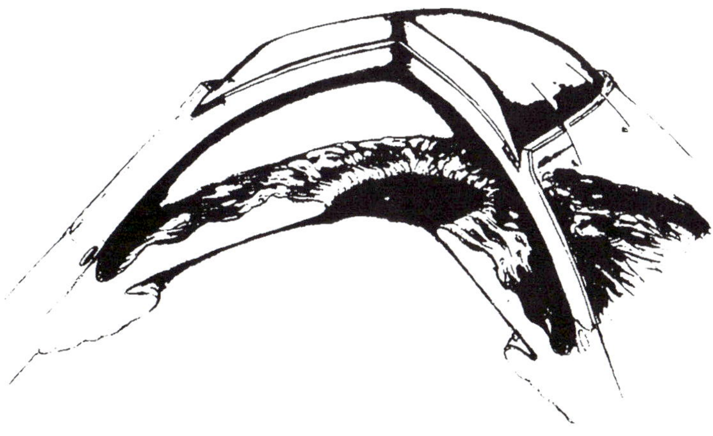

Fig. 10.109 Old-style epikeratophakia using an annular keratectomy and undermining. Note the wide gap required to be crossed by the epithelium.

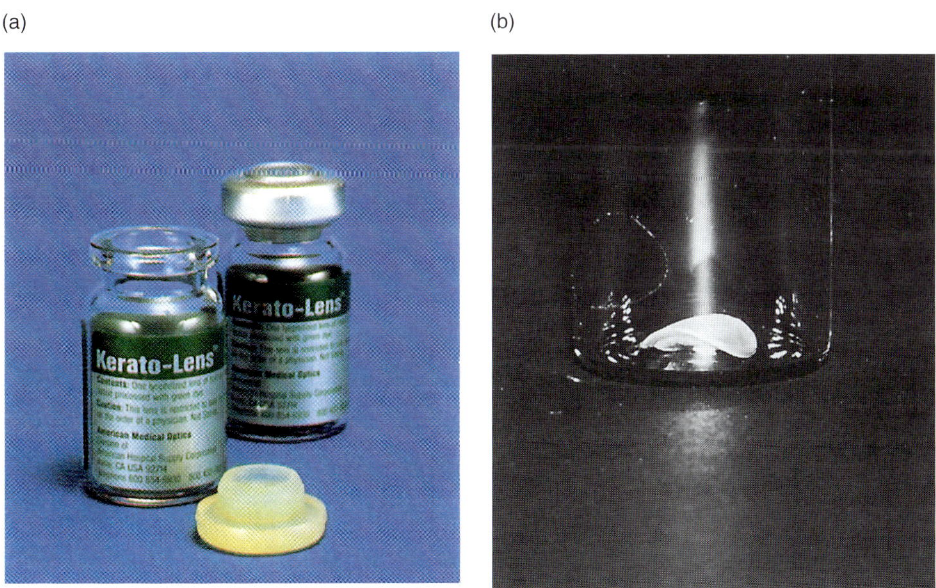

Fig. 10.110 (a,b) Kerato-Lens—lyophilized epilenticule (or "potato chip") as supplied by Alcon.

Early technique and results

The original methodology for EKP was to mark and cut a circle approximately 8.0 mm in diameter through Bowman's layer and partially into the corneal stroma after first removing the epithelium in the center (Figure 10.111a, b). A wedge-shaped tissue annulus was then resected with scissors. The outer edge of the resection bed was then undermined to provide a pocket for the epigraft's "wing." The lenticule was then tucked into the annular resection, whereupon it was sutured in place with 16 interrupted 10-0 nylon sutures so placed as to draw the wing into the prepared pocket (Figure 10.111c, d).

Needless to say, the outcome of the surgery was subject to many variables, not the least of which was the inevitable variable tension applied to the epilenticule by the interrupted sutures. It was found that considerable difference in the ultimate correction depended on the degree of suture tension applied—especially in myopic lenticules [35]. Then, too, postoperative astigmatism was hard to control not only because of the sutures but also because of the irregularity in the hand-cut annular resection. The original technique was then changed to marking and cutting two concentric circles approximately 7.5 and 8.0 mm in diameter, respectively, through Bowman's layer. A wedge-shaped tissue annulus was then resected with scissors between the trephinations. This resulted in a more even annulus but missed the point that a resection of tissue was occurring (Figure 10.112).

Epithelialization was delayed in most cases, sometimes as long as a week or more, for a number of reasons. One of these was the necessity of the new cells to "jump the gap" created by the resected annulus. The problem was more prevalent in aphakic lenticules probably because of their increased thickness. This delay sometimes would precipitate a reaction leading to loss of the lenticule,

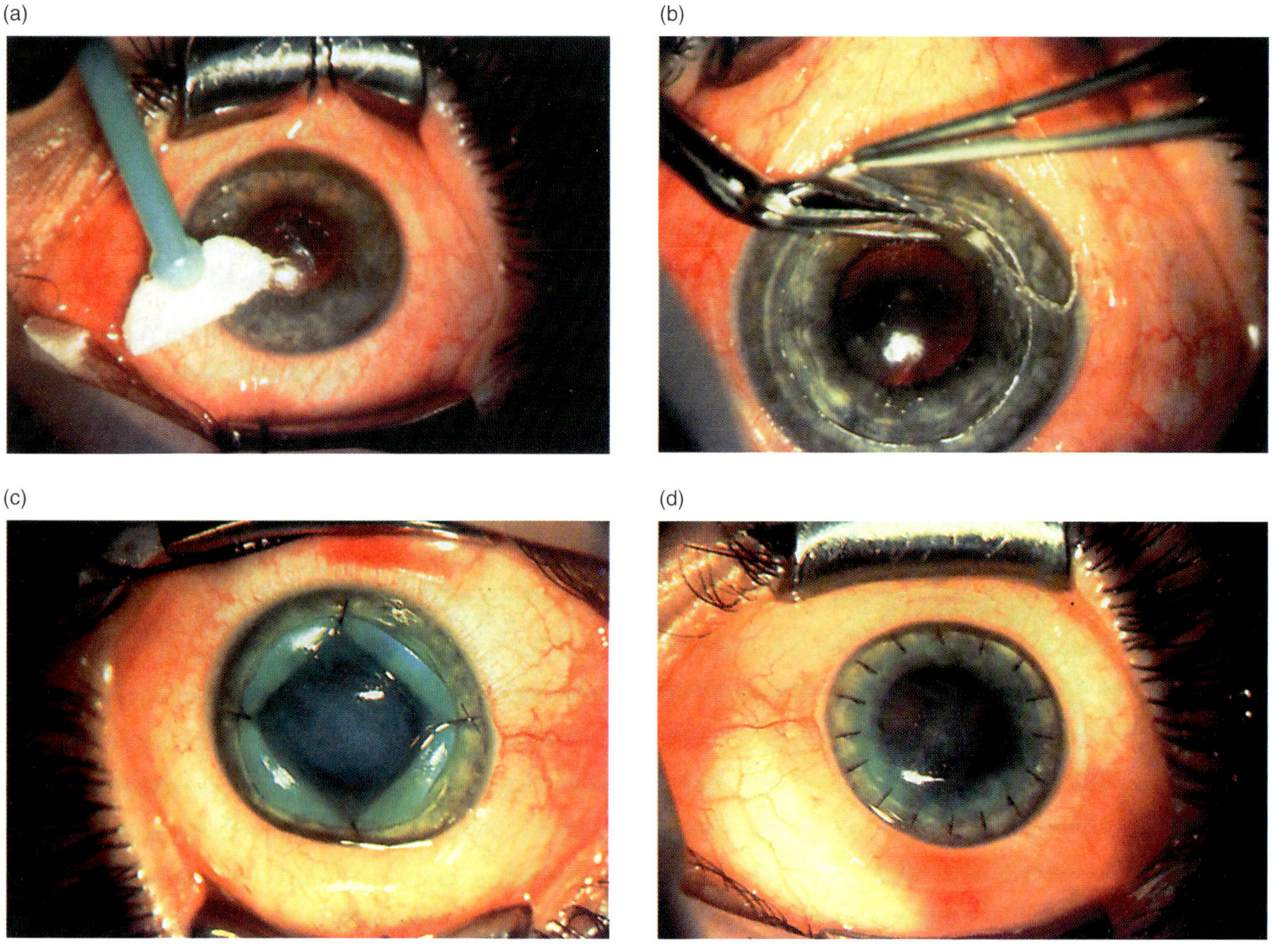

(a) (b) (c) (d)

Fig. 10.111 (a) The epithelium is removed from the surface using a truncated Weck-Cel moistened with 10% cocaine (not alcohol). (b) Shallow trephination is followed by a scissors keratectomy. (c) The reconstituted epilenticule is secured by four cardinal sutures pulling the wing into the undermined cornea incision. (d) Sixteen interrupted sutures are used.

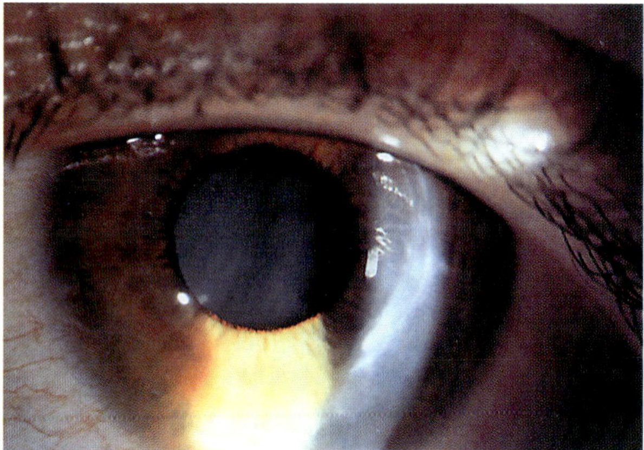

Fig. 10.112 Postoperative old-style epikeratophakia. Note the wide scar associated with the annular keratectomy.

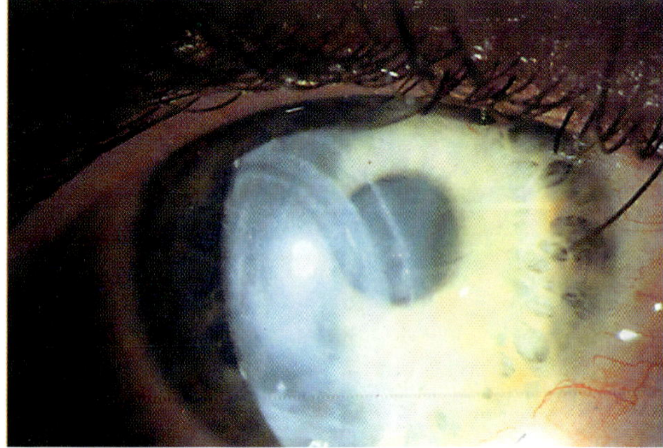

Fig. 10.113 Delayed re-epithelialization is often responsible for lenticular failure in these cases.

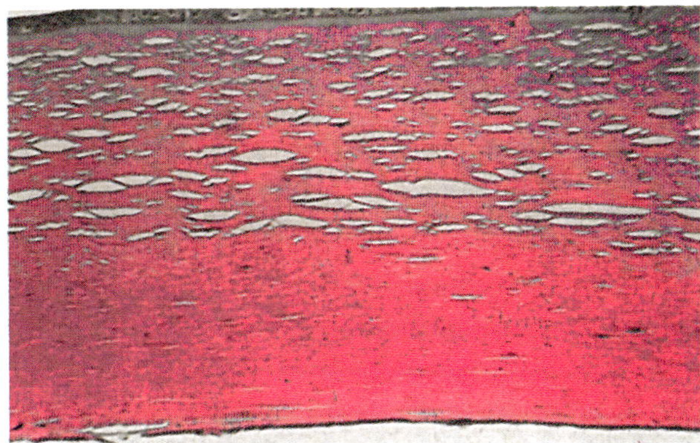

Fig. 10.114 Light microscopic appearance of an epilenticule applied 10 years before.

necessitating repeating or abandoning the procedure [36] (Figure 10.113). Nonetheless, once established, these lenticules are well tolerated by the eye (Figure 10.114).

Wet epikeratophakia

By using freshly frozen and lathed tissue (so-called wet EKP) and a slanted, circular corneal incision, coupled with the Barraquer antitorque suture, the author has accomplished good results with this technique in cases of keratoconus (Figures 10.115 and 10.116). It is not possible, using current methods, to predict the actual postoperative refractive error in these cases, but most result in improvement of both unaided and aided visual acuity, coupled with a strengthening of the central cornea. Sufficient time has not elapsed with these cases to determine long-term corneal stability, but results so far are promising (see below). Re-epithelialization is much more rapid with the new technique, as is visual recovery.

Another area that has shown encouraging results with EKP is in pediatric aphakia [37–39]. Here, the outcome has been universally good and probably will continue to remain so. It is a reasonable alternative to implantation of an intraocular lens in these cases. While good results have been reported in low hyperopia, other techniques, less traumatic and more predictable, have come on the scene [40]. Still, it has been used in RK overcorrections with good results and could be a solution to high irregular astigmatism after RK (Figures 10.117 through 10.119).

This procedure has been touted as reversible. Experience, however, has shown that while the procedure is

(a)

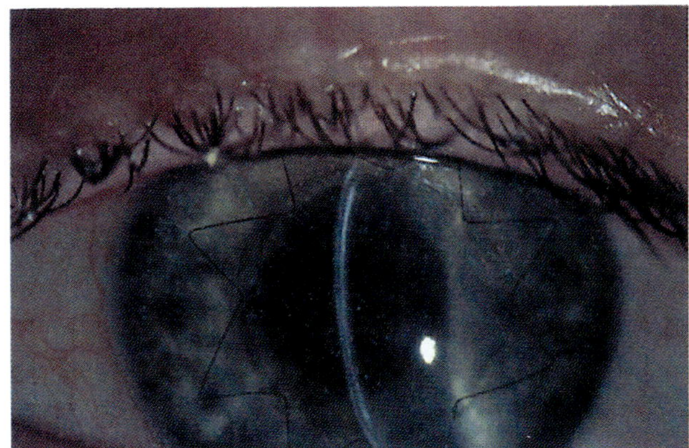

(b)

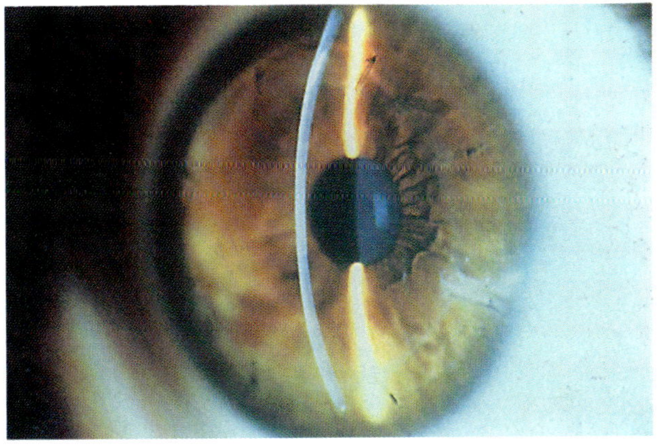

Fig. 10.116 (a) A wet-epi, 2 weeks postsurgery. (b) Myopic epi using the wet technique. Note the almost invisible keratectomy scar. Compare with Figure 10.112.

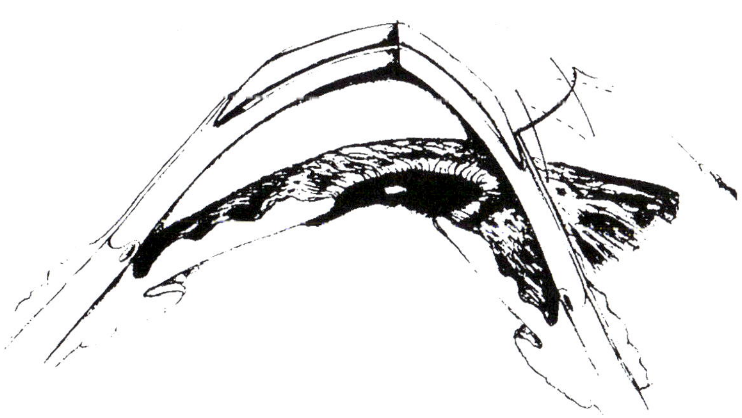

Fig. 10.115 The so-called wet-epi. Note the relatively smooth transition and small gap for the epithelium to bridge.

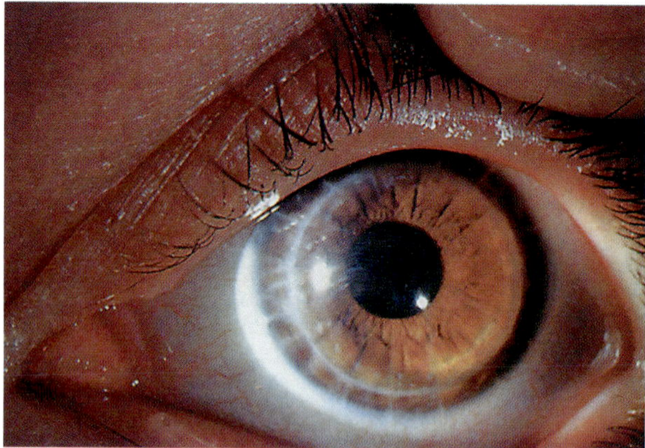

Fig. 10.117 Epilenticule over a radial keratotomy done for keratoconus 6 years before—1 year postepi.

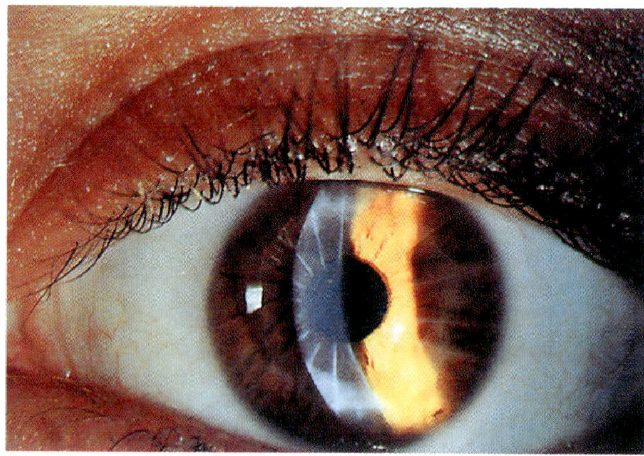

Fig. 10.118 An overcorrected radial keratotomy eye that underwent a lyophilized epi which subsequently failed. The postepi corneal curvature *steepened* in this case—the usual reaction is to flatten.

certainly "redoable"—that is, a lenticule can be removed and replaced—the term *reversible* does not apply. In the author's experience, once Bowman's layer has been severed in this way, permanent changes occur in the central corneal curvature—curiously enough often in the direction of flattening (see Figure 10.118). This effect has been shown experimentally by Gilbert, who made shallow trephinations of eye bank eyes [41]. This is an interesting finding in view of the results obtained by Gills with deep circular-radial incisions and the effect of the hexagonal configuration [42].

Keratophakia—Homoplastic and alloplastic

Keratophakia arose from a need not being adequately met at the time of its inception and predates keratomileusis for myopia. The condition of aphakia, while restoring sight, in many ways left the patient in worse condition than before the surgery. One can only speculate

(a)

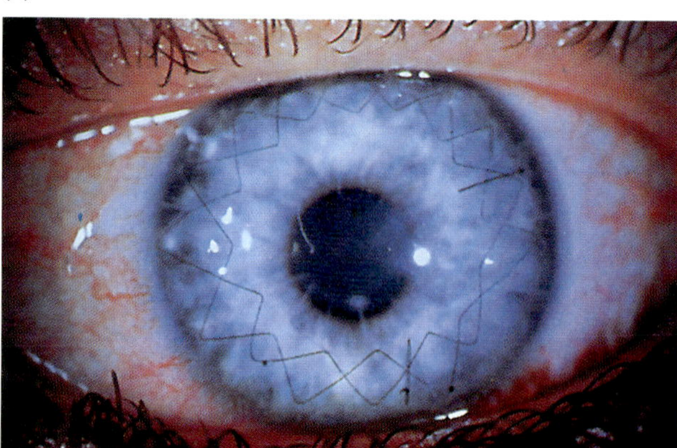

(b)

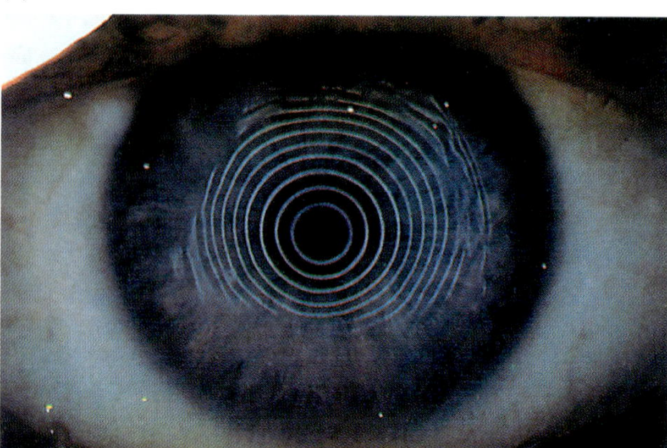

Fig. 10.119 (a) An epilenticule applied to a radial keratotomy overcorrection—1 month postepi. (b) Note the smooth circular photokeratoscopy mires. (Courtesy of S. Slade.)

on the number of hip fractures resulting from the wearing of aphakic spectacles. Casey Wood's classic paper documenting his own experience with aphakia aptly describes the day-to-day existence of a person with that condition; it should be required reading for all cataract surgeons. The procedure is designed for high hyperopia usually associated with cataract surgery. With the advent of intraocular lens implants, the need for this type of procedure has declined. However, it is still indicated in those patients in whom introduction of the intraocular lens is contraindicated—such as severe diabetics. These contraindications—never absolute—are diminishing in number and variety, however.

Homoplastic keratophakia

In this surgery, thick sections of fresh or preserved donor corneal tissue are used (Figure 10.120). Furthermore, tissue not suitable for use as transplant material can be employed, including that which has been cryopreserved for prolonged periods [43,44]. This is fortunate in that no drain is placed on the scanty transplant tissue supply. Fresh tis-

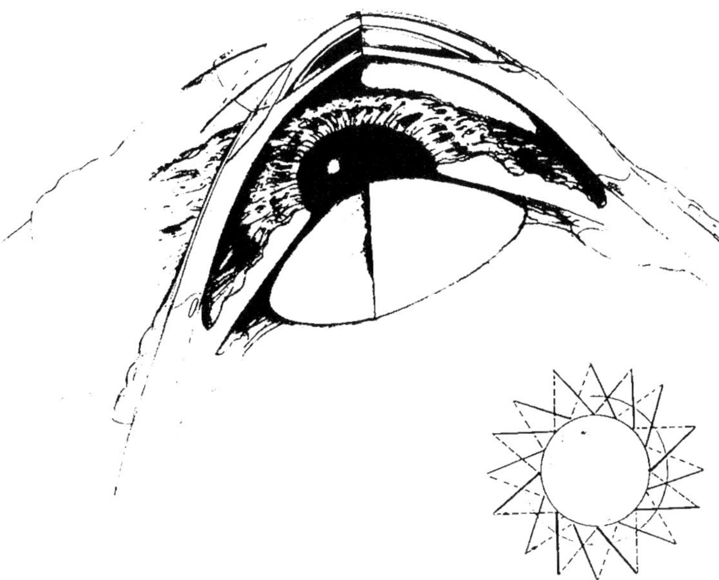

Fig. 10.120 The principle of keratophakia.

sue needs to be desiccated a little before lathing; usually a blow dryer or a stream of anhydrous nitrogen is used.

Planned cases should have small-incision cataract extraction before the keratophakia procedure. Aphakic cases should have had an uneventful healing period of at least 6 months or more. The suction ring drives the intraocular pressure to at least 65 mm Hg—sufficient to rupture an incompletely healed incision. What's more, the wound site must be smooth. Either an incompletely healed or nonsmooth wound area can cause problems with maintaining suction. A break in suction during the keratectomy always results in an irregular section—both in thickness and in shape—which leads to induced astigmatism.

The lathing procedure is similar to that of KM except that the tissue is placed on the base with the *convex side out* so that Bowman's layer is removed entirely (Figure 10.121). The lathing is done in a similar manner and is accomplished before the keratectomy is performed on the patient. In keratophakia, the patient's resection is larger than in KM, and the thickness is determined by the amount of refractive error to be corrected. There is a tendency to adjust the thickness (and consequently the diameter) to make it slightly thinner in higher cases to control the overall central corneal thickness. The lenticule is placed in the bed, and the patient's tissue is placed over it. Cardinal sutures are placed in four quadrants rather than three, as in KM. A double running nontorquing suture is then placed, providing 16 areas of support (Figure 10.122). The cardinals are then removed and the eye treated as in KM.

Postoperative care is similar to that in KM except that the sutures are allowed to remain for a longer period of time. Recovery of vision is quite slow, and a number of patients will never achieve the same level of corrected vision as preoperatively. Nonetheless, the technique is a valuable procedure in indicated cases. Theoretically, there is no upper limit to the amount of hyperopia that one can correct. However, the considerations of corneal physiology and anatomy set an upper limit of 22 D with this surgery.

Allopathic keratophakia

It is probably incorrect to group allopathic corneal stromal implants with homoplastic implants (keratophakia); allopathics should perhaps be called *intracorneal lenses*

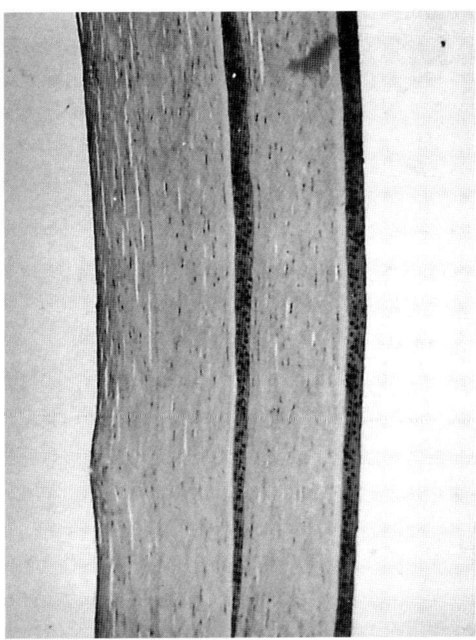

Fig. 10.121 An incorrectly lathed keratophakia lenticule. Note the presence of intact Bowman's and regrowth of epithelium. Note also the viable keratocytes within the lenticule.

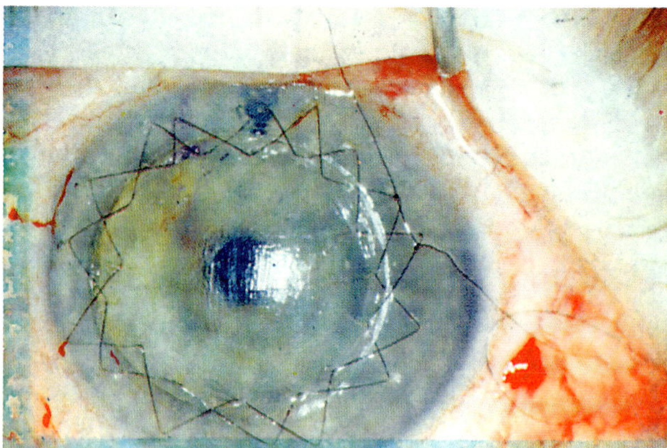

Fig. 10.122 Keratophakia.

(ICL). However, the principles are the same, even though the materials may differ. Barraquer's original work involved the correction of aphakia by the method of stromal implants. During the course of many years, he tried many different materials, finding that human corneal tissue produced the best results [4,45–49]. The objection to the use of other materials was the same, with few variations—namely, that they all interfered with corneal nutrition of either the anterior or posterior stroma or both (Figure 10.123). The course of trial also was the same: Implantation was best done at the junction of the outer and middle thirds, and eventually, all materials (except human and later hydrogel) needed to be fenestrated to improve corneal physiology—all eventually failed [50] (Figure 10.124). The problem with nonpermeable intrastromal implants is that they must live in harmony with a complex environment (Figure 10.125).

Choyce has experimented with allopathic corneal inlays for years [51–55]. He has reported trials with a material known as polysulfone [56]. This original work was expanded by Kirkness, Lane, and others [57–62]. Original results, as in the past, have been reported as favorable.

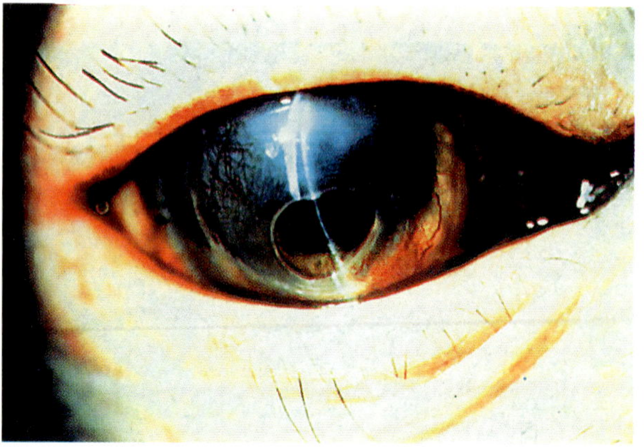

Fig. 10.123 Anterior stromal melting over a nonpermeable intracorneal lens. (Courtesy of B. McCarey.)

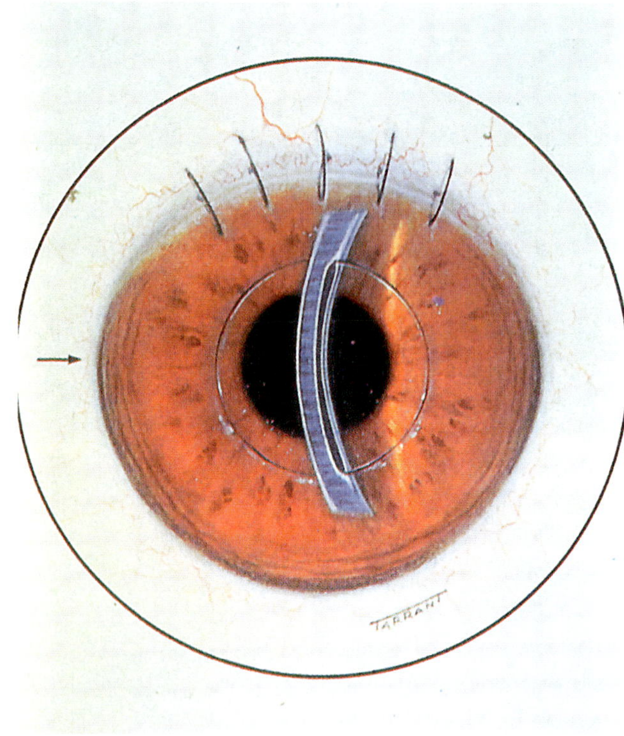

Fig. 10.124 Incorrect position for an intracorneal lens; it should be more anterior than this drawing shows. (Courtesy of R. Lindstorm.)

Significantly, the lenticules, which began as solid, have become fenestrated in the latest versions (Figure 10.126).

Werblin reported greater success with the implantation of hydrogel materials within the corneal stroma of animals, including nonhuman primates [63–70]. This study was expanded to include human aphakes, and the results in the first small group, while promising, failed in the end, and the sponsor abandoned the project (Figure 10.127). The technique, except for the lathing, is the same for alloplastic as for homoplastic keratophakia; the most difficult part is still the keratectomy (Figure 10.128).

Very little intolerance has been shown by the corneal stroma to the hydrophilic material in most cases. An unusual reaction to the material has occurred in the monkey model (Figure 10.129). This exact reaction has not been seen in the human subjects. However, two human cases have shown small granular precipitates that lie on the ICL and accumulate at its edge (Figure 10.130). In the author's case, these precipitates contributed to poor postoperative vision and the decision to remove the implant. Van Rij reported a bilateral case with poor visual acuity in one eye after a year who responded with improved vision to explantation of the ICL and implantation of a Worst Claw lens [71] (Figure 10.131). Time alone will tell whether this or any allopathic material can be implanted safely.

Having an impact on this procedure is the diminishing need for this type of surgery due to improvement in both intraocular lens (IOL) technology and implantation techniques. The hydrogel study has been suspended

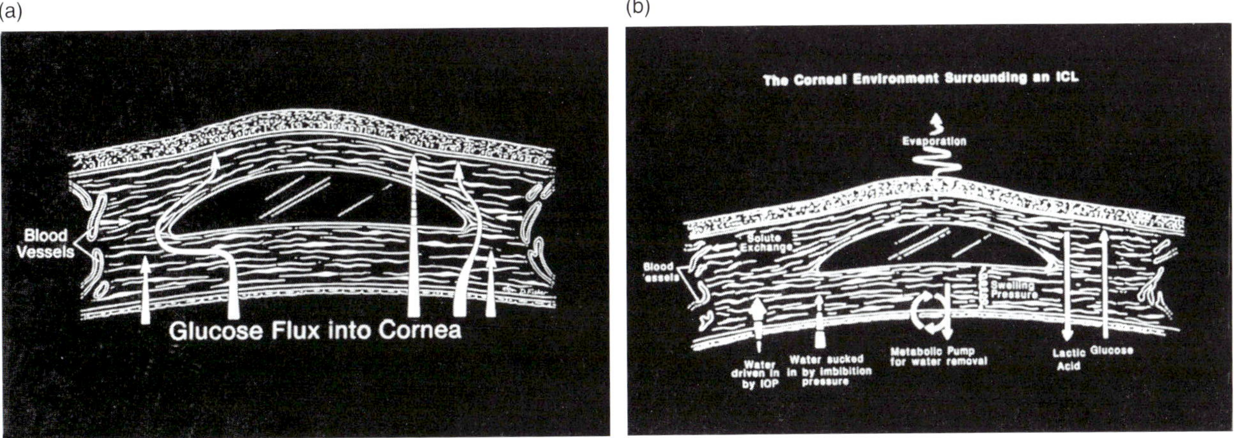

Fig. 10.125 (a) Glucose movement within the cornea; (b) the corneal environment surrounding an intracorneal lens. (Courtesy of B. McCarey.)

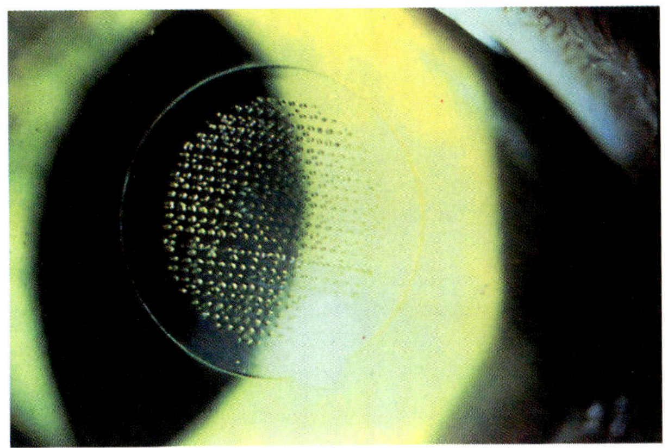

Fig. 10.126 Implanted fenestrated polysulfone intracorneal lens. (Courtesy of R. Lindstrom.)

not because of complications but for want of indications. Whether additional work in this area will continue is moot. The costs of such research continue to increase every year. Federal restrictions have only added to the bill. This fact, coupled with the shortsighted and litigious attitude of many Americans, stimulated by rabid consumerism and "technoterrorism," has encouraged manufacturers to do the initial and clinical trials out of the country—if they do them at all.

Intracorneal ring segments (Intacs)

Contributed by Daniel S. Durrie, M.D. and Trent L. Vande Garde, M.D.

Note by Dr. Bores: *Of all the alloplastic implantation techniques used in attempting to modify the corneal surface shape, the system described here is providing the most successful outcomes of them all. Not the least of its advantages is that the central visual axis is not compromised.*

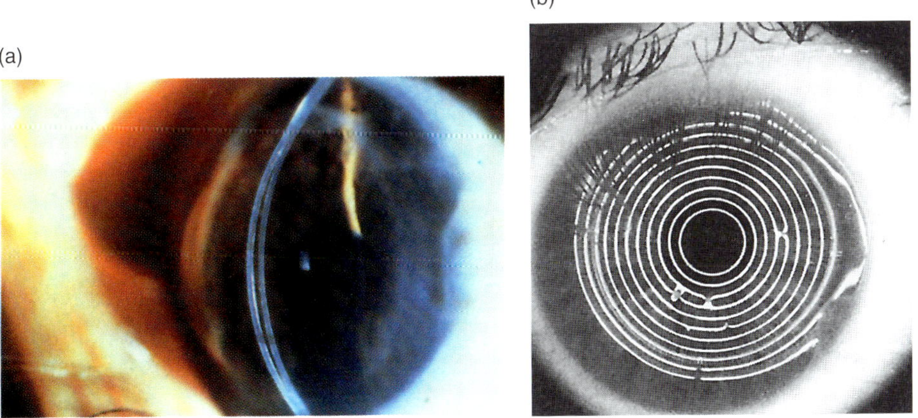

Fig. 10.127 (a) Implanted hydrogel intracorneal lens at 2 months. (b) As this photokeratoscopy shows, the corneas are usually smooth.

(a)

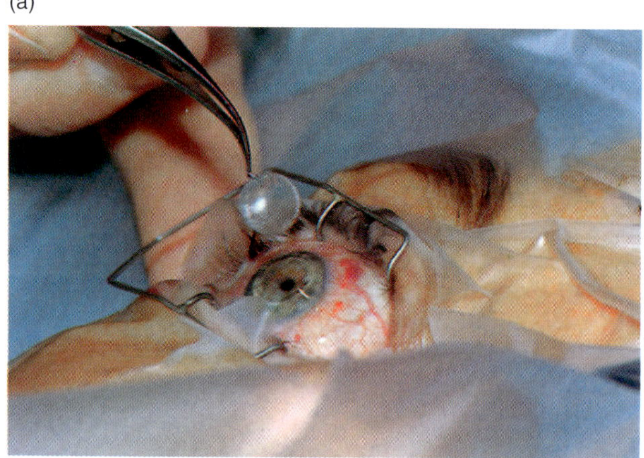

(b)

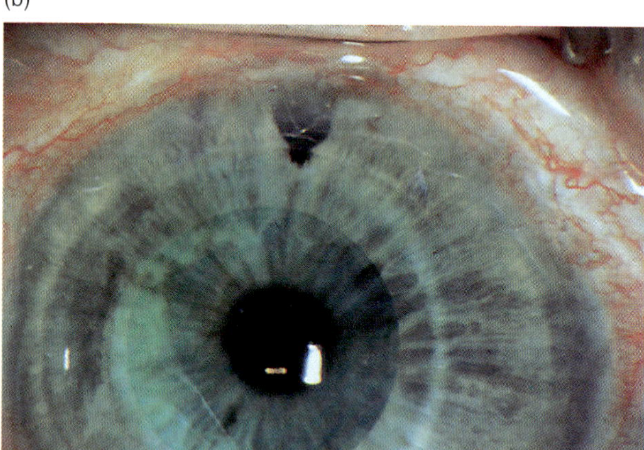

(c)

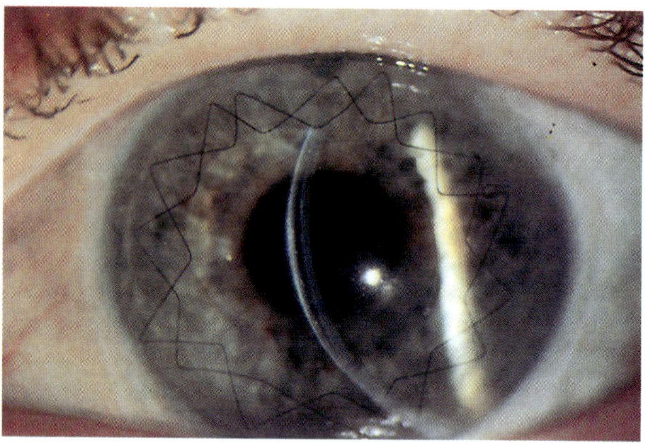

Fig. 10.128 (a) The corneal cap should be at least 8.0 mm in diameter. (b) The hydrogel intracorneal lens has been dyed with kitton green for improved visibility. (c) The usual double-running suture is used to secure the lenticule.

(a)

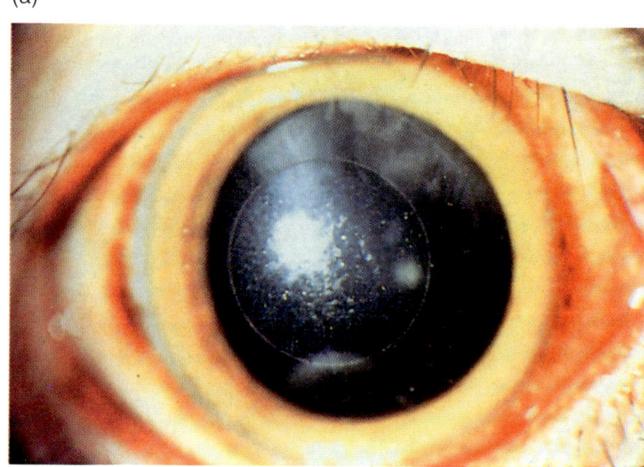

(b)

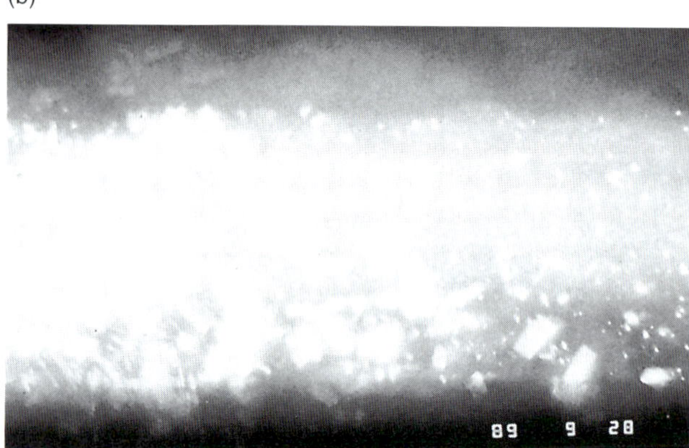

Fig. 10.129 (a,b) An unusual crystalline keratopathy occurring in a monkey with a hydrogel intracorneal lens. (Courtesy of B. McCarey.)

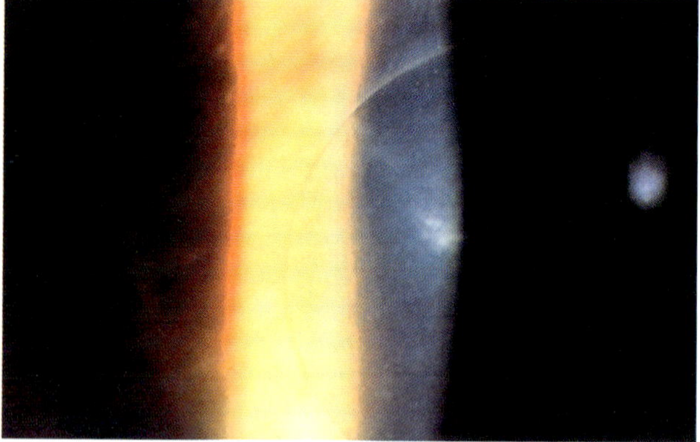

Fig. 10.130 Peculiar granulated material at the interface and edge of a hydrogel intracorneal lens. (Courtesy of F. Price.)

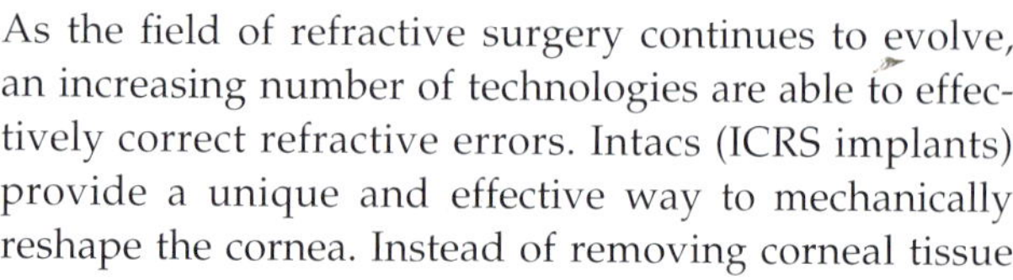

As the field of refractive surgery continues to evolve, an increasing number of technologies are able to effectively correct refractive errors. Intacs (ICRS implants) provide a unique and effective way to mechanically reshape the cornea. Instead of removing corneal tissue from the central optical zone, as is done with excimer laser procedures, placing Intacs is an additive procedure that involves the peripheral cornea. Approval of this procedure by the Food and Drug Administration in April 1999 has given refractive surgeons another option in pro-

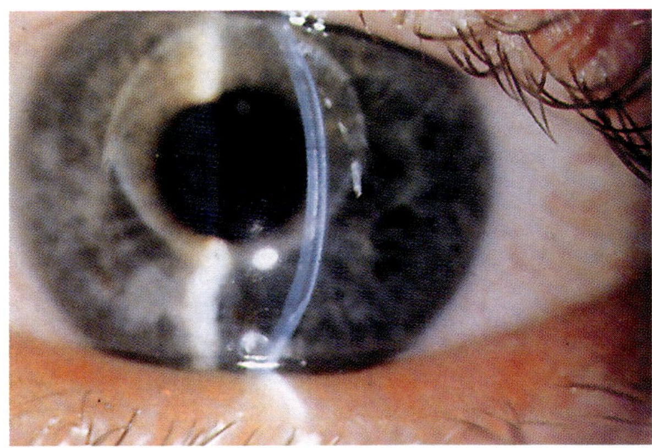

Fig. 10.131 Hydrogel-implanted eye with poor visual acuity at 1 year. (Courtesy of van Rij.)

viding high-quality refractive surgery to their patients with low levels of myopia.

Description

The Intacs corneal implant device consists of two clear, thin polymethyl methacrylate (PMMA) segments, each having an arc length of 150°. Each segment has a single positioning hole at the superior end to aid in surgical manipulation (Figure 10.132). These segments are inserted into the midperipheral corneal stroma, which spares the central cornea and thus the central optical zone. Intacs act as passive spacing elements that shorten the arc length of the anterior corneal curvature and therefore flatten the central cornea. The amount of visual correction achieved relates to the thickness of the insert, with the thicker segments providing greater amounts of correction.

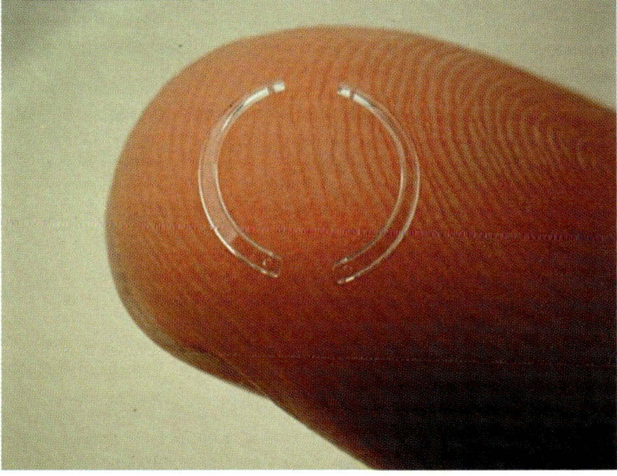

Fig. 10.132 The ICRS implants. These segments are inserted into the midperipheral corneal stroma, which spares the central cornea and thus the central OZ.

Indications

Intacs are currently used for the treatment of myopia from −1.00 to −3.00 D. It is also important to note that they are only used in patients with 1.00 D or less of astigmatism. They are available in 0.25- , 0.30- , and 0.35-mm thicknesses, which give average corrections of −1.30, −2.00, and −2.70 D, respectively. We generally recommend having an upper limit of −2.75 D attempted correction because there currently is not a thicker ring segment to place if a patient with −3.00 D of myopia is undercorrected with the 0.35-mm device. Clinical trials involving Intacs with a wider range of segment thicknesses eventually should increase the treatable range of myopia from −0.75 to 4.50 D.

Intacs are approved for patients who are 21 years of age or older and have a stable refraction. They are not to be placed in patients with known collagen-vascular, autoimmune, or immunodeficiency diseases. Other contraindications include pregnant or nursing women, as well as those with ocular conditions such as keratoconus, recurrent corneal erosions, or corneal dystrophies.

Surgical procedure

The Intacs procedure is performed on an outpatient basis and uses topical anesthesia. The surgery is done in a standard operating room to avoid fibers and particles that can be found in carpeted rooms. Most patients do not require any sedation, and we use 5 mg diazepam (Valium) only if the patient specifically requests it. One drop of 0.5% Tetracaine is placed just prior to entering the operating room.

Once the patient is in the operating room, the eye is prepped with Betadine swabs and draped. A wire lid speculum is placed, and another drop of 0.5% Tetracaine is given after placing a ring sponge on the limbus. The geometric center of the cornea is marked, and then this spot is indented using the end of a Sinskey hook. The incision and placement marker (IPM) is prepared with rose Bengal and used to mark the corneal surface, centering around the geometric center indentation. Rose Bengal is used because it is less toxic to the epithelium. Ultrasonic pachymetry is used to determine corneal thickness at the incision mark, and then a diamond knife is calibrated to 68% of the pachymetry reading. The diamond knife is used to make a 1.8-mm radial incision at the incision mark, which is at the 12 o'clock position. While holding the edge of the incision with 0.12 forceps, a Sinskey hook is used to begin forming stromal pockets on both sides at the base of the incision. It is very important that these pockets are started at the base of the incision so that the channels will be at the desired two-thirds depth of the cornea. This important step prevents the possibility of a shallow implant depth. A stromal spreader is used to further extend the stromal pockets in both directions using a swimming-type motion.

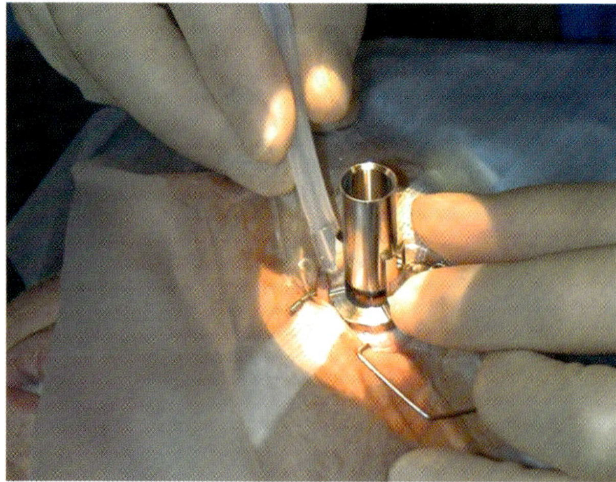

Fig. 10.133 The vacuum centering guide (VCG) and dissector. The dissector is placed in the pocket; the glide (which has acted as a shoehorn) is removed, and the dissector is rotated about 180° until the first stromal channel is made. The same sequence is performed on the second side.

Next, the vacuum centering guide (VCG) is placed, centering around the geometric center mark. The suction is initiated to increase globe rigidity, and a glide acts as a shoehorn to guide the dissector into the pocket. Once the dissector (Figure 10.133) is placed in the pocket, the glide is removed, and the dissector is rotated about 180° until the stromal channel is made. The same sequence is performed on the second side, and then the dissector and VCG are removed. Care should be taken to limit the continuous VCG time to 2 minutes or less. The incision is irrigated, and the Intacs segments are fed into each of the lamellar channels with the positioning holes of the segments adjacent to the incision. It is important to avoid contact of the Intacs segments with the Betadine and the epithelial surface. Once the segments are in proper position, an 11-0 nylon suture is placed to close the initial incision site. This suture should have enough tension to keep the wound edges apposed but should not be overtightened because this can induce astigmatism. It has been found that patients have quicker visual recovery and less visual fluctuation if a suture is placed.

Postoperative care

Immediately after the surgical procedure, Ocuflox is placed in the operative eye. If the epithelium has been disrupted extensively, a bandage contact lens may be applied. A drop of Tobradex is then given before putting a shield over the eye, and the shield is kept in place overnight. The patient should continue to wear the shield at night for 1 week to prevent rubbing the eye, which can induce migration of the Intacs segments within the lamellar channels.

On the first postoperative day, the patient begins a regimen of Ocuflox and Pred Forte, both four times a day for the first week. Patients should be advised that they may experience visual fluctuations, dryness, and halos at night for the first month. There may be an epithelial defect at the incision site on the first postoperative day that only needs a bandage contact lens if it is outside the incision site or the patient has significant discomfort. If there is a large epithelial defect, then the patient is often seen on postoperative day 3 to ensure proper healing and removal of the bandage contact lens. Otherwise, the patient's next visit is 1 week postoperatively.

By the end of the first week, all epithelial defects should be healed, and any residual foreign-body sensation should be resolved. Occasionally, a filament will develop at the incision site causing foreign-body sensation or pain. This can be managed by hypertonic saline drops, debridement, or a bandage contact lens. The patient's uncorrected vision is usually 20/40 or better, and the patient also should be refracted at this visit mostly to check for any suture-induced with-the-rule astigmatism. If there is astigmatism of greater than 1.00 D and the suture appears tight, then the suture should be removed. Occasionally, permanent astigmatism can be induced if this suture remains in place. If there is less than 1.00 D of astigmatism, then the suture is not removed until the 1-month visit. Other reasons for early suture removal are pannus formation and a loose suture. If there are no remaining epithelial defects, the Ocuflox is discontinued, and the Pred Forte is tapered over the next 3 weeks.

The 1-month visit is when the incision suture usually is removed. The visual fluctuations should be decreasing by this point, and the patient should be off of the Pred Forte drops. The vision is usually significantly better at the 1-month visit, and the patient should be encouraged that it will likely continue to improve.

The next scheduled visit is 3 months postoperatively, and the visual acuity often is stable by this point. Occasionally, some residual astigmatism may be present. Experience shows that this continues to resolve over time, even when relatively high degrees of cylinder are present. The 3-month visit is when there can be consideration of implant exchange or removal if the desired refractive change is not attained. Otherwise, the patient is seen at 6 months postoperatively and then routinely thereafter.

Postoperative findings

The initial incision created for the insertion of the dissector can heal in three different ways. It can heal normally, too tightly, or too loosely. The normal response is given a grade of 0, a tight response is graded +1 or +2, and a loose healing response is graded −1 or −2. While a tight incision may induce astigmatism, a loose incision generally results in undercorrection or loss of effect. A loose healing response will appear as a gape in the incision.

The incision is epithelialized, but the edges appear drawn apart and in some cases may be filled with epithelial plugs or cysts. Epithelial plugs are white or opaque in color and usually are small round or elongated opacities. Cysts, on the other hand, are clear. They too may be round or elongated. Cysts and plugs commonly will break up into sections and eventually disappear. A grade of –2 is given when the incision area has obvious gape and an undercorrection of greater than 0.75 D. A grade of –1 has less obvious gape and an undercorrection of 0.75 D or less. Neither cysts nor plugs require any treatment unless they cause incisional gape resulting in a loss of effect.

A similar grading system of –2 to +2 is given to ring-segment location for each segment (Figure 10.134). The normal location with superior ends situated approximately 2 to 3 mm apart and the inferior ends slightly closer is given a grade of 0. If the rings are in a lower position, a grade of –1 or –2 is given. Slight inferior ring-segment displacement is graded as –1, and if the ring segments are touching inferiorly, it is graded as –2. This displacement is usually asymptomatic and does not require repositioning. Slight superior displacement is +1, and significant superior movement is +2 when the segments are under the incision. Repositioning is required if there is +2 displacement because this can result in improper incision healing and localized corneal melting.

A finding common in nearly all Intacs patients is channel haze. This haze is usually seen within the first month and can be graded on a 0- to 4-point scale depending on its severity. A grade of 0 is no haze and crystal-clear lamellar channels. A grade of 1 is translucent haze or mild loss of stromal transparency. A grade of 2 is moderate loss of stromal transparency (Figure 10.135) and usually is visible along the entire ring segment length. Underlying structures are slightly obscured with diffuse illumination. Lamellar channel haze of 3 is moderate to heavy loss of transparency with visible involvement of the stroma anterior and posterior to the ring segment. Grade 4 haze is heavy loss of transparency and completely surrounds the ring segments.

Another common finding is lamellar channel deposits. These usually occur later than haze and may be further classified based on consistency or shape. Deposits are characteristically round and white or yellowish in color. These deposits are thought to be expelled from stromal keratocytes to fill in empty spaces. A similar grading system is used to describe channel deposits. Grade 0 is absent or barely detectable deposits, whereas grade 1 is deposits isolated throughout the channel. Grade 2 is more diffuse deposits with underlying structures being moderately obscured. Grade 3 is moderate channel deposits that are more confluent and underlying structures that are moderately obscured (Figure 10.136). Grade 4 deposits are fully confluent and may completely obscure iris detail. These deposits may involve the entire channel width. Channel deposits do not usually cause symptoms, although occasionally they may contribute to glare and halos in low-light conditions.

The postoperative Intacs eye, like the postoperative LASIK eye, may show exogenous debris such as fibers from sponges or other surgical equipment. Unless an inflammatory response is evident, this finding is insignificant. Channel debris also may include blood, which may occupy the channel after surgery if vascular encroachment is present in the area of the incision. This will resolve over

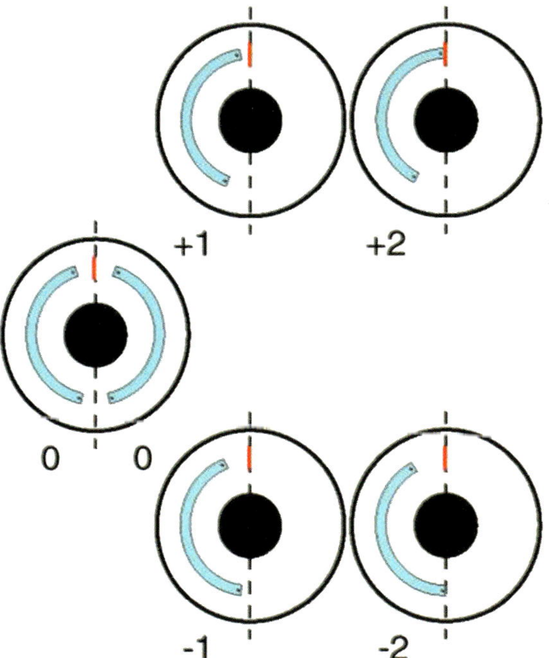

Fig. 10.134 A grading system of –2 to +2 is given to ring segment location for each segment. The normal location with superior ends located approximately 2 to 3 mm apart and the inferior ends slightly closer is given a grade of 0 (see text).

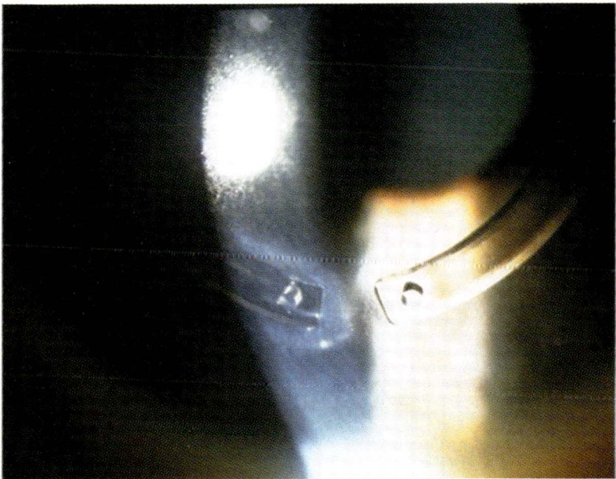

Fig. 10.135 A finding common in nearly all Intacs patients is channel haze. Grade 2 is moderate loss of stromal transparency, as shown here.

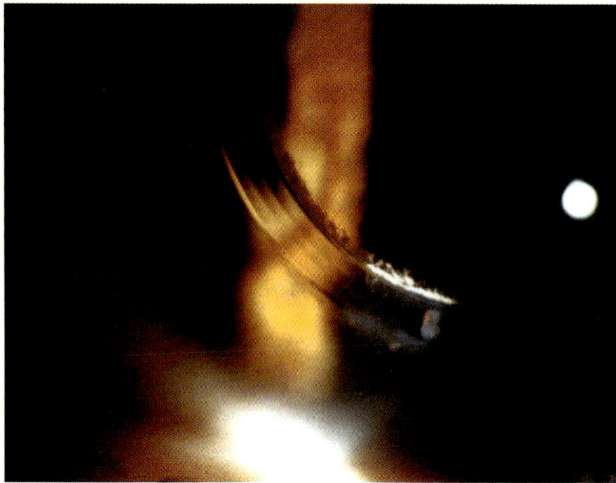

Fig. 10.136 Another common finding is lamellar channel deposits. Grade 3 is moderate channel deposits that are more confluent and underlying structures that are moderately obscured, as shown here.

1 to 6 weeks depending on the amount of blood initially present.

Complications

Most complications associated with Intacs can be prevented with good patient selection, careful surgical technique, and close follow-up. These complications can be divided into mechanical, medical, and optical categories. Most can be managed effectively and result in good visual outcomes for the patients. These aspects will be discussed in Chapter 15.

Conclusion

Classic (cryolathed) MKM

Long-term stability of the correction and vision is excellent with this technique (Figure 10.137). The author's experience with this procedure is somewhat small, not having become involved with lamellar procedures until late 1984. The results in the author's cases are summarized in the scatter plot in Figure 10.138. Of the 72 cases in the author's series with follow-up greater than 1 year, 6 (8.3%) developed astigmatism greater than 1 D postoperatively. In all but 1 of these cases the astigmatism was myopic, reflecting an undercorrection of the patient's myopia. In 2 cases the astigmatism was irregular and required that the surgery be repeated. Four of the regular and both of the irregular astigmatism cases occurred in patients who experienced epithelial ingrowth or cysts. Forty (55.6%) of the cases were undercorrected, of which 15 (20.8%) were undercorrected more than 2 D. Of these 15 cases, 7 had preoperative myopia that exceeded 17 D. In most cases, RK incisions were successful in reducing the undercorrections, except in 1 case in where very little additional flattening occurred. Twenty-five (34.7%) patients were overcorrected, of whom 10 (13.8%) were overcorrected in excess of 2 D. Most of the overcorrections in excess of 2 D received additional surgery (either HKM or HLK) to correct the error. Using Barraquer's limit of accuracy of ±2 D, 46 (63.9%) cases fell within the limit. It would appear from this experience that the greatest accuracy of the calculation formulas lies with cases between 12 and 16 D of preoperative myopia [72]. The low incidence of irregular healing, as evidenced by the small number of cases with irregular astigmatism, bears out the safety of this procedure. The side effects and complications to be expected with this procedure are discussed in Chapter 15.

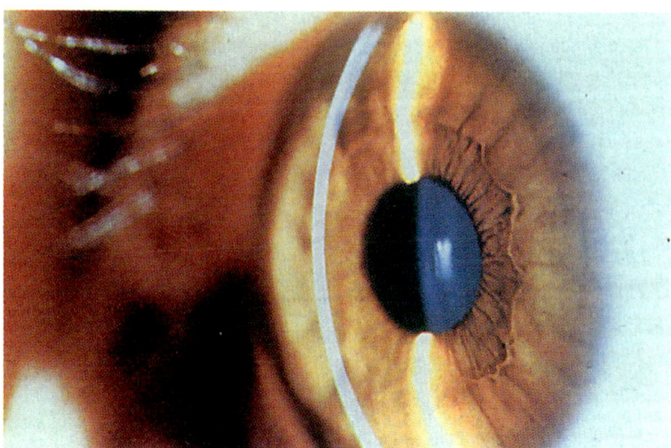

Fig. 10.137 MKM eye 18 years postsurgery.

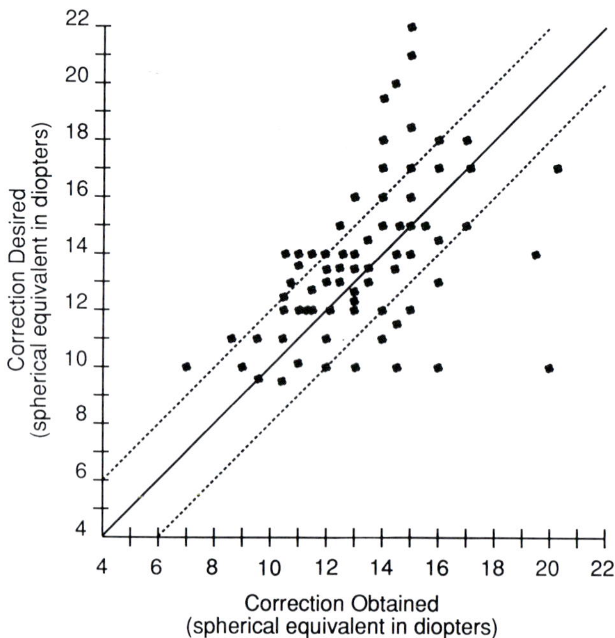

Fig. 10.138 Scattergram showing the author's results with classical MKM in 72 cases.

Epikeratophakia

The author has used the freeze-dried "potato chip" lenticules supplied by AMO and has made his own lenticules for wet epikeratophakia. Table 10.2 summarizes the author's experience with 19 cases of dry epikeratophakia. While the overall uncorrected visual acuity was improved markedly in all cases, the best-corrected vision was not. Almost 40% of the cases had some reduction in best corrected visual acuity after aphakic EKP. In only 5 cases was best-corrected vision attained in the first month; the remainder of the cases experienced prolonged visual recovery—in 1 case lasting 6 months. Two cases required removal of the lenticule—neither case elected to have the surgery repeated. Keratoconus patients fared somewhat better, and in no case was postoperative best-corrected vision less than that seen preoperatively. However, compared with fresh or wet epikeratophakia, visual recovery was markedly prolonged. Fresh epilenticules sutured into a slant-cut circular keratotomy with a non-torquing suture have proven to be most satisfactory in keratoconus cases. The results of such application are summarized in Table 10.3. As in dry EKP, the table does not tell the whole story. Nonetheless, the overall results in the wet cases were markedly better than in the dry ones. Not all eyes escaped without residual astigmatism, however, which in some cases actually helped the overall uncorrected visual acuity (see Chapter 9). Three of the eyes required penetrating keratoplasty within 1 year of the EKP. In each of these cases, the graft was placed through the epilenticule, which was left in place. As in keratomileusis, side effects and complications of this surgery are discussed in Chapter 15. There is not, in the author's opinion, any indication for aphakic epikeratophakia—not even in pediatric patients. The author's excellent experience with IOLs in pediatric cases mitigates against the use of aphakic EPI in these cases [73].

Although epikeratoplasty has been more or less shelved as a primary procedure for routine use, it should be considered as an alternative to PKP in some keratoconus patients. The author has had success in cases with small cones and in those with traumatic ectasia. Others have reported good results in such cases as well [74]. In some cases, the lenticule can be shaped on a cryolathe to assist in correcting any accompanying refractive error; cryolathing is not a dead art by any means. The author has done this successfully in these cases, the only problem being to assess a representative power. A rigid contact lens can help here.

Keratophakia

The author has performed both homoplastic and alloplastic keratophakia procedures with indifferent results. The two cases of homoplastic keratophakia for aphakia had improved vision (as opposed to spectacles) but were a long time in coming right. Epithelialization was prolonged (longer than 2 weeks in both cases), and vision remained below 20/100 for at least 6 months despite the apparent clarity of the lenticule. In neither case was irregular astigmatism present, but low-grade regular astigmatism was—2.25 D in one patient and 1.87 D in the other—after 1 year. Both patients required spectacle correction, remaining moderately hyperopic (+3.25 + 1.87 × 97° in one case and +2.50 + 2.25 × 165° in the other), and had a best-corrected vision of 20/40 and 20/50, respectively, at 2 and 3 years postoperatively.

The author has implanted one hydrogel intrastromal lens as part of the AMO study. After 9 months, the patient's best-corrected visual acuity was 20/80 with considerable ametropia: −7.50 + 4.50 × 88°. The overlying corneal tissue remained clear, but there was a fine refractile crystalline deposit on the lens itself and accumulated along its edge (see above). The lenticule was removed because the vision and the deposits did not clear.

This is a good technique. The hydrogel material is the first of the implanted allopathic materials to retain clear corneas in all examples. The problems are indications and availability. The indications for such use have diminished with the increasing success of IOL implantation. Furthermore, the study has been suspended for reasons mentioned earlier, and it is unlikely that the company will make lenses available on an "if come" basis. Nonetheless, Kaufman is currently examining other materials for use in intrastromal implants.

Conclusion

The approval of Intacs is a significant step forward in providing high-quality refractive surgery for patients. It provides a unique and effective way to correct low amounts of myopia. With continuing clinical trials, Intacs should be able to be used in the treatment of slightly higher levels of myopia. This technology also holds promise for the future treatment of hyperopia (Figure 10.139) and astigmatism.

Baikoff has reported his experience with his first 13 Intacs patients, his first 103 PRK patients, and his first 103 LASIK patients, who had at least 1 year of follow-up [75]. In the long term, he found that the accuracy was less with Intacs. The rate of undercorrection was the highest with that technique compared with the others. Considering the visual acuity, the predictability, the efficiency, and the safety, LASIK and PRK did not show any difference in low myopes. Baikoff noted that the other two refractive procedures were more predictable than Intacs. The rate of enhancements was much higher with Intacs, even for low myopia, for an inexperienced surgeon.

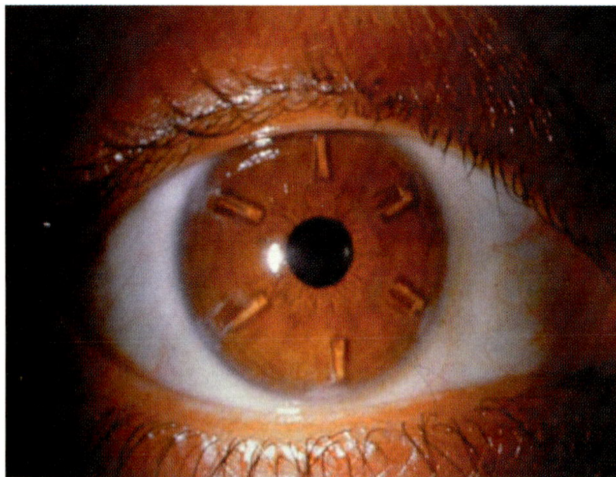

Fig. 10.139 This technology also holds promise for the future treatment of hyperopia and astigmatism.

References

1 Barraquer JI. Queratoplastica refractiva est. Inform Oftal (Instituto Barraquer) 1949; 2: p. 10.
2 Barraquer JI. Queratoplastia. Arch Soc Am Oftal Optom 1961; 3: p. 147.
3 McCarey BE, van Rij G, Beekhuis WH, *et al.* Hydrogel keratophakia: a freehand pocket dissection in the monkey model. Br J Ophthalmol 1986; 70(3): p. 187–91.
4 Barraquer JI. *Queratomileusis y Queratofaquia: C. Clasification de las Queratoplastias Refractivas. II. Metodos que modifican la curva de una o ambas superficies corneales, varaindo la relacion entre ellas.* Instituto Barrquer de America, Bogota, 78–9; 1980.
5 Krwawicz T. Attempted Modification of Corneal curvature by Means of Experimental Plastic surgery [Proby zmiany krzywizny rogowski droga doswiadczalnych operacji plastycznych] <Original> Klin Occna 1960; 30: p. 229–36.
6 Krwawicz T. New plastic operation for correcting refractive error of aphakic eyes by changing corneal curvature : preliminary report. Brit J Ophth 1961; 45: p. 59–63.
7 Krwawicz T. Lamellar corneal stromectomy. Am J Ophth 1964; 57: p. 828.
8 Pureskin NP. [Weakening ocular refraction by means of partial stromectomy of cornea under experimental conditions] <Original> Oslablenie refraktsii glaza putem chastichnoi stromektomii rogovitsy v eksperimente. Vestn Oftalmol 1967; 80(1): p. 19–24.
9 Elstein JK, Sehgal VN, Kaplan MM, et al. Instrumentation and techniques for refractive keratoplasty. Am J Ophthalmol 1969; 68(2): p. 282–91.
10 Hoffmann F and Jessen K. [Keratokyphosis for the optical correction of aphakia] <Original> Keratokyphose zur optischen Korrektur der Aphakie. Fortschr Ophthalmol 1985; 82(1): p. 86–7.
11 Swinger CA, Krumeich J, and Cassiday D. Planar lamellar refractive keratoplasty. J Refract Surg 1986; 2(1): p. 17–24.
12 Binder PS, Krumeich JH, and Zavala EV. Laboratory evaluation of freeze vs non-freeze lamellar refractive keratoplasty. Arch Ophthalmol 1987; 105(8): p. 1125–8.
13 Krumeich JH, and Swinger CA. Nonfreeze epikeratophakia for the correction of myopia. Am J Ophthalmol 1987; 103 (3 Pt 2): p. 397–403.
14 Ruiz LA. Lamellar keratectomy for hyperopia. In: *KeratoRefractive Society.* Dallas, 1987.
15 Bores LD. Hyperopic lamellar keratotomy (HLK). Post-operative results. In: *KeratoRefractive Society Annual Meeting.* Dallas, 1987.
16 Ruiz LA. Personal communication. 1989.
17 Googe JM, Palkama KA, and Werblin TP. The histology of epikeratophakia grafts. Invest Ophthalmol Vis Sci 1981; 20(Suppl): p. 8.
18 Werblin TP, and Kaufman HE. Epikeratophakia: the surgical correction of aphakia. II. Preliminary results in a non-human primate model. Curr Eye Res 1981; 1(3): p. 131–7.
19 Werblin TP, Kaufman HE, Friedlander MH, *et al.* A prospective study of the use of hyperopic epikeratophakia grafts for the correction of aphakia in adults. Ophthalmology 1981; 88(11): p. 1137–40.
20 Werblin TP, and Klyce SD. Epikeratophakia: the surgical correction of aphakia. I. Lathing of corneal tissue. Curr Eye Res 1981; 1(3): p. 123–9.
21 Morgan KS, Werblin TP, Asbell PA, *et al.* The use of epikeratophakia grafts in pediatric monocular aphakia. J Pediatr Ophthalmol Strabismus 1981; 18(6): p. 23–9.
22 Werblin TP, Kaufman HE, Friedlander MH, *et al.* Epikeratophakia: the surgical correction of aphakia. III. Preliminary results of a prospective clinical trial. Arch Ophthalmol 1981; 99(11): p. 1957–60.
23 Berkowitz RA, McDonald MB, and Werblin TP. Epikeratophakia for myopia. Invest Ophthalmol 1982; 22(suppl): p. 201.
24 Werblin TP, Kaufman HE, Friedlander MH, *et al.* Epikeratophakia—the surgical correction of aphakia. Upd1981. Ophthalmology 1982; 89(8): p. 916–20.
25 Kaufman HE, and Werblin TP. Epikeratophakia for the treatment of keratoconus. Am J Ophthalmol 1982; 93(3): p. 342–7.
26 Werblin TP. Epikeratophakia: techniques, complications, and clinical results. Int Ophthalmol Clin 1983; 23(3): p. 45–58.
27 Werblin TP. Epikeratophakia: a new treatment for corneal irregularity and keratoconus. W Va Med J 1983; 79(2): p. 26–8.
28 Werblin TP, and Blaydes JE. Epikeratophakia: existing limitations and future modifications. Aust J Ophthalmol 1983; 11(3): p. 201–7.
29 Werblin TP, Blaydes JE, and Kaufman HE. Epikeratophakia: the surgical correction of astigmatism—preliminary experimental results. CLAO J 1983; 9(1): p. 61–3.
30 Yamaguchi T, Koenig S, Kimura T, *et al.* Histological study of epikeratophakia in primates. Ophthalmic Surg 1984; 15(3): p. 230–5.
31 Goodman GS, Peiffer RLJ, and Werblin TP. Failed epikeratoplasty for keratoconus. Cornea 1986; 5: p. 29–34.
32 McDonald MB, Koenig SB, Friedlander MH, *et al.* Alloplastic epikeratophakia for the correction of aphakia. Ophthalmic Surg 1983; 14(1): p. 65–9.
33 Baumgartner SD, Zavala EY, and Binder PS. A laboratory analysis of lyophilized epikeratophakia lenticules. Invest Ophthalmol Vis Sci 1985; 26(Suppl): p. 204.
34 Arffa RC, Busin M, Barron BA, *et al.* Epikeratophakia with commercially prepared tissue for the correction of aphakia in adults. Arch Ophthalmol 1986; 104 (10): p. 1467–72.
35 McDonald MB, Kaufman HE, Aquavella JV, *et al.* The nationwide study of epikeratophakia for myopia. Am J Ophthalmol 1987; 103(3 Pt 2): p. 375–83.
36 Grossniklaus HE, Lass JH, Jacobs G, *et al.* Light Microscopic and Ultrastructural Findings in Failed Epikeratoplasty. Refractive and Corneal Surgery 1989; 5(5): p. 296–301.
37 Hiles DA. Epikeratophakia—an alternative to glasses, contact lenses and intraocular lens for optical correction of aphakia in children. Trans Pa Acad Ophthalmol Otolaryngol 1986; 38(1): p. 279–85.
38 Morgan KS, McDonald MB, Hiles DA, *et al.* The nationwide study of epikeratophakia for aphakia in children. Am J Ophthalmol 1987; 103(3 Pt 2): p. 366–74.

39 Morgan KS, McDonald MB, Hiles DA, *et al.* The nationwide study of epikeratophakia for aphakia in older children. Ophthalmology 1988; 95(4): p. 526–32.
40 Ehrlich MI, and Nordan LT. Epikeratophakia for the treatment of hyperopia. J Cataract Refract Surg 1989; 15(6): p. 661–6.
41 Gilbert ML, Roth AS, and Friedlander MH. Corneal flattening by shallow circular trephination in human eye bank eyes. Refract Corneal Surg 1990; 6(2): p. 113–6.
42 Gills J. Trephination in combination with radial keratotomy for myopia. In: *Radial Keratotomy,* R Schacher, N Levy, and L Schacher, Editors. LAL, Dennison, 1980.
43 Friedlander MH, Rich LF, Werblin TP, *et al.* Keratophakia using preserved lenticules. Ophthalmology 1980; 87(7): p. 687–92.
44 Maguen K, Pinhas S, and Verity SM. Keratophakia with lyophilized cornea lathed at room temperature: New techniques and experimental surgical results. Ophthalmic Surg 1983; 14: p. 759–62.
45 Barraquer JI. Keratophakia for the correction of high hyperopia. J Cryosurg 1964; 1: p. 39.
46 Barraquer JI. Modification of refraction by means of intracorneal inclusions. Int Ophthalmol Clin 1966; 6: p. 53.
47 Barraquer JI. Keratophakia. Trans Ophthalmol Soc UK 1972; 92: p. 499–516.
48 Swinger CA, and Barraquer JI. Keratophakia and keratomileusis clinical results Ophthalmology 1981; 88(8): p. 709–15.
49 Barraquer JI. *Cirugia Refractiva de la Cornea: Queratofaquia. Vol. 1.* Instituto Barraquer de America, Bogota, Columbia, 328–53; 1989.
50 Beekhuis WH, McCarey BE, van Rij G, *et al.* Complications of hydrogel intracorneal lenses in monkeys. Arch Ophthalmol 1987; 105(1): p. 116–22.
51 Choyce DP. Intra-cameral and intra-corneal implants. A decade of personal experience. Trans Ophthalmol Soc UK 1966; 86: p. 507–25.
52 Choyce DP. Implants and the human body. Lancet 1968; 2(568): p. 633.
53 Choyce DP. The present status of intra-cameral and intracorneal implants. Can J Ophthalmol 1968; 3(4): p. 295–311.
54 Choyce DP. Perforating and non-perforating acrylic corneal implants, including the Choyce 2-piece perforating keratoprosthesis. Ophthalmologica 1969; Suppl: p. 292–300.
55 Choyce DP. Intra-corneal plastic implants. 2. Nurs Times 1970; 66(23): p. 715–8.
56 Choyce DP. The correction of refractive errors with polysulfone corneal inlays. A new frontier to be explored? Trans Ophthalmol Soc UK 1985; 104(Pt 3): p. 332–42.
57 Kirkness CM, Steele AD, and Garner A. Polysulfone corneal inlays. Adverse reactions: a preliminary report. Trans Ophthalmol Soc UK 1985; 104(3): p. 343–50.
58 Lane SS, Lindstrom RL, Williams PA, *et al.* Polysulfone Intracorneal Lenses. J Refract Surg 1985; 1(5): p. 207–16.
59 Lane SS, Lindstrom RL, and Cameron JD. Fenestrated intracorneal lenses. Ophthalmology 1987; 94(Suppl): p. 125.
60 Lindstrom RL, Lane SS, Cameron JD, *et al.* Intracorneal lenses. Vol. 36. New Orleans: New Orleans Acad Ophthalmol. 279–96; 1988.
61 McCarey BE, Lane SS, and Lindstrom RL. Alloplastic correal lenses. Int Ophthalmol Clin 1988; 28(2): p. 155–64.
62 Lane SS and Lindstrom RL. Polysulfone intracorneal lenses. Int Ophthalmol Clin 1991; 31(1): p. 37–46.
63 Werblin TP, Blaydes JE, Fryczkowski A, *et al.* Refractive corneal surgery: the use of implantable alloplastic lens material. Aust J Ophthalmol 1983; 11(4): p. 325–31.
64 Werblin TP, Blaydes JE, Fryczkowski AW, *et al.* Stability of hydrogel intracorneal implants in non-human primates. CLAO J 1983; 9(2): p. 157–61.
65 Werblin TP, Fryczkowski AW, and Peiffer RL. Myopic correction using alloplastic implants in non-human primates—a preliminary report. Ann Ophthalmol 1984; 16(12): p. 1127–30.
66 Werblin TP, Peiffer RL, and Fryczkowski A. Myopic hydrogel keratophakia: preliminary report. Cornea 1984; 3(3): p. 197–204.
67 Peiffer RL, Werblin TP, and Fryczkowski AW. Pathology of corneal hydrogel alloplastic implants. Ophthalmol 1985; 92: p. 1294–304.
68 Werblin TP, Fryczkowski AW, and Peiffer RL. Hydrogel keratophakia: measurement of intraocular pressure. CLAO J 1985; 11(4): p. 354–7.
69 Werblin T, and Patel A. Myopic hydrogel keratophakia. Improvements in lens design. Cornea 1987; 6(3): p. 197–201.
70 Werblin TP, Peiffer RL, and Patel AS. Synthetic keratophakia for the correction of aphakia. Ophthalmology 1987; 94(8): p. 926–34.
71 van Rij G. Personal communication, 1990.
72 Barraquer JI. *Cirugia Refractiva de la Cornea: Resultados. Vol. 1.* Instituto Barraquer de America, Bogota, Columbia, 461; 1989.
73 Bores LD. Intraocular Lenses, Post-operative Management. In: *Intraocular Implants in Children,* D Hiles, Editor. Gruen and Stratton, New York, 1979.
74 Vajpayee RB, Sharma N, Saxena N, *et al.* Epikeratoplasty for traumatic corneal ectasia. Cornea 1999; 18(2): p. 237–9.
75 Baikoff G, Maia N, Poulhalec N, *et al.* Diurnal variations in keratometry and refraction with intracorneal ring segments [see comments]. J Cataract Refract Surg 1999; 25(8): p. 1056–61.

11
Laser Refractive Surgery

Be not the first to set the old aside,
Nor yet the last to leave the new untried.
[Alexander Pope]

In the first edition of this work, it may have seemed presumptuous of me to attempt to write a chapter on laser refractive surgery. Much of the information contained within that work probably will be of historical interest only by the time this revision sees print—an inevitable event considering the rapid pace at which this whole discipline is evolving. Nevertheless, there is still much of value in a study of the investigations that are concurrent with this writing, as well as those of a more historical nature, if for no other reason than to prevent the recurrence of mistakes and spare patients the grief. We can but try to bring some clarity out of the fog of conflicting claims and data and perhaps inject a modicum of sanity into the still current atmosphere of *laser rapture*—a close cousin to *He-Ne rapture*, and just as pernicious. The term *He-Ne rapture* was coined to describe the tendency of the ophthalmic surgeon who—so taken with the sight of a posterior capsule being blasted to bits under his or her He-Ne focus spot—keeps pushing the button on his or her YAG laser until all remnants of the capsule have been totally vaporized.

It is the purpose of this chapter not to view lasers *aenigmate* ("through a glass darkly"), but to shed some light (no pun intended) on these fascinating devices and their possible application in refractive surgery. To this end, we will outline the physical properties of the laser—what makes it go, as it were—and the effect of such amplified light, good and bad, on living tissue. In addition, we will share with you some of the techniques currently being applied to the corneal surface to modulate its shape along with their results, as well as provide a glimpse of some laser technology still to come.

The term *laser* is an acronym for *l*ight *a*mplification by *s*timulated *e*mission of *r*adiation—and it may be the sexiest acronym in the human lexicon. It carries with it visions of *Star Wars,* connotations of unfettered power, and a mystique of benevolent utility. The very nuance of the term is that of something embodying everlasting welfare—*"We don't know what it means, but it sure sounds great!"* It has been made the subject of unprecedented media hype and has acquired a reputation for accuracy and applicability—some of it justified, some not. Many see lasers as the Greek *panacea*—the universal cure, the ultimate liniment. Or the penultimate snake oil—since the term *laser* itself has been used to sell everything from trinkets to automobiles.

There is no question that such devices, through the beam of electromagnetic radiation that they emit, are extremely powerful things. They can, in an instant, vaporize the most refractory of substances. Heady stuff this, both to witness and to contemplate. It is, however, this very power that makes them extremely dangerous devices. Dangerous not only in their manifest (as well as latent) power but also in their ability to fascinate, nay mesmerize, human beings—perhaps into applying them in ways that may prove to be more harmful than beneficial.

The author once made an unfortunate response to an interview question regarding the application of lasers to refractive surgery when he replied, somewhat tongue-in-cheek, that *"lasers are the refractive surgical instrument of the future and are likely to be so for the next 10 years."* This answer was not original; it was, in fact, a paraphrasing of something someone else had said about the same subject. It was, moreover, unfortunate because it was mistaken in some quarters as sour grapes and taken in others as a jest. The author's intent, however, was to point out that the routine use of lasers in refractive surgery was not then routine (however much some individuals and manufacturers would have liked it to be) and that considerable research and trial lay ahead. Considering the power of the term *laser* to stimulate individuals' imaginations, the potential for harm if lasers are applied willy-nilly is still very great—and this is no joking matter. Regardless, that sentence is still applicable for the ultrafast nano-, femto-, and picosecond lasers (see below).

Lest it be said that the author somehow categorically opposed to the use of such devices in refractive surgery, he will go on record by stating that the value of the laser for such use is high. However, let the record also show that none of the early results reported justified the hype surrounding such application. Even with the current upsurge in laser use in laser in situ keratomileusis (LASIK), there are still some shortcomings—not the least of which is overuse. Both the public and ophthalmologists are ill-served by a self-serving media blitz. The question *"Cui bono?"* cannot yet be answered—the patient. The following is a case in point.

The "king" is dead

I have mixed emotions about PRK because it turns out that the Food and Drug Administration (FDA) was right. This is hard for me to admit because I think of the FDA as the paradigm for obstructionist government intervention. Not that the agency planned to be right, mind you—more like right by accident or default. Besides, it is impossible to be wrong all of the time. Why do I say the FDA was right? Because they delayed the approval of widespread use of the PRK procedure in this country—and a good thing too! It does not work that well, you see. The darling of the laser cult turned out to have feet of clay, and while it may not be dead, it is certainly in *extremis.*

I do not say that PRK does not work at all—because it does. But it does not work as well as it was touted, and it does not work very well for the higher degrees of myopia for which it was slated. In fact, most of the "movers and shakers" of the U.S. laser world have pretty much abandoned PRK and have switched over to LASIK for all the reasons that I criticized (and they defended) PRK in the first place: It is not a very good procedure and exposes the eye to serious infection. It is a major surface burn, after all.

It is really problematic both from a predictive standpoint and a complications standpoint in myopia over 5 D (the FDA allows its use to 7 D). It is at its best at under 3 D (but so is a less expensive surgery with quicker recovery—radial keratotomy); even Theo Seiler has said as much. What, then, was all the ballyhoo about? The answer is simple. If you spent $450,000+ for an instrument, wouldn't you want it to pay for itself? It doesn't take a rocket scientist to figure that one out.

Most surgeons have switched over to LASIK, but LASIK requires thinking (see Chapter 10). PRK was the ultimate "no-brainer" at the time. Just feed the patient's refraction into the computer, aim the laser, push the button, and the money rolls in. *Gadzooks! What a neat way to recover the lost revenue from the reduction in cataract fees!* The beauty was that you could get on the refractive surgery "gravy train" with all the rest of the "beautiful people" and not have to retrain. *Great days! Sign me up!* And hundreds did.

Other people played it smarter. They realized that all the "approved" lasers were mostly fluff—or as the Japanese would say—*soup without fish* (we would say *sizzle without steak*). That is, the basic excimer laser beam generator can be bought—off the shelf—for 30 grand retail! So how come it sells for 15 times that? It's called *profit,* grasshopper, only in this case it's "charging what the market will bear." To be fair, there are a few things that must be added to the basic laser to make it capable of delivering a well-behaved column of light in just the right way.

It turns out that in the industry the name for "dirty laser beam" is excimer, and nothing has changed there in all this time. If you look at the beam profile of a typical excimer laser's output, you would see what I mean—not good. Lots of voids, cold spots, hot spots—a mess. So you throw in some diffusers, dove prisms, mirrors, rotating what-nots, and gum wrappers to mix up the beam sufficiently so that what comes out the business end is reasonably homogeneous, but corneal "islands" still occur and in the worst of places (good ol' Murphy). So factoring the "homogenizer" in, the "one-off" price of such a unit will rise to anywhere from $80,000 to $150,000 (depending on the diaphragm mechanism, amount of chrome, air-conditioning, stereo, etc.)—still considerably short of $450,000. Considering that the usual markup for low-ticket items is 2.5 times, this puts the retail price at around $425,000 starting at the top end (throwing in the extra $25,000 for "miscellaneous"). However, high-ticket items typically carry a lower markup, and the base price I quoted was for a "one-off." They get cheaper when you build more of them. Still expensive, but still cheaper as well.

Some folks tried making their own lasers, but the industry, aided and abetted by the FDA, made a fuss, calling them "black boxes" and implying that use of such devices was reckless in the extreme. Only one of these devices ultimately was approved by the FDA. Probably because Kremer hung in there [1], while the rest, scared off by their lawyers (and possibly offered deals by the industry), acquired "legitimate" machines and shelved their units, hence proving that the Golden Rule still operates—*The guy with the gold rules.*

There is a particular photo you should take a look at (see Figure 11.9). The mushroom-shaped cloud you see there is made up of what is called in the trade *ejecta.* That is, debris created by the blast effect of the excimer—as it "disrupts the collagen molecular bounds"—being thrown into the air. McDonald called it "Bowman's Blasting," and an apt name it is. Basically, the surface of the cornea has been blasted—seared if you will—by a miniature atomic explosion which lacks only the radioactive fallout. This results in a burned area some 5–6 mm in diameter on the front surface of the cornea, and all burns are slow to heal, as well as painful. Pain is a real problem with PRK. This was brought under control somewhat by using nonsteroidal anti-inflammatory drugs (NSAIDs) like Acular post-treatment. No one can give me an exact meaning for the term *under control* except to say that pain was less. Less. Does that mean it fell from excruciating to almost tolerable, or? There's the rub. You didn't know until you tried. And it turns out that NSAIDs are not all they are cracked up to be and in some cases can make things worse. If the only postoperative anti-inflammatory used is an NSAID, the buildup of arachidonic acid and the potential shift in the equilibrium toward the leukotriene pathway increases the risk of such conditions as diffuse lamellar keratitis (DLK, "sands of the Sahara"—call it what you will). NSAIDs also have a very modest but real inhibitory effect on epithelial cell migration (see Chapter 15).

It would seem that I am somewhat down on PRK. Guilty as charged. Never was enamored of it. Not likely to be either unless a miracle occurs. That miracle embodies better beam profiles, smoother cutting through scanning, and better centration. Some of these issues have been addressed in the second- and third-generation lasers undergoing trials in the United States and in regular use outside. The fact remains, however, we are disrupting natural tissue relationships. PRK is the only procedure that does this by removing Bowman's layer. Call me old-fashioned, but I am firm in my belief that the human cornea needs Bowman's layer—it is not like the appendix.

Isn't there *anything* good about PRK? Of course! It doesn't weaken the eye as radial keratotomy (RK) very definitely does. RK incisions are also very slow to heal, and they take years to get up to the original strength of the surrounding cornea. The fact is that they may never reach this point. I recently treated a police officer who was kicked in the eye. Despite having had the surgery 13 years before, the nasal incision split open, entrapping the iris. I am of the opinion that had the incision not opened, the globe would have ruptured posteriorly with worse consequences. As it was, I saved the eye. I could argue that the RK saved the eye—but I can't prove it.

Despite all, PRK remains a useful procedure—in some specialized cases. In its incarnation as PTK it has been used successfully to treat corneal nodules (see below). An extension of this technique has been to use it to smooth corneas roughened by irregular wound healing from RK, PKP, and trauma much as "glass rubbers" do today for mirrors and lenses in optical shops. It is probably the treatment of choice for off-centered LASIK procedures rather than repeating the LASIK (an iffy procedure at best); despite the cavalier attitude of some, lifting the LASIK flap (cap) is not a "breeze." PRK is still used occasionally to "touch up" undercorrected RK, a procedure it was supposed to supplant (see also Figure 11.59), and it is being studied as a possible approach to treat hyperopia. And given only the choice between PRK and LASIK for myopes under –4 D, I would choose PRK in a heartbeat (but I would much prefer RK here).

The beginning of lasers

Lasers evolved as an offshoot of work on microwave amplifying devices called *masers*—another acronym, this time meaning *m*icrowave *a*mplification by *s*timulated *e*mission of *r*adiation. At first they were called *optical masers* because they amplified light in much the same way that masers amplified microwaves. Arthur L. Schawlow and C. H. Townes are given credit for the idea, which they originally proposed in 1958, although similar concepts are said to have been under development in the Soviet Union at that time [2]. The first practical laser, using ruby, was built and operated in the United States in 1960 by Theodore H. Maiman [3] (see below). This was followed in 1961 by the first continuous laser—again in the United States—built by Ali Javan. In fact, the United States has led the way in laser research since that time, with semiconductor lasers appearing in 1962 and liquid-dye lasers appearing in 1966 [4,5]. Various other types of gas, solid-crystal, and tunable dye lasers have made their entrance on the scientific stage in the ensuing years.

Fundamentals of laser mechanics

Lasers produce light, as do ordinary lamps, but lasers produce it with such intensity and spectral purity that laser light seems to have properties quite different from ordinary light. We seldom, however, notice the properties of light other than the visual. Even its heating effect, which is noticeable in direct sunlight (especially here in Arizona), is seldom appreciated under conditions of comfortable illumination. Therefore, the fact that certain types of coherent light can burn holes through steel is cause for amazement even among the sophisticated. We have, all of us, been subject to *He-Ne rapture* at one time in our careers.

The reason for this seeming naiveté is that most of our interaction with light has been with its incoherent, or anarchic, form. If ever there was an example of "power through group action," that of laser light fits the bill. But all lasers are not created equal; they differ among themselves even more than ordinary light sources do. To understand the kinds of properties that lasers can have and the properties that some lasers do have, we shall first look at how lasers operate and how they differ from all earlier sources of light.

Before the advent of lasers, essentially all light was generated by hot objects of one kind or another, whether it was the sun, a bonfire, a candle, a lantern, or the filament in an incandescent lamp (see also Chapter 3). The light produced from such sources results from the discharge of energy that occurs when the electrons within the thermally excited atoms change state (Figure 11.1). An atom that is, for an instant, raised to some high-energy level can drop back to a lower one, emitting the stored energy as a burst of light. If the energy released is large, the light quantum has a high frequency and a correspondingly short length. A smaller energy release corresponds to a longer wavelength and lower frequency.

The wavelengths emitted by any particular substance depend on the energy levels of that substance. However, every substance has many energy levels as well, and so it is usual for sources to emit many or even a continuous distribution of wavelengths of light. If a single pure color of light is needed, however, it can only be obtained by filtering out all the rest of the wavelengths. When this happens, usually there is not much power remaining in the narrow region of the desired wavelength. A laser, on the other hand, can emit all its power as a nearly pure single wavelength or frequency.

In ordinary light sources, the individual atoms radiate quite independently as they are excited. This has several consequences, one of which is that a light ray is as likely to emerge in one direction as in any other; and so the light is always emitted nearly equally in all directions. Such light is called *incoherent light,* for obvious reasons. Ordinary light sources are really not very powerful, although some of them appear very bright. Lasers, however, generate light that is highly coherent and hence very intense.

When two light waves arrive simultaneously at the same place, they may add to or subtract from the resulting intensity. This phenomenon, called *interference,* has already been discussed in Chapter 3 and so will not be repeated here. However, as pointed out there, it is this very fact of interference that explains lasers and that drives them. The essence of the laser is to stimulate the emission of light by encouraging constructive or additive interference. It does so because the many individual atoms are forced to emit in phase, instead of being allowed to emit randomly. This forcing is the process of stimulated emission of radiation, which was predicted theoretically by Einstein in 1917 [6]. If during the brief interval that an atom is excited, a photon from a similar atom reaches it, the arriving photon will stimulate the excited atom to emit radiation. The induced radiation will have the same frequency, wavelength, and phase as the stimulating photon or wave. As the wave passes through a medium that contains many excited atoms, the resulting wave becomes amplified by this process of stimulated emission.

The reason that the laser is not found in nature (at least in our current universe) is that the probability of spontaneous emission is usually so high in comparison with that of induced emission that the possibility of an electron staying in an excited level long enough to be induced to a lower level is slight. In the laser, electrons are raised into so-called metastable states—a population inversion is created. These states are of higher energy than the ground state but are restricted by the laws of quantum mechanics so that the probability of spontaneous emission to the ground state is very low—reverse of the normal situation. In fact, transitions to the ground state from these levels are forbidden (see also Chapter 3). Hence the term *metastable*—the atom is in an almost stable configuration. Because the probability of its spontaneously decaying to a lower level is so slight, the probability of induced emission is greater than the probability of spontaneous emission. All that is needed is a supply of photons of the proper wavelength to stimulate the atoms to emit coherent light.

Some substances can either absorb certain wavelengths or amplify them, depending on what fraction of their atoms is excited. If the medium is not excited and all the atoms are in their lower energy states, radiation can only be absorbed. If more than half the atoms are excited into the upper state, amplification exceeds absorption.

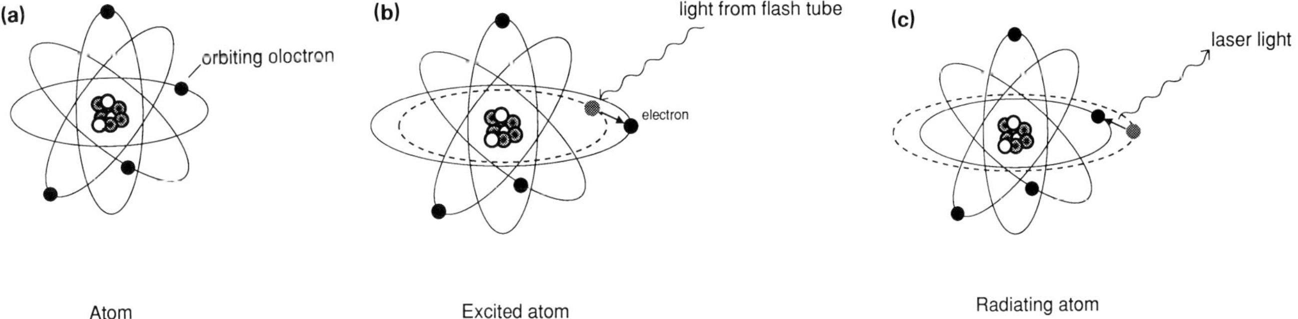

Fig. 11.1 (a) Typical atomic structure; (b) a photon striking an orbiting electron causes it to jump up one level; (c) when the electron spontaneously jumps back to its original level (decays), a photon is emitted.

This phenomenon never occurs for a system of atoms in equilibrium at any temperature, no matter how high, however—otherwise, the universe and everything in it would have burnt to a crisp long ago (see the discussion on ultraviolet catastrophe in Chapter 3). Thermal agitation *does* excite atoms but always leaves more of them in the lower state than in the higher. If the temperature is sufficiently high, significant numbers of molecules will be found in upper levels. The distribution of atoms within these levels is described by Boltzman's distribution—a higher energy level always has fewer atoms populating it than a lower level. Fortunately, it turns out not to be too difficult to force or "pump" most of the atoms into an excited state—akin to beating a wasp's nest with a stick. Once excited, the atoms do not hold their energy for very long—usually for only a small fraction of a second (in contradistinction to wasps)—before losing it by spontaneous or stimulated emission or in some other way. Thus the amplifying stage, with more than half the atoms in the upper energy state, must be created and maintained by some kind of vigorous pumping.

A number of different ways have been found to accomplish this pumping, and they have been applied to many materials. It turns out that it is possible to obtain amplification by stimulated emission of radiation at wavelengths throughout the visible spectrum with some materials and far into the ultraviolet and infrared regions with others. Thus, if we have a coherent light wave, it can be amplified by stimulated emission. However, in almost all lasers, the amplification is used as part of the process of generating a coherent wave from atoms that are randomly excited. To do this, we must enclose the excited atoms in some suitable kind of resonator.

Masers

Masers used a metallic box called a *cavity resonator* that would store (or fit) just one particular microwave and no other. This box can be of a practical size because typical microwaves have a wavelength of 1.0 cm or so. If excited atoms or molecules that can emit this particular wavelength are put into the box, any radiation they emit will be stored within the resonator. This stored radiation (which is ricocheting around within the enclosure) then stimulates other atoms or molecules to emit their energy as radiation at the same wavelength and phase as the stored wave. Soon the stored wave is strong enough that stimulated emission occurs before the atoms have any chance to emit spontaneously, and then essentially all the radiation becomes coherent. A small amount of the radiation is allowed to leak out through a coupling hole to provide the maser's output, but enough is retained in the resonator at any given instant to continue the process as long as excited atoms or molecules are supplied.

Visible light, on the other hand, has a wavelength much shorter—by about some 20,000 times—than the centimeter-length radio waves, so it is not practical to build a resonator as small as the wavelength, and even if it were, the box would not be large enough to hold many atoms. Therefore, the laser's resonator is made to a more convenient size—which can range in length from a millimeter to some meters, but always many times larger than the wavelength of the light itself. Such a box, if it were constructed like the microwave cavity resonator, could sustain waves of almost any length, going in almost any direction, and would not select any waves to store and amplify and hence would be essentially useless for our purposes.

For these reasons, a laser uses a resonator that has convenient dimensions but is of a special kind. It can be thought of as cavity (box) resonator with all the box, except the two end walls, discarded. The laser structure therefore typically is a long rod or column of some active material, with mirrors at the ends of the column. This is a satisfactory resonator for any wave that travels along the long axis of the structure. Such a wave can zip back and forth between the mirrors, gaining energy by stimulating emission from the excited atoms as it goes. If one of the end mirrors has been made partly transparent, some of this stimulated light can leak out through it. This laser structure was first proposed by Schawlow and Townes in 1958 and is used in almost all examples of these devices.

Properties of laser light

From the structure of a typical laser, we can easily deduce the properties of laser light. The light emerging from a laser will be a highly directional beam, since a wave can remain in the active medium long enough to be built up appreciably only if it is traveling along the axis of the resonator. Such a beam is intense because the atoms are stimulated to emit much faster than they ordinarily would. The beam of light is also usually monochromatic because the condition for amplification is satisfied only, or at least most strongly, at a single wavelength. Finally, the laser light beam is coherent because all the atoms are stimulated to emit in synchrony with the photons that are flailing about between the mirrors.

The first laser to be actually built and operated was constructed by Theodore H. Maiman in 1960, who used a solid rod of pink ruby (an aluminum oxide crystal containing 0.05% chromium ions in place of the equivalent number of aluminum ions) [3]. The chromium ions in ruby can absorb and be excited by either green or blue light, and these excited atoms quickly drop down to a resting metastable state (Figure 11.2). This metastable state has a lifetime of about 3 ms at room temperature, and atoms might accumulate for a while when the pumping light is first turned on. However, atoms in the metastable state can spontaneously emit red light at a wavelength of 6943 Å. This is in the very deep red portion of the spectrum at a wavelength so long that the typical eye is only

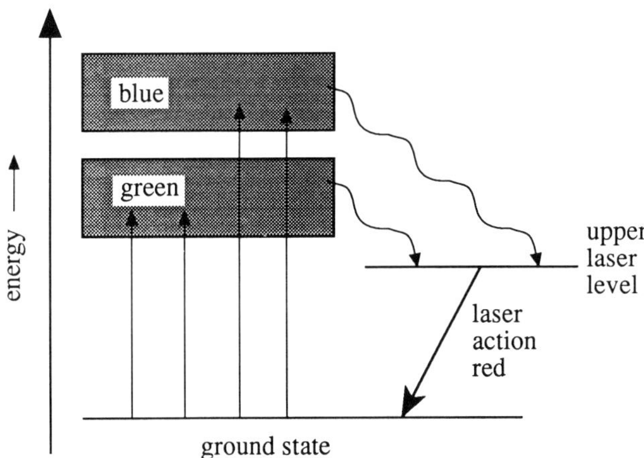

Fig. 11.2 Ruby laser metastable state.

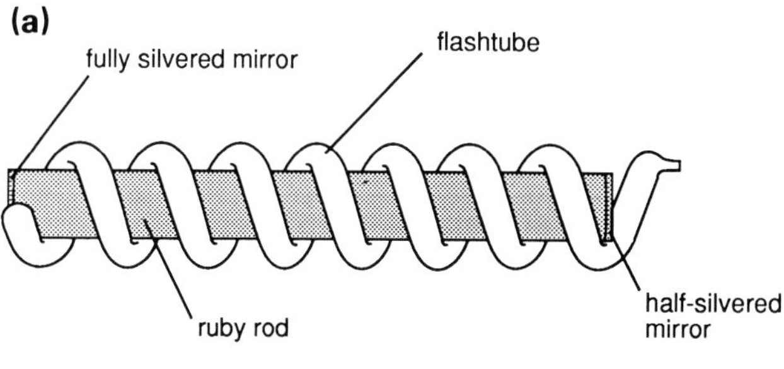

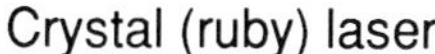

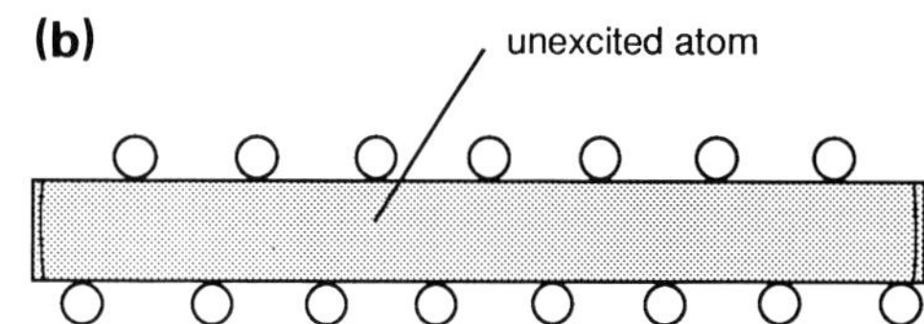

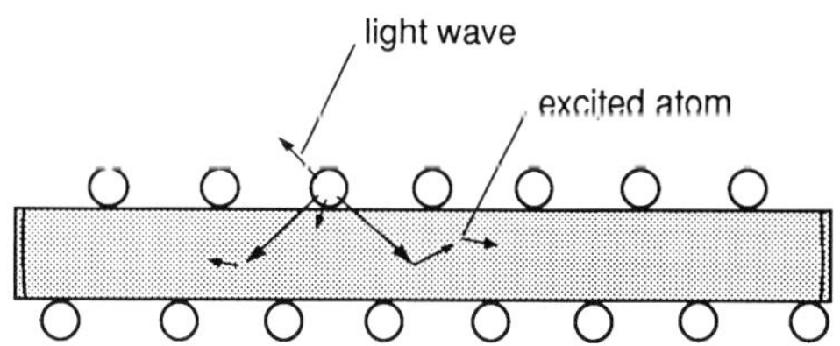

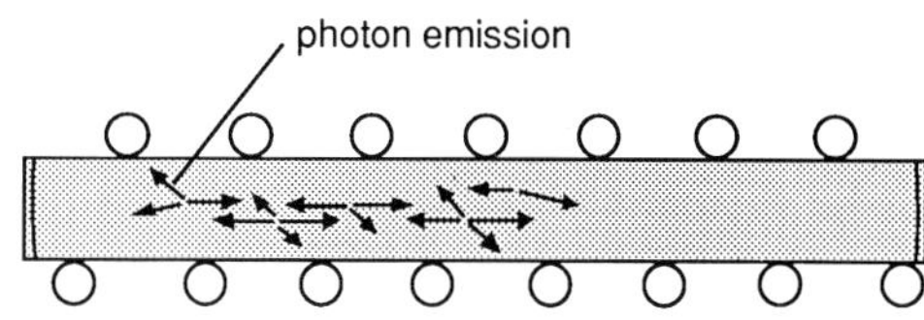

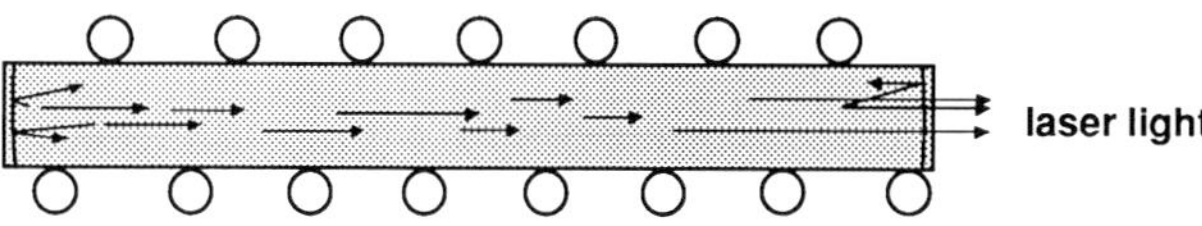

Fig. 11.3 Typical solid or crystalline (ruby) laser construction and action.

about 1/200 as sensitive to it as it is to green. Nevertheless, the pumping process is so efficient and the intensity of the beam so high that the red beam can be seen easily when the laser is operating.

In this as in many other solid-state lasers, the mirrors are placed directly on the ends of the solid rod, which have been polished flat and parallel to each other. The exciting light is an intense flash from a xenon arc lamp, much like those used in a photographer's strobe light. If enough light has been received from the pumping lamp during the few milliseconds that chromium ions remain in the metastable state, enough excited ions are accumulated so that amplification by stimulated emission begins. A laser beam is then set up and emerges through one of the partially silvered ends of the rod. Because a very bright lamp is required to produce enough excited atoms in the short time available, the first ruby laser (and many subsequent solid-state lasers) operated only in a short burst, lasting for about 0.5 ms. However, during this burst, the power output is extremely large, being typically of the order of 1000 to 10,000 W and confined to a relatively narrow beam with a divergence of about 0.01 rad (0.5°).

The construction of a typical optically pumped solid crystalline laser is shown in Figure 11.3. The flash lamps are placed close to the rod and surrounded by a reflector that concentrates the light onto the rod. This same structure can be used to produce different wavelengths and different power levels depending on the individual materials used within the rod. Two of the other commonly used solid-state materials incorporate neodymium ions rather than chromium in either suitably doped glass or a crystal of yttrium-aluminum-garnet (YAG). The neodymium ion lasers emit radiation in the near-infrared range at a wavelength of 10,000 Å (1.06 μm). Both ruby and neodymium lasers produce radiation that can be transmitted through the transparent parts of the eye and so can be used in eye surgery or can cause eye damage if applied carelessly. Some other types of lasers operate far into the infrared range and produce light that is absorbed in the outer parts of the eye and thus are suitable for surface applications.

When the light from such a pulsed laser is focused with a lens, it produces a small spot of very high intensity. For example, if the focal length of the lens is f and the angular divergence of the laser is q, measured in radians (1 rad = 57.3°), the diameter of the spot at the focus is equal to fq. Its area, therefore, is

$$\frac{\pi f^2 q^2}{4}$$

Thus the power density in this focal spot is power divided by the area, that is,

$$\frac{4P}{f^2q^2}$$

As a typical example, if the laser delivers 1000 W during its brief flash, the divergence is 0.01 rad, and the focal length of the lens is 2 cm, then the power density is 3×10^6 W/cm^2. If this focus occurs in a transparent medium, there is negligible absorption, and nothing noticeable happens. However, if the focus occurs on the surface of an opaque medium, the power may be absorbed to a very small depth and consequently in a very small volume. For example, an opaque material such as carbon will absorb the light at a distance of about 10.5 cm, and within the absorbing surface layer the power density would be, in the laser of our example, about 10^{11} W/cm^3. This is a very high value, and the material would be immediately heated to incandescence, and a portion of the surface would vaporize.

Few biologic materials are as opaque as this, however, and the effect of the laser is to heat a small portion of the tissue to some moderately high temperature. For example, when the laser is used in retinal surgery, the light traverses the clear parts of the eye with little absorption until it strikes the pigment epithelium of the retina, where it is absorbed and converted to heat. The degree of heating in this small focal spot can be controlled by adjusting the power of the laser or by defocusing the lens.

The pulse of light from most lasers does not deliver very much energy, but if the power is concentrated, so is the energy. It is the total energy delivered per unit volume that determines the heating effect of the absorbed beam. For example, it requires l cal or 4.18 J to heat 1 cc of water through 1°C. It requires 620 cal or about 2600 J per cubic centimeter to heat water from room temperature to 100°C—to boil it. A typical small pulsed ruby laser might deliver an energy of 0.025 J in a pulse lasting about 0.5 ms. With this as an example, if the laser light pulse is absorbed in a volume of 0.0001 cc, the energy density is 2500 J/cc, which is just sufficient to vaporize most of the water in the target volume. If it is absorbed in a larger volume, the temperature rise will be less, and there will be no boiling.

It is important to note that the effects of pulsed laser heating can be extremely localized. If one were to apply the heat slowly, much of it would be conducted away into surrounding material and would heat a larger volume than was desired. A short pulse, however, can produce its effects by heating the absorbing target so quickly that the event is over before the heat has had a chance to spread out appreciably. It is hard to get used to just how very rapid laser heating can be. Perhaps it is best visualized by noting that the sudden heating can vaporize dark, light-absorbing ink off a sheet of paper without harming the paper underneath or even remove carbon ink from a rubber balloon without damaging the balloon or even human skin when used to remove tattoos or eye liner.

Since biologic tissues have characteristic wavelengths at which they absorb or do not absorb light, it would be desirable to be able to choose the wavelength for the purpose at hand. In principle, this can be done by choosing the right material, although there is no simple rule to say which material will work at which wavelength.

Solid lasers

The reason that solid laser materials are especially effective for pulsed operation is that they have a much higher density than a gas and so can have more active ions and store more energy to be released in the laser pulse. In the sort of laser that has been described, this pulse typically lasts about 0.5 ms, or 500 μs. However, there is a method that permits the energy to be released in a much shorter and therefore much more intense pulse, typically millions of waves for some billionths of a second. This is the technique called *Q-switching*, whereby the quality factor of the resonator is altered during the pumping cycle. It can be visualized as shown in Figure 11.4, where one of the mirrors is removed from one end of the rod and a shutter is interposed between the mirror and the rod. Initially, the shutter is closed as the flash lamp begins to pump light into the rod and thereby excite some of the active ions. After a short interval, enough ions are excited so that laser action would begin except that the mirror is blocked and the laser action is incomplete. It is thus possible to go on exciting more ions without starting the laser action so that a large number of ions can be accumulated in the excited state—a mechanism akin to that of a capacitor. Then the shutter is suddenly opened so that the laser action is complete, and the energy is released in one giant short pulse—capacitor discharge.

There are a number of different ways to make the shutter. It can be a mechanical shutter. For instance, the mirror may rotate so that it is parallel to the other mirror for only a short interval. An electro-optical shutter, such as a liquid Kerr cell or a solid Pockels cell, also may be used. One of the simplest ways to provide Q-switching is to use a bleachable dye, either solid or liquid. For ruby, the dye typically is some blue material such as cryptocyanine in solution contained in a glass cell of optical quality. This dye strongly absorbs the red light and prevents any spontaneous light emitted by a ruby rod from reaching the mirror. However, it is rather easily bleached, and when sufficient spontaneous ruby light has reached the dye cell, it bleaches sufficiently to let the red light pass to the mirror and the giant pulse begins. Q-switched lasers have delivered pulses as high as 1 billion W, with a duration of perhaps 5 to 10 ns (billionths of a second). With some refinements, even shorter pulses, as short as 0.001 ns (1 ps), have been generated by a technique known as *mode locking*.

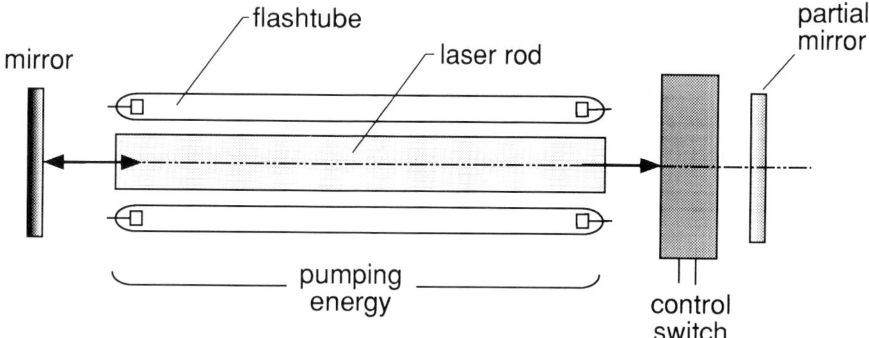

Fig. 11.4 Switched laser.

Mode locking

Despite the purity of the light produced by laser action, the nature of the process is such that inhomogeneity exists within the beam. Regardless that these inhomogeneities may be small, they are sufficient to degrade the quality of the beam. Thus some method must be employed to improve beam quality. One method of doing this is through a process known as *mode locking*. Mode locking is a technique for producing periodic high-power, short-duration laser pulses. It can be either active or passive in nature. Active mode locking uses a shutter mechanism that opens at regular intervals corresponding to the cavity round-trip time of one of the many laser modes—with an Nd:YAG laser, such pulses are about 50 ps in duration. Any other modes are damped.

Passive mode locking is accomplished by using certain dyes whose absorption decreases with increasing irradiance. A dye is chosen with an absorption band at the lasing transition frequency. Such a dye (e.g., cryptocyanine) is called a *saturable absorber*. At low light levels, the dye is opaque. As the number of excited molecules increases, a point is reached where the dye becomes transparent or bleached, and a laser pulse is emitted (Figure 11.5). Initially, the laser medium emits spontaneous radiation, which gives rise to incoherent fluctuations in the beam energy density. Some of these fluctuations may be amplified to such an extent that the peak part of the fluctuation is passed by the saturable absorber with little attenuation. The low-power parts of the fluctuation are more highly attenuated; thus a high-power pulse can grow within the cavity provided the dye has a short recovery period. Typically, when a saturable absorber is used to mode lock a laser, the laser is simultaneously Q-switched.

Q-switching

Q-switching is another technique for obtaining short, intense bursts of oscillation from lasers [7]. First it should be understood that the term Q is used to represent the quality factor of the laser resonating chamber. Q can be defined in general by the expression

$$Q = \frac{2\pi \times \text{stored energy}}{\text{dissipated energy per cycle}}$$

or

$$Q = \frac{\text{resonant frequency}}{\text{linewidth}} = \frac{v}{Dv}$$

Single high-power pulses can be obtained by introducing time- or energy-dependent losses into the cavity. The effects of such losses can be interpreted in terms of spiking oscillations. If there is initially a very high loss in the laser cavity, the gain due to population inversion can reach a very high value—without laser oscillations occurring.

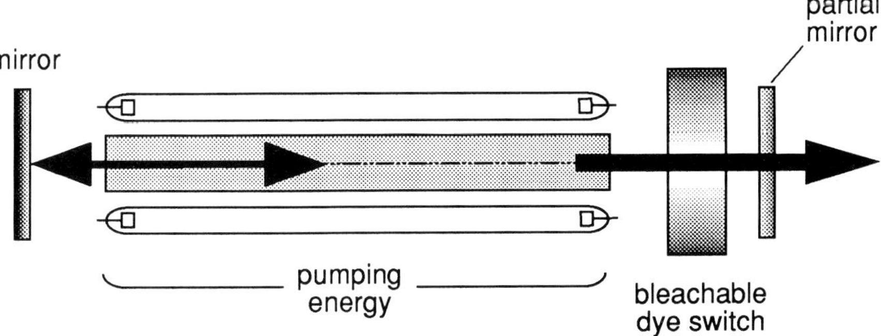

Fig. 11.5 Dye laser.

The high loss prevents laser action while energy is being pumped into the excited state of the medium. If, when a large population inversion has been achieved, the cavity loss is suddenly reduced (i.e., the cavity *Q* is switched to a high value), laser oscillations will suddenly commence. On Q-switching, the threshold gain decreases immediately (to the normal value associated with a cavity of high *Q*), whereas the actual gain remains high because of the large population inversion. Owing to the large difference between the actual and the threshold gain, laser action within the cavity builds up very rapidly, and all the available energy is emitted in a single large pulse. This quickly depopulates the upper lasing level to such an extent that the gain is reduced below threshold, and the lasing action stops. The time variation of some of the laser parameters during Q-switching is shown schematically in Figure 11.6.

Q-switching dramatically increases the peak power obtainable from lasers. In the ordinary pulsed mode, the output of an insulating crystal laser such as the Nd:YAG crystal consists of many random spikes of about 1 ms duration with a separation of about 1 ms; the length of the train of spikes depends principally on the duration of the exciting flashtube source, which may be about 1 ms. Peak powers within the spikes are typically of the order of kilowatts. When the laser is Q-switched, however, the result is a single spike of great power, typically in the megawatt range, with a duration of 11 to 100 ns. It should be noted that although there is a vast increase in the peak power of a Q-switched laser, the total energy emitted is less than in non-Q-switched operation owing to losses associated with the Q-switching mechanism. Q-switching is carried out by placing a closed shutter (i.e., the Q-switch) within the cavity, thereby effectively isolating the cavity from the laser medium. After the laser has been pumped, the shutter is opened, thus restoring the *Q* of the cavity. A little thought reveals that there are two important requirements for effective Q-switching. These are:

- The rate of pumping must be faster than the spontaneous decay rate of the upper lasing level; otherwise, the upper level will empty more quickly than it can be filled so that a sufficiently large population inversion will not be achieved
- The Q-switch must switch rapidly in comparison with the buildup of laser oscillations; otherwise, the latter will build up gradually, and a longer pulse will be obtained, thus reducing the peak power. In practice, the Q-switch should operate in a time less than 1 ns.

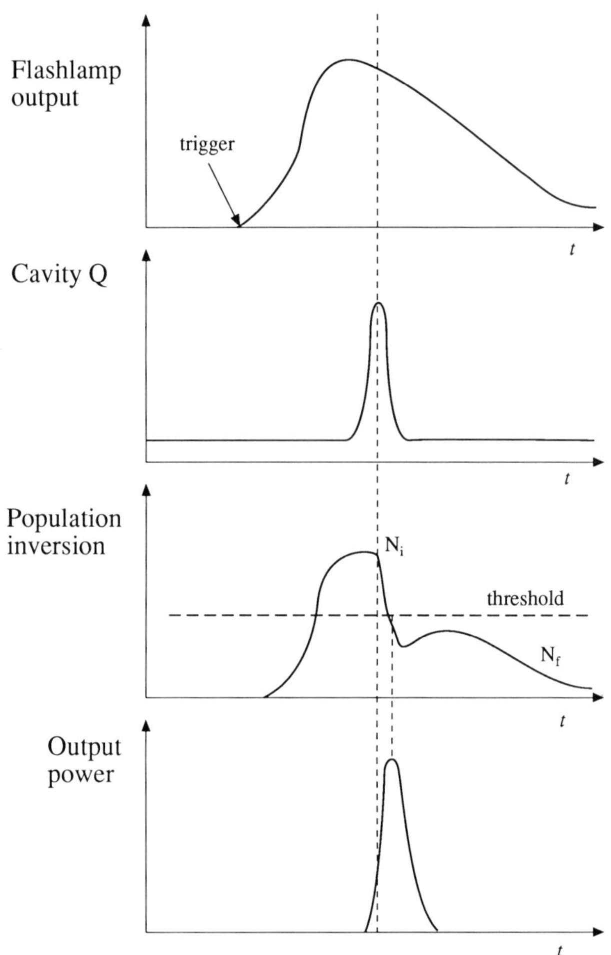

Fig. 11.6 Principle of Q-switching (from Wilson J, Hawkes JFB. *Optoelectronics, An Introduction.* Simon and Schuster, Cambridge, pp 227–230, 1989).

Rotating mirror method

This method, which was the first to be used, involves rotating one of the mirrors at a very high angular velocity such that the optical losses are large except for the brief interval in each rotation cycle when the mirrors are very nearly parallel. Just before this point is reached, a trigger mechanism initiates the flashlamp discharge to pump the laser. Since the mirrors are not yet parallel, population inversion can build up without laser action starting. When the mirrors become parallel, Q-switching occurs, allowing the Q-switched pulse to develop as illustrated in Figure 11.6.

The repetition rate of laser firing is determined by control of the flashlamp and not by the speed of rotation of the mirror, which may be very high. If the laser fired every revolution, the repetition rate would be approximately 1000 times per second, a rate that is prohibitive due to the excessive heating of the laser rod that would occur. Although rotating-mirror-type Q-switches are cheap, reliable, and rugged, the method suffers from the major disadvantage of being slow. This results in an inefficient production of Q-switched pulses with lower peak power than can be produced by other methods.

Electro-optical, magneto-optical, and acousto-optical modulators can be used as fast Q-switches. If a Pockels cell (a doubly refractive crystal whose refractive state changes when an electric current is applied; in a Kerr cell, light produces the change), for example, is used and the laser output is not naturally polarized, then a polarizer must be placed in the cavity along with the electro-optical cell. A voltage is applied to the cell that converts the linearly polarized light into circularly polarized light. The laser mirror reflects this light and in so doing reverses its direction of rotation so that on passing through the electro-optical cell again it emerges as plane-polarized light, but at 90° to its original direction of polarization. This light is therefore not transmitted by the polarizer, and the cavity is switched off. When the voltage is reduced to zero, there is no rotation of the plane of polarization, and Q-switching occurs. The change of voltage, which is synchronized with the pumping mechanism, can be accomplished in less than 10 ns, and very effective Q-switching occurs. Alternative arrangements using Kerr cells and acousto-optical modulators are available. In the case of the acousto-optical modulator, an acoustical signal applied to the modulator deflects some of the beam out of the cavity, thereby creating a high loss. When the sound wave is shut off, Q-switching occurs as before. Acousto-optical devices are often used when the laser medium is continuously pumped and repetitively Q-switched, as is frequently the case with Nd:YAG and CO_2 lasers.

Passive Q-switching

Passive Q-switching may be accomplished by placing a saturable absorber (bleachable dye) in the cavity. At the beginning of the excitation, the dye is opaque, thereby preventing laser action and allowing a larger population inversion to be achieved than would otherwise be the case. Passive Q-switching has the great advantage of being extremely simple to implement, involving nothing more than a dye in a suitable solvent held in a transparent cell. Suitable dyes include cryptocyanine for ruby lasers and sulfur hexafluoride for CO_2 lasers. Lasers that use a saturable absorber for Q-switching are also mode locked if the dye, once bleached, recovers in a short time compared with the duration of the mode-locked pulses (see "Mode locking," above).

Nonlinear laser operation

With the giant pulse from a Q-switched laser, the effects of the light can no longer be considered as simple heat. The light is an electromagnetic wave, and the electrical field at the focus of these intense pulses can be as much as millions of volts per centimeter or even more. This electrical field increases as the square root of the power density and is equal to 1 million V/cm at a power level of 10^{10} or 10 billion W/cm^2. At a power density much above this, and one that can be obtained easily by focusing a Q-switched laser, a spark breakdown can be obtained in open air. Moreover, many otherwise transparent materials act in a manner referred to as *nonlinear* at these power levels. The nonlinearity refers to the relationship between the electrical field and its immediate effect—the electrical displacement. In a nonlinear medium it is possible to generate true optical harmonics that have twice or three or more times the frequency of the incident light with correspondingly short wavelengths. Thus a red light can be converted to ultraviolet, and under some circumstances, a very large fraction of this light can be so converted. Intense high-frequency vibrations may be set up inside transparent media under some conditions. This is all very well except that this nonlinear transformation may be into a frequency range that is more detrimental than useful. Case in point—193 nm ultraviolet. Some investigators have noted that tissue treated with this wavelength often glows with a visible blue color.

The explanation of nonlinear effects lies in the way in which a beam of light propagates through a solid. The nuclei and associated electrons of the solid form electrical dipoles. The electromagnetic radiation interacts with these dipoles, causing them to oscillate, which in turn causes the dipoles themselves to act as sources of electromagnetic radiation. If the amplitude of the vibration is small, the dipoles emit radiation of the same frequency as the inciting radiation. If this radiation is intense (irradiance increases), the relationship between this intensity increase and the induced dipole vibration becomes nonlinear, resulting in the generation of harmonics of the original radiation. Thus frequency doubling or second harmonic generation (or higher) occurs.

Nonlinear optics is a very large and complicated subject, and there are many possible phenomena that have been investigated in some simple materials and are becoming reasonably well understood but that have not been much explored in biologic material. It is quite conceivable that such high-power lasers, emitting red light, could produce the chemical and biologic effects of ultraviolet light inside some material that the ultraviolet itself could not penetrate. Some chemical reactions that ordinarily require ultraviolet light have been demonstrated to be producible by intense red light. Lest anyone think that these effects are to be feared at all power levels, however, it must be pointed out that many of these effects have a threshold, and they do not occur at all below this threshold power level. It seems fairly certain that at power levels of a kilowatt or so, most of the effects observed in most materials can be understood simply as rapid heating effects, without specifically considering the electromagnetic and nonlinear phenomena.

The processes of nonlinear optics can be used to generate new wavelengths from existing lasers. With care, relatively high conversion efficiencies can be obtained even at levels so low that nonlinear effects in most materials are not ordinarily noticeable. Special nonlinear materials such as lithium niobate and barium sodium niobate have been used to generate optical harmonics, producing green light from the infrared neodymium glass or garnet lasers. In this way, continuous or repetitively pulsed lasers with average powers on the order of 1 W in the green can be constructed. The nonlinear material also makes it possible to construct tunable laser-type devices. Basically, these consist of some kind of a driving laser and a converter that converts the light to other desired wavelengths.

Gaseous lasers

One of the simplest kinds of lasers is that using a gas discharge of the sort common to a neon sign or a related electrical discharge at a different pressure and voltage condition. The gas-discharge laser consists of a long, narrow tube containing the gas or a mixture of gases with mirrors at the end of this column. No separate pumping lamp is needed. The first of these gas-discharge lasers pulsed a mixture of helium and neon gas (He-Ne), with about 10 times as much helium as neon. The combined effect of these two gases is to strongly excite a few particular levels in neon during the discharge so that laser action can be obtained at several wavelengths in the infrared and visible regions. The exact wavelength is usually determined by coating the mirrors to be good reflectors for only a particular wavelength and not for other possible wavelengths that the medium can amplify. Most often, these helium-neon lasers are operated in the visible orange-red region at a wavelength of 6328 Å. Helium-neon lasers are used very commonly as aiming beams for other laser systems as well as for other devices and purposes.

Small helium-neon lasers give power outputs on the order of 1 mW, which produces a small, bright-appearing spot on a white surface but is not intense enough to do much burning. For example, such as laser can be used to generate the coherent light beam used to measure an optical surface (see Chapter 6) or serve as a lecture pointer. A continuous beam of even 1-mW power has many other laboratory uses and demonstrates very easily the peculiar properties of coherent light. When the beam from a helium-neon laser or any other continuous visible laser illuminates a surface, the surface has an unusual characteristic grainy, sparkling appearance. This occurs because the light from the laser is coherent, and any part of the wavefront can interfere with any other part of the wavefront constructively (adding up to a higher intensity) or destructively (producing a lower intensity). After the light is scattered by a rough surface, for instance, a wall or a piece of paper, the waves from individual points spread out in all directions and overlap at many places in space and produce a three-dimensional interference pattern that the eye perceives. This complex interference pattern shifts when the eye is moved even slightly, so the surface appears to sparkle. However, if the *surface* is moving, even fairly slowly, the pattern is averaged out so that the graininess and sparkling disappear. The size of the sparkle pattern depends on where the eye is focused; thus the pattern can be used as an indicator of the eye's focus.

Helium-neon lasers can be built with power outputs as high as several hundred milliwatts, or even up to 1 W. However, it is usually easier to obtain such power levels from other gas-discharge lasers by means of higher currents, narrower tubes, and lower gas pressures. These lasers use such gases as argon, krypton, and xenon. The gas is ionized in the electrical discharge, and laser emission occurs from particular energy levels of ions. Krypton can produce a number of wavelengths from the red to the violet. Argon gas lasers can easily give 1 W or more of green light at a wavelength of 4880 Å. Argon lasers have been used for surgery of various kinds because the focal spot is intense enough to produce rapid heating. Moreover, the wavelength of the argon laser is short enough and the power density in the absorbing region is high enough to be strongly absorbed by hemoglobin so that the heating can be much more sharply localized. These gas lasers also can be pulsed either singly or repetitively, but their peak powers are usually not nearly as high as those from the solid-state lasers.

There are many other types of gas lasers that produce light with wavelengths varying from the ultraviolet through the visible and infrared regions out even to the millimeter-wavelength radio region. Most notable of these is the carbon dioxide laser, which operates in the infrared at a wavelength of 10.6 μm (106,000 Å). This laser is relatively efficient, perhaps 30%, and can be made in large sizes. Power outputs from several hundred to many thousand watts can be obtained in a well-directed beam. The carbon dioxide radiation is absorbed by almost every nonmetallic material and can produce extremely intense heating and rapid burning, cutting, or drilling if high powers are used.

There are still other types of lasers, including optically pumped liquids. Some of these use solutions of organic dyes. Since many fluorescent dyes are known, it is possible to select one for any desired wavelength region in or near the visible portion of the spectrum. The output wavelength even can be controlled to some extent by varying the solvent or by mixing two dyes in different proportions. Fine control of the wavelength may require incorporating a prism or diffraction grating in the instrument to limit the wavelength distribution within the beam.

Semiconductor lasers

Semiconductor lasers have the appearance of a small transistor or rectifying diode but are made of materials such as gallium arsenide or indium antimonide (Figure 11.7). They also can be quite efficient, not requiring the pumping action of light but only an electrical pulse; thus they are simpler to construct. Current solid-state diode lasers deliver 808 nm of laser light at various power levels. Most semiconductor lasers operate in the far-red or infrared region. However, semiconductor lasers are usually made only in small sizes; to obtain much power for more than a short instant requires that they be operated in arrays, using a considerable number of them. Some can be operated continuously but most easily when they are cooled to temperatures well below room temperature. A typical

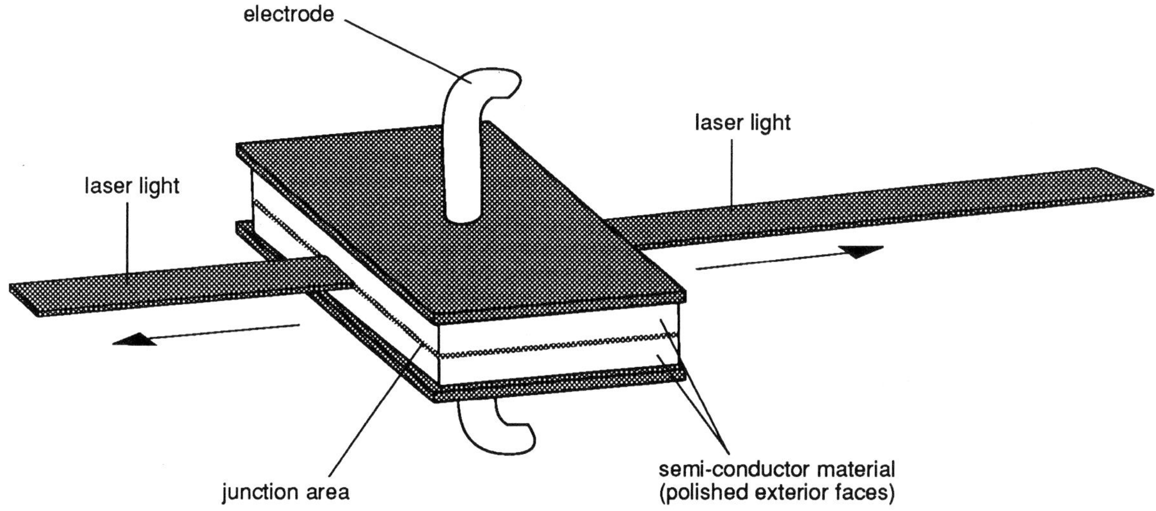

Fig. 11.7 Solid-state laser.

single-diode laser operated at room temperature might give 10,000 pulses per second, each pulse lasting 1000 billionths of a second and having a peak power of about 10 W. The total energy in each pulse is thus about 1 millionth of a joule, and the average power over many pulses and intervals between them is about 0.001 W.

Clinical applications of laser light

Lasers were used in ophthalmology almost as soon as they had become available. In 1961, Campbell and his group began work in New York, and in 1962, my fellow Kresge alumnus Chris Zweng began his work in Pal Alto—both with a pulsed ruby laser [8,9]. In 1966, L'Esperance and his group started with the argon laser in animals, carrying it to humans in 1968. Commercial argon lasers became available in 1971—the author purchased one of the first ones when he was director of the Laser and Fluorescein Angiography Clinic at Harper Hospital in Detroit. The year 1971 also saw the first work being done with the krypton and frequency-doubled neodymium-yttrium-aluminum-garnet (Nd:YAG) lasers at Harkness Eye Institute. In Detroit, Beckman was doing work with the CO_2 laser [10], and in 1972, Krasnov performed the first laser trabeculectomy with a Q-switched ruby laser [11].

Medical laser applications are big business. Millions of dollars have been expended to produce instrumentation to meet (or stimulate) market demand. With the current interest in these devices to modify corneal curvature, the game often has been played with something less than the full spirit of fair play and occasionally divorced from the scientific spirit as well. However, the rapid technological development continues despite the concern expressed that method patents issued to single persons and companies would discourage diverse corporate investment and hamper investigation by a broad range of researchers [12] (Table 11.1).

Tissue response to light energy

Before we get too heavily involved in the details of lasers and their application in ophthalmology, we need to consider the effect of light energy on living tissue. Light, much like oxygen, can produce profound cellular changes—many of them in the "not good" category. Case in point—skin cancer or, less ominous (but more painful), sunburn. Mutagenesis, however, is only part of the spectrum of interactions between cells and light—some reactions are more subtle, and not all are bad.

Currently, we have laser systems that alter tissue using photochemical, photothermal, and photodisruptive techniques. Photocoagulation occurs when light energy is

Table 11.1 The effective output wavelength of various lasers

Laser type	Wavelength (nm)
Excimer (F2)	157
Excimer (ArF)	193
Excimer (KrF)	248
Excimer (XeCl)	308
Helium–cadmium (He–Cd)	325
Nitrogen (N2)	327
Argon (Ar)	488/514.5
Krypton (Kr)	458/548/647
Copper vapor (Cu)	510.6/578.2
Rhodamine G	560–640
Gold vapor	627.8
Helium–neon (He–Ne)	632.8
Ruby	694.3
Gallium arsenide	905
Neodymium:YAG (Nd:YAG)	1064
Erbium	1228
Hydrogen fluoride (HF)	2900
Erbium:YAG (Er:YAG)	2900
Color center	2900
Raman	2900
Carbon dioxide	10600

absorbed by the target tissue and converted to heat. The reaction can be anything from protein denaturization to carbonization to vaporization. Most ophthalmologists are familiar with the effects produced by the argon laser used to treat various forms of retinopathy and in laser trabeculectomy. There are newer laser tissue coagulators—among which are solid-state diode lasers—all providing energy in many forms. Dye lasers are available that have either continuous or pulsed output. Mid-infrared solid-state crystal lasers deliver wavelengths anywhere from 1.96 μm (thulium:YAG) and 2.1 μm (holmium:YAG) to 3 μm (erbium:YAG)—all delivering useful wavelengths and energy fluxes. The range of tunable systems is even wider. In addition, tunable lasers can deliver continuous output or pulsed energy, making them valuable for surgical tasks ranging from coagulation to controlled tissue ablation.

Excimer lasers, with pulsed output in the ultraviolet (UV) range, have a unique combination of properties that makes them suitable for corneal surgery at 193 nm as well as lens fragmentation and tissue drilling at 308 nm. These lasers operate through a singular process known as *ablative photodecomposition*. Because organic materials have a strong absorbance for UV radiation below 300 nm, this part of the light spectrum is very powerful in its ability to produce destructive effects within these tissues (Figure 11.8). UV photons are highly energetic and can directly break chemical bonds, which is the key to their effectiveness, but also to their potential danger. UV radiance breaks protein molecules into diatomic and triatomic fragments, which, because of the tremendous energy transfer taking place, are blown clear of the illuminated area. These particles, by being blown away, take with them much of the surplus energy within the system and thus prevent more than minimal thermal damage to surrounding tissue (Figure 11.9).

The jury is still out on other forms of damage. UV light is well known to be both mutagenic and carcinogenic—We have mentioned skin cancer—its effects in the cornea are only now being examined [13–24]. Seiler's observation of secondary fluorescence of corneal tissue during excimer ablation is troubling, as is Clarke's finding of free radicals following laser angioplasty [25]. Nuss and coworkers concluded that 193-nm UV light has little, if any, mutagenic effect on corneal tissue [27]. However, effects such as cascading could elicit secondary UV wavelengths of a more deleterious nature [28].

Lasers currently under clinical evaluation and testing operate in ranges from the far-ultraviolet to the mid-infrared. Almost every wavelength region in the electromagnetic spectrum has a potential clinical application. Many factors, including variations in wavelength, continuous or pulsed delivery pattern, amount of total energy out of total energy applied, and the delivery system of the laser light, will produce a wide range of clinical effects. Numerous studies examining these potential applications are legion; a few examples:

- Researchers are injecting chromophores (indocyanine green) to enhance retinal vascular coagulation.

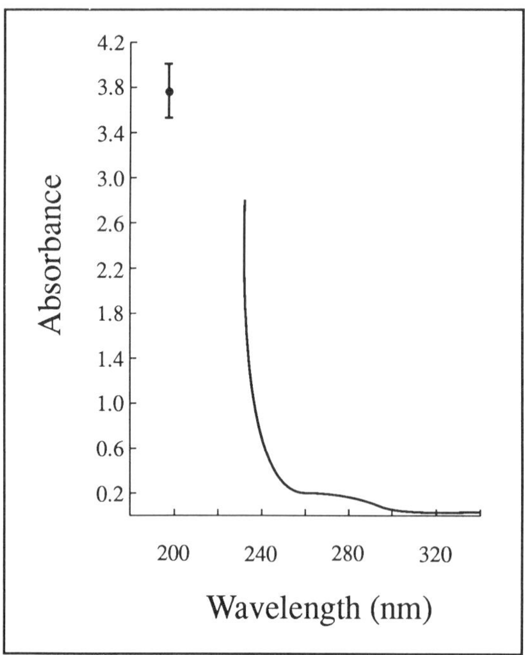

Fig. 11.8 Plot of absorbance versus wavelength in the far-ultraviolet spectrum for bovine cornea. The point at 193 nm represents the average of laser transmission measurements made on eight different 32-μm-thick samples. The error bar indicates 1 s.d. (from Puliafito CA, Steinert RF, Deutsch TF, Hillenkamp F, Dehm EJ, Adler CM. Excimer laser ablation of the cornea and lens. Experimental studies. Ophthalmology 1985; 92:741–748).

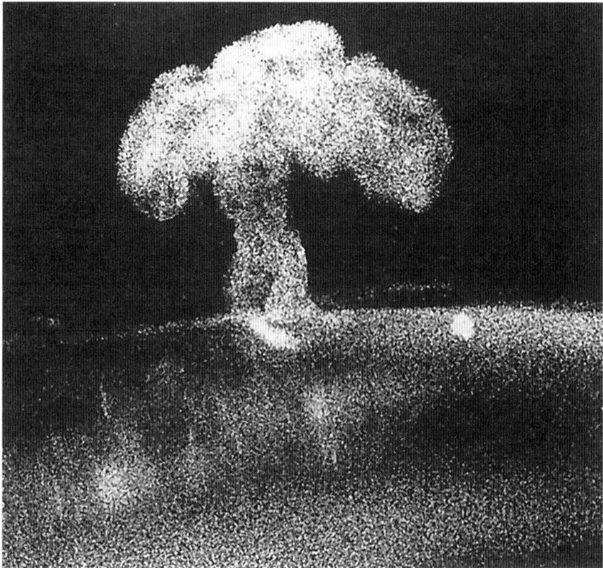

Fig. 11.9 Ablation plume during laser corneal photoablation at 193 nm (from Puliafito CA, Stern D, Krueger RR, Mandel ER. High-speed photography of excimer laser ablation of the cornea. Arch Ophthalmol 1987; 105(9):1255–9).

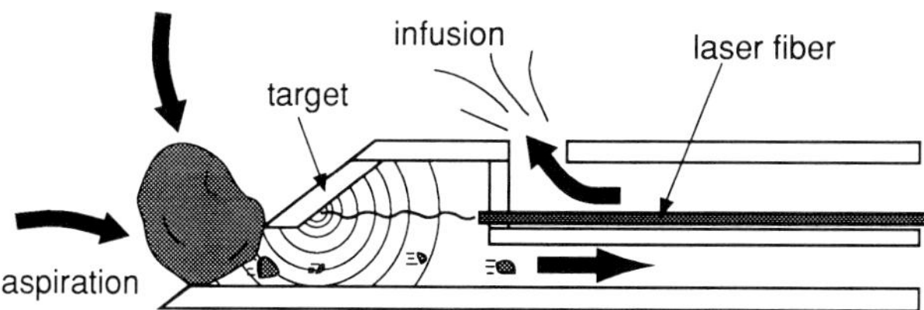

Fig. 11.10 Laser phakolysis.

• Successful filtering procedures are being done using pulsed laser light aimed gonioscopically into the angle, which has previously been saturated with methylene blue dye using iontophoresis. Absorption and ablation are sufficiently enhanced by the presence of the dye and the short laser pulses to produce a draining fistula.
• Investigators seeking applications in general surgery have used light absorption by dye-fibrin mixtures stabilized in a viscous medium to seal blood vessels in animals and humans.
• Reshaping of the corneal surface to change its refracting properties is being done through direct effect or through doping of the tissue with photoreactive materials.
• The laser might also possibly be used to remove cataracts (Figure 11.10; see also below).

Safety

Of course, new technical devices such as lasers also present us with moral, economic, and intellectual challenges. First, we must be mindful that lasers have unique hazards. As new wavelengths evolve, we must study not only unexpected effects of the laser light but also any other hazards associated with use of the instrument (see discussion above on UV lasers). Safety for the surgeon, surgical assistants, and any other operating room staff requires safety glasses tailored to the particular laser wavelength in use. The excimer is a typical example of a laser that introduces a new potential hazard. There is the small matter—with excimer lasers—of the extremely toxic fluorine gas used in these devices. Fluorine gas management is new in the clinical environment and requires special planning and laser design for safe use. Proper venting of the laser and the treatment room are essential—the toxicity of the gas is extremely high.

According to the Occupational Safety and Health Administration (OSHA), delayed effects such as photoretinitis, accelerated aging of biologic tissue, cataractogenesis, and carcinogenesis can result from laser exposure. Depending on the wavelength and exposure dose, these impairments can be irreversible. Laser side effects can be initiated in three ways: thermally, photochemically, or both. They are thermally initiated in the infrared spectrum and photochemically initiated in the ultraviolet spectrum. In the visible blue end of the spectrum, both processes can begin. Factors that can contribute to undesirable effects include total exposure time, pulse duration, the various absorption spectra of different biologic systems, and wavelength. Regardless of the wavelength involved, there is a time-dependent and a wavelength-dependent effect. While exposure time determines the major risk factors for potential thermal damage from infrared laser light, wavelength still determines the relative penetration depth of the energy. Exposure time, by the rule of additivity (which applies to most photochemical damage mechanisms), a very low dose rate, or irradiance may be potentially hazardous when accumulated over a full procedure. The safety limit for all UV lasers with wavelengths less than 311 nm, such as the argon-fluoride or krypton-fluoride laser, is probably at 3 mJ/cm^2 per day.

Pulse duration

Short pulses allow very little time for heat flow; therefore, depth of damage remains wavelength-dependent. However, for continuous-wave lasers, such as the carbon dioxide lasers, heat flow completely masks the selective absorption effects of the laser's very different penetration depths.

Absorption

During photoablation, the cornea absorbs 100 W of the energy from wavelengths shorter than 280 nm. It absorbs more than 90 W of photon energy when the wavelength increases to 300 nm, but about 1 photon in 50 reaches the lens. At 360 nm, the lens absorbs most photons.

Wavelength

Wavelengths much longer than 320 nm are not energetic enough to break bonds, and wavelengths shorter than 300 nm are absorbed by the cornea. Thus an acute cataract can result from only a narrow band of wavelengths. In vitro tests have shown that use of the 193-nm wave (excimer) is associated with very little evidence of mutagenesis or carcinogenesis. Both the penetration depth of the radiation and the absorption spectrum of the DNA in each cell determine how mutagenic a given wavelength of laser light will be, according to Seiler [24]. In theory, he says, the penetration depth of laser radiation should be approximately one-half a cell's diameter to enter the nucleus and to produce mutagenic effects. Seiler further cautions that even though we know that 193 nm is a very efficient wavelength for doing refractive and curative corneal ablation, we still have to keep in mind that while the risk of creating mutagenic effects is very small, it is not zero. The risk is also wavelength-dependent. The risk from 193 nm radiation is 1000 to 10,000 times less than the risk from 248-nm radiation, for example [29].

Although reports on the mutagenicity of short-wave (193-nm) UV laser light are contradictory, no doubts exist as to the potential of 248-nm laser light to induce DNA repair mechanisms [24,27]. Light at 308 nm has a low threshold for the induction of cataract [30]. Since secondary radiation (for reasons governed by physical laws in the longer-wavelength range) is known to be emitted from the area of 193-nm laser light impact, a cataractogenic potential of far-UV light cannot be completely excluded.

The FDA's biggest concern regarding excimer laser treatment of myopia was to rule out any association with excessive scarring, poor healing, or recurrent erosion despite the preclinical research used to establish the fluence levels and repetition rates. Although re-epithelialization has been shown to occur quickly after laser treatment and does not appear to be a problem, the mode of cell attachment is not wholly normal. For example, Bowman's layer does not re-form and is, instead, replaced by a pseudomembrane. Endothelial injury also has been seen [31]. It is unlikely that this will prove to be a problem given the experience with RK. However, it must be remembered that the effects of light on living tissue are insidious and still incompletely understood.

Excimer laser applications

High-power pulsed UV laser light has been shown to precisely etch not only synthetic material [32] but also biologic tissues such as atherosclerotic lesions [33], hair and cartilage [34], and skin [35] and for use in neurosurgery and angioplasty [36–38].

Steve Trokel and the history of the excimer laser in ophthalmology

Author's note: *The author is grateful to Steven Trokel, M.D. for his gracious assistance and permission to use much of the material contained within this history—which is from his personal archives.*

Excimer lasers had their birth in 1975 when two physical chemists, Velazco and Setser, working at Kansas State University, noted that certain physical properties of the metastable states of rare gas atoms resembled those of the alkali metals. They reported that they found a similarity of the chemical properties of metastable xenon atoms (Xe) to sodium and lithium in their ability to react with halogens (such as fluorine) to produce an unstable compound, Xe (fluorine, chlorine, etc.) [39–42]. The halogens fluorine and chlorine exist in a gaseous state under normal temperatures and are highly active. High pressure is necessary, however, because the so-called noble gases are a standoffish lot whose atoms do not mix well with the madding crowd of other atoms—hence the name *noble.* However, under certain circumstances—such as high pressure—they are crowded together, and they knock each other about sufficiently so as to partially ionize. In this state they can be induced to form unstable combinations with other atoms.

This noble gas–halogen compound rapidly dissociates to the ground state of the individual molecules with the release of an energetic UV photon—and therein lies the significance. Velazco and Setser inferred from this that the diatomic noble gas–halides were of special interest because ". . . these bound-free emissions have considerable potential as ultraviolet laser systems for excitation of mixtures of xenon (or other rare gases) and halogen-containing compounds." Such a laser would have widespread application in the plastics industry as well as in designing and building semiconductor systems. It has other intriguing possibilities as well. All that was needed was a big enough stick to get the wasps moving.

A few months following their suggestion that this metastable compound could be used as the basis of a laser, four molecules, XeF, XeCl, XeBr, and KrF, were observed to undergo light amplification by stimulated emission when they were excited by an electron beam under proper conditions. Hoffman, for example, in early 1976 observed laser action at 1933 Å from the ArF molecule [43]. The energy source used to pump this laser was a 2-MeV electron beam with 6 kJ of beam energy—a big stick indeed. This system was cumbersome and of limited practical use for widespread experiments—linear accelerators are somewhat bulky. It was not until later that same year that sufficient experimentation showed that a more practical laser system could be constructed. Instead of requiring a linear accelerator to produce the electron beam, Burnham demonstrated laser action with ArF in a relatively compact device using a transverse electrical discharge akin to lightning [44]. The space required to house such a device was thus brought down from a building to room size.

Preionized discharge had long been used in infrared molecular lasers, and Burnham's demonstration that the technology would work in the UV range led to the development of practical UV lasers. Burnham and coworkers had used a modified Tachisto CO_2 laser for their work, so it was not surprising that Tachisto was the first company to market a laser designed to operate in the UV end of the spectrum. By the close of 1976, laser action had been demonstrated for the biologically important UV wavelengths from 193 nm using ArF to 351 nm using XeF.

As always, once something has been born, it is within the nature of human beings to christen it with a name. Nomenclature for these early UV lasers was mixed. The word *excimer* had been coined by Stevens in 1960 as a contraction of *excited dimer* to describe an energized molecule with two identical components—hence it was a natural for this situation [45]. When analyzing the action of these lasers, it was thought that the argon molecule formed an "excited dimer" during the preionization phase of its excitation. This ultimately was found not to be true, yet the term persisted. Alternative names have been used for these lasers and include *rare gas halide lasers*, which describes the gas mixture in the cavity, and the name of the specific gas mixture (e.g., argon-fluoride laser) to describe a specific system. Another name was suggested when the actual lasing compound was recognized to be an "excited complex molecule" consisting of two different elements, the rare gas and the halide. Some workers suggested that this was best described as an "excited molecular complex," and the word *exciplex* was coined to describe the lasers—but it does not ring, if the truth were told. Excimer won through because it has the virtue of greater simplicity and the perversity of being first, although the other terms continue to be used to describe these laser systems.

Subsequently, the potential medical and industrial applications of these new lasers were the subject of a meeting at the 1977 Optical Society of America. In the next few years, a great deal of discussion began appearing in the optical and electronics literature, as well as in the press [46–49]. By 1978, both Tachisto and Lambda Physik (in Gottingen, Germany) were marketing excimer lasers for laboratory use.

Taboada was the first to investigate the ocular biologic interactions of these new lasers [50]. Tests were made on the response of rabbit epithelium to ArF exposures at the Laser Effects Branch of the Radiation Sciences Division at the USAF School of Aerospace Medicine. Taboada had considerable experience studying damage thresholds within the eye, having investigated the effects of mode-locked and Q-switched Nd:YAG laser pulses on ocular tissues in the past. ArF exposure on the rabbit cornea was noted to produce either opacification or fluorescein staining that took the general shape of the laser beam distribution. In a subsequent study of the damage effects of 193-nm ArF laser light on the eye, Taboada reported the first studies of the interaction of this far-UV light with the cornea, looking for damage similar to that produced by the ArF (248-nm) beam [51].

Steve Trokel, who had, at that time, considerable interest in lasers, especially Nd:YAG systems, was preparing a clinical monograph describing high-powered pulsed Nd:YAG lasers. He invited Taboada to contribute a chapter describing the effects of pulsed lasers on ocular tissues. Taboada accordingly sent him reprints of his published papers and a chapter for the monograph that included a more detailed description of the excimer laser–cornea interaction. Trokel's attention was immediately caught by a phrase Taboada used to describe the effect on the cornea of the ArF laser radiation at varying energy levels:

> At the higher levels, exposures of 27.5 mJ/cm^2 or greater, an immediate indentation of the corneal surface appeared taking the shape of the beam. One hour later, the surface indentation would fill in.

Taboada postulated that the far-UV light "was resonantly captured in random electromagnetic cavities formed by the microprojections of the anterior epithelial cell layer, which may have caused a preferential temperature jump in this thin layer of tissue." This, of course, should have produced a swelling, not an indentation. His observation of an indentation suggested to Trokel that tissue was being removed not heated, and he sought access to an excimer laser to study this phenomenon and to verify his proposition. If his idea was correct, perhaps it would be possible to use this technology to perform more precise RK. It seemed that the technical limits of knife incision technology might be overcome by using a laser technique that would create a more predictable incision to follow the corneal curve. However, Trokel also considered the possibility that laser keratomileusis could be done by directly removing tissue from the corneal surface to modify its curve. This idea was seen as somewhat droll and was not greeted with enthusiasm. Accurate control of tissue removal to the standard of precision that would allow the cornea to heal with normal optical properties was considered somewhat farfetched.

Only experimentation could confirm the surgical potential of these laser systems, and in the beginning of 1983, Trokel spent considerable time seeking access to an excimer laser. His efforts bore fruit when he was introduced to Rameesh Srinivasan, a photochemist working with the argon-fluoride excimer laser at IBM's TJ Watson Laboratories in New York.

Srinivasan showed Trokel his own studies in which he had described the ablation of plastics using 193-nm laser light. Srinivasan discussed the applications of this modality to other organic materials, which included ablating fine grooves in a strand of human hair. Describing the effect of 193-nm light on plastic, Srinivasan wrote: "A threshold . . . for ablative photodecomposition . . . was measured at 10 mJ/cm^2. Thus, one pulse at 16 mJ/cm^2 gave an etch mark that was clearly visible in reflection, whereas 50 pulses at 4 mJ/cm^2 pulse did not leave any etch mark . . ." [52]. At this point, the possibility of optical "fine-tuning" of the corneal surface seemed at once less droll and more reasonable. Only further experimentation would show the utility of this method to cut clear cornea (Figure 11.11).

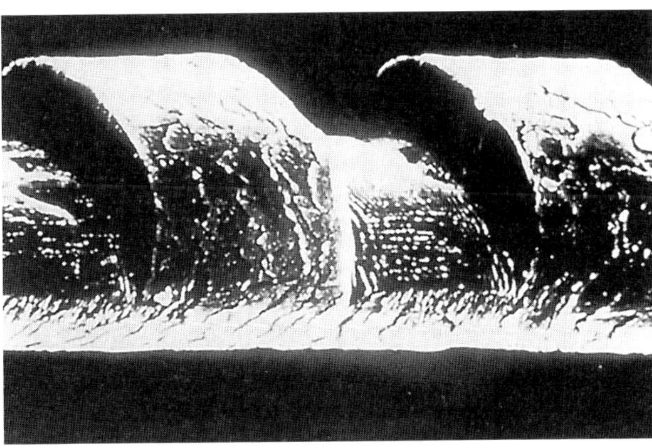

Fig. 11.11 Electron micrograph of grooves cut into a hair by an excimer laser.

Following the first reports by Taboada and coworkers on the response of the corneal epithelium to ArF and KrF excimer laser pulses in 1981, Trokel and colleagues achieved a precise linear ablation of bovine (veal) cornea with 193-nm radiation [53]. The first eye done showed a crisply edged groove, made deeper in successive sections. Histologic analysis showed no collateral damage and a uniquely smooth ablated surface (Figure 11.12). Srinivasan's collaboration proved to be of enormous value. In particular, he was able to define the correct pulse rates and the minimal irradiances necessary to achieve the desired effect. Furthermore, his lasers were fully calibrated, and their beam profiles had been carefully studied, allowing the achievement of particularly clean cuts. Homogeneity of the laser beam is paramount to accurate wide-surface ablation and to depth control—a problem still.

The results of these experiments and the essentials of the ArF excimer laser–cornea interaction were reported in 1983 [53]. The investigators demonstrated that they were able to remove a fraction of a micron of corneal tissue with each pulse of the laser light—data showed a removal rate of about 0.25 mm of tissue per pulse. Further, the resulting surfaces were shown to be extremely uniform and smooth. On biomicroscopic examination and by light microscopy, no damage to the adjacent stroma was observed. Electron microscopy revealed an extremely narrow three-banded zone of damage (each band of 0.07 mm). Lastly, it was possible to control the shape and pattern of tissue removed by adjusting the distribution of the incident laser beam. Possible surgical applications of the ArF laser both to cut slits in the cornea that would resemble an incision and to remove large areas of tissue to produce a controlled laser lamellar keratectomy—laser keratomileusis—were discussed.

Trokel visited the Lambda Physik facility in mid-1983 immediately after the first series of experiments was completed. The people there provided him with a model 102 excimer laser for his laboratory at Columbia, and they showed him how to obtain a 9-mm beam circle of sufficient fluence to ablate tissue. During this trip, Trokel also visited Heroldsberg to discuss these early results with Reinhardt Thyzel, who was then owner of Meditec Laser Company, one of the first companies to produce a clinical Nd:YAG laser. Thyzel believed that this laser–cornea interaction would be the technique for producing an improved version of RK, and he began development of a medical excimer laser project straightaway.

Most of the emphasis at that time was on application of the excimer laser to perform RK. There are obvious limitations to the RK technique, among them incision depth control—still an elusive problem, even for that marvel of human ingenuity, the laser. When Trokel showed slides of these first corneal tissue excisions, the impact was profound, because we had all been accustomed to seeing laser interactions that produced extensive destruction of surrounding tissues [54]. The preservation of the tissue contours was remarkable and strengthened the premise that this modality could be applied in a clinical setting (Figure 11.13). In planning experiments, the necessity for development of an effective delivery system quickly became apparent, as did the realization that this application would

(a)

(b)

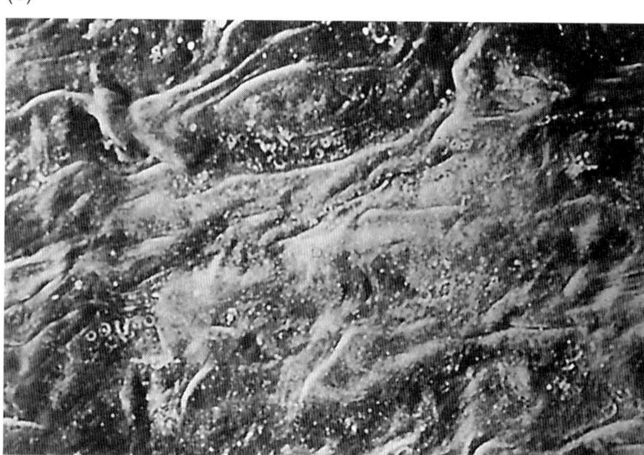

Fig. 11.12 Comparison of a corneal button cut with a trephine (a); and a laser (b).

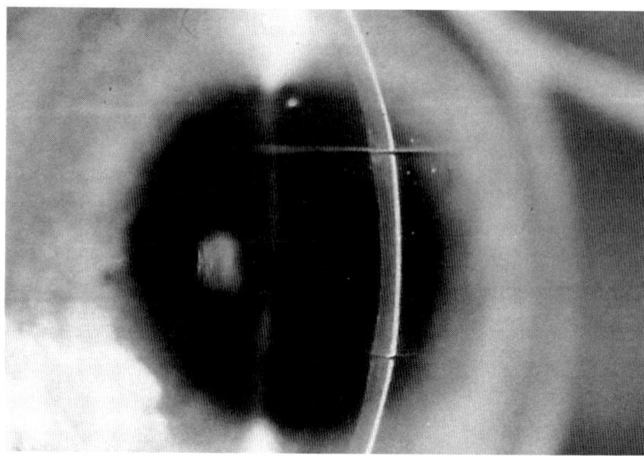

Fig. 11.13 T-cuts made in a human cornea with the excimer laser.

require support and help from industry. Furthermore, there were many questions about excimer laser functions and UV laser optics that required considerable technical expertise.

Earlier attempts had been made to alter the corneal refractive power by direct mechanical tissue ablation techniques [55,56]. However, a strong presumption that maintenance of Bowman's layer was essential to maintain epithelial integrity and thus stromal transparency existed [57,58]. However, no one had as yet been able to cut a completely smooth surface on a cornea—so the jury was still out.

One of the first experiments done with the new Lambda Physik laser was to remove a large, 9-mm-×-9-mm square of corneal stroma from a rabbit cornea. Neal Burstein, who was studying electrical potentials across the corneal endothelium, showed that the treated cornea retained a normal electrical potential across its surface.

In the spring of 1984, Trokel and Marshall did a series of collaborative investigations. Using a crude delivery system, they went on to study the texture of the ablated corneal surface (Figure 11.14), as well as the ultrastructural detail of each layer of the cornea. Animal corneas were exposed to the laser radiation in the New York laboratory and immediately taken to London to Marshall's laboratory. In 1984, Trokel would produce lesions on rabbit and monkey corneas on Thursday mornings, pack the enucleated eyes in ice, and grab a cab to JFK Airport. He would arrive at Heathrow at 7:00 A.M., take the underground to Russell Square, and walk the two blocks to Judd Street, where Marshall's laboratory was located. These studies were first done on rabbit corneas and then in monkey eyes, both acutely and after healing. Most impressive was the smoothness of the ablated area and the optical quality of the re-epithelialized healed surface [59–63].

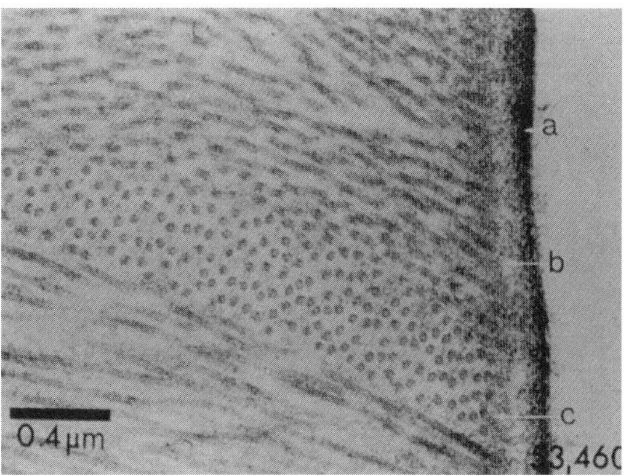

Fig. 11.14 High-power electron micrograph of an excimer laser ablated surface. Three zones of structural abnormalities approximately 0.7 µm in thickness can be identified: (a) an outer densely staining region, (b) a middle lightly staining region; and (c) an inner region showing some increasing staining in an area where the fine structure of the collagen is partially preserved (from Puliafito CA, Steinert RF, Deutsch TF, Hillenkamp F, Dehm EJ, Adler CM. Excimer laser ablation of the cornea and lens. Experimental studies. Ophthalmology 1985; 92(6):741–748).

Meanwhile, in New York, Ronald Krueger, an electrical engineer (then a medical student), helped Trokel investigate the nature of the laser–tissue interaction. They determined thresholds, ablation rates, and healing patterns and measured ablation parameters at all available excimer wavelengths [64–66] (Figures 11.15 and 11.16).

Particularly interesting were the results of studies in which Trokel's group created a fungal corneal ulcer and excised a large circular disk of tissue that healed the ulcer without producing corneal haze [67,68]. This gave impetus to the thought that the excimer, by virtue of its ability

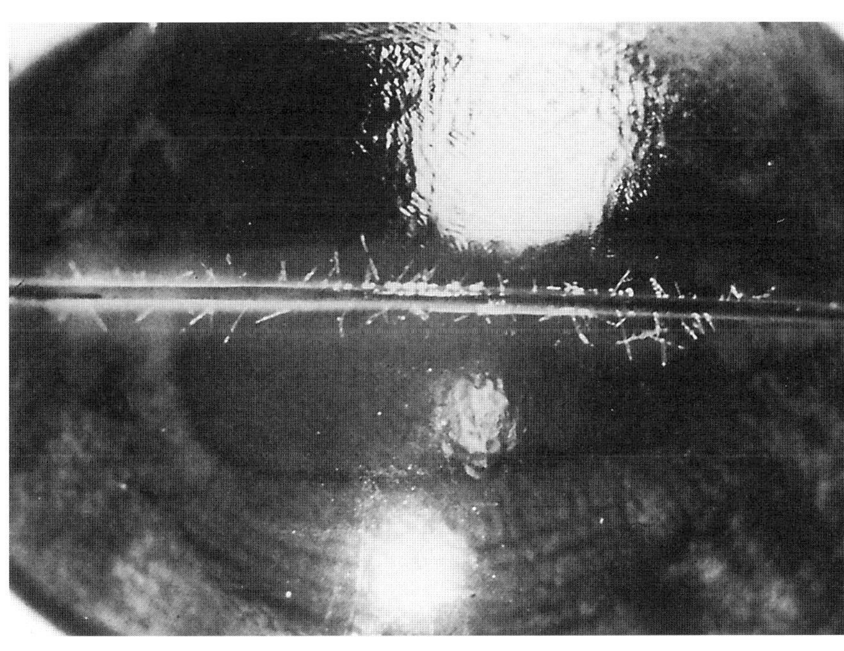

Fig. 11.15 Linear cracks extending laterally from a 249-nm ablated incision. These appear shortly above threshold and disappear at higher irradiances. They have been unique to 249-nm irradiated tissues (from Krueger RR, Trokel SL, Schubert HD. Interaction of ultraviolet laser light with the cornea. Invest Ophthalmol Visual Sci 1985; 26:1455–1464).

(a)

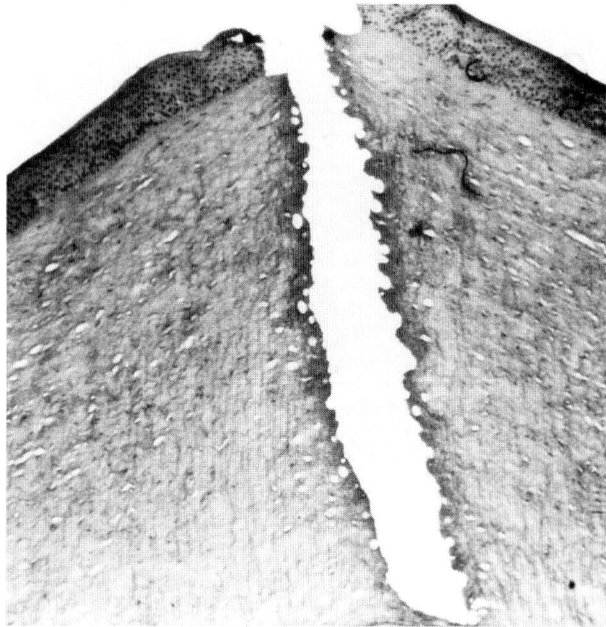

(b)

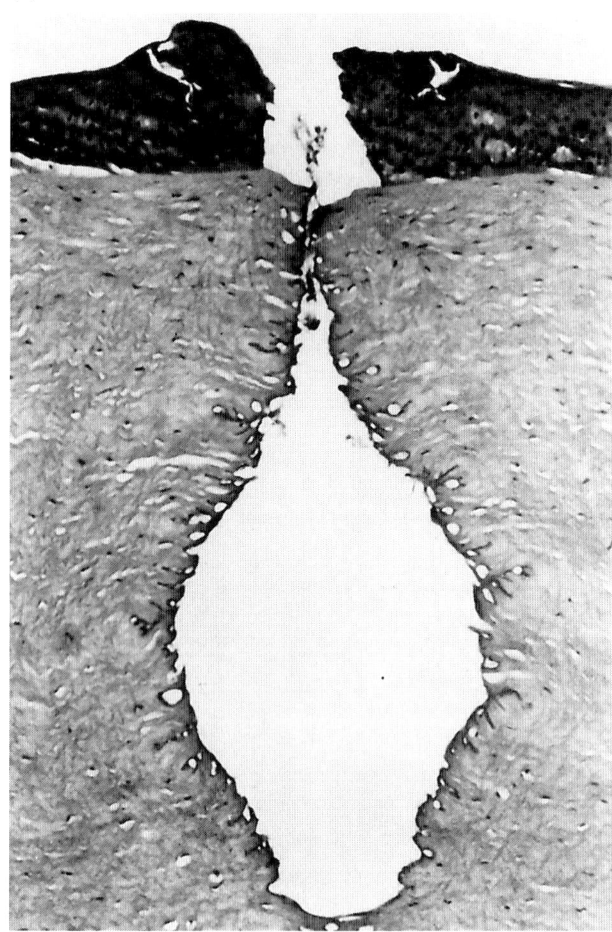

(c)

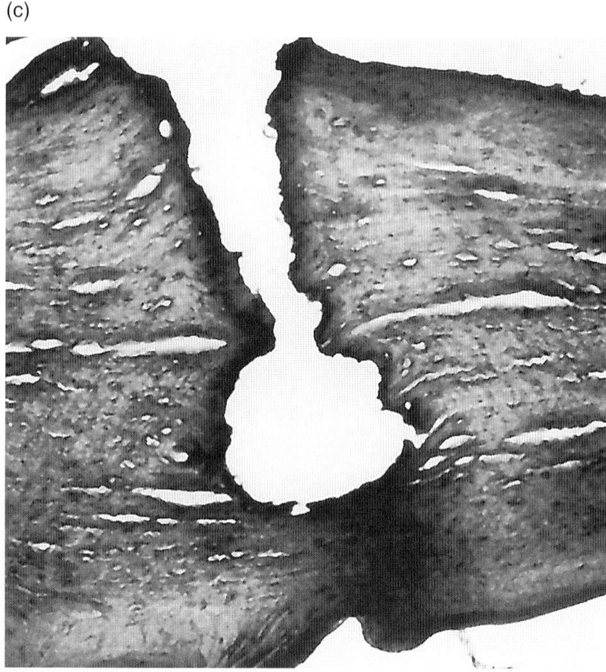

Fig. 11.16 The stromal lesions produced with 249-nm radiation. (a) Linear lesion with parallel walls produced at supra-ablation irradiance. (b) Incision walls bulge as irradiance is increased. The bulging is probably due to gas pressure formed by the greater thermal irradiance. (c) Lesion produced when both irradiance and firing rate are increased. The walls and floor of the lesion show increasing thermal effects with actual melting and dissolution of the stroma. Original magnification ×24 (from Krueger RR, Trokel SL, Schubert HD. Interaction of ultraviolet laser light with the cornea. Invest Ophthalmol Visual Sci 1985; 26:1455–1464).

to produce extremely fine-layered ablations with minimal tissue interaction, could be used therapeutically—perhaps even to excise scar tissue [69,70].

At the same time, Munnerlyn was at work deriving the quantitative relationships associated with removing corneal tissue. He had calculated that for a 4-mm optical zone, only 5 mm of tissue need be removed to reduce the corneal refractive power by 1 D. At Munnerlyn's urging, Trokel ablated a series of 3-mm circles in rabbit corneas to progressively increased depths. Several weeks after they had healed, only the eye with the deepest ablated zone showed any stromal haze; the others had healed without discernible opacification by slit-lamp examination. These experiments gave Munnerlyn and others in the industry the impetus to proceed with the development of clinical excimer laser systems.

Munnerlyn wrote a paper using the results of these early animal studies to show the relationship of tissue removal to optical zone size to achieve a given optical effect. The formula states

$$\text{depth of ablation} = \frac{\text{diopters of change}}{3} \times \left(\begin{array}{c}\text{diameter of}\\ \text{optical zone}\end{array}\right)^2$$

For example, a 6-mm optical zone, 4 D of myopia is corrected with a 48-mm ablation depth [71]. Today, a slightly smaller (5.5-mm) optical zone is used. With this zone size, the ablation rate is 10 mm/D. Thus, in the example cited, 40 mm of tissue will be removed using 166 pulses at 5 Hz.

In this paper, Munnerlyn coined the term *photorefractive keratectomy* to describe this technique [72]. However, it took 4 more years before the paper was accepted for publication because it was deemed "too speculative and of no practical value." The editors of such journals must have that expression on file, since it was that same excuse that prevented the author and others from publishing results of RK in peer-reviewed journals in the early days.

Thus it was that for a time, Steven Trokel's laboratory in New York continued to have the only excimer laser in the world dedicated exclusively to ophthalmic research. This situation changed abruptly, however, in mid-1985 when the interest in ophthalmic and refractive applications of this technology suddenly exploded—simultaneously with the development of commercial interest in excimer laser systems. Attention then became diverted from the laboratory and directed more into the clinical arena.

Being able to ablate polymers in a precise way does not necessarily lead to clinical success. It is one thing to blitz the cornea in animal eyes. It is still another to do it in cadaver eyes or even blind human eyes—such exercises merely prove feasibility. And there is a large gap between feasibility and suitability—an idea is easier to conceive than to execute. Therefore, it should come as no surprise that the clinical application of this modality has some formidable hurdles to overcome, and it is by no means certain that such obstacles will fall.

Overview

The ability to cut precise sections with the argon fluoride (ArF) excimer laser at a wavelength of 193 nm is based on the absorption mode of the high-energy far-ultraviolet photons within the first few microns of the focal point. The ablated particles are ejected at supersonic speed, carrying most of the excess thermal energy with them and thereby producing corneal incisions with an adjacent zone of damage that is in the submicron range (0.1 to 0.3 mm) [59,61,73–75]. Consequent corneal wounds appear to be sealed by a pseudomembrane, and keratocytes appear normal immediately adjacent to the ablation area [76]. In contrast, the use of longer wavelengths (KrF at 248 nm, XeCl at 308 nm, and XeF at 351 nm) always induced ragged incision edges and a comparatively broad zone of tissue damage [65] (Figure 11.17). This is probably a consequence not only of the increased absorption length of these wavelengths in the cornea (as compared with 193 nm) but also of significant thermal loading [24,28]. Furthermore, the energy-absorbing target chromophore may play a role in the various mechanisms of photoablation [27]. Steinert found the threshold for ablation in a human eye at 193 nm to be 46 mJ/cm^2. For KrF (248 nm) it was 58 mJ/cm^2. At all exposures, it required a higher fluence for the 248-nm beam than for the 193-nm beam to obtain comparable results.

Applications

On the therapeutic side, experiments have centered primarily on treating superficial corneal pathology. Glaucoma filtration surgery and trephination of corneal transplants are also on the excimer wish list, although the latter may prove impractical.

The excimer has been used mostly as a refractive tool to date, specifically to correct myopia and astigmatism. Attempts are also being made to correct hyperopia. There had been considerable hype that some day the laser would be used to perform radial keratotomy (RK), but early attempts failed to achieve results that in any way surpassed then-current RK methods.

For refractive surgery with the excimer laser, three basic principles were investigated:

1 Linear or arcuate excisions for the correction of myopia: laser radial keratectomy and astigmatism, laser transverse or arcuate keratectomy

2 Removal of tissue from the central healthy cornea: laser keratomileusis or photorefractive keratoplasty (PRK)

3 Preparation of plano or powered lenticules for epikeratophakia.

Laser radial keratectomy

Laser radial keratectomy followed the approach that has been taken over the last decade with RK for the correction of myopia and astigmatism. Similar to synthetic polymers, the etch depth per pulse depends on laser fluence, and plotting reveals a sigmoid-shaped curve whose steep part shows an almost logarithmic relationship [64,77]. Inflection points in these plots correspond to the fluence levels for the most efficient ablation. In enucleated human eyes, incision depth and flattening were found to correlate well with laser output. Up to 5.35 D of flattening was achieved [75]. Since the pulse-to-pulse amplitude fluctuation is highly variable in all currently available excimer lasers (around 5% to 8%), ablation at the inflection points may be clinically undesirable, since small changes in laser output would significantly alter ablation rate [78]. Ablation at higher fluences may be preferable because there does not appear to be any increase in ultrastructural damage with fluences between 400 and 600 mJ/cm^2 per pulse—at these levels the etch-depth plot has the smallest slope [71]. Other research groups have used the laser attached to a slit lamp to perform in vivo

(a)

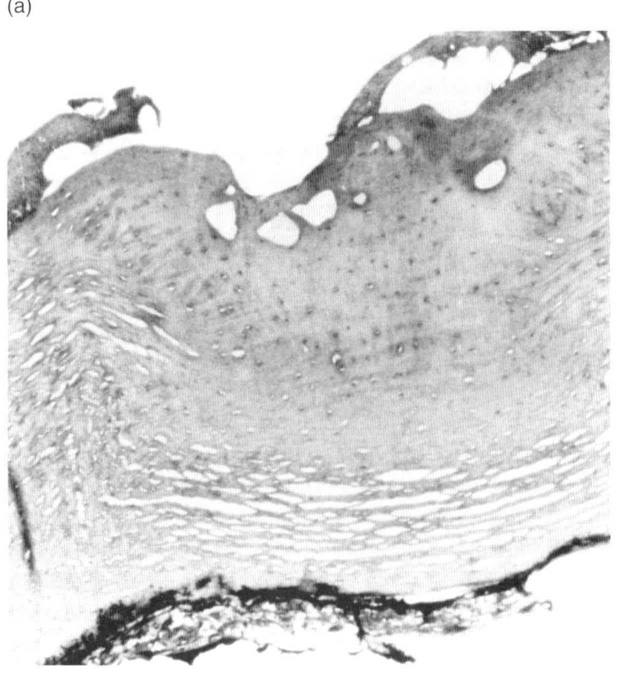

(b)

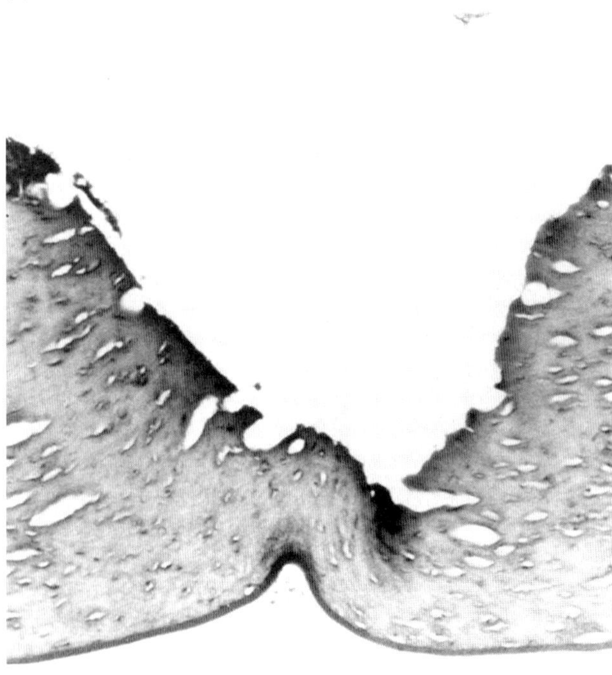

(c)

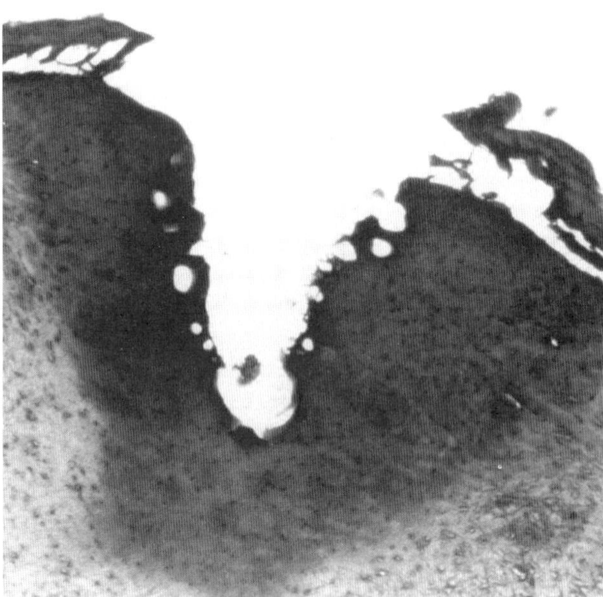

Fig. 11.17 Ultraviolet light (351 nm). (a) Extensive disorganization of the stroma below the ablation threshold. There is widespread heating and destruction of the corneal stroma. (b) A low firing rate above the ablation threshold shows tissue removal with local stromal changes. Gas bubbles can be seen extending into the stroma, and an obvious thermal interaction zone can be identified. (c) Both the firing rate and irradiance are higher, and a broader thermal zone can be seen. Original magnification ×24 (from Krueger RR, Trokel SL, Schubert HD. Interaction of ultraviolet laser light with the cornea. Invest Ophthalmol Visual Sci 1985; 26:1455–1464).

radial keratectomies in experimental animals [79]. Lack of significant corneal inflammation with a possibly weaker wound-healing response as compared with thermokeratoplasty or diamond blade RK is the hallmark of these laser incisions [80].

Theoretically, there are several advantages to use of the excimer laser for radial keratectomy. No direct contact with the cornea is required during the procedure, as with the diamond knife incisions, but is usual when a mask is used. This would allow real-time monitoring of progress during surgery by performing a continuous topographic analysis of the corneal contour (see "LASIX," below). The use of suitably shaped masks allows for simultaneous incisions with a high spatial accuracy and repeatability, thus eliminating some of the variables of conventional radial keratectomy (Figures 11.18 through 11.20). With a repetition rate in the 20- to 50-Hz range, ablation would require only a few sec-

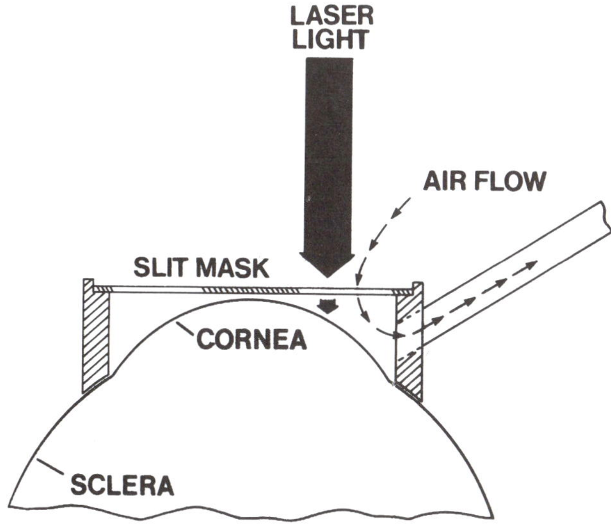

Fig. 11.18 Cross section of typical ablation mask. (Courtesy of MediTec.)

onds, thereby reducing variability caused by dehydration during conventional surgery [81].

It must be realized that while the laser can make a relatively atraumatic cut in the cornea, that cut resembles the cut made by a saw—substance is removed, not cleaved (Figures 11.21 and 11.22). According to Steinert and Puliafito, there are certain practical limits as to the narrowness of the kerf (minimum around 30 mm) that can be created by a laser [79]. Tissue fluid seeps into the space that is created during excision, thus narrowing it. A diamond knife only splits the tissue without removing it. The ablation depth per pulse depends not only on the hydration of the cornea but also on the width of the groove [82].

Because the excimer laser produces an excision rather than an incision, the ingrowth of a broader epithelial plug might result in slower wound healing and thus not only an increased or unpredictable effect (compared with conventional RK) but also prolonged diurnal fluctuations and a diminished long-term stability of the correction

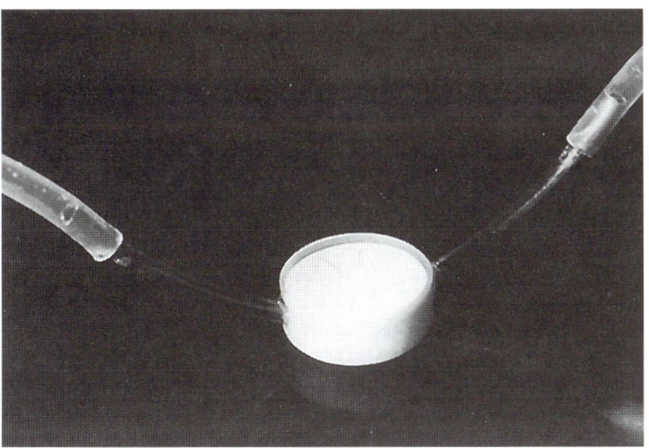

Fig. 11.19 Frontal view of an eight-incision corneal mask. (Courtesy of MediTec.)

(a)

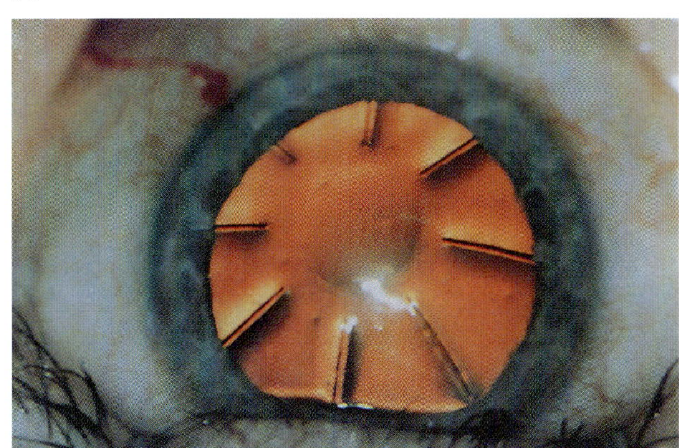

(b)

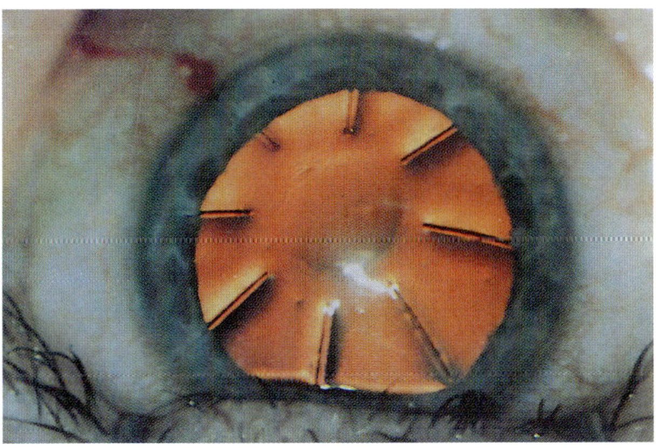

Fig. 11.21 Human eye with excimer laser RK immediately post-ablation. Incision length is 3.0 mm, incision width 70 μm, with an incision depth of 300 μm (60% of central corneal thickness). (Courtesy of MediTec.)

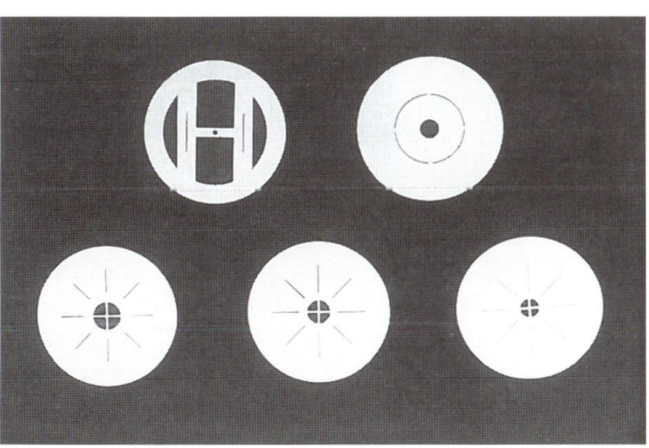

Fig. 11.20 Corneal masks for radial keratotomy, penetrating keratoplasty, and astigmatism. (Courtesy of MediTec.)

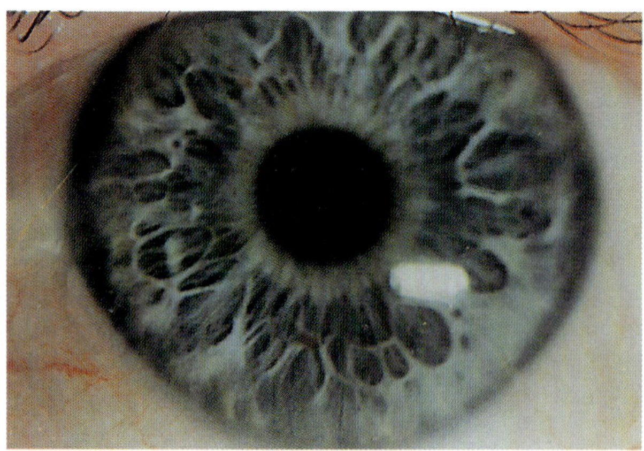

Fig. 11.22 The same eye 1 week postoperation. Diopter change + 2.0 D. (Courtesy of MediTec.)

achieved (Figures 11.23 and 11.24). Are wider scars less flexible, and/or do they somehow convey more resistance to rupture than incisions? Not likely. Thus, while solving one problem (maybe), laser radial keratectomy could possibly create others. Steinert suggests that wider scars might result in greater curvature change, especially if enhanced by pharmacologic wound-healing agents [71]. However, studies to date of agents such as epidermal growth factor (EGF) have been disappointing—it is not possible to overdrive the system. Incisional RK, with its smaller scar, actually might respond better to such agents. Furthermore, comparisons of early steel knife data with those of smoother diamond knife results seem to indicate that the finer incisions of the diamond are accompanied by an improvement in outcome [83,84].

Several technical problems had to be solved prior to widespread clinical use. Although the total duration of

(a)

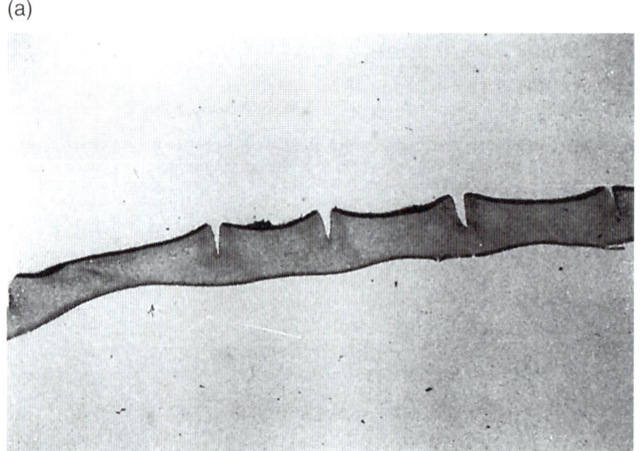

(b)

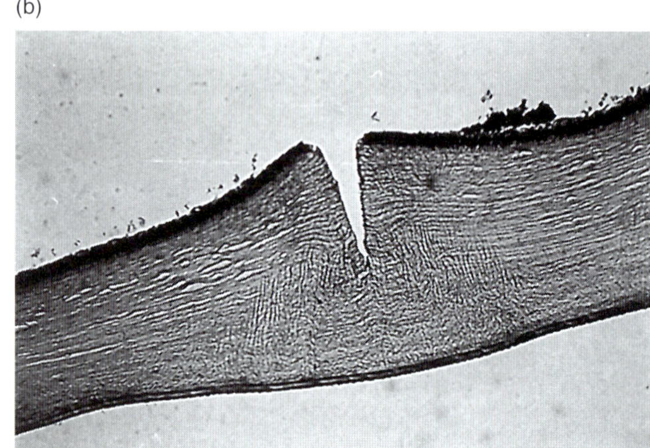

Fig. 11.23 Incision in rabbit cornea immediately postapplication. (Courtesy of MediTec.)

(a)

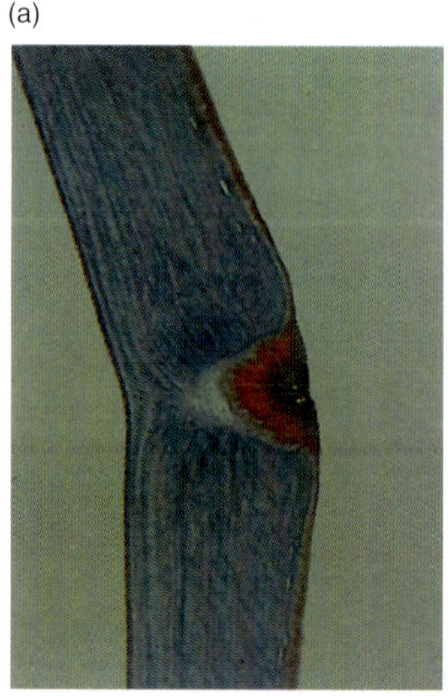

(b)

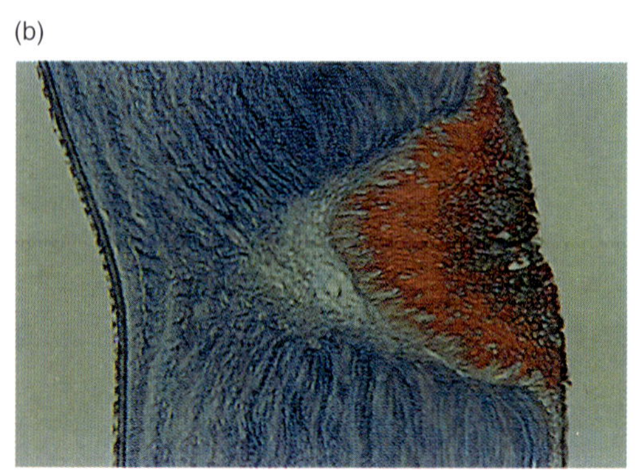

Fig. 11.24 Similar incision in rabbit cornea 2 months postapplication. The epithelial plug is beginning to thin and new stroma is visible. (Courtesy of MediTec.)

(a)

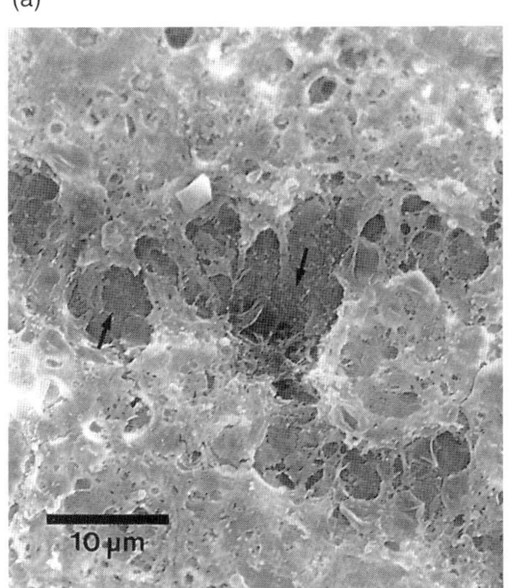

(b)

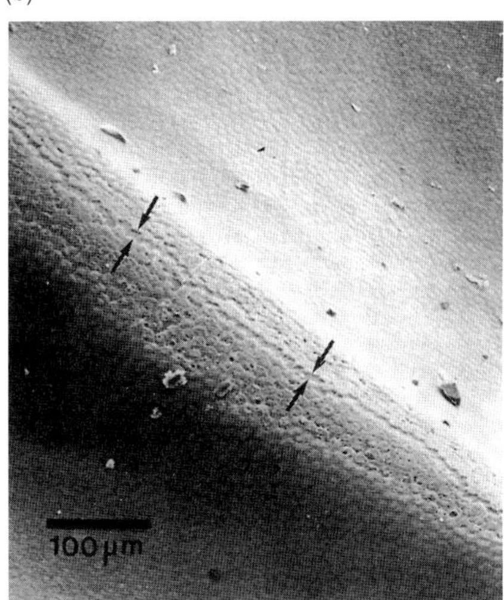

Fig. 11.25 (a) Endothelial surface ridge raised by ablation; (b) damaged endothelium following laser tissue ablation (from Dehm EJ, Puliafito CA, Adler CM. Endothelial injury in rabbits following excimer laser ablation at 193 and 248 nm. Arch Ophthalmol 1986; 104:1364–1368).

surgery is comparatively short, immobilization of the eye and/or coupling of the laser beam to the cornea with protection of areas that should not be irradiated are mandatory. The use of a suction cup with evenly spaced slits and of coated contact lenses had been proposed [85–87].

Real-time monitoring of excision depth eluded technical means, although Stern and coworkers described the femtosecond optical ranging of corneal incision depth with the use of a colliding-pulse-mode locked-ring dye laser [88]. A high rate of corneal perforation was described by several groups, possibly caused by individual response variations in the corneas [89].

Dehm and associates have shown changes to the endothelium following 90% incisions of the corneal depth with 193-nm laser light, similar to those seen after incisional RK. Higher-density exposures led to a denudation of the endothelium under the ablation zone [31,90] (Figure 11.25). Ablations with the KrF laser (248 nm) revealed loss of cells and severe damage to the tissue surrounding the excisions. In addition, ultrastructural changes in Descemet's membrane have been reported, probably as a result of acousticomechanical shock waves or secondary radiation [91,92].

The excimer laser offers several potential technical advantages for radial keratectomy, but these advantages may not appreciably change either the results or postoperative course in the long run. Additionally, both the cost and sophistication of the equipment weigh heavily against the method becoming clinically viable. There has been no further developmental work in this area to my knowledge.

Astigmatism and laser keratectomy

The excimer laser also has been used in a limited number of patients to correct astigmatism in the manner of RK. Here, the laser produces curved excisions that essentially mimic the classic T-incisions made with a knife. A contact lens that has been coated with reflective material and contains small openings or slits is used to permit projection of the laser beam onto the appropriate part of the cornea. Candidates enrolled in the initial phase of study were restricted to those with 3 to 5 D of astigmatism. It may be that the procedure can be used to correct greater amounts of astigmatism, but the clinical study was not expanded [93]. According to Fenzl, the excimer laser not only has produced excellent results but also provides increased predictability compared with conventional surgery. Fenzl claims that the depth predictability achievable with a knife is only 110 to 115 μm but cites no evidence establishing this figure, whereas the accuracy that can be obtained with the laser is 14 μm. Follow-up extending to 18 months in patients enrolled in the initial clinical trial shows that the procedure is associated with stable results and no complications. Using the suction cup–slit technique, Seiler and coworkers have corrected corneal astigmatism of up to 4.16 D. Since small variations in excision depth—within 10%—cause large differences of the resulting astigmatic correction (±2.5 D), reproducibility and predictability depend mainly on the precise control of the ablation depth [82]. Attempts at treating astigmatism through elliptical ablation zones also have been made [94,95] (see below).

Preparation of plano or powered lenticules for epikeratophakia

The method originally described by Barraquer for the shaping of donor tissue (applied in keratophakia and epikeratophakia) or of an anterior lamella from a patient's own cornea (for myopic and hyperopic keratomileusis) makes use of the cryolathe, a sophisticated device that causes cell death of all keratocytes during the procedure unless cryoprotective measures are taken [96]. Despite this fact, histologic examinations of keratomileusis lenticules have demonstrated the presence of living keratocytes, which presumably have infiltrated from the underlying stroma postoperatively [97,98]. It has not been demonstrated conclusively that living keratocytes are necessary for the success of keratomileusis in any event. Still, there are some indications that nondestructive tissue shaping could speed recovery in such cases and perhaps eliminate some of the complications seen with the freeze-lathing technique [99–101]. Lieurance and associates have demonstrated the shaping of unfrozen tissue using the excimer laser at 193 nm, and successful plano lamellar transplants in the human eye have been reported by others [102,103].

Laser in situ keratomileusis (LASIK)

By far the most serious test application of the excimer has been in laser keratomileusis, where it has been used in attempts to correct myopic errors through large-area ablation of the cornea. This type of refractive corneal surgery performed with the ArF excimer laser is based on the expectation that tissue can be removed with submicron precision from the central corneal surface in such a gentle manner that the corneal epithelium heals over the ablated area without hyperplasia and activation of significant repair mechanisms causing scarring. This is known as *photoablative refractive keratectomy* (PRK) (Figure 11.26) (but see "The king is dead," above). The new anterior radius of curvature thus would achieve the desired optical correction in the same way as classic myopic and hyperopic keratomileusis, keratophakia, intrastromal hydrogel implantation, or epikeratophakia [104]. Initial experience with clinical use in partially and fully sighted humans was reported as positive, but several important biologic issues required further study. These included the predictability of the procedure, its long-term stability, and the effect on corneal clarity and regularity.

Laser in situ keratomileusis (LASIK) got started in the late 1980s because some thought that an operation like PRK, in destroying Bowman's membrane, would affect corneal innervation and healing. Both Steven Brint at LSU and Lucio Buratto of Milan performed laser keratomileusis (photokeratomileusis, or PKM) on a loose corneal cap with some success; Ioannis Pallikaris of Crete was the first to do this technique under a corneal flap [105]. Buratto has the longest experience. His technique and results are outlined below [106].

Thirty eyes of 22 patients underwent treatment. All patients had anisometropia that did not respond to glasses and/or contact lenses. All disks were resected with a no. 30 plate and had a diameter of 8.5 mm, reflecting the investigator's experience with the BKS unit used for the keratectomies (Figure 11.27). In freeze-lathing cases, the average disk diameter is 7.0 to 7.5 mm. In 2 cases the disk thickness was less than 240 mm, which created problems postoperatively—which it would in classic MKM.

A Summit Technologies Excimed UV 200 excimer laser was used. The ablations were performed with a repetition rate of 10 Hz, a fluence of 180 mJ/cm^2, and an optical zone

(a)

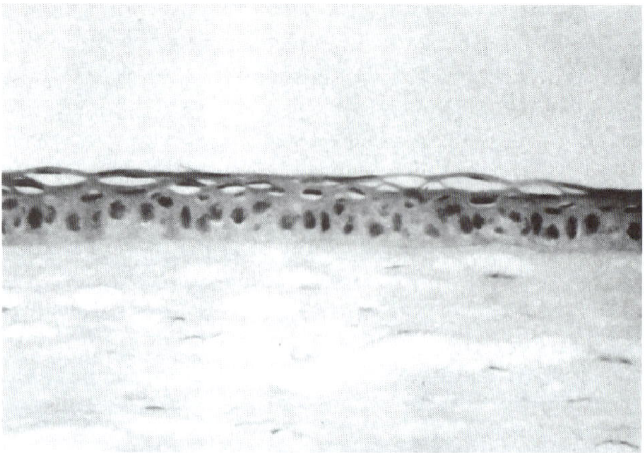

(b)

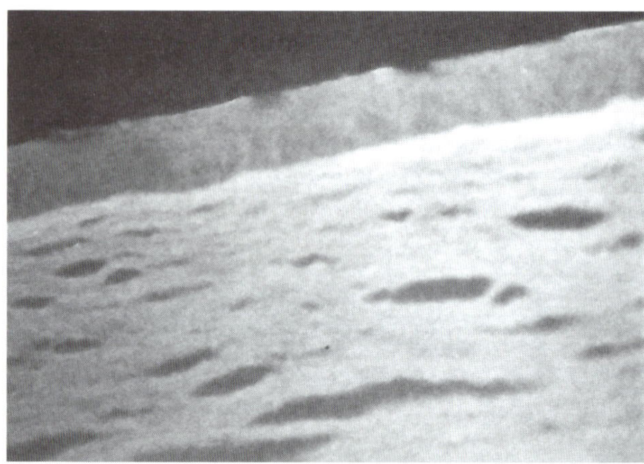

Fig. 11.26 Four weeks after a 2 D, 4.5 mm ablation. (a) Hematoxylin and eosin, original magnification ×475; (b) TEM, original magnification ×60 000. There is re-epithelialization with basement membrane complexes and hemidesmosomes (from Goodman GL, Trokel SL, Stark WJ, Munnerlyn CR, Green WR. Corneal healing following laser refractive keratectomy. Arch Ophthalmol 1989; 107:1799–1803.

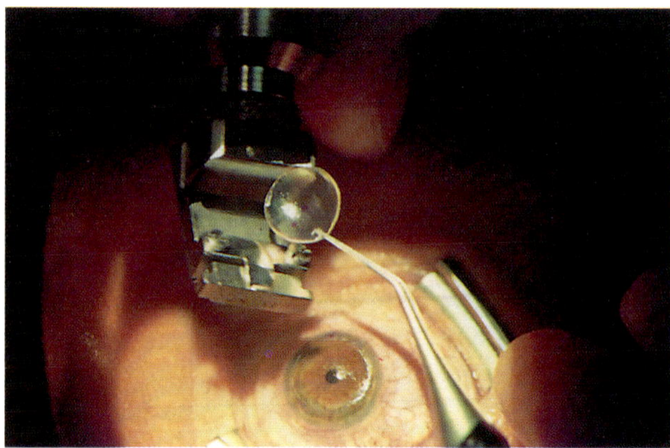

Fig. 11.27 Large keratectomy with the keratome. (Courtesy of S. Brint.)

(a)

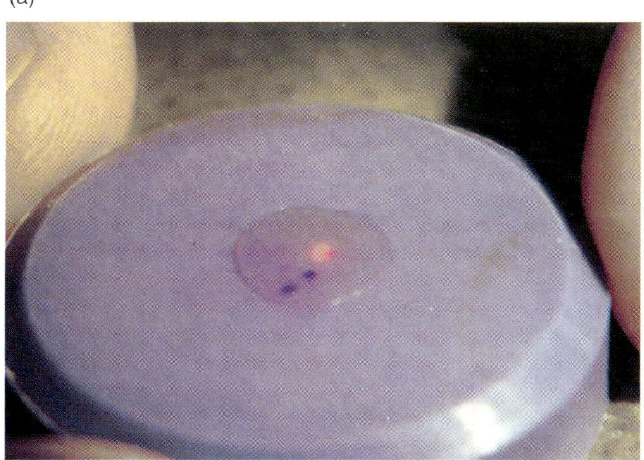

(b)

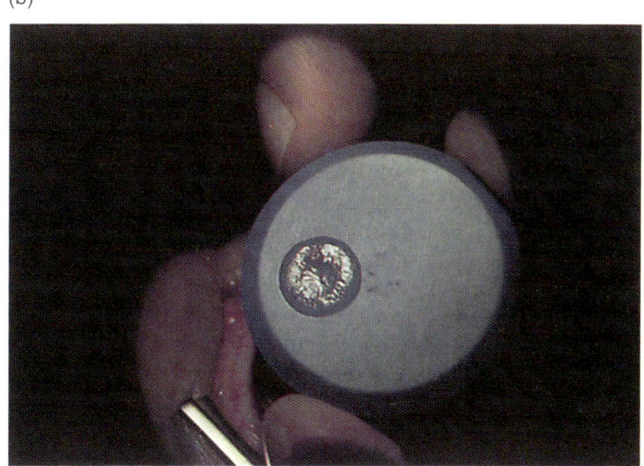

Fig. 11.28 (a) Ablation being performed. Centration is by inspection; (b) ablated tissue disk. (Courtesy of L. Buratto.)

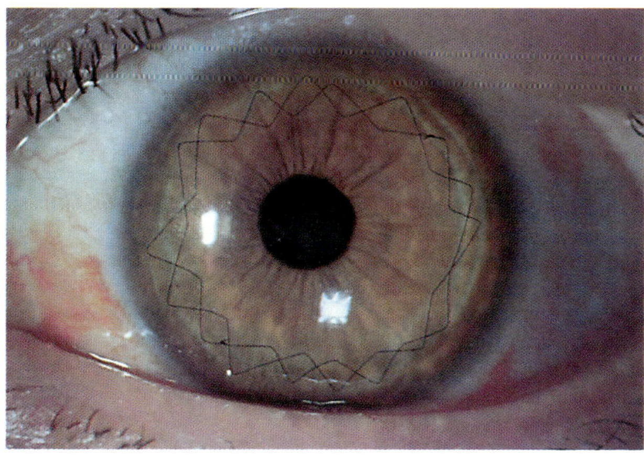

Fig. 11.29 Postoperative laser keratomileusis. (Courtesy of L. Buratto.)

ranging from 3.5 to 4.5 mm. The resected disks were laid flat on a hard rubber base for the treatment (Figure 11.28). Postoperatively, the patients were treated with topical tobramycin five times daily until the corneas had re-epithelialized and with dexamethasone five times daily thereafter (Figure 11.29). Sutures were removed in 14 days.

The average preoperative myopia was –17.875 ± 3.32 D. The mean residual refraction at 6 months was –2.126 ± 1.40 D. Intrastromal haze was observed in 5 cases (16.6%). Best-corrected vision remained at the preoperative level in 74% of the cases, improved in 16%, and declined in 10%. Uncorrected vision was 20/50 or better in 10% and 20/100 in 83.3%. Astigmatism before and after surgery was essentially the same, being 2.02 ± 1.04 D preoperatively and 2.26 ± 1.09 D postoperatively. It should be noted—as pointed out in Chapter 10—that these figures can be misleading presented in this way. It is not known how many of this group actually lost astigmatism, how many gained, and in how many astigmatism was reversed. This caveat is underscored by the fact that Buratto reported that 4 of 30 (13.3%) developed irregular astigmatism. This is higher than the average in freeze lathing. However, if we remove the two thin sections in which such distortion is inevitable, we are left with a 6% incidence of irregular astigmatism. This is more in line with freeze lathing and is better than in keratomileusis in situ (KMIS; see Chapter 10). Such astigmatism is usually related to decentration of the ablated zone within the resected disk and can be minimized with improvements in centration and beam delivery (Figure 11.30). Of this

(a)

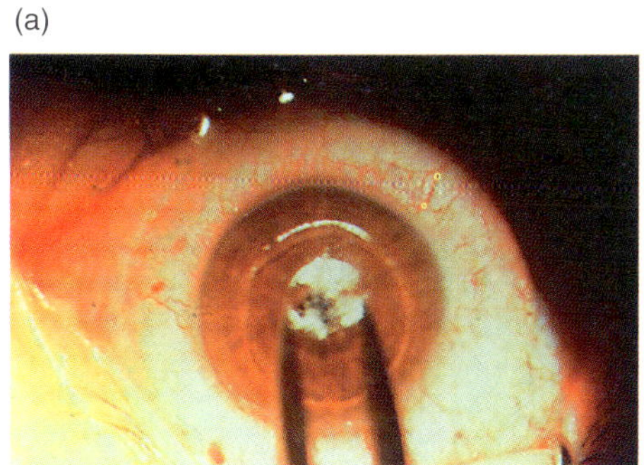

(b)

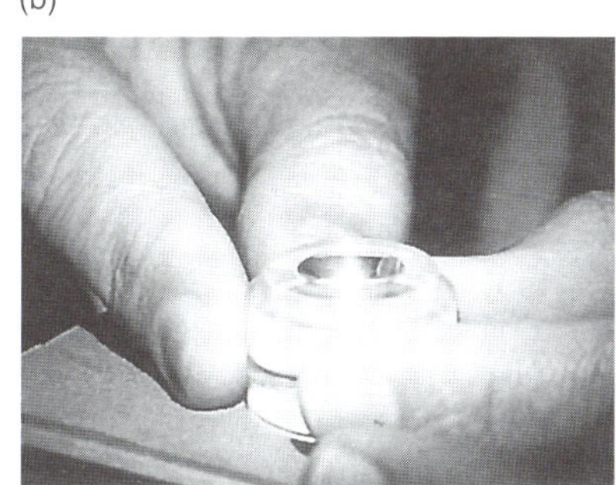

Fig. 11.30 (a) Note decentration of the ablated zone in this case of *in situ* laser ablation; (b) it is difficult to ensure accurate centration when holding the tissue beneath the laser beam.

group, two were thin sections with subsequent wrinkling of Bowman's layer. This also happens in freeze-lathe cases when the central thickness is less than 0.10 mm after lathing. Of these 2 cases, one required a homoplastic graft at 6 months because of extremely poor vision.

The current procedure

LASIK is performed by surgically making a lamellar corneal dissection, followed by excimer laser ablation of the stroma and then replacement of the dissected cornea. It is used in attempts to correct myopia, hyperopia, and astigmatism. LASIK has evolved as the alternative to PRK for several reasons. LASIK offers more rapid visual recovery and much less pain and irritation immediately postoperatively. After LASIK, one does not see the occasional stromal haze or scarring that is seen with PRK. Higher refractive errors can be corrected with LASIK than with PRK. LASIK, when performed properly, offers a very high percentage of success. According to some studies, 96% of patients see 20/40 or better after the procedure.

The microkeratome is used to make a 130- or 160-μm-thick section of corneal stroma and its overlying epithelium (see also Chapter 10). It travels approximately 80% across the cornea to a stop, creating a nasally or superiorly located "hinge" of corneal stroma. This flap is folded away so that photorefractive laser keratectomy may be performed in the stromal bed. The corneal flap is replaced, and the interface is irrigated with sterile balanced saline solution. One usually waits a period of 1 to 4 minutes for the stromal flap to "stick" in position.

The procedure generally is performed as follows: Topical anesthesia is instilled in the conjunctival gutters, and the eyelids are prepped with Betadine Solution. Plastic drapes are placed on the upper and lower eyelids. Alignment marks are made on the cornea with gentian violet (Figure 11.31).

A pneumatic suction ring (Figure 11.32) is seated on the eye at the corneal limbus. The intraocular pressure is checked with a Barraquer tonometer. A microkeratome is inserted into a track on the suction ring. It is advanced across the cornea, making a tissue flap of 130 or 160 μm in thickness (Figure 11.33). The microkeratome and suction ring are removed, and the corneal flap is opened and laid back over its hinge of tissue. The corneal stroma is ablated with the excimer laser, and the corneal flap is irrigated and then closed.

The interface is irrigated with balanced saline solution between the corneal flap and the stromal bed for a few seconds to remove debris, and the corneal flap is wiped into alignment with a wet surgical spear. A 2- to 3-minute waiting period is observed to allow the corneal flap to adhere to the stromal bed. Antibiotic eye drops and steroid eye drops are instilled onto the cornea. The patient is returned to the slit lamp for a final recheck of corneal flap alignment before being discharged.

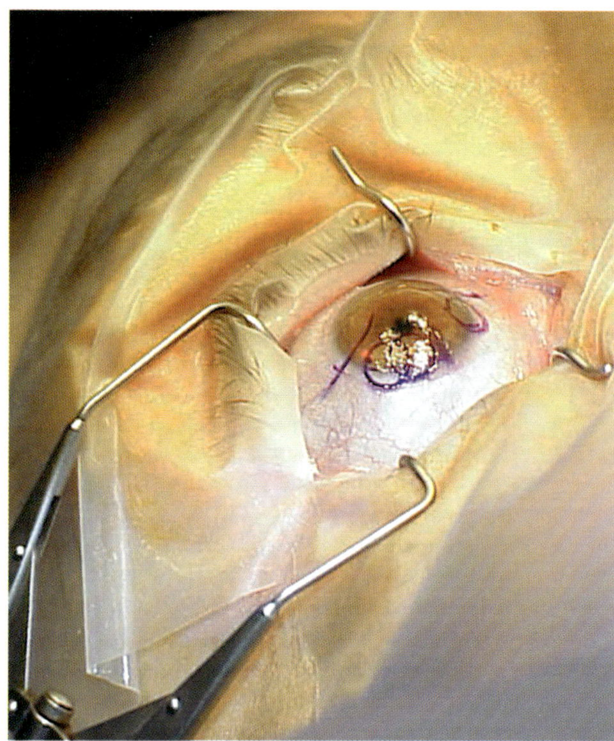

Fig. 11.31 Eyelids prepped and draped with gentian violet alignment marks shown on cornea.

One reason LASIK is so popular with patients is because there is usually minimal irritation during and after the procedure. Most patients have blurry vision immediately after the surgery. They often describe it as if they

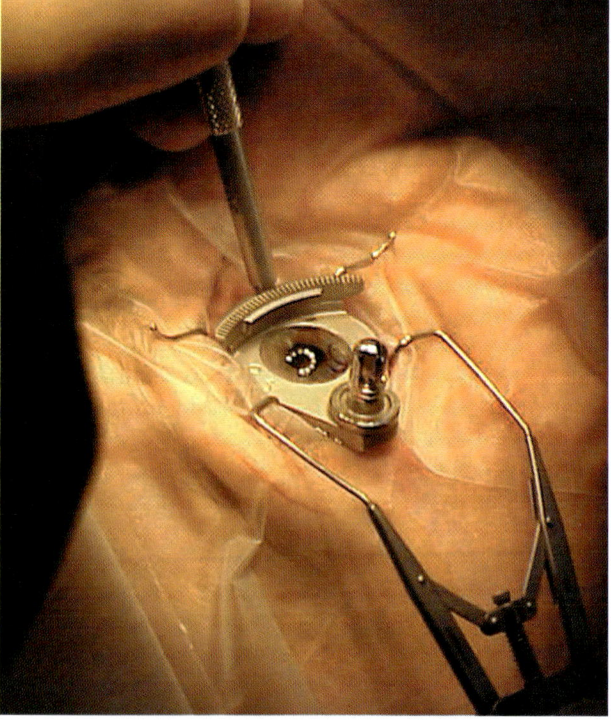

Fig. 11.32 Suction ring in position on the eye.

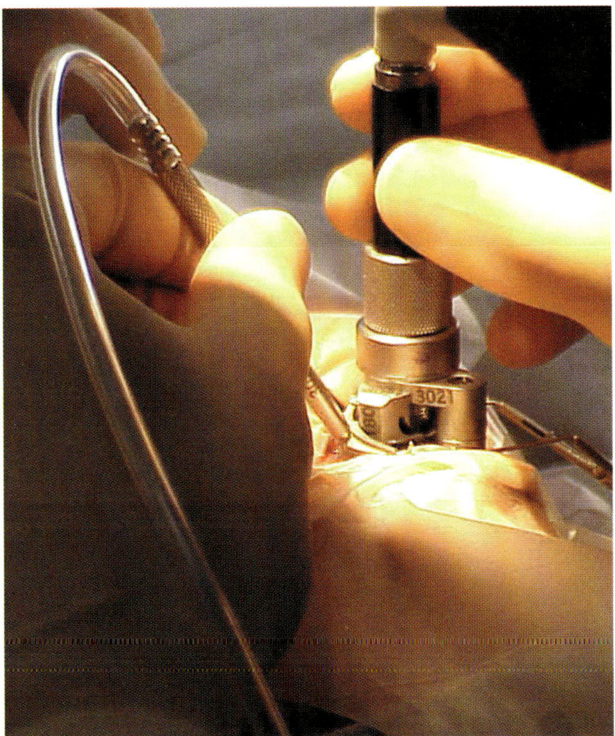

Fig. 11.33 Microkeratome making corneal flap.

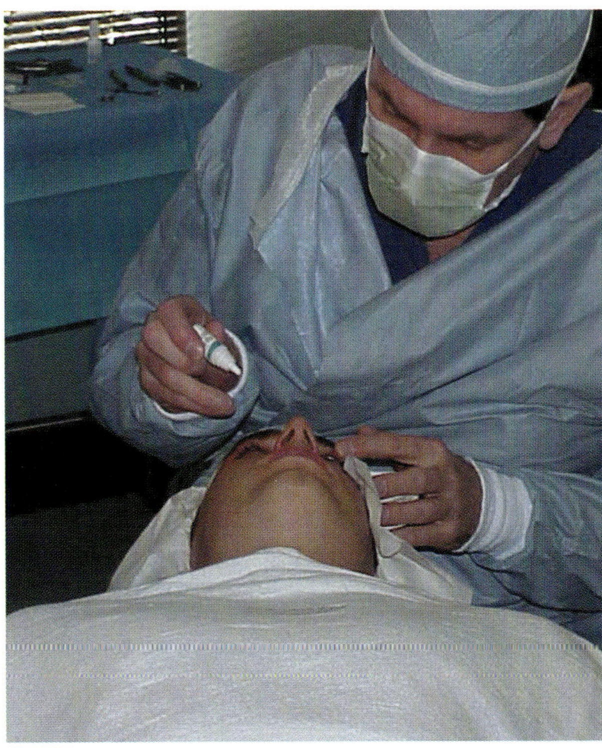

Fig. 11.34 Antibiotic and steroid eyedrops instilled in laser suite at end of surgery.

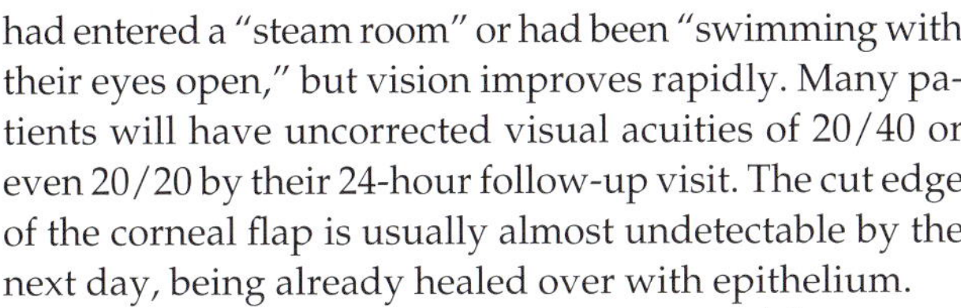

had entered a "steam room" or had been "swimming with their eyes open," but vision improves rapidly. Many patients will have uncorrected visual acuities of 20/40 or even 20/20 by their 24-hour follow-up visit. The cut edge of the corneal flap is usually almost undetectable by the next day, being already healed over with epithelium.

Antibiotic and steroid eye drops are used four times daily for 1 week and then discontinued (Figure 11.34). Lubricant eye drops are often helpful for at least 6 months. The patient should be seen postoperatively at 1 day, 1 week, and 1, 3, and 6 months.

Although there appear to be fewer complications with LASIK than with other refractive procedures, the complications that can occur are usually much more severe (see Chapter 15). Irregular astigmatism, epithelial ingrowth, displaced flaps, stromal melts, and poorly cut flaps can be very hard to manage. Since the complications that occur can be difficult to correct, prevention is the order of the day. This can be accomplished by obtaining the best possible training for oneself and the surgical staff and by paying meticulous attention to the details of laser calibration, setup, and surgical performance.

Today or not today . . .

Simultaneous bilateral LASIK surgery is considered by many refractive surgeons to be within the standard of care [107]. Others feel differently on the matter. Patients seem to prefer the convenience of having both eyes done on the same day, but the ultimate decision lies with the operating surgeon.

I have read and heard all the arguments supporting same-day LASIK, and I do not buy any of them. I see nothing compelling about the anisometropia argument, especially in view of the potential for serious adverse events. RK was and is a far safer procedure than LASIK and I do not condone same-day surgery with that procedure either. There are those who will condemn this point of view, and I am sure that support will be found in the event of what Jaffe used to call a "legal adventure," but this does nothing for the patient who is left handicapped with subnormal vision following an elective surgery—all in the name of expediency. And it is that—make no mistake. Sequential surgery benefits the surgeon most of all.

Pearls and caveats

Use an operating microscope for the keratectomy and to reposition the flap. The excimer laser's poor illumination, minimal clearance, and lack of a foot pedal are not conducive to performing the best keratectomy or for seeing foreign bodies on the stromal surface.

Patients with a high degree of myopia and flat corneas are not good candidates for LASIK. This was equally true with RK, and Barraquer set a lower limit to preoperative corneal curvature for cryo-MKM. Such patients are not common but may represent an incidence of as high as 4%. Moshirfar, at the Moran Eye Center at the University of Utah, Salt Lake City, found that 24 of 948 eyes in his patient group met the criteria—a corneal steepness of 42.5 D or less and myopia of more than 8 D. These patients ended up having worse uncorrected vision, more folds, and more glare and halos at night after LASIK.

To study the effect of corneal curvature on the outcome of LASIK, Moshirfar placed patients into three categories based on the degree of myopia: low, below 4 D; moderate, 4 to 8 D; and high, more than 8 D. The same eyes also were put into categories based on the steepness of the cornea: flat, below 42.5 D; medium, 42.5 to 45.5 D; and steep, more than 45 D.

Results of LASIK for the nine groups of patients were assessed by measurements of pre- and postoperative best spectacle-corrected visual acuity, uncorrected visual acuity, manifest and cycloplegic refraction, corneal topography, changes in astigmatism, biomicroscopy, and subjective scoring of glare and halo disturbances. In the nine groups of patients, eyes with the highest degree of myopia and flattest corneas had the highest rate of undercorrection/regression compared with other groups in the study and were more likely to develop surgically induced astigmatism. They also had the worst visual acuity and the lowest subjective index of daytime and nighttime vision and had more folds, an outcome that was augmented by the flatness of the cornea.

While these results represent the experience of only one practitioner, they should give the refractive surgeon pause. My recommendation would be to consider some other modality—such as phakic IOLs—in lieu of LASIK.

LASIK in low myopes Using LASIK for low myopes is fast becoming an acceptable alternative for high-volume refractive surgeons—a decision I have difficulty with. Stonecipher has performed more than 600 LASIK procedures and prefers LASIK to PRK for low myopes [108]. He says that there is a larger effective optical zone with LASIK versus PRK. His PRK optical zones average about 6 mm or slightly larger, whereas his effective optical zone for LASIK is between 6.5 and 7 mm, which he claims makes for better-quality vision. Perhaps this is true, but this possibility is more than offset by the dangers inherent in performing a lamellar procedure when a less invasive procedure will do. Furthermore, a difference of 0.5 mm is not critical with the shallow ablations used for low myopes; the transition zone is much less likely to produce aberrations. And although Stonecipher states that his PRK patients are more than 10 times more likely to fill their Voltaren and pain prescriptions compared with LASIK patients, this has not been my experience, nor that of others. A disposable high-water-content contact lens will improve not only comfort but also epithelialization and visual recovery as well.

Although patients tend toward LASIK because it is easier to tolerate and the visual rehabilitation is faster, PRK is clearly safer for corrections of up to 4 D, according to Theo Seiler at the University Eye Clinic, Dresden, Germany. The refractive success, as well as visual success, is very similar in PRK and in LASIK low-diopter corrections. Seiler noted that the Dublin group showed that decentration is twice as frequent in LASIK compared with PRK, and double the amount of eccentricity is seen after LASIK compared with PRK [109,110]. Although scarring is one of the most important problems after PRK, the incidence of scarring for corrections up to 4 D is extremely low. Cutting errors and flap problems occur in about 0.5% to 1% of LASIK cases, according to Seiler [111]. In my view, low-tech RK is safer yet.

Laser treatment for hyperopia

Hyperopic PRK

Despite a very appreciative prospective audience, namely, hyperopic patients, who are not nearly as demanding as their myopic counterparts and who equal (if not exceed) their numbers (Figure 11.35), the hyperopic laser show is only now beginning to come into full swing. Less promising results were obtained in limited experiments to correct hyperopia through photoablative means (Figure 11.36). It started in Germany in the early 1990s when Dausch began performing hyperopic PRK to mixed reviews [112].

Dausch had fair results in patients with low hyperopia but not very good results in those above +3 D, with most eyes developing peripheral angular corneal haze. It appears that these attempts have been unsuccessful because the ablation zone is filled in by remodeling of the epithelium, eliminating any effect of the excimer in the midperiphery of the cornea. This phenomenon also seems to be an active factor in the myopic patients as well. Gimbel reported better results in a patient undergoing laser ab-

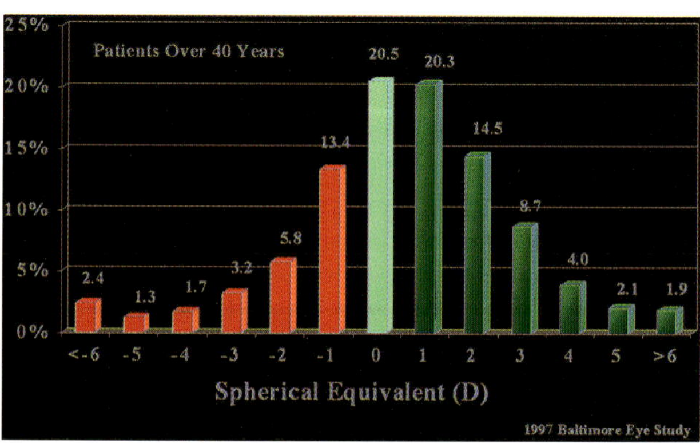

Fig. 11.35 Refractive error demographics. Adapted from the Framingham Study. (Courtesy of Sunrise Technologies.)

(a)

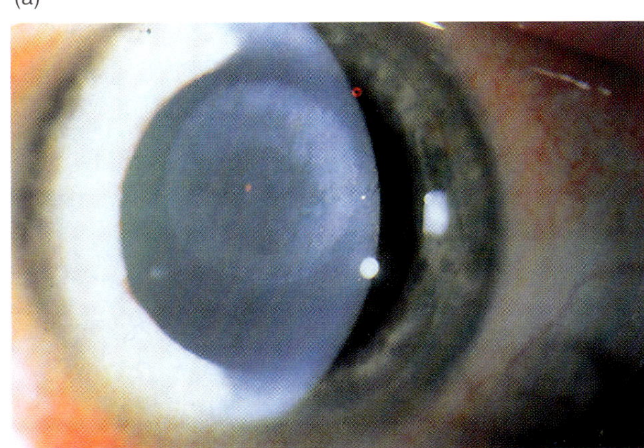

(b)

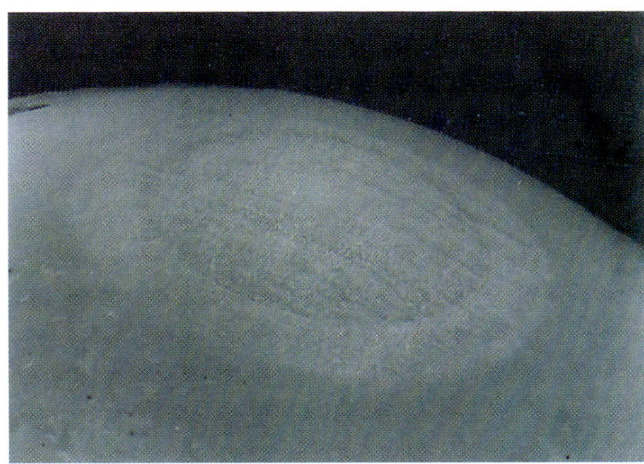

(c)

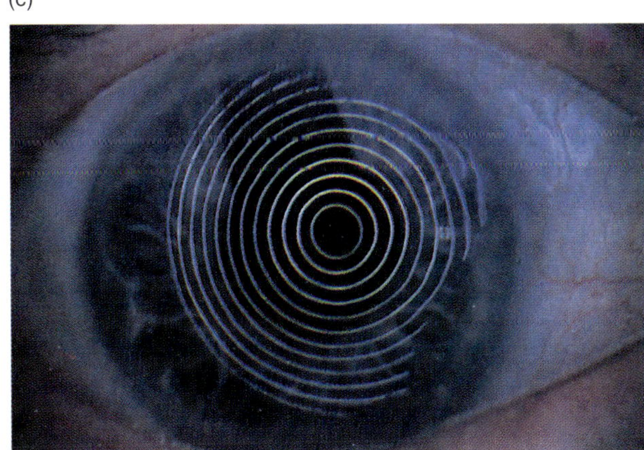

Fig. 11.36 (a) Typical appearance of hyperopic treatment area; (b) SEM of corneal surface after treatment for hyperopia; (c) post-operative topographical appearance after laser treatment. (Courtesy of T. Seiler.)

lation over an epikeratophakia [113]. However, the physical conditions involving the onlay graft in epikeratophakia are not the same as those existing within an integrated structure such as the corneal stroma, and conclusions drawn from results in these cases should not be applied to the results of hyperopic laser ablations in general. Furthermore, patients have been treated with the excimer laser for hyperopia in the past, and results similar to Gimbel's also have been achieved, but these regressed after about 5 months.

It was apparent that better results would require larger optical zones than were available at that time, with especially wider outer zones and better blend zones to improve the outcomes. Today, newer techniques and equipment allow for this. Broad-beam technology has advanced considerably in recent years. VISX recently changed its beam-delivery system to split the beam into seven different components, which are homogenized and, in the case of hyperopia, actually offset to scan out to a maximum diameter of 9 mm. The S2 Smoothscan laser actually has inner and outer zones to consider.

A study of hyperopic PRK data from 222 eyes, in which there was a 5.5-mm inner and a 9-mm outer zone, has been reported [114]. Recovery was slow for the first 3 months and then picked up to a point where 50% of patients achieved 20/20 vision. By 9 to 18 months, 90% of patients reached 20/40. Refractive stability was excellent, with only 1 patient losing two or more lines of best-corrected visual acuity, due to irregular healing. The conclusions drawn were that hyperopic PRK with the S2 laser produces safe results for spherical hyperopic refractive error up to +6 D, although prolonged recovery of uncorrected and best-corrected visual acuity in these patients often remains a problem.

Hyperopia correction with the broad-beam Summit laser is accomplished using an erodible mask known as the *Emphasis disk* that is used to shape the laser beam. The Summit hyperopia procedure, with or without astigmatism, is suited to treat up to 6 D of sphere and 6 D of cylinder. The procedure begins with steepening out to the 6.5-mm optical zone, with a blend zone out to 9.5 mm achieved using a prismatic lens called an *axicon*. In a study involving treatment of up to 6 D of hyperopic sphere and 3 D of cylinder, investigators were impressed with the predictability achieved early on, in which 84% of patients were within 1 D at 6 months, with no retreatments.

Hyperopic LASIK

Hyperopic LASIK, like hyperopic PRK, requires that tissue be ablated surrounding a clear optical zone (Figure 11.37), essentially steepening the central zone after the cap is replaced. The results have been mixed to date—something to be expected at this stage. Talamo presented hyperopic LASIK outcomes from a study of 100 consecutive eyes with up to 1 D of cylinder treated in the last year using the VISX S2 Smoothscan laser. The mean correction was about 0.5 D more than for the PRK group, with patients recovering vision more rapidly. Best-corrected and uncorrected visual acuity recovery was much more rapid than for hyperopic PRK. Day 1 results for the patients with 20/40 vision were near what might be expected at 3 to 6 months with PRK. However, just 46% of patients attained 20/20 at 6 months [115].

Lindstrom and colleagues conducted a 2-year prospective study of hyperopia and hyperopic astigmatism correction with the VISX STAAR S2 excimer laser. The study enrolled 100 patients with up to +6 D of hyperopia and up to +5 D of cylindrical error. A 9.5-mm, 180-μm flap is created using the Hansatome microkeratome. Excimer laser ablation is performed with a 5-mm optical zone and a 9-mm treatment zone.

Thus far, 61 treated eyes have completed 12 months of follow-up. The patients ranged in age from 23 to 66 years and had a mean manifest refraction SE of +2.65 D preoperatively. Mean manifest sphere and cylinder before surgery were +2.28 and +0.74 D, respectively. Follow-up of refractive errors over time showed that there was good stability for cylinder early on, whereas significant regression of the spherical component occurred over the first 6 months. The authors found this pattern to be similar to that associated with LASIK for myopic astigmatism, although the amount of regression in the spherical component was greater for hyperopia than for myopia.

On the first day after surgery, mean SE was near emmetropia, but by 1 month it had increased to +0.63 D, and by 6 months, it was +0.92 D. Mean SE at 12 months was +0.85 D. Overall, at all follow-up visits, about 50% of the eyes were within 0.50 D of emmetropia, and more than three-fourths were within 1 D. By 1 month, 86% of eyes had better than 20/40 uncorrected vision, and 98% saw better than 20/60. The results were similar at 6 months, and at the 12-month visit, uncorrected visual acuity was better than 20/60 in 100% of eyes.

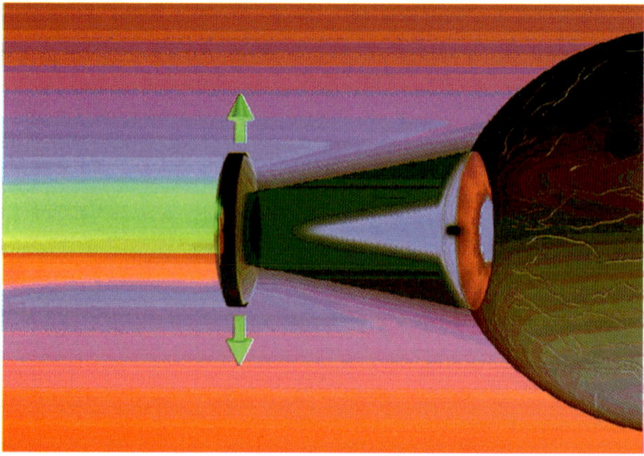

Fig. 11.37 Hyperopic LASIK requires a broad-beam laser and a doughnut-shaped ablation. (Courtesy of VISX.)

Conclusions were that this procedure is not quite as good as myopic LASIK in terms of correction of the spherical error, improvement in uncorrected visual acuity, and predictability. The incidence of epithelial defects was higher in this group than one would expect in a cohort of patients being treated with LASIK for myopia as well. However, patients with hyperopia tend to be older and probably have a higher incidence of subclinical anterior basement membrane dystrophy that contributes to this complication. These patients were, on average, 10 years older than our myopic patients [116].

Laser thermal keratoplasty (LTK)

While LASIK has dominated the refractive field of late, two emerging technologies, namely, laser thermal keratoplasty (LTK) and conductive keratoplasty (CK), are offering less invasive approaches to the correction of hyperopia. Although both techniques administer thermal lesions outside the visual axis, they do it in very different ways.

The procedure of flattening the cornea by surface application of heat is not a new idea, having been employed in the last century to treat astigmatism (see Chapter 9). Nevertheless, it has had a dismal track record (but then, so has so-called radio frequency keratoplasty). The results from Fyodorov's group using a hot wire (so-called infrared thermokeratoplasty) were uniformly good but were matched in no particular by the American experience (see Chapter 14). It should be noted that few, if any, patients in that series were corrected completely, nor were all included; data were patchy. Additionally, stepwise regression analysis of what data were available showed no correlation of preoperative factors with outcome. While 70.8% of the preoperative hyperopia had been decreased at 1 year, only 40% was corrected to less than 1 D of emmetropia in that time [117,118]. I am at a loss to explain the discrepancy, since I know Fyodorov personally and trust his integrity.

The LTK procedure works by the absorption of holmium laser light, primarily by water in the cornea. This light energy is converted to heat, and the heat, in turn, causes collagen contraction, which changes corneal curvature. In an effort to control the amount and extent of stromal thermal damage and thus quantify the procedure, Seiler employed the holmium laser to make the burns with a handheld contact probe [119]. Figure 11.38 illustrates the effect of this application. Summit Technologies conducted extensive U.S. trials with this device, but when reports indicated a high incidence of regression and

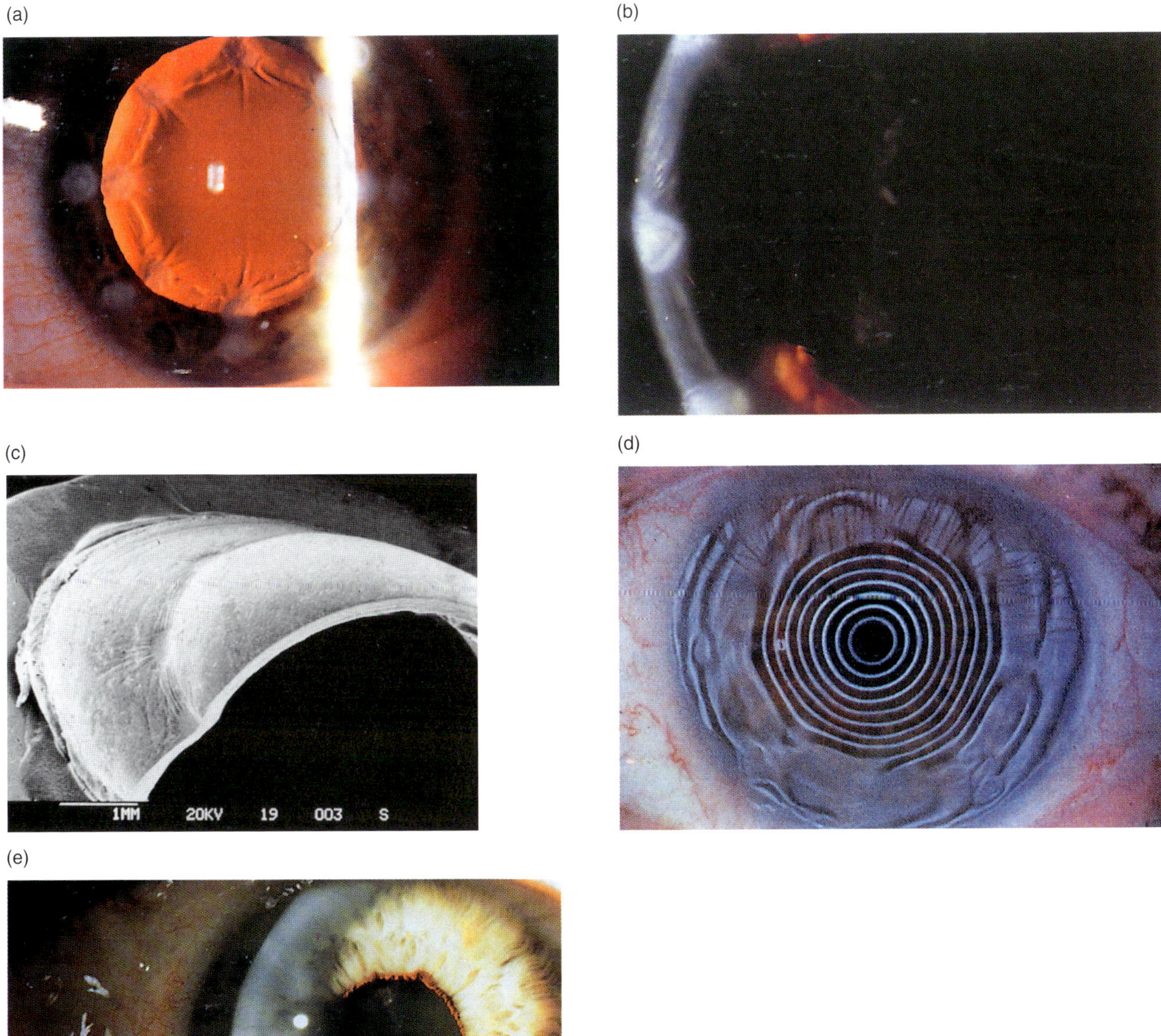

Fig. 11.38 Holmium laser thermokeratoplasty. (a) Note the central steepening of the cornea. (b) The lesions typically are cone-shaped. (c) Scanning electron microscopy of corneal section showing the cinchlike action of the lesions and the profound central corneal steepening. (d) As evidenced by this photokeratograph, central distortion is minimal. (e) The eye in part a 3 months after application (Courtesy of T. Seiler).

surgically induced irregular astigmatism, the study was discontinued.

The Sunrise noncontact LTK procedure provides for symmetrical treatment of the cornea, treating a ring of eight spots at a time, something that conductive keratoplasty does not do. Radial patterns of eight spots, each at 6- and 7-mm diameter, are placed on the cornea for 2.9 seconds (Figure 11.39). The magnitude of correction is largely determined by the laser energy applied. Previous approaches with contact probes have been plagued with problems of irregular astigmatism, because, as you march around the cornea, the cornea is changing each time you get to the next spot. It has been changed topographically, and its hydration properties are also changed. Irregular astigmatism has been a problem with other approaches that use a single spot contact or penetrating treatment.

Koch and colleagues reported on a series consisting of 1 eye in each of 28 patients treated with this method for correction of low to moderate hyperopia (up to +3.88 D). At 2 years follow-up, uncorrected distance visual acuity was improved by 1 or more lines of Snellen visual acuity in 19 (73%) of 26 of the treated eyes. The mean lines gained were 2.5 ± 2.2/3.3 ± 2.7 for one- and two-ring treatment groups, respectively. The mean change in spherical equiv-

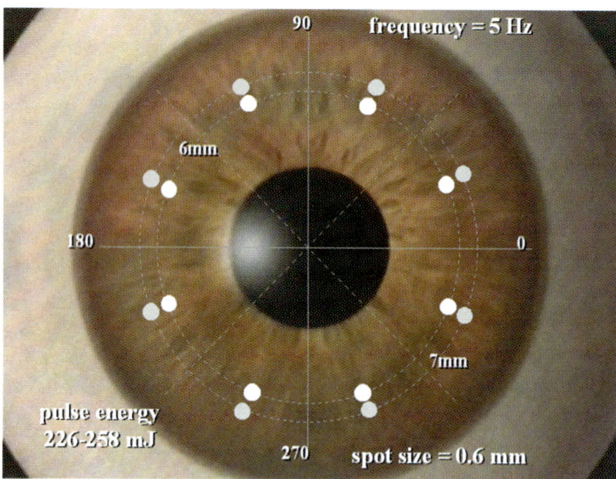

Fig. 11.39 The Sunrise nontouch device lays down a series of simultaneous spots. (Courtesy of Sunrise Technologies.)

alent of the subjective manifest refraction was −0.53 ± 0.33 D/−1.48 ± 0.58 D for one- and two-ring treatment groups. Regression between 1 and 2 years was 0.01 and 0.16 D, respectively, which is an improvement over the regression between 6 months and 2 years of approximately 0.4 to 0.5 D in Koch and McDonnell's early studies [120]. In the one-ring treatment group (18 eyes), 13 eyes (72%) had refractive corrections (range −0.38 to −1.13 D), and 5 eyes (29%) were unchanged (within +0.25 D) relative to their preoperative measurements. In the two-ring treatment group, all eight eyes (100%) had reductions in their hyperopia (range −0.38 to −2.25 D). None of the eyes lost two or more lines of spectacle-corrected distance visual acuity. There were no sight-threatening complications. The authors' conclusions were that this initial U.S. clinical study indicates that noncontact laser thermal keratoplasty treatment of low hyperopia is safe and produces modest but persistent corrections with 2 years of follow-up [121]. A study by Nano, however, reported that 17% of the patients in his group required retreatment at 9 months, having lost 1 D or more of correction in that time [122].

The problem is that we are still burning (coagulating) the cornea. Predictability still remains elusive. The striking thing to note is the extremely localized extent of the corneal burns and the apparent smoothness of the central changes. Whether the effect will remain stable or, like all previous attempts to use heat, gradually diminish over time, remains to be seen. When the FDA first turned down approval of the device, it cited the regression of effect. Patients in the study experienced, on average, 1.5 D of regression at the 2-year mark, with models predicting nearly full regression at 3 to 5 years, although there was evidence that some of the effect may be permanent. The disturbing trend for me is that the first cases started out reporting good results with 8 burns; then they went to 16. Vinciguerra's study used 24 spots in three rings, with the outer one staggered in half the eyes [123]. Now, 32 spots, done in four quick applications, have been advocated so as to reduce the rate of regression.

To be fair, no procedure currently under study for treating hyperopia has shown long-term effectiveness, so it will come down to convenience, rapidity, patient acceptance of the possible need for retreatment, and the physician's wallet (Figure 11.40).

Most experienced physicians take an eclectic approach. Chayet is using hyperopic LASIK in cases with from +1 to +4 D. One of the technique's drawbacks, he finds, is that the perfect ablation profile has not been ascertained, and patients sometimes complain of glare and halos early in the postoperative course. Chayet also has been getting about 20% regression of effect. He is in clinical trials with the Nidek Smoothscan laser, which he hopes will improve hyperopic LASIK outcomes. Chayet also performs laser thermokeratoplasty (LTK) up to +2 D. He finds the nontouch procedure to be quick and painless, with low complication rates, but with 30% regression [124].

Ditzen uses LTK for congenital hyperopic treatment up to +2.5 D. He thinks it is easier on patients than LASIK and that LTK's efficiency is surprising up to +2 to +2.5 D, but for more than this, neither efficiency, stability, safety, nor predictability are good. He also uses the LTK procedure as a secondary operation for overcorrected myopes. This he has found can be effective up to the +4-D range [125].

Discussion of laser applications in refractive surgery

To date, the excimer laser has been used to treat myopia in patients with pretreatment spherical equivalents ranging from −1 to −12 D. Follow-up of the effect on refractive error after PRK has shown a reduction of myopia in most patients, with an initial hyperopic overshoot during the first month after treatment, a shift downward over the next 1 to 2 months due to stromal remodeling,

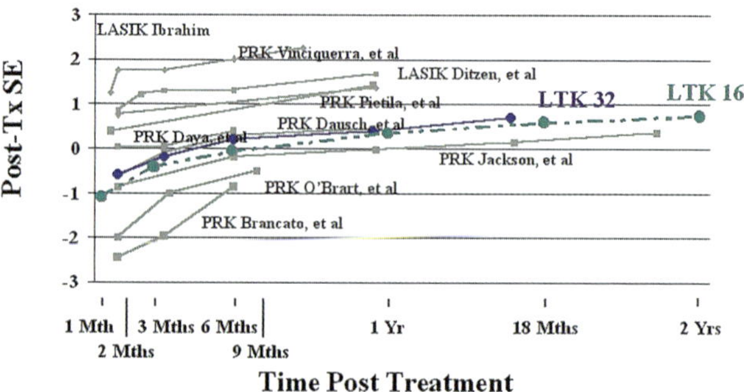

Fig. 11.40 Comparing various techniques for treating hyperopia. (Courtesy of Sunrise Technologies.)

and restabilization of the effect within 3 to 6 months after surgery. Emmetropia has been achieved in some patients who have undergone myopic keratomileusis, but serious undercorrections also have been observed.

The term *dirty beam* is used widely to describe UV lasers [78]. The output of the laser tube is nonhomogeneous, frequently showing *hot spots* [126] (Figure 11.41). Furthermore, the pulse energy shows great variations between single pulses—more so in the low-energy range. The average pulse energy falls off as the number of pulses delivered increases. This fall-off depends on the gas-filling status of the laser tube. Additionally, the laser-induced changes occurring within the delivery system itself as the laser is in use—even when multiple coated optical elements are used in the delivery system—add to the ambiguities [127]. This necessitates integrating monitoring devices into the newer laser systems [128].

Quality of ablation depends not only on the homogeneity of the beam but also on the method of creating smooth transition zones between single pulses so as to avoid the creation of significant steps (Figure 11.42). A major effort is underway to improve the quality of the laser beam prior to ablation of biologic tissue. Circular and rectangular masks have been used for the treatment of myopia, hyperopia, and astigmatism. It has been acknowledged, however, that steps between the zones will still be created [128]. Moving slits, dynamic diaphragm imaging on the cornea, and constricting diaphragms all have been proposed to smooth out this transition [129–131].

It also will be important to determine whether there is a superior delivery system. Use of an ablatable mask surface versus an iris diaphragm may not make a difference clinically. The technique essentially uses the excimer laser to create an impression of a mask onto the cornea. The mask is formed in the same shape as the lens tissue desired to be removed from the cornea and ablates at the same rate as the cornea. The primary theoretical advantage is that it would offer optimal flexibility, since it replaces the moving pads or moving slit beam of the laser with a mask customized to any desirable shape. However, a high-quality laser beam is necessary to produce uniform ablation of the mask, and while ablation of the mask image onto the cornea has been accomplished, it remains to be seen whether or not it is associated with a better refractive result—beam quality is not the excimer's strong suit. Various fluids have been studied for the same purpose [132].

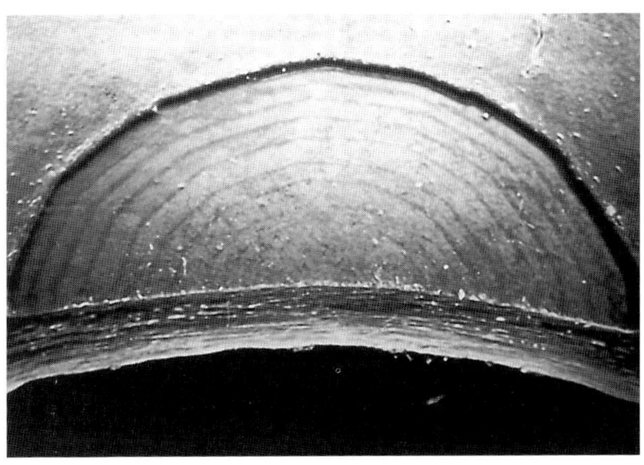

Fig. 11.42 Photoablated corneal surface.

There is still hope that by eliminating the abovementioned variations in homogeneity and transition zones, the healing response of the cornea can be minimized. Epithelia–stromal interactions are probably important but have not been analyzed in detail. Adjustability seems possible theoretically because additional ablations can be performed. The potential risks of infection, additional scarring, and even increased variability remain unaltered, however.

In order to accurately monitor the progress of ablation, a keratoscope has been integrated into one system that was supposed to demonstrate corneal topography during surgery [128,133]. There are formidable obstacles to overcome to make such real-time surface monitoring a functional reality. Photokeratoscopy techniques are of insufficient sensitivity to be used for this purpose. The same can be said for raster stereography. Holographic methods would serve but currently require a tremendous amount of computational time [134,135]. This will become less of a problem now that CPU speeds are approaching the gigahertz range. Still, parallel processors may be needed.

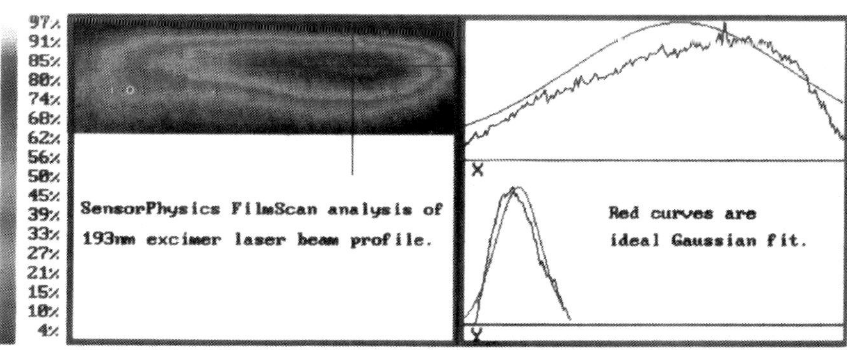

Fig. 11.41 Analysis of 193-nm excimer beam profile shows a maximized beam. (Courtesy of SenssorPhysics, Redwood City, CA—FilmScan Beam Analyzer.)

As Taylor and associates have emphasized, the variability in response from one cornea to another despite reasonably uniform conditions of treatment—the individual biologic variation in wound healing—appears to be the pivotal point of success or failure of laser keratomileusis [136]. This variability must necessarily result in unpredictability of the refractive outcome. Thus tissue response, implicated in RK variability, is not avoided by using the laser.

McDonald noted in her series of partially sighted patients treated with the excimer laser for myopic correction that serious undercorrection primarily affected those individuals whose preoperative refraction was greater than 5 D [137]. It was clear that patients who were high myopes did less well than those whose dioptric error initially was 5 D or less. Since the optimal range of myopia correction for RK is up to –5 D, such results are not good enough to justify use of the laser in these cases. Keratometric studies in these cases have shown that unlike other refractive procedures currently in use, large-area ablation with the excimer laser produces stable central flattening of the cornea and does not induce astigmatism in the vast majority of patients. However, the amount of induced astigmatism following RK is also less among experienced keratotomists. Reporting on a series of 21 sighted patients who underwent myopic ablation with the excimer laser, Deitz noted that only 2 patients had an increase in astigmatism of greater than 1 D [138].

A few years ago, excimer investigators had hoped that corneal tissue could be ablated without eliciting a response from the corneal stroma. However, results from the early studies now demonstrate that this is not true. In both experimental animals and the first series of patients, subepithelial scarring—a faint reticular haze by slit-lamp microscopy—has persisted for many months and sometimes was severe [62,136,139] (Figure 11.43). This fine haze has been noted in virtually all patients who have undergone laser keratomileusis, but at this writing it does not appear to pose a clinically significant problem. The haze develops a month or more after surgery and reaches a maximum at 3 or 4 months, after which it fades to the point where its detection by a trained observer becomes more difficult (Figures 11.44 and 11.45). Steroid drops were useful for improving the quality of corneal clarity but not uniformly so. In McDonald's series, mean corneal clarity was rated good among 10 partially sighted patients who underwent laser keratomileusis and received only steroid treatment at ablation to decrease early iritis. However, when the postoperative treatment regimen was changed to include a tapering dose of topical steroids for 1 month, only trace amounts of haze could be detected among 19 sighted patients.

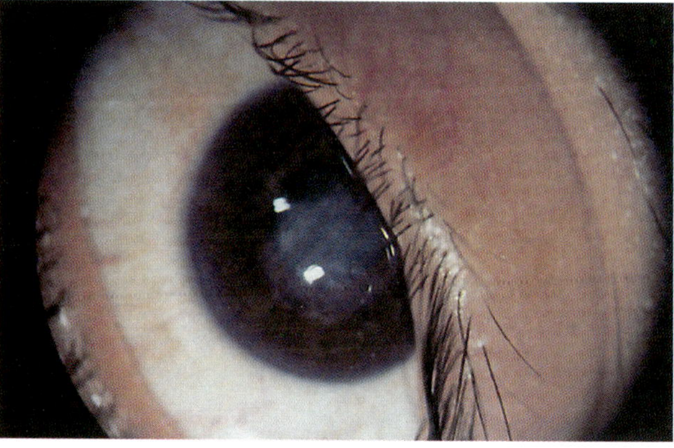

Fig. 11.43 Corneal haze following laser corneal photoablation.

This change may well cause clinically significant light scattering and image degradation and thereby render the procedure unacceptable for use on normal corneas for the correction of ametropia. In troublesome cases, additional laser energy can be used to remove the area of scarring (Figure 11.46). In contrast, others have claimed successful anterior "corneal sculpting" without scarring and stable dioptric correction in 20 of 20 nonhuman primate eyes 12 months after surgery, as well as excellent dioptric correction (within 10%) and clear corneas in three blind human eyes [140]. On histologic examination, a proliferation of keratocytes in the area of ablation with secretion of new extracellular matrix, as well as hyperplasia of the epithelium, was demonstrated, both adding up to a regression of the corneal flattening achieved initially [79,133,141].

A lot of discussion has revolved around the issue of choosing an optical zone when performing PRK and LASIK. The depth of the ablation must be increased for a given dioptric change and ablation zone, but greater ablation depths are associated with greater biologic problems, including increased tendency toward haze and regression. Epithelial gap filling tends to reduce the correction in deeper ablations. Therefore, most protocols have established the use of optical zones that vary with the intended amount of correction in order to maintain constant depth. However, it must first be determined if smaller optical zones are consistent with good, clear vision or whether they result in loss of contrast sensitivity or glare disability. It has been the author's experience that smaller optical zones show increased postoperative problems, including glare and irregular astigmatism. This is especially true with techniques involving lamellar resections [142].

Another issue that needs to be resolved is whether there are systemic factors that can play a role in determining the success of the procedure. For example, Zabel reported complete regression in one patient who was later found to be 2 weeks pregnant at the time of the laser surgery [143]. This particular patient also had previously failed epikeratophakia, and Zabel questions whether epikeratophakia might alter the corneal structure so that the response to refractive keratectomy also may be affected. Reactions such as the one described should not come as

(a)

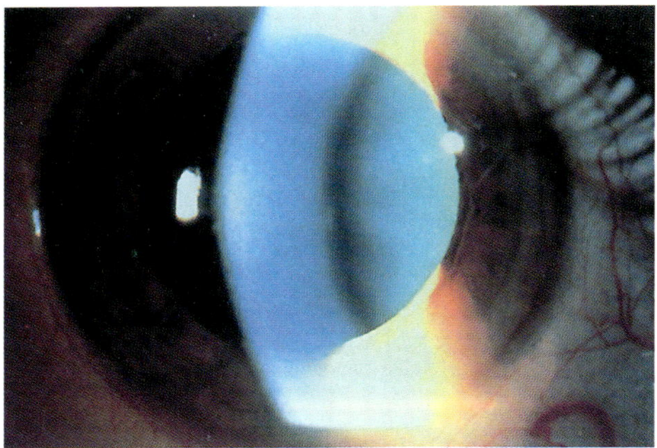

(b)

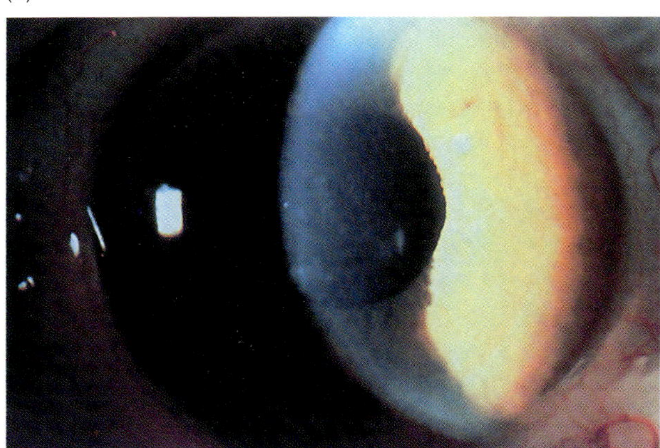

(c)

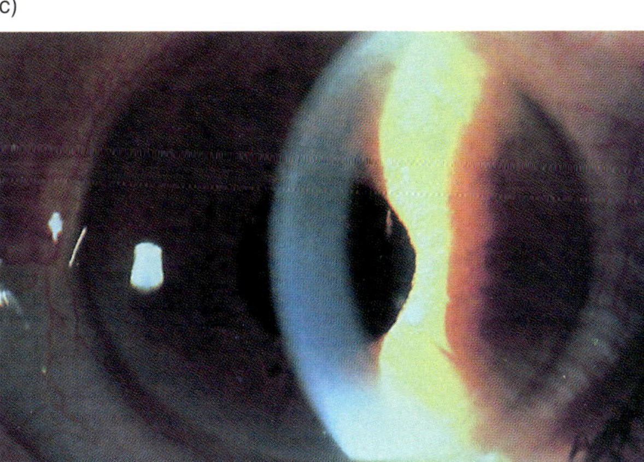

Fig. 11.44 Photoablative refractive keratectomy. (a) 1 month postsurgery; (b) 3 months postsurgery; (c) 9 months postsurgery.

a surprise, however. Experienced contact lens practitioners as well as refractive surgeons often report the same or similar phenomena with pregnant patients. It has ever been the author's practice to recommend that such patients wait at least 3 months postpartum (or after breast feeding) before undergoing any refractive surgical procedure—particularly RK. Such precautions also should be observed in patients either just going on or coming off birth control medication.

In addition to the biologic issues that remain in question, many technical issues regarding the use of laser keratomileusis are still not completely resolved. One of these issues concerns eye fixation and patient positioning. Although total ablation time to achieve significant correction is short, spatial stability of the eye within microns is mandatory, and fixation of the globe with a suction ring has been used [133]. Computerized optical "tracking" of the eye seems to offer some practical advantages—the need for retrobulbar anesthesia (for the placement of the suction ring) with all its attendant hazards in the myopic eye (see Chapter 15) has, at least, been eliminated. The various laser systems available offer different methods of fixation, but it remains to be seen whether any of these is indeed the optimal approach. The Autonomous laser may have the best solution.

Should the challenging problems of wound healing and radiation-mediated cell damage finally be solved, a computer simulation of laser keratomileusis will help not only to understand but also to predict the final outcome of lamellar refractive corneal surgery [144].

Intrastromal ablation

Ablation of tissue within the stroma itself, leaving the superficial layers intact (including Bowman's layer), may answer some of the objections to surface ablation (Figure 11.47). Sort of keratophakia in reverse—instead of putting something in, we take something out. Since no incision is necessary, Bowman's layer is not disturbed. The thought is appealing, but some reflection is in order. No one has as yet answered the question of where the explosive by-products are to go during this procedure (see Figure 11.9). If we hearken back to Puliafito's photographs of the ablation plumes and Trokel's photographs of the expanded wound cavities from gas formation, we are led to ask the question "What happens to all the little

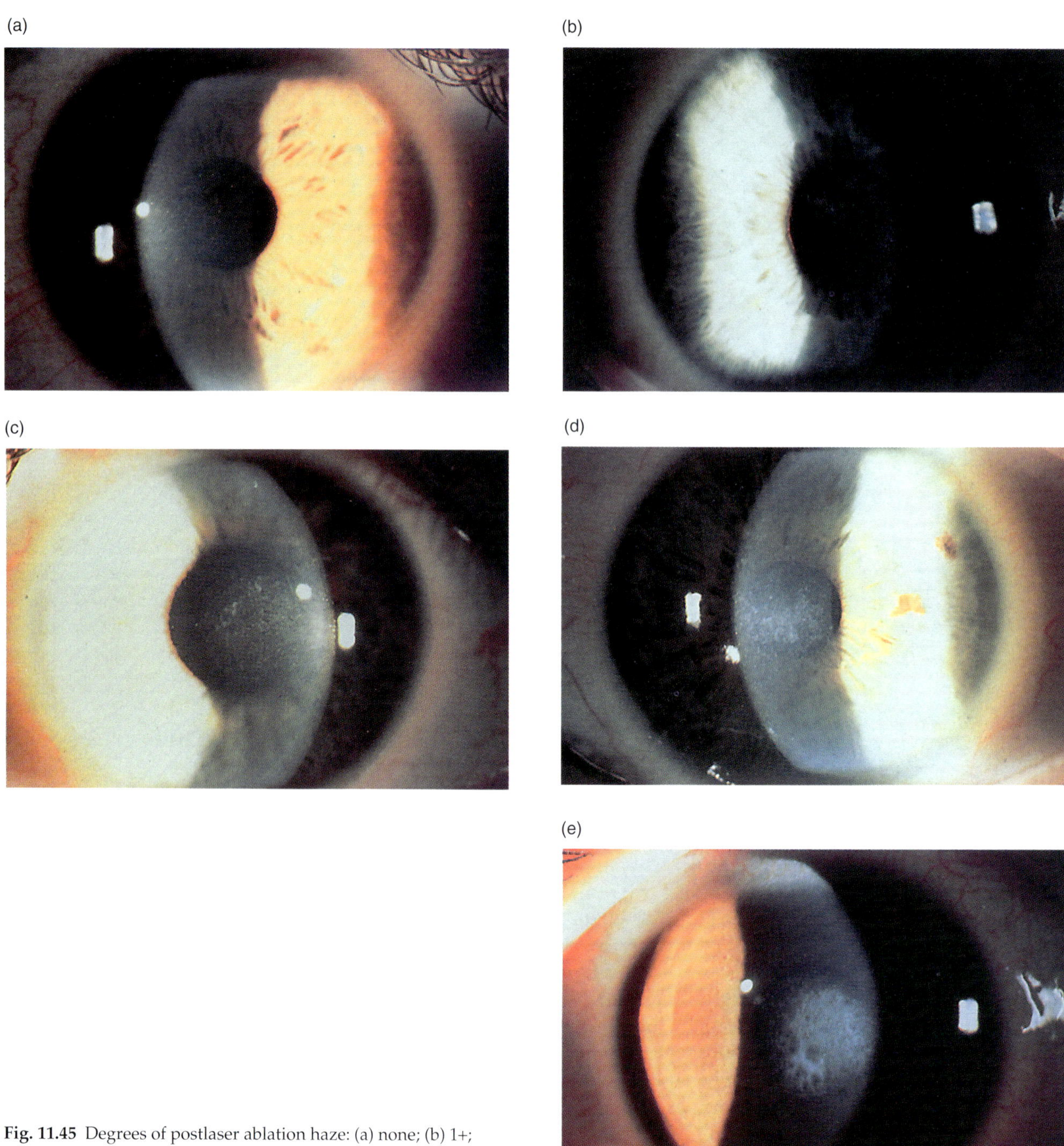

Fig. 11.45 Degrees of postlaser ablation haze: (a) none; (b) 1+; (c) 2+; (d) 3+; (e) 4+. Note the reticular nature of the scarring. (Courtesy of T. Seiler.)

bits?" The gas and by-products of the "blast effect" of photoablation of tissue do not just get "beamed out" of the stroma—they have to go somewhere. Or stay where they are. There are some lingering questions about the carcinogenic effect of such monatomic and diatomic particles left in situ, not to mention the effect of rapidly expanding gases on tissue integrity. Additionally, there is no evidence that the cornea will achieve or retain an altered curvature after such treatment.

However, further work with intrastromal ablation using frequency-doubled YAG lasers has fallen by the wayside as of this writing.

(a)

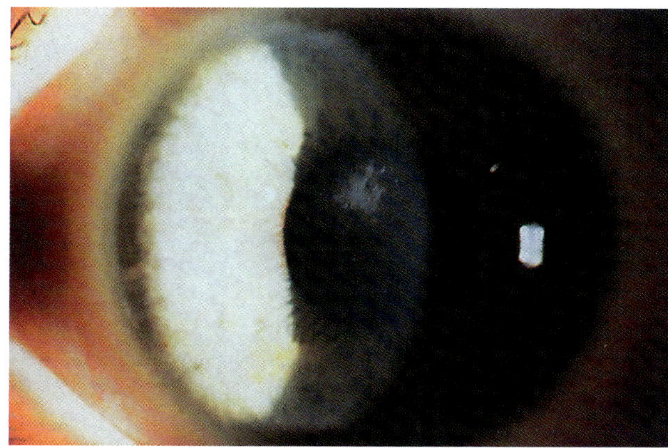

(b)

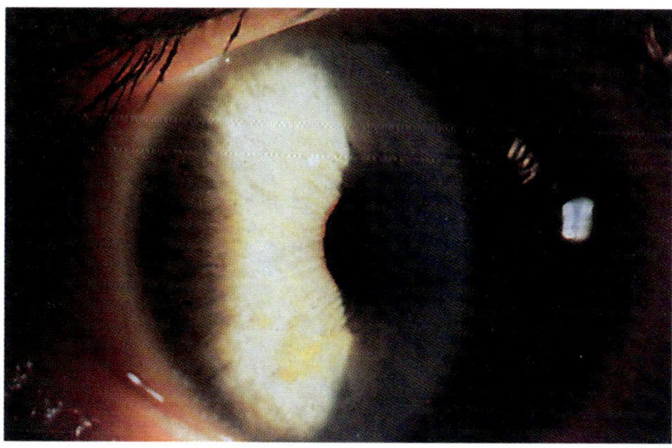

Fig. 11.46 (a) Area of postlaser scarring causing degraded vision; (b) same eye after additional laser energy was used to remove the scar. (Courtesy of T. Seiler.)

Smoothing the corneal surface—Phototherapeutic keratoplasty (PTK)

One of the most exciting uses of such surface ablation is in superficial keratectomy, essentially planing off the roughened corneal surface to promote smoother epithelial regrowth. One of the questions that still remains regarding superficial keratectomy using the excimer laser is whether there is an optimal laser strategy and surfacing agent. In most protocols, a methylcellulose-type preparation is first applied to level the surface of the cornea. This allows removal of the affected areas, or peaks, without injury to the healthy tissue found in the valleys. Fasano and colleagues reported on phototherapeutic keratectomy using a rabbit model (Figures 11.48 and 11.49). In a series of 30 monkeys followed for up to 18 months, Fantes reported that type III collagen and keratin sulfate were found to be deposited in sufficient amounts that they actually filled in the ablated area to some degree [145]. There also appeared to be some biologic variability in the wound-healing response. This implies that it will not be possible to do an exact pretreatment calculation of the amount of cornea to be ablated, since it cannot be predicted how much tissue fill-in will occur. There also can be a regression of effect as a result of the wound-healing response. Topical corticosteroids—which reduce fibroblast production of new tissue—can modulate this to some extent, but they do not provide precise control. Still another effect is the development of glare. The scar tissue that is formed does not have the structure of normal corneal tissue. This is, of course, the precise circumstance with refractive ablation. In these cases, the small amount of persistent corneal haze still allows improved visual acuity above and beyond that of the previous condition, however. Nevertheless, the scarring is not very intense and can be lessened with the use of corticosteroids.

Steinert and Puliafito reported the appearance of a fibroplastic nodule at the apex in a case of with kerato-

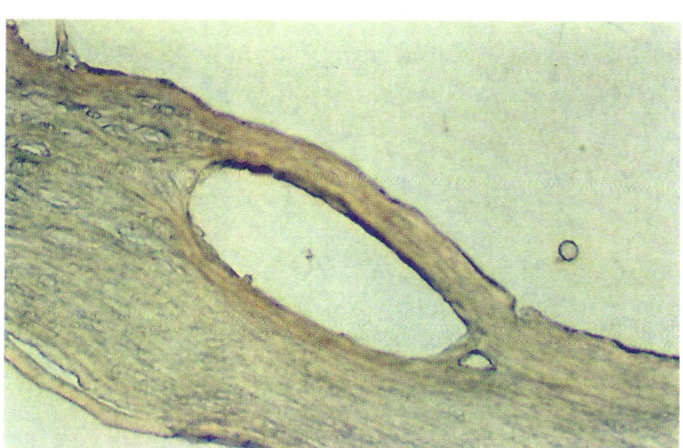

Fig. 11.47 Intrastromal corneal ablation performed using a frequency-doubled YAG system from Intelligent Laser Systems. (Courtesy of S. Brown.)

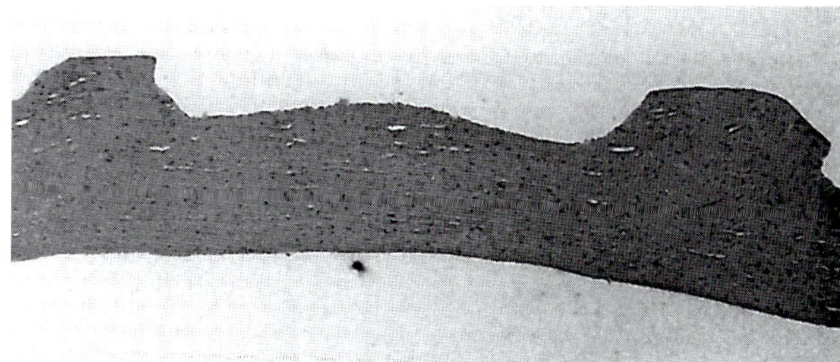

Fig. 11.48 Light micrograph demonstrates surface irregularity achieved using the excimer laser to perform a 50-μm-deep ablation with the cornea partially masked by stainless steel screening. (Hematoxylin and eosin, original magnification ×40) (from Fasano AP, Moreira H, McDonnell PJ, Sinbawy A. Excimer laser smoothing of a reproducible model of anterior corneal surface irregularity. Ophthalmol 1991; 98:1782–1785).

(a)

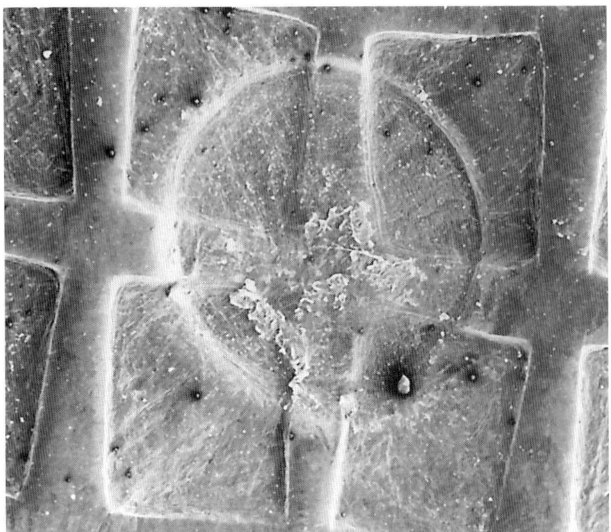

(b)

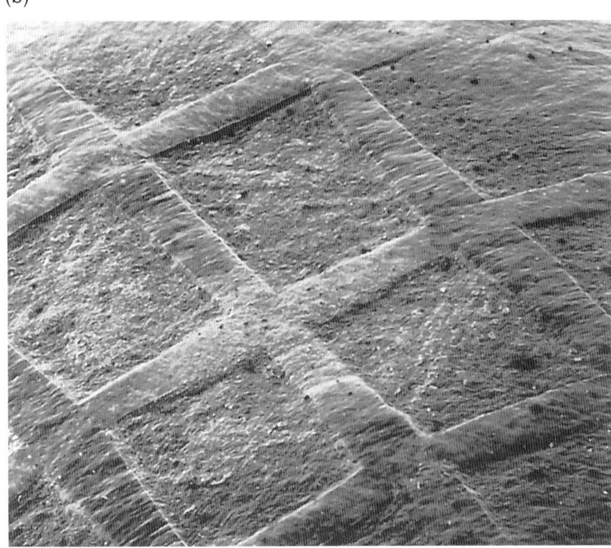

(c)

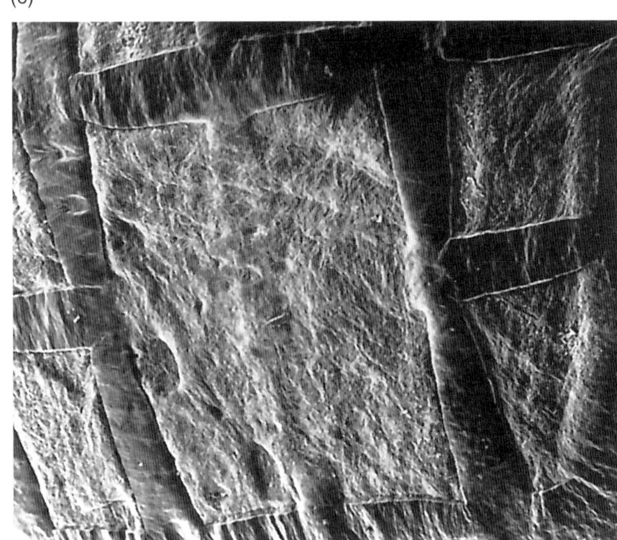

Fig. 11.49 SEM of irregular cornea reablated to a depth of 50 μm, using a repetition rate of 10 Hz, without application of fluid to the surface. (a) Depressions and elevated ridges persist (×35). (b) SEM of similarly reablated cornea after application of fluid shows surface irregularity to be decreased relative to the original model (Fig. 11.48) and (a), above. Original magnification ×35. (c) SEM of cornea reablated as in (b) but with a reduced repetition rate of 2 Hz. Surface irregularity is minimal compared with the preablation model and with (a) and (b), above. Original magnification ×35.

conus removed by excimer ablation [70]. Despite previous surgical keratectomy, the keratoconus had recurred over a few months (Figure 11.50). Using an energy level of 180 mJ/cm², a 1.0-mm zone, and a repetition rate of 10 Hz, 242 pulses were applied. Methylcellulose was applied to adjacent cornea to limit exposure damage. Contact lens tolerance returned to 8 hours within 2 weeks of the treatment. The nodule has shown no signs of returning.

PTK with Biomask

Treating patients with irregular corneal surfaces presents a challenge for ophthalmologists. However, new developments may make it easier. One potential option may be PTK performed with Biomask, a liquid collagen-derivative gel used to smooth the corneal surface. The material is heated to a liquid state, placed on the corneal surface, and covered by a rigid contact lens, providing a template for the desired curvature. The lens is removed when the material has solidified. Then a large excimer laser beam is used in the PTK mode to ablate the corneal surface and Biomask, which is ablated at the same rate as the corneal tissue. As the laser ablates the mask, it trims the steeper areas of the cornea, which break through first. During this process, the curvature of the front of the mask is transferred to the cornea. Kremer has found so far that in certain types of settings (e.g., Salzmann's nodular dystrophy) and following refractive surgery, "we see very significant improvement." He is also studying the material in patients with corneal scars and other dystrophies [146]. Sur-

(a)

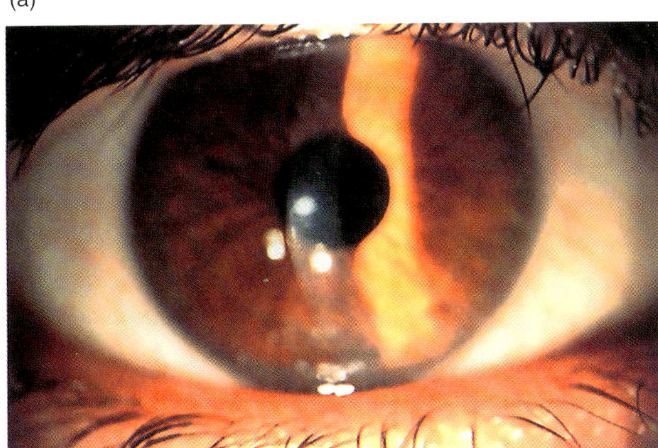

(b)

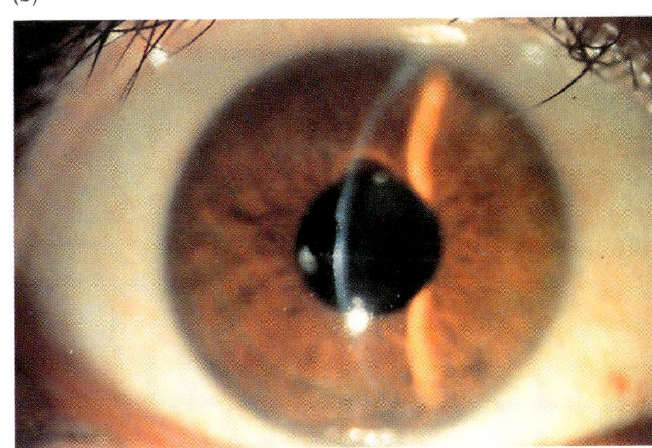

(c)

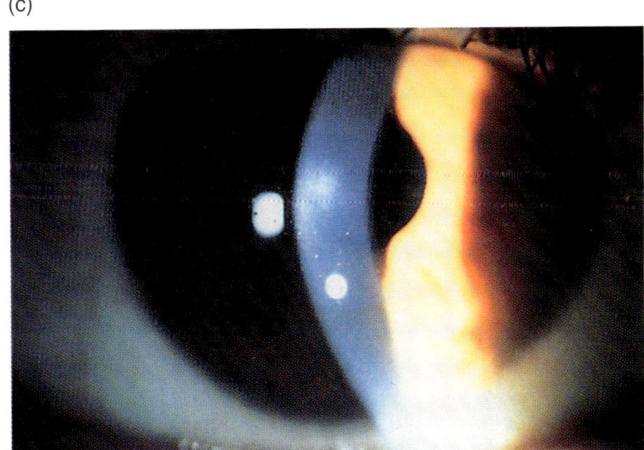

Fig. 11.50 (a) Fibroplastic corneal nodule; (b) immediately after treatment with the laser; (c) smooth postoperative surface with mild reticular haze. (Courtesy of Steinert.)

geons must be careful not to tilt the contact lens when covering the Biomask, which would affect the results.

During PTK with Biomask, Kremer uses ultraviolet light to help delineate where the Biomask ends and the cornea begins. He recommends turning off the room and microscope lights, positioning the laser's aiming beam, and allowing time for the surgeon's eyes to adapt to the dark. "The most elevated part of the cornea that peeks through first will start to fluoresce first, and the surgeon can observe the fluorescence as it corresponds to the elevation in the topography. . . . As you go deeper and deeper in the mask, the area of fluorescence will get larger. When you get through the epithelium, the area in which you first go through the epithelium will stop fluorescing. . . . When the fluorescence has completely gone, that means you're totally through the epithelium and you're into either Bowman's membrane or stroma. We stop when there's still a little bit of fluorescence."

Autofluorescence-guided PTK

Investigators also are studying how epithelial autofluorescence can be used to guide transepithelial PTK to treat mild overcorrection resulting from PRK or LASIK.

Because the VISX 2020B and STAAR PTK beams tend to produce midperipheral epithelial breakthrough, this tendency can be used to reverse low to moderate overcorrections. To observe the autofluorescence, all the lights on the operating room microscope are turned down, and the room lights are turned off. Fluorescence is lost in the periphery first, because that's the way the laser beam is breaking through; the epithelium is leaving there first. The laser is activated until almost all the central epithelium is removed. If you do not follow the epithelial fluorescence, you do not really know when to stop the laser.

In a study of this method, all 12 patients had a reduction in their induced hyperopia and improved uncorrected visual acuity. The advantages of this technique are that the desired effect is achieved with minimal tissue removal, it does not require laser software upgrades, and it produces a smaller epithelial defect. In addition, this technique can be used without raising the flap in LASIK patients. However, it can be used only for mild to moderate overcorrections. You cannot get much more than 1.25 D, so if someone is massively overcorrected, this is not the technique [147].

Decentered ablations

One means used to treat irregular astigmatism is to decenter the ablation over the irregularity, based on corneal topography. This deviates from more conventional excimer ablations, which are usually centered over the pupil or the light reflex.

The first physicians to publish findings on decentration treatment of irregular astigmatism were Gibralter and Trokel [148]. They published results of two patients in whom multiple eccentric ablations, 4 mm in diameter, were made in a C pattern. Focal treatments were done first, followed by the standard ablations for refractive error, with an intentional undercorrection to prevent hyperopic shift. Uncorrected visual acuity improved from count fingers and 20/200 preoperatively to 20/50 postoperatively in both patients.

Gustavo E. Tamayo, of Bogota, Colombia, has presented findings from localized PRK excimer laser ablations with the VISX STAAR S2 Smoothscan [149]. With this experimental technique, Tamayo was able to effectively ablate the most elevated areas of the cornea by manually decentering the excimer laser beams and reducing the diameter of the myopic ablation to correspond with that of the irregularity. He used this technique on the eight corneas with irregularities caused by prior LASIK procedures, keratoconus, or penetrating keratoplasty. At a follow-up period of 2 to 12 months, all eyes had improved uncorrected visual acuity, and no eyes lost any lines of best-corrected visual acuity.

VISX has developed a software package that assists in this decentration process through its contoured ablation pattern (CAP) method, which is investigational in the United States. This method allows physicians to center on the cornea, as usual, and program offset refractive ablations at varying depths and sizes of ellipses, circles, and cylinders. The CAP method allows the surgeon to control the ablation size, depth, and shape but leaves decentration to the security of the computer.

Custom ablations

With the emergence of flying-spot scanning lasers, custom ablations promise to play a significant role in the treatment of irregular corneal surfaces (see above). One example is a LaserSight Technologies' research-and-development project focusing on custom corneal ablations performed with a flying-spot scanning laser guided by tomographic, topographic, and other data. While not specifically a PTK application, the system is expected to cover a range of indications such as corneal scars, irregular astigmatism, overcorrections, undercorrections, and nodules.

Ditzen presented data on this technology, called Topolink. Using a Technolas laser that employed data from the C-Scan Placido-based videokeratography machine from Technomed, he treated 13 eyes in the study. Monocular diplopia disappeared in all cases. Enlargement of the optical zone occurred in eight eyes, yet five eyes lost two lines of best-corrected visual acuity due to irregularities that could not be ablated. More blurring and color effects occurred in nearly all eyes. These data demonstrated that the Topolink spot with a Placido-based system seems to be effective about 60% of the time [150]. However, Ditzen also stated that there must be an intensive cooperation between the excimer laser and topography companies to develop this technology.

Placido-based videokeratography may be part of the problem. Looking at power maps for custom ablations is worthless. Elevation maps are needed because the laser requires height or Z data to place ablations accurately. This is not obtainable with sphere-based topographic systems of any stripe (see Chapter 6).

The future of laser refractive corneal surgery

Aberration-guided photoablation

Resurfacing a cornea based on measurements of the total optical aberration of an eye may be the answer to the less than totally satisfactory results with current surface methods. By adapting our surgical modifications in such a way as to compensate for such aberrations, visual acuities in excess of 20/20 (6/6) may be possible (Figure 11.51).

The operative word here is *may*, because the niggling old axiom remains: *Just because we can do a thing does not signify that we should do a thing*. Newly developed devices using adaptive optics measure the total aberration of the optical system of the eye. The problem here is that all the aberrations are measured, including those caused by internal lens opacities/cataract changes. Such aberrations will be dynamic—changing over time. Winnowing these out may prove to be a larger task than anticipated. It is still unclear whether the wavefront map will pick up a keratoconus suspect. And there are other aspects to

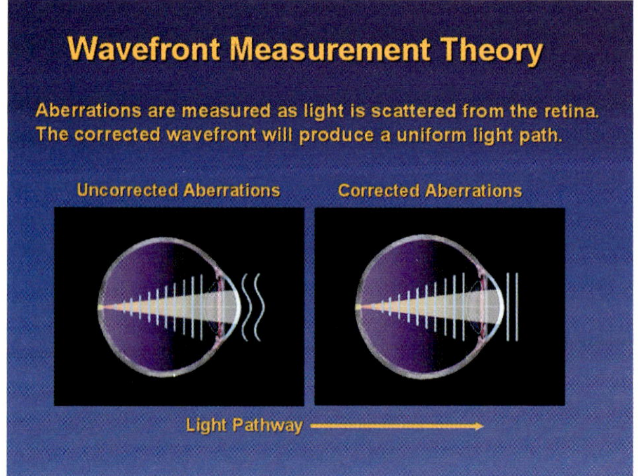

Fig. 11.51 Wavefront technology measures aberrations in reflected light. (Courtesy of VISX.)

be considered as well, such as structural factors—constitutive properties (for a more complete discussion of wavefront/adaptive optics technology, see Chapter 6).

Wavefront technology is now positioned as the hottest new thing in refractive surgery. Whether "supernormal" or "super" vision will be possible, however, is still something that only time will reveal. What should concern most ophthalmologists is why they were surprised by this new technology, and they should ask themselves why they have not been paying attention. Wavefront technology is not new. Holographic and interferometric technology has been used in lens design for years—onto a century (see Chapter 6)—and devices for correctly measuring the corneal surface appeared on the scene some 12 years ago.

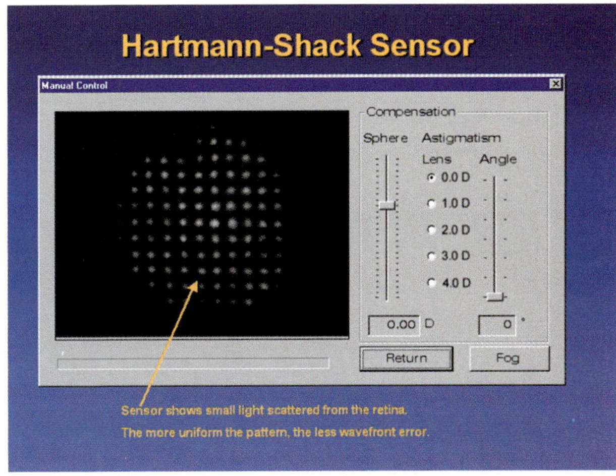

Fig. 11.52 This is the return from an eye with few, if any, aberrations. (Courtesy of VISX.)

Why wavefront?

One common misconception right now is that wavefront technology is supposed to supersede and replace corneal topography. Rather, the measurements that wavefront systems provide are used in addition to those yielded by corneal topography and refraction. I like to think of wavefront technology as another piece of the puzzle, with the puzzle being the physics of vision.

Corneal topography provides us with invaluable information, but only about the anterior surface of the cornea. Wavefront technology, in turn, allows us to measure more of the optical system in order to determine what exactly distorts a ray of light during its journey from the front to the back of the eye. With more parameters to enter into the laser, we should be able to achieve better outcomes.

When a ray of light enters the eye, whatever is between the origin of the light and the middle of the retina (e.g., cornea, lens, aqueous, vitreous) distorts it. Wavefront technology detects these so-called higher-order aberrations. First, wavefront systems project light rays into the eye (Figure 11.52). Next, the technology measures how much the patient's optical system distorts this wavefront by comparing it with the original wavefront that was perfect before it hit the eye (Figure 11.53). The system then determines what adjustments must be made to the subject's corneal surface to produce a crisply focused image on his or her retina (Figure 11.54).

The correction of higher-order aberrations can increase our ability to see "out," thereby offering the possibility of increased visual acuity, perhaps beyond the typical limit of 20/15. In theory, diffraction-limited optical cutoffs for 3- and 8-mm pupils would be high enough to yield retinal images of letter targets as small as 20/6.7 and 20/2.5, respectively. Improving the quality of the retinal image is an important first step toward achieving supernormal visual acuity, but it may not be sufficient. This is so because when optical limitations have been removed, visual performance now becomes constrained by neural factors. Specifically, the spacing between retinal photoreceptors represents a neural limitation to visual resolution that is only slightly higher than the normal optical limit. Consequently, increasing the quality of the retinal image probably will not yield a major increase in resolution acuity, although it could have a large impact on detection acuity.

By using adaptive optics that can be adjusted to correct the aberrations, a masking system could be constructed to permit precise laser contouring that may correct the eye to "super" vision. Supernormal vision will not be possible in everyone because of biologic limitations and other factors. In ideal patients, however, a key will be to tailor the ablation profile to each eye rather than to a patient's prescription.

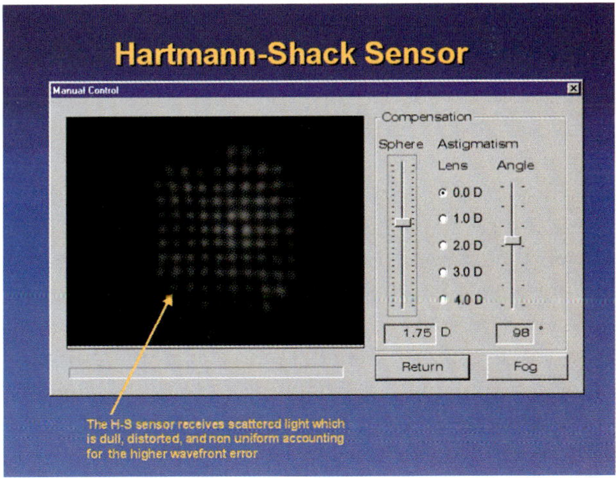

Fig. 11.53 This pattern shows pincushion distortion typical of higher-order astigmatism. The same pattern can be derived using ray tracing from data derived from interferometry of the corneal surface. (Courtesy of VISX.)

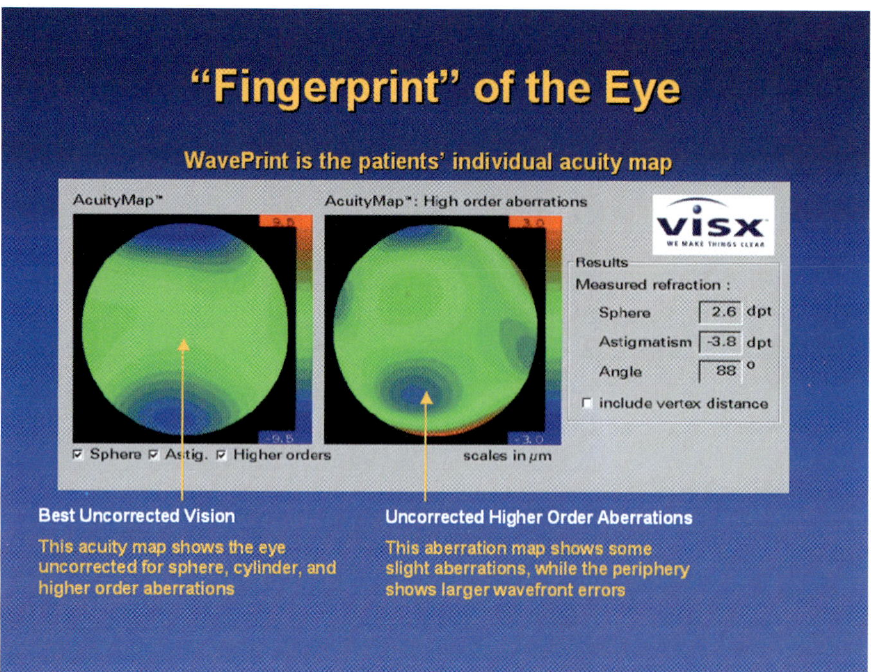

Fig. 11.54 Maps can then be constructed showing both low- and high-order aberrations (missed with conventional systems using sphere-based technology). (Courtesy of VISX.)

Customized corneal ablation

In the world of LASIK vision correction, no topic is drawing more attention than customized ablation that would give a unique shape to each individual cornea. If two eyes have +2 D of hyperopic astigmatism, we might consider them optically the same, and certainly today if both were treated with the same excimer laser, both would receive the same pattern and depth of ablation (Figure 11.55). Thus, doing a +2-D LASIK procedure on each eye is likely to give a good refractive and visual acuity outcome (e.g., –0.25 D manifest refraction 20/20 uncorrected visual acuity).

However, the outcome would fall short of the ideal, which would be 20/10 uncorrected visual acuity with a plano manifest refraction and a reduction in destructive optical aberrations, because these two eyes are not optically the same. Topographically, each would have a different corneal shape; the basic pattern would be prolate, steeper centrally and becoming flatter paracentrally and peripherally, but the exact topographic shapes would be different. Optically, both eyes would have an average of 5 D of myopic defocus. But the actual image pattern striking the retina would be different, because the defocus might be somewhat asymmetric—maybe a little more out of focus superiorly and a little less inferiorly, without the presence of measurable astigmatism. The wavefront aberration patterns of the two eyes would be different, with slightly more spherical aberration in one and slightly less coma aberration in the other and with similar differences in higher-order aberrations (Figure 11.56).

The importance of being prolate

Right now, refractive procedures entail the flattening of the central cornea, which creates an oblate shape. Wavefront technology will benefit the majority of patients if it can enable surgeons to maintain a prolate corneal shape postoperatively. The reason a prolate shape is favored, of course, is that the cornea's natural design is what helps to focus peripheral light rays on the center of the retina. The biggest criticism of wavefront technology has been that although it can produce very fine measurements of the optical system, most current lasers are not able to produce such submicron-level changes. Newer guided lasers, however, such as Autonomous's LADARVision, Wavelight's Allegretto laser, and LaserSight's LaserScan LSX, can make these smaller incremental alterations. They also feature an eye tracker, which compensates for saccadic movements by signaling back to the laser when and by how much the eye has moved.

Additionally, wavefront technology should enable us to fix our previous mistakes, namely, all our patients with oblate corneas who complain about glare and halos. Wavefront technology should let us determine which parts of these patients' optical systems are distorted and help us to reduce those aberrations, perhaps even to create prolate corneas in these patients (see the discussion on phototherapeutic keratectomy, or PTK, above).

Modifying the contour of the cornea is part and parcel of refractive correction and results in an oblate corneal curvature as opposed to its original prolate shape and that tends to enhance spherical aberration. Could maintaining

(a)

(b)

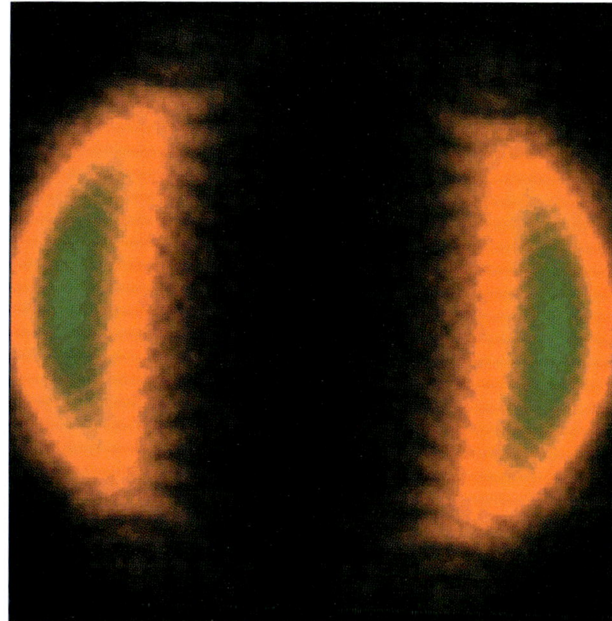

(c)

Fig. 11.55 (a) This is a topographic map of a cornea with somewhat asymmetrical hyperopic astigmatism. (b) This is the normal pattern for an eye being treated for astigmatism. (c) The outcome using "normal" LASIK technique. Note the area of paracentral aberration. (Courtesy of Autonomous Systems.)

the eye's natural prolate shape, as occurs with intracorneal ring segments (ICRSs), give patients better acuity?

It is all a matter of optics. With an oblate or spherical cornea, the peripheral cornea focuses light rays in front of the area where it is focused by the central cornea. Thus, instead of all your light being focused into one point, especially with a dilated pupil, the peripheral cornea is actually focusing light rays anterior to the light rays that are focused from the central cornea. This reduces fine two-point discrimination and contrast sensitivity. With the prolate cornea, however, where it is steeper centrally than by the periphery, outer area light rays are converged more closely together with the innermost ones, which improves the resolution of the eye.

(a)

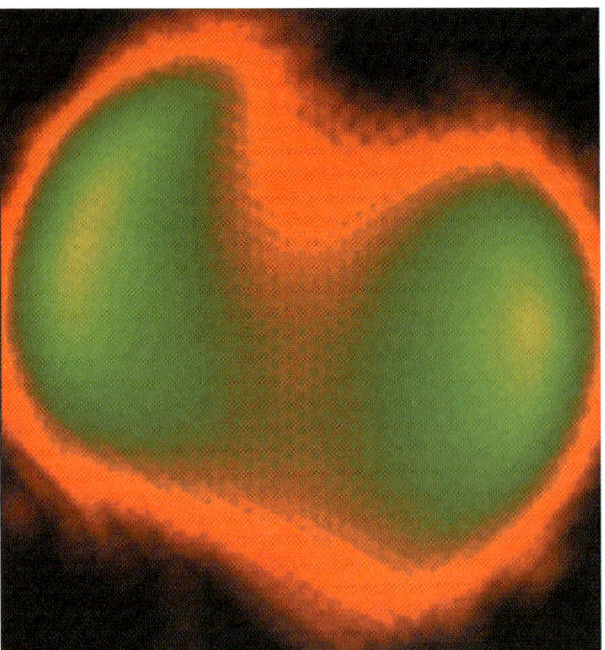

(b)

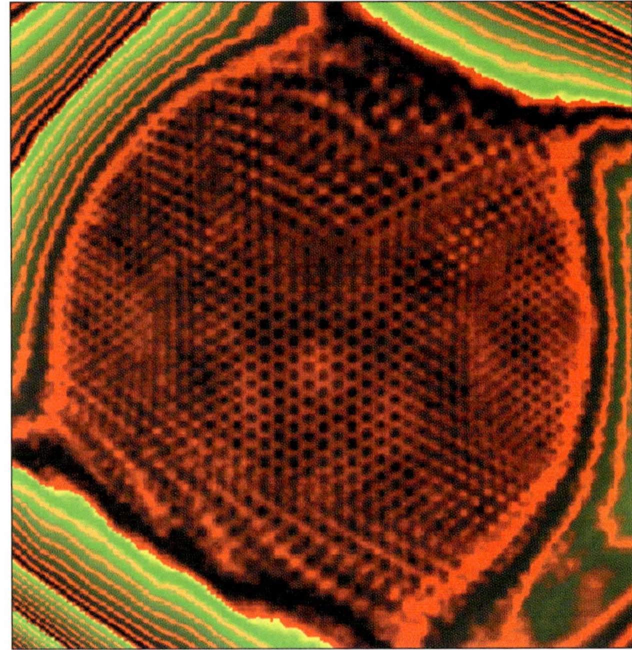

Fig. 11.56 (a) A customized treatment pattern of the same cornea accounts for smaller high-order aberrations, which make each ocular system unique. (b) The result is a much smoother refracting surface. (Courtesy of Autonomous Systems.)

The only widely used refractive procedure that results in a prolate cornea for myopic patients is the use of Intacs (see Chapter 10), which work by adding material to the cornea's midperiphery, which is flattened along with the central cornea, but to a greater degree, thereby preserving the cornea's prolate shape and conceivably improving vision [151].

The ideal corneal asphericity (Q) of eyes, compared with between 0 and −0.25 for normal preoperative eyes, has not been convincingly established. However, increasing the prolate asphericity (Q) to −0.50 (as suggested by some authors) could result in diminished vision due to loss of contrast sensitivity in mesopic conditions [152]. While there are some benefits to an increased prolate shape, there are some drawbacks as well. With a dilated pupil, while the more prolate-shaped cornea may better balance the spherical aberrations of the lens, this is by no means a night-vision panacea. For those who have very large pupils, for example, there can be an extremely abrupt transition with intracorneal ring segments, since a deep trough is needed in the periphery to maintain the change in curvature between the outlying area and the center. Such abrupt transitions potentially can cause patients with very large pupils more trouble than what they would have had just based on the fact that they had gone to a more oblate shape with LASIK. At the levels of myopia for which intracorneal ring segments are applicable (from −1 to −3 D), glare and contrast sensitivity really have not been a concern for LASIK patients. Problems with night vision in general with LASIK are probably due to a combination of factors, as well as the cornea's shape. These include the size of the optical zone, how well centered it is, and how much irregular astigmatism results from the ablation. This also may be true for the intracorneal ring segments (Intacs). Even if you have a good prolate shape, if you have decentration of the intracorneal ring segments, if you have edema around your incision, and if the segments slip downward or upward, you can have asymmetric astigmatism.

The aberroscope and its ilk

Theo Seiler and colleagues developed the Dresden wavefront analyzer based on Tscherning's aberroscope [153,154]. The system uses a frequency-doubled Nd:YAG laser emitting at a wavelength of 532 nm and a mask system for creating 128 equidistant and parallel light rays that are projected through the cornea. Via optical imaging, the system focuses these rays onto the retina. A computerized low-light closed-circuit device (CCD) camera then uses indirect ophthalmoscopy to measure the deviation of the spots as they appear on the retina (see Figure 6.48a). The system reconstructs the wavefront using Zernike polynomials.

The Dresden wavefront analyzer is linked to Wavelight's Allegretto laser. In Germany, Dr. Seiler has shown improved outcomes when using the wavefront-guided laser versus conventional laser systems with and without eye trackers. He treated his first patients in June 1999. Myopic sphere ranged from –1.5 to –6.5 D, with less than 1.0 D of astigmatism. Preoperative best-corrected visual acuities ranged from 20/25 to 20/8 for all patients. Postoperative uncorrected visual acuities ranged from 20/20 to 20/8 with an observable reduction in higher-order aberrations. Postoperatively, 26% of patients had the same best-corrected vision, 61% experienced an improvement of one or two lines, and 13% gained three or more lines. Scotopic vision either remained unchanged or improved. Seiler found that reductions in wavefront aberrations correlated with improved uncorrected visual acuities [155].

Numerous companies are developing aberrometers to link to excimer lasers: Bausch & Lomb's Zywave instrument with the Technolas 217C, Autonomous's Hartmann-Schack waveform sensor used in the custom cornea system, VISX's 20/10 instrument with the STAAR S2, the Emory Vision Correction Center with the spatially resolved refractometer, Nidek with its ARC-10,000 linked to the Nidek EC-5000, the Tscherning aberrometer with the Wavelight flying-spot laser, and possibly others.

VISX's and Autonomous Technologies' analyzers rely on a Hartmann-Shack wavefront sensor to detect optical aberrations (see above). The systems direct an eye-safe probe laser beam into the patient s eye to illuminate a small spot on the retina. A fraction of the probe light re-emerges from the eye but is distorted by the aberrations in the optical system. The system's measurement devices contain optics that convey the wavefront to the Hartmann-Shack sensor's entrance face, which in turn contains an array of microscopic optical lenses or "lenslets." These lenslets then divide the wavefront into a number of sub-apertures. Next, the analyzer focuses each part of the wavefront onto a CCD chip. It reconstructs the wavefront and measures the shift in these points caused by aberrations, again using Zernike polynomials.

VISX has teamed up with Bille to incorporate wavefront analysis [156] into a VISX laser system. The 20/10 Perfect Vision system features a closed-loop system that allows patients actually to experience what it would be like to see after undergoing wavefront-based correction. It does so based on the principle of adaptive optics, which enables the system to adjust the distorted wavefront emerging from the patient's s eye back into perfect alignment. It is this perfected image that the patient then sees. At present, VISX is at work on its own version of a scanning-spot laser with an automated eye tracker to be used in conjunction with its wavefront technology.

At Autonomous, Pettit and colleagues have designed the CustomCornea accessory device. Their preclinical studies confirmed that wavefront analysis is an effective and repeatable measure of visual optics. Company data presented at the 1999 meeting of the Association for Research in Vision and Ophthalmology (ARVO) showed that wavefront measurements of standard spherocylindrical errors were consistent with those obtained with a phoropter. The data also demonstrated that these measurements can reveal significant aberrations not seen with conventional phoropter measurements.

Pettit outlined an FDA feasibility trial that was begun in conjunction with Marguerite McDonald in October 1999. Subjects included 20 patients undergoing bilateral LASIK surgery and 20 patients undergoing bilateral PRK surgery. Myopic sphere ranged from –2.00 to –3.75 D, and cylinder ranged from 0 to –1.25 D. Hyperopic patients with sphere between +0.25 and +4.25 D and cylinder ranging between 0 and –3.25 D of astigmatism are also being followed.

In the study, investigators randomly selected one eye for CustomCornea and the other for conventional treatment with the LADARVision surgery system (see above). Although 1-week postoperative data revealed no statistically significant difference between the two groups, all patients had visual acuities between 20/16 and 20/32. Pettit notes that these are initial patients and early results—before nomograms could be refined. As refinements to the nomogram have been implemented at each progressive stage of the study, investigators have found improved visual outcomes for the CustomCornea patients (especially the myopes) over those receiving conventional techniques.

Wakil and Pallikaris are currently working with the Tracy ray-tracing refractometer (Figure 11.57). Rather than projecting a grid pattern of light rays on the eye, the refractometer measures the eye's refractive power on a point-by-point basis. For this reason, the system will not be subject to the potential problem in a highly aberrated eye of crisscrossing data points, as the three other wavefront systems could be. The refractometer rapidly fires a series of very small parallel light beams one at a time through the entrance pupil of the eye in an infinite selection of software-selectable patterns. Unlike other wavefront technologies, the Tracy system therefore is capable of probing particular areas of the eye's aperture, not just the entire aperture at once.

The system features semiconductor photodetectors, which can detect where each light ray strikes the retina and provide raw data that actually measures the (x–y)

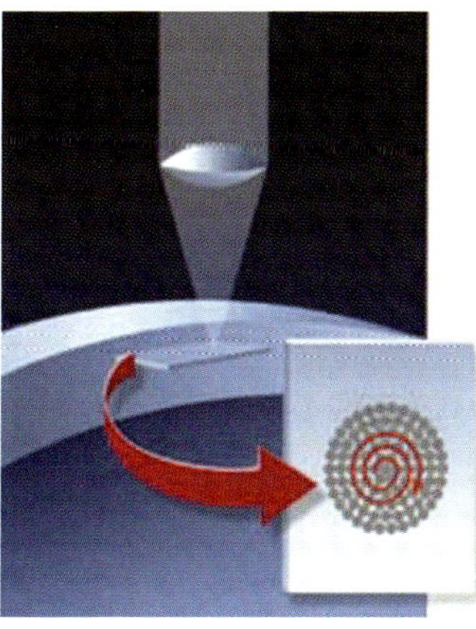

Fig. 11.57 Tracy system uses a single flying spot to measure aberrations via rapid ray-trace processing. (Courtesy of Tracy.)

error distance from the ideal conjugate focal point. The manufacturer states that the refractometer functions with exceptional speed, which will compensate for saccadic movements, unlike other systems.

All wavefront technologies, whether the aberroscope, the Hartman-Shack sensor, or interferometrically derived, depend on the laser ablation being controllable. This constraint practically demands that the laser energy be delivered point by point—something called *pointillism* and which is the hallmark of the flying-spot lasers.

One of the benefits of the flying-spot laser is that the stress waves caused by the shock of the beam hitting the cornea and blasting away tissue are minimized (Figure 11.58). This goes far to reduce collateral damage to the endothelium demonstrated by some studies (see Figure 11.25). Another valuable feature of such lasers is that the spot pattern can be controlled by software, making these systems a natural for routine and custom ablations (Figures 11.59 and 11.60).

Where are we headed?

Before LASIK surgeons begin advertising custom, individualized treatments, before companies begin promoting aberrometers, and before patients begin expecting individualized treatment, a number of challenges must be overcome, such as

• What is the desired shape of the cornea? A totally spherical cornea is, of course, undesirable, because the eye is an aspheric optical system. What are the ideal aspheric optics to be created in correcting refractive errors and optical aberrations? How much asphericity should remain? If this asphericity creates some optical aberrations, how much is desirable?

• In analyzing optical aberrations, the equation that is used most commonly to quantify the aberrometry data can be expanded up to 30 terms. How many of these terms have a clinically useful effect on visual function? How many of the terms could be incorporated into computer programs that would create an "ideal" optical surface?

• Is one type of aberrometer better than another, and should there be standardization in the field? Does the subjective visual response of the patient achieved with the spatially resolved refractometer give more psychophysical information than the objective information obtained with a Hartmann-Schack aberrometer?

• Can the aberrometer stand alone? How can we act on a surface when its exact shape is unknown? Will ablating by aberrometer alone without the input of a non-sphere-based topographic surface measurement create more problems than it solves?

• Do we need to attend to subtleties such as the Stiles-Crawford effect and the directionality of the cones in understanding and analyzing wavefront aberrations and

(a)

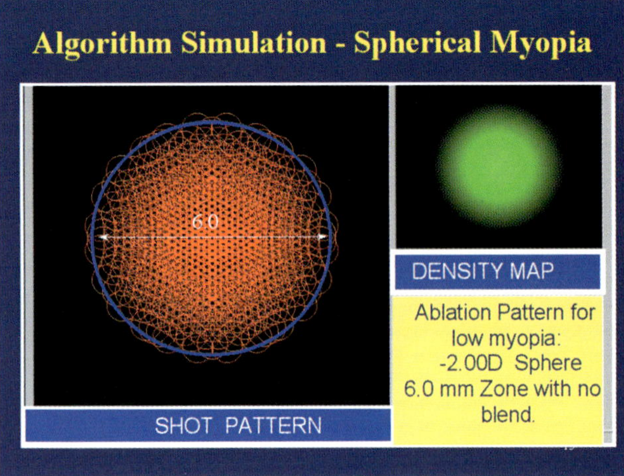

(b)

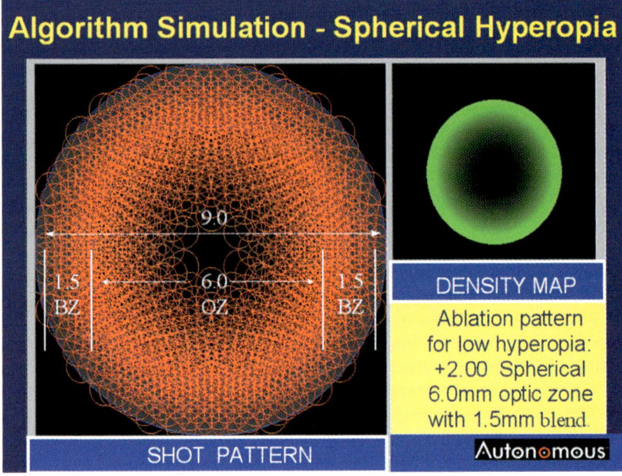

Fig. 11.59 (a) Flying-spot pattern for spherical myopia. (b) Flying-spot pattern for spherical hyperopia. (Courtesy of Autonomous Systems.)

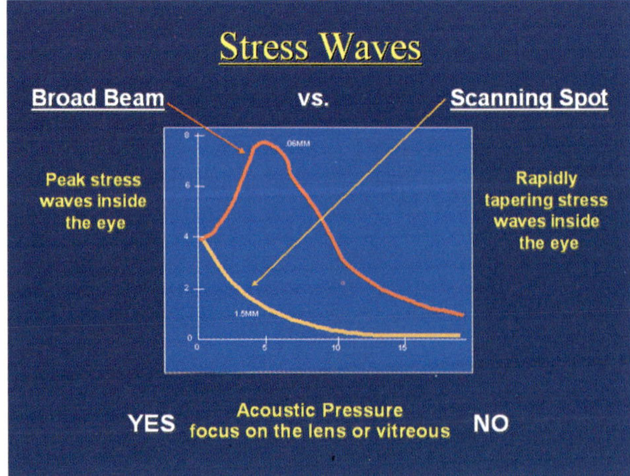

Fig. 11.58 Graph comparing broad-beam excimer ablation and flying-spot stress waves. (Courtesy of Autonomous Systems.)

(a)

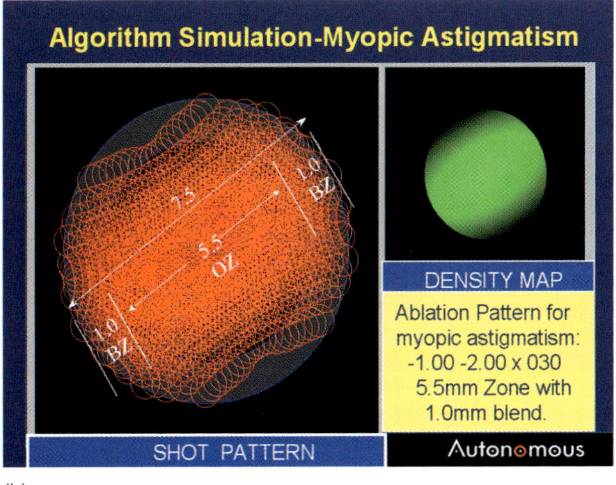

(b)

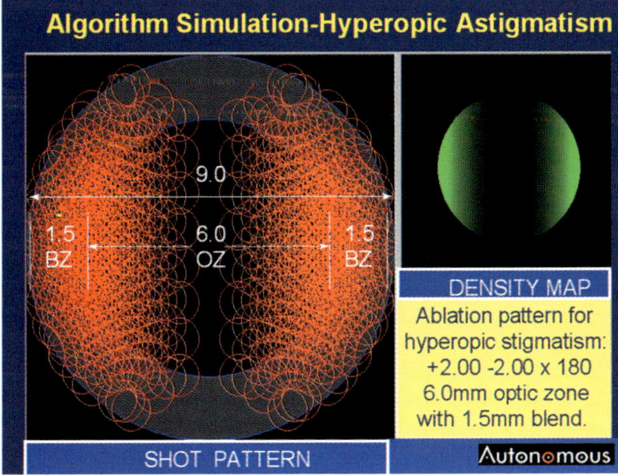

Fig. 11.60 (a) Flying-spot pattern for myopic astigmatism. (b) Flying-spot pattern for hyperopic astigmatism. (Courtesy of Autonomous Systems.)

"best-possible visual acuity"? What exactly will be the relationship between the refractive and aberrometry data and the programs that guide the spatial distribution of the laser? What kind of ablation patterns are needed? Can larger-area ablations with a scanning slit or 2-mm scanning spot be done, followed by a "fine tune"? What kind of an eye tracker is necessary to ensure proper placement of the small laser spots?

• How smooth a surface must be made by the microkeratome (whether metal-bladed, waterjet, or laser) to accommodate the refined shape changes needed? Will standard mathematical optical equations suffice to create the desired changes, or will a more refined approach, such as fractals, be necessary?

• Can a large enough ablation diameter be achieved to eliminate the aberrations that cause night halos, night glare, and night myopia without creating ablations that are so deep they violate the structural integrity of the cornea?

Most of the thinking concerning wavefront aberration-guided correction of vision concerns excimer lasers and the LASIK technique, but it is certainly possible to create an aspheric, aberration-correcting phakic intraocular lens (IOL). Indeed, it might be much easier to create the ideal shape in plastic than it is to create it in the living human cornea. Optical engineers have been creating marvelous optical systems that greatly reduce aberrations in cameras, telescopes, and other devices, so creating phakic IOLs could be an extension of this known technology guided by the new physiologic aberration measurements. Of course, such an IOL would have to be placed in the eye exactly in the required position and not change that position, something that has been shown to be difficult to achieve [157,158]. Corneal astigmatism created by implantation incisions are not completely stable either [159]. Advantages over LASIK might include a better quality of vision and certainly exchangeability or removability if needed.

Similarly, could a keratophakic lenticule be shaped with the subtle changes proposed to correct optical aberrations as well as defocus? This would make the manufacturing easier, would allow placement under a corneal flap, would allow exchangeability and removability, and potentially could allow laser refinement and shaping of the lenticule in situ to correct aberrations that either persisted or arose after the original lenticule implantation within the cornea.

These considerations paint a very bright future for the continued rapid development and refinement of refractive surgery. They may help us reach our goal of having 90% of refractive surgery patients seeing 20/10 without optical corrections by the year 2010.

Short-pulse lasers

Intensive research is still being performed on the application of the excimer and other types of lasers to refractive corneal surgery. Improvement of the current experimental and early clinical results—mainly as far as subepithelial scar formation is concerned—is mandatory for acceptance in widespread clinical use and could come from applying less laser energy (per volume of tissue removed).

There are some promising areas for exploration. First is the use of shorter excimer laser pulses now available (in the 300-fs versus the usual 11- to 20-ns range), since it has been shown that the etching behavior of PMMA could be improved significantly and that materials such as Teflon and plain salt (NaCl) could be structured by controlled ablation for the first time [82]. This last sentence was written almost 10 years ago, and these lasers are still "promising." It isn't that they do not work—they do. In fact, they carry advantages in that less energy needs to be used, and consequently, there is considerably less heating of the cornea. The difference in ablation reaction, however, is not that great, but the price differential is; these things are more expensive than conventional excimers. Unless the prices come down and/or the benefits can be shown to be a quantum advance over current techniques, these fast lasers will continue to be a "tool of the future."

Biocompatible dopants

Second, the use of biocompatible dopants (such as oxybuprocain or fluorescein) that can act as additional chromophores and absorb photon energy at even higher wavelengths seems possible [77]. A similar mechanism has been described for a variety of synthetic polymers [160]. Both methods could help to further reduce the penetration depth of those photons of the UV laser pulse that do not etch away corneal layers (for lack of sufficient bond-breaking energy) but still may adversely affect and thereby stimulate stromal cells. Similarly, in synthetic polymers, chemical processes can occur even below the bottom of ablated areas [161]. Some of the problems possibly could be eliminated by tangential corneal ablation, as patented by Belgorod.

Alternative-wavelength lasers

Since the evaluation of potential UV-induced mutagenesis and cataractogenesis has not yet come to a definite conclusion, as detailed earlier, researchers have continued to evaluate the corneal ablation characteristics of laser sources emitting photons at higher wavelengths. In the visible range Troutman and coworkers have reported attempts to create an intralamellar stromectomy without affecting Bowman's layer on Descemet's membrane using a pumped-dye laser system (at 595 nm) that creates an optical breakdown within the tissue [82,162]. Whether a nondisrupted Bowman's membrane allows for refractive changes similar to the effect found in RK remains to be investigated. Excisions made with picosecond and femtosecond lasers at 532 and 625 nm showed almost as little tissue damage as excisions made with excimer lasers at 193 nm [163].

Following previous work with the CO_2 laser (emitting at 10.6 mm) in the middle-infrared spectrum (with the water molecules of the cornea strongly absorbing this radiation), newer attempts have investigated the potential use of the hydrogen fluoride laser (3.0 mm), a Raman-shifted neodymium:YAG laser (2.80 and 2.92 mm), and an erbium:YAG laser (2.94 mm) for corneal surgery—water shows absorption peaks in this range as well [54,164,165].

Laser-adjustable synthetic epikeratoplasty (LASE)

The concept of LASE has been presented in order to avoid some of the problems inherent in direct laser ablation of the corneal surface. Since the central host cornea is covered by the synthetic epikeratophakia lenticle that is to be shaped by the laser beam, the risk of irreversibly damaging the patient's optical zone is minimized. Stromal regeneration and scarring in the ablation zone do not occur, and multiple ablations can be carried out if the correction is unsatisfactory or changes over time. If necessary, the lenticule could be replaced, as is sometimes the case in epikeratophakia. The stable attachment of the epithelium to the surface of the artificial lens—an indispensable requirement for LASE—has not yet been solved despite numerous attempts, however.

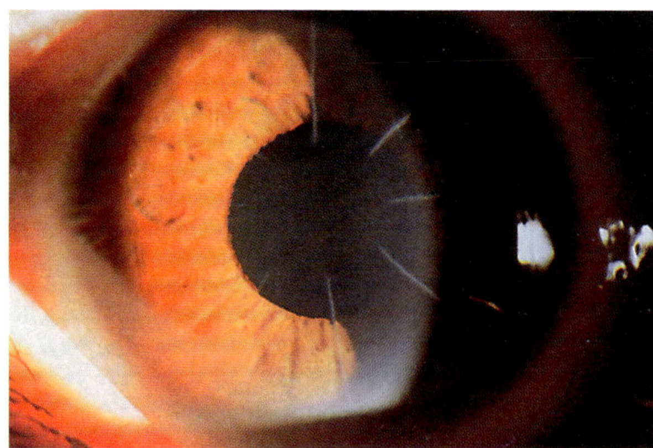

Fig. 11.61 An eight-incision RK patient 6 months postlaser ablation for undercorrection. (Courtesy of T. Seiler.)

Another concept is the use of the excimer laser to treat an RK undercorrection. This is especially of value in cases that have already received the maximum number of incisions. An even more exciting possibility is the use of the excimer laser in combination with conventional RK to correct higher degrees of myopia. A 10-D myope could have eight incisions to reduce his or her refractive error to 5 D with RK, followed a few months later by excimer photoablation to remove the remaining ametropia—thus combining the best of both worlds (Figure 11.61).

There is no doubt that laser corneal surgery still holds great challenges, but it also holds greater promises for patients, investigators, and corneal surgeons alike. Wavefront technology can determine exactly what final corneal shape would produce an eye with 20/10 vision. However, there is much yet to be learned about the basic biologic mechanisms of LASIK surgery and their effect on the cornea before we can accurately achieve the ideal change in corneal shape. It looks like the dawn of a new era in refractive surgery to me.

References

1 Kremer FB. Kremer defends laser [letter; comment]. J Refract Surg 1996; 12(3): p. 330.

2 Schawlow AL, and Townes CH. Infrared and optical masers. Phys Rev 1958; 112: p. 1940.

3 Maiman TH. Stimulated optical radiation in ruby masers. Nature 1960; 187: p. 493.

4 Siegman AE. *Introduction to Masers and Lasers.* McGraw–Hill, New York, 1971.
5 Wilson J, and Hawkes JFB. *Lasers: Principles and Applications.* Prentice–Hall, New York, 1987.
6 Einstein A. Zur Quantentheorie de strahlung. Phy Z 1917; 18: p. 121.
7 Wilson J, and Hawkes JFB. *Optoelectronics, an introduction.* Simon and Schuster, Cambridge, 461; 1989.
8 Kapany NS, Peppers NA, Zweng HC, *et al.* Retinal photocoagulation by laser. Nature 1963; 199: p. 146.
9 Koester CJ, Snitzer E, Campbell CJ, *et al.* Experimental laser retina coagulator. J Opt Soc Am 1962; 52: p. 607.
10 Beckman H, Barraco R, Sugar HS, *et al.* Laser iridectomies. Am J Ophthalmol 1971; 72(2): p. 393–402.
11 Krasnov MM. [Laser puncture of the anterior chamber angle in glaucoma (a preliminary report)]. Vestn Oftalmol 1972; 3: p. 27–31.
12 McDonald MB. Future of R&D jeopardized. J Refract Surg 1987; 3: p. 207.
13 Chilbert MA, Peak MJ, Peak JG, *et al.* Effects of intensity and fluence upon DNA single-strand breaks induced by excimer laser radiation. Photochem Photobiol 1988; 47(4): p. 523–5.
14 Ediger MN. Excimer-laser-induced fluorescence of rabbit cornea: radiometric measurement through the cornea. Lasers Surg Med 1991; 11(2): p. 93–8.
15 Gebhart E, Lang GK, Tittelbach H, *et al.* [Chromosome mutagenicity of a 193 nm Excimer laser]. Fortschr Ophthalmol 1990; 87(3): p. 229–33.
16 Green HA, Margolis R, Boll J, *et al.* Unscheduled DNA synthesis in human skin after in vitro ultraviolet-excimer laser ablation. J Invest Dermatol 1987; 89(2): p. 201–4.
17 Green H, Boll J, Parrish JA, *et al.* Cytotoxicity and mutagenicity of low intensity, 248 and 193 nm excimer laser radiation in mammalian cells. Cancer Res 1987; 47(2): p. 410–3.
18 Kochevar IE. Cytotoxicity and mutagenicity of excimer laser radiation. Lasers Surg Med 1989; 9(5): p. 440–5.
19 Kochevar IE, and Buckley LA, Photochemistry of DNA using 193 nm excimer laser radiation. Photochem Photobiol 1990; 51(5): p. 527–32.
20 Kochevar IE, Walsh AA, Held KD, *et al.* Mechanism for 193-nm laser radiation-induced effects on mammalian cells. Radiat Res 1990; 122(2): p. 142–8.
21 Kochevar IE, Walsh AA, Green HA, *et al.* DNA damage induced by 193-nm radiation in mammalian cells. Cancer Res 1991; 51(1): p. 288–93.
22 Matchette LS, Waynant RW, Royston DD, *et al.* Induction of lambda prophage near the site of focused UV laser radiation. Photochem Photobiol 1989; 49(2): p. 161–7.
23 Rimoldi D, Miller AC, Freeman SE, *et al.* DNA damage in cultured human skin fibroblasts exposed to excimer laser radiation. J Invest Dermatol 1991; 96(6): p. 898–902.
24 Seiler T, Bende T, Winckler K, *et al.* Side effects in excimer corneal surgery. DNA damage as a result of 193 nm excimer laser radiation. Graefes Arch Clin Exp Ophthalmol 1988; 226(3): p. 273–6.
25 Clarke RH, Nakagawa K, and Isner JM. The production of short-lived free radicals accompanying laser photoablation of cardiovascular tissue. Free Radic Biol Med 1988; 4(4): p. 209–13.
26 Bende T, Seiler T, and Wollensak J. [Superficial ablation of the cornea using the excimer laser (193 nm)]. Fortschr Ophthalmol 1989; 86(6): p. 589–91.
27 Nuss RC, Puliafito CA, and Dehm E. Unscheduled DNA synthesis following excimer laser ablation of the cornea in vivo. Invest Ophthal & Vis Sci 1987; 28(2): p. 287–294.
28 Bende T, Seiler T, and Wollensak J. Side effects in excimer corneal surgery. Corneal thermal gradients. Graefes Arch Clin Exp Ophthalmol 1988; 226(3): p. 277–80.
29 Trentacoste J, Thompson K, Parrish RK, *et al.* Mutagenic potential of a 193-nm excimer laser on fibroblasts in tissue culture. Ophthalmology 1987; 94(2): p. 125–9.
30 Zigman S. Light damage to the lens. In: *Clinical Light Damage to the Eye,* D Miller, Editor. 1987, Springer–Verlag, New York, p. 65–78, 1987.
31 Dehm EJ, Puliafito CA, and Adler CM. Corneal endothelial injury in rabbits following excimer laser ablation at 193 and 248 nm. Arch Ophthalmol 1986; 104: p. 1364–8.
32 Srinivasan R, and Mayne–Banton R. Self developing photoetching of poly (ethyleneterephthalate) films by far–ultraviolet excimer laser radiation. Appl Phys Lett 1981; 41: p. 576–8.
33 Linsker R, Srinivasan R, Wynne JJ, *et al.* Far–ultraviolet laser ablation of atherosclerotic lesions. Laser Surg Med 1984; 4: p. 201–6.
34 Srinivasan R, Wynne JJ, and Blum SE. Far–ultraviolet photoetching of organic materials. Laser Focus 1983; 19: p. 62–6.
35 Lane RJ, Linsker R, Wynne JJ, *et al.* Ultraviolet-laser ablation of skin. Arch Dermatol 1985; 121(5): p. 609–17.
36 Lane RJ, and Wynne JJ. Medical applications of excimer lasers. Lasers and Appl 1984; 3: p. 59–62.
37 Grundfest WS, Litvack F, and Forrester JS. Laser ablation of human atherosclerotic plaque without adjacent tissue injury. J Am Coll Cardiol 1985; 5: p. 929–33.
38 Muller D, and Svrluga R. Excimer lasers offer promise in surgical applications. Laser Focus 1985; 21: p. 71–81.
39 Velasco JE, and Setser DW. Bound–free emission spectra of diatomic xenon halides. J of Chemical Physics 1975; 62: p. 1990–1.
40 Searles SK, and Hart GA. Appl Phys Lett 1975; 27: p. 243.
41 Ewing JJ, and Brau CA. Appl Phys Lett 1975; 27: p. 350.
42 Brau CA, and Ewing JJ. Appl Phys Lett 1975; 27: p. 435.
43 Hoffman JM, Hays AK. and Tisone GC. High–power UV noble–gas–halide lasers. Appl Phys Lett 1976; 28: p. 538–9.
44 Burnham R, and Djeu N. Ultraviolet–preionized discharge–pumped lasers in XeF, KrF, and ArF. Appl Phys Lett 1976; 29: p. 707–9.
45 Stevens B, and Hutton E. Radiative lifetime of the pyrene dimer and the possible role of excited dimers in energy transfer processes. Nature 1960; 186: p. 1045–6.
46 Eden J, Burnham R, Champagne LF, *et al.* Visible and UV lasers: problems and promises. Inst of Electrical and Electronic Eng 1979; 16: p. 50.
47 Huestis DL. The excimer age: lasing with the new breed. Optical Spectra 1979; 13: p. 51.
48 Rhodes CK. *Excimer Lasers: Topics in Applied Physics.* Springer–Verlag, New York, 30; 1979.
49 Ruderman W. Excimer laser in photochemistry. Laser Focus 1979; 15: p. 68.
50 Taboada J, Mikesell GW, and Reed RD. Response of the corneal epithelium to KrF excimer laser pulses. Health Phys 1981; 40: p. 677–83.
51 Taboada J, and Archibald CJ. An extreme sensitivity in the corneal epithelium to far–UV ArF excimer laser pulses. In: *Proc Sci Prog Aero Med Assoc,* San Antonio, 1981.
52 Srinivasan R. Kinetics of the ablative photodecomposition of organic polymers in the far–ultraviolet (193–nm). J Vac Sci Tech 1983; 4: p. 923–6.
53 Trokel SL, Srinivasan R, and Braren B. Excimer laser surgery of the cornea. Am J Ophthalmol 1983; 96(6): p. 710–5.
54 Keates RH, Pedrotti LS, Weichel H, *et al.* Carbon dioxide laser beam control for corneal surgery. Ophthalmic Surg 1981; 12(2): p. 117–22.
55 Olson RJ, Kaufman HE, and Rheinstrom SD. Reshaping the cat corneal anterior surface using high speed diamond fraise. Ophthalmic Surg 1980; 11(12): p. 784–6.
56 Mueller FO, and O'Neal P. Some experiments on corneal grinding. Exp Eye Res 1980; 6(12): p. 42–7.

57 Barraquer JI. Bases de la keratomileusis. Excerpta Medica International Congress Series 1963; 148: p. 85.
58 Barraquer JI. Modification de la refracction por medio de inclusiones intracorneales Arch So Am Oftal Optom 1963 4 p. 229
59 Marshall WJ, Trokel SL, Rothery S, *et al.* An ultrastructural study of corneal incisions induced by an excimer laser at 193 nm. Ophthalmology 1985; 92 (6): p. 749–58.
60 Marshall WJ, Trokel SL, Rothery S, *et al.* A comparative study of corneal incisions induced by diamond and steel knives and two ultraviolet radiations from an excimer laser. Br J Ophthalmol 1986; 70 (7): p. 482–501.
61 Marshall WJ, Trokel SL, and Rothery S. Photoablation reprofiling of the cornea using an excimer laser photorefractive keratectomy. Lasers in Ophthalmology 1986; 1: p. 21–48.
62 Marshall WJ, Trokel SL, and Rothery S. Long-term healing of the central cornea after photorefractive keratectomy using an excimer laser. Ophthalmology 1988; 95: p. 1411–21.
63 Kerr-Muir MG, Trokel SL, Marshall WJ, *et al.* Ultrastructural comparison of conventional surgical and argon fluoride excimer laser keratectomy. Am J Ophthalmol 1987; 103(3 Pt 2): p. 448–53.
64 Krueger RR, Trokel SL, and Schubert HD. Interaction of ultraviolet laser light with the cornea. Invest Ophthalmol Vis Sci 1985; 26(11): p. 1455–64.
65 Krueger RR, and Trokel SL. Quantitation of corneal ablation by ultraviolet laser light. Arch Ophthalmol 1985; 103: p. 1741–1742.
66 Trokel SL. The cornea and ultraviolet laser light. In: *Laser in der Ophthalmologie.* Enke–Verlag, Stuttgart, 1988.
67 Serdarevic O, Darrell RW, Krueger RR, *et al.* Excimer laser therapy for experimental Candida keratitis. Am J Ophthalmol 1985; 99(5): p. 534–8.
68 Serdarevic O, Darrell R, Krueger R, *et al.* [The ultraviolet laser in the treatment of keratomycoses] <Original> Le laser ultraviolet dans le traitement des keratomycoses. Bull Mem Soc Fr Ophtalmol 1986; 97: p. 227–8.
69 Jacques SL, McAuliffe DJ, Blank IH, *et al.* Controlled removal of human stratum corneum by pulsed laser. J Invest Dermatol 1987; 88(1): p. 88–93.
70 Steinert RF, and Puliafito CA. Excimer laser phototherapeutic keratectomy for a corneal nodule. Refract Corneal Surg 1990; 6(5): p. 352.
71 Steinert RF, and Puliafito CA. Laser corneal surgery. Int Ophthalmol Clin 1988; 28(2): p. 150–4.
72 Munnerlyn CR, Koons SJ, and Marshall J. Photorefractive keratectomy: a technique for laser refractive surgery. J Cataract Refract Surg 1988; 14(1): p. 46–52.
73 Puliafito CA, Stern D, Krueger RR, *et al.* High-speed photography of excimer laser ablation of the cornea. Arch Ophthalmol 1987; 105(9): p. 1255–9.
74 Aron-Rosa DS, Boerner CF, Bath P, *et al.* Corneal wound healing after excimer laser keratotomy in a human eye. Am J Ophthalmol 1987; 103(3 Pt 2): p. 454–64.
75 Cotliar AM, Schubert HD, Mandel ER, *et al.* Excimer laser radial keratotomy. Ophthalmology 1985; 92(2): p. 206–8.
76 Serdarevic ON, Hanna K, Gribomont AC, *et al.* Excimer laser trephination in penetrating keratoplasty. Morphologic features and wound healing. Ophthalmology 1988; 95(4): p. 493–505.
77 Husinsky W, Mitterer S, and Grabner G. Photoablation by UV and visible laser radiation of native and doped biological tissues. Appl Physics 1989; 49: p. 463–7.
78 Kermani O, Koort HJ, Roth E, *et al.* Mass spectroscopic analysis of excimer laser ablated material from human corneal tissue. J Cataract Refract Surg 1988; 14(6): p. 638–41.
79 Steinert RF, and Puliafito CA. Corneal incisions with excimer laser. In: *Refractive Corneal Surgery,* R Hofman and JJ Salz, Editors. Slack, Thorofare, p. 401–10, 1986.
80 Binder PS. What We Have Learned About Corneal Wound Healing From Refractive Surgery (Barraquer Lecture). Refractive and Corneal Surgery 1989; 5(2): p. 98–120.
81 Villasenor RA, Salz J, Steel D, *et al.* Changes in corneal thickness during radial keratotomy. Ophthalmic Surg 1981; 12(5): p. 341–2.
82 Grabner G. The future for excimer–laser in refractive corneal surgery. European J Impl Refract Surg 1990; 2(6): p. 135–40.
83 Deitz MR, Sanders DR, and Raanan MG. A consecutive series (1982–1985) of radial keratotomies performed with the diamond blade. Am J Ophthalmol 1987; 103(3 Pt 2): p. 417–22.
84 Bores LD. Historical review and clinical results of radial keratotomy. Int Ophthalmol Clin 1983; 23(3): p. 93–118.
85 Schroder E, Dardenne MU, Neuhann T, *et al.* An ophthalmic excimer laser for corneal surgery. Am J Ophthalmol 1987; 103 (3 Pt 2): p. 472–3.
86 Seiler T, Bende T, Wollensak J, *et al.* Excimer laser keratectomy for correction of astigmatism. Am J Ophthalmol 1988; 105(2): p. 117–24.
87 Seiler T, Bende T, and Wollensak J. Klinische aspekte der laserchirurgie der hornhaut. In: *Laser in der ophthalmologie,* J Wollensak, Editor. Enke–Verlag, Stuttgart, p. 134–47, 1988.
88 Stern D, Lin WZ, Puliafito CA, *et al.* Femtosecond optical ranging of corneal incision depth. Invest Ophthalmol Vis Sci 1989; 30(1): p. 99–104.
89 Puliafito CA, Wong K, and Steinert RF. Quantitative and ultrastructural studies of excimer laser ablation of the cornea at 193 and 248 nanometers. Lasers Surg Med 1987; 7: p. 155–9.
90 Berns MW, Liaw LH, Oliva A, *et al.* An acute light and electron microscopic study of ultraviolet 193-nm excimer laser corneal incisions. Ophthalmology 1988; 95(10): p. 1422–33.
91 Burstein N, Gaster R, and Binder PS. Wound healing after excimer laser photoablation in the rabbit. Soc Photo Inst Eng 1988; 98: p. 57–64.
92 Gaster RN, Binder PS, and Coalwell K. Corneal surface ablation by 193 nm excimer laser and wound healing in rabbits. Invest Ophthalmol Vis Sci 1989; 30: p. 90–8.
93 Fenzl RE. Personal communication, 1991.
94 Lang GK, Schroeder E, Koch JW, *et al.* Excimer laser keratoplasty. Part 2: Elliptical keratoplasty. Ophthalmic Surg 1989; 20(5): p. 342–6.
95 Lang GK, Naumann GO, and Koch JW. A new elliptical excision for corneal transplantation using an excimer laser [letter]. Arch Ophthalmol 1990; 108(7): p. 914–5.
96 Lee TJ, Wan WL, and Kash RL. Keratocyte survival following a controlled rate freeze. Invest Ophthalmol Vis Sci 1985; 26: p. 1210–5.
97 Zavala EV, Binder PS, and Deg JK. Refractive keratoplasty. Lathing and cryopreservation. CLAO J 1985; 11: p. 155–162.
98 Binder PS, Krumeich JH, and Zavala EV. Laboratory evaluation of freeze vs non-freeze lamellar refractive keratoplasty. Arch Ophthalmol 1987; 105(8): p. 1125–8.
99 Bores LD. Shortened recovery from keratoplasty and epikeratoplasty [letter]. Arch Ophthalmol 1989; 107 (2): p. 167.
100 Bores LD. Mechanical modulation of the corneal surface. Int Clinics Ophth 1991; 31(1): p. 25–36.
101 Zavala EY, Binder PS, and Rock M. Light and electron microscopy of nine failed epikeratoplasty for keratoconus cases. Ophthalmol 1990; 97(9): p. 137.
102 Lieurance RC, Patel AC, Wan WL, *et al.* Excimer laser cut lenticules for epikeratophakia. Am J Ophthalmol 1987; 103 (3 Pt 2): p. 475–6.
103 Gabay S, Slomovic A, and Jares T. Excimer laser-processed donor corneal lenticules for lamellar keratoplasty. Am J Ophthalmol 1989; 107(1): p. 47–51.
104 Brightbill FS. *Corneal Surgery.* C.V. Mosby, St Louis, 1986.
105 Pallikaris IG, Papatzanaki ME, Stathi EZ, *et al.* Laser in situ keratomileusis. Lasers Surg Med 1990; 10(5): p. 463–8.

106 Buratto L. personal communication, 1991.
107 Gimbel HV, van Westenbrugge JA, Penno EE, *et al.* Simultaneous bilateral laser in situ keratomileusis: safety and efficacy. Ophthalmology 1999; 106(8): p. 1461–7; discussion 1467–8.
108 Stonecipher KG. *LASIK for low myopia,* 2000.
109 Mulhern MG, Foley-Nolan A, O'Keefe M, *et al.* Topographical analysis of ablation centration after excimer laser photorefractive keratectomy and laser in situ keratomileusis for high myopia. J Cataract Refract Surg 1997; 23(4): p. 488–94.
110 Sano Y, Carr JD, Takei K, *et al.* Videokeratography after excimer laser in situ keratomileusis for myopia. Ophthalmology 2000; 107(4): p. 674–84.
111 Petersen H, and Seiler T. [Laser in situ keratomileusis (LASIK). Intraoperative and postoperative complications]. Ophthalmologe 1999; 96(4): p. 240–7.
112 Dausch D, Klein R, and Schroder E. Excimer laser photorefractive keratectomy for hyperopia. Refract Corneal Surg 1993; 9(1): p. 20–8.
113 Gimbel HV. Personal communication, 1991.
114 Talamo JH. Hyperopic PRK. In: *American Academy of Ophthalmology.* Orlando, 1999.
115 Talamo JH. Hyperopic LASIK. In: *American Academy of Ophthalmology.* Orlando, 1999.
116 Lindstrom RL, Hardten DR, Houtman DM, *et al.* Six-month results of hyperopic and astigmatic LASIK in eyes with primary and secondary hyperopia. Trans Am Ophthalmol Soc 1999; 97: p. 241–55.
117 Neumann AC, Fyodorov SN, and Sanders DR. Radial thermokeratoplasty for the correction of Hyperopia. Refract Corneal Surg 1990; 6: p. 404–12.
118 Neumann AC, Sanders D, Raanan M, *et al.* Hyperopic thermokeratoplasty: clinical evaluation. J Cataract Refract Surg 1991; 17(6): p. 830–8.
119 Seiler T, Matallana M, and Bende T. Laser thermokeratoplasty by means of a pulsed holmium:YAG laser for hyperopic correction. Refract Corneal Surg 1990; 6(5): p. 335–9.
120 Koch DD, Kohnen T, McDonnell PJ, *et al.* Hyperopia correction by noncontact holmium:YAG laser thermal keratoplasty. United States phase IIA clinical study with a 1-year follow-up. Ophthalmology 1996; 103(10): p. 1525–35; discussion 1536.
121 Koch DD, Kohnen T, McDonnell PJ, *et al.* Hyperopia correction by noncontact holmium:YAG laser thermal keratoplasty: U.S. phase IIA clinical study with 2-year follow-up. Ophthalmology 1997; 104(11): p. 1938–47.
122 Nano HD, and Muzzin S. Noncontact holmium:YAG laser thermal keratoplasty for hyperopia. J Cataract Refract Surg 1998; 24(6): p. 751–7.
123 Vinciguerra P, Kohnen T, Azzolini M, *et al.* Radial and staggered treatment patterns to correct hyperopia using noncontact holmium:YAG laser thermal keratoplasty. J Cataract Refract Surg 1998; 24(1): p. 21–30.
124 Chayet AS. Distant visions: How practitioners outside the United States are treating hyperopia. In: *EyeWorld Online,* 1999.
125 Ditzen K. Distant visions: How practitioners outside the United States are treating hyperopia. In: *EyeWorld Online,* 1999.
126 Kahlert HJ, Sowada U, and Basting D. Excimer laserstrahlen quellen för ophthalmologische Anwendungen. In: *Laser in der Ophthalmologie,* J Wollensak, Editor. Enke–Verlag, Stuttgart, p. 161–165, 1988.
127 Bende T, Matallana M, and Seiler T. [Calibration of the 193 nm Excimer laser beam]. Biomed Tech (Berlin) 1990; 3(14): p. 14–5.
128 L'Esperance FJ, Warner JW, Telfair WB, *et al.* Excimer laser instrumentation and technique for human corneal surgery. Arch Ophthalmol 1989; 107(1): p. 131–9.
129 Hanna K, Chastang JC, Pouliquen Y, *et al.* A rotating slit delivery system for excimer laser refractive keratoplasty. Am J Ophthalmol 1987; 103(3 Pt 2): p. 474.
130 Arneodo J, Azema A, Botineau J, *et al.* Corneal optical zone reshaping by excimer laser light photoablation (PKM method), in Laser Technology in Ophthalmology, J. Marshall, Kugler, and Ghedini, Editors. 1988: Amsterdam. p. 205–11.
131 Missotten L, Boving R, Francois G, *et al.* Experimental excimer laser keratomileusis. Bull Soc Belge Ophtalmol 1986; 220(103): p. 103–20.
132 Kornmehl EW, Steinert RF, and Puliafito CA. A comparative study of masking fluids for excimer laser phototherapeutic keratectomy. Arch Ophthalmol 1991; 109(6): p. 860–3.
133 L'Esperance FA, Jr., Taylor DM, Del Pero RA, *et al.* Human excimer laser corneal surgery: preliminary report. Trans Am Ophthalmol Soc 1988; 86: p. 208–75.
134 Bores LD. Corneal Topography: The Dark Side of the Moon. In: *Ophthalmic Technologies.* SPIE–The International Society for Optical Engineering, Los Angeles, 1991.
135 Gross GW, Baker P, and Bores LD. Corneal Topography via Two Wavelength Holography. In: *Soc Photo Inst Eng.* SPIE–The International Society for Optical Engineering, Los Angeles, 1990.
136 Taylor DM, L'Esperance FA, Jr., Del Pero RA, *et al.* Human excimer laser lamellar keratectomy. A clinical study. Ophthalmology 1989; 96(5): p. 654–64.
137 McDonald MB, Frantz JM, Klyce SD, *et al.* Central photorefractive keratectomy for myopia. The blind eye study. Arch Ophthalmol 1990; 108(6): p. 799 808.
138 Deitz MR. Personal communication, 1991.
139 Aron-Rosa D, Carre F, Cassiani P, *et al.* Keratorefractive surgery with the excimer laser. Am J Ophthalmol 1985; 100(5): p. 741–2.
140 McDonald MB. The future direction of refractive surgery. Refract Corneal Surg 1988; 3: p. 158–67.
141 Tuft S, Marshall J, and Rothery S. Stromal remodeling following photorefractive keratectomy. Lasers Ophthalmol 1987; 1: p. 177–83.
142 Barraquer JI. Basis of refractive keratoplasty. Arch. So. Am. Oftal. Optom. 1967; 6: p. 21.
143 Zabel RW, Sher NA, Ostrov CS, *et al.* Myopic excimer laser keratectomy: a preliminary report. Refract Corneal Surg 1990; 6(5): p. 329–34.
144 Hanna KD, Jouve FE, Bercovier MH, *et al.* Computer simulation of lamellar keratectomy and laser myopic keratomileusis. J Refract Surg 1988; 4: p. 222–231.
145 Fantes F, Hanna KD, Waring GO, *et al.* Wound healing after excimer laser keratomileusis (photorefractive keratectomy) in monkeys. Arch Ophthalmol 1990; 108: p. 665–675.
146 Kremer FB. *Phototherapeutic keratectomy,* 2000.
147 Belin MW. *Autofluorescence-guided PTK,* 2000.
148 Gibralter R, and Trokel SL. Correction of irregular astigmatism with the excimer laser. Ophthalmology 1994; 101(7): p. 1310–4; discussion 1314–5.
149 Tamayo GE. Localized photorefractive keratectomy excimer laser ablation. In: *American Society of Cataract and Refractive Surgery (ASCRS).* Seattle, 1999.
150 Ditzen KN. Computed topography guided ablations using Topolink. In: *American Society of Cataract and Refractive Surgery (ASCRS).* Seattle, 1999.
151 Holmes-Higgin DK, Baker PC, Burris TE, *et al.* Characterization of the aspheric corneal surface with intrastromal corneal ring segments. J Refract Surg 1999; 15(5): p. 520–8.
152 Collins MJ, Brown B, Atchison BA, *et al.* Tolerance to spherical aberration induced by rigid contact lenses. Ophthalmic Physiol Opt 1992; 12(1): p. 24–8.
153 Mierdel P, Kaemmerer M, Krinke HE, *et al.* Effects of photorefractive keratectomy and cataract surgery on ocular optical errors of higher order. Graefes Arch Clin Exp Ophthalmol 1999; 237(9): p. 725–9.

154 Seiler T, Kaemmerer M, Mierdel P, *et al.* Ocular optical aberrations after photorefractive keratectomy for myopia and myopic astigmatism. Arch Ophthalmol 2000; 118(1): p. 17–21.
155 Mrochen M, Kaemmerer M, and Seiler T. Wavefront-guided laser in situ keratomileusis: early results in three eyes [In Process Citation]. J Refract Surg 2000; 16(2): p. 116–21.
156 Liang J, Grimm B, Goelz S, *et al.* Objective measurement of wave aberrations of the human eye with the use of a Hartmann-Shack wave-front sensor. J Opt Soc Am A 1994; 11(7): p. 1949–57.
157 Frohn A, Dick HB, and Thiel HJ. Implantation of a toric poly (methyl methacrylate) intraocular lens to correct high astigmatism. J Cataract Refract Surg 1999; 25(12): p. 1675–8.
158 Korynta J, Bok J, Cendelin J, *et al.* Computer modeling of visual impairment caused by intraocular lens misalignment. J Cataract Refract Surg 1999; 25(1): p. 100–5.
159 Drews RC. Five year study of astigmatic stability after cataract surgery with intraocular lens implantation: comparison of wound sizes [see comments]. J Cataract Refract Surg 2000; 26(2): p. 250–3.
160 Srinivasan R, and Braren B. Ultraviolet laser ablation and etching of polymethylmethacrylate sensitiled with an organic dopant. Appl Physics 1988; 45: p. 289–92.
161 Srinivasan R. Ablation of polymer and biological tissue by ultraviolet lasers. Science 1986; 234: p. 559–65.
162 Troutman RC, Veronneau TS, Jakobiec FA, *et al.* A new laser for collagen wounding in corneal and strabismus surgery: a preliminary report. Trans Am Ophthalmol Soc 1986; 84(117): p. 117–32.
163 Stern D, Schoenlein RW, Puliafito CA, *et al.* Corneal ablation by nanosecond, picosecond, and femtosecond lasers at 532 and 625 nm. Arch Ophthalmol 1989; 107(4): p. 587–92.
164 Keates RH, Levy SN, Fried S, *et al.* Carbon dioxide laser use in wound sealing and epikeratophakia. J Cataract Refract Surg 1987; 13(3): p. 290–5.
165 Codere F, Brownstein S, Garwood JL, *et al.* Carbon dioxide laser treatment of the conjunctiva and the cornea. Ophthalmology 1988; 95(1): p. 37–45.

12
Lenticular Refractive Surgery

Things done well, and with a care, exempt themselves from fear.
[Henry VIII]

History of clear lens extraction

We have already alluded to the initial suggestion of Boerhaave in 1708 in which he proposed clear lens removal for high myopia [1] (see Chapter 2). It is commonly believed that it took nearly 200 years before this idea was implemented in the work of Fukala and Vacher. It has usually been assumed that the technique was introduced—*de novo*—by Fukala in 1889. This, however, is clearly not the case, since Vacher published in close proximity to Fukala. Scholars may argue about who—Fukala or Vacher—should receive primacy for clear lens extraction for myopia, but the argument is moot considering the evidence of history. Vacher in particular would like to give credit to a fellow countryman—the Abbé Desmonceaux—and bask in reflected glory as the "rediscoverer" of the method [2]. Vacher states:

> The myopia operation, i.e., the extraction of a clear lens, is now a century old and was invented by a Frenchman, the Abbé Desmonceaux; all honor belongs to him. . . . Just as the extraction of a cataract is the invention of a Frenchman [here he is probably referring to Jaques Daviel], so is the extraction of a clear lens for curing high myopia the idea of a Frenchman and should be called the Desmonceaux operation. . . . I congratulate myself that I have contributed to the rehabilitation of an operation of French origin; it is the merit of the ophthalmologist Desmonceaux to have announced its advantages and to have performed it regularly as of 1776.

There is a serious flaw in this reckoning, however. The Abbé (in his own words, "because of lack of courage") did not operate and was an indifferent physician by all accounts; in fact, he may have referred such cases to Janin (see below).

Janin reported in detail the case of an elderly woman who had been myopic since childhood such that she could only read at a distance of 2½ in.; she developed a cataract when she was 70 and had an extraction performed by Janin in 1769. After the operation, the patient could see much better at distance than before the cataract had developed. She could read at a distance of 15 to 16 in. without glasses [3].

Otto argues, persuasively, that Janin's true purpose was to correct the myopia per se, not just remove the cataract [4–6]. The author is inclined to agree with him after reading Janin's published descriptions. It is clear that Janin intended to operate for the myopia. He stresses the necessity of operating on young patients, that the myopia has to be high, and that "the clear lens is best for most favorable surgical results." It appears likely that the self-effacing Abbé referred such patients to Janin, whom he describes as *"occuliste le plus experimente."* Whatever the circumstances, clear lens extraction was precisely described in 1713 by Heister—27 years before Desmonceaux and Janin in any event [7].

Albrecht von Haller, himself a myope, in his famous and generally well-known work *Elementa Physiologiae*, states

> The myope can be improved . . . by extracting or couching the clear lens thereby decreasing considerably the refractive power of the eye [8].

Von Haller did not perform surgery either, saying that he was more likely to do harm than good. He was, instead, a philosopher, a physician, a poet, and a writer whose book was, during the 18th century, quoted by nearly every medical author writing at the time. Haller, in no manner an intellectual thief, further writes that he got the idea from a monograph by Woolhouse (*De cataracte et glaucome*) and also writes in his *Bibliothek Chirurgische*:

> Joseph Higgs, Chirurg. Birminghamensis, a practical essay on the cure of venereal, scorbutic, arthritic, leprous, scrophulous and cancerous disorders. In a method entirely new. London 1745. The myopia was cured by couching the lens [9].

The following paragraph from Higgs' book (page 37) is of interest:

> Some years ago I proposed to Dr. Desaguliers a method for relieving nearsighted persons, by depressing the crystalline humour, as in couching; inasmuch as, when that medium is removed, one of a less density will succeed, which will supply the place of glasses. But the experiment I have never as yet tried.

Desmonceaux (1734–1806) published his *Traite des maladies des yeux et des oreilles, considerees sous le rapport des quatre ages de la vie de l'homme* (Treatise on the diseases of the eye and the ear, considered in correlation with the four ages of man) in 1786 [10]. In it he wrote:

> Myopes with a far point at 2–3 in. are very unhappy because they see what is at their feet very indistinctly; they are not suitable for performing any work. Therefore I recommend to extract the lens while these patients are still young. This will decrease the extension of the cornea and sharpen the image of objects. This I have shown in a small monograph of 1776: this operation is less dangerous than a cataract extraction. The lens which is still clear will easily be extracted after the capsule has been opened. This method to help myopes of high degree was heretofore unknown as it developed from the cataract extraction. It will only be of use to those who have to work [II, p. 140].

Since Desmonceaux did no surgery whatsoever, this advice has the flavor of "Go right ahead, I'll hold your coat." He goes on:

> The cataract is not the only indication to perform a corneal incision. It may be indicated for severe myopes as we assume that the cause of this disease is a too voluminous lens. I have observed this operation often and it was often successful. Every lens in whichever condition it may be can easily be extracted. The high myope will obtain a true advantage from this operation and will improve his vision considerably [I, p. 406].

The mystery is whom did he watch "do it often"? Probably Janin, with whom he maintained a correspondence, but we do not know with certainty. The monograph referred to above, *Lettres et observations . . . sur la vue enfants naissants* (Paris, 1776), contains the following sentence on page 5:

> This surgical procedure seems to be new but it can be successful and will nearly always be successful when performed by the skillful hands of Baron Wenzel. He has proven this several times and he has been most charitable when operating on poor patients who come to me for help [11].

It is not clear who, if anyone, may have performed this procedure often (specifically to reduce myopia) following these suggestions despite Desmonceaux's observations. It is highly likely, however, that someone did in view of Desmonceaux's comments to the effect that a Baron Wenzel had done so. In any case, the reference is probably to Wenzel Sr. because Jr. wrote his thesis in 1779. Hirschberg notes that Wenzel Jr. does not mention this procedure in either his *Traite de la Cataract* (Paris, 1786) or his *Manual d' Oculistique* (Paris, 1808). Hirschberg tends to favor von Haller for primacy in precisely describing the operation. Notwithstanding, it is likely that von Haller would have been the first to deny this—he credits the original idea to Woolhouse [12]. Here, Hirschberg does what, unfortunately, he frequently does—steps out of scholarly mien. He obviously dislikes Woolhouse but is ambivalent, naming him a charlatan from one side of his pen and a brilliant surgeon from the other. He then goes on to further damn Woolhouse with faint praise [11].

Richter [13] mentions cataract extraction for myopia but is cautiously ambivalent:

> The only method would be the extraction or couching of a lens; but this procedure is, even in patients with the highest degree of myopia, of little benefit as it may lead to complete loss of vision . . . but should one not attempt in a case of severe myopia to couch or extract the lens in order to decrease the refractive power of the eye? [III, pp. 489–496].

Beer [14] is more forthright but still cautious:

> Is it not possible to help a patient with an extremely severe myopia by extracting the lens? The success of a cataract extraction in patients who before the cataract had a high myopia would speak for such an approach; no other patient has such a good vision after the operation than the myope. His vision improves after the cataract operation to an extent that he could not imagine. What is, however, the success rate of this operation? Especially when we extract a clear lens? It is possible that the myopic patient who sees quite clearly all the instruments which approach his eye becomes apprehensive and resistant. Would this

> not make the final result more uncertain than in a usual cataract extraction? Is it not difficult to extract a lens that has not become opaque? Somebody who has never tried it can really not evaluate it. It does, however, seem worthwhile to try this procedure at least on one eye of highly myopic patients [II, p. 659].

Hirschberg insists, despite what appears to be strong evidence that such surgery was indeed carried out, that no such operation was performed up until the latter 19th century. Yet he says in the same section that in 1858, Weber and Mooren cautiously attempted it. Although he promises to discuss it "later," this author is unable to discover where Hirschberg's "later" is. That he is clearly opposed to such surgery is evident in his stating flatly: *"During the 18th century mankind was still spared the scourge of the myopia operations"* [11, p. 341].

Nevertheless, the first unambiguous report of actual cases of clear lens extraction for myopia was apparently made by Fukala in 1889, and history will not be harmed by assigning the credit to him, rather than Vacher, who has the aroma of a "wanna-be" [15]. Or, if the reader is of a fairer mien, to both Fukala and Janin. However, as Darwin stated, *". . . in science the credit goes to the man who convinces the world, not to the man to whom the idea occurs."*

Modern clear lens extraction

It would be a mistake to assume that clear lens extraction for myopia is merely a matter of removing the lens itself. Eyes that are candidates for this surgery are high myopes with all that this term implies. They are long, they are thin-walled, and they are prone to developing glaucoma and retinal detachments as well. Many of them will already have poor visual acuity secondary either to posterior pole changes or to the inevitable minification of images. As many as 22% will not have binocular vision [16]. The visual field will likely be restricted with scotomas and night blindness. Color vision also may be impaired.

Merely plucking out the lens—whether it is done intracapsularly or, preferably, with phakoemulsification—will destabilize the eye sufficiently to invite either of the major complications mentioned. Glaucoma is one thing, but a retinal detachment in a high myope is bad news. It is the consensus among those of us who perform this surgery that the implantation of an intraocular lens—even one with no power—is therefore a must. The placement of a posterior chamber lens, whether "in-the-bag" or in the sulcus, serves to stabilize the eye by preventing the vitreous from moving forward. Detachments appear to occur less often under these circumstances; getting the correctly powered lens is the problem.

Intracapsular cataract extraction (ICCE) carries with it a high incidence of retinal detachment (RD)—1% to 3%, as opposed to 0.005% to 0.01% in unoperated eyes [17–21]. In myopes, this incidence increased to 6% [22,23]. The incidence of this complication following extracapsular cataract extraction (ECCE) has been decidedly reduced—1.4% to 1.7% in the general population—it is probably less with an implant. The data for myopic ECCE procedures are somewhat blurred, however. Praeger, using phakoemulsification and standard ECCE techniques, reported an incidence of 18 (6.5%) retinal detachments in 278 cases—which is high. Among those 18 eyes, 11 (15.5% of all cases) had experienced loss of vitreous (out of a total of 14 such cases) [24]. Another way to look at these figures is to state that this series had a 78.5% incidence of retinal detachment in myopic eyes experiencing vitreous loss during cataract surgery, and 61.1% of the detachment cases followed vitreous loss. The whole idea of ECCE is to avoid vitreous loss, however, which is more easily managed with phakoemulsification—especially with small incisions. Verzella, in a series of 1047 cases of myopic clear lens extraction, reported only 8 (1% incidence) RDs using just this technique [16].

The patient selected for clear lens extraction requires more of a workup than the normal "run through" for routine cataract extraction. Besides the usual A-scan biometry, intraocular pressure (IOP) determination, and K-readings, the author adds a B-scan, gonioscopy, indirect ophthalmoscopy, retinal photography, an Ishihara color perception examination, and an Amsler grid and fluorescein angiography—the latter if there are some posterior fundus indications.

This situation is a natural for a small incision with capsulorhexis and flexible or narrow optical lens procedures primarily because of wound size. Standard ECCE procedures are not recommended. One reason for advocating the first approach is the higher skill levels required for small-incision procedures—purely and simply stated. As the incision gets smaller both in the sclera and in the capsule, the margin for operator error gets smaller as well. Working "in-the-bag" to remove the lens material keeps trauma of the anterior chamber structures to a minimum. Additionally, it forces the surgeon to work slowly and carefully and pay attention to the eye.

The other reason is that capsule rupture is more likely to occur in high myopes with nuclear expression techniques. These typically require large incisions that are inherently destabilizing for the eye. The larger incision takes longer to heal and, in the author's experience, so do ECCE eyes generally. These patients are also prone to be steroid responders, so the less time they are on anti-inflammatories the better (see also Chapter 13). Clear lens extraction is a viable option for high myopes despite the potential hazards. Modern techniques can reduce the morbidity considerably.

Sutureless lens surgery

Since Kelman first introduced phakoemulsification in 1965 and extracted a cataract through a small opening, surgeons have looked forward to the day when visual rehabilitation could be accomplished through that same small incision. It was not until the late 1980s, when reliable foldable lenses made out of silicone material became available for general use, that ophthalmologists could begin to accomplish this dream. With the use of small-incision lenses, surgery could be carried out through a 4-mm incision or smaller, and visual recovery decreased from the usual time of 6 to 12 weeks to as early as 1 to 2 days—with a stable refraction in 7 to 14 days. In early 1990, McFarland discovered a patient whose single suture became untied the day after surgery. There was neither a leak nor a shallowing of the anterior chamber despite the obvious loss of support from the absent suture. Many surgeons became intrigued with this phenomenon and felt that the size, shape, and configuration of the scleral incision, as well as its distance from the surgical limbus, were important factors in obtaining a watertight seal. The author is grateful for the following contribution by Paul Ernest—a noteworthy pioneer in small-incision, sutureless lens surgery:

> When I began performing sutureless surgery in February of 1990, it was my feeling that the key factor in watertight wounds was not the size, shape or configuration of the scleral incision, but the creation of an internal corneal lip incision which acts as a one-way valve.

Technique

A one-third to one-half depth scleral incision is made 1 to 2 mm posterior to the surgical limbus, 4 mm in width, with an angled Alcon crescent blade. Using the same blade, starting at the lateral margin, a dissection is carried forward toward the surgical limbus and into clear cornea approximately 1 mm beyond the capillary arcade. The same blade is used to widen the tunnel and corneal incision to a full 4 mm without entering the chamber (Figure 12.1).

A 15° razor knife is used to make a counterpuncture at 3 o'clock, following which a 3.2-mm angled keratome

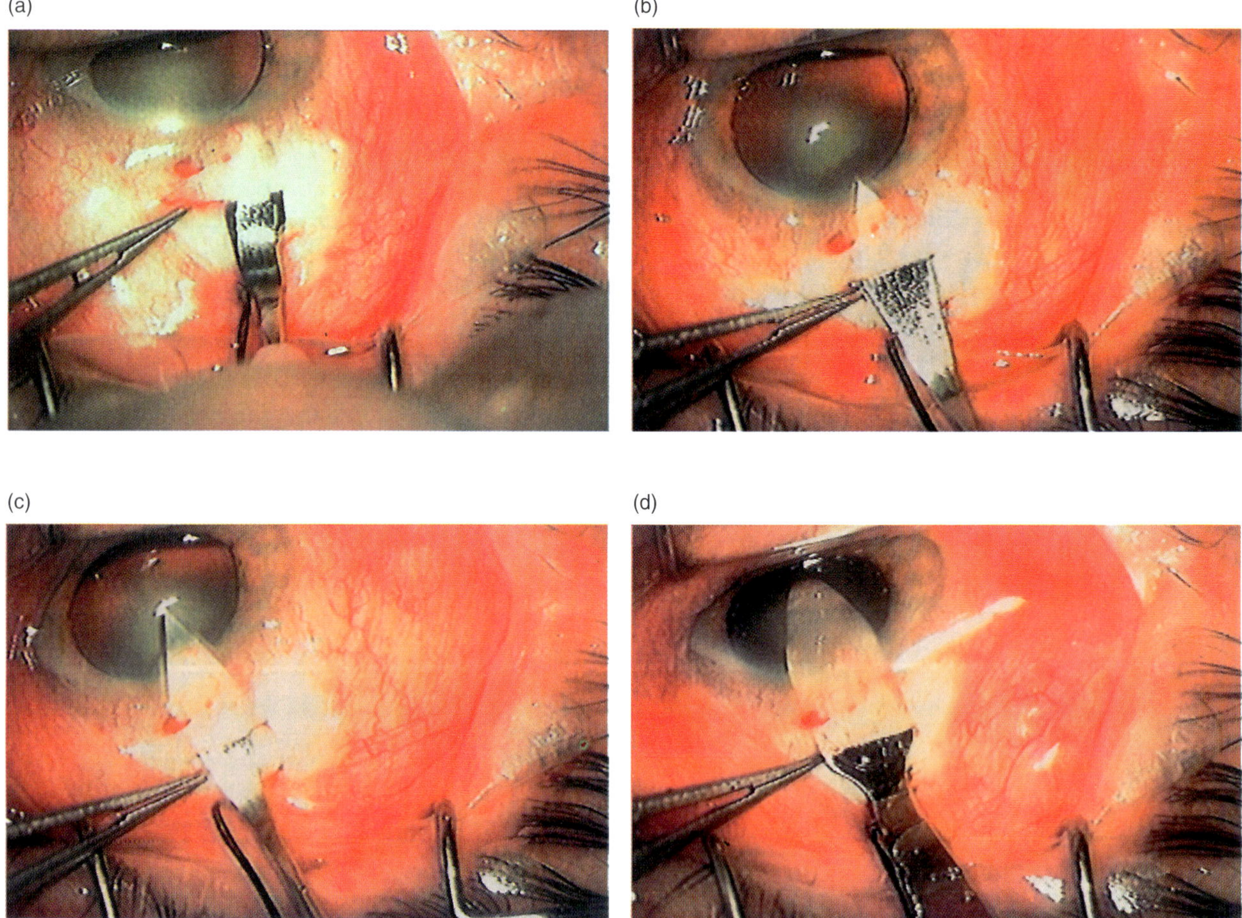

Fig. 12.1 Ernest's method of sutureless cataract surgery adapted by the author. (a) 4-mm tunnel incision is made beginning 2 mm from the limbus; (b) a phakotome is then introduced into the tunnel; and (c) then enters the anterior chamber approximately 1.5 mm in clear cornea; (d) a blunt-tipped, bevel-down keratome completes the incision. (Courtesy of P. Ernest.)

(a)

Capsule Cortex Outer nucleus Inner nucleus

(b)

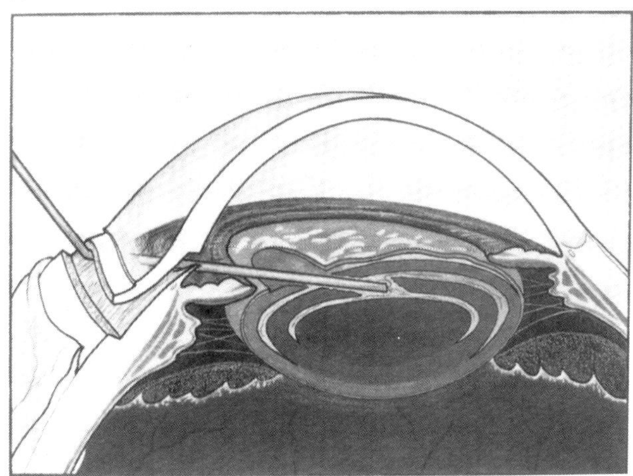

Fig. 12.2 (a) A small opening or capsulorhexis is made and hydrodissection of the nucleus is performed; (b) hydrodelineation of the nucleus follows. (Courtesy of J. Singer.)

blade is passed into the scleral tunnel to the end of the corneal dissection. The keratome blade is passed slowly into the anterior chamber, angling the tip downward, so as to ensure a linear incision. The blade is then removed, viscoelastic material is instilled in the anterior chamber, a blunt-tipped keratome blade is substituted, and the internal incision is widened to 4 mm. The purpose of the blunt-tipped keratome blade is to protect against a false passage through the already-made corneal incision. On completion of the internal wound, standard capsulorhexis is performed. The nucleus of the cataract can be emulsified within the posterior capsule using a standard central debulking technique and rotation of the peripheral nuclear rim, which is removed in segments (Figures 12.2 through 12.5).

Author's note: *The method of Ernest is preferred to remove the nucleus. In Ernest's technique, great care is taken to ensure that the nucleus is freely mobilized within the lens before proceeding. If, as someone once said, the genius is in the details, then the success of phakoemulsification (especially through a long tunnel incision) lies in careful preparation of the hard nuclear material for extraction. Ensuring that the nucleus is free within the epinucleus allows extraction without excess movement of the probe tip and the attendant danger of irrigation sleeve obstruction and chamber collapse. During extraction, the epinuclear material provides an additional cushioning effect to prevent capsular damage.*

Viscoelastic material is introduced into the anterior chamber, completely filling it. A 15° phako tip is then used to groove the nucleus to a depth of 1.5 times the diameter of the probe. A cyclodialysis spatula through the side port assists the phako probe in rotating the nucleus to produce the cross-shaped groove (Figure 12.6). A Dodick nuclear cracking forceps is then introduced into the anterior chamber, and the nucleus is split, using the forceps to rotate the nucleus twice—cracking each quadrant in turn (Figure 12.7a). Additional viscoelastic material is instilled into the chamber, and the nuclear fragments are removed piecemeal (see Figure 12.7b). Figure 12.8 compares the phako energy required with sculpting and cracking (a) and the mean endothelial cells counts (pre- and postoperatively) in each method (b).

On removal of all cortical material (leaving the cortex at 12 o'clock) using an automated I&A handpiece, viscoelastic material is reinstilled into the anterior chamber. A three-piece AMO silicone lens is folded in a McDonald forceps (model 2), the support loops are tucked into the crease, and the lens is passed through the scleral tunnel into the anterior chamber. Special care is taken to ensure that the leading as well as the trailing edges of the lens does not engage Descemet's membrane. Once the lens is completely inside the anterior chamber, the forceps is rotated, directing the folded loops against the posterior capsule. The lens is opened in a two-stage manner—first releasing the loops and then the optic of the lens. The two-step release is important to prevent a sudden explosive movement that can tear the posterior capsule.

Following insertion, the lens is rotated within the capsular bag both to ensure centration and to free up the remaining cortical material at the 12 o'clock position. Any residual cortex left at 12 o'clock is removed at this time, employing the implant as a protective barrier against tearing the posterior capsule. Viscoelastic material is carefully removed from the anterior chamber using the I&A unit. The implant is rotated and tapped posteriorly (balotted) with the I&A tip to cause any trapped viscoelastic material to extrude from behind the implant.

The wound is tested, at both high and low pressure, to be sure that no leakage of fluid occurs. Fluid is then re-

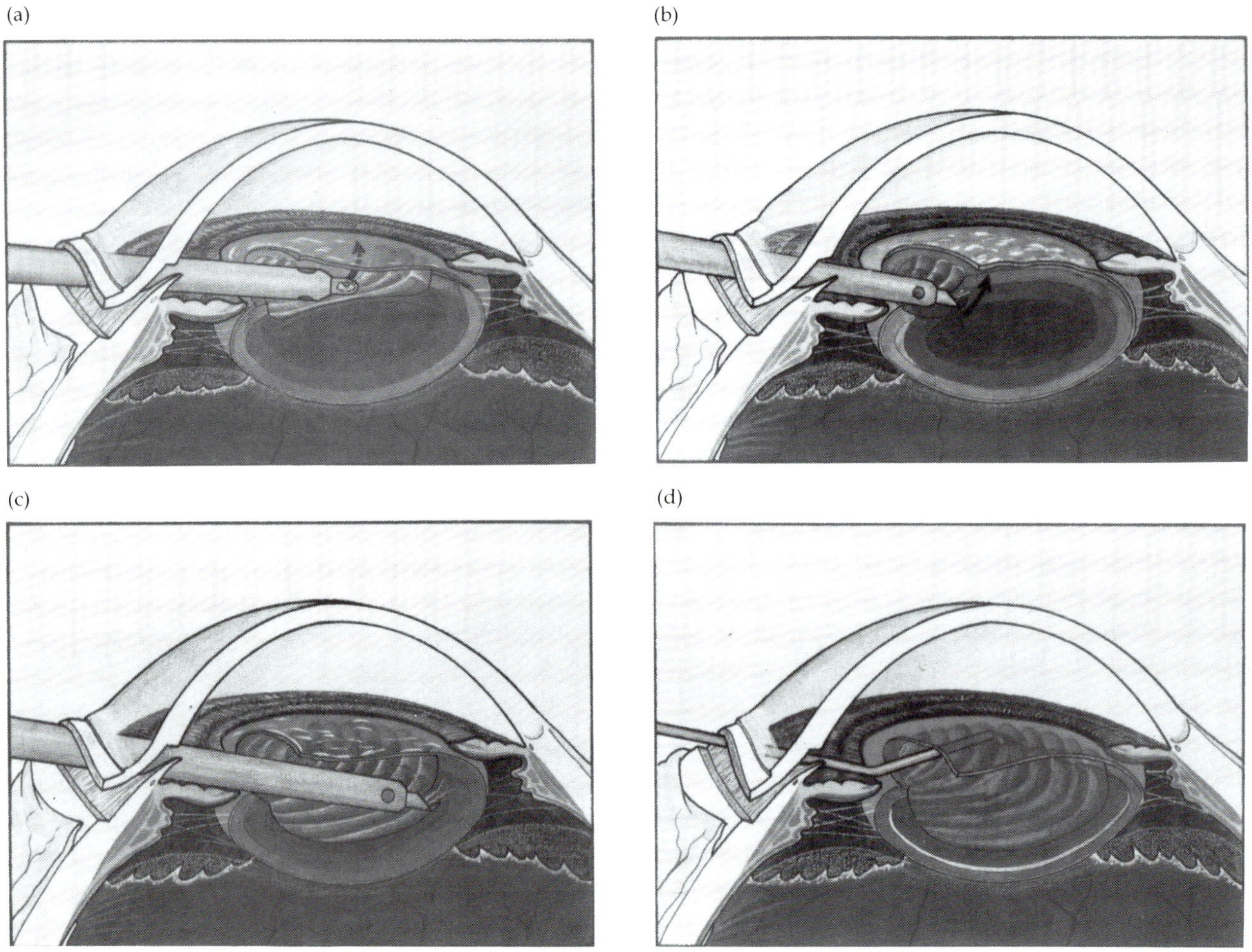

(a)

(b)

(c)

(d)

Fig. 12.3 (a,b) Thinning of the anterior cortex/nucleus is followed by (c,d) debulking of the central nucleus. (Courtesy of J. Singer.)

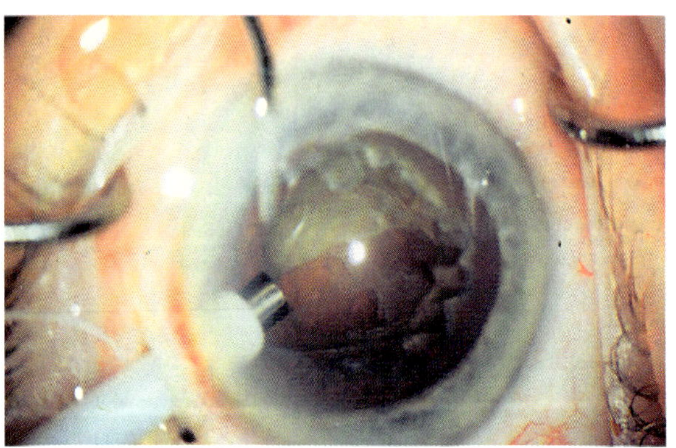

Fig. 12.4 Further dissection of the posterior nucleus is accomplished.

moved from the anterior chamber via the counterpuncture to ensure that the eye is soft postoperatively. The conjunctiva is closed over the wound using light cautery. Subtenon's injection of a steroid (such as DepoMedrol) and an antibiotic (such as Garamycin) is optional.

Results

In 1500 consecutive cases, no shallowing of the anterior chamber nor hyphemas occurred. No delayed filtering blebs were seen. Gonioscopy of the superior angle revealed no signs of peripheral anterior synechiae. Occasional patients experienced an increase in IOP after surgery due to the tightness of the corneal lip incision and the presence of residual viscoelastic material. This was treated successfully (in extreme cases) with a sterile paracentesis through the previously made counterpuncture incision. Figure 12.9 shows the incidence of induced astigmatism following this technique using vector analysis. There was no increase in corneal astigmatism on the day after surgery due to any residual corneal edema. Recovery time is equal to previously made tunnel incisions using the horizontal-stitch closure advocated by John Shepard. Patients without surgical complications were able to receive their final prescriptive lenses within 14 days. Figure 12.10 shows the resulting visual acuities following four different wound-closure methods.

No limitation of patient activity nor protective eye wear was necessary, either during daylight or at night,

(a)

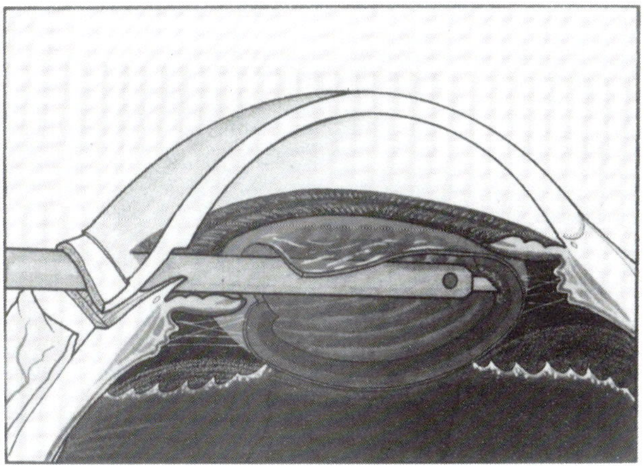

(b)

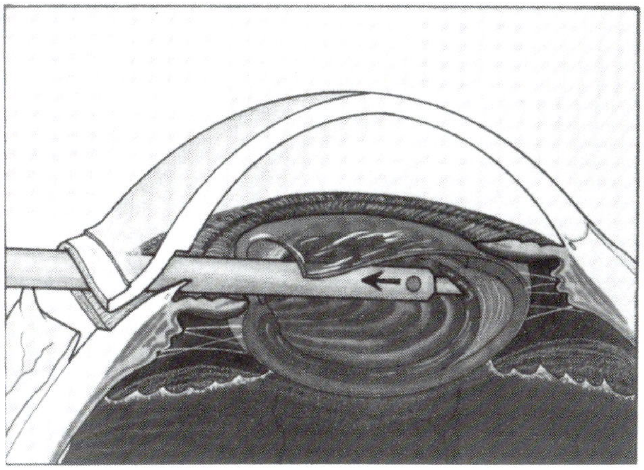

(c)

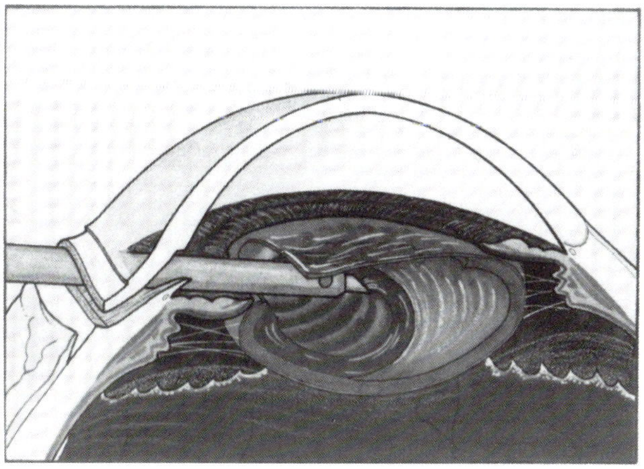

(d)

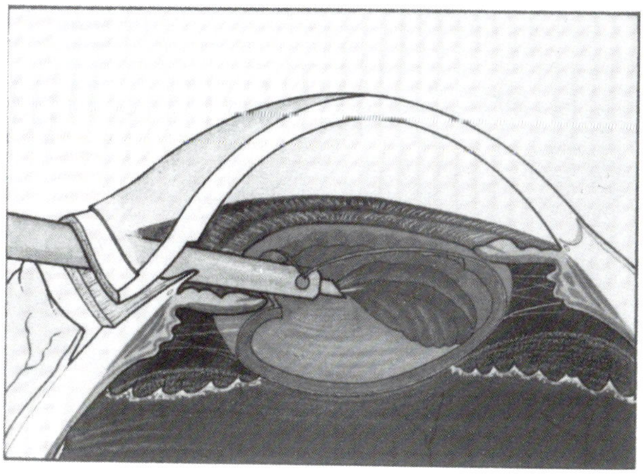

(e)

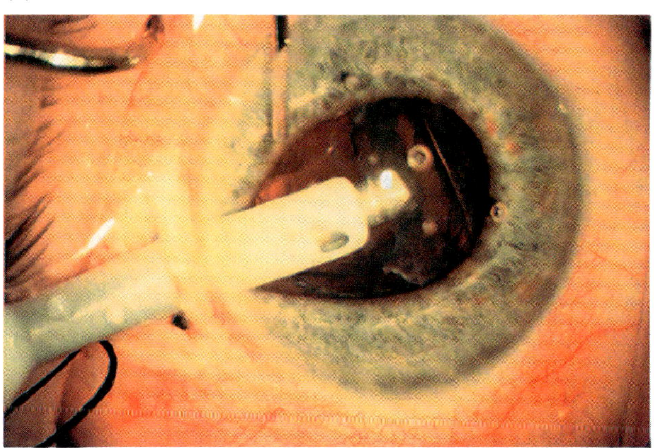

Fig. 12.5 (a,b) Using suction and low-power phako, the nucleus is engaged in the phako tip and dislocated. (c,d) By keeping the suction on and phako power low, the nucleus is captured and removed. Cortical cleanup is accomplished with the I&A tip. (Courtesy of J. Singer.)

and patients were able to rub their eyes after surgery without fear of wound leaks. Patients on anticoagulants, including aspirin, Persantine, and Coumadin, were able to maintain a full dose of medication, including the day of surgery, without any risk of hyphema—due to the construction of the corneal lip incision. Patients were advised of an increased risk of periocular and subconjunctival hemorrhaging, however.

Reduced visualization of the 12 o'clock nuclear cortical material occurred due to infolding of the cornea. This problem was reduced by enlarging the wound to 4 mm prior to performing phakoemulsification. If the corneal incision was carried beyond 1.5 mm, an increase in hydration of the stroma would obscure visualization of the superior cortical remnants. Any corneal hydration that did occur resolved within 48 hours. An occasional small

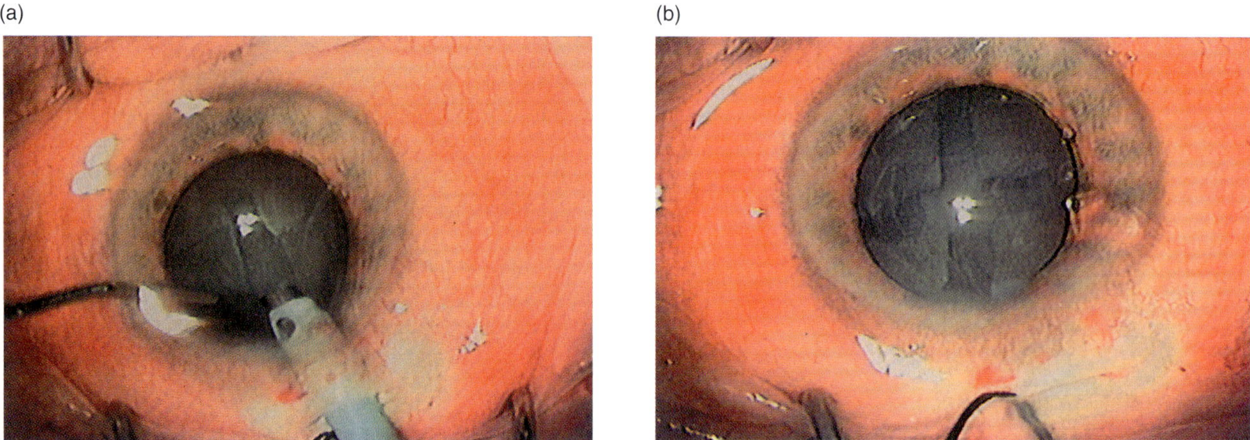

Fig. 12.6 The nucleus is grooved to 1.5× the phako tip diameter (a) using a cyclodialysis spatula through a side port to help rotate the nucleus into position (b). (Courtesy of P. Ernest.)

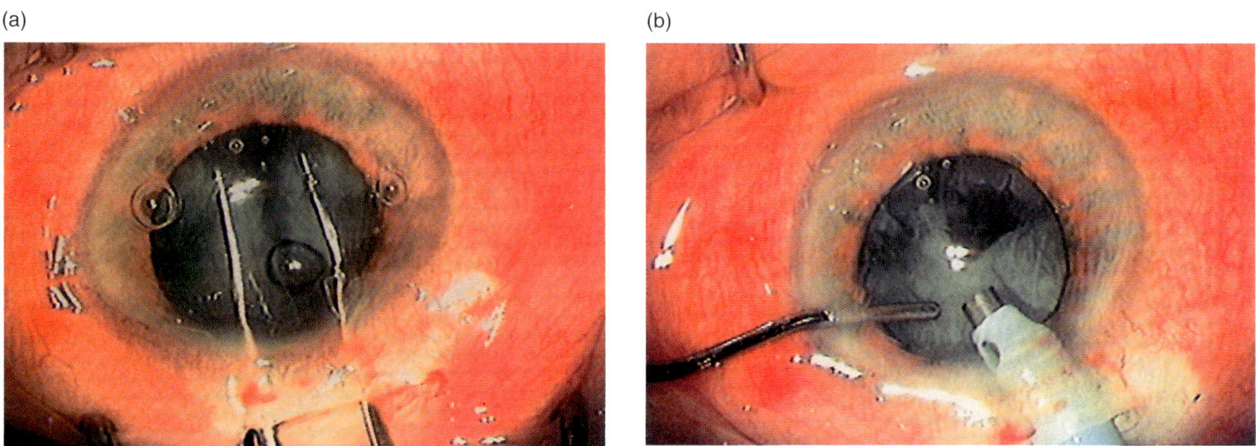

Fig. 12.7 A Dodick nuclear cracker is used to split the nucleus into four pieces (a) which are then extracted piecemeal (b). (Courtesy of P. Ernest.)

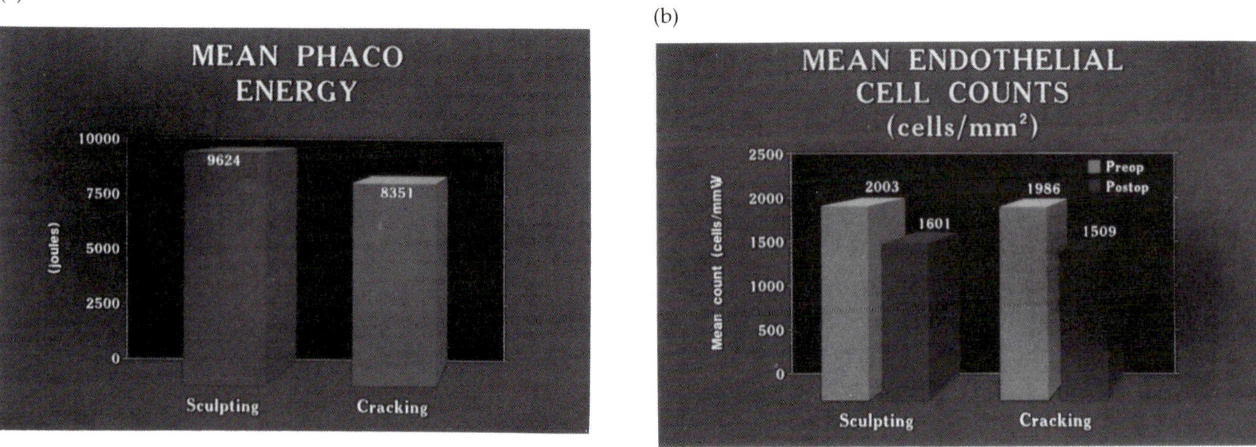

Fig. 12.8 (a,b) Phako energy required and endothelial cell counts in both the nuclear sculpting and cracking techniques.

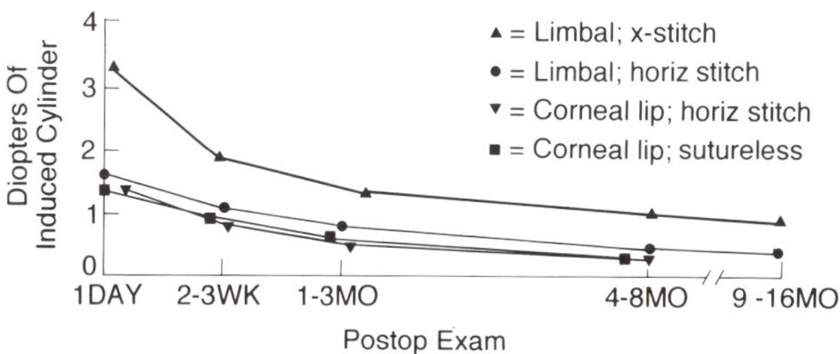

Fig. 12.9 Induced astigmatism following sutureless lens surgery. (Courtesy of P. Ernest.)

(a)

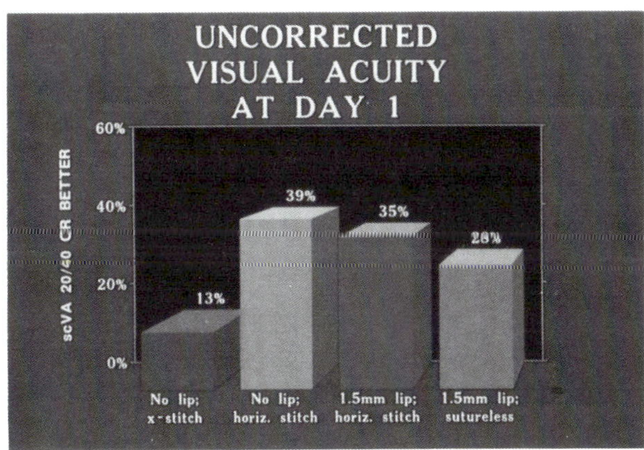

(b)

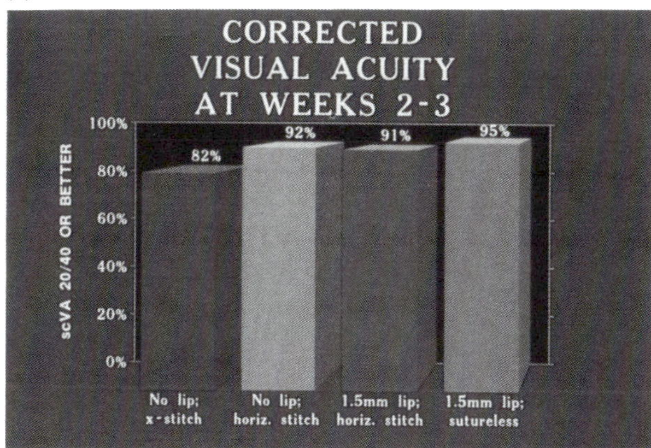

Fig. 12.10 Visual acuities following four different wound-closure techniques. The slight decrease in vision at 1 day for sutureless surgery is attributed to the small amount of corneal edema which occurs at the wound site. (Courtesy of P. Ernest.)

flaplike dehiscence of Descemet's membrane was seen. This usually happened in patients receiving high-diopter silicone lenses prior to the use of the McDonald forceps, which gives much better compression of these thicker implants. With lens powers in excess of 21 D, an SI20 silicone lens could be used, taking advantage of its increased refractive index. The SI30 lens may eliminate explosive release and endothelial rubbing entirely.

Experimental verification of sutureless wound strength

Using a corneal lip incision, it is possible to construct a sutureless wound that is a three-step incision in nature and that is stronger than the standard two-step incisions closed with sutures (Figures 12.11 through 12.13). A number of incisions were made in human cadaver eyes using the corneal lip incision as well as standard incisions of 4, 5, 7, and 12 mm in length, closed with interrupted 10-0 nylon sutures. A transducer attached to a 23-gauge needle was inserted into the eye at the 6 o'clock position. A needle puncture incision was made through cornea at 3 o'clock, and a balanced salt solution was injected into the anterior chamber. Careful measurement of the IOP was done, and any change in wound integrity was observed. It was found that even at pressures exceeding 400 mm Hg, the corneal lip incision did not show any leakage or change in shape. However, at 200 to 400 mm Hg in all sutured wounds with vertical closure and running 10-0 nylon sutures, the wounds ruptured, sutures broke, and chambers collapsed. Even 5- and 7-mm incisions closed with horizontal and infinity sutures demonstrated leaks at 400 mm Hg.

(a)

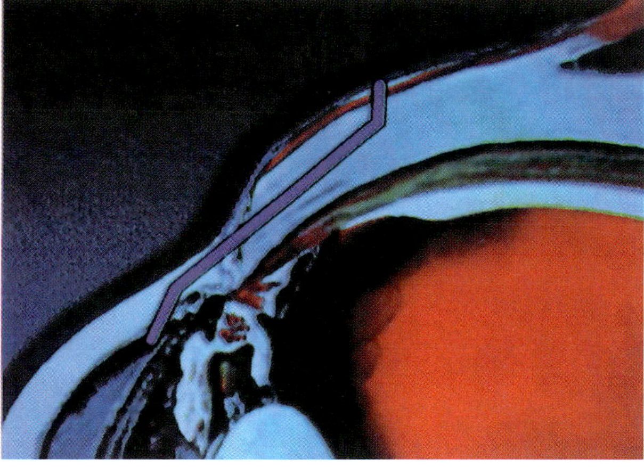

(b)

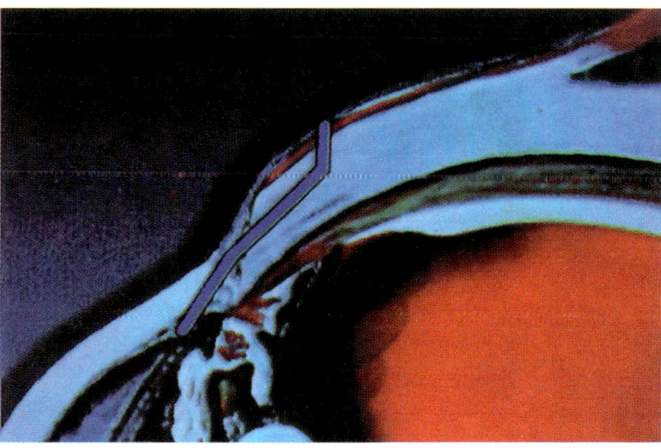

Fig. 12.11 (a) The three-step incision of sutureless surgery; (b) the standard two-step incision. (Courtesy of P. Ernest.)

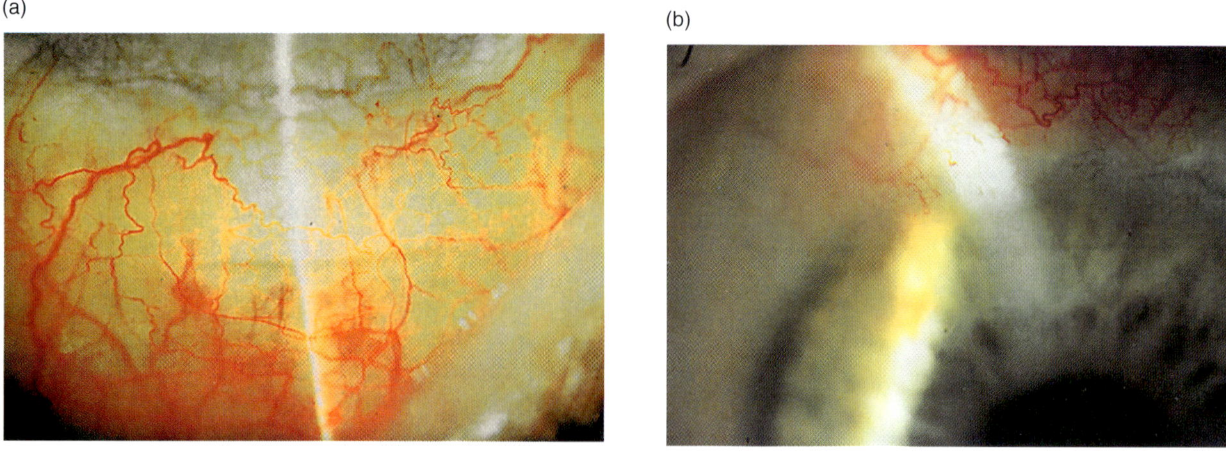

Fig. 12.12 (a) The scleral portion of the wound; (b) the corneal portion.

(a)

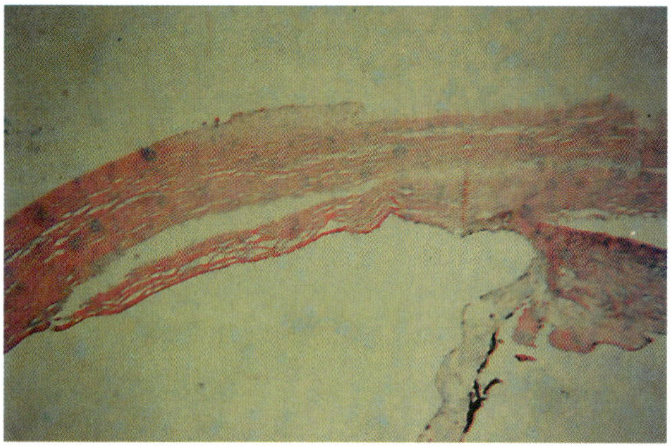

(b)

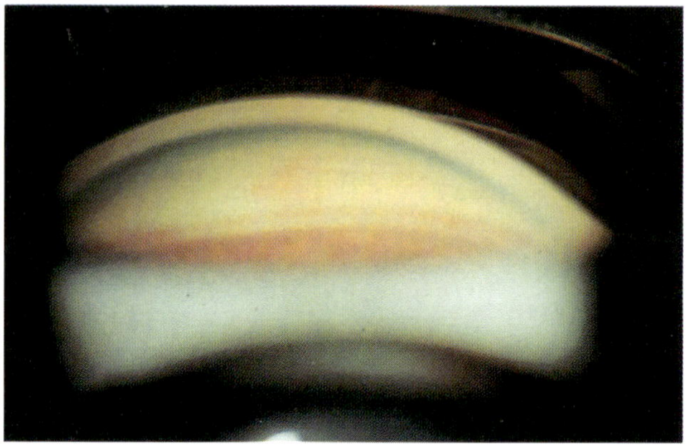

(c)

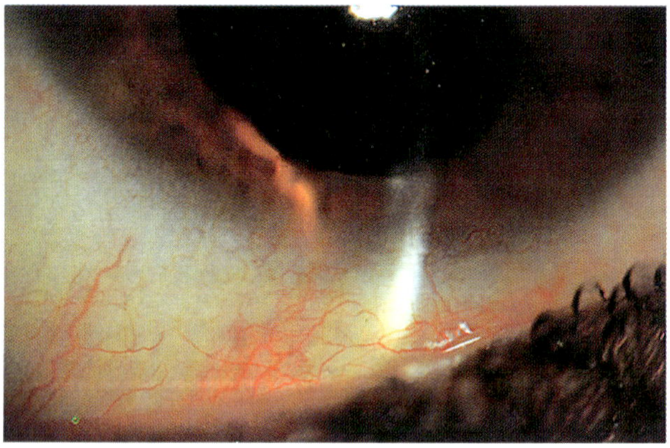

Fig. 12.13 (a) Histologic section showing the extent of the three-step wound; (b) gonioscopic view showing the inner aspect of the wound—well clear of the angle; (c) frontal view of the incision (note the anterior position of the entry). (Courtesy of P. Ernest.)

It is easy to see how such a valvelike wound (as advocated by Ernest) would tend to remain sealed with increased IOP. However, some authors have suggested that such wounds may increase the risk of ocular infection through external forces [25,26]. To test how such a wound would withstand direct external pressure, Ernest and colleagues devised an additional study with cadaver eyes [27]. Ten different wound types were tested. The results are summarized in Figure 12.14. The data supported the following conclusions:

- 4-mm incisions with 1.5-mm internal corneal lips withstood external pressures of up to 525 lb/in^2 for initial IOPs of 10 to 25 mm Hg.
- Other wounds (larger or with shorter lips) leaked and did not withstand external forces as well when the initial IOP was lower.

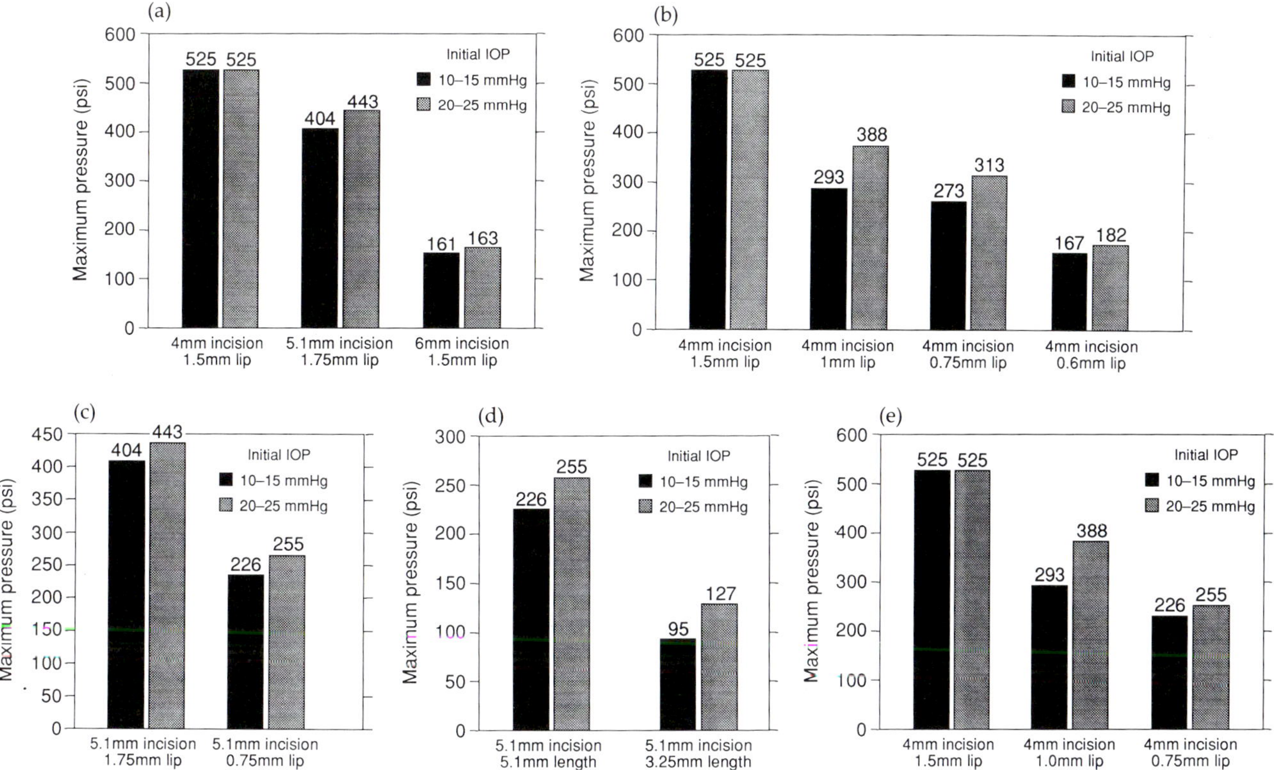

Fig. 12.14 Wound strength as a function of (a) incision width, (b,c) size of internal lip, (d) width/length ratio, (e) varied initial intraocular pressure. (Courtesy of P. Ernest.)

One patient with a sutureless incision received a blow from a golf ball (driven from a distance of 150 yards) to his operated eye 9 days postoperatively. The impact was sufficient to almost knock the patient unconscious, but the eye remained intact with no sign of any wound dehiscence. Conversely, two patients 6 months to 1 year after cataract surgery using the planned extracapsular technique and interrupted suture closure suffered falls with trauma to the operated eye. In both cases the cataract wound ruptured with expulsion of the intraocular lens, iris, and vitreous (Figure 12.15).

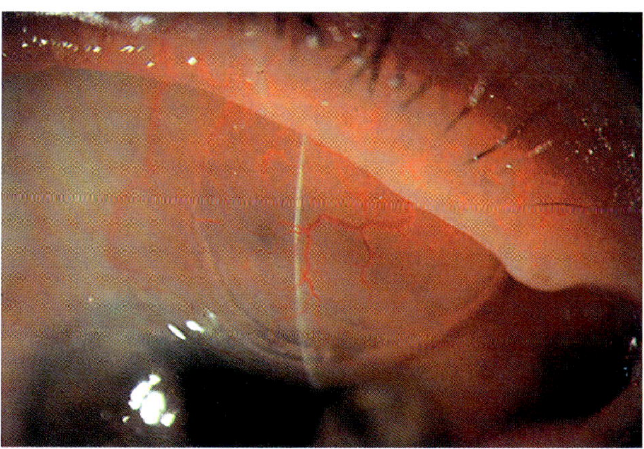

Fig. 12.15 A subconjunctival posterior chamber IOL following blunt trauma in an eye having had a planned ECCE surgery with sutures. (Courtesy of P. Ernest.)

Fyodorov has a group of 94 patients with follow-up ranging from 2 to 6 years in whom clear lens extraction had been performed [28] (Table 12.1). In 72% of the cases, best-corrected visual acuity was 0.5 or greater. Preoperative treatment included scleroplasty and retinal photocoagulation. The incidence of RD in this group was less than 2%. This points up the importance of careful surgical technique as well as dealing with the myopic eye as a pathologic entity.

Franco Verzella has the largest experience with this technique to date, and his data are impressive (Figures 12.16 through 12.20). The author's experience follows

Table 12.1 Clear lens extraction for myopia

Variable	Value
Number of patients	94
Age range	18–56 years
Refraction range	15–34 D
Mean preoperative vision	
Uncorrected	0.02
Corrected	0.0–0.6
Mean postoperative vision	
Uncorrected	0.40
Corrected	0.16–1.00

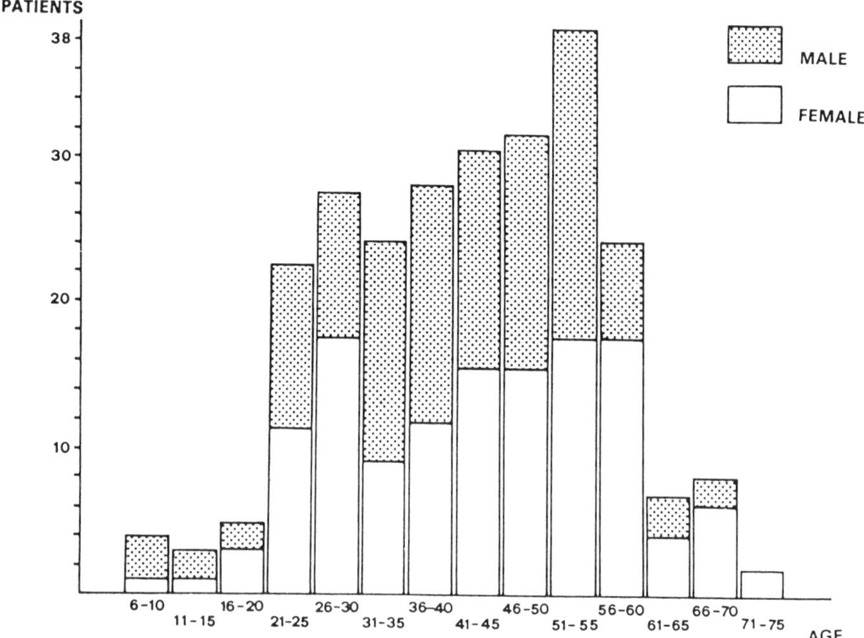

Fig. 12.16 Sex and age distribution of 458 eyes followed for 6 years. Range 6–71 years; 89% 21–60 years. (Courtesy of F. Verzella.)

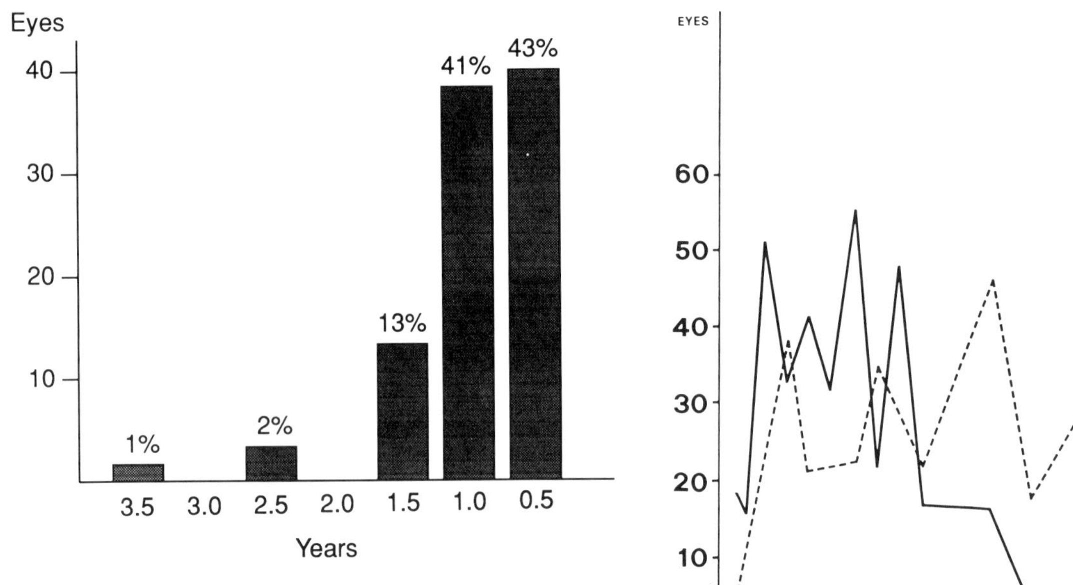

Fig. 12.17 Interval between lens extraction and posterior capsulotomy. (Courtesy of F. Verzella.)

Fig. 12.18 Best-corrected visual acuity before and after clear lens extraction. Preoperative range 0.04–0.95; postoperative range 0.04–1.2. (Courtesy of F. Verzella.)

(Table 12.2). The author has not had any cases of RD in his small series, whereas Verzella reported only 3 (0.66%), a truly impressive result.

RD seems to be the most feared complication. Many authors report less than a 1% incidence in small series followed for a few years. Colin reported a series of clear lens extractions with a 7-year follow-up using small, sutureless incisions and PCL implants for myopia of greater than 12 D.

Patients with lattice degeneration, a retinal tear, or a hole underwent photocoagulation before clear lens extraction. The author's performed phakoemulsification through a 3.2-mm-wide incision using primary irrigation and aspiration, widened the incision to 6.5 mm, and implanted a one-piece polymethyl methacrylate intraocular lens (IOL). At 7 years, the SEs of 29 eyes (59.1%) were within ± 1.0 D of emmetropia, and 42 eyes (85.7%) were within ± 2.0 D. Mean SE was −1.01 D (±0.94 D). At 7 years, mean uncor-

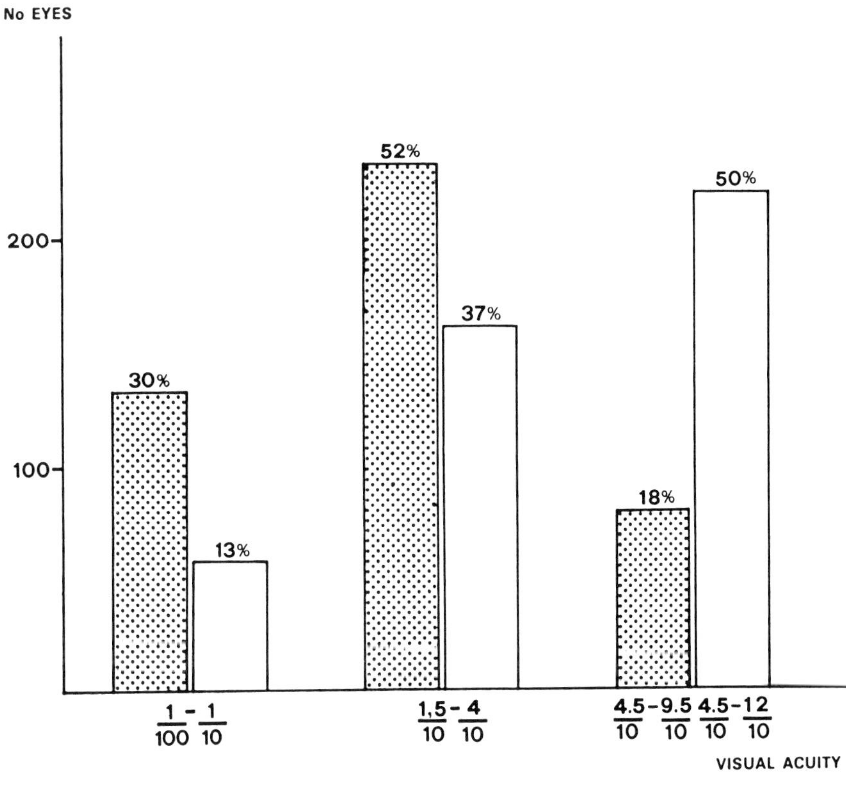

Fig. 12.19 Comparison of pre- and post-operative vision by vision groups. For example, 30% of the patients had a best-corrected preoperative vision between 0.01 and 0.1, whereas only 13% were in that group post-surgery. (Courtesy of F. Verzella.)

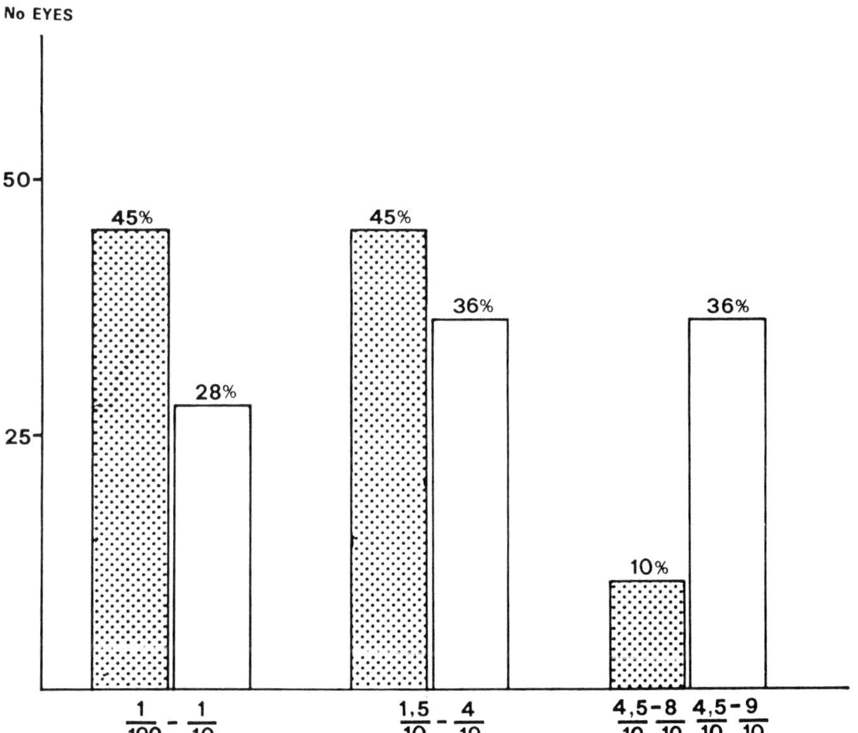

Fig. 12.20 The same comparison made with patients giving evidence of myopic maculopathy. (Courtesy of F. Verzella.)

rected visual acuity was 20/80, compared with 20/66 at 1 year. Best-corrected and uncorrected visual acuities were better in eyes with open capsules versus intact capsules. During the 7 years, 30 eyes (61.2%) required capsulotomy for opacification. Mean time for capsulotomy was 48.4 months after clear lens extraction. The authors performed 10 argon laser retinal treatments after surgery, with all but one in the first postoperative year. The overall incidence of posterior vitreous detachment was 16.3%. The incidence of RD during the 7 years was 4 of 49 eyes, or 8.1% (versus 2.0% at 4 years)—all the eyes had axial lengths of more than 8 mm [29].

Table 12.2 Results of clear lens extraction in the author's small series

Variable	Value
Number of patients	37
Age range	28–58 years
Refraction range	9–21 D
Mean preoperative vision	
Uncorrected	0.1–0.5
Corrected	0.5–1.0
Mean postoperative vision	
Uncorrected	0.4–1.0
Corrected	0.5–1.0

There is a category of eye between −6 and −9 D that supposedly has a higher incidence of RD than one with a higher degree of myopia, but there are no scientific or epidemiologic data to answer this question. The jury is still out. Despite advances in surgical technique, retinal detachment remains a major concern after clear lens extraction for high myopia. In Colin's series, the incidence of RD after clear lens extraction was nearly double that estimated for persons with myopia greater than −10 D who do not undergo surgery. Although clear lens extraction has advantages, including rapid and predictable visual rehabilitation, stable refraction, the ability to replace the IOL, and often superb optical quality with no irregular astigmatism, it is invasive and can result in severe vision loss. Long and continuous follow-up of the outcomes of clear lens extraction for high myopia is absolutely necessary before the authors can consider the procedure a routine option for patients with high myopia. Active searching and prophylactic laser treatments for retinal tears developed before and after cataract extraction in patients with high myopia are recommended. This may lower the incidence of postoperative RD.

Laser phakolysis

Since the early 1990s, Dodick has been studying the use of the Q-switched, pulsed 1064-nm Nd:YAG laser for one-stage direct photolysis of cataractous lenses [30,31] (Figure 12.21). The probe, similar to a standard I&A handpiece, consists of an irrigation and aspiration port chamber that contains a 300-μm quartz-clad fiber. The proximal portion of the 300-μm fiber is attached via a standard laser connector to the laser source. The fiber enters the probe through the infusion cannula and terminates approximately 2 mm in front of a titanium target inside the probe tip. The pulsed laser energy is transmitted via the quartz fiber and is focused on the titanium target, thus enabling optical breakdown and plasma formation to occur at very low energy levels. This, in turn, produces shock waves, which propagate within the aspiration chamber toward the mouth of the probe, where the nuclear material is held in approximation by the suction created by the aspiration port. The shock waves disrupt the nuclear material, and

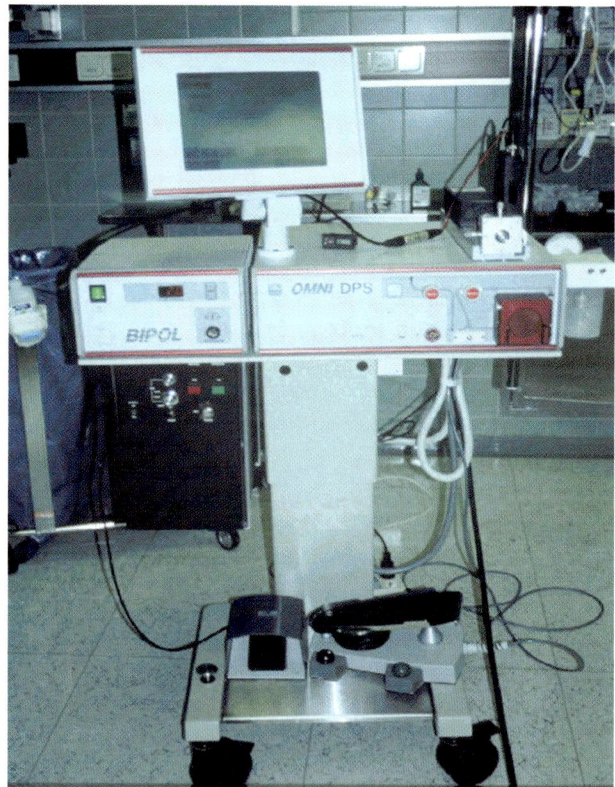

Fig. 12.21 Dodick laser phakolysis unit. (Courtesy Dr. J. Dodick, New York.)

the fragments are aspirated [30,31] (Figure 12.22). The titanium target is the essential element of this device, since the metal target, with its low ionization potentials, acts as a transducer in converting light energy to shock waves at low laser energy levels. Because there is no direct contact between the laser energy and the target tissues, the shock waves generated here are more controlled so that only the area in contact with the tip of the device is disrupted. In effect, the titanium target shields the nontarget tissues such as the endothelium and the retina, as well as the surgeon's eyes, from direct laser light. The quartz-clad fiber and the titanium targets are relatively inexpensive, making disposable handpieces a possibility. The same tip may be used for I&A.

Recently, several other devices using laser energy to emulsify and remove the human lens have undergone tests. Although they are unlikely to replace ultrasound phako systems in the near future, laser phako systems do have several advantages over ultrasound systems. First, the probes are typically smaller in diameter. More recently, Kanellopoulos reported results from a series of 100 consecutive patients treated at four surgical centers throughout the United States and Europe. For this series, the measures of outcome used were improvement in visual acuity, endothelial cell loss, change in IOP, total energy used, and intra- and postoperative complications.

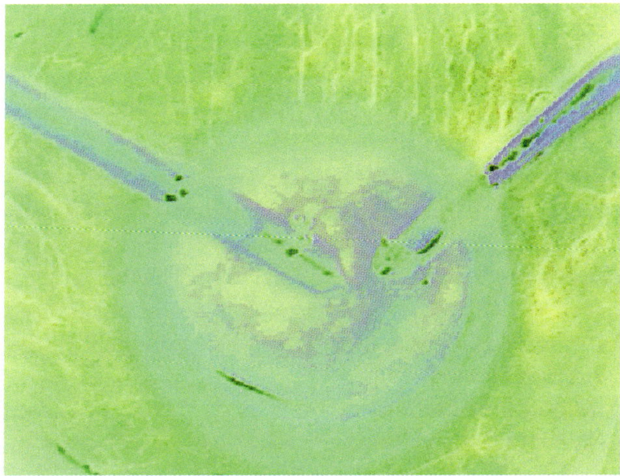

Fig. 12.22 Laser phakolysis in action. (Courtesy Dr. J. Dodick, New York.)

The lens density in this series ranged from 1 to 4+. The mean visual acuity improved from 20/46.5 (0.43) to 20/26.6 (0.75). The mean decrease in endothelial cell count was 7.55% (177 cells/mm), while no significant changes in IOP were noted. The mean number of laser pulses used per case was 555 pulses at 12 mJ per pulse, translating into a total average energy of 6.7 J per case. While posterior capsular rupture occurred in 3 cases, only 1 was during the laser photolysis portion of the procedure. In 8 cases, conversion to ultrasound phakoemulsification was necessary. It was noted in this study that lenses of 1 to 2+ density were removed with comparable efficiency as compared with phako. However, denser lenses required significantly longer operative times. In this series, a Venturi pump system with vacuum settings of 250 to 300 lb/in^2 was used. Incision size prior to IOL implantation was 1.4 mm, whereas a 0.9-mm incision was used for the irrigation handpiece. Newer probe designs (0.9 mm diameter) undergoing clinical testing eventually would be able to pass through a 1.0-mm corneal incision.

Because the laser probes produce no clinically significant heat, there is no risk of corneal and scleral burns. Studies have demonstrated that after 30 seconds of continual use under standard conditions, a temperature increase of 2.6°C was noted with a laser probe, compared with an increase of 30°C with an ultrasound probe. Furthermore, the water temperature in a 2.5-cc closed chamber increased by 1°C with a laser probe versus 9.5°C with an ultrasound probe. The minimal heat generated by the laser probes eliminates the need of a water bath around the probe, thus enabling the separation of irrigation from the laser/aspiration and thereby reducing probe and incision size.

Furthermore, unlike ultrasound phako handpieces, the laser probes do not house motors and do not require electrical voltage to drive vibrating needles, both of which are subject to wear and tear. In addition to being lighter and easier to handle, the components of the laser probes are relatively cheap, thus making disposable handpieces a possibility.

A notable problem with current laser systems is that dense nuclei still present a challenge. One can expect that with further refinements in fluidics and laser parameters, this problem will be overcome in the near future.

Intraocular implants for ametropia

We learn wisdom from failure much more than success; we often discover what will do, by finding out what will not do; and probably he who has never made a mistake never made a discovery. [Samuel Smiles]

In recent years, the surgical correction of refractive errors has concentrated primarily on corneal surgery. Procedures such as photorefractive keratectomy with the excimer laser, lamellar procedures such as automated lamellar keratectomy or laser in situ keratomileusis, and radial keratotomy change corneal curvature and, therefore, refraction.

Another way to change the eye's refractive status is to implant an intraocular lens (IOL). Phakic IOLs originated in the 1950s and early 1960s when myopic anterior chamber lenses were designed. Later, iris-fixated lenses and angle-supported phakic IOLs were developed. In 1991, the use of a phakic posterior-chamber IOL to correct high myopia was introduced in Russia. Since then, phakic IOLs have received increasing attention for correcting high myopia and hyperopia.

Phakic IOLs have potential advantages over conventional corneal refractive surgery. Unlike most corneal refractive procedures, which permanently alter corneal curvature and can be difficult to modify, phakic IOLs are potentially adjustable (via IOL exchange) and reversible (via IOL removal). The techniques for phakic lens implantation, similar to methods for inserting standard IOLs, are familiar to most ophthalmologists. In addition, visual rehabilitation is faster because the postoperative refraction tends to stabilize earlier than with most corneal procedures.

The best candidates are presbyopic aged patients who are beyond accurate and safe laser in situ keratomileusis (above +4 D and above −9 D). For hyperopes, very small incision may not be possible because the silicone lenses do not come higher than +30 D. Bausch & Lomb makes a lens up to +45 D, but you need a 5.5- to 6-mm incision to implant it. If you need low power or minus lenses for high myopes, you run into the same problem. These lenses are not usually available in low powers or minus powers, although the Alcon AcrySof now goes to +6 D at this writing.

However, implanting an IOL is not a new idea. In fact, it is centuries old.

Tadini and Casaamata

Ask the average ophthalmologist who Sir Harold Ridley is, and you will get a knowing smile. Ask the same ophthalmologist who Alessandro Tadini and Giovanni Virgilio Casaamata were, and the smile disappears. Which is a pity because these gentlemen anteceded Mr. Ridley by some 200 years—albeit not successfully. This is not to take anything away from Sir Harold Ridley. He, after all, did something about it, while Tadini only made the suggestion and Casaamata carried it out—half-heartedly.

Not much is known about Casaamata and even less about Tadini. Most of what we do know about the latter is through the memoirs of that notorious rake—Casanova. Casaamata was an ophthalmologist of Italian birth, who at the time of the event alluded to, was court physician to Friedrich III (later the Polish King August II), Elector of Saxony. It is curious that despite his having held this obviously honorable position, Hirschberg dismisses him as a mere itinerant surgeon and deigns to give him a mere 13 lines in his *History of Ophthalmology* [11]. During this period, Casaamata established one of the first eye hospitals in Germany. While he did travel extensively to operate, this was the custom of the time. His permanent residence was Dresden. Casaamata obviously deserves more than the few lines Hirschberg gives him. For one thing, he was well trained. For another, he established—in 1782—what was probably the very first eye hospital—in his home. Beer, in his *Bibliotheca Ophthalmica*, describes him as an innovative and talented surgeon who had an unusual method of operating—he sat on the table, and the patient occupied the chair (actually three chairs were used, one for the patient and one each for Casaamata's feet). Beer mentions that Casaamata once substituted a glass lens for the extracted one but gave no details [33].

A contemporary, Rudolph Schiferli, also had published a small handbook entitled, *Theoretisch-praktische Abhandlung über den grauen Starr* (A Theoretical and Practical Dissertation on Cataract), in 1797. He observed and wrote about the techniques of many surgeons of his day. In the chapter "Post-Operative Treatment" of this handbook, he writes

> ... Casaamata made the attempt to insert a glass lens through the operative wound and under the cornea. He found that this lens could not take the place of the original because it fell to the bottom of the eye. He therefore decided that the idea had no merit. This attitude prevails today as a corollary to the NIH (Not Invented Here) syndrome. That is—"we can't (or didn't) do it; therefore, nobody can." But one has another way to replace the loss of the lens and this is the best and common one: they are namely, convex lenses worn before the operated eye, as spectacles [34].

Nevertheless, further investigation reveals that this idea was not original to Casaamata. It seems to have come from another Italian citizen—Tadini.

Of Tadini little is known except that he was one of that singular class of physicians known as the itinerant ophthalmologist. Most of these were indifferent surgeons at best and charlatans at worse. Tadini may well have been both—he certainly thought well of himself. Of course, so did Giacomo Casanova. His memoirs, nonetheless, contain more than just an inventory of his amorous conquests; he included an abundance of historical information, including medical anecdotes [35]. He had met both Boerhaave and von Haller and writes jocularly about another eye physician of his acquaintance—Alessandro Tadini—whom he had met twice.

The first of these meetings was in Warsaw, Poland. There he was asked to mediate a dispute between the vagabond Tadini and an established surgeon of the city whom Tadini had labeled a dunce after the failure of the latter to completely remove a lady's cataract. Casanova writes:

> I was, with the greatest pleasure, ready to listen to the two hostile doctors. The old one was German, though he spoke French relatively well. He attacked Tadini in Latin but the latter interrupted him immediately, by saying, the lady (who was also present) has to be able to understand what they were saying. Obviously Tadini didn't understand a word of Latin. The German eye doctor tried to reason with him. He said: "It is true that the incising of the cataract gives both the patient and the surgeon the certainty that the cataract will not return; but that surgery is less safe and puts the patient in danger of going blind when losing the irreplaceable crystalline lens."
>
> Whereupon Tadini committed the stupidity of pulling out a small box containing small glass balls resembling the crystalline [The human lens was often called the crystalline in the older literature. It is still referred to as that even today in some cultures.] "What is that supposed to mean?" said the old surgeon. "I," said Tadini, "possess the skill to insert these glass lenses through the cornea." At this the old surgeon laughed so hard and long that the lady couldn't help but join in. I would liked to have laughed as well, but was embarrassed to be taken for an ignoramus and kept still. Tadini undoubtedly thought that my silence was a rebuke to the German and hoped to bring on a thunderstorm when he turned to me.
>
> I answered: "Since you wish to know my opinion, I'll tell you. There is a very big difference between a tooth and the crystalline of the eye and you are wrong to suppose that one could fit a glass lens into the eye between the cornea and retina like pulling out an old tooth and replacing it with a false one. Sir, I have never fitted a person with a

false tooth which is possible; but surely an artificial crystalline is not."

Tadini left the meeting in disgrace. The old professor published an article in the *Warsaw News* ridiculing Tadini and managed to persuade his cronies on the faculty to insist that Tadini take an examination in his professed métier. Tadini responded by attacking the professor physically and had to flee the city.

Casanova met Tadini again in Barcelona, where the former was incarcerated for his philandering. It seems that Tadini had arrived in town without credentials. Refusing to submit to an examination (in Latin) prior to setting up shop, he was inducted into the army *instanter* and assigned a job more suited to his talents—that of a jailer. At the end of their meeting, Casanova asked:

"So, what did you do with those glass lenses?"

"After Warsaw, I gave them up, though I am sure they would have been a success."

It seems that he had never really tried them.

Thus Casaamata is established as the first to attempt to insert a pseudophakos. It is unlikely, though, that Tadini had ever met Casaamata—they moved in somewhat different circles. Casaamata could certainly not have read the memoirs of Casanova, since they were published in 1818, twenty years after Casanova's death and eleven years after his own. It is possible that the Warsaw episode mentioned above came to Casaamata's attention in his role as court physician. There is, however, another, simpler explanation. In those days, Dresden was one of the most opulent capitals of Europe. The Elector was, as were so many other nobles, a patron of the arts and drew many talented people to his court. Among these were the actress Gianetta Casanova, the mother of Giacomo, and his younger brothers Francesco and Giambattista, who were painters. From 1785 Casanova himself served as the librarian of the Count Waldstein in Dux (not far away), where he wrote his memoirs. There was plenty of opportunity for him to visit his family at the Saxon court, where he undoubtedly told and retold the story of the ridiculous Italian ophthalmologist and his glass lenses.

Despite the benefits of phakic IOLs, a number of concerns exist. Foremost is the risk of intraocular surgery, with its attendant complications. Phakic IOL design also presents challenges because these lenses must rest safely between the corneal endothelium and crystalline lens for several decades. This is especially a problem with hyperopic lenses, which typically are heavier and convex, making contact with the central corneal endothelium a potential hazard.

Three types of phakic IOLs are under investigation: anterior-chamber designs, iris-fixated IOLs, and posterior-chamber designs (implantable contact lenses). Although each phakic lens design shows promise, significant issues need to be resolved for them gain wide acceptance.

Anterior-chamber lenses

Angle-supported lenses

The main problems associated with the anterior-chamber angle-supported phakic lens are intermittent touch with the endothelium and angle, rotation of the lens, ocular pain, pupil ovalization, and glare. Lens designers have addressed the first problem by modifying haptic angulation and optical thickness, and recent studies with the Baikoff model suggest that endothelial cell loss may no longer be a problem [36]. Inaccurate sizing of the implant leads to implanting an undersized lens, predisposing to excessive rotation in the anterior chamber, or an oversized lens, causing ovalization of the pupil and globe tenderness. Angle-supported lenses have been used following cataract surgery for years with more or less success, the more modern versions being considerably safer than the older models such as the Strampelli and the Dannheim lenses. It should not be thought, however, that it is the rigid lenses alone that have produced the complications reported. The Dannheim (and the later Leiske) lenses have resulted in their share of iridocyclitis, hyphema, glaucoma, and corneal decompensation. Because of this, it cannot be said that the concept of an angle-supported myopic implant has been proven [37]. On the contrary, experience with lenses of this type has shown just the opposite—in phakic eyes.

Notwithstanding the opinion of some, the implantation of IOLs into the phakic eye to treat myopia has a disastrous history. Strampelli implanted lenses of his own design in 1953 with indifferent results [38]. The most notorious example, however, is that of Joaquin Barraquer's experience in 1959 [39]. Iridocyclitis, recurrent hyphema, secondary glaucoma, and corneal decompensation necessitated removal of most of the lenses implanted. While some blame can be laid to the fact that the surgery was performed with loupe magnification only, the lenses used were principally the cause of the corneal and anterior-chamber problems encountered. That these complications were caused chiefly by the lenses is shown clearly by Drews, who examined a group of 162 such IOLs—some of which had been removed from phakic myopes [40] (Figure 12.23).

That current lenses are considerably better in both design and fabrication than their predecessors is not in dispute. That these same lenses are likewise more suited for implantation into the phakic eye is a question whose resolution is not as yet complete. Still, some work is ongoing to test this premise—some using silicone-type construction and others PMMA. The most noteworthy of the latter is the Worst-Fechner iris claw lens (see below).

Georges Baikoff has been one of the leading exponents of angle-supported IOLs to correct myopia. He reported on a series of 163 myopic implants of a multiflex-design PMMA minus lenses with 2 years of follow-up (Table 12.3 and Figures 12.24 through 12.28). In almost 3% of

(a)

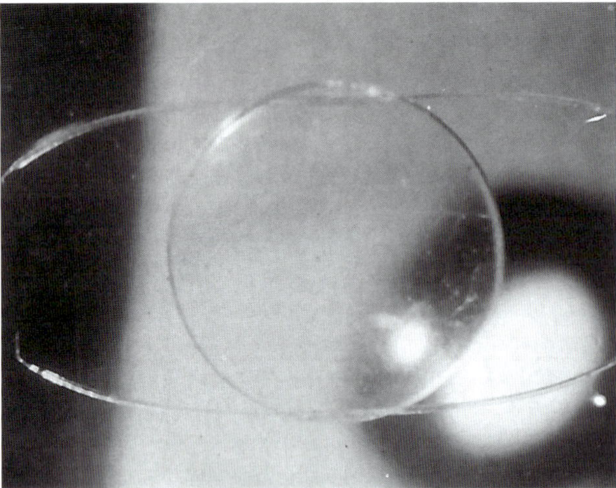

(b)

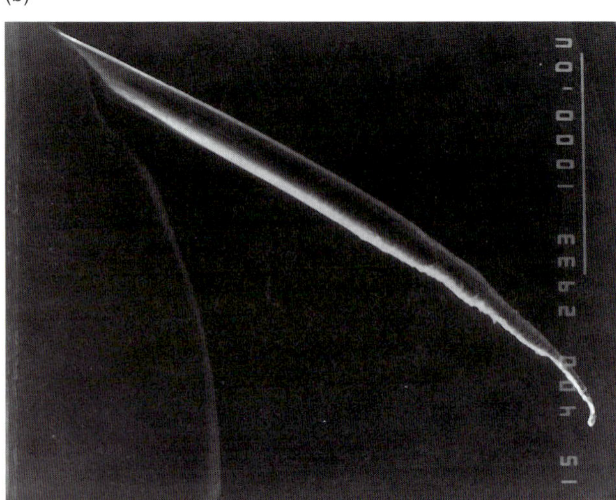

Fig. 12.23 Dannheim lenses from the Barraquer series. (a) This minus lens shows typical loss of the loop ends. (b) SEM confirms the loss due to biodegradation (from Drews RC. The Barraquer experience with intraocular lenses. Ophthalmology 1982; 89:386–393).

Table 12.3 Visual results following phakic anterior intraocular lens implantation for myopia

	Preoperative visual acuity	Day 1–2	Day 15–30	2–3 months	5–6 months
Myopia (D)*	−14.94 ± 4.68	−0.17 ± 1.25	−0.04 ± 1.33	−0.17 ± 1.11	−0.22 ± 1.08
	(154)	(94)	(115)	(118)	(74)
Best-corrected visual acuity†	0.47 ± 0.26	0.52 ± 0.23	0.61 ± 0.23	0.64 ± 0.25	0.62 ± 0.26
	(163)	(108)	(127)	(128)	(92)

* Numbers in parentheses represent number of eyes.
† Snellen ratios (e.g., 0.5 = 20/40).

cases the implant required removal primarily for power error within the first 2 postoperative days. Rotation of the lenses (due to small size) was seen in 4% of cases. All these lenses were reported to have stabilized in their new positions, however. This phenomenon has been reported in anterior-chamber lenses used for aphakia and almost always requires removal some time in the postoperative course. Although 1 case is reported to have developed a cataract subsequent to the IOL implant, cases in which some opacification of the lens preceded the surgery have not shown progression of those changes [36,41,42].

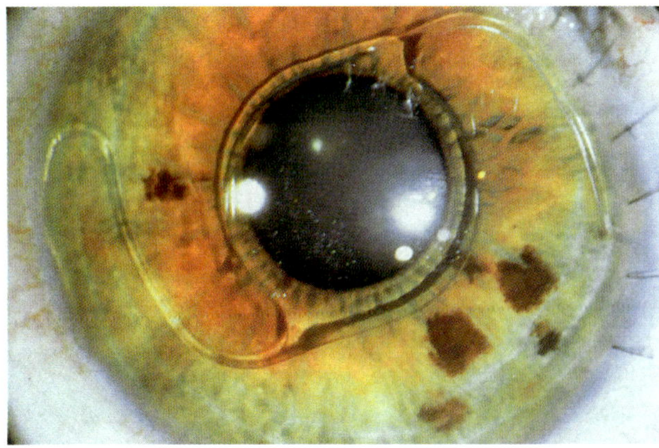

Fig. 12.24 ACL lens in a phakic eye for myopia. (Courtesy of G. Baikoff.)

Progressive endothelial cell loss following implantation of angle-supported IOLs has been reported elsewhere [43]. Baikoff reports no evidence of endothelial cell loss at 1 year. However, that study was retrospective; thus no proper baseline has been established from which to measure cell loss. How many cells were lost at the time of surgery, for instance? Sargoussi and Lesure, nonetheless, reported substantial endothelial cell damage at the footplates of the implant [44,45] (Figure 12.29). These lenses are being implanted in the United States under an investigative protocol (Figure 12.30).

Worst-Fechner biconcave iris claw lens

Although the Worst-Fechner iris-supported lens is more difficult to implant than an angle-supported IOL, good initial results have been reported. The greatest concern is long-term safety. Since few reports have shown ongoing

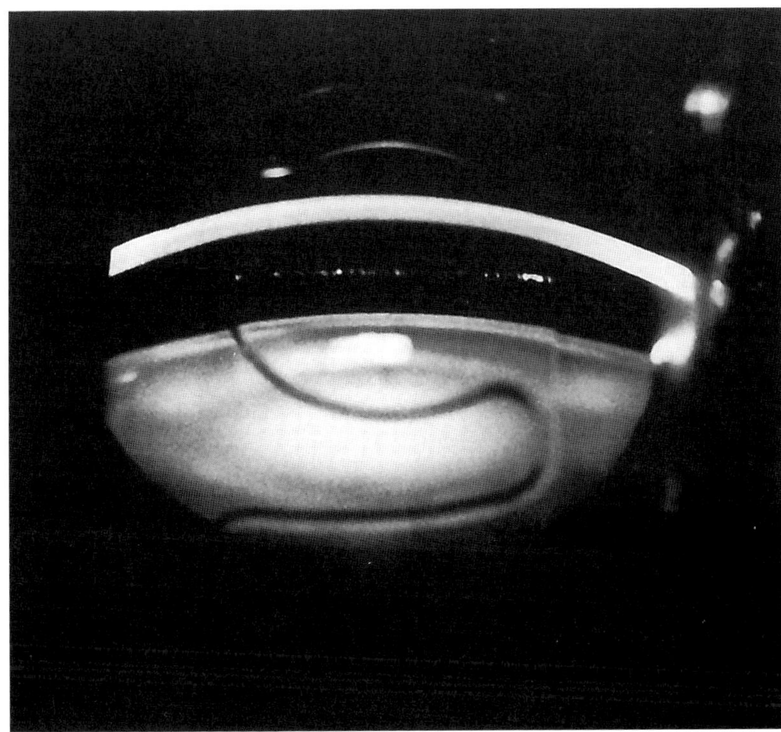

Fig. 12.25 This slit-lamp photo shows the space between the lens and the endothelium. (Courtesy of G. Baikoff.)

(a)

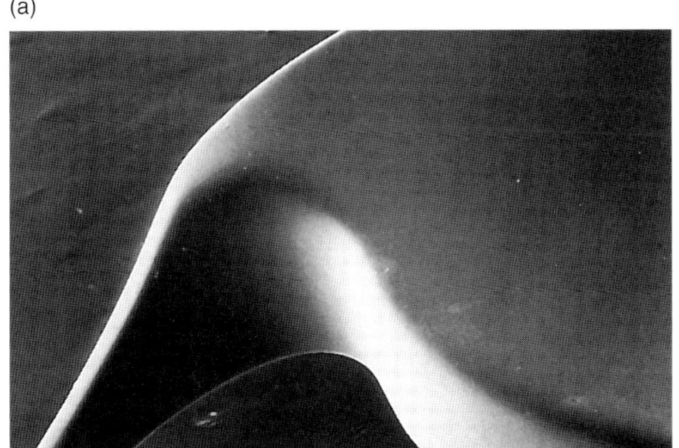

(b)

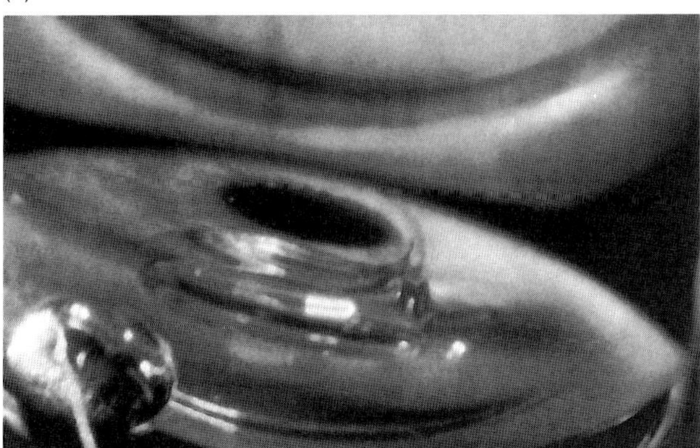

Fig. 12.26 (a) The smoothness of finish of the lens used by Baikoff is evident in this photo. (b) Gonioscopic view of first-generation implant. (Courtesy of G. Baikoff.)

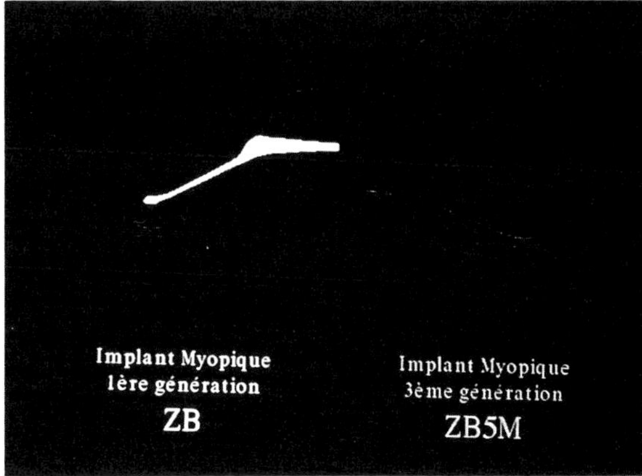

Fig. 12.27 The design change between the first and third generation of lenses. (Courtesy of G. Baikoff.)

corneal endothelial cell loss (as a function of anterior-chamber depth) and elevated anterior-chamber flare at 2 years postoperatively, long-term controlled multicenter trials are needed to better assess this lens.

This lens has had a good track record in aphakic eyes—some 40,000 having been implanted since 1979 [46]. Some fewer of these lenses have been implanted in phakic eyes—chiefly by Fechner—since the first one in 1980 [47]. Worst and Fechner changed the lens to a biconcave design in 1986—available from Ophtec BV, the Netherlands [48,49]. Figures 12.31 through 12.34 demonstrate the method of

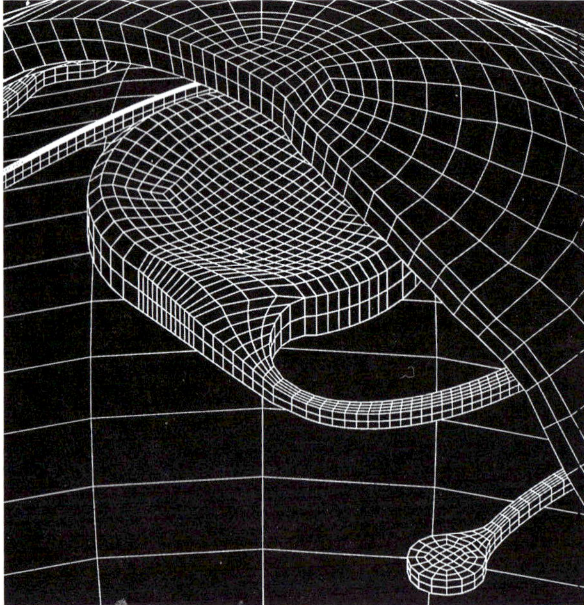

Fig. 12.28 Computer-simulated study of the functioning of a myopia-correcting implant within the eye. (Courtesy of Hanna.)

implanting this lens. Some of the results obtained are shown in Table 12.4. The essential points are

• The anterior chamber has to be filled with viscoelastic material.

• Make a small nasal incision before making the larger temporal one.

• Make a peripheral iridectomy to avoid pupillary block.

• Use traction sutures or a Flieringa ring.

This lens is also being used for some cases of hyperopia with mixed results (see also below) [50].

Posterior-chamber lenses

Even though excellent clinical results have been presented with posterior-chamber IOLs recently, the major unresolved issues with the plate-haptic posterior-chamber lenses are cataract formation, long-term stability of lens position, and the risk of chronic breakdown of the blood-aqueous barrier.

Phakic IOL implantation is undergoing intense research and growth because of the promise of stability, predictability, and reversibility; the avoidance of surgical modification of the optical axis—hallmark of the laser in situ keratomileusis (LASIK) and PRK procedures—and preservation of corneal asphericity and accommodation. However, the safety of phakic IOLs can be confirmed only by long-term, controlled multicenter trials.

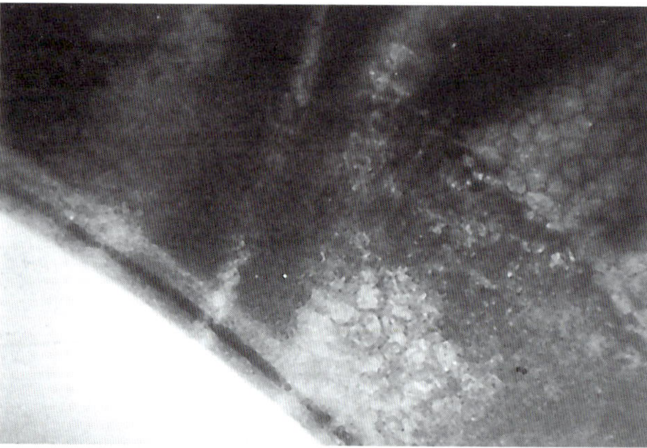

Fig. 12.29 Endothelial damage secondary to angle-supported lens (from Sargoussi *et al.*)

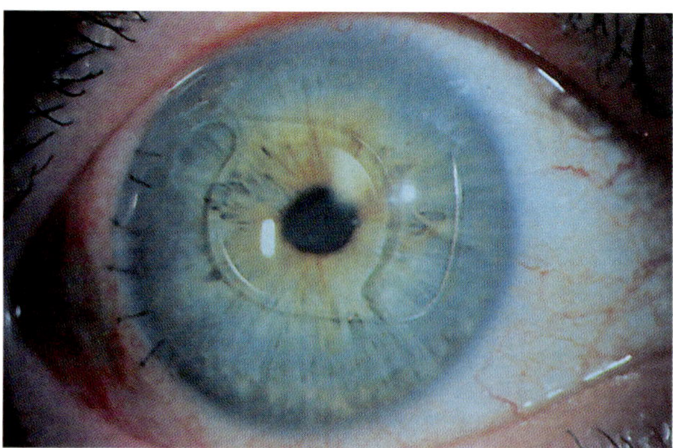

Fig. 12.30 First such lens to be inserted in the USA. (Courtesy of H. Kaufman.)

Posterior-chamber (epilenticular) lenses for myopia

The use of semielastic silicone material to construct IOLs is not new. Ruedemann reported on a series of such lenses implanted in rabbits—a project begun in 1975 [51] (Figure 12.35). Little if any reaction was noted in these notoriously reactive eyes. Shortly after this experience, Ruedemann inserted at least two such lenses into humans in the author's presence—in late 1976. Both were

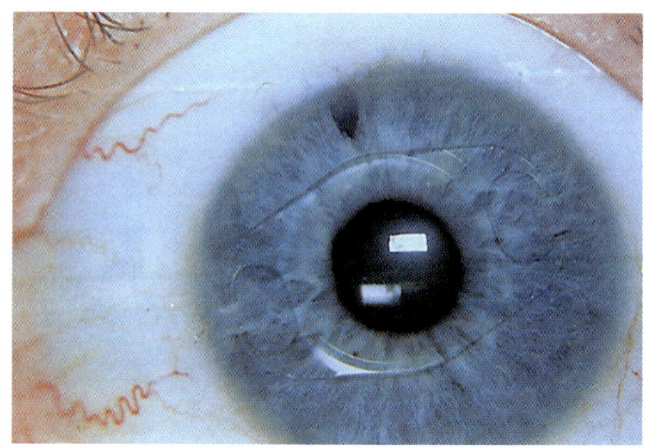

Fig. 12.31 Worst-Fechner claw lens. (Courtesy of G. van Rij.)

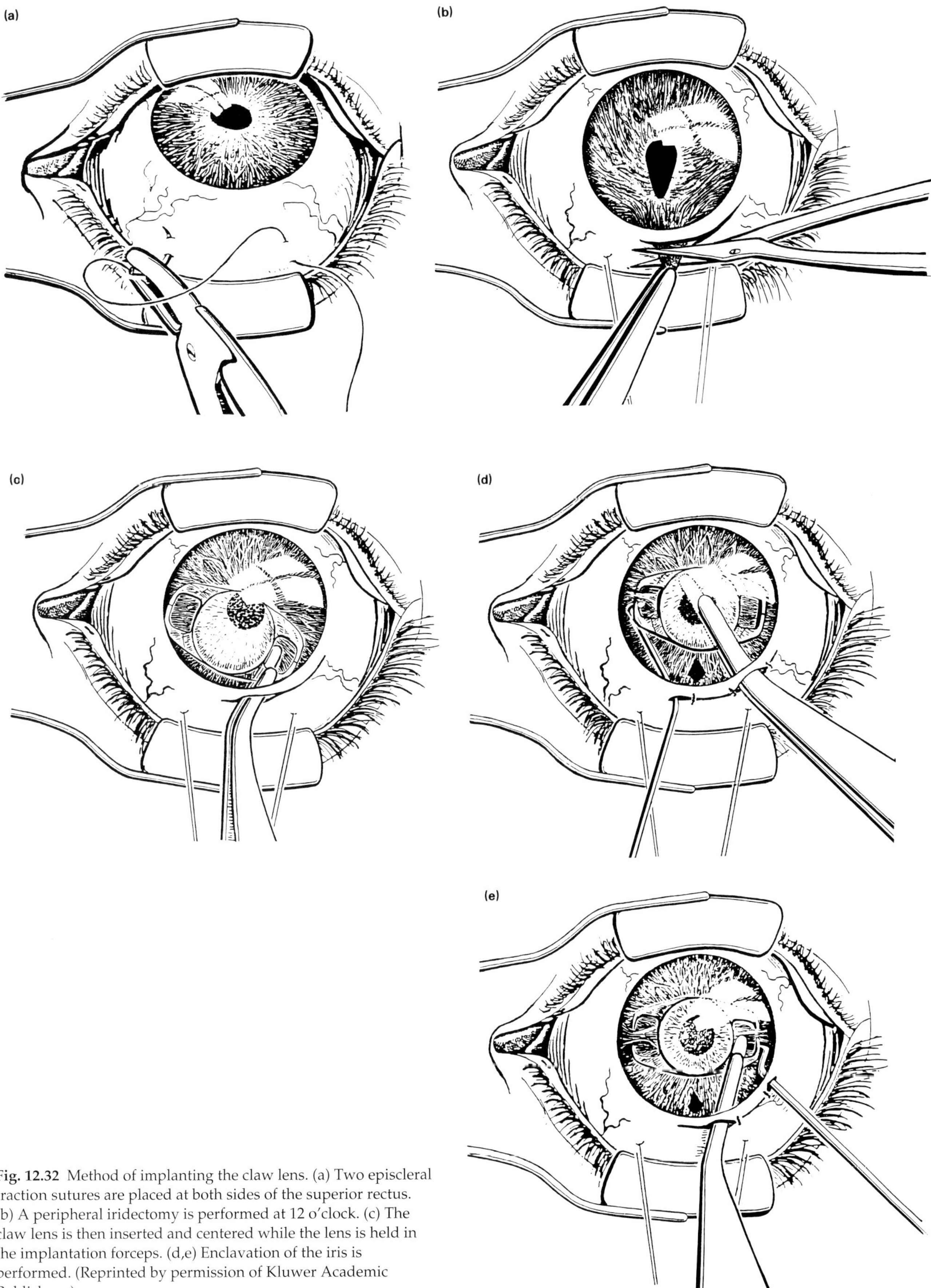

Fig. 12.32 Method of implanting the claw lens. (a) Two episcleral traction sutures are placed at both sides of the superior rectus. (b) A peripheral iridectomy is performed at 12 o'clock. (c) The claw lens is then inserted and centered while the lens is held in the implantation forceps. (d,e) Enclavation of the iris is performed. (Reprinted by permission of Kluwer Academic Publishers.)

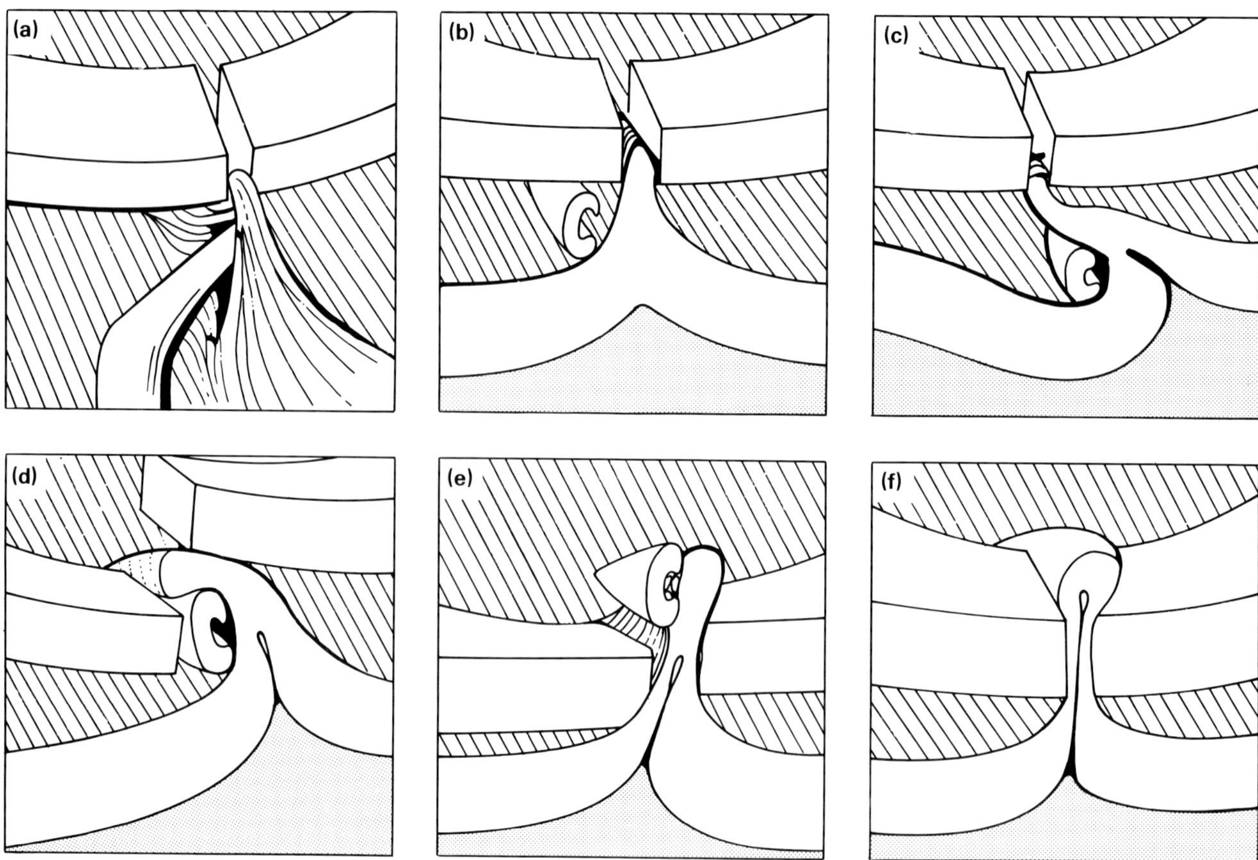

Fig. 12.33 The technique of enclavation. (a) The iris is looped up under the lens; (b) the "knuckle" of iris is pressed up into the haptic, engaging it; (c) the spatula is dropped down to pick up more iris; (d) the lens is supported with another tool while the spatula and iris are pressed up into the split haptic; (e,f) the iris is trapped within the haptic. (Reprinted by permission of Kluwer Academic Publishers.)

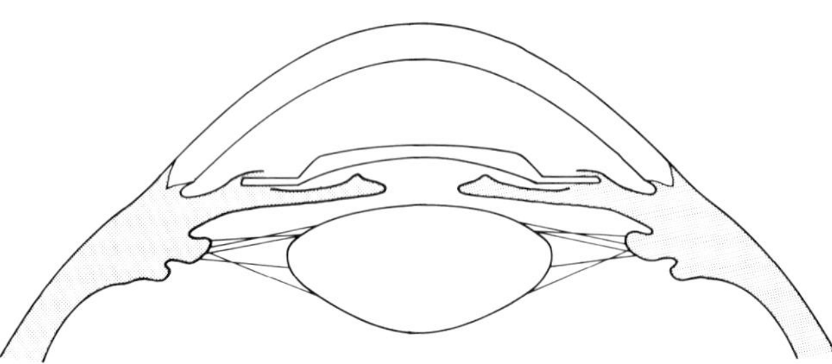

Fig. 12.34 Position of the claw lens within the AC. (Reprinted by permission of Kluwer Academic Publishers.)

angle-supported, and one of these was placed through a small opening (the previous incision having been partially sutured closed) and the lens unrolled in the anterior chamber with a spatula. Ruedemann commented at the time that the elasticity of the silicone material lent itself to this kind of implantation but that the problem was making it stiff enough. This problem has since been solved, and the relative nonreactivity of the material is remarkable. The other point in its favor is the low specific gravity in aqueous. This means that there is less inertia to damage delicate ocular structures during the nearly constant ocular movement. The author has noted in a study of PMMA iris-fixated lenses that lens weight—both in air and in aqueous—is related to the frequency of postoperative complications.

Fyodorov has proposed and tested a silicone collar-button type of lens in a number of myopes. Implantation of this particular lens has been fraught with difficulty [52]. Additionally, monocular diplopia has been reported at night, and opacification of the natural lens has resulted in some cases [53]. In 1990, Fyodorov and his group began implanting a newly designed lens of a more elastic nature (Figure 12.36). The lens is of one-piece design with a slightly narrower haptic and a 5.5- to 6.0-mm optic that does not protrude through the pupillary opening. The lens is somewhat easier to implant, not requiring viscoelastic material. A 1-year follow-up of 43 highly myopic eyes has been satisfactory, with uncorrected visual acuity ranging from 0.5 to 1.0 and no serious or vision-threatening complications [53]. Recently, Fyodorov and his group also began implanting a similar lens made from highly polymerized collagen material (Figure 12.37).

Table 12.4 Results of clear lens extraction in eight myopes (from Worst JG, van der Veen G, Los LI. Refractive surgery for high myopia. The Worst–Fechner biconcave iris claw lens. Doc Ophthalmol 1990; 75:335–341)

Patient no/eye	Sex (M/F)	Age (years)	Intraocular lens (D)	Spherical equivalent		Visual acuity		Follow-up (months)
				Preop.	Postop.	Preop.	Postop.	
1 OD	M	21	−15.00	−18.00	−2.00	0.4	0.5	22
OS			−15.00	−18.00	−3.00	0.4	0.5	15
2 OD	M	35	−14.00	−14.00	0.50	0.3	0.5	14
OS			−14.00	−11.50	0.00	0.15	0.5	13
3 OD	M	57	−15.00	−15.00	0.50	0.4	0.5	9
OS			−16.00	−16.00	−0.50	0.5	0.6	8
4 OD	M	42	−17.00	−12.00	−1.00	0.4	0.4	1
OS			−13.00	−14.00	0.00	0.4	0.4	1
5 OD	F	35	−10.00	−10.00	0.00	0.3	1.25	3
OS			−9.00	−9.00	0.00	0.4	0.8	3
6 OD	M	56	−19.00	−18.50	0.00	0.25	0.4	2
OS			−19.00	−18.00	0.00	0.5	0.4	0.25
7 OD	M	35	−9.00	−8.00	0.00	1.0	1.25	3
8 OD	M	30	−14.00	−13.50	1.50	0.4	0.5	3
OS			−14.00	−13.50	2.00	0.6	0.8	0.25

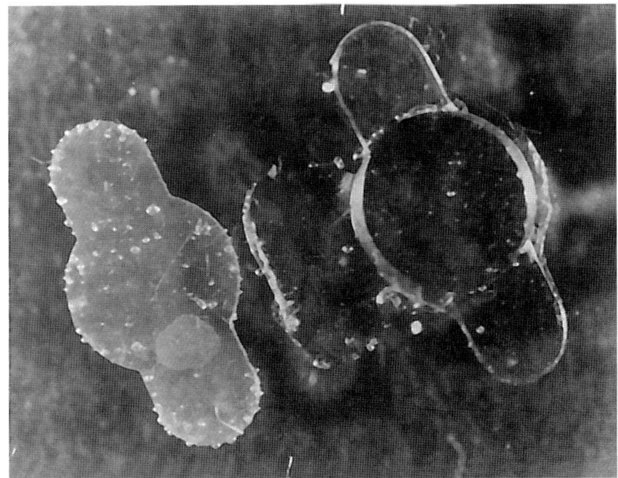

Fig. 12.35 Ruedemann's flexible silicone intraocular lenses.

Posterior-chamber lenses for hyperopia

Hyperopia correction with IOLs has been performed on a regular basis since the late 1960s to correct the severe hyperopia (12 to 14 D) following cataract extraction. However, we hardly think about this procedure as a refractive procedure, but in the strictest sense it is. Nevertheless, it is only recently that surgeons have considered implanting lenses solely for this purpose. Patients with high hyperopia are still subject to a certain amount of ametropia following normal extraction of their cataracts, even with the availability of high-plus (+26 D) IOLs.

Gayton may have been the first to solve the problem of the high hyperope when he piggybacked two plus-power IOLs in a 31-year-old patient to correct 46 D of hyperopia [54]. With a successful outcome in this case, he continued to perform this type of surgery and found that even when higher power lenses were available, piggybacking the lenses resulted in greater visual acuity, probably through reduction of the spherical aberration that accompanies high-diopter lenses (see Chapter 3). In a recent series, he found that while only 7% of patients had 20/40 or better uncorrected vision before surgery, after surgery, 50% had this level of vision [55]. However, to avoid the disturbing and difficult-to-treat development of an interimplant cellular infiltrate, it is advised that only one of the IOLs be implanted within the bag and the other into the so-called ciliary sulcus. Furthermore, it is advised that the implants be arranged so as to have the convex surfaces facing one another (Figure 12.38; see also Chapter 15).

The lurking problem with phakic IOLs is what to do with them when a cataract inevitably forms—a cataract not necessarily caused by the implant—and highly myopic eyes develop cataracts earlier than normal eyes, perhaps 10 to 15 years earlier. All these IOLs probably will have to be removed, and all of them, save perhaps the more flexible posterior-chamber lenses (except that the STAAR has no holes in the haptic, but this material does not appear to develop adhesions like silicone does), will require large extraction incisions with all that such incisions imply.

Lens implantation for age-related macular degeneration

While implantation of a lens to treat a medical problem may not seem like refractive surgery, the author has chosen to include it because the ultimate effect is to change—dramatically—the refractive workings of the eye. Unlike cataract surgery, which merely replaces a cloudy element, the implantation of a catadioptric lens, much like

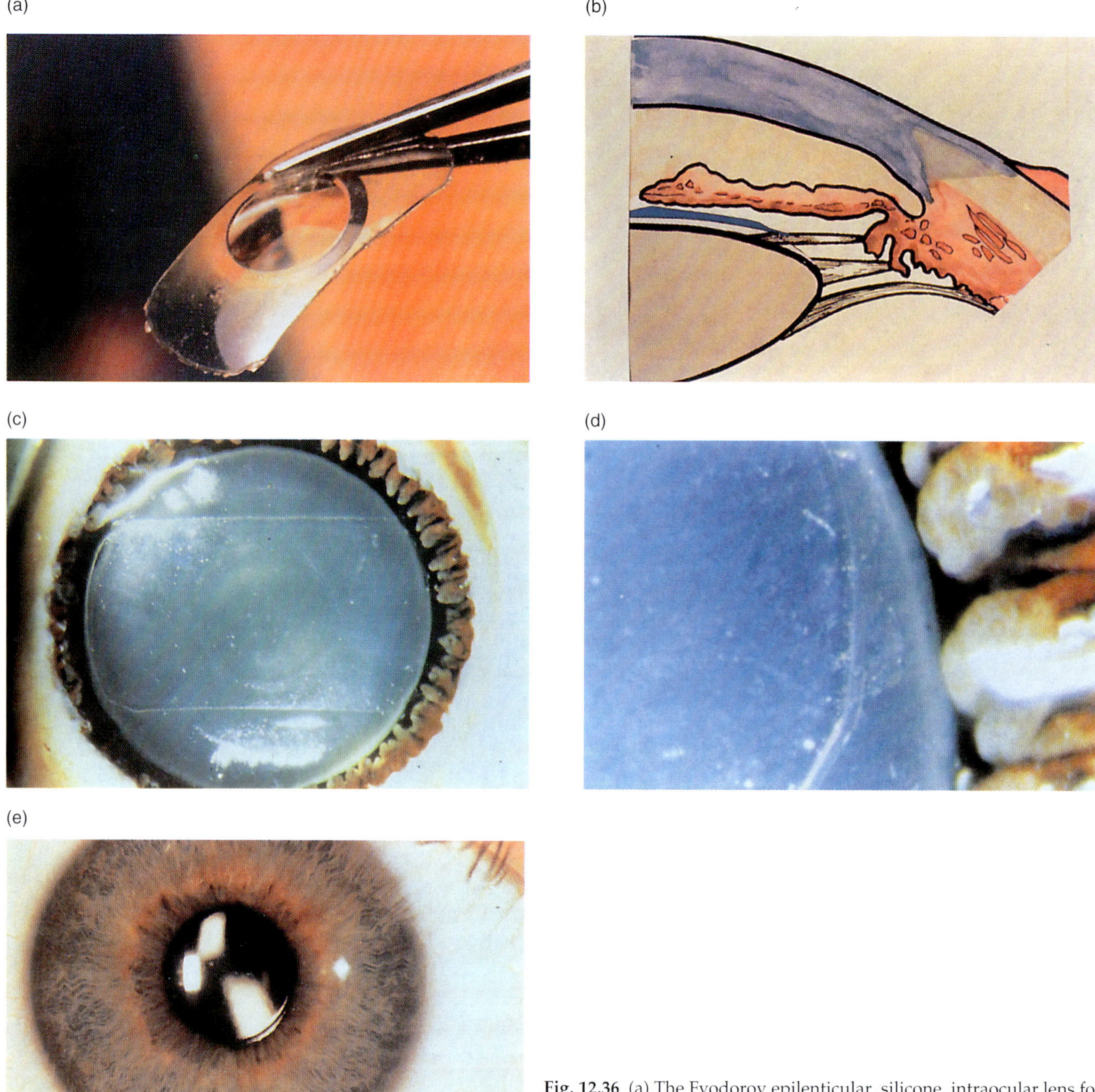

Fig. 12.36 (a) The Fyodorov epilenticular, silicone, intraocular lens for myopia; (b) cross-section showing the position of the haptic; (c,d) a cadaver eye with the iris stripped away to show the position of the lens on the crystalline surface; (e) postsurgical eye. (Courtesy of S.N. Fyodorov, M.D.)

an anterior-chamber phakos for myopia, changes the entire optical character of the eye.

Age-related macular degeneration (ARMD) is the leading cause of visual loss in adults aged 60 years and older and, as our population ages, will become an even greater problem [56,57]. After age 60, the incidence increases to 28% of the adult population between the ages 75 and 85 years. Two clinical types of ARMD are recognized: the dry or atrophic form, making up 90% of cases, and the neovascular or wet form. Visual loss in the dry form is mild and slowly progressive, but it is severe in the wet type. Soft *drusen* seem to be associated with the onset of ARMD, whereas the more discrete, hard type do not. There is a 14.5% cumulative risk over 5 years that patients with bilateral soft *drusen* will develop macular neovascularization [58–61].

Until fairly recently, the treatment for wet ARMD was the laser, when possible. Experiments are underway using special dyes that take up the laser energy more effectively [62]. Short of transplanting the macula, or translo-

(a)

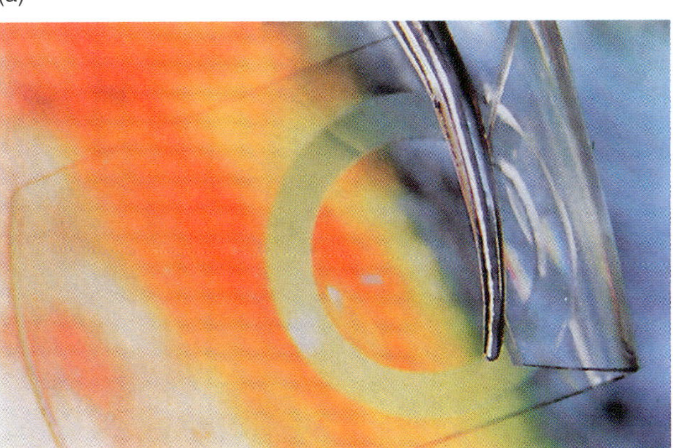

(b)

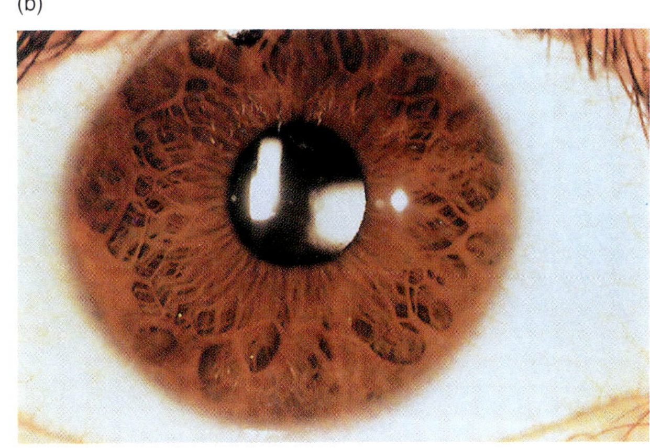

Fig. 12.37 (a) The Fyodorov collagen implant for myopia; (b) postimplant eye (Fyodorov).

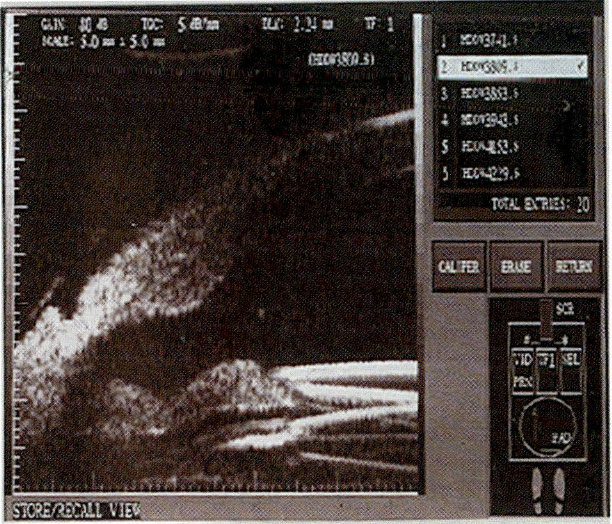

Fig. 12.38 B-scan showing planoconvex piggyback IOLs in situ. (Courtesy Dr. B. Kraemer, Los Angeles.)

cation [63], the only treatment for the dry type has been vitamin and zinc therapy.

Low-vision aids

According to the Snellen chart, 20/20 visual acuity is normal; thus anything less than this is, by definition, subnormal. For practical purposes, however, ophthalmologists consider loss of visual acuity in the range of 20/50 to 20/80 to be a serious handicap. Reading becomes difficult when visual acuity is less than 20/70, and low-vision aids are prescribed for patients with this acuity if it has not responded to conventional therapy—such as cataract surgery. Although a variety of low-vision aids are available, all are based on the same principle: increasing retinal image size through magnification of the object.

The *magnification power* of a given vision aid is defined as the ratio of image size to object size. For the eye, the magnifying power is 1 for an object 25 cm from the eye. This value is logically assigned because the average eye can focus to a distance of 25 cm (4 D of accommodation).

Two types of low-vision aids are currently in use: telescopes and convex lenses. Telescopes have a two-lens system in which one lens produces an image near the eye, and the other lens focuses the image on the retina. Convex lenses simply bring into focus objects that are closer than 25 cm to the eye. For example, an object held 6.25 cm from the eye would require 16 D of accommodation (100 cm divided by 6.25 cm) to bring the object into focus to produce 16/4, or four times, magnification.

Telescopes

Both Galilean and astronomical telescopic systems have been used as low-vision aids. Both models use a con-

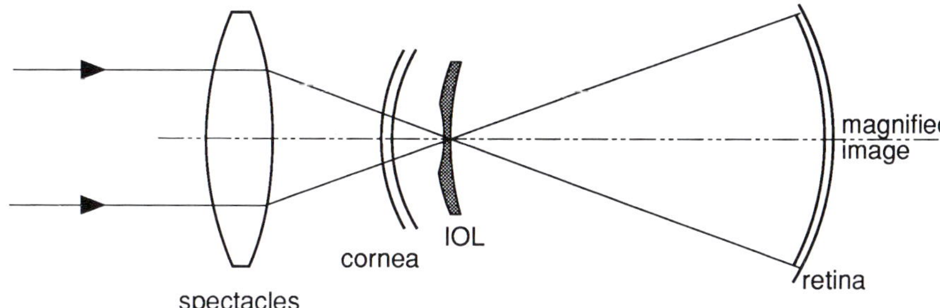

Fig. 12.39 Schematic of the Donn-Koester intraocular lens producing a Galilean telescope when a plus lens is placed before the eye (from Peyman G, Koziol J. Age-related macular degeneration and its management. J Cataract Refract Surg 1988; 14:421–430).

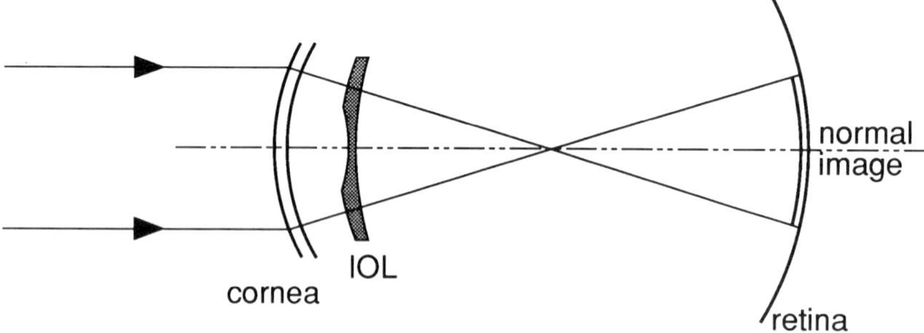

Fig. 12.40 Schematic of a ray passing through the plus (peripheral) portion of the Koziol–Peyman lens. Note the normal image size produced on the retina (from Peyman G, Koziol J. Age-related macular degeneration and its management. J Cataract Refract Surg 1988; 14:421–430).

verging lens as the objective lens to create an image close to the eye. The astronomical telescope then uses a plus-lens ocular that is separated from the plus objective lens by a distance equal to the *sum* of their focal lengths (see Chapter 3). The image is inverted, however, and requires a prism to be seen upright. In the Galilean telescope, a minus ocular is separated from the plus objective lens by the *difference* in the absolute values of their focal lengths. This places an upright image formed by the objective lens at the focal point of the ocular.

The advantage of telescopes is their long working distance. When telescopes are used as low-vision aids, close work can be brought into focus without bringing the material close to the eye. The image, instead of the object, is focused near the eye, and this image is then seen through the ocular of the telescope. The disadvantage of the telescope is the restricted field of view—4° to 10°. This makes walking or reading difficult.

Convex lenses

With a convex lens, the size of the retinal image increases as the object is brought nearer the eye. An object at 8.25 cm produces a retinal image four times greater than at 25 cm and requires a 16-D (100 cm divided by 6.25 cm) lens to focus the image onto the retina. Because the rays are parallel when they emerge from the magnifying lens, the eye can be any distance behind the magnifier. However, the distance of the lens to the object always must be at the focal length; thus the patient would need to move closer to a magnifying lens to take advantage of the wider field of view.

Historical background

Choyce [64] and later Donn and Koester [65] proposed using a high-minus intraocular lens (Figure 12.39) as the ocular of a Galilean telescope in 1984. A high-plus spectacle lens would then be the objective lens. The advantage of this system is the enlarged visual field that results as the ocular lens of the telescope is placed within the eye. Koester calculated that a ×3 telescope produced with this system would yield a visual field of 37°, or three times the visual field of a conventional telescope. Furthermore, the field of vision and the amount of magnification obtained can be changed by adjusting the power and vertex distance of the spectacles without altering the implant.

This system has several serious disadvantages, however. First, without spectacle lenses, the implanted eye has an uncorrected hyperopia of 60+ D. In addition, when plus-lens spectacles are used, a magnified image is produced on the retina, but peripheral vision is substantially reduced. The magnified image will not fuse with the image in the fellow eye, so that eye must be occluded when using magnification.

Teledioptric and catadioptric IOLs

To eliminate the disadvantages of external telescopes or high-minus intraocular lenses, two new IOLs have been designed by Koziol and Peyman [66]. The Koziol-Peyman teledioptric lens has a one-piece optic with both plus and minus portions (Figures 12.40 through 12.42). The plus portion provides normal phakic vision and a full visual field and preserves any preexisting central vision. The

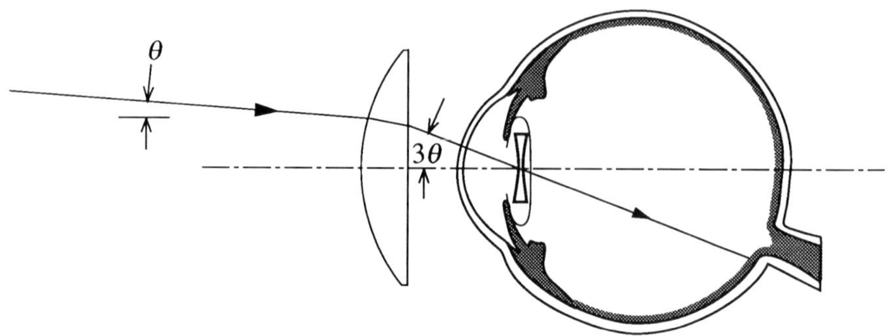

Fig. 12.41 Schematic of a ray passing through the central (minus) part of the same lens, forming a Galilean telescope when a plus lens is placed before the eye. Note the magnified image size produced on the retina (from Peyman G, Koziol J. Age-related macular degeneration and its management. J Cataract Refract Surg 1988; 14:421–430).

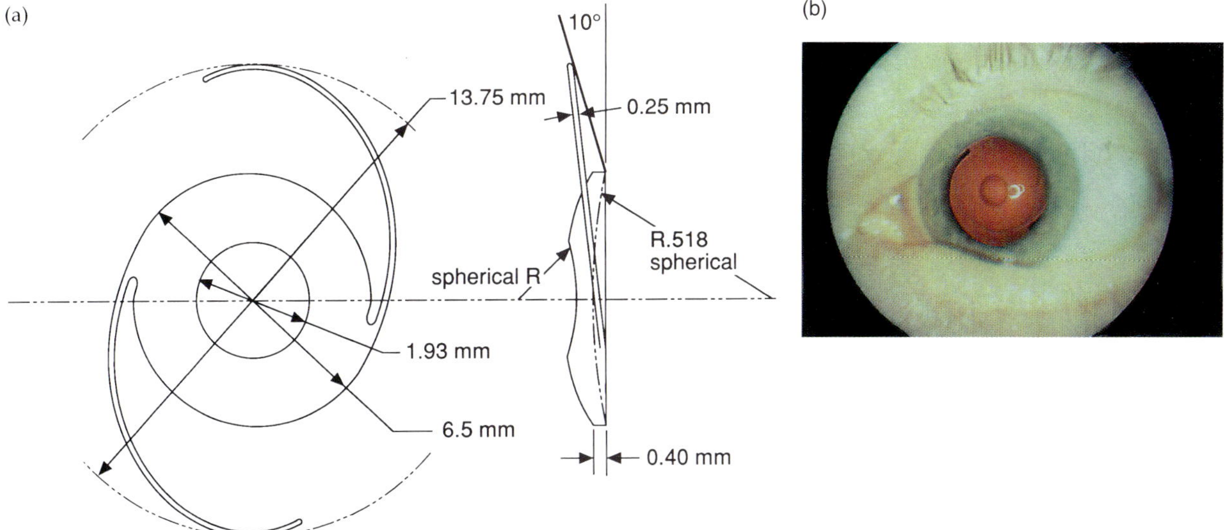

Fig. 12.42 (a) Schematic of the bioptic AMD-100B implant. (b) Photo of the implanted lens (from Willis TR, Portney V. Preliminary evaluation of the Koziol–Peyman teledioptric system for age-related macular degeneration. Eur J Implant Refract Surg 1989; 1:271–276).

high-minus (center) part of the lens acts as the ocular of a Galilean telescope when used with high-plus spectacles. A patient can then use special glasses whenever a magnified image is needed, such as for reading, or remove them when a full field is required, such as for walking. The visual field is approximately 80°, large enough to permit normal ambulation even with a magnified field of view. This currently discontinued lens had a very high resolution (Figure 12.43). The visual results in four patients are shown in Figure 12.44. Alignment problems with the spectacle portion of the complex were not satisfactorily solved.

A suggested catadioptric lens (Figure 12.45) would use mirrored surfaces to produce a magnified image without an external spectacle lens. To date, this lens is not being manufactured/implanted.

Lipshitz and his group have designed a new IOL with an entire telescope in its center and have begun implanting it [67].

Fig. 12.43 (a) Resolution of a standard intraocular lens. (b) Resolution of the AMD-100B lens with spectacles. (Courtesy of American Medical Optics.)

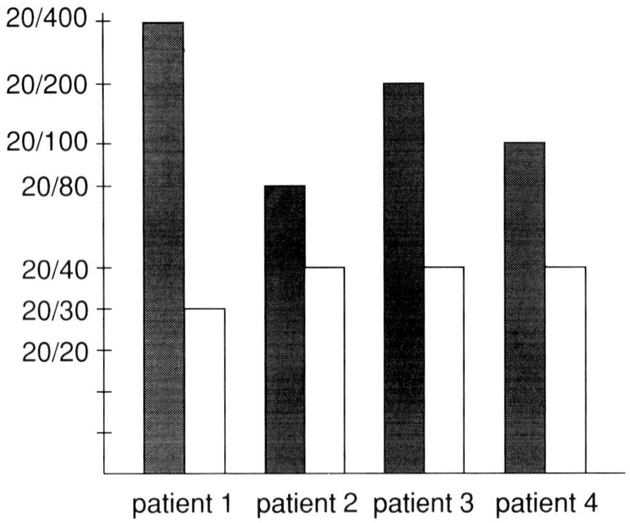

Fig. 12.44 Visual acuity in four subjects before and after implantation of the AMD-100B intraocular lens and fitting with dual-element spectacles. Near vision assessed in patients 2–4, and far vision in patient 1. (Courtesy of Willis.)

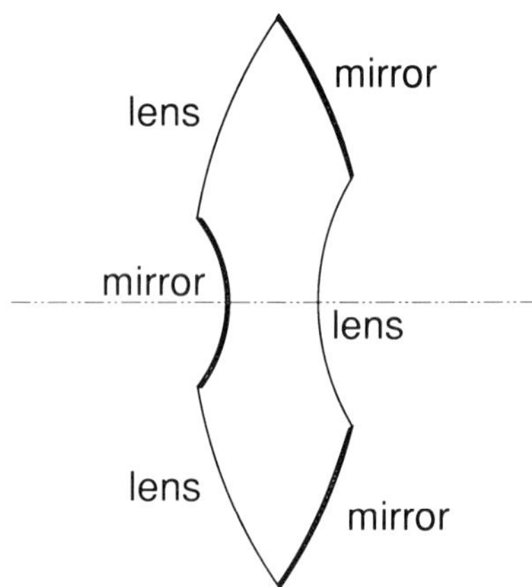

Fig. 12.45 Cross section of a catadioptric lens with a mirrored surface. (Courtesy of Willis.)

References

1 Boerhaave H. *Prælectiones publicæ, de morbis oculorum.* A. Vandenhoeck, Göttingen, 1746.
2 Vacher L. An operation for myopia. Annales d'Oculistique 1896; CXVI(1): p. 8,19.
3 Janin de Combe–Blanche J. *Memoires et observations anatomiques, physiologiques et physiques sur l'oeil.* Didot, Paris 429; 1772.
4 Otto F. I.Beobachtungen uber hochgradige Kurzsichtigen und ihre operative behandlung (Observations of high myopia and its surgical treatment. I). Arch f Ophth 1898; XLIII(2): p. 324 8.
5 Otto F. II. Beobachtungen uber hochgradige Kurzsichtigen und ihre operative behandlung (Observations of high myopia and its surgical treatment. II). Arch f Ophth 1898; XLVII(1): p. 242–8.
6 Otto F. Berichtigung der sogenannten Richstellung des Herrn Dr. Fukala zu meiner Abhandlung uber Behandlung hochgradiger Kurzsichtigkeit. Albrecht von Graefes Arch Ophthalmol 1898; XLVII(1): p. 224–8.
7 Heister L. *A General System of Surgery in Three Parts.* 7th ed. J Clarke (etc), London, 1759.
8 Haller Av. *Elementa Physiologiae Corporis Humani.* Vol. 5. Francisci Grasset, Lausanne, 516; 1763.
9 Haller Av. *Bibliothek Chirurgische.* Vol. 2. Geissner, Fuessli, Orell, Tiguri, 405; 1774–7.
10 Desmonceaux A. *Traite des maladies des yeux et des oreilles, considerees sous le rapport des quatre ages de la vie de l'homme. (Treatise on the diseases of the eye and the ear, considered in correlation with the four ages of man).* Vol. 2. Lottin de S. Germain, Paris, 1786.
11 Hirschberg J. Vol.3 *The Renaissance of Ophthalmology in the Eighteenth Century, part 1, in The History of Ophthalmology,* F. Blodi, Editor. Bonn, Wayenborgh Verlag, p. 28–36, 1984.
12 Woolhouse JT. *Dissertations scavantes sur la Cataract et le Glaucome.* Chez Bonaventure de Launoy, Offenbach sur la Main, 1717.
13 Richter AG. *Chirurgische Bibliothek.* Vol. 3. L B F Gegels, Frankenthal, 489–98, 1790.
14 Beer J. *Lehre von den Augenkrankheiten.* Vol. 2. Heubner & Volke, Wein, 1813.
15 Fukala V. Surgical Treatment of High Degrees of Myopia through Aphakia [Operative Behandlung der hochstgradigen Myopie durch Aphakie]. Graefes Arch Ophth 1890; 36: p. 230–244.
16 Verzella F. *High Myopia: Microsurgical Extracapsular Extraction of the lens for optical purposes.* Lens Editions, Keratorefractive Society, Chicago, 72; 1983.
17 Muller H, and Papastylianos S. [3000 cataract extractions: complications and results]. Klin Monatsbl Augenheilkd 1968; 152(4): p. 476–87.
18 Liu CH. Cryoextraction of cataracts in high myopes. Eye Ear Nose Throat Mon 1973; 52(2): p. 53–5
19 Mickiewicz L, and Balmuchanow A. [Cataract extraction in myopic patients] <original> Krioekstrakcja zacmy u osob krotkowzrocynch. Klin Oczna 1974; 44(2): p. 141–5.
20 Edmund J, and Seedorff H. Retinal detachment in the aphakic eye. Acta Ophthalmol (Copenh) 1974; 52(3): p. 323–33.
21 Clayman HM, Jaffe NS, Light DS, *et al.* Intraocular lenses, axial length, and retinal detachment. Am J Ophthalmol 1981; 92(6): p. 778–80.
22 Jaffe NS, Clayman HM, and Jaffe MS. Retinal detachment in myopic eyes after intracapsular extraction: A ten year study. Ophthalmology 1984; 97: p. 48–52.
23 Jaffe NS, Clayman HM, and Jaffe MS. Retinal detachment in myopic eyes after intracapsular and extracapsular cataract extraction. Am J Ophthalmol 1984; 97(1): p. 48–52.
24 Praeger D. Five years' follow-up in the surgical management of cataracts in high myopia treated with the Kelman phacoemulsification technique. Ophthalmology 1979; 86(11): p. 2024–33.
25 Hessburg TP, Maxwell DP, and Diamond JG. Endophthalmitis associated with sutureless cataract surgery [letter]. Arch Ophthalmol 1991; 109(11).
26 Stonecipher KG, Parmley VC, Jensen H, *et al.* Infectious endophthalmitis following sutureless cataract surgery. Arch Ophthalmol 1991; 109(11): p. 1562–3.
27 Ernest PH, Kiessling LA, and Lavery KT. The effect of external pressure on sutureless cataract wounds. J Cataract Refract Surg 1992; to be published.
28 Fyodorov SN. Personal communication. Unpublished data 1991.
29 Colin J, Robinet A, and Cochener B. Retinal detachment after clear lens extraction for high myopia: seven-year follow-up. Ophthalmology 1999; 106(12): p. 2281–4; discussion 2285.
30 Dodick JM, and Christiansen J. Experimental studies on the development and propagation of shock waves created by the interaction of short Nd:YAG laser pulses with a titanium target. Possible implications for Nd:YAG laser phacolysis of the cataractous human lens. J Cataract Refract Surg 1991; 17(6): p. 794–7.
31 Dodick JM. Can cataracts be removed using laser technology? Ophthalmology Clinics of North America 1991; 4: p. 355–64.

32 Kanellopoulos AJ, Dodick JM, Brauweiler P, *et al.* Dodick photolysis for cataract surgery: early experience with the Q-switched neodymium: YAG laser in 100 consecutive patients. Ophthalmology 1999; 106(11): p. 2197–202.
33 Beer GJ. *Bibliotheca Ophthalmica*. Vol. 2. Carl Schaumburg, Wein, 1799.
34 Schiferli RA. Theoretisch–praktische Abhandlung über den grauen Starr. (A theoretical and practical dissertation on cataract). In: *Zur Geschichte der intraocularen Korrektur der Aphakia*, W. Munchow, Editor. Jena and Leipzig, Gabler, 1797.
35 Casanova G. *History of My Life*. 1818.
36 Baikoff G, Arne JL, Bokobza Y, *et al.* Angle-fixated anterior chamber phakic intraocular lens for myopia of −7 to −19 diopters [see comments]. J Refract Surg 1998; 14(3): p. 282–93.
37 Baikoff G, and Colin J. Damage to the corneal endothelium using anterior chamber intraocular lenses for myopia. Refract Corneal Surg 1990; 6(5): p. 383.
38 Strampelli B. Sopportabilita di lenti acriliche in camera anteriore nella afachia e nei vizi di refrazione. Atti Soc Oftal Lomb 1953; 8: p. 292.
39 Barraquer J. Anterior chamber plastic lenses. Results and conclusions from 5 year's experience. Trans Ophthalmol Soc (UK) 1959; 79: p. 393–424.
40 Drews RC. The Barraquer Experience with Intraocular Lenses. Ophthalmology 1982; 89(4). p. 386–93.
41 Baikoff G. The refractive IOL in a phakic eye. Ophthalmic Practice 1991; 9(2): p. 58–61.
42 Baikoff G. Phakic anterior chamber intraocular lenses. Int Ophthalmol Clin 1991; 31(1): p. 75–86.
43 Ellingson FT. The uveitis-glaucoma-hyphema syndrome associated with the Mark VIII anterior chamber lens implant. J Am Intraocul Implant Soc 1978; 4(2): p. 50–3.
44 Lesure P, Bosc JM, George JL, *et al.* [Our experience with myopic implants. Initial optical results] Bull Soc Ophtalmol Fr 1990 90(1) p. 87–91.
45 Saragoussi JJ, Puech M, Assouline M, *et al.* Ultrasound biomicroscopy of Baikoff anterior chamber phakic intraocular lenses [published erratum appears in J Refract Surg 1997 Jul–Aug; 13(4):329]. J Refract Surg 1997; 13(2): p. 135–41.
46 Worst JG, van der Veen G, and Los LI. Refractive surgery for high myopia. The Worst-Fechner biconcave iris claw lens. Doc Ophthalmol 1990; 75(3–4): p. 335–41.
47 Fechner PU. Die Irisklauene–Linse. Klin Monatstbl Augenheilkd 1987; 191: p. 26–9.
48 Fechner PU, Haubitz I, Wichmann W, *et al.* Worst-Fechner biconcave minus power phakic iris-claw lens [published erratum appears in J Refract Surg 1999 May–Jun;15(3):following table of contents]. J Refract Surg 1999; 15(2): p. 93–105.
49 Fechner PU, van der Heijde GL, and Worst JG. [Intraocular lens for the correction of myopia of the phakic eye] <original> Intraokulare Linse zur Myopiekorrektion des phaken Auges. Klin Monatsbl Augenheilkd 1988; 193 (1): p. 29–34.
50 Fechner PU, Singh D, and Wulff K. Iris-claw lens in phakic eyes to correct hyperopia: preliminary study. J Cataract Refract Surg 1998; 24(1): p. 48–56.
51 Ruedemann ADJ. Silicone intraocular implants in rabbits. Trans Am Acad Ophthalmol Otolaryngol 1977; 75: p. 436–55.
52 Fyodorov SN, Zuev VK, and Tumanian ER. [Intraocular correction of high-degree myopia] <original> Intraokuliarnaia korrektsiia miopii vysokoi stepeni. Vestn Oftalmol 1988; 104(2): p. 14–6.
53 Fyodorov SN, Zuev VK, and Aznavayev VM. [Intraocular correction of high myopia with negative posterior chamber lens] Intraokuliarnaia korrektsiia miopii vysokoi stepeni zadnekamernmi otritsatelimi linzami. Oftalmochirugia 1991; 3: p. 57–8.
54 Gayton JL, and Sanders VN. Implanting two posterior chamber intraocular lenses in a case of microphthalmos. J Cataract Refract Surg 1993; 19(6): p. 776–7.
55 Gayton JL, Sanders V, Van der Karr M, *et al.* Piggybacking intraocular implants to correct pseudophakic refractive error. Ophthalmology 1999; 106(1): p. 56–9.
56 Leibowitz HM, Krueger DE, Maunder LR, *et al.* The Framingham Eye Study monograph: An ophthalmological and epidemiological study of cataract, glaucoma, diabetic retinopathy, macular degeneration, and visual acuity in a general population of 2631 adults, 1973–1975. Surv Ophthalmol 1980; 24(Suppl): p. 335–610.
57 Klein BE, and Klein R. Cataracts and macular degeneration in older Americans. Arch Ophthalmol 1982; 100(4): p. 571–3.
58 Folk JC. Senile macular degeneration. Prim Care 1982; 9(4): p. 793–9.
59 Sarks SH, Van DD, Maxwell L, *et al.* Softening of drusen and subretinal neovascularization. Trans Ophthalmol Soc U K 1980; 100(3): p. 414–22.
60 Strahlman ER, Fine SL, and Hillis A. The second eye of patients with senile macular degeneration. Arch Ophthalmol 1983; 101(8): p. 1191–3.
61 Smiddy WE, and Fine SL, Prognosis of patients with bilateral macular drusen. Ophthalmology 1984; 91(3): p. 271–7.
62 (TAP) Study Group. Photodynamic therapy of subfoveal choroidal neovascularization in age-related macular degeneration with verteporfin: one-year results of 2 randomized clinical trials—TAP report. Treatment of age-related macular degeneration with photodynamic therapy (TAP) Study Group [see comments]. Arch Ophthalmol 1999; 117(10): p. 1329–45.
63 Akduman L, Karavellas MP, MacDonald JC, *et al.* Macular translocation with retinotomy and retinal rotation for exudative age-related macular degeneration. Retina 1999; 19(5): p. 418–23.
64 Choyce DP. Galilean telescope using the anterior chamber lens as eyepiece, ed. DP Choyce. HK Leivia, London, 156–61, 1964.
65 Donn A, and Koester CJ. An ocular telephoto system designed to improve vision in macular disease. Clao J 1986; 12(2): p. 81–5.
66 Peyman G, and Koziol J. Age-related macular degeneration and its management. J Cataract Refract Surg 1988; 14(4): p. 421–430.
67 Lipshitz I, Loewenstein A, Reingewirtz M, *et al.* An intraocular telescopic lens for macular degeneration. Ophthalmic Surg Lasers 1997; 28(6): p. 513–7.

13
Scleral Reinforcement

Somebody said that it couldn't be done
But he with a chuckle replied
That maybe it couldn't, but he would be one
Who wouldn't say so till he'd tried.
[Edgar A. Guest]

Despite the reluctance of some individuals in the contemporary medical community to accept myopia as a disease or affliction, as it once had been in the past, the fact remains that it is the fifth or sixth leading cause of blindness in the world today—which, if one gives it a moment's thought, is remarkable for a process considered a nondisease. Additionally there appears to be very little, if anything, that can be done to prevent it and even less to treat it—other than surgery—once established.

It should be clear by now (see Chapter 2) that occupational or environmental factors play a role in the evolution of myopia, however small that role may be. If that is true, then alteration of these factors should have some effect on either eliminating or at least slowing the progressive myopic process. Depending on whose philosophy one adopts, such treatment can range from chemical to mechanic [1,2]. For example, some investigators believe that excess accommodation contributes to the observed progression of the myopic state [3,4].

McCollim conducted a unique experiment wherein pressure was applied to the globe of the eye by artificially induced contracture of the superior oblique muscles [5]. One of the two effects produced was 5 D of myopia; the other was dual vision which took years to subside, even after the pressure was released. It was surmised that the pressure, transmitted through the sclera to the vitreous, forced the vitreous against the back of the lens, flattening the periphery but not the axial (central) region, resulting in a high degree of negative spherical aberration, combined with increased accommodation. The author concluded that this suggests that accommodation can be actuated by contraction of the extraocular muscles. He further noted that when the lens is allowed to relax after a long period of accommodation, the return to the unaccommodated state is extremely slow, indicating that a significant factor in the etiology of myopia is repeated long periods of accommodation in which periods of rest are insufficient to allow the lens to return completely to the unaccommodated state. Thus the elastic memory of the natural lens is somehow impaired.

The Russians (among others) have attempted to interfere with the myopic process by prescribing low-plus glasses for *skolniki* (school children) along with base-in prism. There are some rather severe problems associated with conducting such studies and despite study design flaws, the Russians have claimed that this mode of treatment has reduced the number of cases of progressive myopia in their series [6].

Other investigators have posited that this progression in myopia occurs through elevation of the intraocular pressure (IOP), which has been shown to occur during accommodation [7,8]. Fledelius demonstrated the strong myopigenic effect of elevated IOP in young eyes suffering from traumatic secondary glaucoma [9]. Another study reported significantly greater axial changes in the affected eye of children with monocular congenital glaucoma. This elongation was beyond that which could be attributed to normal growth. Successful surgery in these cases produced an early decrease in mean axial length of 0.8 mm [10]. There is a tendency for a higher mean IOP in myopes in any event [4,11–13]. Tomlinson and Phillips found that in patients aged 18 to 27, the average IOP was highest in myopia (15.49 ± 2.85 mm Hg) and lowest in hyperopia (13.91 ± 2.28 mm Hg). They found a strong correlation between applanation and both axial length and refraction [14]. Accordingly, antiglaucomatous medications have been prescribed in an effort to keep the IOP below certain levels and hopefully prevent progression of the myopia. Unfortunately, the drugs employed carry with them sufficient hazard to make their use in children problematic, and the side effects—not to mention lack of compliance—have proved to be troublesome. Furthermore, the results of such usage have been equivocal. Despite the pressure-lowering effects of pilocarpine, the induced accommodation caused by the drug may itself stimulate myopia, making its use for this purpose illogical. Still, some feel that it is reasonable to keep the IOP in high myopes below 20 mm Hg [15]. Nonetheless, the subject of ocular hypertension is still in flux. Perkins suggests that while the myopic eye is significantly more at risk of developing glaucoma, it is less likely to have ocular hypertension [16]. It should be noted in addition that the myope is more likely to be a steroid responder, which has considerable significance in refractive surgery (see also Chapter 9). Podos and colleagues tested a number of myopic patients and found that 88% of the cases in their series responded to steroid administration with IOPs in excess of 20 mm Hg or more; in 29% of these the IOP exceeded 31 mm Hg [17]. Amba and associates have suggested a genetic linkage between glaucoma and myopia [18,19].

Surgical techniques to produce ocular hypotension such as repeated paracentesis [20,21], iridectomy [22], sclerotomy [22,23], cyclodialysis [24], and myotomy or recession of the extraocular muscles [25], have all failed to yield impressive results and all seem to have a low benefit-risk ratio and hence are not recommended.

A few simpler techniques that were intended to improve the circulation of the eye or strengthen the sclera are noted here, more for historical completeness than for any other reason. Among these are such treatments as the use of mild ocular compresses [26] and compression of the eye into the orbit [27,28]. This latter regimen appears to increase IOP, an event of no particular benefit and of some potential harm to the myopic eye (see the discussion on glaucoma, above). Massage of the eyes also has been suggested [29–31] as well as, more recently, ultrasound [32,33]. There is no scientific evidence, however, that any of these measures has been effectual in reducing or halting the progression of myopia.

Regardless of such claims and the "feelings" of practitioners as to the effect of certain factors on myopic progression, the medical treatment of myopia is, on balance, not a part of standard medical care—thus the progress of the affliction is left to chance. For the most part, this element of chance typically leads to an eventual stabilization of the growth of the eye in most, but unfortunately not all, myopes. This stabilization may not come, however, until the eye is severely myopic and showing all the signs and symptoms of pathologic myopia along with serious reduction in vision or worse. In these cases, the incidence of retinal detachment is high and the risk of total visual loss significant. Rarely, stabilization does not occur at all, eventually leading to total blindness—*malignant* myopia.* Additionally, staphylomatous eyes present unique impediments to normal visual acuity, visual field, binocularity, and stereopsis. They are also prone to premature cataract formation, glaucoma, and retinal detachment.

Pathology

The pathology of the ametropic (usually myopic) eye has been described in more detail elsewhere [15] and therein it was noted that posterior scleral elongation and thinning (posterior staphyloma) are the hallmark of severe as well as pathologic myopia. The basic pathology of high myopia is the gradual enlargement and elongation of the entire globe (Figure 13.1). The tunics of the eye (sclera, choroid, and retina) become stretched. The sclera in pathologic myopia is underdeveloped in both quantity and quality. The scarce and thin scleral fibers in the high myope can no longer support the globe sufficiently. Serious architectural abnormalities can be seen in the fiber bundle arrangement. The bundles themselves show disorganization. Electron microscopy shows the collagen fibrils to be of smaller diameter, and abnormal forms of these fibrils can also be observed. The ectasia of the thin posterior sclera, notably in the area of the staphyloma, tends to be progressive, especially during the first three decades of life. This ectasia is accompanied by an increasing incidence of degenerative changes in the fundus. The eye enlarges posteriorly, losing its spherical shape as it does so. The choroid becomes consequently thinner; its vessels become sclerotic and attenuated, resulting in decreased circulation. This enlargement does not progress at a uniform rate and may ultimately result in localized staphyloma formation (Figure 13.2).

Hence staphylomata can occur in any portion of the globe. They may appear at the equator or anterior to it, especially in highly myopic eyes that have developed retinal tears, holes, or retinal detachments. These staphylomata may make the placement of an encircling silicone band or segmental silicone explant extremely difficult because of the thin underlying sclera. Erosion of such explants into the vitreous is not unknown.

* It seems remarkable that a "nondisease" can become malignant.

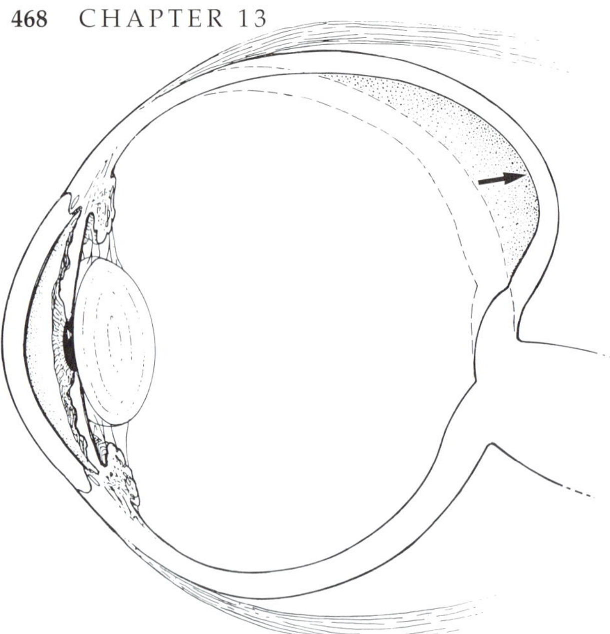

Fig. 13.1 Localized staphyloma characteristic of moderate to low high myopia.

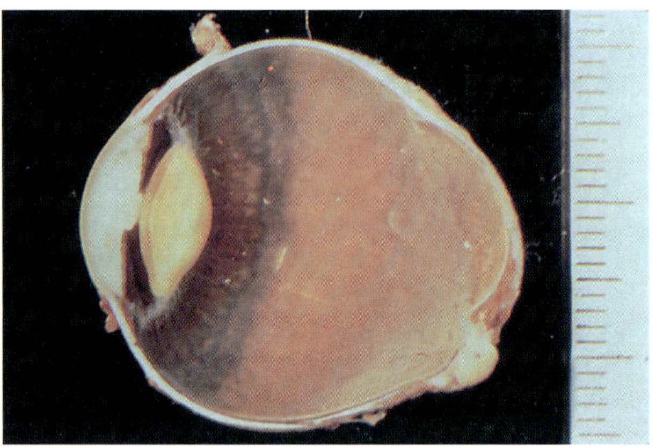

Fig. 13.2 Autopsy specimen clearly demonstrating a staphyloma and general enlargement of the globe associated with progressive myopia. (Courtesy of A. Momose.)

Von Ammon first suggested congenital weakness of the posterior sclera as causative [34]. He described an area of localized ectasia in the embryonic eye which he termed the *protuberantia scleralis*. This area is contiguous to the optic nerve, and it was thought to be caused by an embryonic opening of the sclera on the cerebral side. Normally closed at birth, this defect could produce staphylomata in the absence of normal development. Sondermann, studying fetal eyes, also found a scleral ectasia which developed at the fourth month of gestation and which gradually diminished as the embryo matured [35–37]. Such a fetal sclerectasis posterioris has not been corroborated by other investigators, however.

Grading changes for staphylomata formation in highly myopic eyes have been developed by Curtin and others [15]. However, these grading systems have involved the changes which can occur in all areas of the myopic eye. A system for specifically grading the progression of posterior macular staphylomata has long been needed. Such a grading system is presented here courtesy of Frank Thompson, in which posterior temporal and macular staphylomata are divided into two types and 10 grades (Figure 13.3 and Table 13.1).

In many cases staphylomata develop on the nasal side of the optic nerve posterior to the equator. These staphylomata usually do not cause severe visual loss since they are not within the central visual axis. Those posterior staphylomata which develop in highly myopic eyes and involve the macula usually begin in the inferior temporal quadrant, anterior to the retinal arcades around the macula, and then progress into the macular area. They may be seen with indirect ophthalmoscopy as pale yellow areas with prominent choroidal vessels (Figure 13.4). Their appearance in the inferior temporal quadrant accompanies the characteristic development of peripheral retinal paving-stone degeneration in the anterior inferior temporal quadrant (Figure 13.5). Both this paving-stone degeneration and the staphylomata are frequently located near the inferior temporal vortex vein and the insertion of the inferior oblique. This may be due to torsional effects from the insertion of the inferior oblique, leading to further weakening of the already thinned scleral and choroidal tissues.

As the staphyloma progresses from the inferior temporal quadrant to involve the central macular and foveal area, the sclera between the disk and macula may become so weakened that an apparent tilting of the optic nerve occurs. This can sometimes be mistaken for neurologic disease when in reality the patient simply may have staphylomatous changes.

As the posterior staphyloma enlarges over the macular area, the choroidal tissue becomes thinned and pale yellow in appearance (Figure 13.6). Eventually breaks in Bruch's membrane or lacquer cracks may invest the macula. As these breaks evolve, encroaching vessels from the underlying choroid can lead to the formation of a neovascular membrane adjacent to or actually involving the capillary free zone of the fovea (Figure 13.7). Once the neovascular membrane develops, macular or perimacular hemorrhages may occur. These may progress into Fuch's spots with consequent retinal gliosis and chorioretinal atrophy. If these hemorrhages develop in the foveal area, the visual acuity loss may be sudden and permanent.

After the development of lacquer cracks and hemorrhages, chorioretinal atrophy progresses until, at the end stage, the entire posterior pole of the eye becomes devoid of choriocapillaris, retinal pigment epithelium, lamina vitrea, and outer retinal elements. The posterior

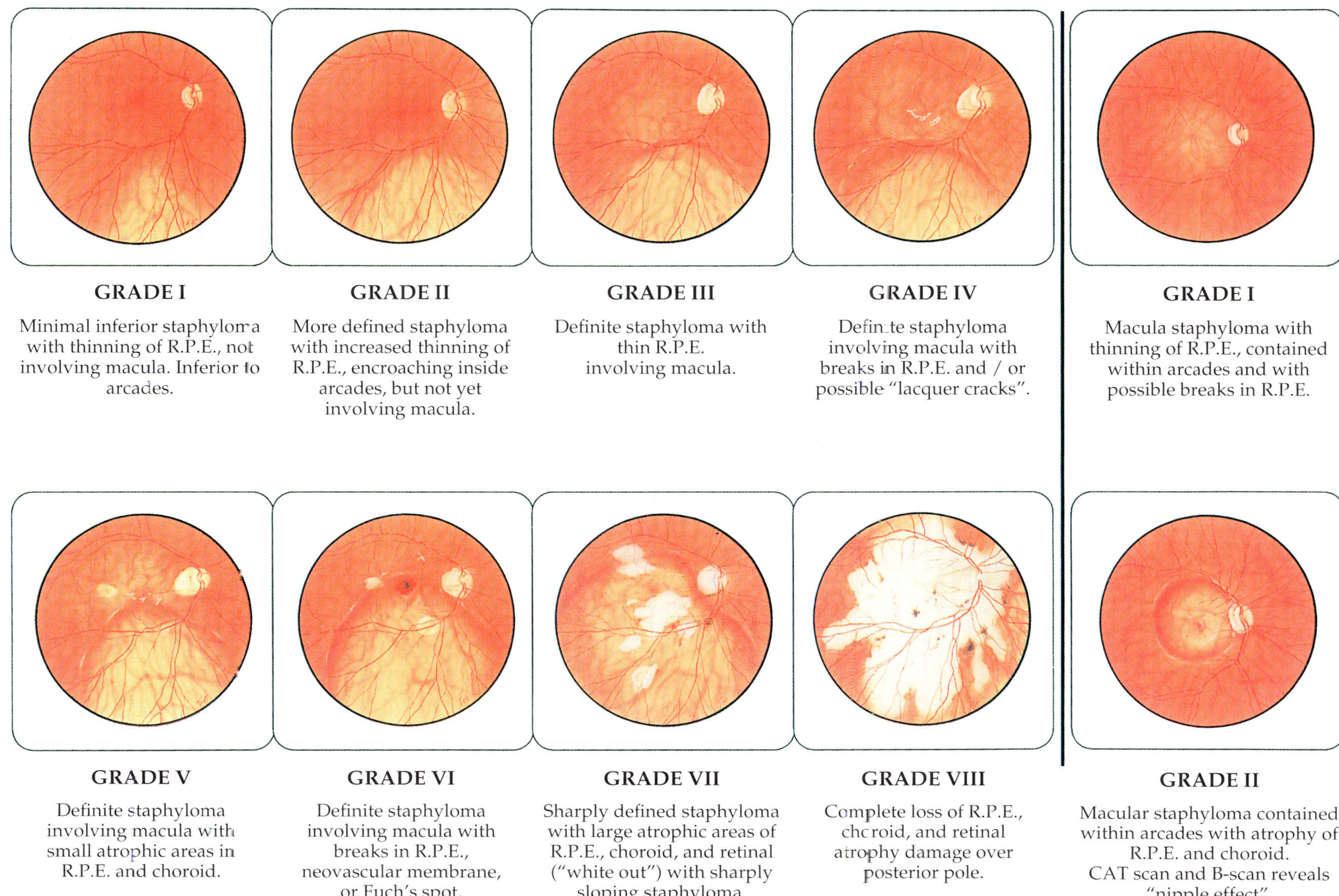

Fig. 13.3 Thompson's classification of myopic staphylomata. (from Thompson FB. Scleral reinforcement. In: *Myopia Surgery, Anterior and Posterior Segments,* FB Thompson (ed). Macmillan, New York, 1990).

Table 13.1 Grading system for temporal staphyloma in high myopia. Adapted from Thompson FB. Scleral reinforcement. In: *Myopia Surgery. Anterior and Posterior Segments*, FB Thompson (ed). Macmillan, New York, 1990

	Type I—Inferior temporal staphylomata
Grade I	Minimal staphyloma, inferior to arcades, with thinning of RPE not involving macula
Grade II	More defined staphyloma encroaching within arcades, with increased thinning of RPE. No involvement of macula
Grade III	Well-defined staphyloma with thin RPE involving macula
Grade IV	Well-defined staphyloma involving macula with breaks in RPE and/or "lacquer cracks"
Grade V	Well-defined staphyloma involving macula with small atrophic areas in RPE and choroid
Grade VI	Well-defined staphyloma involving macula with breaks in RPE and associated neovascular membrane or "Fuch's spot"
Grade VII	Sharply defined staphyloma with large atrophic areas of RPE, choroid and retina
Grade VIII	Sharply sloping staphyloma. Complete loss of of RPE and choroid, and retinal atrophy over entire posterior pole—"white-out" phenomenon
	Type II—Macular staphylomata
Grade I	Macular staphyloma with thinning of RPE contained within the vascular arcades. Possible breaks in RPE
Grade II	Macular staphyloma contained within the vascular arcades with atrophy of RPE and choroid. Computed tomography scan and B-scans reveal "nipple" effect

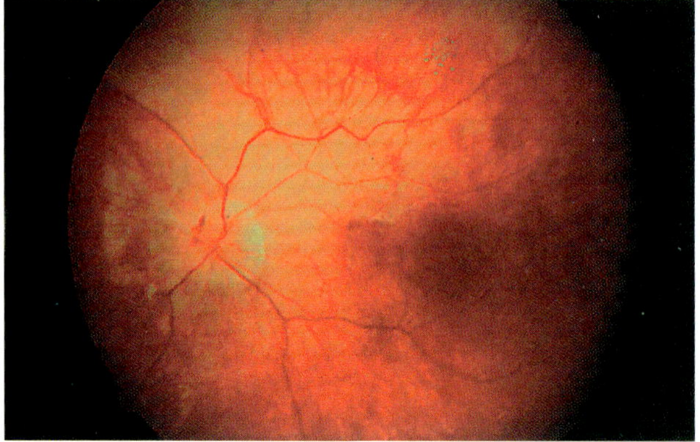

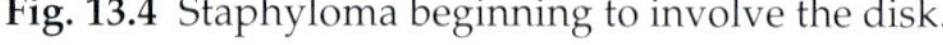

Fig. 13.4 Staphyloma beginning to involve the disk.

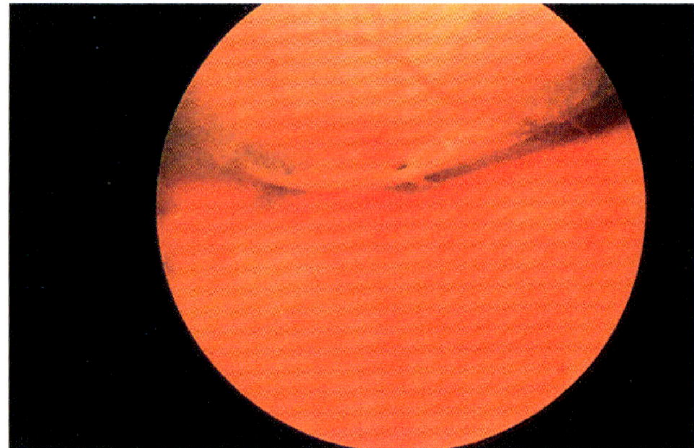

Fig. 13.5 Paving-stone degeneration with retinal hole.

pole subsequently takes on a characteristic white-out appearance (Figure 13.8).

Retinal degeneration is accompanied by degradation of the vitreous. This can lead to peripheral holes and tears with subsequent detachment of the retina (Figure 13.9).

The degree of myopia is responsible for two separate clinical pictures. Those patients with higher degrees of myopia tend to develop more acute retinal and visual changes at a younger age. In contrast, those with a lower degree of myopia tend to present as older patients in whom the visual loss is more subtle and of slower onset. These patients have suffered the gradual destruction of the chorioretinal tissue at a much lower level of myopia but over a longer period of time.

Those patients who range in age from 70 to 90 years old (with as little as 4.0 to 8.0 D of myopia) can suffer deterioration of the chorioretinal tissue over smaller posterior staphylomata. It is unusual but not rare to see younger

(a)

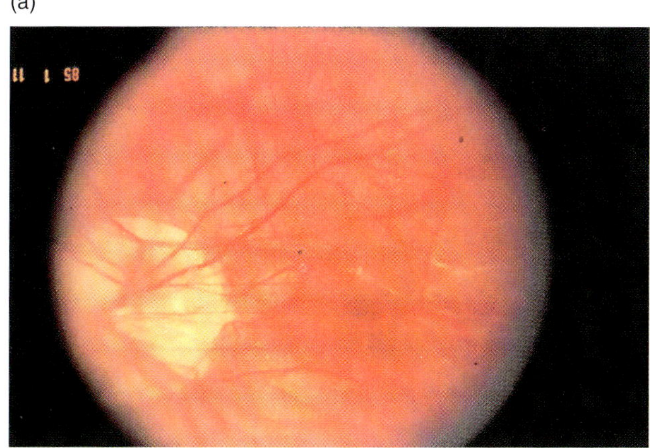

(b)

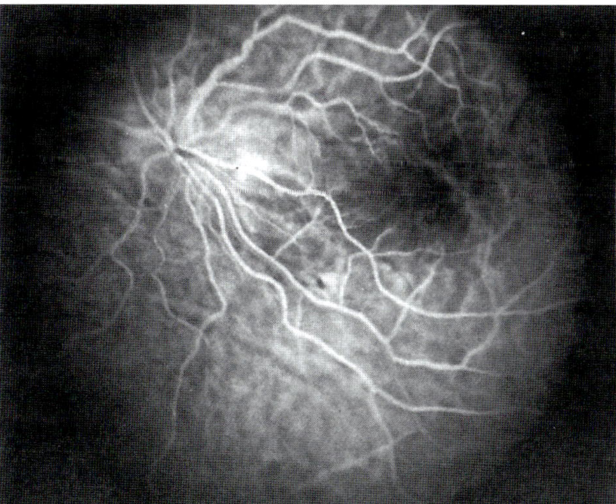

Fig. 13.6 (a) Lacquer cracks developing in macular area; (b) fluorescein angiogram showing lacquer cracks. (Courtesy of F. Thompson.)

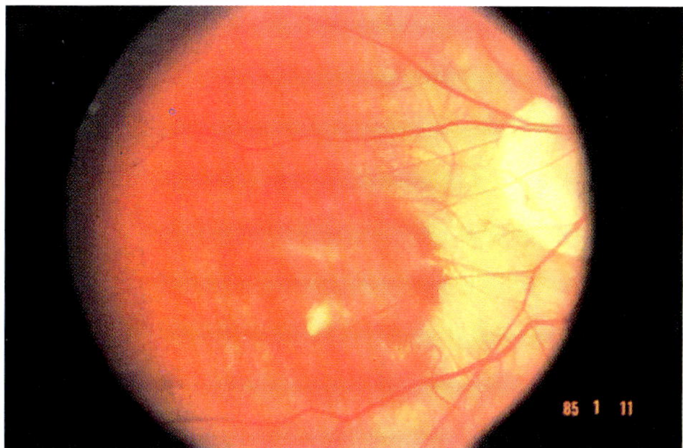

Fig. 13.7 Fuch's spot associated with subretinal neovascularization and gliosis.

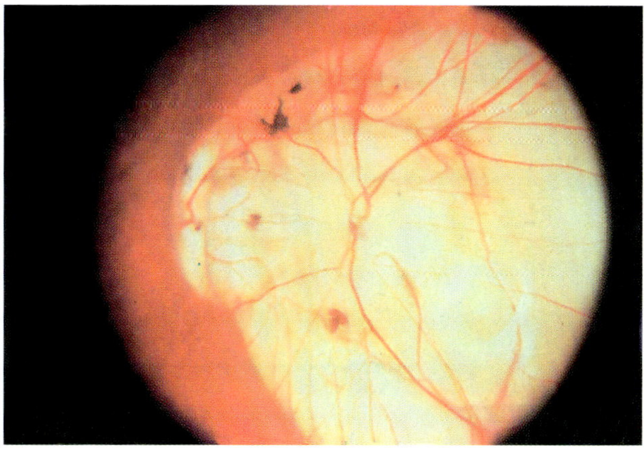

Fig. 13.8 Retinal white-out in advanced progressive myopic degeneration.

patients with central staphylomata at lower levels of myopia (4.0 to 6.0 D). No studies demonstrate the reason why the posterior scleral fibers are more prone to the formation of central staphylomata in these particular patients. Speculation associates this with other systemic problems, such as a deterioration of elastic collagenous material in other parts of the body (see also Chapter 2). Scleral reinforcement surgery is an attempt to support these macular staphylomata with some type of grafting material.

History of scleral reinforcement surgery

This posterior staphyloma formation in high myopia remains a therapeutic challenge despite the fact that the condition was identified and described anatomically almost 200 years ago by Scarpa in 1801 [38]. In 1856, von Arlt [39] showed that increases in axial length and myopia were related to staphylomata involving the posterior pole of the eye. The observation, however, was not correlated with pathologic myopia until the work of von Ammon [40], von Graefe [41], and von Jaeger [42], later in the 19th century. Speculation about reinforcement of the eye began even then.

Scleral augmentation has a sound scientific basis and such reinforcement of the posterior sclera early in the course of the disease is a sound therapeutic goal. This has been amply demonstrated in animal models as well as clinically in a large number of case reports describing the use of patch grafts of homologous fascia lata or sclera for anterior scleral disease [43–45]. In his discussion of surgery for refractive errors, Rubin noted that scleral reinforcement "is probably the only one of all the surgical techniques [for myopia] which attempts to correct a cause, rather than an effect" [46].

Various modalities to treat the sclera in myopia have been reported in the early literature—most aimed at modifying the axial length—the first by Muller in 1903, wherein he described a method of shortening the eyeball by resecting a ring of sclera at the equator [47].

Overlying grafts of dense collagenous tissues can give added support to the sclera. While surgical treatment for

(a)

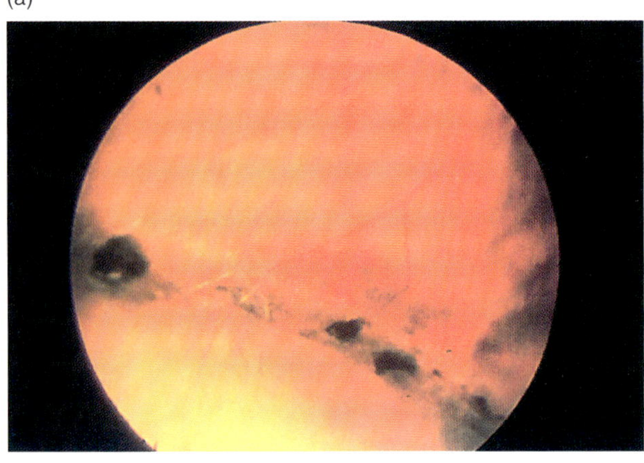

(b)

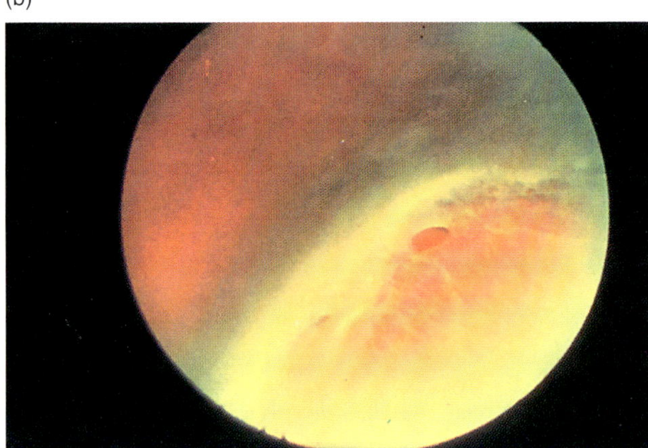

(c)

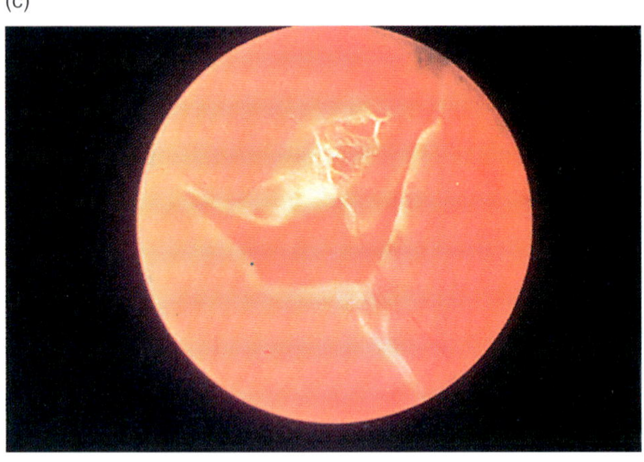

Fig. 13.9 (a) Lattice and pigment degeneration; (b) atrophic retinal hole; (c) large retinal tear.

the strengthening of the back of the eye and reinforcement of the posterior staphyloma in highly myopic eyes had been discussed in the early medical literature for many years, the first scientific report appeared in the Russian literature in the 1930s when Shevelev published a paper on the use of fascia lata to support the posterior sclera in dogs [48]. No further articles on the subject appeared until 1954 when Malbran reported on the use of periscleral explants in 21 human cases [49]. Scleral resection also was performed in 7 (33%) of these patients. Malbran's object was to support the posterior sclera, preferably early in the course of high myopia, with the purpose of preventing further expansion of the posterior segment. Malbran's original series used homologous fascia lata, although he had earlier experimented with equine and human tendon.

A number of different collagenous tissues have been used for reinforcement in a variety of ways. Most investigators in the United States have used homologous sclera in the form of a belt or cinch placed vertically over the posterior pole, under the inferior and superior oblique muscles and sutured to the anterior sclera. Borley and Snyder first used the technique in the United States as a separate procedure as well as in combination with scleral resection [50]. The nine cases presented in their pioneering study combined a scleral homograft with lamellar scleral resection to shorten the axial length of the eye and included penetrating diathermy to treat areas of peripheral degeneration and retinal holes. This combination approach reduced the amount of nearsighted correction but unfortunately induced significant complications which included retinal detachment. Consequently the combination technique was abandoned.

Miller and Borley subsequently reported two large follow-up series summarizing surgeries in which scleral reinforcement alone was performed. An occasional patient in this group underwent additional scleral resection, however. This approach appeared to be effective in halting the progress of the posterior staphyloma and the pathology of degenerative myopia in those cases [51,52].

The indications for surgery in these patients included rapid progression of childhood myopia, retinal detachment in the highly myopic eye, and visual loss in degenerative adult myopia. In reviewing the case reports in all these studies, it appears that the primary indication for surgery in the majority of patients has been deterioration of central vision in adults with myopia.

The procedures of Borley, Snyder, and Miller involved the detachment of the extraocular muscles—primarily the lateral rectus muscle—for better visualization of the

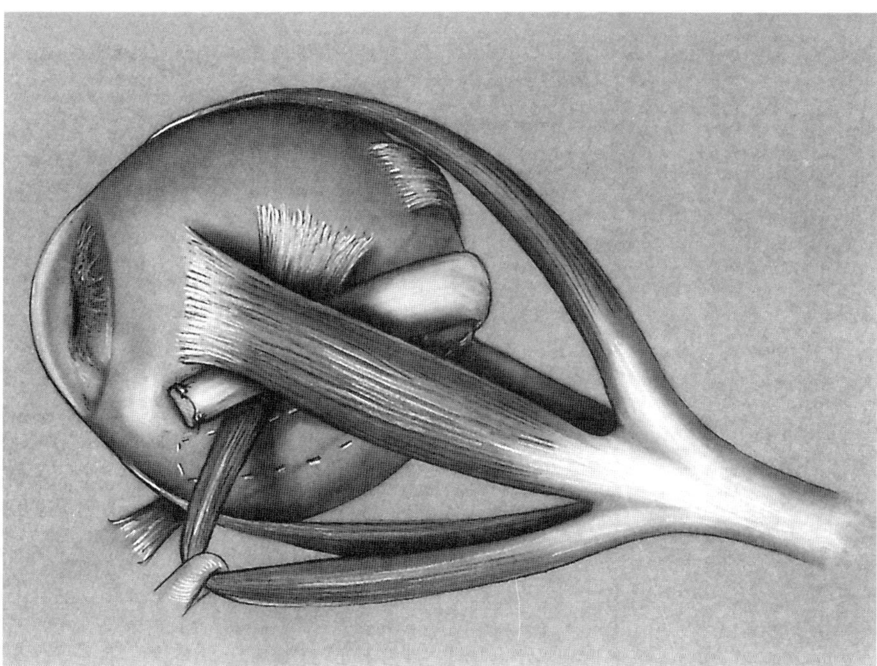

Fig. 13.10 Simplified technique for scleral reinforcement as described by Snyder and Thompson (see text).

posterior pole. They also placed the scleral strip *under* the superior oblique muscle. These two aspects of the surgery, however, increased the possibility of muscle imbalance and anterior segment complications.

In 1972, Snyder and Thompson described a simplified treatment for scleral reinforcement [53] (Figure 13.10; F. B. Thompson, 1990, personal communication). They placed the strip *over* the superior oblique muscle without removing any of the extraocular muscles using an Arruga spoon to provide visualization of the posterior pole. Cryotherapy, instead of thermal cautery, was used to treat the peripheral retinal degeneration and holes. This approach eliminated many of the complications noted with this procedure, as previously reported. This simplified technique, involving placement of the strip over the superior oblique, could, theoretically, prevent the proper apposition of the graft to the host sclera [15]. Nonetheless, experience with the single-strip method and postoperative follow-up to 20 years has shown that there has been excellent adherence of the strip to the host sclera in all cases observed (F. B. Thompson, 1990, personal communication).

Curtin, in 1961, described the use of homologous scleral support of the posterior segment in young patients [54]. Miller published his experience with the procedure in 1974 in cases uncomplicated by retinal detachment [55]. In 1978 Thompson gave an account of nearly 200 cases of scleral reinforcement using human sclera and the simplified technique [56]. The indications were a myopia of 10 D or more, decreasing vision, the presence of a posterior staphyloma, and incipient or established macular degenerative changes. In the majority of adults with degenerative myopia surgically treated, such surgery has been found to produce stabilization of the myopia, and improvement in vision has been obtained.

Mechanism of action

It is difficult to explain the manner in which this improvement in vision is achieved. Malbran, at the outset, clearly indicated that "this therapeutic method does not pretend to be a panacea for the myopic alterations of the posterior segment of the eye" [49]. Myopic degenerative changes at the macula are basically abiotrophic but can be either ischemic or neovascular in nature. The mere physical support of the ectatic sclera has no known beneficial effect upon any of these pathogenic processes—the pathologic process is not reversed. It is likely that the strain on the retina, choroid, and sclera at the posterior pole is reduced by the addition of an explant—the thicker the wall, the less the strain imparted by a given stress—in accordance with Laplace's formula. Laplace's formula refers to pressure within a hollow sphere: Internal pressure is transmitted to the wall as a force that produces tangential, and therefore circumferential, stress. Factors modifying this effect are the radius of curvature of the sphere and the wall thickness; thus $S = pr/2t$, where S = stress in g/mm^2, p = intrasphere pressure in g/mm^2, r = radius of curvature in mm, and t = wall thickness, also in mm. This is a phenomenon known to every child with a balloon. It takes more force to start blowing up the balloon than it does to continue blowing it up. Furthermore, once blown up and then allowed to empty, the balloon is easier to blow up the next time—the wall is weaker.

However, for periscleral reinforcement to have any effect, it seems logical to institute early application of such explants before ischemic and neovascular changes cause irreparable loss of retinal cells. In view of this, scleral reinforcement has been recommended only as a preventive measure, to be used early on in the course of progressive pathologic myopia and before the advanced stages of posterior staphyloma development [57].

All current techniques for scleral reinforcement attempt to arrest the deterioration resulting from the pathology occurring in highly myopic eyes with posterior staphylomata. Our discussion herein will limit itself to an elaboration of the simplified Snyder-Thompson technique using harvested human scleral explants.

Graft shapes

There are three basic graft shapes (Figure 13.11): cruciate with four arms extending anteriorly, Y-shaped (placed both vertically and horizontally), and the single strip anchored anteriorly on the nasal side of the superior and inferior rectus muscles. The single strip is held in place over the posterior pole both by the optic nerve and by the posterior insertion of the inferior oblique muscle. A fourth type, the calotte, is used by few.

Curtin has used the cruciate type of explant with the ends of the graft sutured anterior to both sides of the superior and inferior rectus muscles. This type of graft tends to ride very close to the optic nerve and the ciliary arteries, increasing the likelihood of optic nerve impingement and posterior ischemia. This danger, coupled with the more difficult placement of this type of graft, has persuaded the author to favor the Snyder-Thompson procedure in his few cases. The use of this cruciate-shaped explant was further described by Curtin and Whitmore in a follow-up of some of their earlier surgeries [58]. Their report of cases from 5 to 16 years (median 8 years) of follow-up indicated that only 10 of 23 patients (44%) failed to show significant progression of myopia postoperatively. Additionally, only two of nine of these eyes failed to

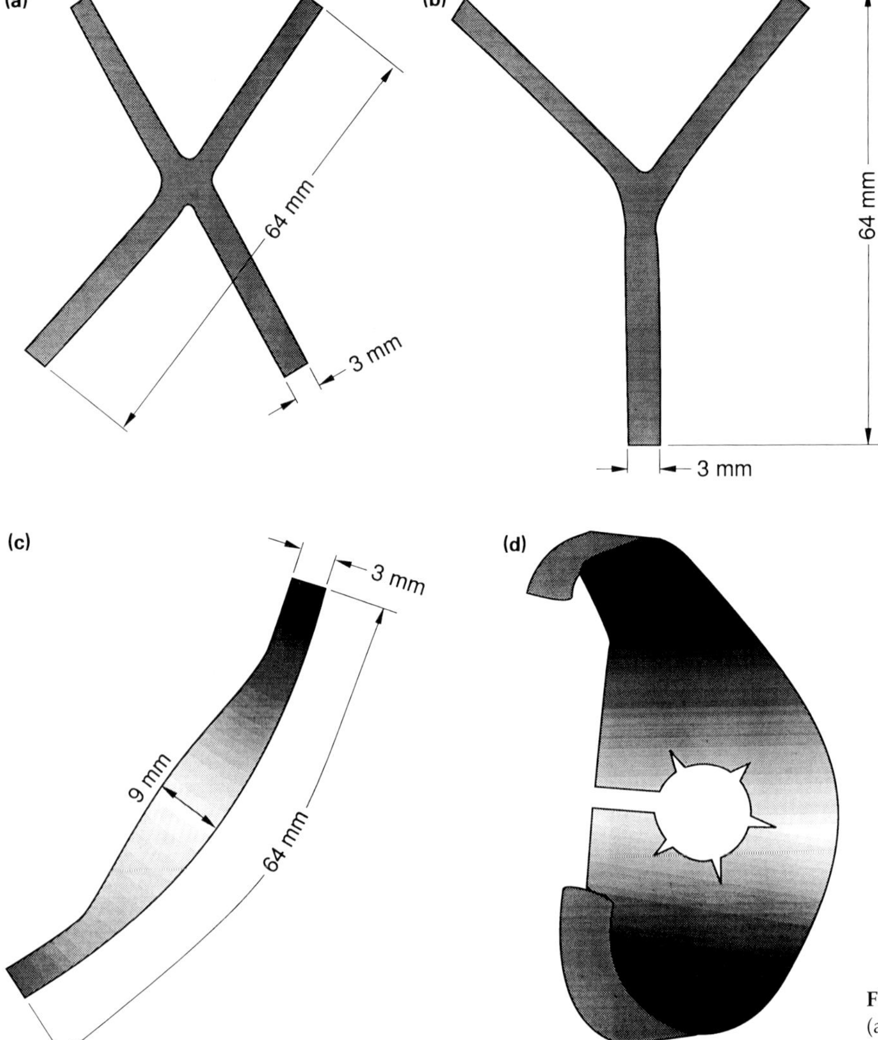

Fig. 13.11 The four explant shapes: (a) cruciate; (b) Y-shaped; (c) single strip; (d) calotte (skull cap) graft.

demonstrate increased axial lengths after surgery. This increase was nearly the same as that seen in the fellow, unoperated eye that was used as a control. The stabilization of refraction seen in these patients could as well be ascribed to the natural course of the disease as to any specific effect of the periscleral graft. The increase in axial length, it appears, was adequately compensated for by changes in total refractive power of the eye. In contrast to these unimpressive results, the effects of scleral reinforcement surgery in eastern European studies could hardly be better [59–63]. Alberth and colleagues, for example, reported a 7-year experience with 400 patients who had undergone fascia lata periscleral reinforcement along with laser photocoagulation [64]. The degree of myopia was decreased by a mean value of 3.0 D in 90%, while the visual acuity improved by a mean value of 0.15 in 70% of the patients treated. No retinal detachments or other serious complications were reported in this series.

Hanczye used a Y-shaped graft positioned both horizontally and vertically and has published the most extensive series of articles on this subject [65]. He used the meridional circumligation technique of Starkiewicz in which a horizontal autologous fascia lata graft was placed over the posterior sclera at the macula in 44 patients, the majority of whom were under 20 years of age [66,67]. An improvement in vision was usually noted, together with an average reduction in myopia of 1.5 D. A reduction in ocular axial diameter, averaging 1.5 mm, also was obtained. In 40% of patients a significant increase in visual fields also was noted, along with the disappearance of isolated scotomata. There was deterioration of the field in 13%, however. In this series a reduction in the ocular tension also was found postoperatively. Again, no serious complications were observed.

Nesterov and coworkers also have contributed extensively to the literature on this subject [68–70]. In a more recent report they summarize the results of 756 scleral reinforcement procedures in which horizontally oriented autologous fascia lata was used [71]. They obtained a reduction in myopia that ranged from 0.5 to 8 D in 86% of these eyes. The axial length decreased an average of 1.47 ± 0.51 mm. Long-term follow-up (mean 6.8 years) in 244 eyes found that these earlier results were stable. Complications included compression of the optic nerve in one case and compression of vortex veins with choroidal hemorrhage in five cases.

The striking differences in results between these studies of Hanczye and Nesterov and those reported by Curtin are difficult to reconcile. The surgical techniques in general are similar—the skill of the surgeon is, of course, an important variable. It would appear, however, that the principal difference rests in the snugness with which the graft has been applied to the sclera. In the eastern European technique, considerable traction appears to have been placed on the graft. This was deliberately not done in the cases reported by Curtin because rabbit studies had indicated that shrinkage of the periscleral graft ensued postoperatively [43]. However, Curtin's cases were almost all children in whom there can be a general enlargement of the globe despite the flattening of the posterior staphyloma. In these cases the criterion for success was refraction. Furthermore, there are theoretic arguments that can be made against the efficacy of overlying grafts of the macular region in posterior staphyloma development.

The most common type of staphyloma, that of the posterior pole, type I, originates nasal to the optic nerve and involves the macular area by expansion. If effective prevention of staphyloma formation is to be achieved, this nasal area also must be reinforced [57]. This has been done in two clinical studies with encouraging early results. Zarkova and Negoda [72] in Russia and Whitwell [73] in Britain have contributed two large studies, each comprising over 40 patients, in which a calotte of homologous sclera was placed about the optic nerve. There can be little question that this approach is a distinct improvement in the reinforcement effect of the surgery but this improvement is obtained at a greater risk of vascular accidents, as evidenced by the inadvertent occlusion of the superotemporal vortex vein in two patients in the British study. This resulted in intraocular hemorrhage and blindness. Additionally, whether placed horizontally or vertically, the Y-shaped graft may press on the optic nerve at the junctions of the arm of the Y, resulting in optic nerve atrophy.

Momose has reported a number of cases using Y-shaped grafts associated with lens extraction [74]. He noted the occurrence of secondary glaucoma and one case of optic atrophy among the 50 eyes in which he used the Y-shaped explant. Because of the increased risk of complications, Momose no longer uses this type of explant, preferring instead to use the single-strip type of support in his last 2000 cases (A. Momose, 1990, personal communication).

Most ophthalmic surgeons, particularly those in the United States, currently use the single-strip support technique whether using fascia lata, lyophilized dura, or sclera. The single strip offers the easiest method for placement, along with the widest area of support over the macula—the main objective of the operation. This approach significantly reduces the incidence of optic nerve impingement. No cases of optic atrophy or damage have been reported using this technique to date (F. B. Thompson, 1990, personal communication).

Curtin correctly points out that the single scleral strip has the disadvantage of only reinforcing the macular staphyloma and does not prevent development of staphylomata in other areas (B. J. Curtin, 1990, personal communication). It should be noted, however, that macular staphylomata are the ones associated with the most profound and permanent visual loss—most of the visual elements required for fine vision, including reading and driving, are contained in this area. For this reason the sole compelling indication for a posterior scleral graft is the developing presence of a macular staphyloma.

Materials

There is much work that has yet to be done with both materials and techniques. Other grafts using different shapes and materials may someday prevent the development of staphylomata in other areas of the globe. A future technique may not only protect the central visual elements but at the same time prevent stretching and elongation of the entire eye.

In the 60 years since Shevelev's paper, a variety of dense collagenous materials have been employed for the reinforcement of the posterior staphyloma. These materials range from fascia lata to lyophilized dura to human donor sclera. Homologous human donor sclera is mainly used for the reinforcing material, particularly by U.S. surgeons, partly because of its ready availability. In addition, sclera is easy to work with and does not tend to develop folds posteriorly, as is the case with other materials. When properly removed from the donor eye, sclera conforms to the contour of the host eye more readily than any of the other reported materials. Furthermore, it is strong and holds sutures well.

In other parts of the world, alternative materials are often used. Human sclera is avoided because of cultural, religious, or technical reasons. Momose in Japan published an optimistic report on over 2000 cases of scleral reinforcement using lyophilized (freeze-dried) dura for posterior support (Figure 13.12) [75]. In 1984, Nesterov and coworkers [71] reported on the use of fascia lata in 756 operations, while Fyodorov in Moscow uses human donor sclera in his scleral explant patients (S. N. Fyodorov, 1990, personal communication). However, one of the problems with fascia lata is that it requires a second surgical procedure on the patient to harvest the tissue. This prolongs the surgery and affords no opportunity for the preservation or sterilization of the harvested material.

The use of equine or porcine tendon has been proposed but not effected. To date, a single strip of homologous human sclera appears to offer the best support with the fewest complications of all the biologic materials.

As for allopathic materials, silicone and nylon are not recommended. The sclera of the highly myopic patient is extremely thin. Any pressure from these highly elastic materials can erode the underlying tissue, as has been noted after their use in retinal detachment surgery on both myopic and nonmyopic patients.

The ideal material would be one that is firm yet has the correct amount of flexibility and elasticity. A suitable artificial material would also eliminate the need for harvesting human tissue, ensure proper and complete sterilization, be readily available, and would not compress the underlying sclera. Such a material is polytetrafluorethylene, commercially available under the trade name Gore-Tex. This material was originally employed as a fabric but has been used for years by vascular surgeons in repairing aortic grafts. It offers promise as a material

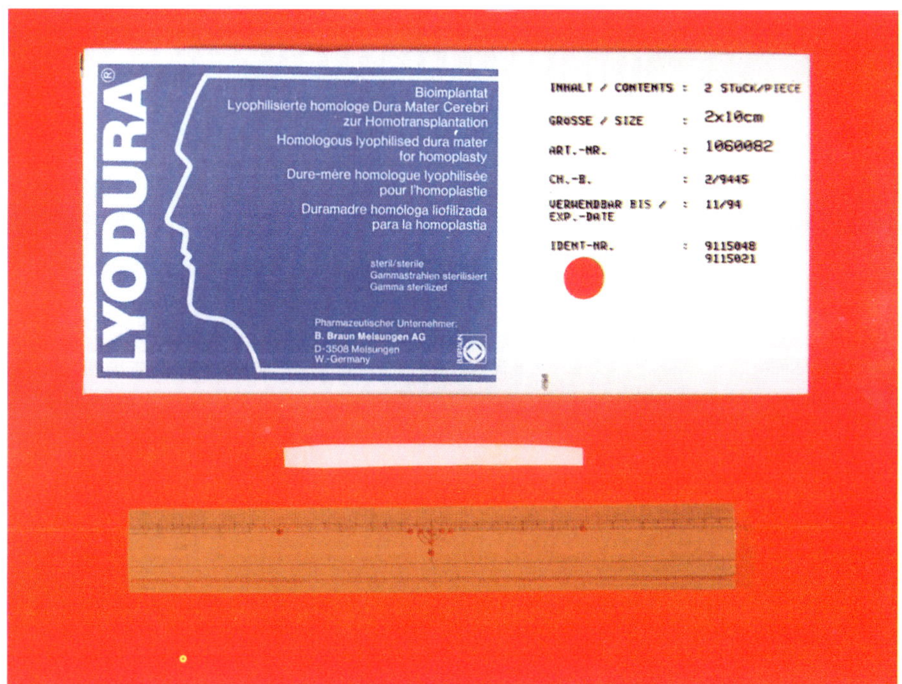

Fig. 13.12 Momose uses lyophilized human dura for his explants.

which can be easily obtained, sterilized, and stored and also provides some give without too much stretch. The experience with it is minimal at this time but some patients have recently undergone scleral reinforcement surgery with this material in the United States (F. B. Thompson, 1990, personal communication).

Preparing the graft

A whole frozen donor eye is the source of scleral grafts—two such strips can be cut from each globe. When the donor eyes have been obtained, they should immediately be frozen. The strips should be cut from them within 1 to 2 weeks after freezing to avoid potential explant weakening resulting from deterioration of the donor sclera. The globes must remain frozen all during this time. Because the eyes of a high myope are much larger than average, the prepared scleral strip must include sufficient corneal tissue so that the explant is long enough to reach around the entire circumference of the host eye. If corneal tissue is not included, the graft may be too short, making placement of the strip much more difficult, if not impossible. The sclera of highly myopic eyes should not be used for grafting because it is too thin and does not offer adequate support over the affected area. Since it is impossible to know the refractive status of most donor eyes, some globes will necessarily be found to be unsuitable during harvesting.

The strips are removed under sterile conditions. The instruments used are a methylene blue marking pen, a Bard-Parker knife with a no. 15 blade, rat-toothed forceps, sterile cotton-tipped applicators, sterile 4 × 4 gauze patches, and a Wescott-type scissors.

To make handling easier, the globes are only partially thawed before removing them from the storage containers. The optic nerve is cut flush with the sclera, and excess orbital fat and connective tissue removed. The donor globe is positioned so that the superior rectus muscle is up. The areas to be cut are marked using the methylene blue marking pen (Figure 13.13). The first mark is placed at the limbus carried posteriorly just adjacent to the optic nerve and brought in a curvilinear path to the opposite limbus nasal to the insertion of the inferior rectus. Two other dotted marks are made parallel to the original marks so as to delineate the path to be cut. The strip that incorporates the optic nerve is made slightly wider posteriorly.

An incision is made tangentially across the cornea in line with the center mark. Grasping the incision with a toothed forceps and using the Wescott-type scissors, the surgeon cuts along the initial middle dotted line circumferentially. The incision is continued around the eye until the globe is separated into two halves. The lines are again followed posteriorly and circumferentially until two scleral strips are obtained. The resulting strips should be in the shape of a boomerang, though not so abruptly curved. The resected strips should be at least 8 mm wide at their center but may be as narrow as 3 to 4 mm at the ends. The length of the strip as measured along the curve should be at least 60 mm.

At this point, the surgeon uses the cotton-tipped applicators to roll up and remove the retinal and choroidal tissue from the inner side of each strip. Excess pigmented

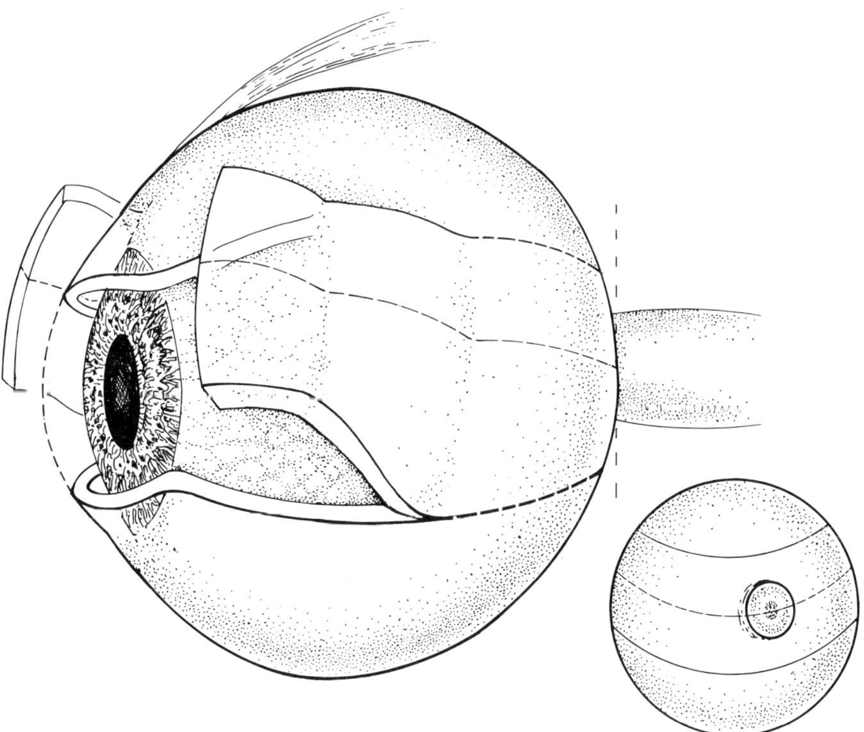

Fig. 13.13 Method for harvesting scleral explants.

tissue is completely removed by scraping with the blunt side of the Bard-Parker knife. It is not necessary, nor is it desirable to depigment the sclera with iodine (as in eviscerations) in preparing these strips. Surplus Tenon's capsule and connective tissue on the external side of the strip, if any, should be removed.

The strips are stored submersed in a solution consisting of two-thirds saline and one-third Neosporin (polymyxin B sulfate–neomycin sulfate–bacitracin zinc) within test tubes fitted with rubber stoppers or caps. An air pocket is left at the top of the tube to allow for expansion of the solution when it is frozen. The stopper is sealed and an adhesive label is placed on one side of the test tube. Each tube is marked with the date of harvesting, the length of the strip, and other pertinent details (e.g., the strip is slightly short, a little thin, more curved than normal). The test tubes are supported vertically in a test tube rack placed in a freezer and kept until surgery. Theoretically, as long as the strips are kept continuously frozen, they should remain viable. Thompson prefers to use them within 1 year of the date of freezing, however (F. B. Thompson, 1990, personal communication).

Patient selection

The primary candidate for surgery is a patient who has progressive posterior staphyloma on the temporal side of the optic nerve involving the macula. This condition can occur in any patient from 2 to 80 years of age and from −4.00 to −40.00 D of myopia. Indications for surgery are myopia greater than 7 D with

1 Decreasing best-corrected vision.

2 Documented increasing axial length (more than 1.0 mm of axial length progression per year for 2 to 3 years).

3 Progressive macular changes on fluorescein angiography.

4 Indirect ophthalmoscopy indicating a posterior staphyloma (evidence of thinning of the retinal pigment epithelium posteriorly).

Pruett correctly points out that there is a trend toward recommending refractive surgery for young patients with high degrees of progressive myopia [76]. Although many can benefit from certain procedures, staphylomatous eyes present unique impediments to normal visual acuity, visual field, binocularity, and stereopsis. They are also prone to premature cataract formation, glaucoma, and retinal detachment. An initially good surgical result can be utterly negated by continued scleral expansion along with posterior retinal degeneration. A review of these limitations should be included in discussions with patients considering refractive surgery.

Many patients will present with already well-developed staphylomata, angiographic evidence of chorioretinal atrophy or "lacquer cracks," and axial lengths measuring over 29 to 30 mm. In these cases, scleral reinforcement should be considered without waiting for further changes. If possible, surgery should be performed prior to the development of a subretinal neovascular membrane so as to reduce the risk of bleeding during the operation. While preventing further enlargement of the staphyloma, scleral reinforcement surgery does not always prevent additional progression of an existing subretinal neovascular network with its subsequent hemorrhage and visual loss.

If initial fluorescein angiography reveals a subretinal neovascular network and the membrane is at least 20 μm outside the capillary free zone, adjunctive laser therapy may be indicated. The laser, however, is contraindicated in the presence of subretinal neovascular membranes in the central foveal area. Current techniques of laser therapy have not been particularly successful in the treatment of membranes, even outside the capillary free zone. The membranes frequently re-form in any event, and treatment of neovascularization may itself produce further bleeding.

Preventive therapy is always controversial. For example, laser therapy is presently being performed much earlier in patients with diabetic retinopathy to prevent the changes seen in the later stages of the disease. However, if scleral reinforcement is as effective and safe as some believe it to be, then it may make sense to perform prophylactic surgery on highly myopic patients who fit the above criteria. This will prevent them from developing the complications resulting from the advanced stages of the disease.

There are an increasing number of geriatric patients being seen in Western society and an increasing longevity being projected for the future. Because of this, we may anticipate seeing more elderly patients who develop posterior staphylomata along with the typical changes of pathologic myopia at much lower levels of myopia than have been seen in the past. If these patients have either a nondilated funduscopic examination or are examined without an indirect ophthalmoscope, they may be misdiagnosed as having age-related macular degeneration (ARMD). It is imperative that these older myopic patients undergo indirect ophthalmoscopy for detection of any late staphyloma formation.

The practitioner must then make a differential diagnosis between the much more commonly seen ARMD and the late cases of myopic degeneration. Some aging patients will not develop the central pigment clumping, gliosis, and deterioration seen in late wet ARMD. Instead they will present with a progressive atrophy of Bruch's membrane, the pigment epithelium, and the retina and choroid over the posterior pole. Finally they may exhibit the typical white-out appearance seen in the high degrees of myopia in younger age groups. To add to the matter, the differential diagnosis between myopic degeneration and dry ARMD is frequently a difficult one (Figure 13.14).

Scleral reinforcement should be seriously considered in some of these older patients. This is particularly appropriate for those who have lost central vision in one eye

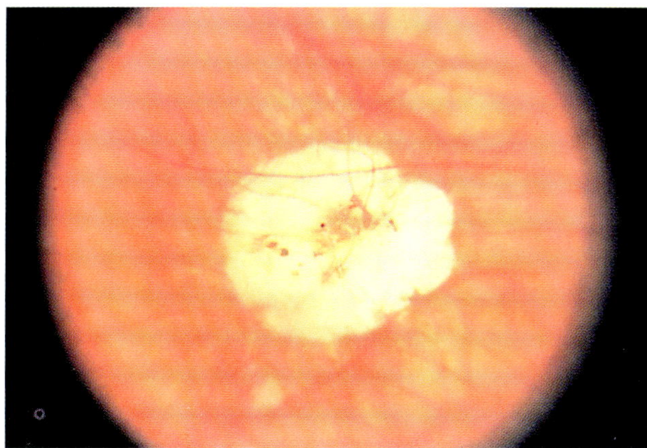

Fig. 13.14 Myopic degeneration is often difficult to distinguish from ARMD.

because of increased staphyloma formation and deterioration of the retinal elements but maintain some reasonable level of visual acuity in the remaining eye. Surgery may be the only recourse for preservation of vision in these cases.

Patient examination—Preoperative and postoperative

Highly myopic patients undergo a thorough eye examination which includes a complete ocular and medical history. In the younger patient particular attention is paid to recent or precipitous changes in the patient's refraction. For all patients, the examiner checks for recent decrease in the best-corrected visual acuity. This is followed by near/distance visual acuity, a glare test, careful dilated slit-lamp examination, refraction, and measurement of IOP. Slit-lamp examination of the younger patient may reveal posterior subcapsular cataracts.

Indirect ophthalmoscopy is particularly useful for observing posterior staphylomatous changes. Those beginning in the inferior temporal quadrant should be carefully documented. In addition, the peripheral fundus is inspected as the younger patient is much more likely to exhibit lattice degeneration and peripheral retinal breaks, holes, or tears. In the highly myopic patient, the examiner should carefully inspect the inferior temporal peripheral retina for paving-stone degeneration. While the indirect ophthalmoscopic view moves from the periphery toward the posterior pole of the eye, a sudden edge or drop-off, indicating a staphyloma, can easily be seen.

Computerized visual fields are performed and are especially useful in these cases. Many of these patients will be found to have central scotomata because of the previously described pathology. Static, computerized perimetry makes repeat comparison studies much easier and enhances their value in earlier detection of advancing changes.

Fluorescein angiography establishes the degree of loss of posterior pigment epithelium and the amount of choroidal and retinal deterioration. This technique is useful for delineating lacquer cracks and early development of subretinal neovascular membranes.

The examiner performs A-scan measurement of the axial length over both the macula and the deepest portion of the eye. The macular measurement and the greatest length of the eye may not necessarily coincide since posterior staphylomata are frequently off-center, particularly in the early stages.

Axial lengths must be measured carefully by an experienced ophthalmic technician as the presence of staphylomata in many cases makes precise measurements extremely difficult. Since the slope of the posterior staphylomata may be rather sharply delineated, variations in the axial length are frequently encountered. The technician must be sure to read the longest part of the eye. A combination of fluorescein angiography and axial length measurements offers the most accurate diagnosis in the highly myopic patient.

B-scan ultrasonic measurements of the eye are not very good for following the progress of staphylomata. It is frequently difficult to get a clear static picture for subsequent evaluation and comparison. However, the so-called Z or isometric examination mode may be invaluable in locating staphylomata accurately for subsequent A-scan measurement.

As yet, there is no standardized measurement of scleral reinforcement surgery results. Because the disease progresses slowly, follow-up needs to be done for a number of years to demonstrate long-term stabilization. There are problems and drawbacks with all of the measurements mentioned above, both as preoperative indicators for surgery and as postoperative evaluations of results.

Refraction is not useful for following the progress of myopic staphylomata because factors other than staphyloma enlargement may influence refractive error. Many highly myopic, middle-aged patients tend to develop cataracts, lenticular swelling, and changes in refractive error from induced myopia. This can occasionally add –5 to –6 D of myopia. If these patients undergo cataract removal (eventually becoming aphakic or pseudophakic), the refraction can change drastically, rendering difficult preoperative and postoperative comparisons. In other cases, especially in children, the entire eye size may enlarge slightly to increase the refractive error though no posterior staphyloma may develop. After surgery, younger patients can have an increase in axial length (and therefore myopia), even though the macular staphyloma may have been stabilized. This autoadjustment in total refractive error may occur in adults as well.

Computed tomography or magnetic resonance imaging scans of the globe are often helpful, although cumbersome and expensive. Many patients are reluctant to repeat the scans because of this. Computer scans do, however, provide excellent imaging confirmation of scleral strip placement and can establish temporal strip integrity as well (Figure 13.15). Such a loss of integrity should always be suspected when advancing axial length is seen postoperatively.

Visual acuity measurements are somewhat subjective for both patient and examiner. Similarly, fluorescein angiography requires some subjectivity in determining further deterioration. Since fluorescein angiography requires an injection, many patients are reluctant to have it repeated at frequent intervals. Not a few patients will experience nausea and/or other unpleasant side effects. Some can even develop a reaction to the fluorescein dye, which fortunately, although uncomfortable, is not usually serious. Anaphylactic-like reactions have, however, been reported.

Ultrasound measurements of axial length seem the most objective method of measuring the efficacy of the procedure. Often ultrasound is the only frequently repeatable diagnostic technique acceptable to the patient. As mentioned above, A-scan measurements of the length of the eye are difficult in patients with sharply sloping staphylomata. Only a practiced technician familiar with the highly myopic eye can obtain an accurate and reproducible axial length measurement.

Increase in axial length is not always a hallmark of progressive staphyloma, however. Younger patients may exhibit a growth of the entire axial length of the eye, even though the scleral reinforcement procedure has stopped the progression of the macular portion of the staphyloma. Such growth may not even be suspected as there is often a compensatory adjustment in other refractive components (emmetropization), as noted in Chapter 2.

Preoperative preparation

The patients are started on Tobrex (tobramycin 0.3%) antibiotic drops 2 days prior to surgery. The operative eyes are dilated with 10% Neo-Synephrine (phenylephrine hydrochloride), 1% Mydriacyl (tropicamide), and 1% atropine drops instilled every 10 minutes four times, beginning 1 hour prior to surgery. It is recommended that the lashes be clipped before surgery and the eyelids carefully scrubbed with half-strength Betadide (povidone-iodide *solution*, not preparation) for 2 to 3 minutes. Betadine preparation contains soap, which can damage the corneal epithelium and irritate ocular tissue.

Surgical technique

The following description is provided courtesy of Frank Thompson: The surgery is preferably performed under general anesthesia. Retrobulbar or peribulbar anesthesia is not recommended because the accompanying edema frequently distorts the periocular tissue posteriorly, making placement of the scleral strip difficult. Additionally, these patients occasionally have areas of scleral ectasia or anterior staphylomata. Because of the thin globe, there is a possibility of ocular perforation, either anteriorly or posteriorly. If local anesthesia is necessary, the surgeon should use a blunted, 25-gauge, Atkinson-type retrobulbar needle to administer it with the patient looking down (toward) the needle. This will swing the thinner posterior pole of the eye up and away from the needle tip (see also Chapter 11 for more details of this technique).

A conjunctival incision is made in the superior temporal quadrant, approximately 4 to 5 mm posterior to the limbus. A fornix-based incision is preferred to a limbal

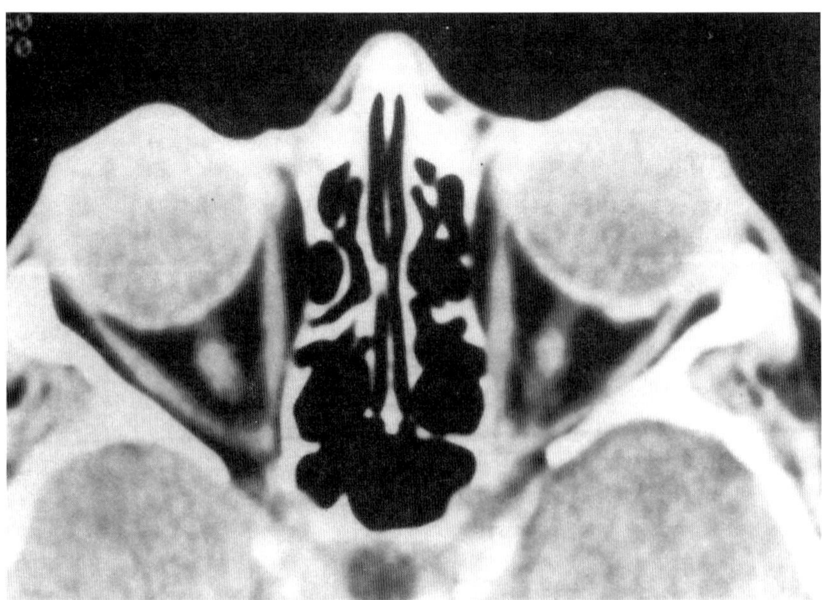

Fig. 13.15 Computed tomography scan showing scleral explant in one eye near the optic nerve. (Courtesy of F. Thompson.)

incision because it allows more exposure of the posterior pole. In addition, later cataract surgery is less difficult because the limbal-based flap leaves the surgical limbus undisturbed.

The incision is extended into both the superotemporal and inferotemporal quadrants, leaving a small amount of conjunctival tissue overlying the medial rectus muscle. Since highly myopic eyes are very large, the extraocular muscles also may be attenuated; therefore, care must be taken when making the conjunctival incisions so as not to sever or damage these muscles.

The underlying Tenon's capsule is incised and the sclera exposed. In younger patients this capsule is usually very thick, very vascular, and difficult to manipulate. In contrast, older patients may have subconjunctival tissue that is extremely thin and atrophic. In any event bleeding must be completely controlled with wet-field cautery to ensure good visualization.

The superior, lateral, and inferior rectus muscles are isolated using muscle hooks. Care must be taken that the check ligaments and adhesions to the overlying conjunctiva and underlying sclera are stripped. Traction sutures of 4-0 black silk are placed beneath these muscles (Figure 13.16) and their ends secured with alligator clamps.

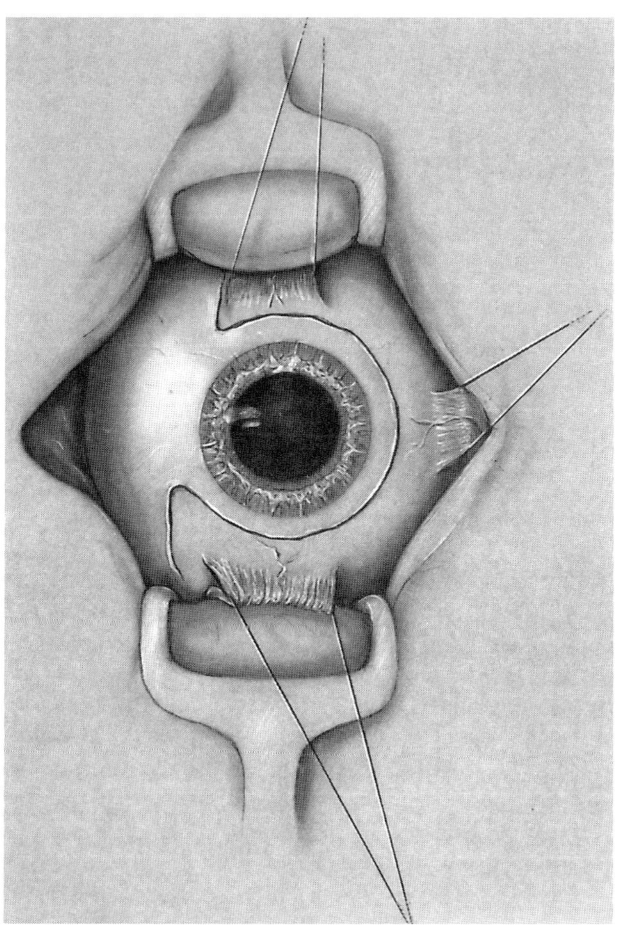

Fig. 13.16 The superior, inferior, and lateral recti are isolated.

The traction sutures around the inferior rectus and lateral rectus muscles are grasped and the eye rotated *medially*. A muscle hook is passed parallel to the globe, hugging the sclera in the inferotemporal quadrant. The tip of the hook is then rotated outward and anteriorly to isolate the inferior oblique. Using a combination of blunt and sharp dissection, the inferior oblique is separated from the orbital septum and connective tissue surrounding the muscle—the orbital septum itself should not be incised. If orbital fat is allowed to come forward, later visualization will be more difficult.

Take care during this step that all fibers of the inferior oblique muscle are brought forward. The muscle may occasionally divide into two parts and sometimes there are muscle fibers which tightly hug the globe posteriorly. These must be brought forward as well, taking care not to tear them. Since the explant must be placed posterior to all the fibers of the posterior insertion of the inferior oblique muscle (ensuring that the strip will not ride too far forward, be positioned accurately over the posterior pole, and be held firmly in place), no muscle fibers can be missed. Repeat surgery may be necessary if the explant splits the anterior and posterior fibers of this muscle. In that event, the explant will inevitably shift anteriorly and create a bothersome muscle imbalance.

Once all fibers of the inferior oblique have been carefully isolated, an additional traction suture of 4-0 black silk is placed around this muscle. Next, passed posteriorly beneath both the superior and inferior rectus, a muscle hook is carefully used to strip away any adhesions extending from the muscles to the globe. The hook is passed gently under the lateral rectus muscle with the eye rotated medially. The adherent fibers are gradually stripped away until the hook can be pushed no further. At this point, the instrument should lie against the fat pad surrounding the optic nerve. There are important blood vessels in this area so gentleness is the order of the day. These adhesions will occasionally resist the hook sufficiently that cutting with scissors will be required. If the patient has a preoperative subretinal neovascular membrane, extreme care must be taken to prevent rupturing this membrane and causing subsequent macular bleeding. This can occur through too vigorous manipulation of the globe—remember the sclera is very thin in this area. The surgeon can easily visualize any posterior adhesive fibers with an Arruga spoon.

After the muscles are isolated and traction sutures placed around them, the periphery of the retina is inspected with the indirect ophthalmoscope and scleral depression is gently performed. Keep in mind always that the myopic sclera is abnormal and thin. The surgeon must work carefully to avoid tearing the vortex vein. Any atrophic holes or retinal tears can be treated cryosurgically under direct visualization with the indirect ophthalmoscope. The inferonasal and inferotemporal quadrants are the most common sites for retinal tears, holes, and paving-stone degeneration. This is in contrast to the moderately myopic patient who demonstrates a tendency for retinal tears and holes in the superotemporal quadrant.

The scleral strip, which has previously been thawed and soaked in an antibiotic solution, is now examined. The surgeon excises any excess connective tissue remaining on the strip and shapes it with the scalpel. The inner portion of the scleral strip is placed against the sclera of the host eye, *beneath* both the superior and lateral rectus muscles (Figure 13.17). As the inferior oblique muscle is pulled forward, the surgeon, using forceps, draws the strip through the opening made by tenting up the muscle. When the muscle is released, the posterior fibers of the inferior oblique will drag the strip backward toward the optic nerve (Figure 13.18). The scleral strip is then tucked under the inferior rectus muscle. The strip is then sutured to the sclera in the superior temporal quadrant, just posterior and nasal to the insertion of the superior rectus and at a 45° angle to the muscle insertion. The superior oblique muscle need not be isolated, however; the strip can be placed over the superior oblique without risking complication (Figure 13.19).

The traction suture around the inferior oblique muscle is now cut and removed, allowing this muscle to retract. The strip is then secured superiorly with two sutures of 5-0 collagen, Vicril (synthetic adsorbable polyglactin 910), or nylon.

With the *left hand,* the assistant grasps the end of the strip (in the inferior nasal quadrant) with a toothed forceps (such as a Bishop-Harmon). The traction suture around the lateral rectus muscle is held with the assistant's *right hand*—this suture is used to rotate the eye medially.

Using an Arruga spoon to visualize the posterior pole of the eye, the surgeon pulls the posterior conjunctiva anteriorly. The strip is placed over the posterior pole either with a fine, smooth forceps or with a custom-designed, curved repositioning instrument (Figure 13.20b). In the first step, the assistant pulls on the lateral rectus insertion to rotate the eye medially for greater exposure over the posterior pole. If the strip is too long and too loose posteriorly, the scleral graft is pulled forward in the inferior nasal quadrant and the excess trimmed away.

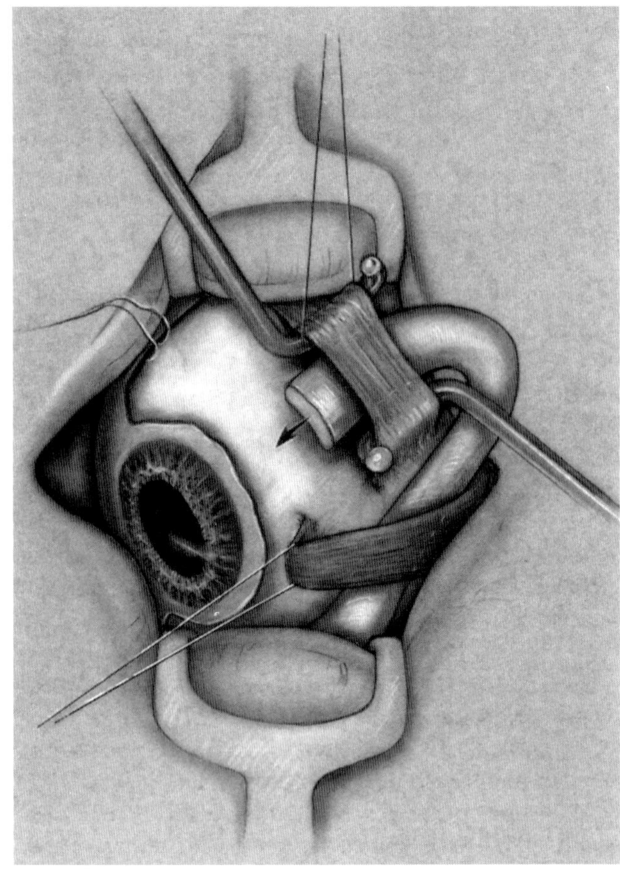

Fig. 13.17 Placement of the strip beneath the superior and lateral recti.

(a)

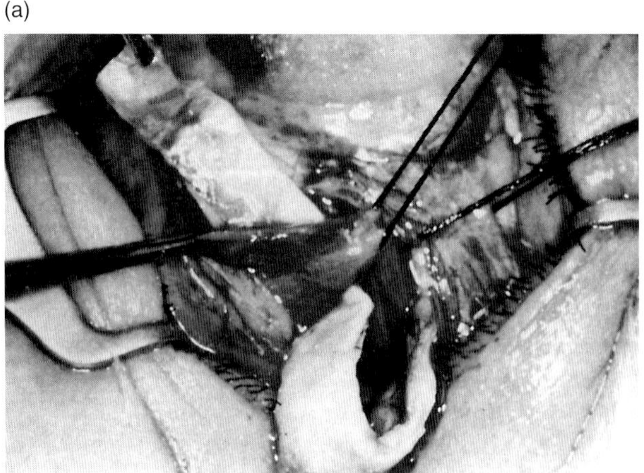

(b)

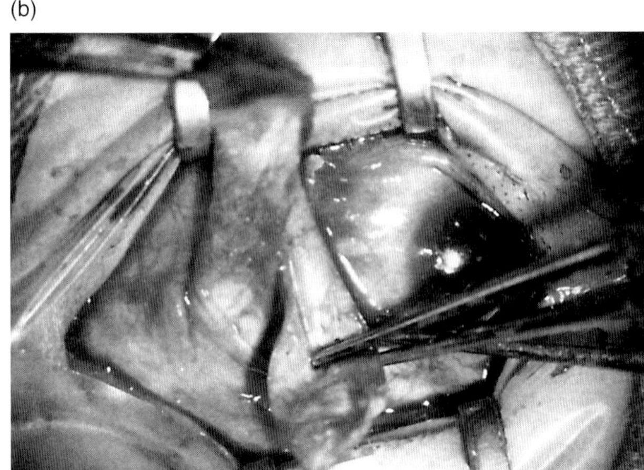

Fig. 13.18 (a) The strip is drawn under the isolated inferior oblique. (b) If the strip is long enough, crossing the ends over the medial rectus lightly helps seat the posterior part. (Courtesy of A. Momose.)

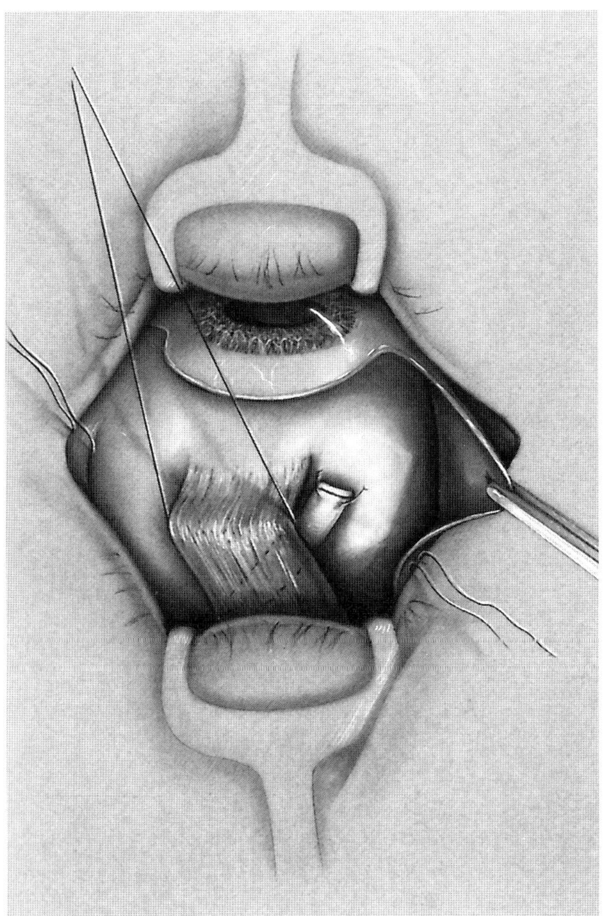

Fig. 13.19 The strip is passed beneath the superior rectus and over the superior oblique and sutured to the globe.

As the Arruga spoon is shifted from just superior to just inferior to the lateral rectus muscle, the scleral strip is checked to ensure that it is positioned correctly over the posterior pole. In this maneuver, only the very anterior edge of the strip should be seen. In the inferior temporal quadrant the strip should be clearly located posterior to the insertion of the posterior fibers of the inferior oblique. The surgeon will need to inspect this region several times to ensure proper placement of the strip. In some older patients, the inferior oblique is very flaccid and may not contract sufficiently. In this case the anesthesiologist will need to administer intravenous succinylcholine chloride to cause contracture of the extraocular muscles.

The traction suture around the lateral rectus is released by the assistant and the eye rotated superiorly. The explant is allowed to lie naturally against the globe in the inferior temporal quadrant. Often the strip will be seen to be too long, necessitating further excision of any excess. The strip is then sutured (with one suture of 5-0 collagen or Vicril) at a 45° angle just nasal and posterior to the insertion of the inferior rectus muscle (Figure 13.21). The needle is placed through the sclera slightly anterior to the position where the strip has been lying against the sclera. This ensures that some tension will be placed on the explant and that it is tight posteriorly when the suture is tied.

With the Arruga spoon, the surgeon once again examines the posterior pole, superior and inferior to the lateral rectus muscle. If the strip is tending to slide forward, it may be necessary to reposition it over the posterior pole. This is easier once the strip has been secured with a suture inferiorly. If the strip is still not fitting snugly against the sclera, the inferior suture can be removed. After an additional portion of the excess strip is excised, it can be resutured to the sclera in the manner previously described. The surgeon may need to perform this resuturing several times to achieve proper placement and tension of the scleral strip over the posterior pole. Again, only the anterior edge of the strip should be visible during maximum nasal rotation of the globe once its proper placement is assured. An extra suture is then placed through the strip in the inferior nasal quadrant (Figure 13.22).

The fundus is again inspected with the indirect ophthalmoscope. Occasionally, a slight indentation over the posterior pole can be seen but this may not appear until several months after the surgery. The surgeon inspects the optic nerve head, and central retinal artery and vein to make sure that the scleral strip has not compromised the blood supply to the optic nerve and retina. The macula is inspected for hemorrhage which can occur as a result of manipulation during the surgery, particularly in those cases where a subretinal neovascular membrane is present.

The IOP is checked with a Schiøtz tonometer. If the strip has been placed tightly over the posterior pole, the IOP may be elevated. Sometimes a partial temporary occlusion of the vortex veins may elevate the IOP as well. In these cases, intravenous mannitol 20% may be administered by the anesthesiologist to soften the eye.

The surgeon should make a final inspection of the posterior pole and scleral strip with the Arruga spoon. Once the strip is confirmed to be in position, the traction sutures around the extraocular muscles are removed. A small amount of Garamycin (gentamicin sulfate) is irrigated posteriorly. The conjunctival incision is closed with a running suture of 6-0 plain gut or 8-0 Vicril. Gentamicin sulfate is injected subconjunctivally along with 1.0 ml of Celestone (betamethasone sodium).

Normally, a canthotomy is not necessary in performing scleral reinforcement. However, in some oriental eyes or in eyes with very small palpebral fissures, it may be necessary to perform a lateral canthotomy to ensure adequate visualization over the posterior pole. If this has been done, the canthotomy is closed routinely. The lid speculum is removed and Cortisporin (polymyxin β sulfate–bacitracin zinc–neomycin sulfate–hydrocortisone) oint-

(a)

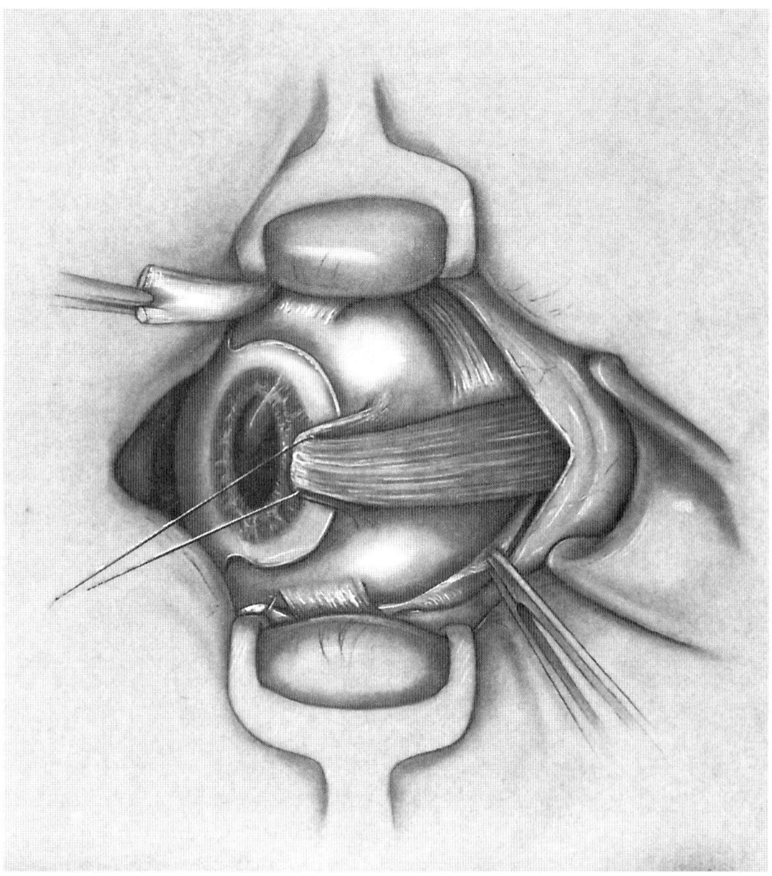

(b)

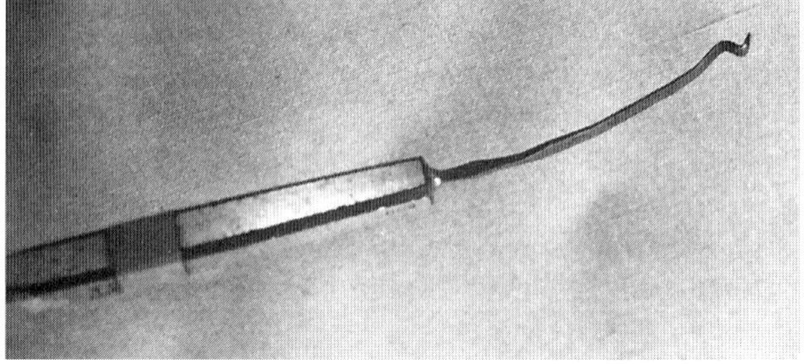

Fig. 13.20 The strip is positioned over the posterior pole with forceps (a) or with a specially bent iris spatula (b).

ment is instilled in the cul-de-sac. Benzoin is placed along the skin of the forehead and cheek; Elastoplast is applied over several eye patches as a pressure dressing.

Postoperative care

The patient remains in the hospital overnight for observation because there may be symptoms of pain, nausea, and vomiting similar to that experienced after retinal detachment surgery. Additionally, 8 mg of Decadron (dexamethasone sodium phosphate) *push* is administered intravenously immediately postoperatively and repeated 6 hours later. A final 8-mg dose is injected the morning following the surgery. That morning the dressing is changed, and the eye is inspected. There is usually a considerable amount of chemosis and lid edema despite the administration of the steroids—patching with ointment is repeated until this chemosis subsides and the lids close normally.

If 1% atropine or 5% homatropine drops were given preoperatively, the pupil should be dilated sufficiently for the fundus to be inspected the day following surgery. It is not crucial if the indentation from the scleral strip cannot be seen, however. Often some degree of choroidal edema or hemorrhage is present, particularly in the inferior temporal quadrant, although there have been no occurrences of vitreous hemorrhage reported following the surgery at this writing.

(a)

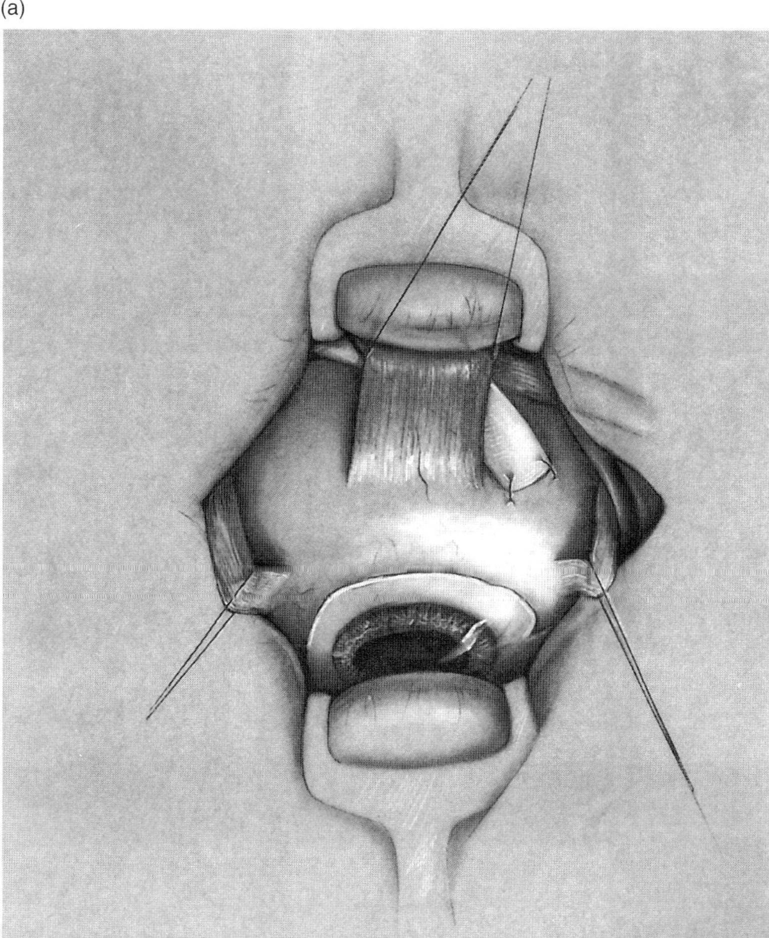

(b)

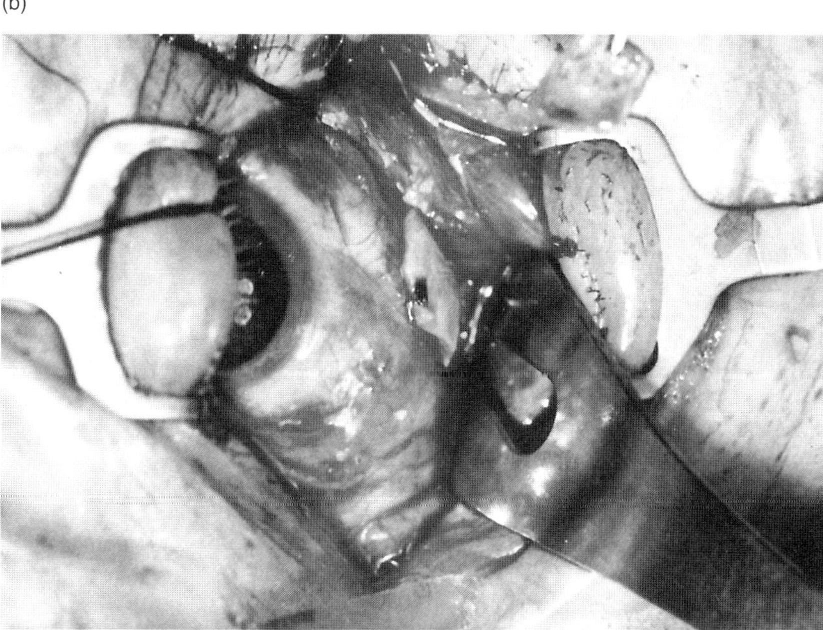

Fig. 13.21 (a,b) When the strip is correctly positioned, it is sutured just nasal, posterior to the insertion of the inferior rectus.

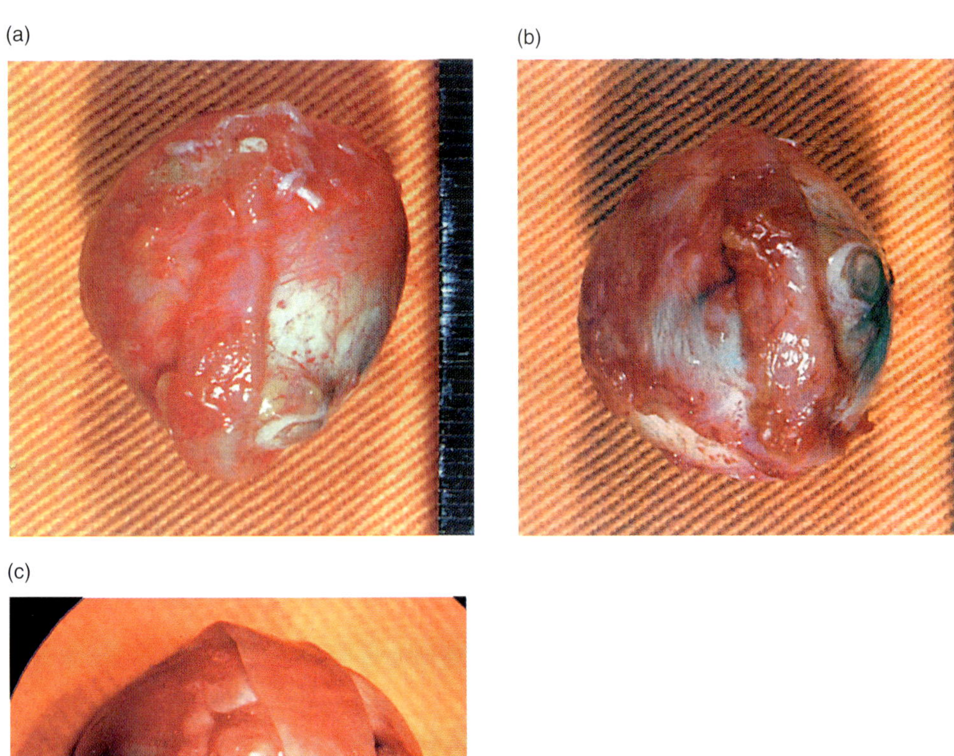

Fig. 13.22 (a–c) The proper positioning of the strip demonstrated on an enucleated eye. (Courtesy of A. Momose.)

Steroid ointment is again instilled and the eye repatched with a pressure dressing. The eye remains patched for 2 to 3 days following surgery depending on the degree of chemosis, lid edema, and discomfort.

The patient is examined again at 3 days, 1 week, 3 to 4 weeks, and then as indicated. Depending on the degree of chemosis and inflammation around the eye, the patient is prescribed 15 to 20 mg of oral prednisone to be continued in a tapered dosage for 2 to 3 weeks postoperatively. The dosage of prednisone may be changed depending on the degree of postoperative inflammation and choroidal edema and/or hemorrhage. Choroidal edema usually resolves 4 to 5 weeks following the surgery.

When the patch is discontinued, the patient is placed on steroid and antibiotic drops four times daily. The antibiotic drops are continued for a week postoperatively, while the steroid drops continue for 3 to 5 weeks following surgery.

A moderate degree of pain may persist for 2 to 3 days postoperatively. The patient can resume normal activities within 1 week from the date of surgery. Beginning 4 to 5 days postoperatively, the patient begins eye exercises consisting of looking as far as possible in the eight cardinal directions without moving the head. This may be quite uncomfortable for the first few days because the extraocular muscles are inflamed. The exercises are to be done for 1 min three times a day for 3 to 4 weeks. These exercises help prevent later adhesions and muscle imbalance. Because of conjunctival irritation and chemosis, contact lens wearers must be cautioned not to wear their contacts on the operated eye for at least 2 to 3 weeks following surgery. The patient should have spectacles to wear. If not, he or she must be certain before the surgery that he or she can function with a monocular contact lens.

Refraction and A-scan measurements can be made 6 to 8 weeks following surgery and are repeated at periodic intervals. This technique provides the most objective assessment of staphyloma stabilization or flattening (Figure 13.23).

(a)

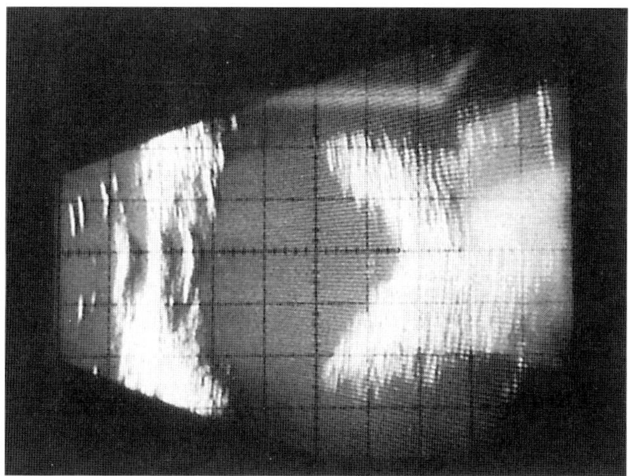

(b)

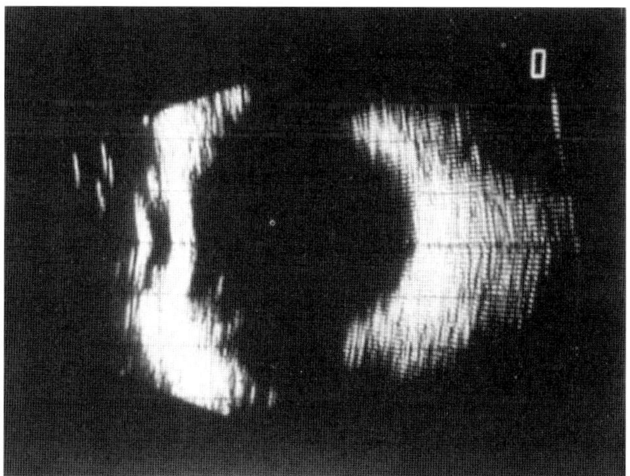

Fig. 13.23 B-scan of an eye before (a) and after (b) scleral reinforcement, demonstrating the flattening of the posterior pole.

If surgery on both eyes is indicated, the second is operated on 2 to 3 months after surgery on the fellow eye, providing stabilization has occurred before proceeding.

If there is any question about subsequent placement, relocation, or viability of the explant, computer scans (computed tomography or magnetic resonance imaging) can be of assistance. A computer scan provides clear imaging of the strip posteriorly. The graft's location and thickness can be easily seen. Because scans are expensive and tedious to the patient, they are indicated only in those cases where there is doubt about the placement or durability of the strip.

Complications

The discussion of complications which follows is taken from Thompson's study of 264 eyes (Table 13.2). The long-term complication rate for scleral reinforcement has been low using the single-strip approach. Short-term complications of marked chemosis and conjunctival injection occur almost without exception, and in all series. These are benign and quickly subside, although the chemosis may persist for 2 to 3 weeks. In some patients with small palpebral fissures, the conjunctiva may protrude between the lids during the first week.

Table 13.2 Complications in 264 scleral reinforcements followed from 6 months to 18 years of age. Adapted from Thompson FB. Scleral reinforcement. In: *Myopia Surgery. Anterior and Posterior Segments*, FB Thompson (ed). Macmillan, New York, 1990

Complication	Eyes
Choroidal edema or hemorrhage (resolved without therapy)	10
Corneal dellen (resolved within 6 weeks)	2
Chemosis	264
Retinal detachment	2
Optic atrophy	0

There has been a 3% to 4% incidence of postoperative choroidal edema or hemorrhage, usually in the inferior temporal quadrant. This is probably secondary to compression of the inferior vortex vein by the strip, resulting in choroidal congestion.

In some cases damage to the vortex vein may occur during the surgery itself because the exit of the vein is very close to the area where the inferior oblique is isolated. This is especially true for some oriental eyes that have narrow palpebral fissures. In these cases, the surgeon may have difficulty visualizing the exit of the vein while isolating the inferior oblique, and damage to the vein can result. These cases have resolved with systemic steroid therapy and have shown no incidence of retinal or vitreous hemorrhage. There are no cases of postoperative infection or instances where the strip has had to be removed.

A few patients will have transient motility problems following the surgery, but these normally resolve within 2 to 4 weeks. There is a low incidence of such problems because the extraocular muscles are not removed during the surgery and the superior oblique muscle is left untouched. The muscle exercises begun 4 to 5 days following the procedure have most likely contributed to the good result.

The only long-term problems involved two patients with preexisting muscle imbalances. Both had preoperative exophoria and hypertropia which had been corrected with prisms. These patients experienced a mild increase in their exophoria and hypertropia which required additional prismatic correction. Such patients should be warned that such problems may worsen following surgery.

Several instances of small corneal dellen have occurred in the temporal limbal margin anterior to the insertion of the lateral rectus muscle. This probably reflects temporary interference with the circulation of the anterior segment. It also should be noted that the surface of the anterior globe has been greatly disturbed, and tearing will not be normal during the first few weeks. All such cases cleared within 4 to 6 weeks of ocular lubricant therapy.

Two cases of retinal detachment are reported in Thompson's series. One of these presented at 10 years postoperatively and the other at 7 years. These were not deemed complications of the reinforcement surgery itself, however. Both occurred as a consequence to the later development of lattice degeneration and of retinal tears and holes not present at the time of surgery. An 8% incidence of retinal detachment following scleral surgery is less than that reported for such complications occurring among high myopes at large.

The few published reports of optic nerve damage following scleral reinforcement have all used a Y-shaped or a cruciate graft instead of the single scleral strip. Using either a Y- or cruciate-shaped graft can lead to the graft pulling too tightly against the optic nerve, which may then occlude the posterior ciliary vessels. The competence of the short and long posterior ciliary vessels and of the vortex veins must always be respected. The use of a horizontal band of donor sclera that fits closely about the optic nerve produced serious complications in one small series because of circulatory decompensation [77].

There have been no cases of optic nerve damage or optic atrophy among Thompson's cases. This can be explained by the fact that a large cushion of fat and connective tissue surrounds the optic nerve at its exit from the globe, protecting the nerve head. Furthermore, the single scleral strip does not press tightly enough against the optic nerve to cause permanent damage.

Theoretically, IOP could be elevated long enough postoperatively to occlude the central retinal artery. This can be a potential problem for the older patient with poor arterial circulation. Because of this, the surgical team should carefully monitor IOP before, during, and immediately after surgery. This monitoring is especially important for the eye with a tight orbit. In this case, retroorbital bleeding can significantly increase pressure on the posterior vessels and nerve.

Results

All scleral reinforcements included in Thompson's series were performed on patients who had deteriorating vision, fluorescein angiographic evidence of pathology, and increasing axial length. Among the 264 scleral reinforcements, 16 eyes were lost to follow-up. Figure 13.24 shows the visual acuity results of 224 patients with an average follow-up of 5.63 years. A decrease in acuity was defined as a loss of two Snellen lines on the visual chart. The findings show 26 (11.6%) of the patients had a decrease in acuity, while 198 (88.4%) either stabilized or showed improved acuity. Of these 198, 143 (63.8%) were stable and 55 (24.6%) had improved vision.

The frequency distribution seen in Figure 13.25 has an abscissa representing the number of lines of acuity change.

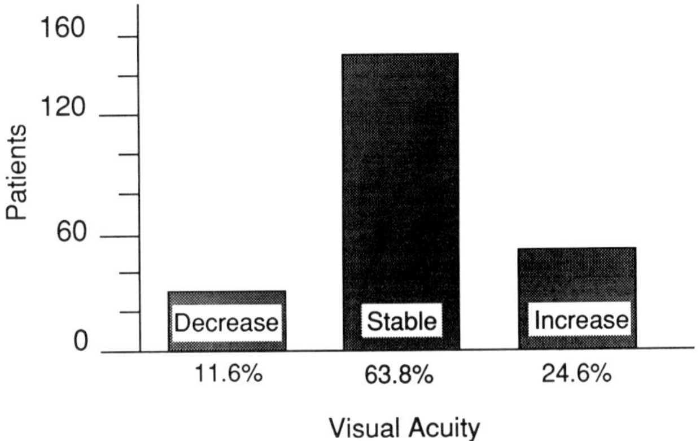

Fig. 13.24 Effect of scleral reinforcement on the visual acuity in Thompson's series.

The curve is skewed to the right, indicating an influencing factor toward improved acuity in these patients. This is contrary to the usual, natural course in pathologic myopes. Among those who had preoperative and postoperative fluorescein angiography, approximately 90% exhibited stabilized angiographic changes.

The data provided in Figure 13.26 summarize the changes in axial length of a group of 77 patients with an average follow-up of 3.54 years. The criterion for judging an eye to have changed in length was the repeatable measurement of a change of 0.3 mm or greater. This represents the smallest change which can reasonably be expected to be discriminated ultrasonically as an indication of lengthening or shortening of the eye.

At this level of statistical significance of 0.3 mm the results showed an increase in axial length in 16 (20.8%) out of 77 eyes. Stability or decrease in axial length was found in 61 (79.2%) eyes.

The frequency distribution of axial length changes presented in Figure 13.27 uses axial length change as the abscissa. The skew to the left indicates a force for stabilization or decrease in axial length which is equal to or greater than the force for elongation in the majority of eyes followed. Again this is contrary to the expected findings in any group of highly myopic eyes left to evolve naturally.

A scatterplot showing a linear regression of pre- and postoperative measurements is presented in Figure 13.28. The efficacy of scleral reinforcement surgery provided to the eye is suggested by the simple regression line slope of 0.976. In the author's two cases, both eyes retained stable axial lengths, as measured by A-scan and refraction.

Discussion

High myopia, defined as greater than –8.00 D, is diagnosed in 3% to 5% of all myopic patients. The condition is the fourth to seventh leading cause of blindness, depending on the geographic area surveyed. High myopia is the seventh leading cause of blindness in the United States

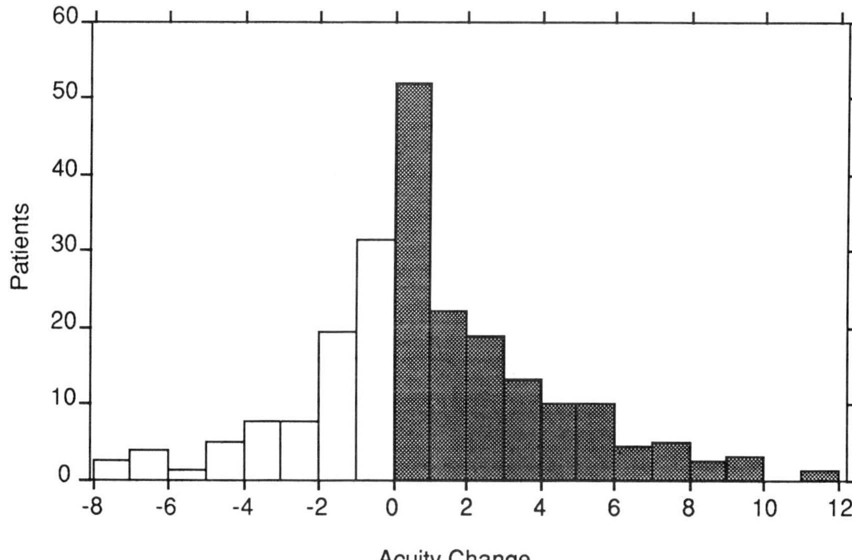

Fig. 13.25 Distribution of the visual acuity changes in this group.

[15]. The incidence of myopic blindness increased from 0.1% in children under 5 years of age to 0.6% in the aged in Kahn and Moorhead's study [78]. The sharpest increase was noted to occur in the middle of the fifth decade. This, unfortunately, coincides with that period of life in which the talents and productivity of those affected are at a maximum, as well as with that time at which there is a peak in financial responsibility; thus, the impact of this blindness upon the family is particularly severe.

In some areas of the world high myopia is much more common than it is in the United States. There appears to be a high concentration of high myopia in northern Italy and Sicily, for example. The data from the United Kingdom are of particular note because of Sorsby's interest in myopia [79]. In an early survey of blindness in England and Wales, he found myopia to be the second most frequent cause of blindness in persons between the ages of

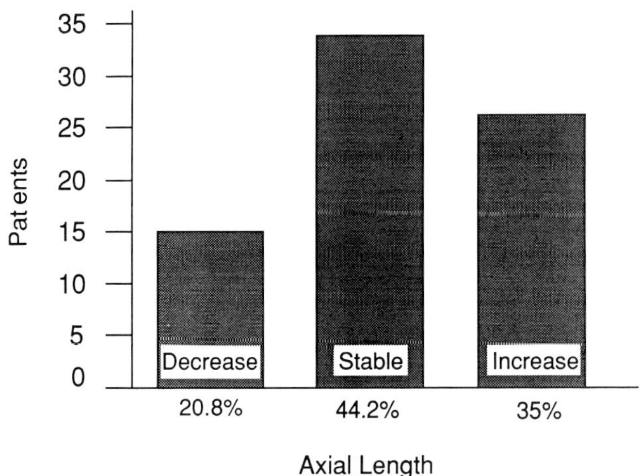

Fig. 13.26 The effect of scleral reinforcement on the axial length of 77 patients in Thompson's series.

30 and 49 years. In the next age group (50 to 69 years) it ranked second only to cataract. Certain areas in Asia, such as China and Japan, report a prevalence of this condition in 15% to 20% of the population. In some Japanese prefectures, high myopia and its complications are the most common cause of blindness recorded. In China and Japan, ophthalmologists attribute high myopia among students (in their late teens to early 20s) to the intensive study of small printed characters. However, this has not been substantiated by formal study.

The prevalence of ametropia also varies with age. The typical incidence of myopia at age 6 months is 4% to 6%. The overall incidence of myopia among school children ranges from 4% in ages 4 to 14 in England to 25% in the same age group in Japan. In the United States, the large HANES study examined the incidence of myopia among youths aged 12 to 17 and found that the incidence rose from 29.3% at age 12 to 33.2% at age 17 (see also Chapter 2) [80].

The principal cause of permanent blindness from high myopia is the development of posterior staphylomata with subsequent choroidal and retinal deterioration. In highly myopic eyes, staphylomata occur in areas nasal and temporal to the optic nerve, and occasionally posterotemporal and anterotemporal.

Scleral reinforcement offers the only treatment for the posterior staphyloma which destroys the retinal pigment epithelium, choroid, and retinal tissue in these highly myopic patients. The aims of this treatment are to:

1 Stop progression of the disease process.
2 Maintain and/or improve vision (especially in younger patients).
3 Reduce staphyloma formation.
4 Reduce or stop further macular damage.

The results reported in Thompson's 264 patients over a 20-year period are good, whether measured by visual acu-

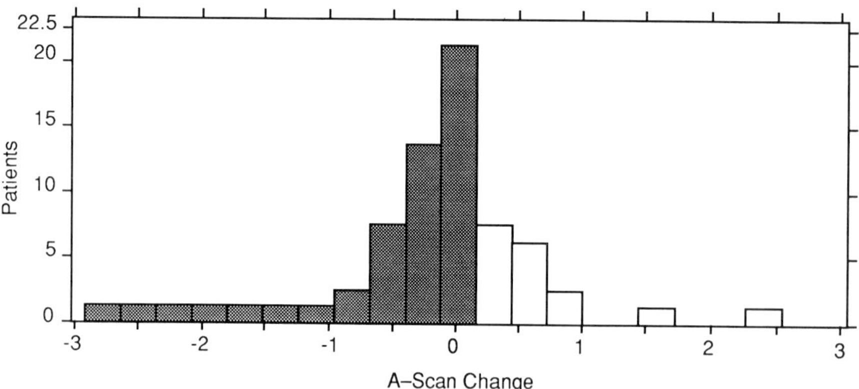

Fig. 13.27 Distribution of the effect on axial length.

ity, fluorescein angiographic changes, or axial length measurements. All the data show the treatment to be effective in a high percentage of cases. Also, the complication rate is low. There have been no serious vision-threatening complications either during the surgery or in the immediate postoperative period.

Despite the good results reported in the series of Thompson [56], Miller [81], Borley [82], and Snyder [83], scleral reinforcement remains a controversial and ignored treatment in the United States. Scleral reinforcement is performed on a much more frequent basis by Fyodorov (6000 cases) and Krasnov in the former Soviet Union, Momose in Japan, Brian and Hollows [84,85] in Australia, and Hanczye et al. [86] in Poland, among others.

Acceptance of scleral reinforcement in the United States has been slow, partly because of unfamiliarity with the procedure and the scarcity of published clinical studies in the United States. Curtin's earlier series of scleral reinforcements using the cruciate graft approach has recently been reevaluated. Using refraction as the method of measurement, the authors reported discouraging long-term results in these patients. Several of these patients were adolescent, however, and younger patients can yield an inaccurate measurement of staphyloma stabilization. Yet, despite his disappointing analysis of the results,

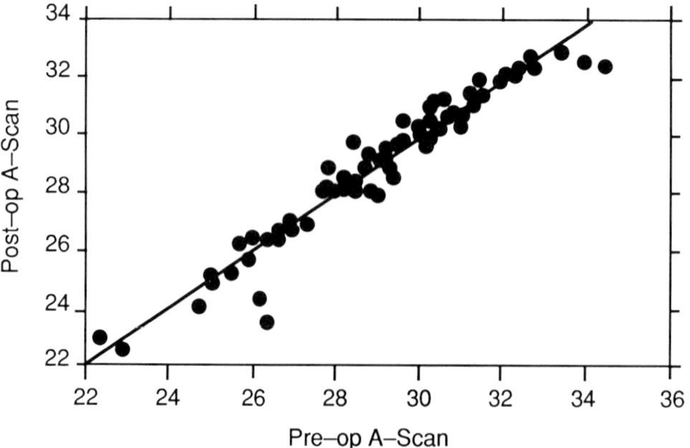

Fig. 13.28 Linear regression of preoperative versus postoperative axial lengths in 77 patients.

Curtin states that scleral reinforcement is the only rational method presently available for treating macular staphylomata [15].

Acquiring and storing sclera presents difficulties, especially to those doing a relatively small number of these cases per year. Additionally, human sclera varies in quality depending on the donor eye from which it was obtained. The search for an adequate artificial material as a replacement of sclera for reinforcement until recently has been disappointing. Kaufman has suggested Gore-Tex as a possible replacement for human sclera (H. E. Kaufman, 1990, personal communication). If a synthetic material provides a satisfactory substitute, it could be sterilized and stored without freezing. The synthetic strips could be a standard size, length, and thickness and, with this in mind, a template has been developed to ensure uniformity (F. B. Thompson, 1990, personal communication).

Until now, other materials have been more difficult than human sclera either to work with or place in situ. Artificial materials such as Silastic or silicone bands are unsatisfactory because these materials erode the already thin sclera under the band or strip. When reoperating for retinal detachment even in normal eyes, it is not uncommon to see that the sclera is thinned under a silicone sponge or band. This could be devastating to the existing thin sclera over the posterior pole of the myopic eye. Gore-Tex may avoid this problem, since it is more flexible than silicone.

American ophthalmologists seem to be reluctant to accept the efficacy of scleral reinforcement until there is a prospective, controlled study. Scleral reinforcement has been performed over 6000 times in the former Soviet Union by Fyodorov's team (S. N. Fyodorov, 1990, personal communication). Momose in Japan has performed between 1000 and 2000 scleral reinforcements, most of them using a similar single-strip technique (A. Momose, 1990, personal communication). The extensiveness of the follow-up of these international series is unknown, but published results are similar to American studies.

Although the type of measurements and criteria used to determine efficacy can vary from surgeon to surgeon, the results seem to indicate prevention of further visual loss from myopic degeneration. A universal protocol needs to be established to measure the success and complication rate for this surgery.

In the United States, a multicentered investigation, being developed by Thompson, the LSU Eye Center in New Orleans, and Retinal Associates in Boston, proposes to conduct a randomized study of scleral reinforcement. Surgery would be performed on one eye and compared with the contralateral eye to evaluate long-term results. Gore-Tex and other artificial materials would be compared to human sclera. The study would be designed to follow patients for a period of 5 to 10 years. It will involve a long-term control study with strict criteria of pre- and postoperative measurements to evaluate the effectiveness of scleral reinforcement surgery. This study should finally settle the 60-year-old question about the value of scleral reinforcement.

While there may be controversy over this methodology or whether our current techniques are effective over the long haul, the fact remains that scleral reinforcement remains the only rational method of increasing scleral resistance in eyes with progressive myopia and posterior staphyloma formation. Patients will continue to suffer further damage to their retinas and posterior circulation from progression of their pathologic myopia in the absence of a mode of reinforcing their "blown-out" scleras. While waiting for the control study, ophthalmic surgeons may want to seriously consider implementing scleral reinforcement therapy for highly myopic patients, since there is currently no effective or alternative treatment. The option is watchful waiting and sympathy, neither of which is of much benefit to the patient and of even less effect on the pathology.

References

1 Algan B. (The treatment of progressive malignant myopia with magnesium chelates of flavones. Apropos of 400 cases.) Bull Soc Belge Ophtalmol 1981; 192:103–112.

2 Smelovaskii AS, Golychev VN, Khomullo GV. Ob ispol'zovanii kal'tsitonina pri progressiruiushchei blizorukosti. (Use of calcitonin in progressive myopia.) Vestn Oftalmol 1988; 104:45–47.

3 Armaly M, Burian H. Changes in the tonogram during accommodation. Arch Ophthalmol 1958; 60:60

4 Abdulla MI, Hamdi M. Applanation ocular tension in myopia and emmetropia. Br J Ophthalmol 1970; 54:122–125.

5 McCollim RJ. On the nature of myopia and the mechanism of accommodation. Med Hypotheses 1989; 28:197–211.

6 Bubolts L. Medvetskaia G. Opyt organizatsii pionerskikh lagerei sanatornogo tipa dlia detei s blizorukost'iu na baze obshcheozdorovitel'nykh lagerei i rezul'taty lecheniia v nikh. (Experience in organizing sanatorium-type pioneer camps for children with myopia based on general health-improvement camps and the results of their treatment.) Vestn Oftalmol 1980; 2:69–71.

7 Diaz-Dominguez D. Mas sobre miopia e hipertension ocular. Arch Soc Oftalmol Hisp-Am 1966; 26:935.

8 Diaz-Dominguez D, Montero Marchena J. Miopia media y tension ocular. Arch Soc Oftalmol Hisp-Am 1966; 26:241.

9 Fledelius HC. Distensibility of the young eye. Doc Ophthalmol 1981; 28:117.

10 Tarkkanen A, Uusitalo R, Mianowicz J. Ultrasonic biometry in congenital glaucoma. Acta Ophthalmol (Copenh) 1983; 61:618.

11 Kamali K, Hamdi M. Relation between applanation tonometry and errors of refraction. Ain Shams Med J 1969; 20:235.

12 Burton EW. Progressive myopia: A possible etiologic factor. Trans Am Ophthalmol Soc 1942; 40:340.

13 Bedrossian EH. Progressive myopia with glaucoma. Am J Ophthalmol 1952; 35:485.

14 Tomlinson A, Phillips CI. Applanation tension and axial length of the eyeball. Br J Ophthalmol 1970; 54:548–553.

15 Curtin BJ. *The Myopias: Basic Science and Clinical Management.* Harper & Row, New York, 1985.

16 Perkins ES. Morbidity from myopia. Sight Sav Rev 1979; 49:11–19.

17 Podos SM, Becker B, Morton WR. High myopia and primary open-angle glaucoma. Am J Ophthalmol 1966; 62:1038–1043.

18 Amba SK, Jain IS, Gupta SD. Topical corticosteroid and intraocular pressure in high myopia: I. Study of pressure response. Ind J Ophthalmol 1973; 21:102.

19 Jain IS, Amba SK, Gupta SD. Topical corticosteroid and intraocular pressure in high myopia: II. Study of pressure response to age, dioptric power, degenerative changes in the eye and scleral rigidity. Ind J Ophthalmol 1973; 21:108.

20 Grunert K. Verhutung und Behandlung der Kurzsichtigkeit und ihrer Folgeerscheinungen. Klin Monatsbl Augenheilkd 1928; 81:521.

21 Landolt E. *The Refraction and Accommodation of the Eye.* Young J. Pentland, Edinburgh, 1886.

22 Dransart H. Traitement du décollement de la rétine et de la myopie progressive par l'iridectomie, la sclérotomie et la pilocarpine. Ann Oculist (Paris) 1884; 92:30.

23 Holth S. Neue operative Behandlung der Netzhautablosung und der hochgradiger Myopie. Ber Zusammenkunft Dtsch Ophthalmol Ges 1911; 37:293.

24 Freide R. A modified cyclodialysis and its use in the treatment of juvenile progressive malignant myopia. Ophthalmologica 1959: 137:282.

25 Harlan GC. Rapidly progressive myopia permanently checked by division of the external rectus. Trans Am Ophthalmol Soc 1885; 4:24.

26 Donders FC. *On the Anomalies of Accommodation and Refraction of the Eye,* WD Moore (transl). Hatton Press, London, 1864.

27 Bourdeaux. Le traitment des myopies extremes. Bull Soc Ophtalmol Fr 1914; 31:670.

28 Ivashina AI, Mikhailova GD, Balashova NV, Ioffe DI, Nikitin IM: Vazokompressiia glaza pri progressiruiushchei blizorukosti i kontrol' za ee effektivnost'iu (predvaritet'noe soobshchenie). [Ocular vasocompression in progressive myopia and the follow-up of its efficacy (preliminary report).] Vestn Oftalmol 1988; 104: 31–34.

29 Bates WH. *The Bates Method for Better Eye Sight without Glasses.* Henry Holt, New York, 1943.

30 Dianoux. Myopie et myotiques. Clin Ophthalmol 1912; 18:68.

31 Domec M. Massage. Pression. Myotiques. Myopie. Arch Ophthalmol 1912; 32:391.

32 Yamamoto Y. Hand ophthalmic supersonic therapeutic instrument. Jpn J Clin Ophthalmol 1963; 17:295.

33 Yamamoto Y. Ultrasonic treatment of acquired myopia. Ganka 1964; 6:935

34 von Ammon FA. Die Entwickelungensgeschicte des menschlichen Auges. Albrecht Graefes Arch Ophthamol 1858; 4:1.

35 Sondermann R. Beitrag zur Frage der Myopie-genese. Klin Monatstbl Augenheilkd 1950; 117:573.

36 Sondermann R. Zur Frage der Myopiaprophylaxe. Klin Monatstbl Augenheilkd 1951; 119:178.

37 Sondermann R. Beitrag zur Genese und Prophylaxe der Myopie. Ber Zusammenkunft Dtsch Ophthalmol Ges 1951; 56:96.

38 Scarpa AA. *A Treatise on the Principal Diseases of the Eye.* J. Bregg, London, 1818.

39 von Arlt CF. *Ueber die Ursachsen und die Entsehung der Kurzichtigkeit.* Wilhelm Braumuller, Vienna, 1856.

40 von Ammon FA. Uber die angebornen Spaltungen in der Iris, Chorioidea und Retina des Menschlichen Auges. [About congenital colobomas of the iris, choroid and retina in the human eye.] Ophthalmologie 1831; 1:55.
41 von Graefe A. Zwei Sektionbefunde von Scleratio-Chronivites posterior und Bermerbegen uber diese Krankeit. Arch Ophthalmol 1854; 1:390.
42 von Jaeger E. *Beitrage zur Pathologie das Auges.* Kaiserlich-Konigliche, Hof-und Staatsdruckerei Vienna, 1870.
43 Curtin BJ. Surgical support of the posterior sclera, Part I, Experimental results. Am J Ophthalmol 1960; 49:1341.
44 Johnson WA. Transplantation of homografts of sclera on eye of dog, including volume determination: experimental study. Thesis, 1961.
45 Johnson WA, Henderson JW, Parkhill EM. Transplantation of homografts of sclera. Am J Ophthalmol 1962; 54:1019.
46 Rubin ML. Surgical procedures available for influencing refractive error. In: *Refractive Anomalies of the Eye,* US Government Printing Office, Washington, 1966.
47 Muller. Eine neue operative Behandlung der Netzhaut abhebung. Klin Monatstbl Augenheilk 1903; 41:459.
48 Shevelev MM. Operation against high myopia and sclerectasia with the aid of transplantation of fascia lata on thinned sclera. Russian Ophthalmol J 1930; 11:107.
49 Malbran J. Una nueva orientacion quirurgica contra la miopia. Arch Soc Oftalmol Hisp-Am 1954; 14:1167.
50 Borley WE, Snyder AA. Surgical treatment of high myopia. Trans Am Acad Ophthalmol Otolaryngol 1958; 62:791.
51 Miller WW, Borley WE. Surgical treatment of degenerative myopia. Trans Pac Coast Otoophthalmol Soc 1963; 44:155–171.
52 Miller WW, Borley WE. Surgical treatment of degenerative myopia. Am J Ophthalmol 1964; 57:796.
53 Snyder AA, Thompson FB. A simplified technique for surgical treatment of degenerative myopia. Am J Ophthalmol 1972; 74: 273–277.
54 Curtin BJ. Surgical support of the posterior sclera, Part II, clinical results. Am J Ophthalmol 1961; 52:853.
55 Miller WW. Surgical treatment of degenerative myopia; scleral reinforcement. Trans Am Acad Ophthalmol Otolaryngol 1974; 78:896.
56 Thompson FB. A simplified scleral reinforcement technique. Am J Ophthalmol 1978; 86:782.
57 Curtin BJ. The natural history of posterior staphyloma development. Doc Ophthalmol 1981; 28:207.
58 Curtin BJ, Whitmore W. Long-term results of scleral reinforcement surgery. Am J Ophthalmol 1987; 103:544.
59 Andrzejewska W. Further therapeutic results in progressive myopia by means of meridional cicumligation. Klin Oczna 1972; 42:263.
60 Belyaev VS. Some possibilities of treatment of high progressive myopia. In *Proceedings of the Third All-Russian Congress of Ophthalmologists.* Tipographia Vashnil, Moscow, 1975.
61 Belyaev VS, Ilyina TS. Late results of scleroplasty in surgical treatment of progressive myopia. Eye Ear Nose Throat Mon 1975; 54:109–112.
62 Eroschevskii TI, Panfilov NI. Meridional'noe ukruplenie sklery shirokoi fastsiei bedrapri progressiruiushchei blizorukosti. [Meridional reinforcement of the sclera with femoral fascia lata in progressive myopia.] Vestn Oftalmol 1970; 2:19–23.
63 Panfilov NI, IuV S. Otdalennye rezul'taty operatsii meridional'nogo ukrepleniia sklery skirokoi fastesiei bedra pri progressiruiushchei blizorukosti. [Remote results of the operation of meridional fixation of the sclera with broad fascia of the hip in progressive myopia.] Oftalmol Zh 1974; 29:130–133.
64 Alberth B, Nagy Z, Berta A. Combined surgical procedure for the prevention of blindness caused by progressive high myopia. Acta Chir Hung 1988; 29:3–13.
65 Hanczye P. Surgical treatment of progressive high myopia: I. age of patients, observation, time and visual acuity. Klin Oczna 1972; 42:269.
66 Starkiewicz W. Meridional circumligation: a new method of surgical treatment of progressive myopia. Klin Oczna 1965; 35:363.
67 Starkiewicz W, Markiewicz-Jablonska E. Pierwsze wyniki leczenia postepujacej krotkowzrocznosci za pomoca circumligatio meridionalis. [First results in the treatment of progressive myopia by means of circumligatio meridionalis.] Klin Oczna 1967; 37:831–838.
68 Nesterov AP, Libenson NB. Ukreplenie sklery shirokoi fastsiei bedra pri progressiruiushchei blizorukosti. [Stengthening of the sclera with the broad fascia of the hip in progressive myopia.] Vestn Oftalmol 19667; 80:15–19.
69 Nesterov AP, Libenson NB. Strengthening the sclera with a strip of fascia lata in progressive myopia. Br J Ophthalmol 1970; 54: 46–50.
70 Nesterov AP, Libenson NB, Svirin AV. Early and late results of fascia lata transplantation in high myopia. Br J Ophthalmol 1976; 60:271–272.
71 Nesterov AP, Svirin AV, Antipova OA. Scleral reinforcement. J Ocular Ther Surg 1984; 3:255.
72 Zarkova MV, Negoda VI. Grafting of homologous sclera in progressive myopia. Vestn Oftalmol 1970; 49:16.
73 Whitwell J. Scleral reinforcement in degenerative myopia. Trans Ophthalmol Soc UK 1971; 91:79–86.
74 Momose A. Posterior scleral support operation combined with extraction of lens in high myopia, two stage operation. Excerpta Medica 1979; 2/450:1232.
75 Momose A. Surgical correction of myopia. J Korean Ophthalmol 1983; 24:717.
76 Pruett RC. Refractive surgery: psychophysical considerations in progressive myopia. Ann Acad Med Singapore 1989; 18: 131–135.
77 Barraquer T, Barraquer JI. Nueva orientacion terapeutica en la miopia progresiva. Arch Soc Oftal Hisp-Am 1956; 16:137.
78 Kahn H, Moorhead U. *Statistics on Blindness in the Model Reporting Area.* US Government Printing Office, Washington, 1970.
79 Sorsby A. The incidence and causes of blindness: an international survey. Br J Ophthalmol 1950; 34 (suppl):13–14.
80 Sperduto R, Seigel D, Roberts J, Rowland M. Prevalence of myopia in the United States. Arch Ophthalmol 1983; 10: 405–407.
81 Miller WW, Borley WE. Surgical treatment of degenerative myopia. Trans Pac Coast Otoophthalmol Soc 1963; 44:155–171.
82 Borley WE, Snyder AA. Surgical treatment of high myopia. Trans Am Acad Ophthalmol Otolaryngol 1958; 62:791.
83 Snyder AA, Thompson FB. A simplified technique for surgical treatment of degenerative myopia. Am J Ophthalmol 1972; 74: 273–277.
84 Brian GR, Hollows FC. Sling markers in scleral reinforcement surgery. Ophthalmic Surg 1988; 19:647–648.
85 Coroneo MT, Beaumont JT, Hollows FC. Scleral reinforcement in the treatment of pathologic myopia. Aust NZ J Ophthalmol 1988; 16:317–320.
86 Hanczye P, Uher M, Koziorowska M. Circumligatio meridionalis. Uwagi dotyczace techniki operacyjnej oraz powikLan drugiego etapu operacji. [Meridional circumligation. Observations on the surgical method and the complications in the second stage of the operation.] Klin Oczna 1982; 84:325–327.

14
Surgery for Hyperopia

. . . we have come to rely upon a comfortable time lag of fifty years or a century intervening between the perception that something ought to be done and a serious attempt to do so.
[H. G. Wells]

Refractive surgery seems to be about myopia and myopic astigmatism. In a review of existing literature, less than 10% of the articles dealing with the surgical treatment of ametropia—excluding aphakia—are about hyperopia. Although the first spectacles were prescribed in 1290 for hyperopia (actually, for presbyopia) not myopia, it was not until almost 300 years later that myopes had some relief from their affliction in the form of glasses.

Perhaps it is because myopes need a correction most of the time, or perhaps it is because they are more vociferous [1–3]. Whatever the reason, myopia has received the lion's share of attention, and hyperopia, at least as far as surgical correction is concerned, is the orphan child. Yet a significant number of the world's population (almost 50% or more in most countries) are hyperopic *de novo*, not to mention those cases iatrogenically produced through one means or another [4]. Grosvenor maintains that hyperopia represents a significant impediment to the learning process [5]. Evidence exists connecting it with behavioral problems as well as low academic standing among elementary school children (see Chapter 2).

In addition, while simple procedures for myopia abound, those for hyperopia are, however, like they said in the *Wizard of Oz*, a horse of a different color. Radial keratotomy (RK) for myopia is a cinch compared with the problem of hyperopia. Here, the challenge is to induce *steepening* of the central cornea instead of merely flattening it—not a simple matter. Flattening is practically automatic; with relaxing incisions, the intraocular pressure (IOP) does the job for you—not so for steepening.

Hyperopia is difficult to treat surgically. Nearly a dozen techniques strive toward safe, effective outcomes. And all techniques face three challenges:

1 The need for accurate centration over the pupil of a steeper central optical zone approximately 5 mm in diameter

2 The potential decreased visual acuity caused by image size [6,7]

3 The creation of corneal contours with physiologic characteristics able to minimize optical aberrations and regression of initial refractive effect

Excimer laser photorefractive keratectomy (PRK) and laser in situ keratomileusis (LASIK) for hyperopia are being developed with ongoing changes in ablation algorithms [8,9] (see Chapter 11). Thermal keratoplasty with a pulsed holmium:YAG laser has been plagued by marked regression of effect when attempting to treat more than approximately +1.00 D of hyperopia [10,11]. An infrared continuous-wave diode laser (wavelength of 1.9 μm) is also being studied in clinical trials [12]. Plus-power phakic intraocular lenses (IOLs) face the design challenge of being placed in hyperopic eyes that often have shallower anterior chambers and less surgical space for implantation than do myopic eyes [13]. Variable grating-type lenses or lens with higher indices of refraction may help surmount some of these problems. Clear lens extraction for high hyperopia with placement of one or two IOLs in the capsular bag or ciliary sulcus has successfully treated some patients who otherwise would have had considerable visual disability [14]. Intracorneal lenses have a 50-year history of unsuccessful clinical trials in the treatment of hyperopia and aphakia [15] (see Chapter 10). Newer surgical techniques, however, such as radially placed intracorneal polymethyl methacrylate stents (see Chapter 10) and keratophakia with new synthetic lenticules, may be the answer. Intracorneal lenses with small diameters and high indices of refraction were studied in a small number of eyes, but decreased quality of vision led to termination of the research without publication of results [16].

Some other methods for surgical correction of hyperopia have experienced transient popularity until the high rate of complications and lack of predictability caused them to fade quietly away: *hot-needle thermal keratoplasty*, which produced focal corneal necrosis and an unstable refraction; *hexagonal keratotomy*, which commonly produced irregular astigmatism; and *hyperopic automated lamellar keratoplasty* (see Chapter 10), which produced progressive corneal ectasia in some eyes (see also Chapter 15).

While this chapter will try to make some sense of it all, it is more historical and somewhat cautionary. Hyperopia remains an elusive problem to solve.

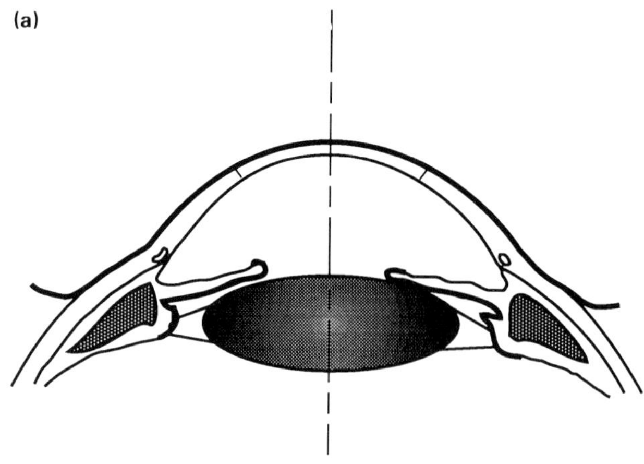

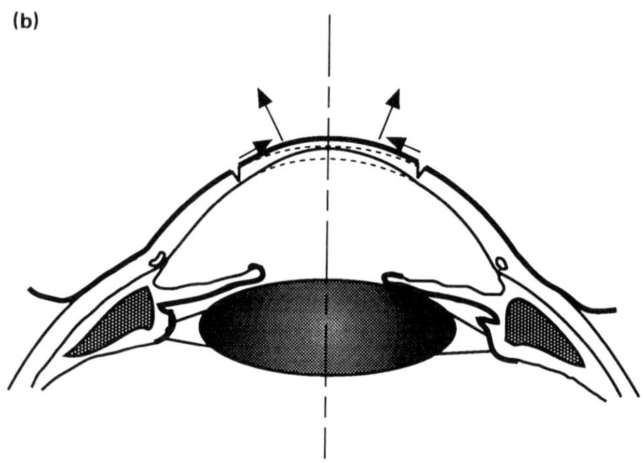

Fig. 14.1 Mechanism of hexagonal keratotomy. (a) The incisions weaken the corneal stroma cutting off all connection with the periphery. (b) The incisions gape, shortening the chord length. That plus the intraocular pressure increases the arc height.

Hexagonal keratotomy (HK)

In 1979, Yamashita, building on the work of Sato and the experience of Gills, experimented with closed-ended incisional configurations in rabbits [17–19]. He found the optimal configuration to be that of six incisions arranged and connected in the shape of a hexagon. By varying the diameter of the hexagon, he was able to induce an increase in the central corneal curvature proportional to the size of the hexagon, the mean change being 2.20 D. The mechanism is simply that of complete relaxation of the corneal cap. This allows the natural elasticity of the cornea and the IOP to increase the arc height of the apex (Figure 14.1).

These cases were first presented at the Keratorefractive Society in 1983, and Yamashita suggested that this technique might be a practical way to eliminate RK overcorrections [20–23]. Encouraged by this work, Mendez applied the technique to human corneas the same year [24]. By varying the size of the hexagon from 7.5 to 4.5 mm, up to 4 D of hyperopia could be reduced. Mendez found that a 6.0-mm hexagon resulted in a reduction in hyperopia of 1.50 D. A mean of 2.0 ± 0.75 D of correction resulted with a 5.5-mm hexagon and 3.0 ± 0.75 D with a 5.0-mm hexagon. The corneas remained fairly stable, and Mendez states that the overall patient complaints were less than with RK [25]. However, others reported that in some cases extreme gaping of the incisions occurred with resulting marsupialization and instability, as well as astigmatism [26]. In at least one case, severe central corneal edema with subsequent sloughing of tissue occurred, necessitating a penetrating keratoplasty. Predictability was only fair, and no account was taken of sex, age, or corneal elasticity in establishing the hexagon size, unlike RK.

In an effort to eliminate some of the postoperative complications, several authors advocated variations in the incision pattern ranging from open hexagons to overlapping apices [27]. The procedure quickly underwent a series of modifications aimed at decreasing the complications of poor wound healing, including anterior displacement of the central cornea, excessive scarring, and induced astigmatism. The modifications went from the initial intersecting hexagonal pattern to nonintersecting patterns and then to nonintersecting patterns with paracentral transverse incisions [25,27–29]. Many of these changes occurred as the procedure was promulgated in commercially sponsored RK skills-transfer courses with the enthusiastic endorsement of refractive surgeons who had extensive clinical experience, such as Mendez [25],

(a)

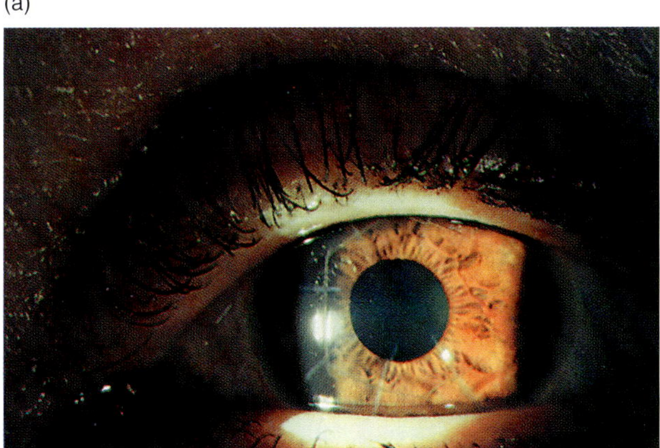

(b)

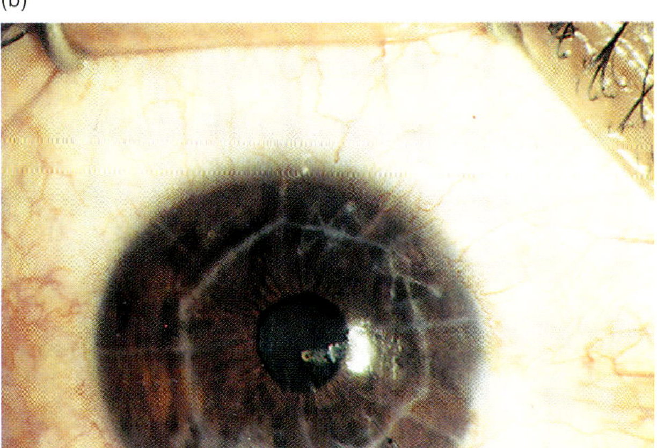

Fig. 14.2 (a) Hexagonal over radial keratotomy. Note the fairly clean intersection of the sides of the hex with the radials (see text). (b) Another case: note the sutures.

Jensen [30], and Casebeer and Phillips [29]. Many of the student ophthalmologists failed to ask: "*If the results reported in the presentations are so good, why are the surgical techniques changing so much?*"

Results

The author had six cases of HK in which moderate depth incisions were made with joined apices and whose hexagons were all 6.0 mm (see also Epilogue). Every one of these cases had severe central corneal instability, requiring suturing in one case, very like a corneal transplant, which instability lasted, in one form or another, for at least 5 years in each case. While this could be construed as an indictment against joining up of the incisions, this same phenomenon has occurred with the newer techniques, especially with smaller-diameter patterns.

Despite repeated removal and/or addition of sutures, each one of these cases demonstrated variable astigmatism (sometimes reaching as high as 7 D), and all required contact lenses, which were a "joy" to both fit and wear. Eventually, they all came right, thankfully. Other refractive surgeons using this technique experienced much the same thing, especially in cases of overcorrected RK [31] (Figure 14.2). Even waiting for at least 6 months before adding the hexagon over the RK radials did not save patients from the problems of instability and high astigmatism. Seemingly perfect cases eventually decline into episodes of unstable astigmatism (Figure 14.3).

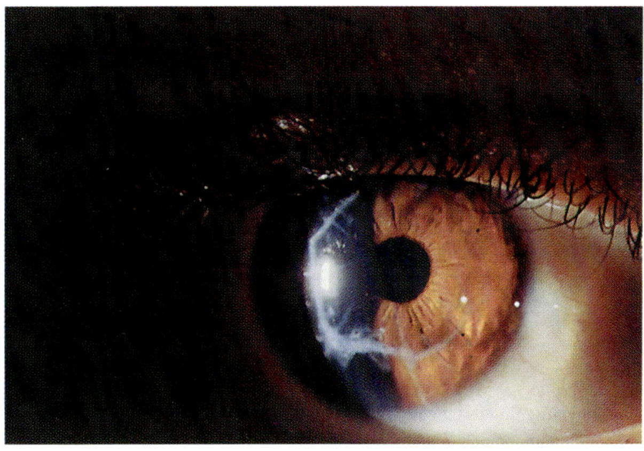

Fig. 14.3 A "run-of-the-mill" hexagonal keratotomy over RK. This patient eventually needed sutures.

Thermokeratoplasty

Is the cornea burning?

Never one to mince words (subtlety is not, alas, my strong suit), I will put it to you this way: I don't care a fig for these procedures, whether they use hot wires [32], lasers [33], or microwaves [34]. This attitude earned me some good-natured browbeating from Fyodorov after I refused to do his procedure, but the fact is that the track record for thermocoagulation techniques of any stripe has been dismal from the time of Lans to date. And I do not expect this to change. I again found myself in agreement with the Food and Drug Administration (FDA) when, at first, they refused to approve the Sunrise Technology procedure. The FDA has since given the company the green light (actually a kind of pistachio) to market the device. However, I predict that the device will fail.

I could turn out to be wrong, but even so, thermokeratoplasty will become moot because there are better procedures out there and they all have a head start. By the time thermokeratoplasty comes up to speed (if it ever does), it will be irrelevant. It is not titratable to any degree of comfort in my view; it is a "slam-bang" technique. No one can predict ahead of time how a particular cornea will respond to denaturization of its protein except to say that eventually the cornea re-forms itself.

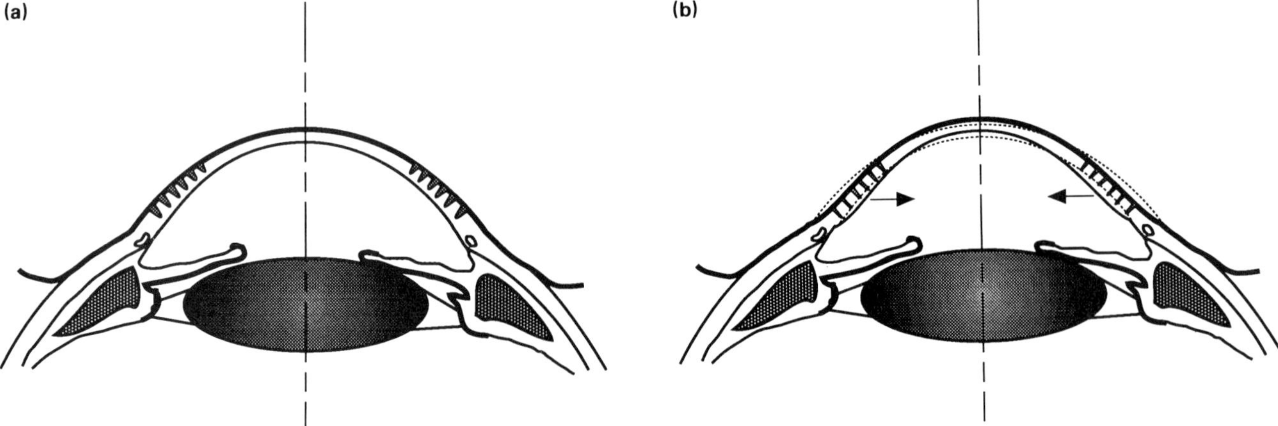

Fig. 14.4 Mechanism of thermokeratoplasty. (a) A series of deep punctate burns is made in the corneal periphery. (b) Shrinkage of the periphery occurs with concomitant increase in the central corneal curvature. This increase in arc height may also be accompanied by an increase in the depth of the anterior chamber, quite apart from that contributed by the steepening arc.

Keratoconus

Keratoconus differs from other forms of ametropia/ astigmatism in that the cornea is indisputably abnormal, suffering from a thinning and an anterior protrusion that often produces a high degree of myopia with associated visual distortion. Fitting of contact lenses is a challenge, and corneal transplantation, while highly successful, does not eliminate astigmatism. Almost all patients will continue to wear contacts after surgery. Therefore, it makes sense to delay keratoplasty until vision is no longer satisfactorily served by appliances.

The procedure of flattening the cornea by surface application of heat is not a new idea, having been employed in the last century (see Chapter 9). It was revived with new technology to facilitate contact lens fitting and to reduce the need for or at least delay corneal transplantation. The early report of success in 59 eyes observed from 2 months to 2 years was followed by observations of inadequate visual improvement in the majority of cases, and the procedure fell into disuse in America, although it stayed in active use in Japan, where donor tissue for corneal transplantation is scarce and religious prohibitions are still an obstacle [35–39].

In 1981, Fyodorov and his group expanded on the earlier work of Gudechkov by applying radial, partial punctiform burns to the peripheral cornea for hyperopia thermokeratoplasty (TKP) (Figure 14.4). Some investigators in the United States have reported success in treating hyperopia with this technique as well [40–44]. Applied with a specially designed, computer-controlled probe, these partial-thickness burns were said initially to have corrected up to 5 D of hyperopia.

The pattern of the burns is similar to RK in that the lesions are placed in a radial pattern (for spherical hyperopia) up to a premarked central optical zone (OZ) diameter. Only the peripheral cornea is treated, and the effect is titrated by varying the diameter of the OZ and the number of radials. Unlike RK, the burns flatten the corneal periphery in the area where they are placed and steepen the central cornea, thereby reducing or eliminating hyperopia (Figures 14.5 through 14.11).

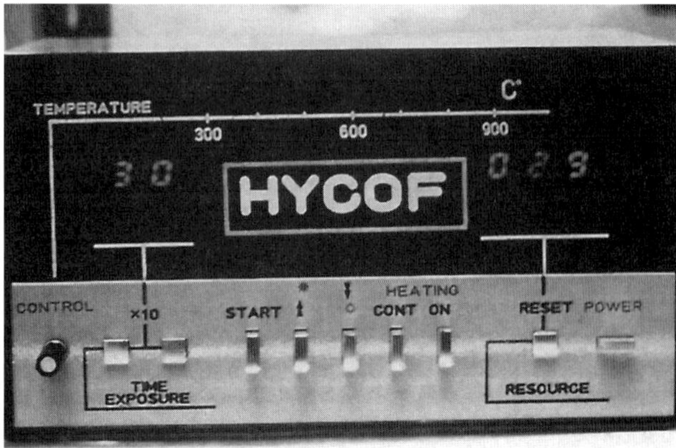

Fig. 14.5 Power unit for the thermokeratoplasty of Fyodorov.

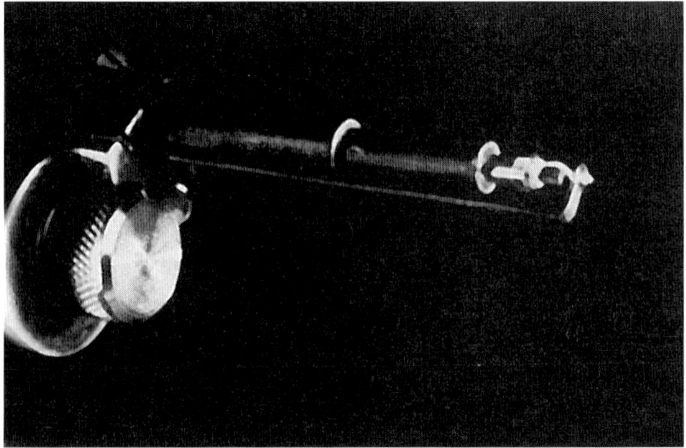

Fig. 14.6 Applications are with a computer-driven handpiece and guarded tip.

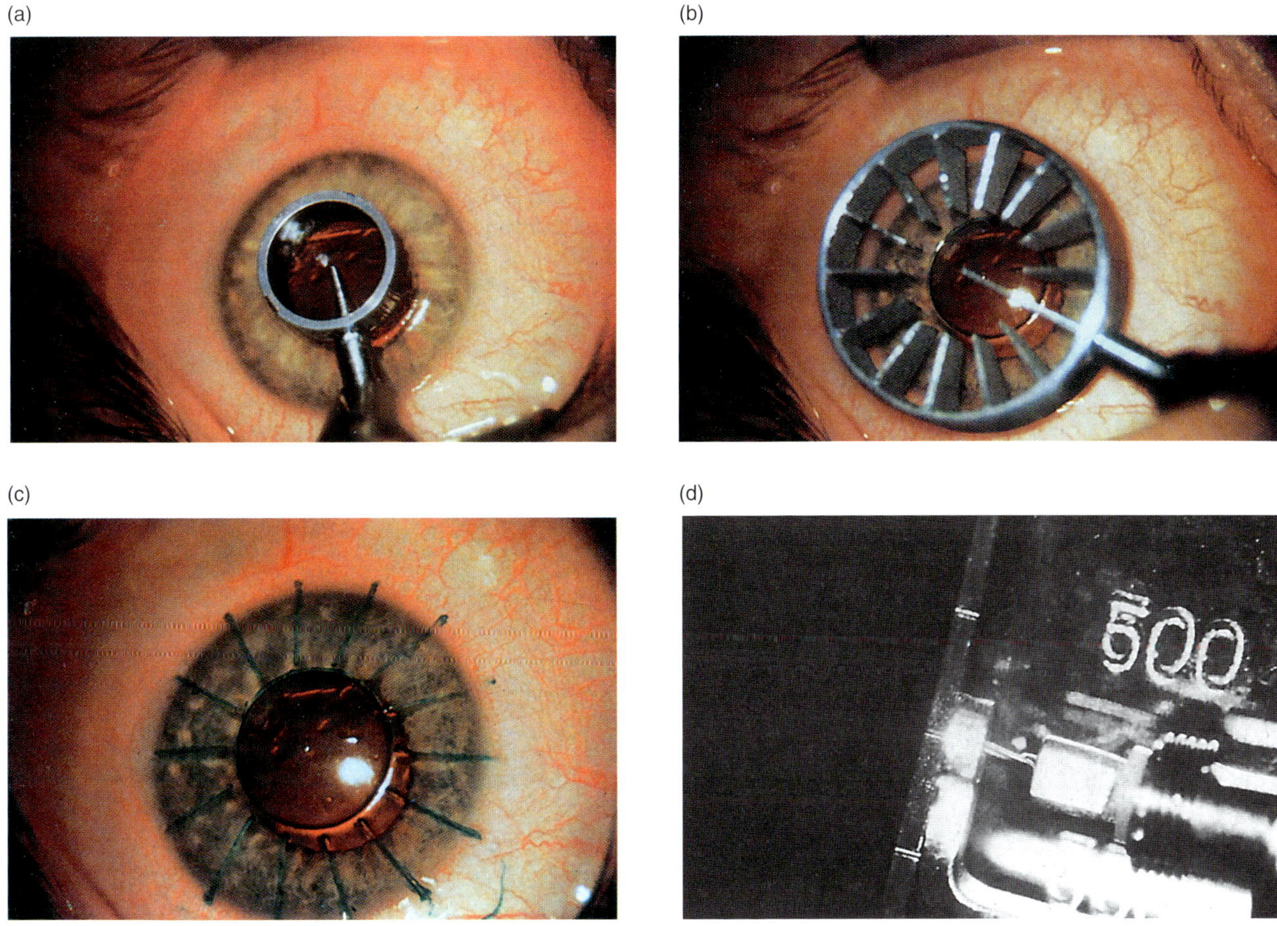

Fig. 14.7 (a) The central optical clear zone is marked; (b,c) followed by the radial application pattern; (d) tip is preset to the required depth using a standard RK knife gauge. (Courtesy of R. Marmer.)

Subsequent reports were not as enthusiastic, and results were mixed [45,46]. The effect is variable and not well controlled and seems to decline over time, with some cases reverting entirely. Scars can still be seen as long as 4 years later, and recurrent erosions have been reported. Many of the previous practitioners stopped performing this procedure [47].

Reports from Fyodorov's group were uniformly good, with little or no regression noted [32]. In 197 eyes of 137 patients followed for a period of 5 to 7 years and reported by Fedchenko, the refraction had stabilized at 1 year. The mean refractive change in patients with preoperative hyperopia ranging up to 13 D was 1.6 D. Mean preoperative unaided vision was 20/70. At 1 year it had improved to 20/40, and at 5 years it dropped to 20/50. In patients whose hyperopia ranged from 3.25 to 6.00 D, the average change was 3.3 D, decreasing to 1.63 D at 5 years. In higher hyperopes, ranging from 6.25 to 9.00 D, the average decrease in refraction at 1 year was 4.93 D, regressing to 3.75 D at 5 years. Unaided visual acuity at 5 years had improved from 20/250 to 20/70.

In 75% of all cases treated at the Moscow center, the reported error of the predicted effect did not exceed 1 D. Average loss of corneal endothelial cells did not exceed 2.5%, and no inflammatory or degenerative changes were noted. At 1 year, biomicroscopy could still detect a slight cloudy and clinically insignificant opacification in the area where the probe had been applied.

The discrepancy between these results and those of some American investigators is difficult to explain and parallels the situation in scleral reinforcement surgery (see Chapter 13). A review of the scatter plots based on the Russian data and reported by Neumann shows a somewhat less optimistic result [44]. It should be noted that few, if any, patients in that series were completely corrected, nor were all included, data were patchy. Additionally, stepwise regression analysis of what data were available showed no correlation of preoperative factors with outcome. While 70.8% of the preoperative hyperopia had been decreased at 1 year, only 40% was corrected to less than 1 D of emmetropia in that time.

Based on what this author has seen of these patients, Neumann's report (and those of others), and the degree of corneal damage induced, it is the author's suggestion that there are, perhaps, less sanguinary ways to correct hyperopia, particularly RK overcorrections.

(a)

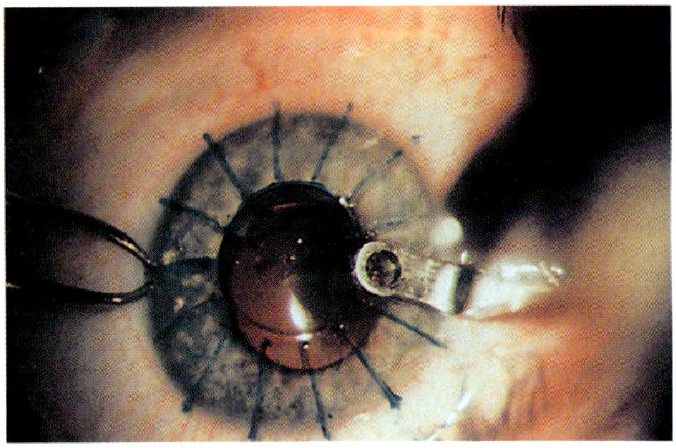

(b)

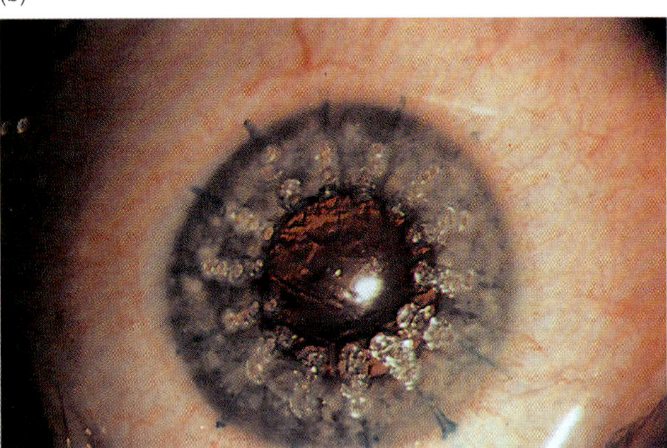

(c)

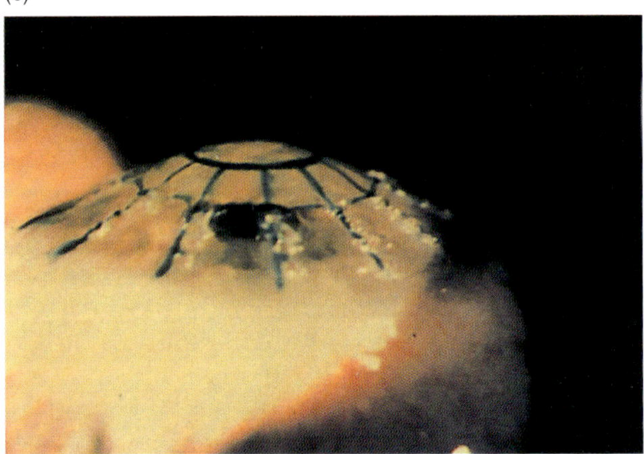

Fig. 14.8 (a) Three to four applications are made along each radial, starting at the optical clear zone; (b) completed treatment; (c) side view of treated cornea. Note the evident steepening of the central cornea.

(a)

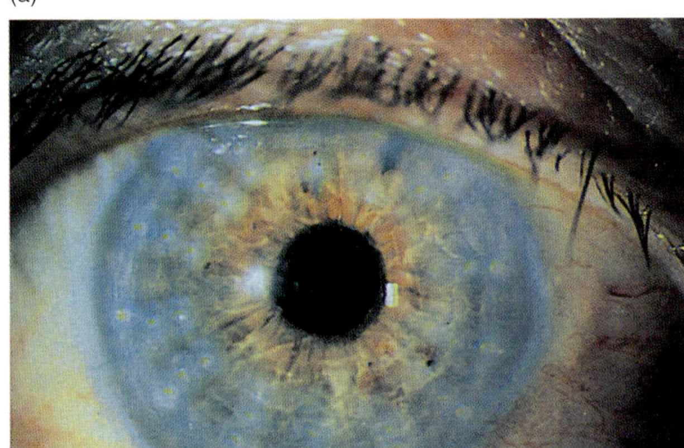

(b)

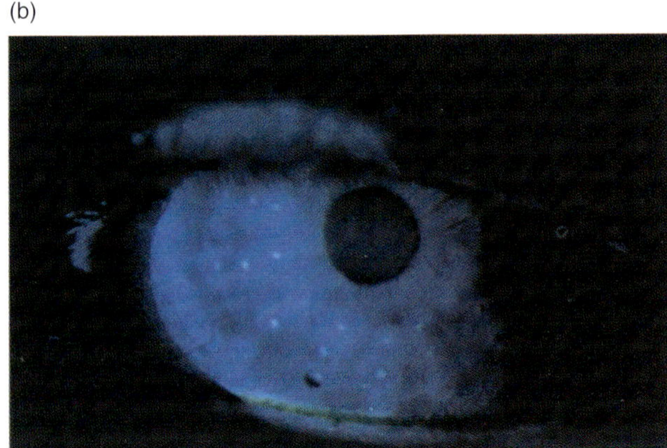

Fig. 14.9 (a) Thermokeratoplasty at 1 week; (b) note the pooling of fluorescein dye in the treatment sites.

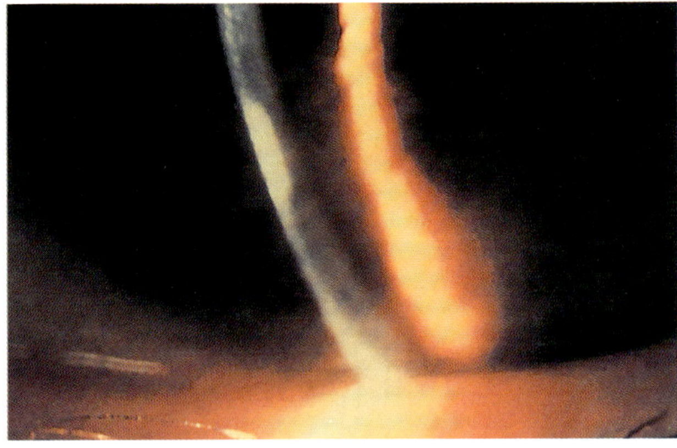

Fig. 14.10 Note the width and depth of scars.

Presbyopia

If hyperopia is the orphan child of refractive surgery, then presbyopia was separated at birth (see also Chapter 2). Loss of accommodation, the curse of all humans over the age of 40 (with rare exceptions), has been seemingly out of reach of corrective measures save spectacles (bifocals—and thank you, Ben Franklin). This is partly due to the current belief that the mechanism of accommodation, as propounded by Helmholtz, is the correct one.

Helmholtz's theory of accommodation

For more than 150 years, the progressive decrease in accommodation was thought to be a loss of lens

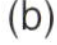

(a)

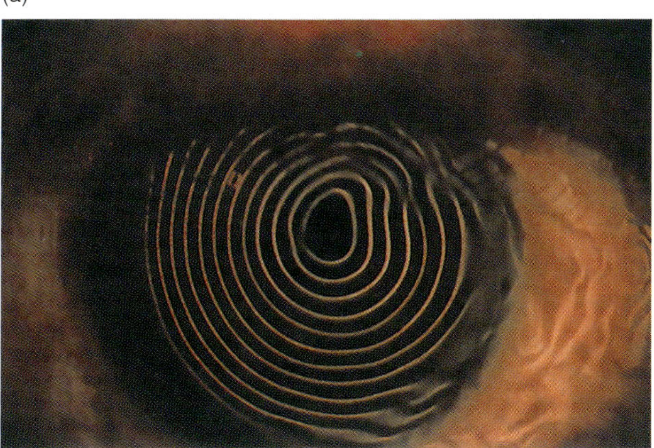

(b)

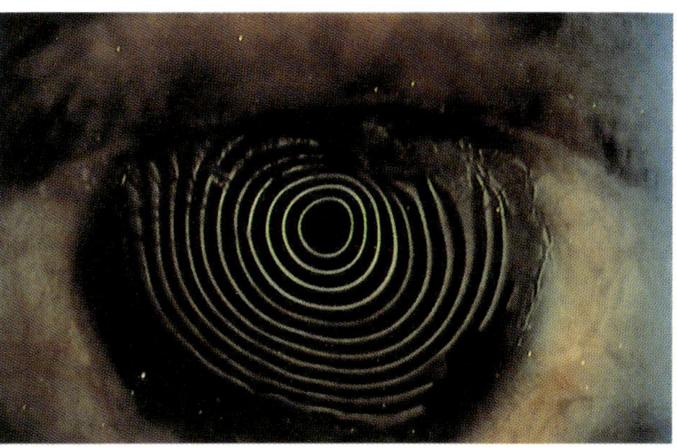

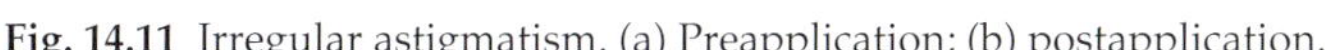

Fig. 14.11 Irregular astigmatism. (a) Preapplication; (b) postapplication.

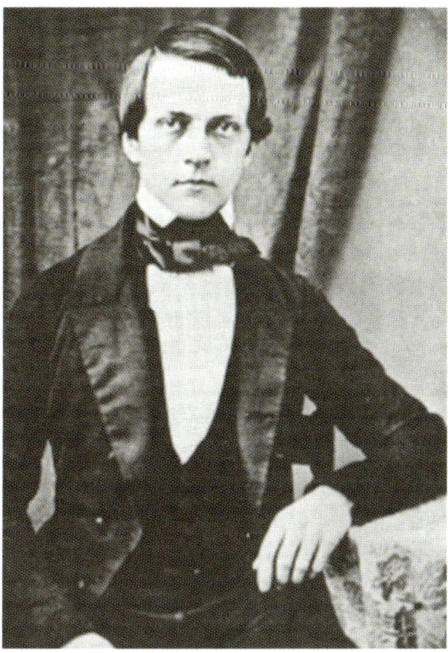

Fig. 14.12 Hermann von Helmholtz.

flexibility [48]. Helmholtz's hypothesis states that in distant vision, the ciliary muscle is relaxed, and the zonules of the lens are under tension. When the eye accommodates, the muscle contracts, reducing the tension on the zonules [49]. This reduced tension allows the elastic capsule of the lens to contract, causing a decrease in equatorial diameter, a decrease in radii of curvatures of the anterior and the posterior surfaces of the lens, with an increase in central thickness. According to Helmholtz, presbyopia results from the loss of the lens with age. When the zonules are relaxed, the lens does not change its shape; therefore, presbyopia is an aging process that can only be reversed by changing the elasticity of the lens or its capsule. Some modern methods have been used to investigate this hypothesis [50].

Schachar's counterhypothesis of accommodation

Much of what Helmholtz propounded is at odds with how the human body functions generally and the reality of lens aging. In 1994, Schachar, disturbed by the inconsistencies in Helmholtz's theory and what seems to actually be happening within the eye, caused him to examine the issue more thoroughly. Schachar's first concern was that the muscles in Helmholtz's eye would be acting indirectly, something that does not seem to be the case generally. When we move our arms or when our irises contract or dilate, the changes are the direct action of a muscle. There does not seem to be a system in the human in which contraction of a muscle results in less tension on attached tissue. Further, according to Helmholtz, during accommodation, when the optical power of the eye is greatest, the zonules are relaxed, and the lens can shift; that is, the lens would not be stable while reading or examining close objects.

However, when viewing through an optical system, the higher the magnification, the more stable the system needs to be. According to Helmholtz's hypothesis, since the equatorial lens diameter increases with age (i.e., the lens equator is getting closer to the ciliary muscle), the zonules should relax. This means that as you age, the power of the lens should increase while viewing distant objects; that is, you should become more myopic, and the lens should become more unstable. In fact, however, you become slightly hyperopic (*senile hypermetropia of Straub*), and the lens remains stable. In addition, Helmholtz attributes the universal linear decrease in the amplitude of accommodation with age to hardening of the lens. Helmholtz's theory implies that the lenses harden in a uniform way. However, during cataract extraction, it is commonly observed that lenses have different degrees of hardness, and no uniform loss of water content of the lens with age has been demonstrated [51–53].

Schachar looked at other possibilities for the accommodative mechanism [54,55]. His conclusions from this were that presbyopia is due to normal equatorial lens

Table 14.1 Results of the Schachar method of treating presbyopia

Institutional comparisons (Accommodation [diopter] changes)					
Operated	N	Mean	Std. Dev.	Median	Range
PV-M	28	3.11	1.62	2.75	0.89 : 7.73
Fra	21	2.47	1.18	2.23	0.37 : 4.58
T-M	7	4.25	3.53	3.59	0.21 : 9.47
Nonoperated					
PV-M	20	0.65	0.61	0.58	–0.55 : 2.28
T-M	7	2.49	1.40	2.33	0.50 : 4.61

By one-way analysis of variance, $P = 0.082$ (operated) and $P < 0.001$ (nonoperated).

growth interfering with ciliary muscle function. The continually growing ectodermal structure, the lens, is reducing the effective function of a mesodermal structure, the ciliary muscle.

Scleral expansion bands (SEBs)

As a consequence of this work, Schachar developed a method of implanting segments of PMMA over the ciliary body to expand the diameter of the eye in that area and increase the efficiency of the ciliary muscles [56]. When the four SEBs are placed through "belt loops" in the sclera, they cause the tissue in the region of the lens equator between the limbus and the belt loop to expand, eliminating the crowding that Schachar theorizes is at the root of accommodation loss. Schachar maintains that the SEBs increase the working distance between the ciliary muscle and the lens equator, which allows the muscle to pull with increased force and actually work again. (See Figures 14.13–14.15.)

The implantation technique involves opening the sclera and making a 4-mm-long belt loop at each of the 45° meridians and then inserting each of the four 5.5-mm implants into the belt loop. Part of the implant sticks out through the belt loop onto the sclera and pulls up the anterior portion in front of the belt loop. When the sclera is pulled up, it lifts the attached ciliary muscle, increasing the distance between the muscle and the lens equator.

Naturally enough, this theory has received some mixed responses. Mathews claims that his use of an infrared optometer shows that accommodation is not enhanced through scleral expansion [57]. Ludwig found evidence, using high-resolution ultrasound biomicroscopy (UBM), that under conditions of near accommodation, the zonular fibers showed signs of relaxation, hence supporting Helmholtz's theory. On the other hand, Strenk, using a GE 1.5-T magnetic resonance imager and a custom-designed eye imaging coil, collected high-resolution MRI images from 25 subjects 22 through 83 years of age. He found that ciliary muscle contraction was present in all subjects and reduced only slightly with advancing age. A decrease in the diameter of the unaccommodated ciliary muscle ring was highly correlated with advancing age, however, lending weight to Schachar's proposal. Lens

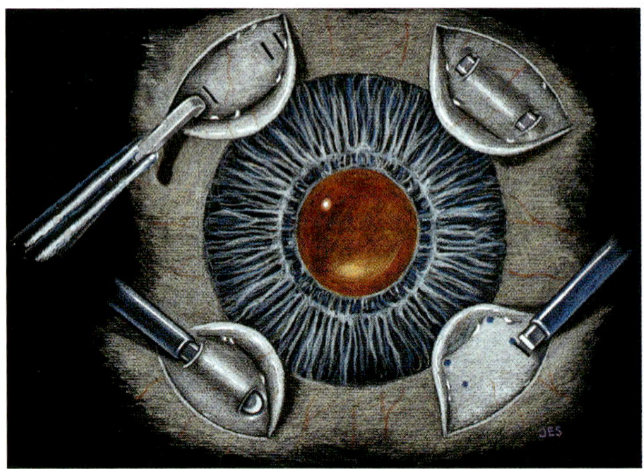

Fig. 14.13 The four steps in inserting the expansion bands.

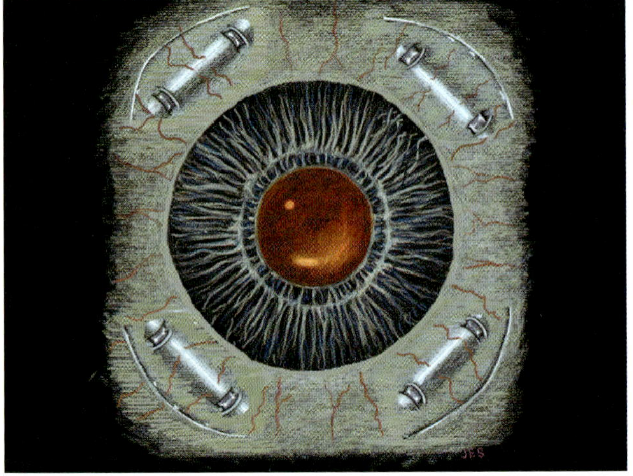

Fig. 14.14 The four expansion bands in place.

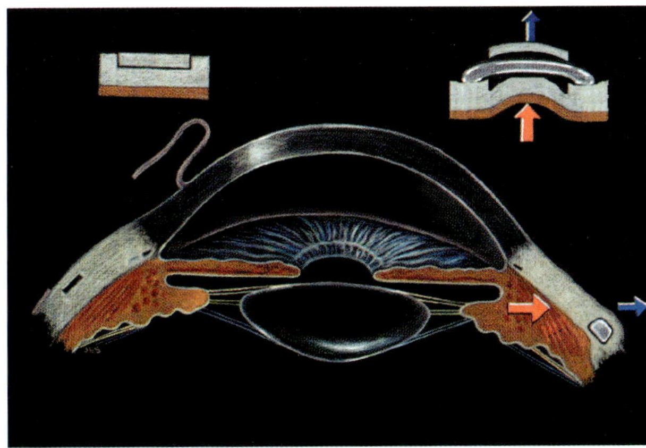

Fig. 14.15 The implanted bands expand the ocular diameter over the ciliary body, improving the presbyopic patient's ability to see close objects.

equatorial diameter does not correlate with age for either accommodative state. Although unaccommodated lens thickness (i.e., lens minor-axis length) increases with age, the thickness of the lens under accommodative effort is only modestly age-dependent.

Whatever the mechanism, the results of this method are interesting. At this writing, approximately 300 patients have received SEBs in progressively improved iterations, which ranged from one continuous fused band early on to the four partial segments now used. With current SEBs, 28 patients achieved a mean accommodation of 3.11 D, with a range from 0.89 to 7.73 D, whereas 7 others had mean results of 4.25 D, with a range from 0.21 to 9.47 D. While problems with the early SEB full-band prototype caused most to be removed, two patients have retained their bands for more than 5 years without problems. In cases where the implants were removed, the eyes returned to their original state, making the procedure reversible. No lost eyes, changes in refraction, or loss of best-corrected visual acuity have been reported to date.

Anterior ciliary sclerotomy (ACS)

ACS, originally proposed by Thornton, uses radial incisions to ease posterior-chamber crowding. This typically requires cutting back the conjunctiva, which means considerably more bleeding than with RK. The technique is still evolving. Incisions in the first phase began outside the limbus, resulting in more regression. In the second phase, incisions began in the limbus and were carried to, but not over, the pars plana [58].

Outcomes from 157 eyes, in which a 6- to 12-month follow-up had been completed, showed an average increase in accommodation of 1.2 D in phases I and II, despite regressions noted in phase I with the early ACS procedure. The average regression of effect for all cases was 2.7 D, and the average reading ability with distance correction in place was J7. Thornton notes that while there were some intraoperative complications, including hemorrhage, lowered IOP, transient IOP elevation in a couple of cases, and limbal perforation with an irregular pupil in one case, there was no visual loss or infection. A weakness of the study was that techniques varied and measurements of accommodation remain largely subjective [59].

While the ACS procedure does not restore all accommodation and is not a cure for presbyopia, there is evidence that it improves accommodation and, as such, can play an important role in refractive surgical treatment. On average, it can restore about 1.5 D of accommodation and may be best suited for early presbyopes who are just beginning to require reading glasses or for older patients who wish to restore intermediate vision.

Zonal excimer laser PRK

Zonal excimer laser PRK was done in three eyes of three presbyopic patients using a specially designed mask with a minimum follow-up of 24 months [60,61]. The procedure was performed with a mask consisting of a mobile diaphragm formed by two blunt blades applied to the Aesculap-Meditec Mel 60 excimer laser. After an initial regression of 1.00 D, the presbyopic correction remained stable during the 36-month follow-up. The patients read at least J3 at normal reading distance without correction. Since the ablated zone was only about 15% of the total area of a 3.0-mm pupil, all three patients also were able to read with their preoperative presbyopic correction (using the untreated 85% of the pupillary area). Although only three eyes were treated with the zonal presbyopia mask, the authors concluded that the visual and refractive outcome appeared promising in view of the relatively long follow-up time.

Presbyopia may be the last frontier of refractive surgery—one that could receive the lion's share of attention in the next 10 to 20 years. No one can predict which of these techniques may turn out to be the long-term survivors, but they are certainly an important first step.

Overcorrections from RK

This properly falls under the category of complications following RK surgery and is discussed in Chapter 15.

Phakic IOLs and laser techniques

Other methods of treating hyperopia such as *hyperopic keratomileusis* and *keratophakia* are discussed in Chapter 10; *laser keratomileusis* and *laser thermokeratoplasty* are discussed in Chapter 11; and phakic IOLs are discussed in Chapter 12.

References

1 Tassman I. Frequency of the various kinds of refractive errors. Am J Ophthalmol 1932; 15: p. 1044.

2 Tenner AS. Refraction in school children: 4800 refractions tabulated according to age, sex and nationality. NY Med J 1915; 102: p. 611.

3 Stenstrom S. Untersuchungen uber die Variation und Kovariation der optischen Elemente des menschlichen Auges. Acta Ophthalmol (suppl) 1946; 26: p. 7.

4 Tielsch JM, Sommer A, Witt K, *et al.* Blindness and visual impairment in an American urban population. The Baltimore Eye Survey [see comments]. Arch Ophthalmol 1990; 108(2): p. 286–90.

5 Grosvenor T. The neglected hyperope. Am J Optom 1971; 48(5): p. 376–82.

6 Applegate RA, and Howland HC. Magnification and visual acuity in refractive surgery. Arch Ophthalmol 1993; 111(10): p. 1335–42.

7 Applegate RA, and Chundru U. Experimental verification of computational methods to calculate magnification in refractive surgery. Arch Ophthalmol 1995; 113(5): p. 571–7.

8 Dierick HG, and Missotten L. Corneal ablation profiles for correction of hyperopia with the excimer laser. J Refract Surg 1996; 12(7): p. 767–73.

9 Göker S, Er H, and Kahvecioglu C. Laser in situ keratomileusis to correct hyperopia from +4.25 to +8.00 diopters. J Refract Surg 1998; 14(1): p. 26–30.

10 Koch DD, Kohnen T., Anderson JA, *et al.* Histologic changes and wound healing response following 10-pulse noncontact holmium:YAG laser thermal keratoplasty. J Refract Surg 1996; 12(5): p. 623–34.

11 Koch DD, Kohnen T, McDonnell PJ, *et al.* Hyperopia correction by noncontact holmium:YAG laser thermal keratoplasty: U.S. phase IIA clinical study with 2-year follow-up. Ophthalmology 1997; 104(11): p. 1938–47.

12 Jean B, Oltrup T, Derse M, *et al.* Hyperopia and astigmatism correction using a continuous wave diode laser (1.9 μm) [abstract]. Invest Ophthalmol Vis Sci 1997; 39(suppl): p. S497.

13 Davidorf JM, Zaldivar R, and Oscherow S. Posterior chamber phakic intraocular lens for hyperopia of +4 to +11 diopters [see comments]. J Refract Surg 1998; 14(3): p. 306–11.

14 Siganos DS, and Pallikaris IG. Clear lensectomy and intraocular lens implantation for hyperopia from +7 to +14 diopters. J Refract Surg 1998; 14(2): p. 105–13.

15 Steinert RF, Storie B, Smith P, *et al.* Hydrogel intracorneal lenses in aphakic eyes. Arch Ophthalmol 1996; 114(2): p. 135–41.

16 Lindstrom RL. Small diameter intracorneal inlay lens for the correction of presbyopia. In: *Surgery for Hyperopia and Presbyopia*, NA Sher, Editor. Williams & Wilkins, Philadelphia, p. 195, 1997.

17 Akiyama K. Posterior corneal incision for hyperopia in rabbits. Nippon Ganka Gakkai Zasshi 1952; 56: p. 11–42.

18 Sato T. Correspondence, a reply on surgical correction of myopia. Am J Ophthalmol 1954; 36: p. 280–282.

19 Gills J. Trephination in combination with radial keratotomy for myopia. In: *Radial Keratotomy*, R Schacher, N Levy, and L Schacher, Editors. LAL, Dennison, 1980.

20 Gaster R, and Yamashita T, Circumferential keratotomy to reduce hyperopia in rabbits. Invest Ophthal 1983; 24: p. 149.

21 Yamashita T, and Gaster R. Experimental hyperopia correction. Parts I and II. In: *Keratorefractive Society*. LAL Publishing, Chicago, 1983.

22 Yamashita T. Hexagonal incision to reduce RK overcorrection. Experimental study. In: *Keratorefractive Society*. LAL Publishing, Atlanta, 1984.

23 Yamashita T, Schneider ME, Fuerst DJ, *et al.* Hexagonal keratotomy reduces hyperopia after radial keratotomy in rabbits. J Ref Surg 1986; 2: p. 261–264.

24 Mendez A, Personal communication, 1991.

25 Mendez A. Correcao da hipermetropia pela ceratotomia hexagonal. In: *Cirugia Refractive*, R Guimarares, Editor. Piramide Livro Medico Editora Ltd, Rio de Janeiro, p. 267–79, 1987.

26 Basuk WL, Zisman M, Waring GR, *et al.* Complications of hexagonal keratotomy. Am J Ophthalmol 1994; 117(1): p. 37–49.

27 Jensen RP. Hexagonal Keratotomy: Clinical Experience with 483 Eyes. In: *Refractive Surgery*, MH Friedlander, Editor. Little, Brown and Co, Boston, p. 69–74, 1991.

28 Gilbert ML, Friedlander MH, and Granet N. Corneal steepening in human eye bank eyes by combined hexagonal and transverse keratotomy. Refract Corneal Surg 1990; 6(2): p. 126–30.

29 Casebeer JC, and Phillips SG. Hexagonal keratotomy: an historical review and assessment of 46 cases. Ophthalmol Clin North Am 1992; 5: p. 727–44.

30 Jensen RP. Hexagonal keratotomy: clinical experience with 483 eyes. Int Ophthalmol Clin 1991; 31(1): p. 69–73.

31 Tamura M, Mamalis N, Kreisler KR, *et al.* Complications of a hexagonal keratotomy following radial keratotomy [letter]. Arch Ophthalmol 1991; 109(10): p. 1351–2.

32 Fedchenko OT. Infrakeratoplasty for the treatment of hyperopia. In: *Ninth International Congress of Eye Research*. Helsinki, 1990.

33 Seiler T, Matallana M, and Bende T. Laser thermokeratoplasty by means of a pulsed holmium:YAG laser for hyperopic correction. Refract Corneal Surg 1990; 6(5): p. 335–9.

34 Rowsey JJ. Radio frequency probe keratoplasty. In: *Kerato–Refractive Society Annual Meeting*. San Francisco, 1979.

35 Gasset AR, Shaw EL, Kaufman HE, *et al.* Thermokeratoplasty. Tr Am Acad Ophth & Oto 1973; 77: p. 441–54.

36 Gasset AR, and Kaufman HE. Thermokeratoplasty in the treatment of keratoconus. Am J Ophthalmol 1975; 79: p. 226–232.

37 Mandelberg AI, Rao GN, and Aquavella JV. Penetrating keratoplasty following thermokeratoplasty. Ophthalmology 1980; 87(8): p. 750–2.

38 Keates RH, and Dingle J. Thermokeratoplasty for keratoconus. Ophthalmic Surg 1975; 6 (3): p. 89–92.

39 Arentsen JJ, and Laibson PR. Thermokeratoplasty for keratoconus. Am J Ophthalmol 1976; 82(3): p. 447–9.

40 McDonnell PJ, Neumann AC, Sanders DR. *et al.* Radial Thermokeratoplasty for Hyperopia (opinion). Refractive and Corneal Surgery 1989; 5(1): p. 50–4.

41 McDonnell PJ. Radial thermokeratoplasty for hyperopia. I. The need for prompt prospective investigation. Refract Corneal Surg 1989; 5: p. 50–2.

42 Neumann AC, Sanders DR, and Salz JJ. Radial thermokeratoplasty for hyperopia: II. Encouraging results from early laboratory and human trials. Refract Corneal Surg 1989; 5(1): p. 55–9.

43 Neumann AC, Sanders DR, Salz JJ, *et al.* Effect of thermokeratoplasty on corneal curvature. J Cataract Refract Surg 1990; 16(6): p. 727–31.

44 Neumann AC, Fyodorov SN, and Sanders DR. Radial thermokeratoplasty for the correction of Hyperopia. Refract Corneal Surg 1990; 6: p. 404–12.

45 Feldman ST, Ellis W, Frucht-Pery J, *et al.* Regression of effect following radial thermokeratoplasty in humans. Refract Corneal Surg 1989; 5: p. 288–91.

46 Feldman ST, Ellis W, Frucht-Pery J, *et al.* Experimental radial thermokeratoplasty in rabbits. Arch Ophthalmol 1990; 108(7): p. 997–1000.

47 Ellis W. Personal communication, 1991.

48 Adler-Grinberg D. Questioning our classical understanding of accommodation and presbyopia [published erratum appears in Am J Optom Physiol Opt 1987 Jan;64(1):75]. Am J Optom Physiol Opt 1986; 63(7): p. 571–80.

49 Helmholtz HLF. Üeber die Accomodation des Auges. Graefes Arch Ophthalmol 1855; 1(2): p. 1–74.

50 Glasser A, and Campbell MC. Biometric, optical and physical changes in the isolated human crystalline lens with age in relation to presbyopia. Vision Res 1999; 39(11): p. 1991–2015.

51 Bours J, Fodisch HJ, and Hockwin O, Age-related changes in water and crystallin content of the fetal and adult human lens, demonstrated by a microsectioning technique. Ophthalmic Res 1987; 19(4): p. 235–9.

52 Bettelheim FA, Castoro JA, White O, *et al.* Topographic correspondence between total and non-freezable water content and the appearance of cataract in human lenses. Curr Eye Res 1986; 5(12): p. 925–32.

53 Huizinga A, Bot AC, de Mul FF, *et al.* Local variation in absolute water content of human and rabbit eye lenses measured by Raman microspectroscopy. Exp Eye Res 1989; 48(4): p. 487–96.

54 Schachar RA, Cudmore DP, and Black TD. Experimental support for Schachar's hypothesis of accommodation. Ann Ophthalmol 1993; 25(11): p. 404–9.

55 Schachar RA, Huang T, and Huang X. Mathematic proof of Schachar's hypothesis of accommodation. Ann Ophthalmol 1993; 25(1): p. 5–9.

56 Schachar RA, Cudmore DP, Torti R, *et al.* A physical model demonstrating Schachar's hypothesis of accommodation. Ann Ophthalmol 1994; 26(1): p. 4–9.

57 Mathews S. Scleral expansion surgery does not restore accommodation in human presbyopia [see comments]. Ophthalmology 1999; 106(5): p. 873–7.

58 Fukasaku H, and Marron JA. Surgical correction of presbyopia. In: *ASCRS Symposium on Cataract, IOL, and Refractive Surgery.* Seattle,1999.

59 Thornton SP. Anterior ciliary sclerotomy correction of presbyopia. In: *ASCRS Symposium on Cataract, IOL, and Refractive Surgery.* Seattle, 1999.

60 Vinciguerra P, Nizzola GM, Bailo G, *et al.* Excimer laser photorefractive keratectomy for presbyopia: 24-month follow-up in three eyes. J Refract Surg 1998; 14(1): p. 31–7.

61 Vinciguerra P, Nizzola GM, Nizzola F, *et al.* Zonal photorefractive keratectomy for presbyopia. J Refract Surg 1998; 14(2 Suppl): p. S218–21.

15

Adverse Events Associated with Refractive Surgery

Life is just one damned thing after another.
[Frank Ward O'Malley].

All surgical procedures, regardless of how benign or "safe," carry with them certain side effects and complications. Refractive surgery is, of course, no exception. *Side effects*, for the purposes of this discussion, are defined as the usual, or expected, sequelae of a surgical procedure that disappear with time and with minimal or no treatment. These effects are usually self-limiting but for the time that they are present can create severe problems for the patient and may, subsequently, have to be dealt with by the surgeon.

Complications are unexpected and/or deleterious side effects that require medical or surgical intervention and which may leave permanent effects. These effects, while fortunately quite rare, are usually those associated with any eye surgery and are dealt with in the same manner. Some are unique to this surgery and must be dealt with uniquely.

We will begin this discussion with radial keratotomy (RK) because the side effects and complications occurring with this surgery encompass problems encountered with almost all other forms of refractive surgery. We will then follow with a section on those peculiar problems associated with lamellar corneal surgery, including those peculiar to laser in situ keratomileusis (LASIK). Problems unique to a specific procedure will be detailed either in a separate section or can be found within the chapter or section dealing with the specific modality. We will not cover in depth those complications which are seen during or following cataract surgery—these have been more than amply discussed in the various textbooks on the subject. The reader is referred to these for edification.

Radial keratotomy (relaxing incisions)

Side effects—Intraoperative

Epithelial stripping

In approximately 6% of cases in the author's experience, stripping of the epithelium in one or more areas will occur when making incisions. This phenomenon is more likely to occur after using topical anesthetics such as cocaine or 4% tetracaine but also can occur after use of buffered 0.5% tetracaine or Proparacaine. In almost all cases, these same patients will have given a history of extreme intolerance to contact lenses or foreshortened wearing time, even of soft lenses. In a few cases the entire epithelial surface "ripples" when touched. In some of these same cases large quadrantal sections of tissue stripped off the corneal surface. The incidence of this side effect was almost double during the time the corneas were kept wet during the surgery and seems to be caused by swelling of the epithelial cells in response to anoxia.

Generally speaking, small triangular areas of stripping (called *concordes* when first encountered because of their resemblance to that aircraft in overhead view) occur along

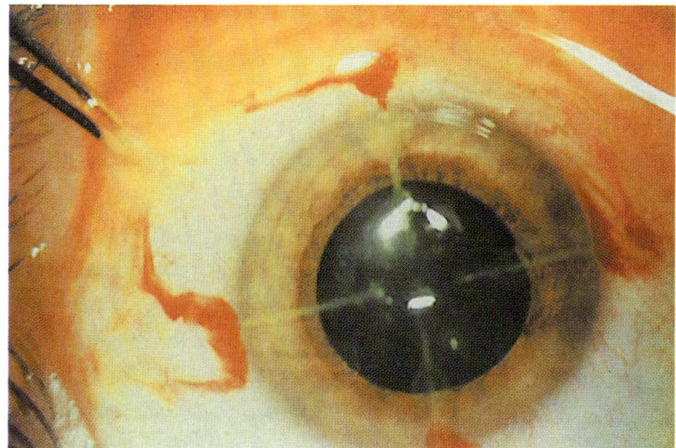

Fig. 15.1 Epithelial stripping—so-called concordes.

the incision line, with the apex of the triangle directed away from the direction of incision (Figure 15.1). They are more frequently encountered, even in "dry" surgeries, with "dull" blades and/or incompletely cleaned or poorly polished footplates. They also can occur if the knife handle is tipped forward and pressure is applied to the front of the footplate causing it to "dig in" (Figure 15.2).

This phenomenon can be minimized by using super-sharp blades such as the XTAL sapphire in handles with highly polished footplates, by keeping the cornea dry, and by using only enough pressure on the knife to keep the footplate in contact with the corneal surface. The appearance of a prominent "motorboat wake" with the newer knifes is an indication of too much pressure and/or a dull blade.

When stripping occurs, gently wipe away the loose tissue from the cornea with a moistened microsponge, taking care not to make it worse. Clean debris away from the blade and off the bottom of the footplate. If it appears that more tissue is going to come away, remove as much peripheral epithelium as you can before proceeding. Do not take off the central epithelium or you will lose your optical zone (OZ) mark. Naturally, if this is a case of stepped incisions, you will not be able to do this. The author has not found it necessary to change the blade setting in these cases to compensate for any possible change in corneal thickness even when the stripping is extensive.

At the close of the surgery, remove any loose tags of epithelium to ensure smooth edges, and then gently irrigate the interior of the incisions. Replacing the epithelial tags has not, in this author's experience, increased anything but the patient's postoperative discomfort. A pressure patch may increase patient comfort during the first 12 to 24 hours, but it may become necessary to remove it before then—2 to 4 hours is usually sufficient. These patients normally require more or stronger postoperative analgesics.

Side effects—Postoperative

Glare

The most common side effect and one that occurs in most RK patients is glare. Glare or dazzle is produced by the corneal scars and is especially noted at night when the pupil will dilate to 5 to 6 mm, exposing the ends of the incisions, making night driving difficult and sometimes impossible (Figure 15.3). A related side effect is photophobia. Glare is usually self-limiting, beginning to diminish at 3 to 4 months, and is gone for the most part within the year. The PERK study noted that glare, as measured by the Miller-Nadler glare tester, was not significantly different at 1 year postoperatively as compared to the preoperative measurements [1].

In general, the best treatment for glare is to take steps to minimize it by careful preoperative planning. The proper combination of incision number and OZ size should be chosen from the computer-generated surgical table. Choose the largest OZ with the least number of incisions even if it means having to use multiple steps or redeepening to achieve the correction desired.

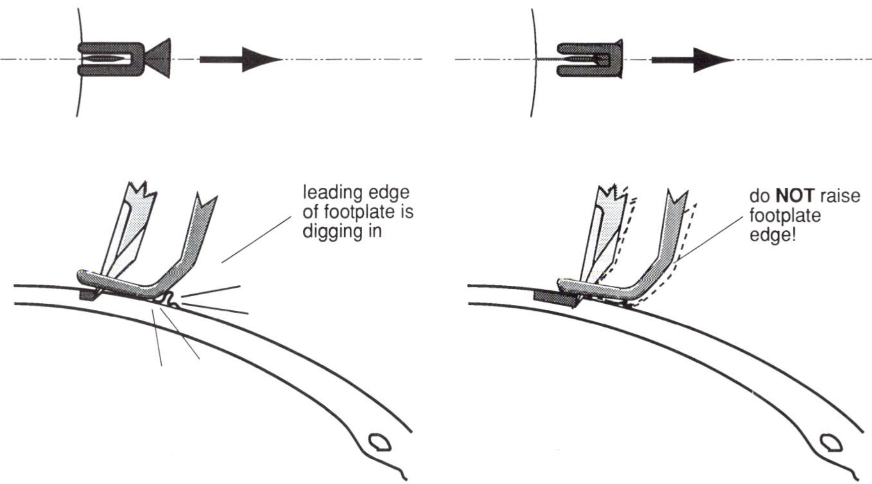

Fig. 15.2 Cause of concordes and the wrong way to deal with them.

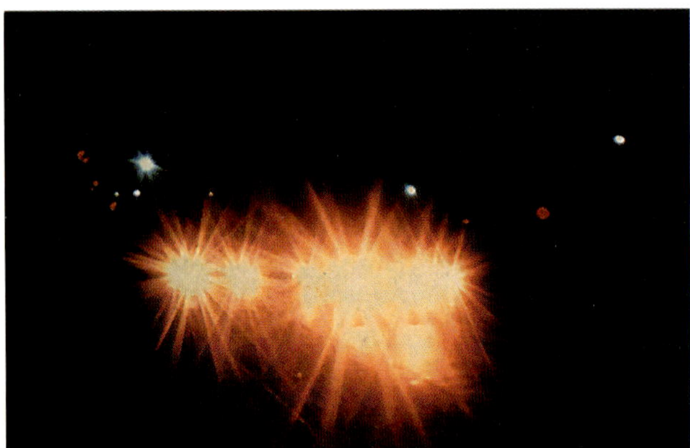

Fig. 15.3 Typical post-RK glare.

The use of the newer ultrathin, ultrasharp blades will produce extremely fine incisions and scars, further reducing the amount of glare. Also, newer techniques in deepening incisions and reoperations have reduced the severity and longevity of the symptoms.

The treatment of glare can take many forms, with the main object that of diminishing its effect on the patient. It is not possible to totally eliminate glare, and patients vary in their response both to glare and its treatment. Some patients never complain at all. Preoperative testing with a device such as the Miller-Nadler glare tester, while alerting the surgeon to a possible problem, has not proven useful in screening out patients with increased glare sensitivity. It is not unheard of for patients to complain of less glare postoperatively and show this in their test results. Some glare is associated with residual myopia or "against-the-rule" astigmatism and can be treated simply by fitting temporary spectacles.

Commercially available absorptive lenses will reduce the amount of visible light reaching the retina and may reduce some of these symptoms. The following may be of value:

1 Antireflective coatings, typically consisting of an ultrathin layer of magnesium fluoride, create light wave interference, thus reducing reflected light. This will improve the optical performance of any spectacle lens and may reduce the multiple image reflections caused by oncoming headlights and other point sources of light.

2 Tinted spectacles are popular with the public for glare reduction, although their effectiveness may be minimal. In the truly light-sensitive (or photophobic) individual, a dense pink tint allowing approximately 52% light transmission (cruxite C) may be of value. Neutral gray tints are available in densities as dark as 12% transmission. These absorb as much as 98% of ultraviolet light, along with infrared, and do not distort colors. If a significant reduction in light intensity during the day is required, such lenses are satisfactory. Green tints may be used similarly but do not reproduce colors as well. Brown tints also may be of value, have some cosmetic appeal, and do slightly enhance contrast. They cause color distortion, however. Yellow-tinted spectacles absorb 100% of ultraviolet and transmit infrared and about 83% of the visible spectrum. They tend to absorb heavily in the blue region and therefore reduce haze and enhance contrast slightly.

3 Polaroid sunglasses, alone or in combination with a dense neutral gray coating, are of value in reducing total incident light as well as eliminating annoying surface reflections such as occur on water or snow. Such lens are particularly effective in treating both glare and photophobia.

4 Photochromic lenses darken when exposed directly to ultraviolet light and lighten when ultraviolet light is withdrawn. In patients exposed to particularly bright sunlight on snow or water, a combination of photochromic glass and a Polaroid filter, as found in photopolar glasses, may be helpful.

5 Special lenses such as the NOIR are available that will absorb varying proportions of the visible spectrum and most ultraviolet and infrared radiation.

Topical pilocarpine in dilute strength (0.25% to 0.50%) also may be used to reduce glare or dazzle symptoms through pupillary miosis. However, such use is of limited value, and some patients will experience brow ache or difficulty in reading.

Often patients will complain of "glare" at night when what they are really experiencing is an enlarged blur circle resulting from the natural shift toward myopia experienced late in the day. In these cases, the problem might be eliminated by fitting the patient with spectacles to be worn only when driving at night. Sometimes repeat surgery may be necessary.

Photophobia

Photophobia is a short-lived side effect usually lasting no more then 14 days. It is associated with corneal edema and diminishes as the edema subsides. It usually does not require any treatment. For those patients with extreme photophobia, temporary spectacles of the type described under glare can be used. The postoperative use of low-concentration steroid drops during the first 2 weeks seems to diminish this side effect.

The author has personal knowledge of at least one RK case which came to penetrating keratoplasty because of glare.

Corneal edema

Corneal edema is seen in 93% of patients in the immediate postoperative period (Figures 15.4 and 15.5). It usually extends from the bottom of the incisions anteriorly, spares the area within the OZ, and is of mild degree. Greater edema is seen most often in cases which have had 12 or more incisions and in those cases in which the in-

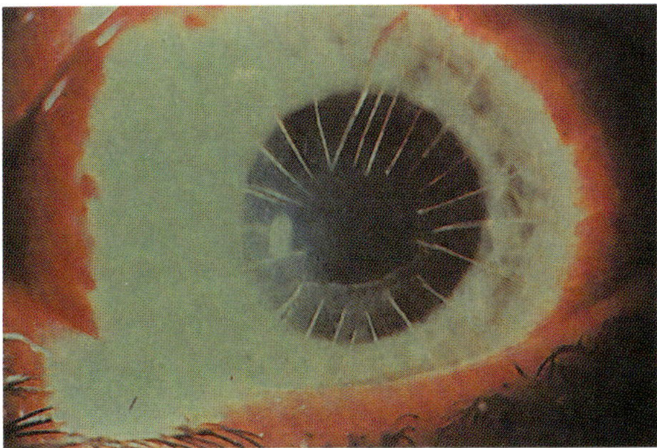

Fig. 15.4 Typical corneal edema seen during the wet surgery era. Note that the edema is present only in the incision areas.

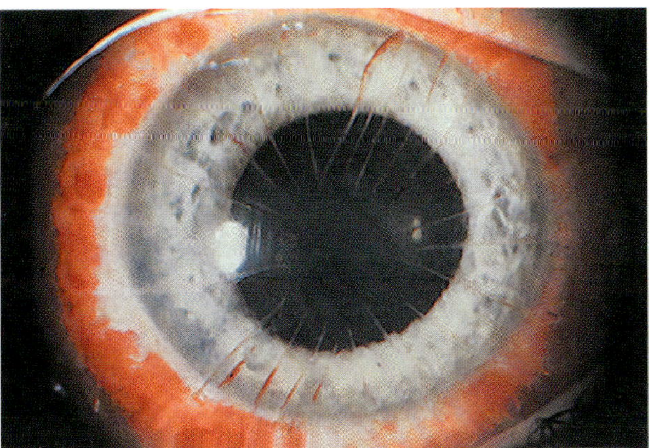

Fig. 15.5 Same cornea at 24 hours postsurgery. These two figures are also representative of the subconjunctival hemorrhaging accompanying incisions that extend across the limbus.

cisions have been stepped or otherwise redeepened or manipulated. It also will occur in those cases in which the cornea has been kept wet or which have have received excess irrigation of the incisions following the surgery [2]. The use of hypertonic saline solutions has been suggested (and tried by some investigators), but they have not proven to be of much help. Such treatment is quite uncomfortable for the patient and of questionable value. Generally, the edema subsides rapidly without treatment and is completely gone within 2 weeks.

Punctate keratopathy

Punctate staining of the cornea along the incisions is seen in all cases in the immediate postoperative period. The staining pattern is linear and begins to disperse at 48 to 72 hours. Some clusters of punctate staining can be seen grouped near the inner ends of the incisions for as long as 14 days (Figures 15.6 and 15.7). Persistent punctate (non-dispersed) staining is associated with tearing, increased photophobia, and a foreign-body sensation and is self-limited (see also "Recurrent corneal erosion," below).

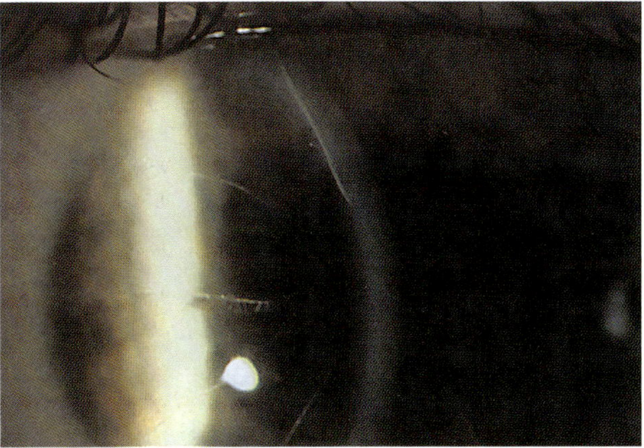

Fig. 15.6 Typical punctate epithelial disturbance seen in RK cases during the initial postoperative period.

Ghost images

In some patients there is a complaint of ghost images or, rarely, discrete monocular diplopia. Usually the patient describes images as having an associated secondary image best described as similar to an out-of-convergence television picture. Occasionally, these secondary images will be sufficiently separate to produce frank diplopia. In all occurrences of this phenomenon, vertical folds in Descemet's membrane can be faintly seen within the OZ (Figure 15.8). These are more prominent in cases of diplopia and are closer to the optical center (Figure 15.9). Circumferential folds also may be found between the incisions outside the primary OZ. If these are prominent, they may add to the complaint of glare. The circular folds spread centrifugally and usually disappear by 4 months. On their disappearance, the vertical folds also leave, taking the diplopia with them. Contrary to the case with glare, correcting any residual myopia may make the symptoms worse. The problem is compounded by the presence of "against-the-rule" astigmatism, either preexisting or iatrogenic. In the latter case, the symptoms may diminish as the astigmatism "perambulates" or disappears.

Binocular diplopia

This symptom usually will occur between surgeries as a result of anisometropia. Treatment is surgery of the fellow eye. Transitory binocular diplopia may occur shortly after surgery in young individuals. This may be as a result of overconvergence associated with overaccommodation. No cases of persistent binocular diplopia following this surgery have been reported to date.

Perambulating astigmatism

In those cases with preexisting astigmatism or in "spectacle sphere" cases with corneal astigmatism and occasionally in purely spherical cases, induced regular astig-

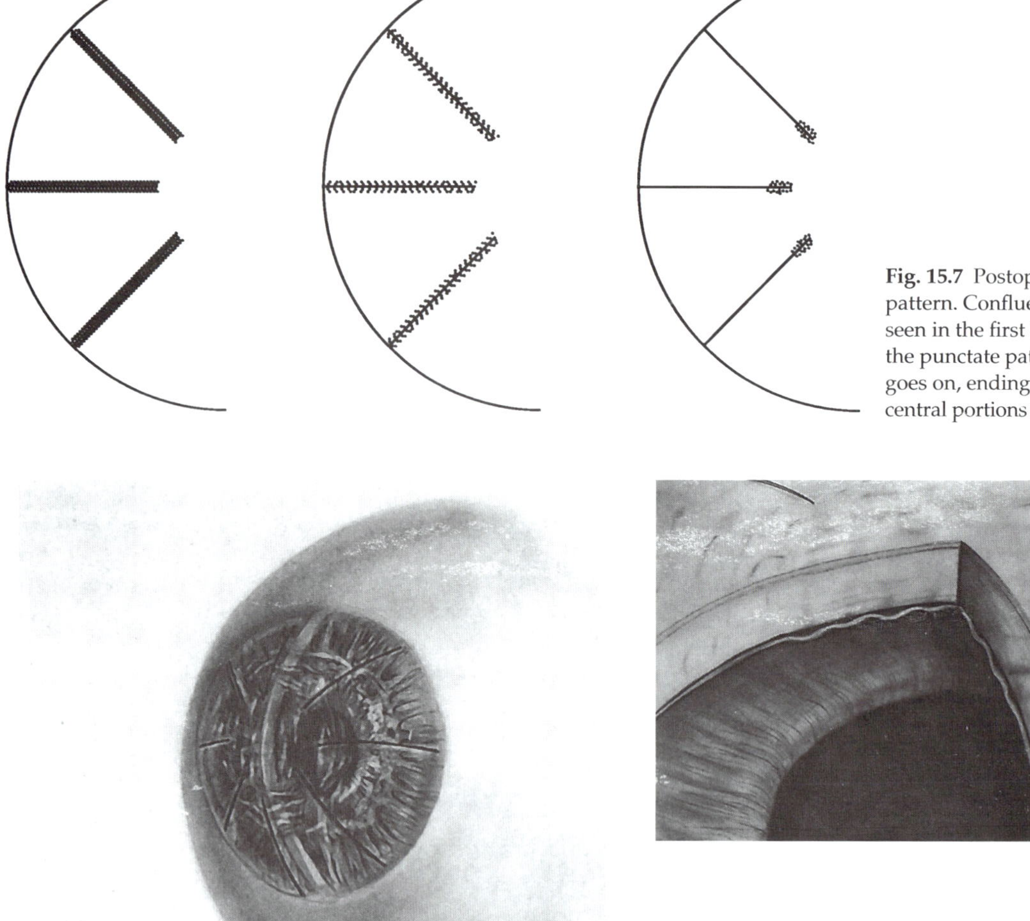

Fig. 15.7 Postoperative punctate staining pattern. Confluent punctate staining is seen in the first 24 hours. The density of the punctate pattern becomes less as time goes on, ending as clumping around the central portions of the incisions at 60 hours.

Fig. 15.8 Descemet's folds near the optic center.

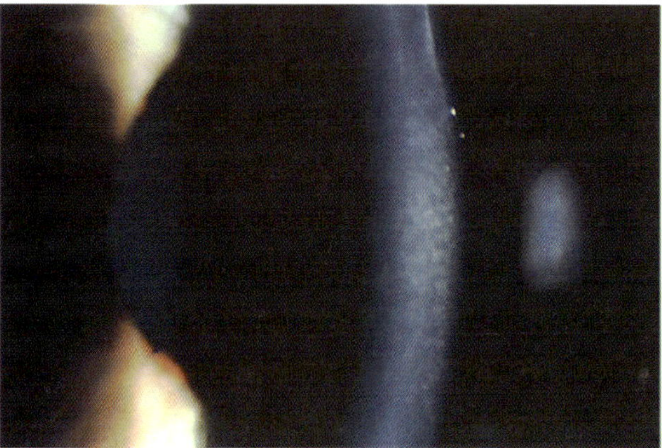

Fig. 15.9 Distribution of folds in Descemet's following RK surgery.

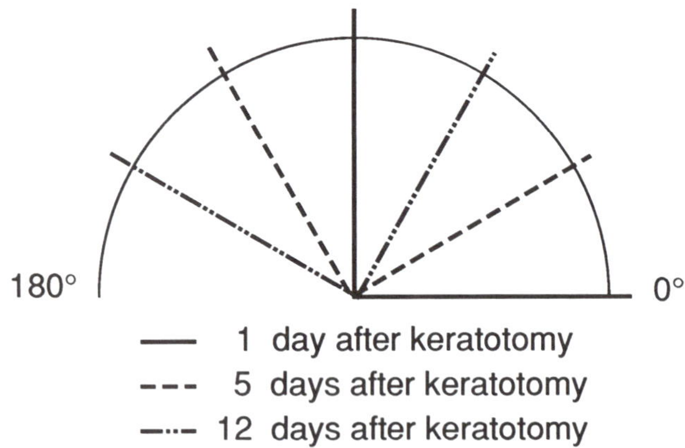

Fig. 15.10 Perambulating or wandering astigmatism following RK.

matism may be seen postoperatively. The axis of this astigmatism will change from day to day toward "with-the-rule" but may change course willy-nilly—hence its name: *perambulating* (or *wandering*) *astigmatism* (Figure 15.10). By itself, it is a transient problem and in operated astigmatism cases is a good prognostic sign. Associated with residual myopia, it accounts for much of the fluctuation seen in these cases. It may aggravate other side effects, notably glare and ghost images. Unless severe, treatment is not recommended and of little use because the situation is rapidly changing. Furthermore, reoperating on astigmatism under these circumstances is highly dangerous (see also Chapter 9).

Asthenopia

Certain patients, particularly those in their early thirties, will complain of some difficulty with "tired" eyes or intermittent blurring while reading. These symptoms are generally seen in cases of preoperative myopia greater than 4 D. These patients may have normal near points of accommodation on initial testing both preoperatively and postoperatively but tire on repeated testing. Consequently, these patients will be unable to perform close work or to read comfortably for a time. The treatment is reassurance—reading glasses are not recommended unless the patient is in the presbyopic age range. The problem can be likened to that of a short distance runner being suddenly expected to run 10 km or more. These patients have not been called on to fully use their accommodation until now—some "getting into shape" is what's required. Recall (Chapter 2) that the accommodative effort is increased in contact lens–wearing myopes [3].

Premature presbyopia

This is actually a misnomer. A better term perhaps would be *unmasked presbyopia*. True premature presbyopia has not been reported following this surgery—the lens is not being altered by the surgery, the cornea is. Causing the confusion has been the complaint by some patients that they can no longer read without their glasses as they had been accustomed to before the surgery. Careful questioning usually reveals that these same patients were not able to read comfortably before the surgery while wearing their distant correction either—especially if they were contact lens wearers. In fact, some of these same patients were able to read only slightly better without their glasses than with them. It is not unusual to have to fit a myope with bifocals sooner than a hyperope.

It also should be borne in mind that many myopes experience some degree of asthenopia for near when wearing contact lenses (see Chapter 2). Such patients should be warned that after a successful RK procedure (or, for that matter, any procedure for myopia), some difficulty with near vision—particularly reading—may be experienced. Interestingly, some patients who were unable to read comfortably previously while wearing a distant correction are able to read after having their myopia fully corrected by the surgery. This could be as a result of a multifocal condition of the cornea occurring after surgery [4,5]. The author reported a series of cases in which the cause for the seeming "loss" of presbyopia appeared to be pseudoaccommodation, wherein the pliable post-RK cornea was flexed by the ciliary muscles [6]. Helmholtz demonstrated that the corneal curvature does change slightly in the normal during accommodation—the incised cornea could be more susceptible to this effect [7]. The author's findings are summarized in Figures 15.11 through 15.14.

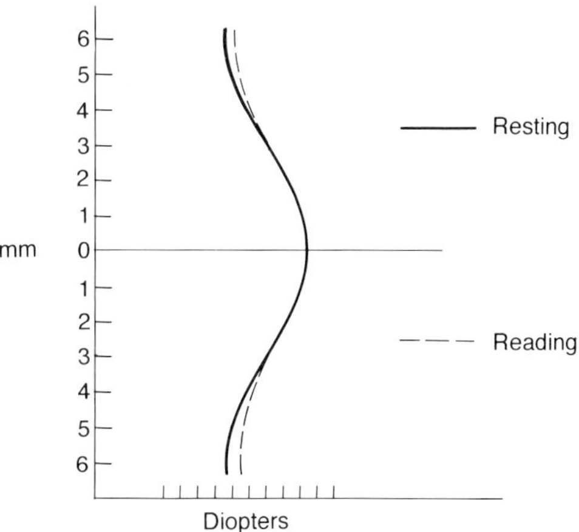

Fig. 15.11 Preoperative central corneal curvature—distance and near.

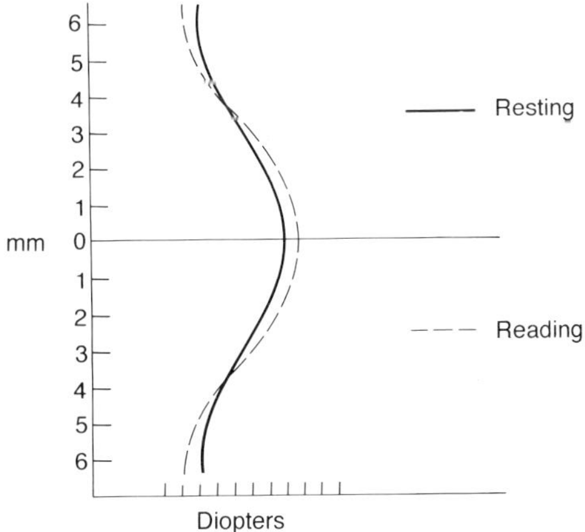

Fig. 15.12 Postoperative central corneal curvature—distance and near.

Treatment consists of reassurance and having the patient review the informed consent tape. Fitting of a proper reading spectacle also may be necessary as well. Most patients accept the situation with good grace, saying that half a loaf is better than none. While not a preventative, proper informed consent (perhaps in the form of a videotape) will go a long way toward softening the blow.

Fluctuation of vision

More than 80% of all RK patients will experience some degree of fluctuating vision throughout the day for the first 4 to 6 months. This phenomenon is seen infrequently in eight-incision cases and is undoubtedly related to the diurnal variation in intraocular pressure (IOP) seen in the human eye [8]. Other factors such as splinting of the malleable cornea by the lids during the night may be a

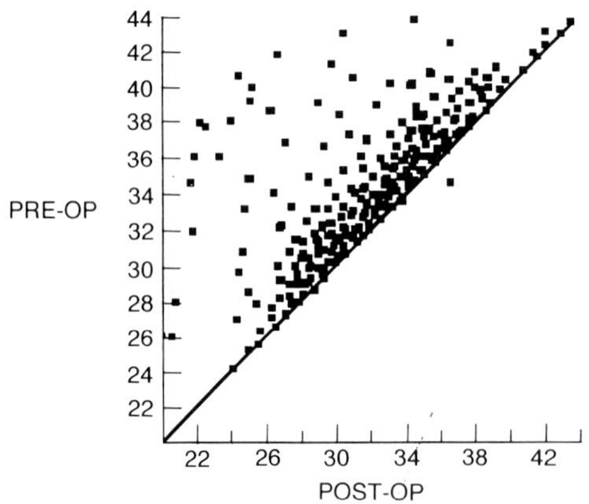

Fig. 15.13 Scattergram of near point of accommodation—pre- and postoperation.

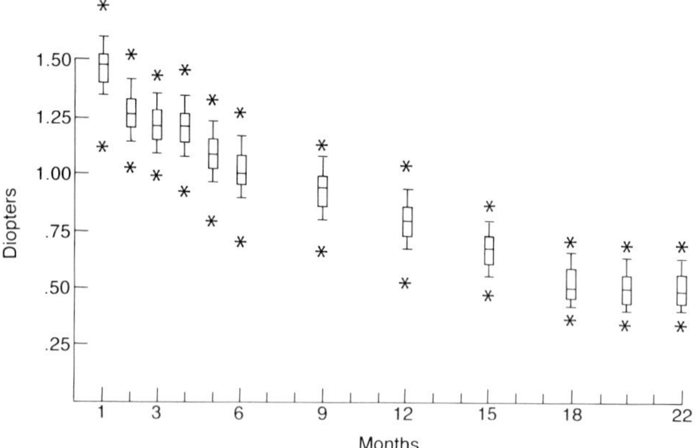

Fig. 15.14 Degree of pseudoaccommodation demonstrated over time.

factor as well. Corneal edema occurring during the night has been suggested as an underlying cause [9,10]. This has not been borne out by repeated ultrasonic thickness measurements carried out on randomly selected patients at different hours of the day—although such changes in thickness have been seen in patients with severe epithelial disease. While the cornea is increased in thickness postoperatively to some degree, no significant changes in this thickness have been found to occur diurnally (see "Undercorrections (residual myopia)," below).

Some studies have suggested that corneal shape changes due to diurnal pressure fluctuation are not a factor by demonstrating no significant corneal curvature changes through the day [11–13]. In a series of patients examined by the author in 1979 over a period of 3 months, applanation pressures were measured on both the operated and unoperated eyes at varying times during the day, including late evening and early morning. In addition, ophthalmometry was performed on each eye. It was found that it was possible to detect small changes in the central corneal curvature by this method. While not conclusive because of the inherent inaccuracies within the method of measurement and the smallness of the changes, these changes were, nevertheless, significant in their own right. In every case in which the visual acuity was affected, the K-readings were measurably different in the operated eye versus the nonoperated eye for a given time period. In those patients, for example, who stated that their vision was better in the morning as opposed to the evening, the central corneas were uniformly flatter centrally in the morning than in the control eye. This observation was well demonstrated by Deitz [14] in a series of patients in whom the IOP was increased by the use of topical steroids and has been corroborated by Fyodorov and coworkers [15] as well as Feldman and coworkers [8].

The *Bates effect* [16] or *phenomenon* has not been suggested as a possible causative agent but may well play a part because the corneas of these patients are extremely malleable. It has been observed that many patients demonstrate good unaided postoperative visual acuity despite their having a residual myopia that ordinarily would drop the vision to 20/100 or less. If the lids are held away from the eye in these same patients, their vision falls to the expected levels. It is possible that varying degrees of orbicularis spasm or lid pressure exerted during the day (with more in the morning when fresh) produce varying amounts of flattening and hence varying acuity.

This side effect, like glare, is self-limited, but it may not go away completely for a number of years [17]. Large fluctuations—those inclined to induce patient complaints—last for a much shorter time and usually subside by 4 to 6 months. The fitting of a hard contact lens to reduce the fluctuation has been tried with limited success. These patients are often lens intolerant in the first place. Further, an exact corneal curvature measurement, required in hard lens fitting, often is not possible during this period. The fitting of a soft contact lens for the same purpose is not recommended before 8 weeks because of the danger of neovascularization of the incisions. Since the lens is extremely flexible, its effect on the variation in vision is small, but some patients notice a diminution of visual variation.

Treatment is "tincture of time" and reassurance. The fitting of any visual appliance for this purpose before 12 weeks is an exercise in futility and in any case unnecessary unless there is significant residual myopia and/or astigmatism. In such cases, the patient should be told that he or she may require additional changes somewhere down the line.

Upper lid edema

Approximately 16% of patients who have corneal abrasions demonstrate edema of the upper lid within 24 hours. The incidence of this side effect after RK is approximately the same, and no special significance is placed on its occurrence. It lasts—for the most part—only for a few days and rarely becomes severe enough to produce complaints.

On such occasions, cool compresses and aspirin analgesia suffice. Tylenol (acetaminophen) does not seem to be as effective.

Increased color saturation

Along with the reduction in myopia and/or astigmatism, this is one of the pleasant side effects of this surgery and was first described by the author in 1979. It is experienced as an increase in the brightness and density of color in objects. Vision is described as "less pastel" in nature. Patients rarely complain of this, and all exclaim about it. One such patient described it as "Dorothy walking out into the Land of Oz"—hence its more popular name: "the *Wizard of Oz* phenomenon."

Spatial displacement

This side effect is a psychological reaction that occurs most often in patients who have had successful surgery in one—usually the nondominant—eye. They describe scenes as if they were viewing them from one side (usually the operated side) and slightly above their actual position. Usually very transitory, disappearing when the second eye has been operated on, it occasionally occurs even then. Sometimes the displaced feeling is sufficiently strong as to produce vertigo. Vertiginous patients may need medication. Fortunately, the phenomenon occurs very rarely and produces no lasting effects.

Complications—Intraoperative

Divots (see also "Side effects—Epithelial stripping," above)

This complication is seen universally as a consequence of incisions being made with a dull blade or the back side of any blade (Figures 15.15 and 15.16). These will still occur if an attempt is made to make incisions with the back of a single-edged blade. They are transverse tears through Bowman's membrane. The triangles point in the direction of the incision, are smaller than the concordes, and result in permanent scarring that may increase both the intensity and the persistence of glare (Figure 15.17). There is no effective treatment other than symptomatic (see "Glare," above). The solution is prevention by using sharp, double-edged blades for the surgery.

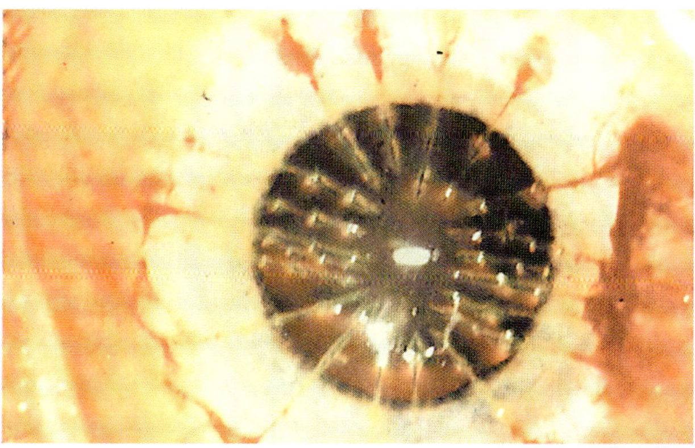

Fig. 15.15 Divots or tears in the corneal stroma—secondary to a poor blade.

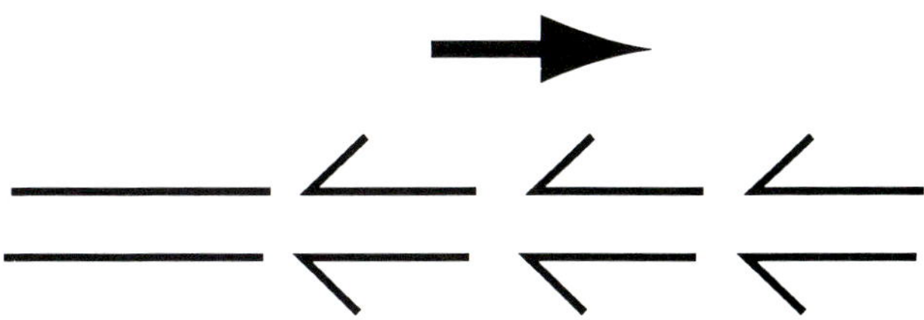

Fig. 15.16 Tears are angled away from the direction of blade travel.

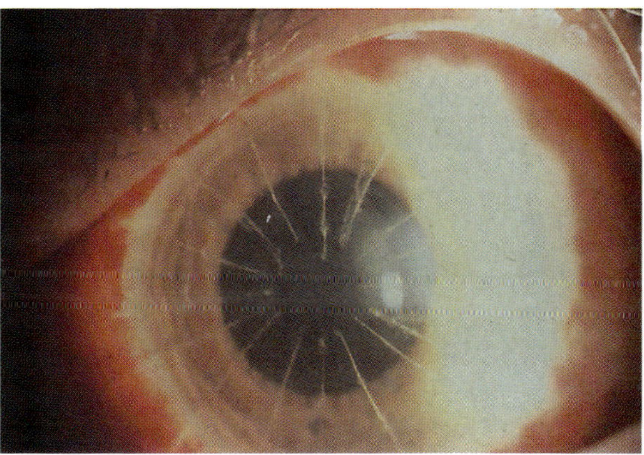

Fig. 15.17 Irregular scarring from transverse tears in Bowman's can increase the problem with glare.

Corneal perforation

There are two types of perforation, micro, in which only the very tip of the blade has entered the anterior chamber, and macro, in which the opening is a frank incision involving the anterior chamber (Figures 15.18 through 15.20). The latter occurs either because the incision is being made too rapidly when a thin spot or "dimple" is encountered or the microperforation went unnoticed and the incision was extended. Perforations may occur initially at the edge of the OZ with the first entry of the blade—in which case the blade obviously was set too long—or anywhere along an incision. The more likely spot for the latter event will be in the inferotemporal quadrant, where such dimples are encountered frequently (Figure 15.21). The most common place along the incision for this to occur is at the midperiphery, especially at the beginning of the second stepped incision in a multistepped incision case.

The incidence of surgical invasion of the anterior chamber in RK has been reported to vary from 6% to 33% [18].

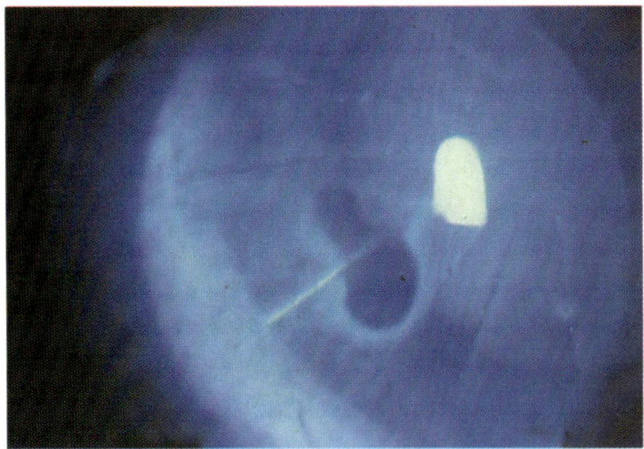

Fig. 15.18 Positive Seidel's sign, indicating an active leak—the sign of a microperforation.

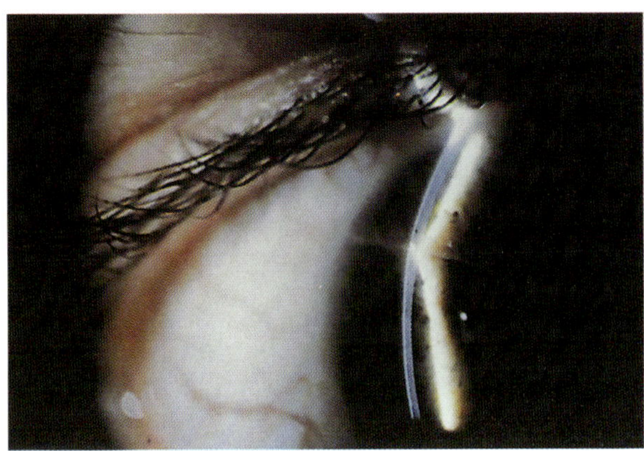

Fig. 15.20 Adherent leukoma—macroperforation.

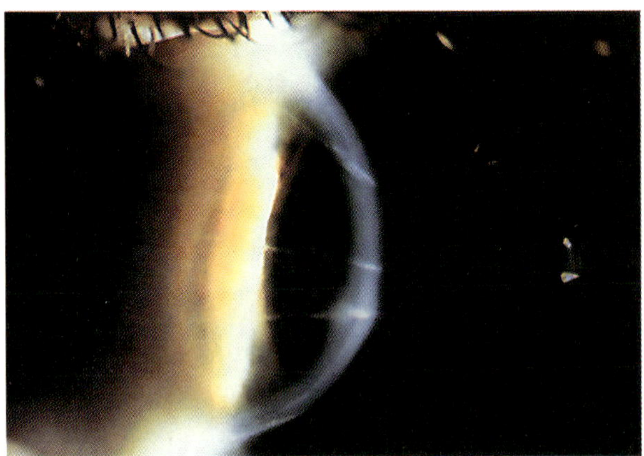

Fig. 15.19 Self-sealed leak—hallmark of a microperforation.

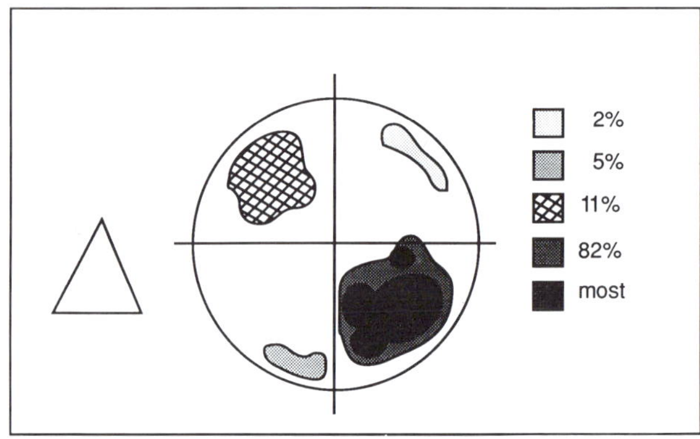

Fig. 15.21 Distribution of corneal "dimples" or thin areas.

The author has found the incidence to vary depending on the blade used, the position of the surgeon on the learning curve for that blade, and the degree of myopia present. The highest incidence of penetration in the author's series occurred with the use of Sputnik steel blades about 1 month after beginning the use of ultrasonic pachymetry. This was 23% and occurred because of the practice of oversetting the blade 10% to 15% in each case. It also could have been due to an erroneous setting for the speed of sound through the cornea. When the author switched to the sapphire blade, the incidence dipped to 8% after only a few months of trial-and-error adjustment of the blade depth to obtain the optimal settings.

Do not be quick to envy the surgeon whose reported perforation rate is low without examining his or her technique and results. It is a small thing to obtain a zero incidence of microperforation—simply set the blade too shallow. There are those who advocate just such an approach [19]. The problem with perforations is not the perforation itself, but the failure to accord sufficient significance to the puncture—it is a potentially serious invasion of the body's defenses. A small number of microperforations, however, is acceptable as an indication that the blade depth is close to optimal. The surgery works best with deep incisions, and each surgeon should make the deepest incisions possible without incurring too great an incidence of perforation. In this author's opinion, an 8% to 10% incidence of microperforation is acceptable for an average surgeon. For an expert, it could be slightly higher.

Unless the perforation has occurred at the beginning of a multistep 16-incision case, it is not necessary to abandon the case, provided that the leak can be stopped or has occurred after the initial incisions have been made (in a stepped procedure) and the surgeon is using an ultrasharp crystalline blade. At the first sign of a perforation—which in most cases will be the sudden appearance of aqueous just behind the blade—the blade should be removed from the cornea immediately to prevent extension of the perforation. Sometimes a microperforation will show itself by a bead of aqueous appearing in one incision during the incising of another part of the cornea.

Perforations occurring while making the initial incisions should be sutured. For this, 10-0 nylon on a fishhook needle is placed approximately 0.5 mm behind the end of the incision (toward the optical center). This is done

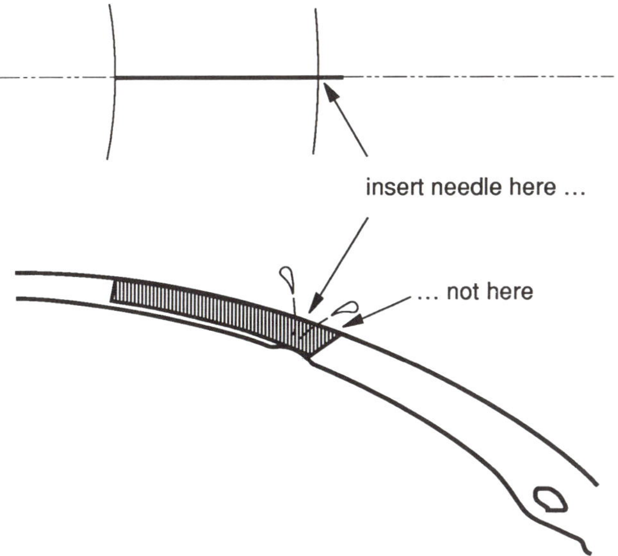

Fig. 15.22 Suture is placed before the end of the incision.

because the leading edge of the incision is slanted backward from the surface of the incision (Figure 15.22). One suture is sufficient if it is placed very deep or above Descemet's membrane. Complete the remainder of the incisions, leaving the sutured one until last. Perform all tag removal and free-hand redeepening (if the chamber is not flat and the pupil is not dilated) before removing the suture. Do not leave the suture in place, and do not cut it with your RK blade. Leaving the suture in place will cause gaping of adjacent incisions and is likely to result in the formation of irregular astigmatism (Figure 15.23).

In cases of microperforation, pressure patching overnight is usually enough to allow the perforation to seal and the leak to stop (see Figure 15.19). In most cases, the anterior chamber is of normal depth and absolutely quiet the following day. In those eyes which show a positive Seidel's sign (leakage demonstrated after topical fluorescein), repeat patching will solve the problem in the majority of instances. The author had to resort to use of a "bandage" contact lens in the face of persistent leak twice and sutures once in over 15 years of experience with this surgery.

A macroperforation will announce itself by a sudden gush of aqueous and collapse of the anterior chamber. More than one suture may be needed to close such an incision. In rare cases, such sutures may have to be left in place after the surgery. However, it is not recommended that they be left longer than 1 week. They should then be removed one at a time, allowing any subsequent leak to seal before removing another one. In no case should less than 24 hours elapse between removals.

Once the primary incisions have been made in a stepped case, the remaining portions of the incisions can be completed with the newer crystalline blades with confidence that the incisions will be of adequate depth. This is not true of steel blades or the older diamond blades.

Most of these perforations will seal off spontaneously with a deep chamber forming within the first 24 hours. Attempting to reinflate the anterior chamber using BSS or Healon (or other viscoelastic material) is not recommended for the reason that there is a risk of introducing contamination. Further, there is a good possibility that this manipulation may cause the wound to leak even more. In addition, the risk of injuring internal structures is increased as well as the possibility of creating an epithelial downgrowth (Figures 15.24 and 15.25). If the leak is bad enough to require refilling the anterior chamber, it is time to abort the surgery and possibly introduce sutures. Most of these perforation spots heal without excessive scarring. However, an occasional small area of subendothelial fibrosis may be seen (Figure 15.26). This process, fortunately, is self-limited and only rarely interferes with vision.

This complication can be minimized by careful ultrasonic pachymetric "mapping" of the cornea, the use of

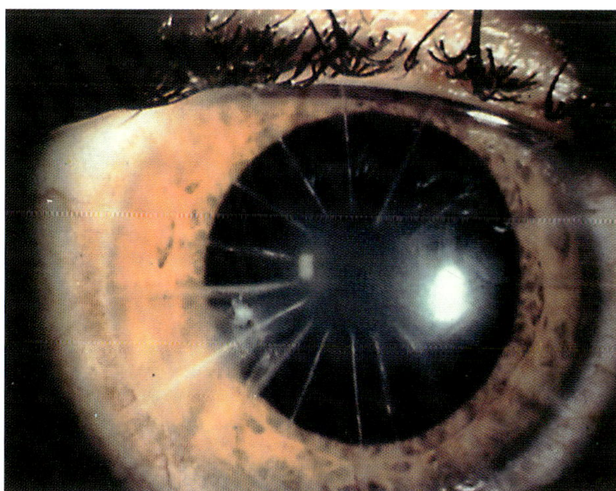

Fig. 15.23 Repaired macroperforation. Note spreading of adjacent incisions.

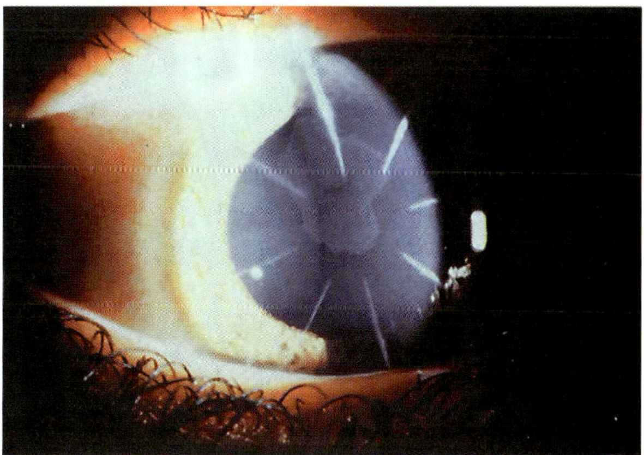

Fig. 15.24 Epithelial downgrowth following a microperforation. (Courtesy of P. Binder.)

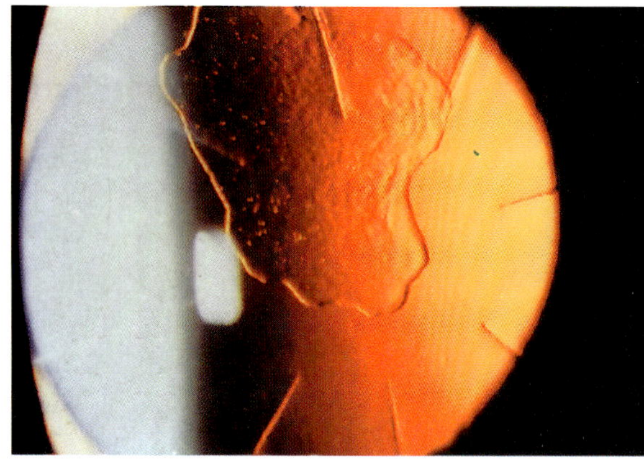

Fig. 15.25 Closer view of an epithelial downgrowth. The patient responded to cryotherapy of the lesion. (Courtesy of P. Binder.)

Fig. 15.26 Fibrous proliferation under Descemet's is sometimes seen after a microperforation.

ultrasharp blades that plunge and cut to a known setting, and precise blade setting. Gauges used to set blades should be checked with known standards to "calibrate" each one individually. An optical or shadowgraph gauge (such as the DGH-800) will help to reduce the incidence of such perforations.

It is recommended that all patients in whom perforations have occurred be started on oral broad-spectrum antibiotics such as cephalosporin for a period of 5 to 7 days (see also "Infection," below). If the chamber has been opened widely, or if influx of fluid has occurred or is suspected (such as by seeing blood in the anterior chamber), it is advised that a subtenon injection of gentamycin (or equivalent) be done on the operating table at the close of the surgery.

Incision abnormalities

These complications are a manifestation of "pilot error" and generally can be avoided. Incision abnormalities include obliquely incised cuts caused by failure to control the perpendicularity of the blade. Despite wider footplates, this is still a problem, especially in soft eyes. Irregular incisions or "dog-legs" are a result of blades being moved too slowly through tissue, sudden patient movement, loss of fixation, torquing of the eye due to incomplete fixation, oblique fixation, or blade-handle footplates that are too short, too narrow, or offset (Figure 15.27). The sharper the blade, the less "forgiving" of slight lateral or torquing movements it will be. These irregularities are more unsightly than harmful, but the causation can lead to confluent incisions. Confluent or joined incisions can occur while making parallel cuts. If care is not taken and/or a dull blade is used, one or more of the incisions can run into the adjacent ones (Figure 15.28). Oblique fixation is the most common cause because it permits the eye to rotate and the incision to drift sideways. When this occurs, the travel of the blade has to be adjusted to curve the blade path away from the adjacent

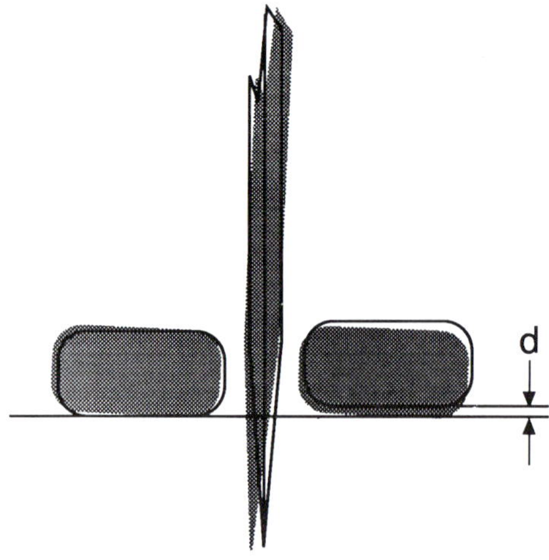

Fig. 15.27 An angled footplate can cause oblique incisions which in turn increase scarring and glare. The shaded figure represents the proper configuration.

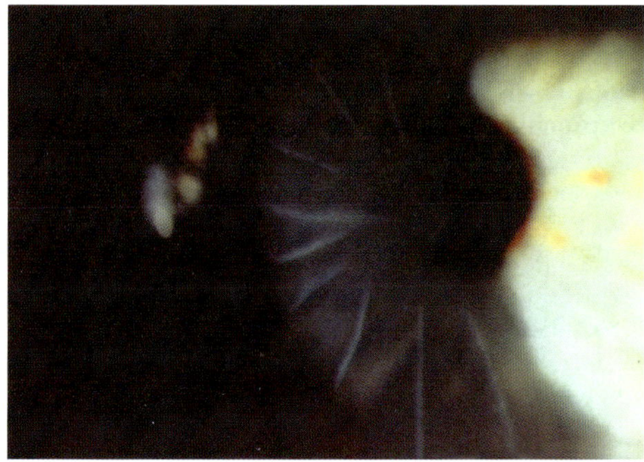

Fig. 15.28 Incisions made from the limbus have a tendency to wander as they approach the center. Sometimes they will join another incision or extend into the optical zone.

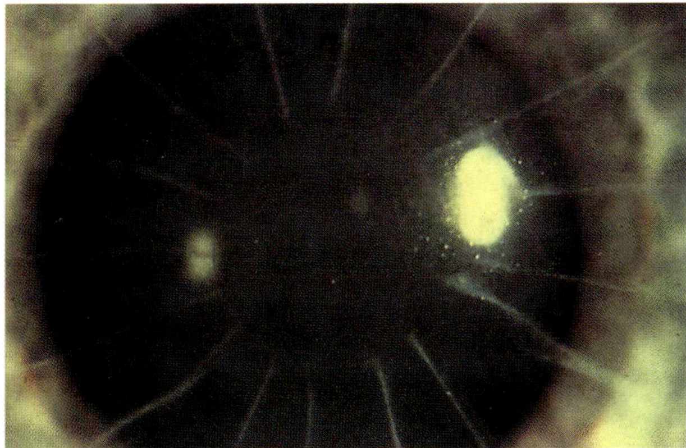

Fig. 15.29 Irregular and oblique incisions.

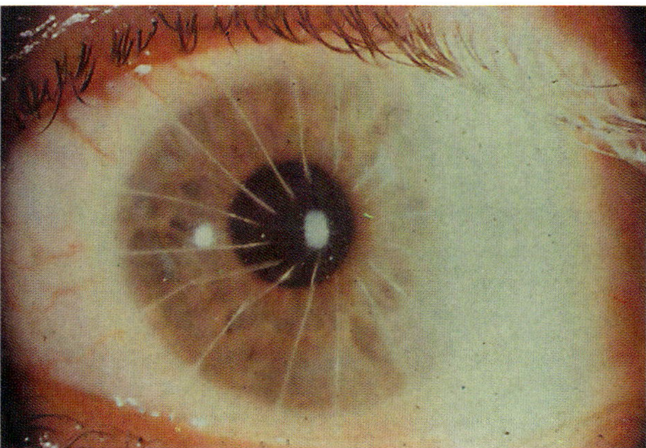

Fig. 15.30 Not only are the incisions irregular in this case, but so is the optical zone.

incision. If two incisions do become joined, the short incision has to be recut so as to extend it to the limbus. There is a possibility of developing astigmatism due to irregular healing in these cases. In small zone cases, less than precise placement of the blade at the edge of the OZ may join incisions. This also can occur when using the limbus-to-center (Russian) incision technique. There is no recovery from this. Occasionally, the very tip of the tissue triangle that results retracts or gets dissolved in the healing process, producing a depressed scar area and permanent glare.

Separated incisions or tissue "stalagmites" can occur during stepping of incisions (Figure 15.29). This is caused by imprecise placement of the blade at the beginning of the secondary incision. These errors prevent the complete outward movement of the cornea in this area—consequently, the tissue is flatter here. Subtle irregular astigmatism results with degradation of best visual acuity, with or without correction. This complication can be prevented by using ultrasharp blades, precision blade implantation, a light touch on the cornea, and proper fixation (see also Chapter 8).

Invasion of the optical clear zone is a much more serious complication that can result in an increase in glare at the least and frank loss of vision at the most. There are two ways in which the visual center can be compromised in this surgery. The first, and by far the most common, is decentration of the OZ (Figure 15.30).

OZ decentration

Decentration of the optical clear zone is clearly a result of surgeon error. This can occur through inattention, failure to obtain cooperation by the patient, or marking concentrically to the pupil. By following a few simple rules (outlined under "Surgery—The technique of RK" in Chapter 8), this complication can be avoided. Displacement of the optical clear zone by inaccurate or careless marking of either the visual axis, the clear zone, or both can lead to incisions in the clear zone or even across the visual axis. In cases of astigmatism, decentration of the optical clear zone inevitably will lead to irregular astigmatism. When in doubt that the patient is cooperating in fixating on the microscope light, have the patient look down, right, left, up, and then back at the light. Turn the microscope light way down if necessary, and dim the room lights so as to be able to see the light reflex. Obey the old surgical adage: *"When in doubt—don't!"*

There is no treatment for this error other than symptomatic. Some cases have required keratoplasty for this specific reason (see also Chapter 6 for a discussion of surface curvature anomalies following OZ decentration).

Invasion of the optical axis or optical clear zone

This complication is almost exclusively confined to the Russian or centripetal incision technique and is always caused by surgeon error (Figure 15.31). Cutting from limbus to center is a hazardous undertaking at all times. The patient has only to look toward the blade to cause it to move into the OZ. A dull blade will contribute to this complication as well by making the speed of the cut dif-

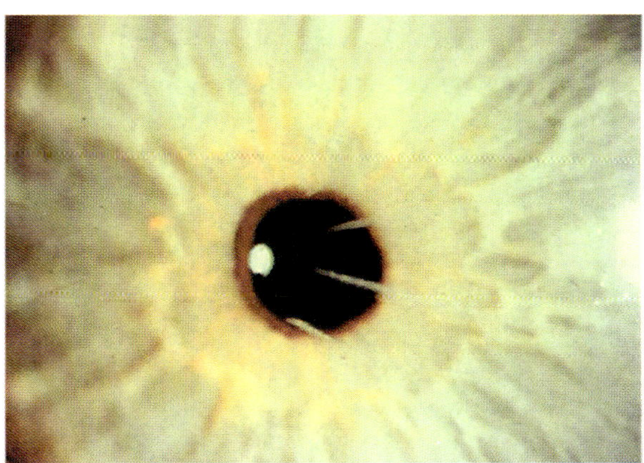

Fig. 15.31 Decentered optical zone.

ficult to control. Precise control and timing are necessary to stop the blade exactly on the edge of the clear zone. If the surgeon is inexperienced and/or the blade is dull, it is very likely that blade movement will cease before the edge of the clear zone is reached. If movement of the blade stops before reaching the edge of the clear zone, it will take more force to get it moving again than it did to keep it moving. In this event, entry into the clear zone is enhanced. This difficulty is enhanced further if the cornea is soft. Sometimes the force is sufficiently disproportionate that the blade "jumps" forward and enters the clear zone before it can be controlled or stopped.

This same scenario can be seen when backing up a double-edged blade to deepen the incision at the primary OZ. It is less likely in this situation because Bowman's layer has already been incised, and therefore, tissue resistance will be markedly less. Still, care must be taken to prevent a disaster.

Consequently, with the centripetal or Russian technique, it is not possible to have a precise OZ margin and for the same reason [20]. Fixation must be behind the knife, and the blade must be exquisitely sharp to perform this method safely. With certain blades, the setting must be modified to prevent perforating into the anterior chamber. All in all, this is an unsafe and unsatisfactory methodology best reserved for redeepening of shallow incisions after the fact and only in experienced hands.

Such an event can be prevented in a number of ways. First, the surgeon should have considerable experience with RK before attempting limbus-to-center incisions. Next, the blade used for this type of incision must be very sharp. A sharp blade is more controllable and easier to start or stop. However, in a soft cornea, transverse folds can occur that can impede forward progress of the knife footplate. In this event, fixation behind the blade at the limbus will give the surgeon more control and may cause the folds to flatten.

Complications—Postoperative

Astigmatism

The incidence of induced irregular astigmatism following RK is, fortunately, quite rare [21,22]. When it is seen, its cause usually can be traced to a problem with the incisions, as described earlier (see "Corneal perforation" and "Incision abnormalities," above). Regular astigmatism that remains after surgery is most often a result of an incomplete correction or residual myopia either through failure to correct for the astigmatic portion or ignoring it. While it is true that up to 1.50 D of astigmatism may disappear after operating for the sphere alone in 16-incision cases, this is not true for incisions less than 16 in number. The rule of thumb for the author is to compensate for the astigmatism when that component equals or exceeds 20% of the spherical myopia and/or when the astigmatism is

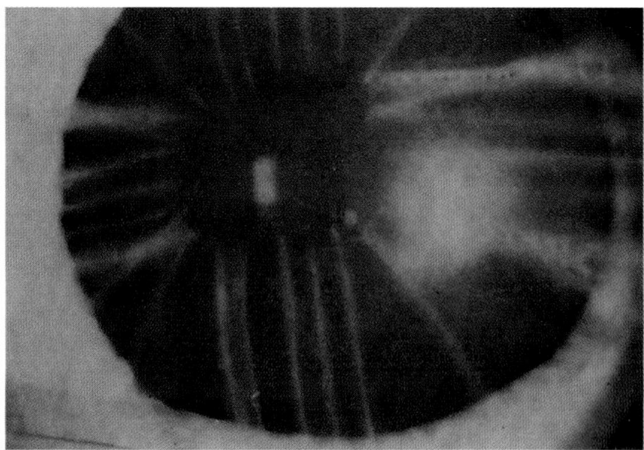

Fig. 15.32 Results of choosing the wrong initial astigmatic axis.

"against-the-rule" (see also Chapter 9). Patients will tolerate surprisingly large values of "with-the-rule" astigmatism postoperatively. It is the author's considered opinion that a small residual "with-the-rule" astigmatism is not a bad thing and actually may improve the patient's visual perception.

One common cause of induced regular astigmatism is making astigmatism incisions in the wrong axis (Figure 15.32). This has happened to experienced surgeons as well as neophytes. It is a very real danger, and the risk of this happening should not be minimized. This can occur as a result of a misunderstanding of the principles of astigmatic correction and confusion of the axis with the meridian. All practitioners are advised to map out the incisional configuration well before, and not during, the day of surgery. If changes are believed to be required at the time of surgery, be sure that such a change is absolutely correct before proceeding. If still confused, or if any doubt exists, do not do the surgery. In fact, a good watchword for this surgery is: *"When in doubt—don't!"*

Use an optical device such as an eyepiece reticle or surgical protractor to mark the plus axis with the marker designed for this purpose. Before making the first incision, double-check the axis, preferably with one of your knowledgeable staff. When in doubt—bail out.

In cases of irregular astigmatism, the cause of the irregularity must be addressed directly (Figure 15.33). If the problem is due to shallow incisions or some other incisional problem, and if the case is less than 1 month after the original surgery, the offending incision should be deepened, or the tag should be removed, or the incision should be lengthened (or whatever)—immediately. If more than 1 month has elapsed since the surgery, then the surgeon is advised to wait a minimum of 4 to 6 months to reoperate—preferably the latter. Sutures or intraincisional debris should be removed immediately and the epithelium allowed to heal completely before proceeding. In unusual cases it may be necessary to perform additional incisions to relax or further modify the corneal shape to

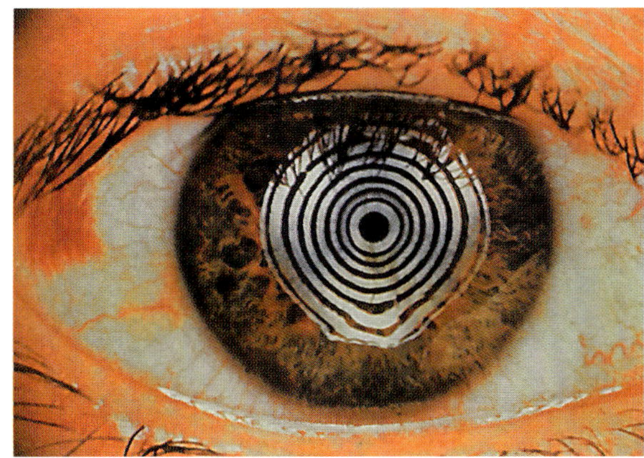

Fig. 15.33 Irregular astigmatism following RK. (Courtesy of A. Neumann.)

relieve the irregularity. Corneal topography is helpful here. In these cases, the full waiting time of 6 months should be allowed to elapse before further surgery is done. It should be apparent that the timing of any additional surgery is predicated on stability of the cornea. If change is still occurring, then further waiting is mandatory.

It may be necessary to curette and suture tightly the incisions in the axis of greatest flattening to reduce the chord length, thereby steepening the corneal curvature (Figure 15.34). This is especially helpful in cases involving T (transverse) incisions (see also "Overcorrections (induced hyperopia)," below).

The correction of induced irregular astigmatism is a specialized problem requiring tailored approaches based on extensive experience. The less experienced surgeon is advised to seek consultation in all such cases.

While waiting for the cornea to stabilize or as an alternative to further surgery, it may be advisable to fit a hard or gas-permeable contact lens. The usual rules apply. However, such a fitting should be delayed until 6 to 8 weeks have elapsed. This delay will minimize any tendency toward developing neovascularization.

Residual or induced regular myopic astigmatism can be treated as outlined in "Undercorrections (residual myopia)" (see below). The best treatment is, as always, prevention by careful preoperative evaluation and planning and the use of ultrasharp blades set at maximum depth with careful blade placement and incision control.

Ax (flat)

X–type suture placed in **FLAT** axis to steepen it.

Ax (steep)

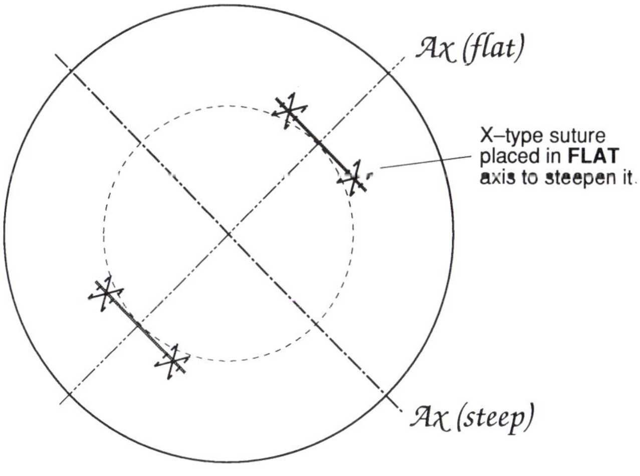

Fig. 15.34 Correcting an over-corrected T-cut with sutures.

Undercorrections (residual myopia)

Despite the best planning, some cases will end up with residual myopia. In the majority of these cases the cause will be incisions that are too shallow, too few, or too short (OZ too big) [23–25] (Figure 15.35). All these problems can be solved for the most part by correcting the deficiencies. Timing is the essence, however, in these corrective efforts.

Generally speaking, shallow incisions should be recut and deepened within the first month of the initial surgery. If not done within the first 30 days, then the deepening should be delayed for at least 4 months—waiting at least 6 months is better. When deepening incisions, the straight or vertical-edged blade should be used, and the incisions should be deepened starting at the limbus and moving toward the center using the previous incision as a guide. Doubled incisions, with infolding of epithelium, can occur when trying to recut incisions from the center to the periphery. As Figures 15.36 and 15.37 illustrate, it is not possible to keep the blade within the old incision track unless the incision is made from the limbus to center. The knife footplate straddles the old incision—the surgeon using it as a guide. Figures 15.38 through 15.40 show the aftermath of incorrect technique. These types of incisions are notoriously unstable.

No more than eight incisions should be deepened at any one sitting. The eye becomes soft very quickly—thus there is a tendency for the blade to wander when approaching the center (Figures 15.41 and 15.42). Corneal pachymetry

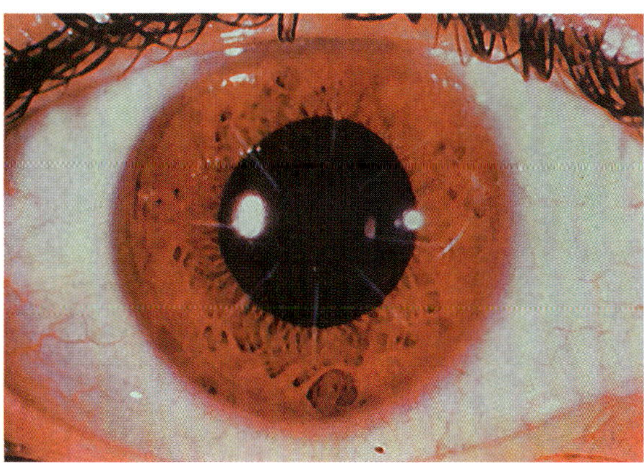

Fig. 15.35 Very short RK incisions. More than 20 incisions can produce the same effect—undercorrection.

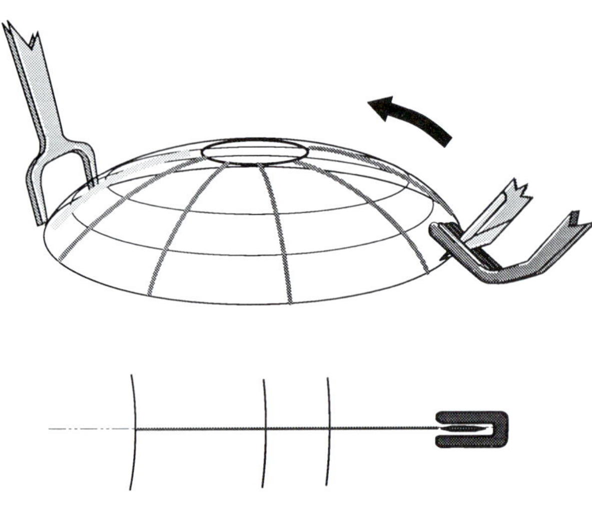

Fig. 15.36 An incision is recut from the limbus to the center.

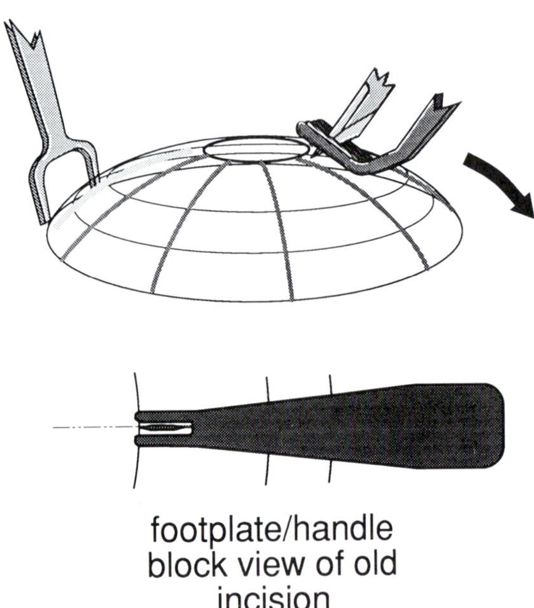

Fig. 15.37 Attempting to recut from the center results in blade wander—the old incision is obscured by the knife handle.

must be repeated because the cornea is always somewhat thicker postoperatively for some months—possibly a year or more [15,26] (Figure 15.43). Mapping can be done again between the previous incisions, but it is usually enough to get the central pachymetry, adding the increase to the original preoperative readings.

The decision to add incisions should be delayed until the corneas have become stabilized (around 4 to 6 months).

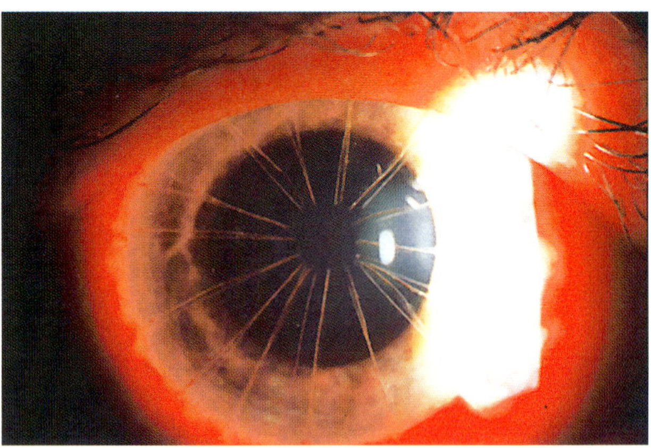

Fig. 15.38 Doubled incision—best case.

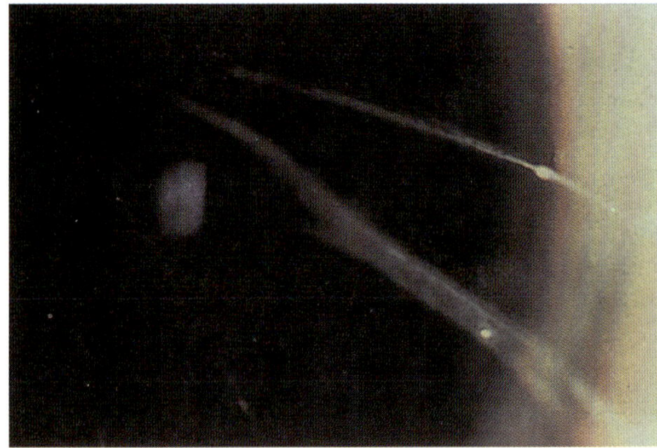

Fig. 15.39 Doubled incision—worst case.

The patient should then be reexamined and the parameters recalculated using the preoperative K-readings. This holds for astigmatic as well as spherical cases. Expect a correction of between 80% and 90% of the residual myopia and/or astigmatism.

It is wise to wait a minimum of 2 weeks before fitting spectacles. There will be a small percentage of patients who will require a change of lenses within 6 months. Contact lens fitting should be delayed for at least 6 weeks for hard lenses and 8 weeks for soft lenses (including extended wear). There is an increased risk of developing neovascularization if soft lenses are fitted before this time.

Overcorrections (induced hyperopia)

The author reported an incidence of postoperative hyperopia of less than 1% in a series of patients [27]. This phenomenon is more likely to occur in patients over 40 years of age with myopia of less than 3 D [28–30]. It is also more likely to occur with cases calculated using nomograms that do not take age or scleral rigidity into consideration. It is not unusual, even in well-calculated cases using

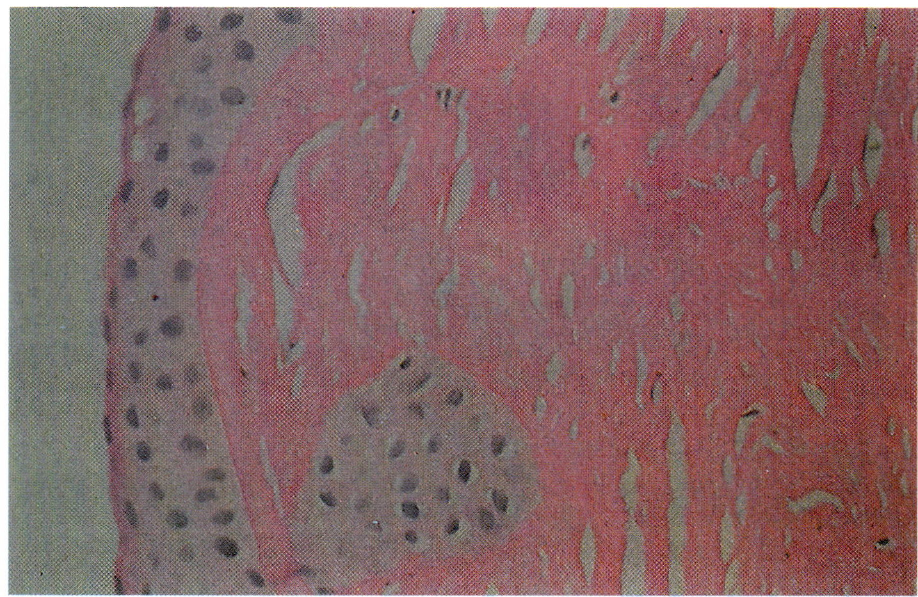

Fig. 15.40 Epithelium "plowed under" the stroma. (Courtesy of P. Binder.)

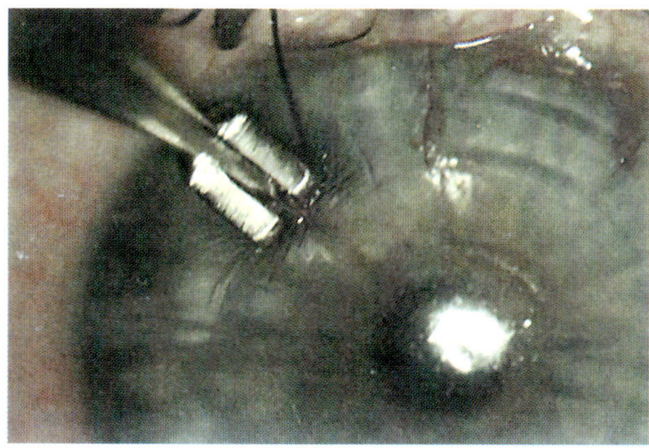

Fig. 15.41 The eye gets soft quickly in repeat operations. Note the wrinkles or furrows ahead of the footplate.

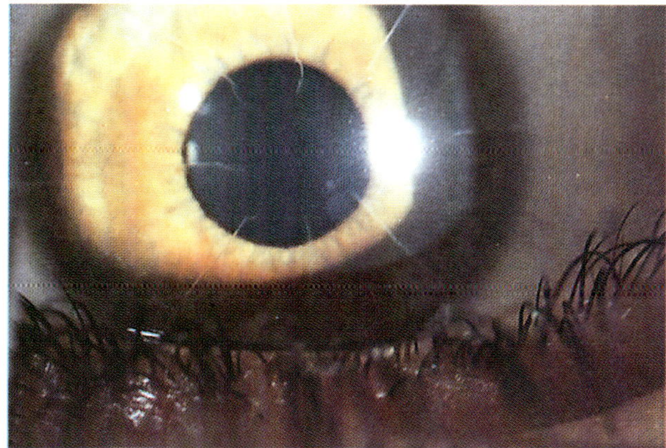

Fig. 15.42 Incisions tend to wander near the center.

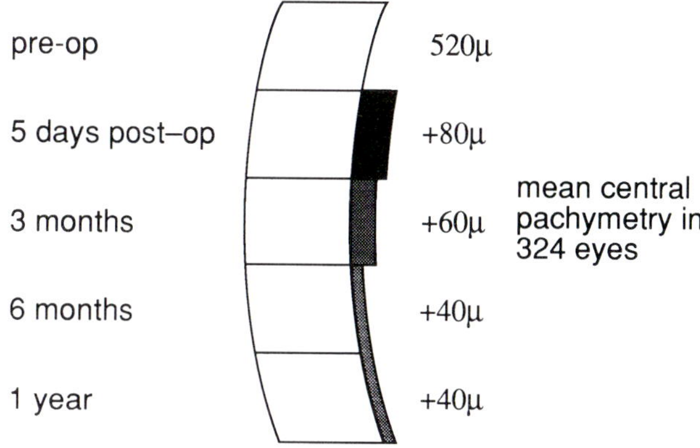

Fig. 15.43 Corneal thickness increases after RK surgery.

regression formulas, for patients to show an initial overcorrection lasting upwards of 3 to 4 weeks. Deitz and Waring have noted that a certain percentage of patients undergoing RK have shown a progression of effect, some of whom have shifted to the hyperopic side—others also have reported a sporadic incidence of this complication [28,31–33]. The author has a few patients within his practice who also have shown a shift to the hyperopic side 4 years after RK, but it is less than the 30% reported by Deitz and Waring. As a matter of fact, some of this so-called progression may be a result of a normal fluctuation in K-readings seen in normal, unoperated patients. Figures 15.44 through 15.48 and Tables 15.1 through 15.4 illustrate this phenomenon.

This problem is difficult to recover from, although if the hyperopia is less than 1 D, it may well be lost eventually through a process called *emmetropization* (Figures 15.49 and 15.50). Any hyperopia greater than 1 D and lasting

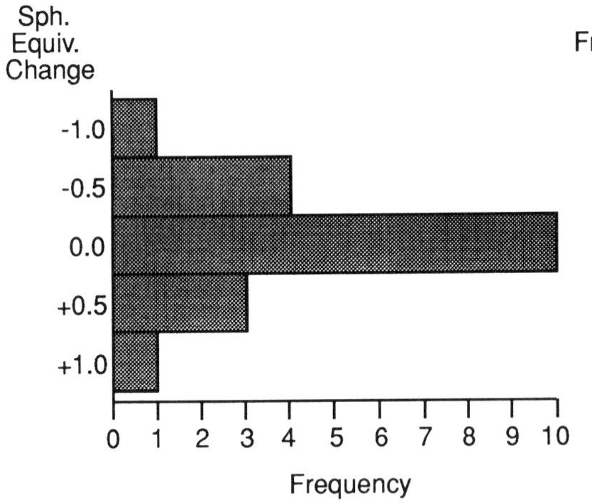

Sph. Equiv. Change	Freq.	Cum. Freq.	%	Cum.%
-1.0	1	1	5.263	5.26
-0.5	4	5	21.053	26.32
0.0	10	15	52.632	78.95
+0.5	3	18	15.789	94.74
+1.0	1	19	5.263	100.00

Frequency

Fig. 15.44 Change in spherical equivalent in RK cases over 3 years. (Courtesy of S. Grandon.)

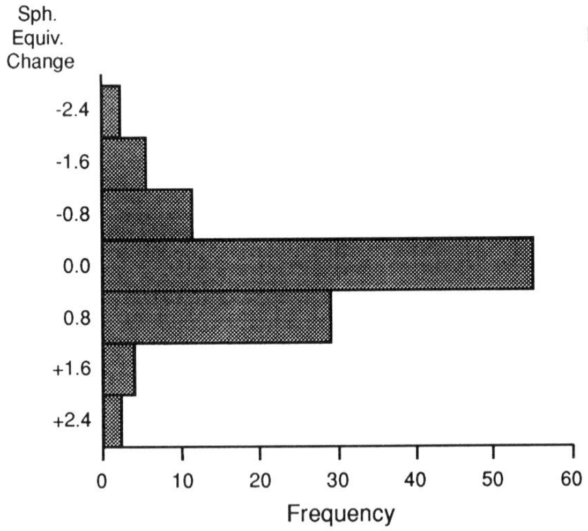 Sph. Equiv. Change	Freq.	Cum. Freq.	%	Cum.%
-2.4	1	1	1.064	1.064
-1.6	5	6	5.319	5.383
-0.8	11	17	11.702	18.085
0.0	54	71	57.447	75.532
0.8	19	90	20.213	95.745
+1.6	3	93	3.191	98.936
+2.4	1	94	1.064	100.000

Frequency

Fig. 15.45 Change in spherical equivalent in control (no surgery) cases over 3 years. (Courtesy of S. Grandon.)

RK cases 3 – 12 mnths 91.9%
RK cases 3 – 24 mnths 87.8%
RK cases 3 – 36 mnths 89.6%
Control cases 3 – 36 mnths 76.9%
0% 100%
Cases

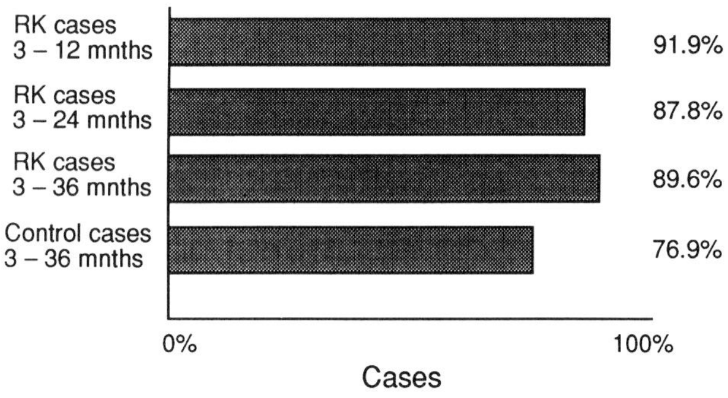

Fig. 15.46 Comparison of spherical equivalent changes in both groups. (Courtesy of S. Grandon.)

RK cases 3 – 12 mnths 2.0% (4 cases)
RK cases 3 – 24 mnths 5.1% (5 cases)
RK cases 3 – 36 mnths 5.2% (5 cases)
Control cases 3 – 36 mnths 10.6% (3 cases)
0% 10%
Cases

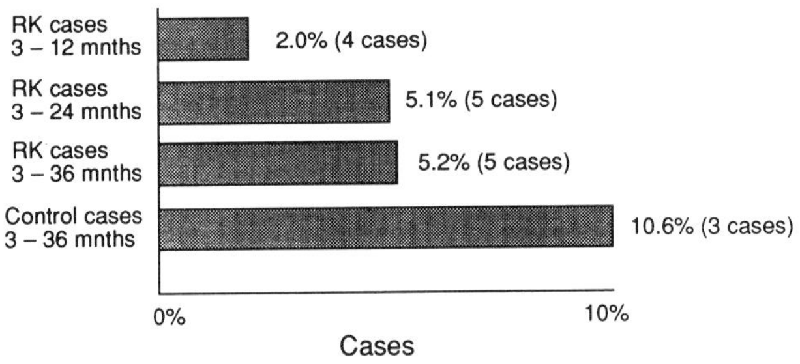

Fig. 15.47 Hyperopic shifts in both groups. (Courtesy of S. Grandon.)

more than 6 to 8 weeks is likely to remain and poses a problem, especially for older patients. The administration of steroid drops (such as 1% Pred-Forte) four times daily for a period of weeks starting at about 8 weeks has, in some cases, reduced the overcorrection by as much as 1 D.

In the past it had been recommended that deep incisions, beginning at 9 mm and extending across the limbus approximately 1.0 mm, be made so as to cause central steepening of the cornea (as demonstrated experimentally) [34]. The author has performed this procedure on

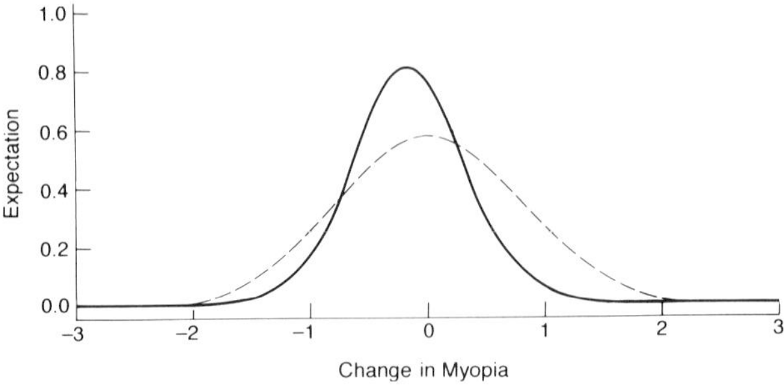

Fig. 15.48 Mean changes in spherical equivalent. (Courtesy of S. Grandon.)

Table 15.1 Preoperative patient statistics in Grandon's study

	Mean	s.d.	Min	Max
Age (years)	34/42	9.59	17	64
Spherical equivalent	−4.58	1.89	−1.12	−13.13
Corneal diameter	11.86	0.49	10.50	13.50
Axial length	25.00	1.01	22.40	28.20
Mean keratometry	44.23	1.45	40.44	47.81

Total number of patients, 335; number of male patients, 136 (40.6%); number of female patients, 199 (59.4%).

Table 15.2 Surgical technique used in Grandon's study

Variable	Value
Topical anesthetic	4.0% Xylocaine
Clear zone size range	3–6 mm
Knife used	Diamond set to 90–100% + 30 μm thinnest pachymetry
Incisions made	8
Redeepening done in high myopic cases	
Postoperative antibiotics	12 days
Topical steroids	0–6 weeks
Timoptic gtts used in some cases	

Table 15.3 Mean changes in spherical equivalent in Grandon's study

	RK cases			Control cases		
Year	*n*	Mean	s.d.	*n*	Mean	s.d.
1	212	−0.12 D	0.68			
2	90	+0.64 D	0.64	94	+0.011 D	0.411
3	19	−0.13 D	0.47	94	+0.016 D	0.724

Table 15.4 Conclusions of the Grandon study

Variation in RK patients does occur over time, but not more than the control group
There is no predominant hyperopic shift in the cases over time
The vast majority of cases remain stable over time
Statistical analysis of changes in myopia over time indicates that preoperative myopia may be a contributing factor

Refraction Dynamics
3.0 D myopia — 12 eyes

Refraction	Observation Period (in years)						
	1/12	0.5	1	2	3	4	4.5
− 1.0 D	2	1	—	—	—	—	—
− 0.5 D	1	2	2	1	2	2	2
0	4	6	9	10	10	10	10
+ 1.0 D	3	3	1	—	—	—	—
+ 2.0 D	2	—	—	—	—	—	—

Fig. 15.49 Emmetropization in 12 eyes. (Courtesy of S.N. Fyodorov.)

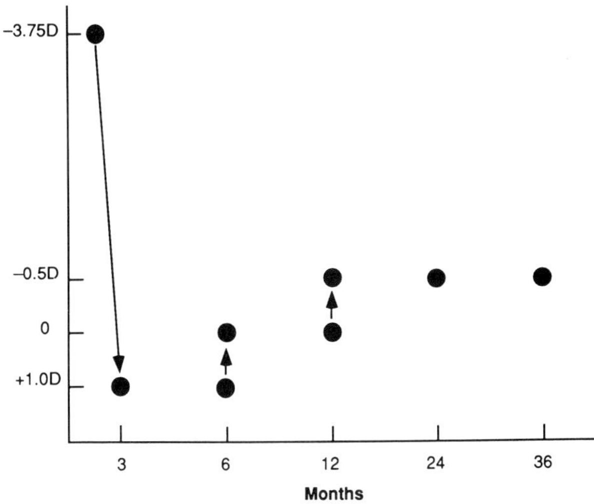

Fig. 15.50 Typical emmetropization pattern. (Courtesy of S.N. Fyodorov.)

two eyes with good results. After 34 months of follow-up, each eye has retained approximately 1 D of steepening. However, the end result is not in any way predictable, and additional experience with this method by the author and others has not supported the initial optimism. Additionally, there is a real danger of inflicting serious damage to the angle structures.

The use of antiglaucomatous medication, such as beta blockers, has proven to be of some value in reducing overcorrections of up to 2 D. It may be necessary to continue the use of such therapy for as long as a year. Even then, some cases have been reported in which the hyperopia has returned upon discontinuation of the medication. Furthermore, not all normal individuals will respond to beta blockers with a reduction in IOP. Such response as there is will be variable. However, if there are no contraindications, it may be worth trying.

Hexagonal incisions (HK) have been advocated for overcorrections up to 4 D of hyperopia [35,36]. The author has used a hexagonal pattern of 6 mm in diameter for hyperopia up to 1.75 D. While recovery of vision is rapid, it is often unstable. In these cases it is necessary that the hexagon sides join or cross the radials. In such cases, the objectionable gaping that usually accompanies small-diameter hexagons is seen often. Splitting of the junction of the transverse and radial incisions has occurred even after 1 year. Consequently, a minimum of 6 months (preferably more) should elapse before these incisions are

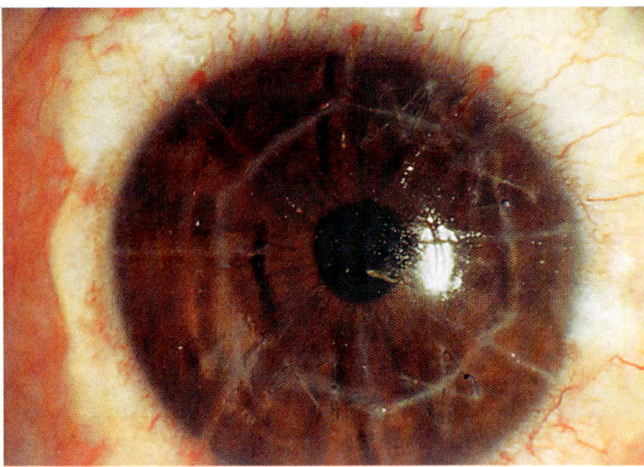

Fig. 15.51 Hexagonal procedure over RK. Despite a delay of 8 months between procedures the incision junctions required suturing to reduce fluctuation of vision and gross overcorrection (too much myopia).

made to avoid gaping at the interstices. However, despite initial and favorable reports of HK over RK, the author does not recommend use of this technique in RK overresponders (Figure 15.51; see also Chapter 14).

Likewise, the author does not recommend the use of thermokeratoplasty, as advocated by Schachar [37]. Placing the burns in the RK incisions results in a variable outcome often associated with induced astigmatism. This occurs because denaturation of the scar tissue does not appear to be a uniform process, and scarring is often much greater than anticipated. Placing the burns between radial incisions often leads to splitting and/or widening of the adjacent incisions. Such splitting or widening also results in unpredictable astigmatism—sometimes of the irregular variety.

Recently the author has used the method of hyperopic lamellar keratotomy (HLK) performed with the Barraquer microkeratome to correct induced hyperopia. By making a section of at least 80% in depth and by varying the diameter of the disk of tissue excised, hyperopia of up to 6 D has been predictably reversed. The procedure has the advantage that the cornea has not been materially weakened, as is the case in HK. A nontorquing 14-point suture is placed at the time of surgery and is removed within 7 to 14 days. The incidence of induced astigmatism is low. Since no freezing or lathing is involved, visual recovery is rapid (see Chapter 10).

In cases of reversal of the astigmatism where the axis has rotated 90°, other methods must be used. This complication is seen mostly in cases where trapezoidal keratotomy (Ruiz procedure) has been used. Invariably, the T-incisions are found to be too long or gape during healing, producing wide, soft scars. The recommended approach is to strip out the old scar and suture it tightly closed with one or two X-type sutures of 10-0 nylon (Figure 15.52). The sutures must be placed symmetrically—one on each side of the optical center—otherwise, gaping may occur in the unsutured T-cut. The sutures close the gap and reduce the chord length, consequently increasing corneal steepening in that meridian.

Such sutures placed at the ends of long T-cuts effectively shorten them and thus can reduce "coupling" and, at least theoretically, flatten the opposite meridian. The author prefers not to rely on theory and suggests employing the clinically proven method of suturing the incision in the flat meridian, as described above, one pair at a time.

The same basic procedure can be employed to correct spherical overcorrections. In these cases, three or four X-type sutures of 10-0 nylon (Ethicon, CUM-5, or similar) are placed symmetrically across the radial incision. These are placed between a 6- and 8-mm OZ mark made on the cornea in the usual fashion, and the knots are pulled below the corneal surface (see Figure 15.52a). The sutures are tightened sufficiently to produce very slight striations around the suture. These are best seen if the cornea is dry. An overcorrection of mild degree is the norm. This reverts within 7 to 10 days. Sometimes it is necessary to remove and replace sutures that are too tight or loose.

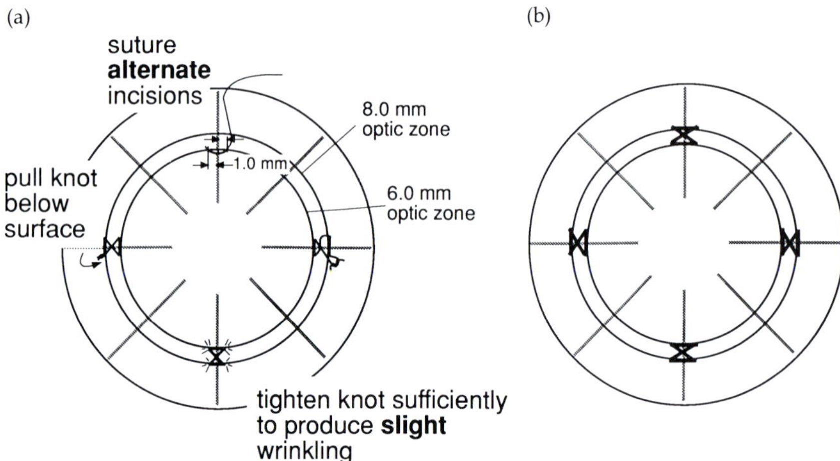

Fig. 15.52 (a,b) X-type sutures are placed symmetrically to steepen the cornea, thereby reducing induced hyperopia.

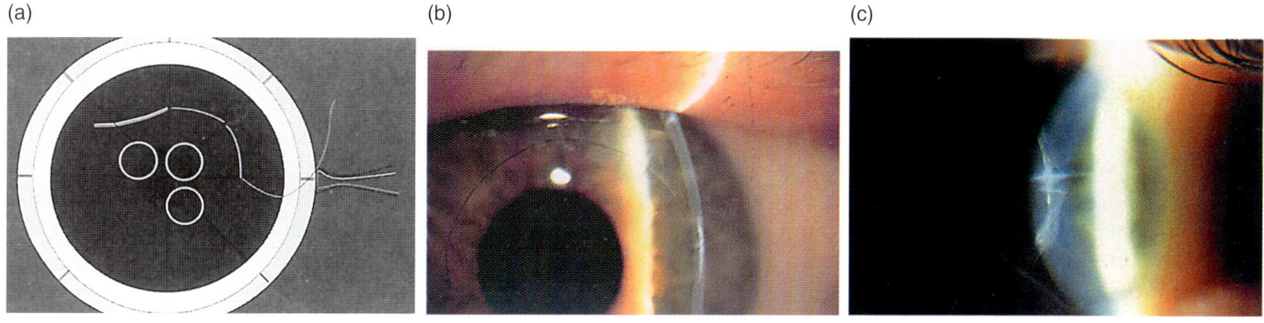

Fig. 15.53 (a) Method of placing the pursestring suture. (b) Suture in place in a human cornea. (c) Cheese-wiring is inevitable as the suture ligature takes a natural curved position within the stroma. (Courtesy of Robert Hoffman.)

These can be removed in 9 to 12 months, but if the patient is comfortable, the author leaves them in.

Starling and Hoffman have advocated the use of pursestring intrastromal sutures as a way of reducing induced hyperopia [38] (Figure 15.53a,b). Such a suture is technically difficult to place and inevitably results in some "cheese-wiring" with resulting loss of effect and induced scarring (see Figure 15.53c). While no cases of erosion of this suture into the anterior chamber have as yet been reported, the possibility of such a complication exists, particularly if the suture is drawn too tightly.

As always, the best treatment of any complication is prevention. Educated guesswork and making surgical decisions using tables based on one or two preoperative parameters is not the best way to optimize this surgery for each patient. Only the use of computer programs employing algorithms derived from regressive analysis of actual cases can be relied on to correlate the numerous parameters required for the successful outcome of this surgery.

Neovascularization

The author was the first to report the occurrence of this complication following the use of a soft contact lens immediately after surgery to stabilize the cornea [39] (Figures 15.54 and 15.55). This complication is evidenced by vessels running along incisions in the superficial part of the scar [20]. Typically, the encroachment is no more than 1 mm central to the capillary arcade. However, one case has occurred in which the vessels reached the edge of the OZ [40] (Figure 15.56). There have been few reported cases of neovascularization after RK except those associated with early contact lens wearing [2]. With the exception of the one case reported by Fyodorov, all have responded to removal of the lenses and application of topical steroids. All patients eventually have been able to wear contact lenses on a limited basis [41].

Neovascularization is not inherent to the procedure of RK even in cases where incisions crossed the limbus.

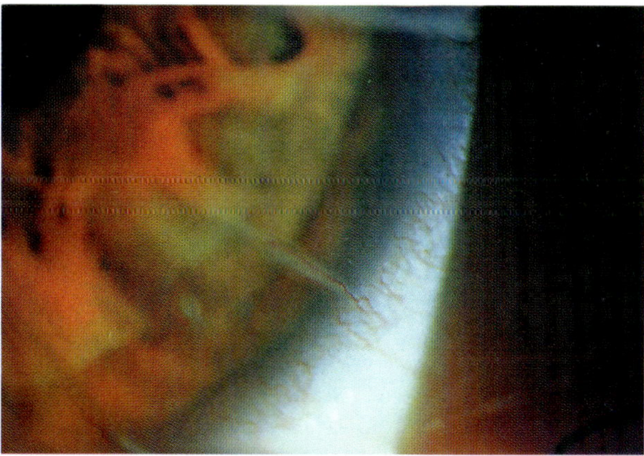

Fig. 15.54 First case of neovascularization reported after RK.

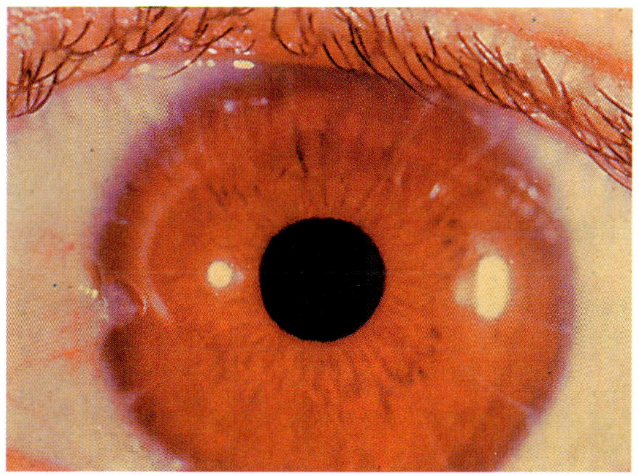

Fig. 15.55 Another, more advanced, case of neovascularization.

Except for some conjunctival "peaks" (Figure 15.57), in the absence of some inciting factor, neovascularization does not occur. The author has performed RK in two cases of superior limbic pannus after performing superficial keratectomies of the pannus. The pannus has not recurred, nor has there been any evidence of new vessel growth in the area.

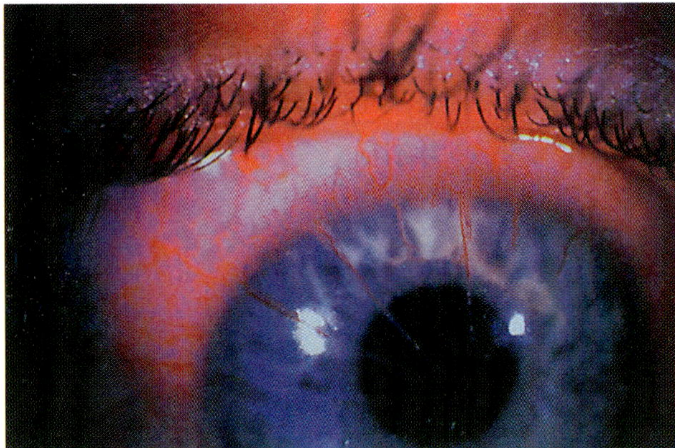

Fig. 15.56 Corneal limbal "peak" appearing when incisions cross the limbus.

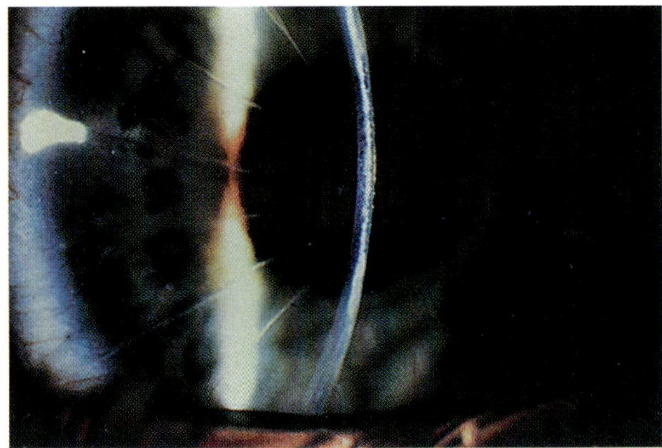

Fig. 15.58 Stromal reaction following RK in a patient with history of herpes keratitis. (Courtesy of M. Dietz.)

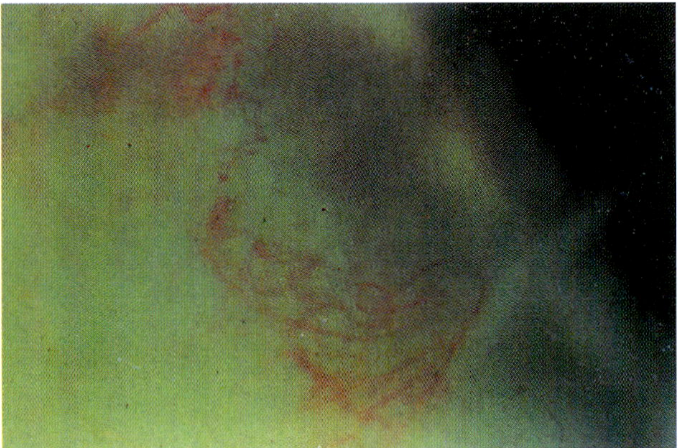

Fig. 15.57 Pseudopterygium after RK.

Infection

Fortunately, this is a rare problem, possibly because we have tended to be cautious in our follow-up—placing all patients on antibiotic drops following the surgery and covering, with oral antibiotics (in some cases, subtenon injection), those patients in whom perforations have occurred. It is also a rare happening undoubtedly because we are dealing with young, healthy eyes whose tear complex is alive and well. Still, the occasional infection does occur and ranges from small areas of epithelialitis to frank endophthalmitis. In 1980, Gelender reported a case of endophthalmitis immediately following RK in a patient in whom a perforation into the anterior chamber had occurred and who had not been placed on antibiotics [42]. Fortunately, the eye was saved by timely intervention with antibiotics and eventually a vitrectomy-lensectomy. At last report this eye had recovered a corrected visual acuity of 20/30.

Another patient was not so fortunate, developing an endophthalmitis 24 hours after surgery. Despite timely intervention, the eye was lost—surely not an expected sequela. Another patient developed a corneal infection approximately 1 month after RK following a hair-brush injury. This infection went on to become a frank endophthalmitis without subsequent loss of the eye.

Deep intrastromal keratitis was reported in three cases by Deitz, as well as Nirankari, in 1983 [14] (Figure 15.58). One of these cases was later shown to have had a history of previous herpetic keratitis. All these eyes sustained a profound loss of vision (less than 20/200) associated with the onset of central stromal clouding some 3 to 4 months after RK. All cases eventually responded to topical steroid therapy over an 8- to 10-week period, with no recurrence reported to date. For this reason, any eye in which previous herpes keratitis has been documented or suspected is not considered a candidate for this surgery [43,44].

Several cases of localized disease seemingly limited to the epithelium have been seen. Some of these occur as persistent optical clear zone marks, implying that the marker has either damaged the basement membrane or implanted some foreign substance (Figure 15.59). Other

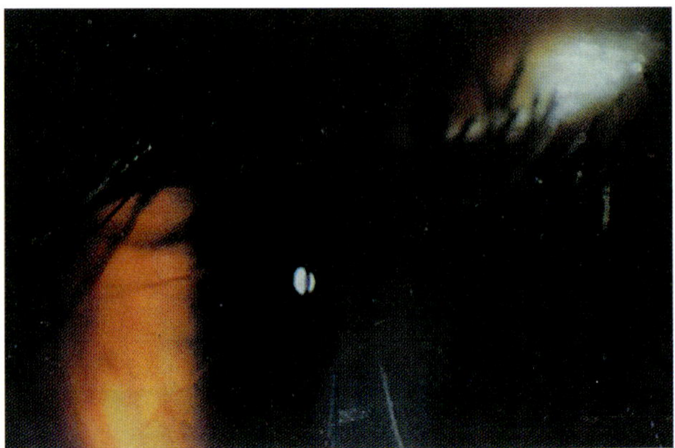

Fig. 15.59 Epithelial reaction at optical zone mark post-RK.

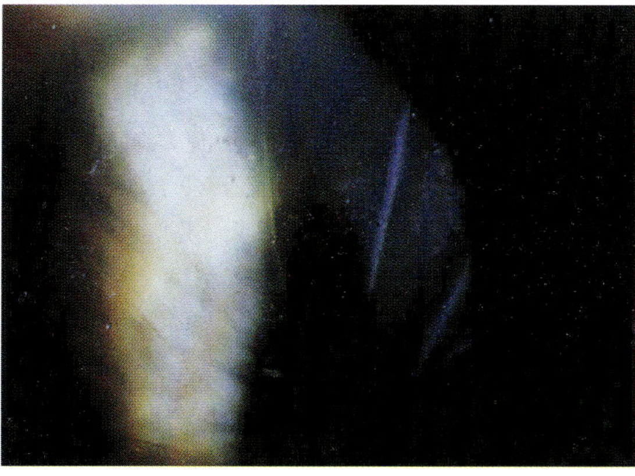

Fig. 15.60 Epithelialitis with a filament following RK.

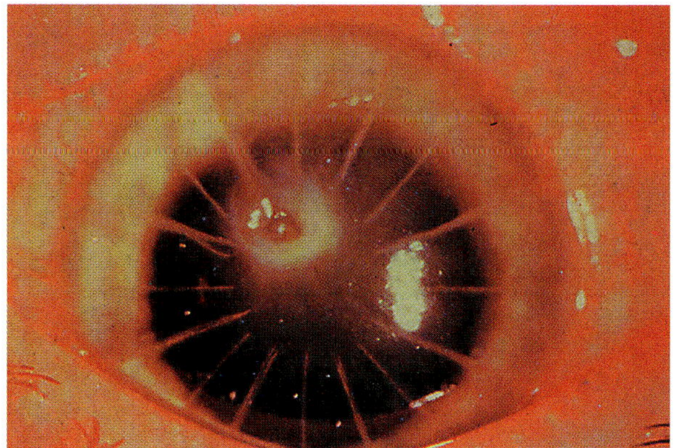

Fig. 15.61 Staphylococcal corneal ulcer.

times the inflammatory process lies between the incisions, and filaments may develop (Figure 15.60).

Fyodorov and his group have reported a case of staphylococcal corneal ulcer occurring in an incision following a reoperation [45] (Figure 15.61). This patient responded to antibiotics and debridement but was left with a wide scar causing increased glare. No astigmatism resulted, and the visual acuity was said to have returned to 20/25.

Iritis beyond a few cells with a trace of cells is unusual in this surgery, but of course, hypopyon has been reported in the presence of corneal ulcers.

The PERK study has reported on two cases of postoperative intracorneal abscesses occurring some 2 years after the initial surgery (Figure 15.62). Both patients eventually responded to conventional therapy as well [46–48]. Geggel reported a case of sterile keratitis which eventually required a penetrating keratoplasty (Figures 15.63 through 15.65). The author has also seen one case in which an intraincisional abscess formed approximately 3 years after RK. The infection cleared within 3 days with Ciloxan (topical ciprofloxacin) (Figures 15.66 and 15.67). Since then, 2 other cases have appeared, one occurring

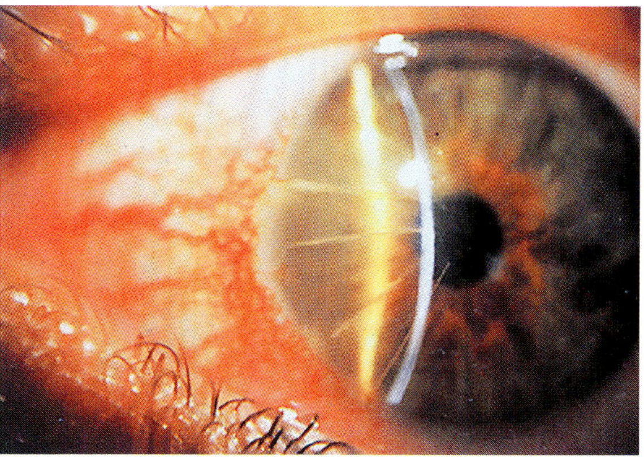

Fig. 15.62 Sterile keratitis surrounding an RK incision (from Geggel H. Delayed sterile keratitis following radial keratotomy requiring corneal transplantation for visual rehabilitation. Refract Corneal Surg 1990; 6:55–58).

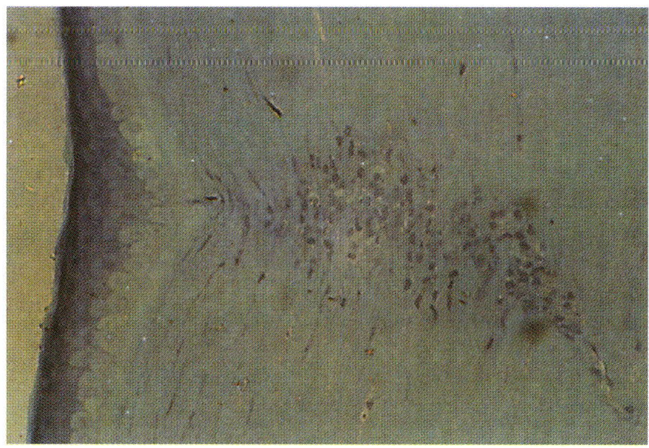

Fig. 15.63 Histologic section of incision area. (Courtesy of H. Geggel.)

at 5 years and the other at 7 years postoperatively (Figures 15.68 through 15.70).

It is obvious, since most of these cases involve the incisions initially, that the scar formed after an incision of this type is soft and offers little resistance to invasion for some years. It has been suggested that the epithelium over RK scars is somehow abnormal and perhaps more susceptible to the occurrence of infection (see Chapter 4). How this can be has never been adequately explained, nor has why these incisions should differ markedly from lacerations or PKP scars. However, there does appear to be, at least initially, disturbance of the corneal wetting mechanism after RK [49]. While the BUT seems to return to normal in most cases the author has examined, it is possible that this might play a role in allowing an invading organism a foothold. It is evident that the appearance of iron lines in these corneas is somewhat higher than in the general population—thus it could be that the mechanism is simply that of a sufficiently irreg-

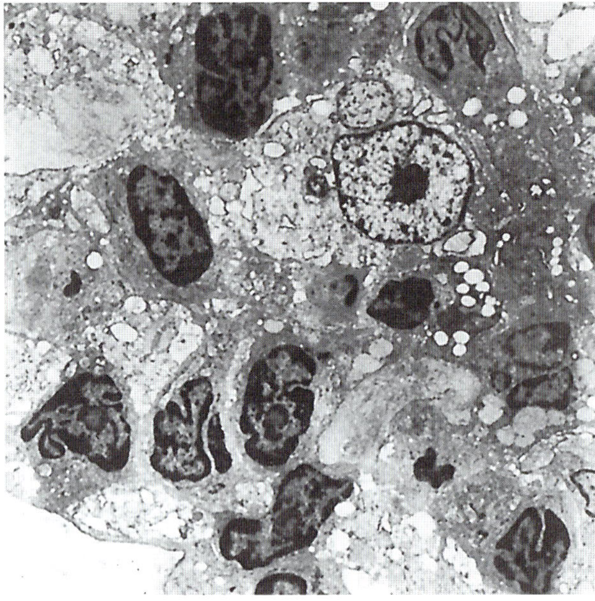

Fig. 15.64 Microscopic smear of the exudate. Note the absence of micro-organisms. (Courtesy of H. Geggel.)

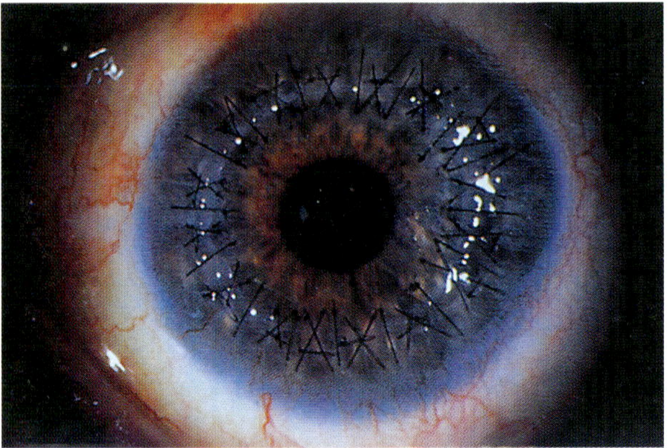

Fig. 15.65 Keratoplasty following a case of sterile keratitis. Note the use of X-type sutures to prevent incisions opening. (Courtesy of H. Geggel.)

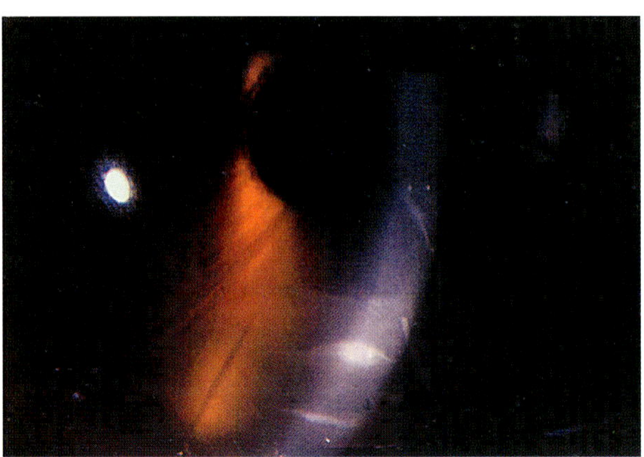

Fig. 15.66 Bacterial keratitis occurring 3 years after RK.

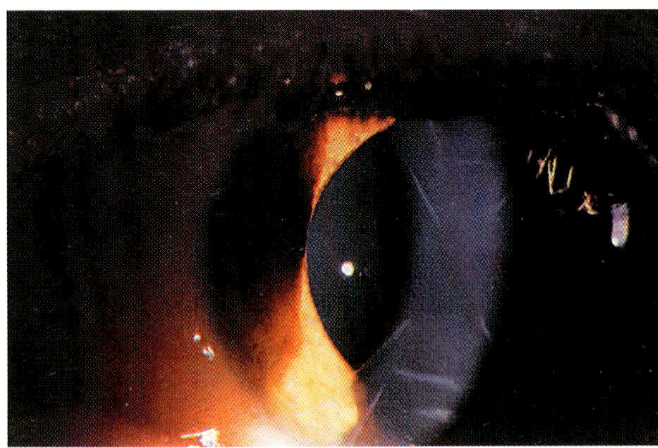

Fig. 15.67 Same case 72 hours after treatment with ciprofloxacin.

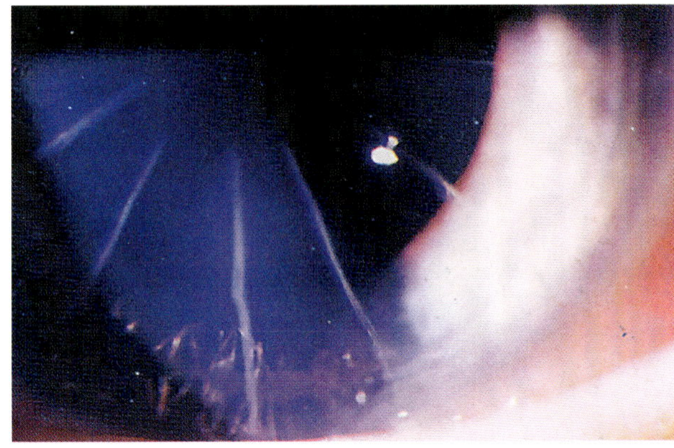

Fig. 15.68 Bacterial keratitis occurring 7 years after RK.

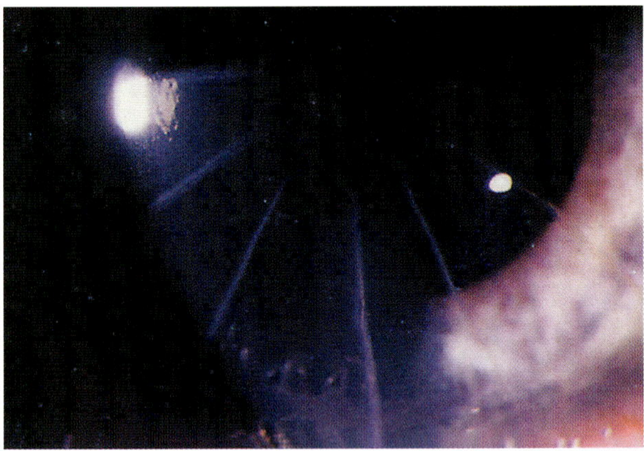

Fig. 15.69 Same case after 48 hours of treatment with ciprofloxacin.

ular surface for organisms to adhere to [50]. Whatever the mechanism, it is evident that these patients may be at slightly greater risk for infection and should be advised accordingly. It is not just RK patients who have difficulty with dry eyes and hence are vulnerable to infection (see "Laser in-situ keratomileusis [LASIK]," below).

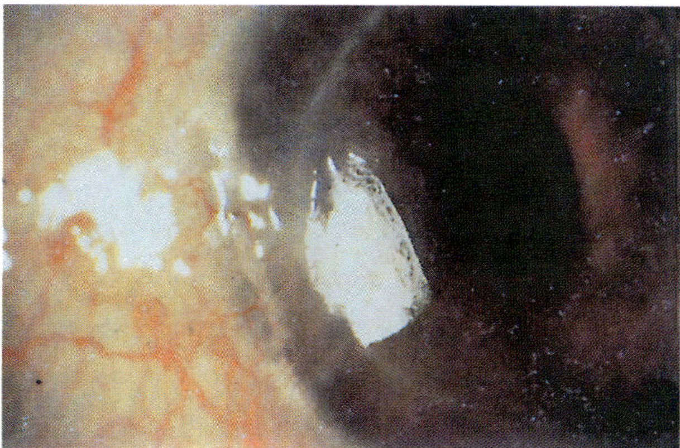

Fig. 15.70 Bacterial ulcer in a post-PKP relaxing incision.

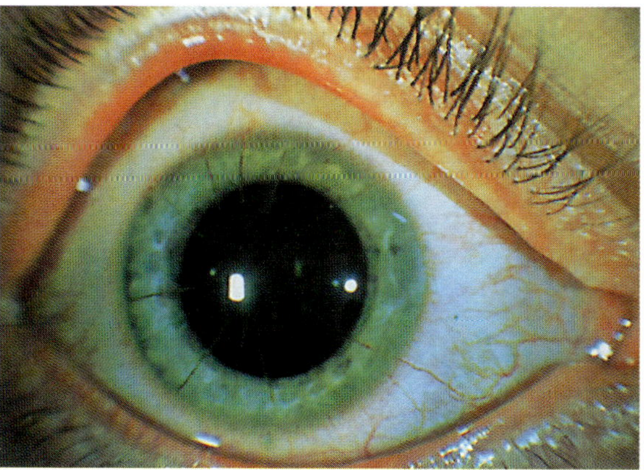

Fig. 15.71 Leaving blood in the incisions can lead to difficulty later on.

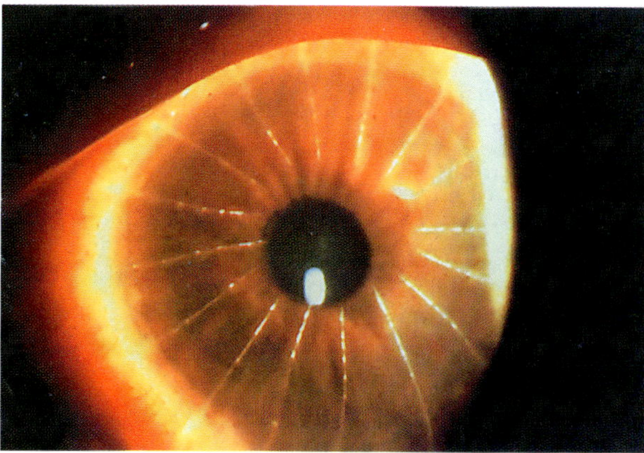

Fig. 15.72 Lipoid deposits appearing where red blood cells were not irrigated from the incisions.

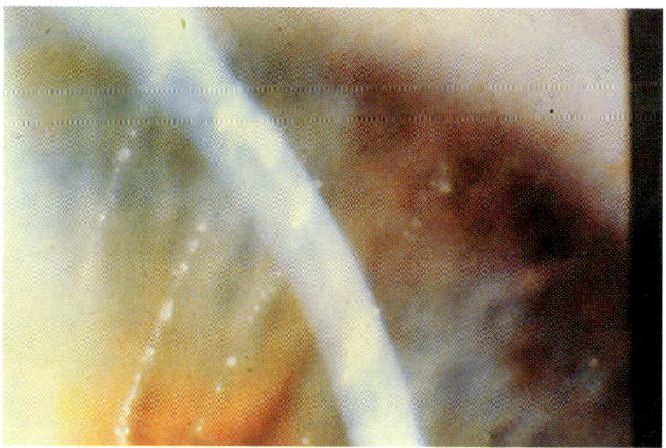

Fig. 15.73 Close-up of these lipoid deposits.

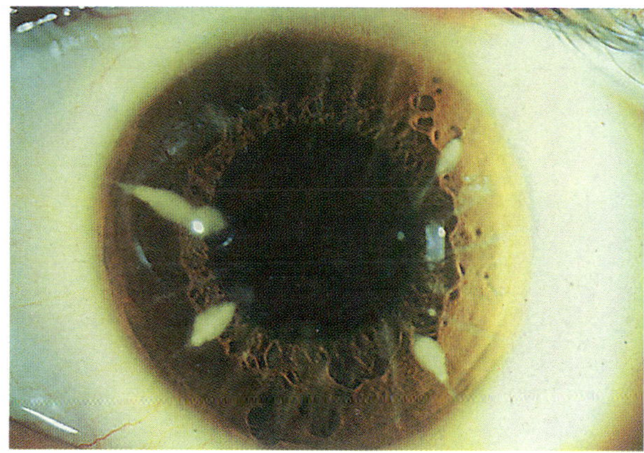

Fig. 15.74 Giant intra-incisional lipid deposit. (Courtesy of S.N. Fyodorov.)

Intraincisional opacities

These have been reported with decreasing frequency as more attention has been paid to postoperative incision irrigation and the practice of keeping the cornea dry during surgery [51]. If blood is left within the incisions, it is possible that the keratocytes will break it down into refractile lipid deposits. Generally, these are unsightly but pose no problem. Occasionally, it has been necessary to remove these deposits with a sharp blade to reduce the glare they can produce. Sometimes they can become quite large (Figures 15.71 through 15.77). If air is left within the wounds, encysted areas will result (Figure 15.78). These collapse in time but may need to be assisted by decompression with a needle tip. Rarely, Meibomian secretions as well as other things can find their way into a partially open incision (Figures 15.79 and 15.80). These may have to be excised as well.

Marsupialization

This very rare phenomenon has been reported only in conjunction with circular-radial keratotomy (and recently with the Mendez operation) [52]. Some numbers of these cases were performed on patients, with the result that large gaps appeared between incisions, particularly at crossing points, that then became lined with epithelium, producing small blind pockets or pouches (Figures 15.81 through 15.83). In addition, the myopia was found to have

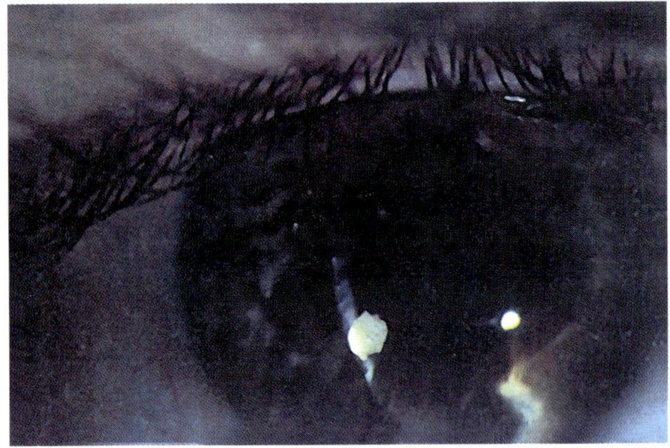

Fig. 15.75 Giant lipid deposit in an RK wound.

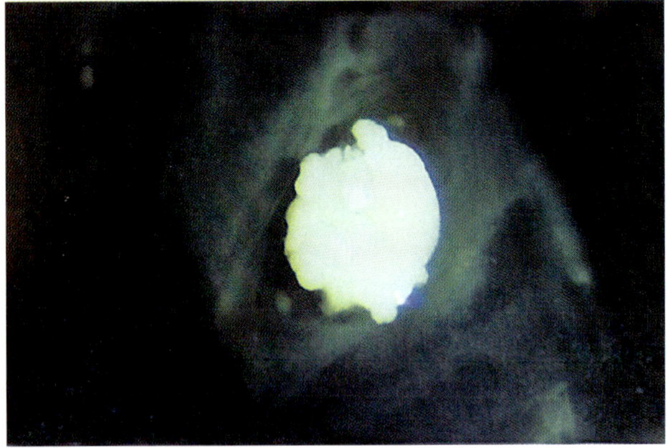

Fig. 15.76 Close-up of the lesion.

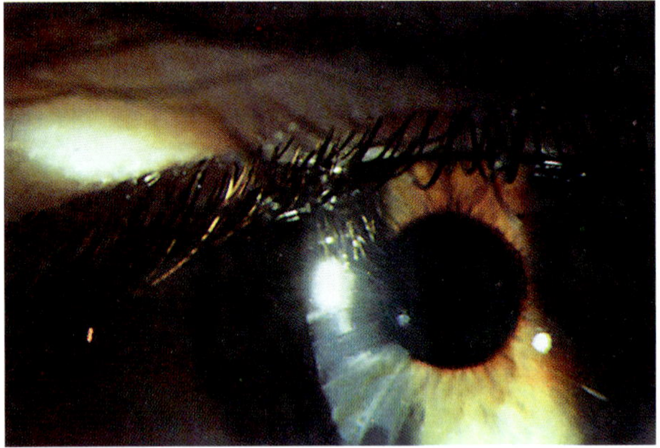

Fig. 15.77 Cornea after removal of the deposit. Note the shallow pocket remaining.

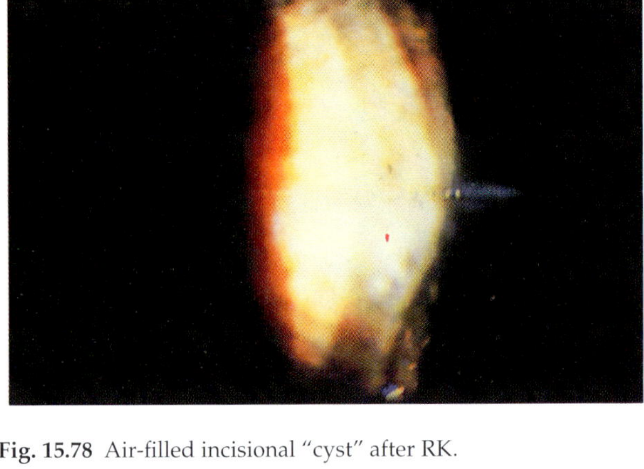

Fig. 15.78 Air-filled incisional "cyst" after RK.

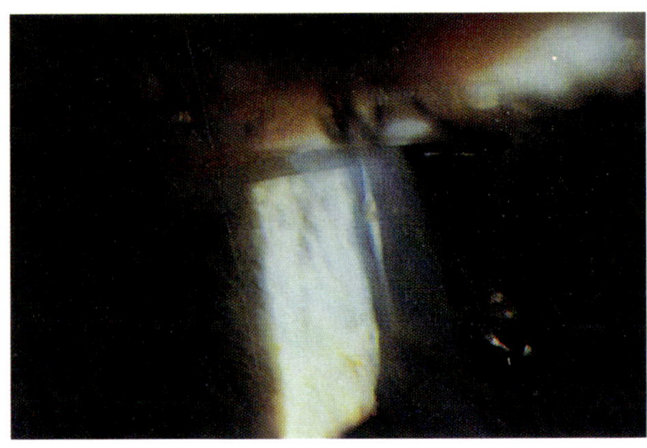

Fig. 15.79 Foreign body in an RK incision.

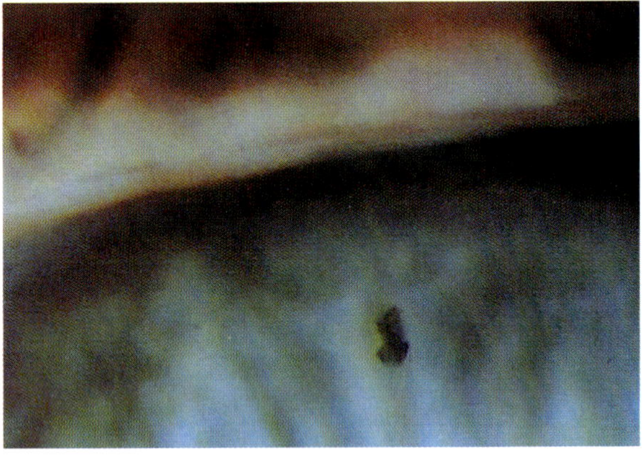

Fig. 15.80 Close-up of the intruder which turned out to be mascara.

increased in all cases along with extreme fluctuation of the vision through the day.

This is a potential problem with any incision that crosses another. The intersected area retracts, sometimes producing a large gap that then becomes only partially filled with the normal mucoepithelial plug. Sometimes the tips of the incision will be lost in the repair process, further increasing the gap to be filled. Retraction of this scar will, in time, induce localized flattening with the potential of creating irregular astigmatism.

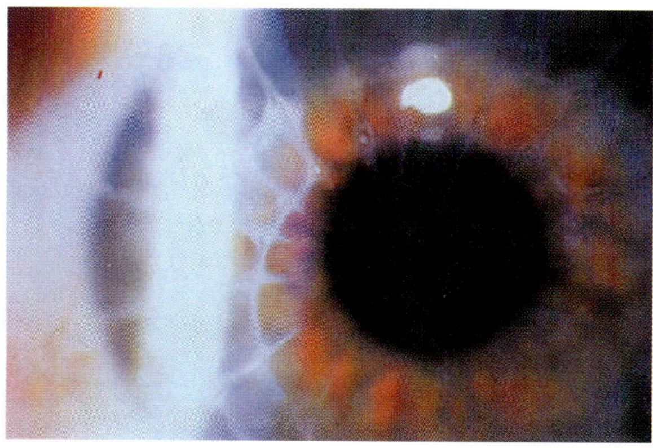

Fig. 15.81 Circular-radial keratotomy. This case resulted in marsupialization of the wounds, a "flail" cornea, and increased myopia. (Courtesy of R. Villasenor.)

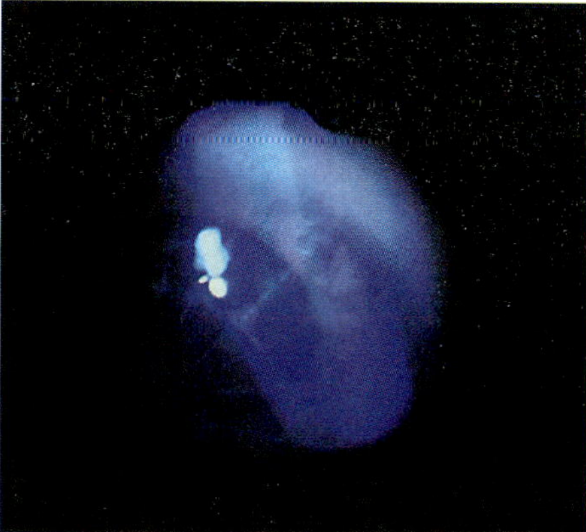

Fig. 15.82 Note the rings of dye demonstrating how tears are pumped out of the pockets with each heart beat. (Courtesy of R. Villasenor.)

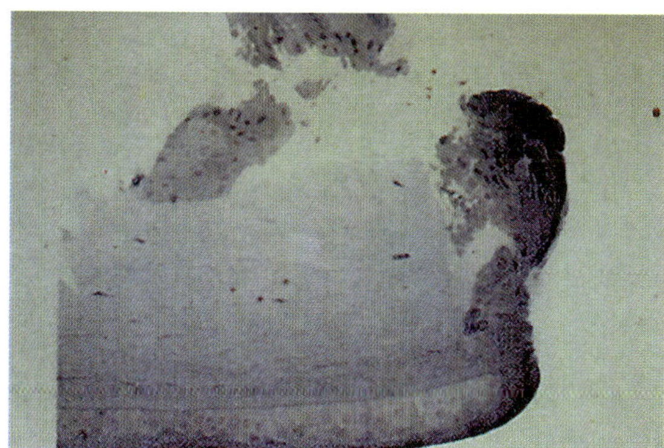

Fig. 15.83 Histologic section of one of the pockets showing marsupialization. (Courtesy of R. Villasenor.)

Therefore, any procedure that requires that incisions cross should be done in two stages with at least 6 months allowed to elapse between stages. In the Ruiz procedure, the radial incisions should not connect with the interior ladders for the same reason.

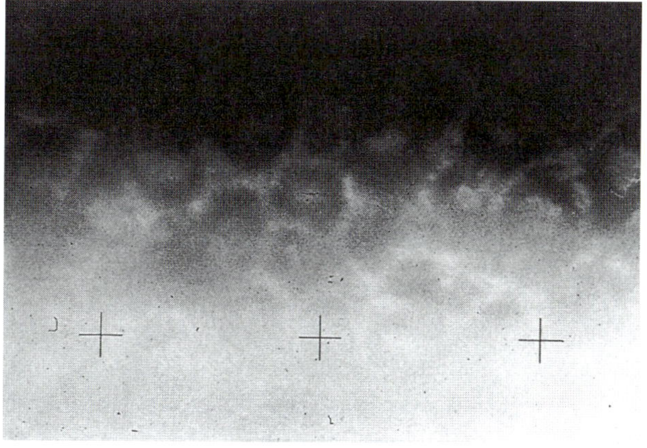

Fig. 15.84 Endothelial microscope picture of one of Sato's cases. (Courtesy of A. Momose.)

Endothelial cell loss

Recent studies have shown no significant endothelial cell loss following RK surgery—unlike that seen in the Sato operation (Figure 15.84). Earlier reports of as many as 22% of cells lost were later shown to be instances clearly related to excess trauma during performance of the surgery. In another report, cells were later found to have been counted incorrectly. Endothelial effects related to surgery in monkey eyes have not been duplicated in humans [2,53].

Microbullous keratopathy

Persistent microbullous keratopathy has not been reported with this surgery to date. The author has had five cases of localized microbullous keratopathy following RK surgery in older patients, however (Figures 15.85 and 15.86). In all cases the endothelial cell counts showed no significant cell loss after RK, with an initial count in the normal range for patient age. In each case the patients had prominent arcus senilis with some increase in corneal shagreen preoperatively but no epithelial abnormalities. All cases were high myopes requiring triple-step procedures, with three having had free-hand deepening. Two had self-sealing microperforations. All cases cleared spontaneously within 2 weeks, and none has shown any sequelae. One case required a second-stage procedure but did not demonstrate a recurrence of the microbullous keratopathy.

No cases of decompensation of the cornea as a result of this surgery have been reported to date. However, it is possible that the application of this technique to corneas that are unhealthy could precipitate such a calamity. An example of what can happen in a case having normal endothelium but abnormal epithelium and/or stroma has been demonstrated experimentally on a human volunteer (Figures 15.87 and 15.88).

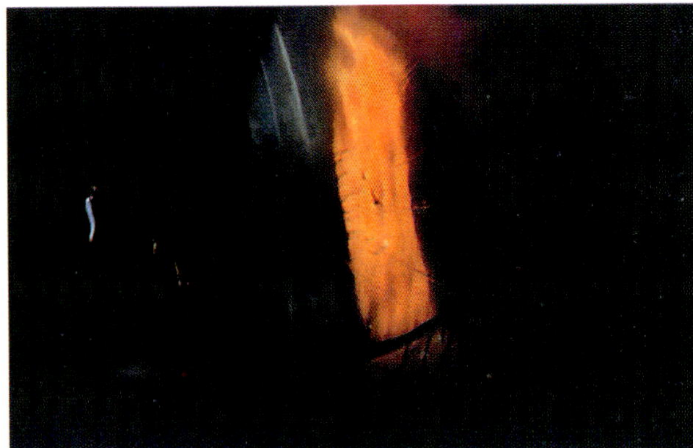

Fig. 15.85 Pseudobullous keratopathy. This wound communicates with the anterior chamber. The bullae are caused by aqueous under the epithelium.

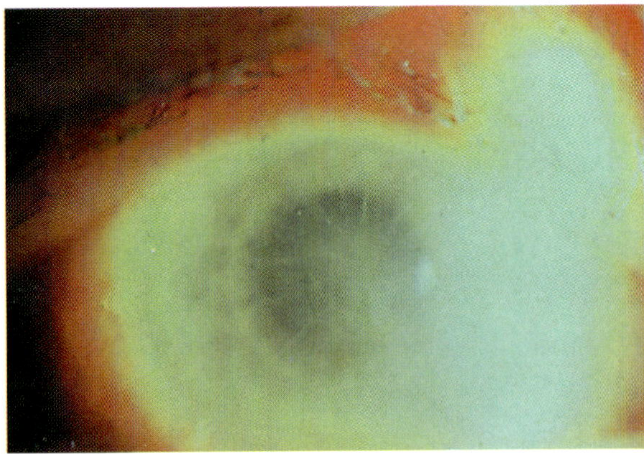

Fig. 15.87 Corneal decompensation in an eye with a history of interstitial keratitis and shallow incisions, immediately postsurgery

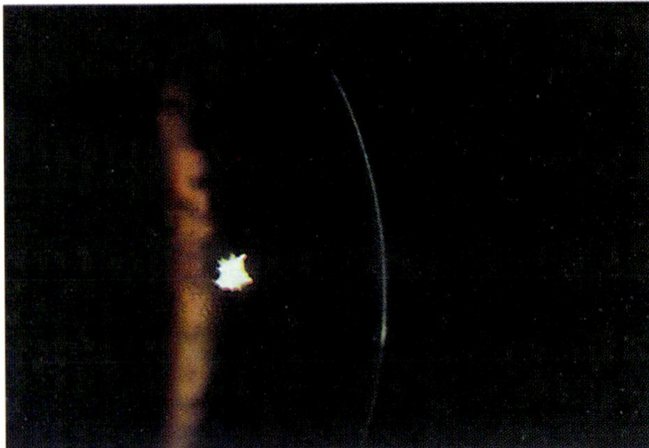

Fig. 15.86 Small area of true bullous keratopathy—the only known case following RK.

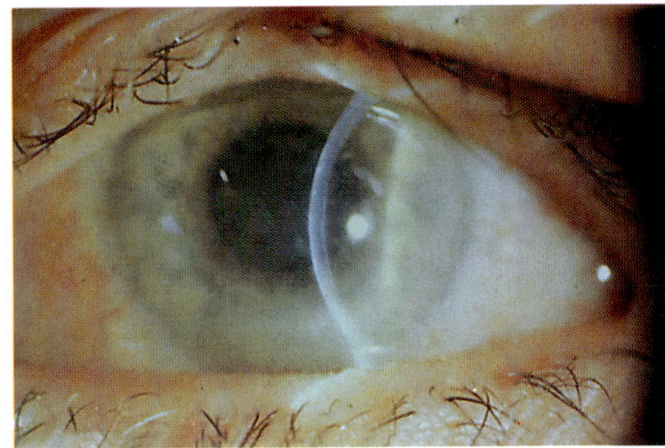

Fig. 15.88 Same eye as above, 5 months postsurgery

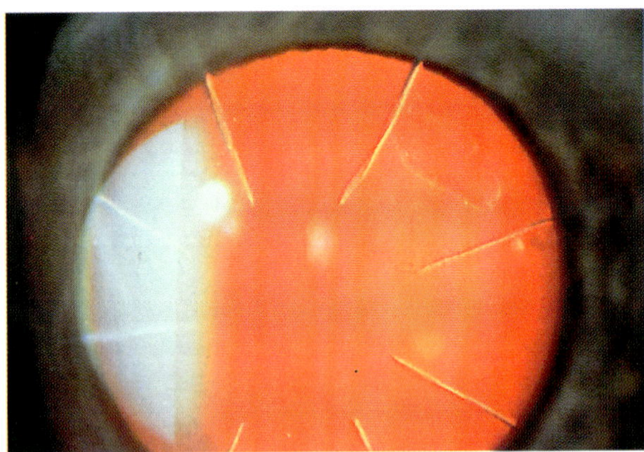

Fig. 15.89 Map-dot corneal changes supposedly not present before the RK.

Recurrent corneal erosion

Epithelial defects associated with basement membrane disease—such as recurrent corneal erosion and map-fingerprint-dot changes—have been reported following RK [32,54]. It is unclear what mechanism would account for the appearance of map-dot changes—the one case can be seen to exist between incisions (Figure 15.89). No note was made as to whether or not stripping of epithelium had occurred during surgery. As to the recurrent erosions, these are often associated with foreign material embedded in Bowman's layer—which probably explains why many patients respond to mechanical or chemical debridement. Some of the microwipes used in RK surgery are notorious for leaving behind particles of cellulose or other material. Perhaps such detritus is responsible for the incomplete detachment of the epithelium in these cases.

Corneal rupture

Numerous cases of severe trauma occurring to eyes at various periods postoperatively have been reported following RK [55–62]. One such case involved a direct hit from a racket ball in an eye 1 month postoperatively. The patient sustained a mild hyphema and a recession of the angle [62]. There was a transient decrease in visual acuity secondary to an associated corneal abrasion. No incisions

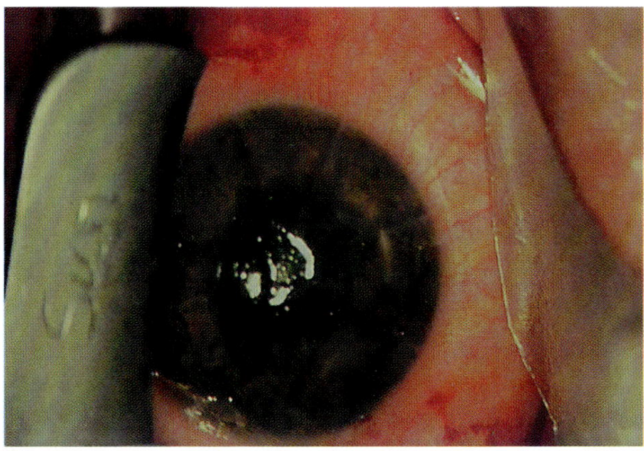

Fig. 15.90 Corneal laceration following blunt trauma (auto accident). The cornea ruptured from limbus to limbus along two RK incisions.

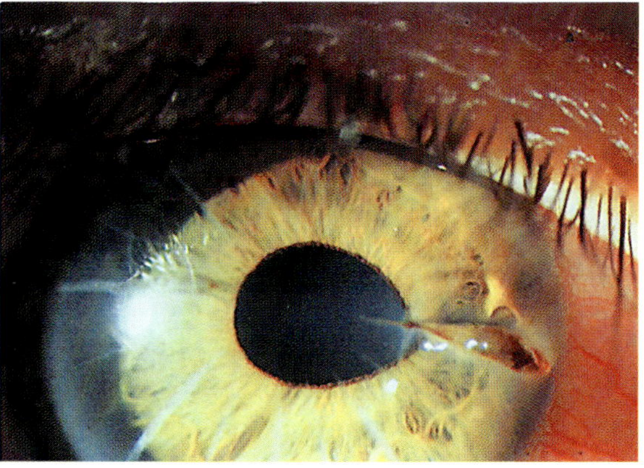

Fig. 15.91 Iris prolapse through RK incision after blunt trauma.

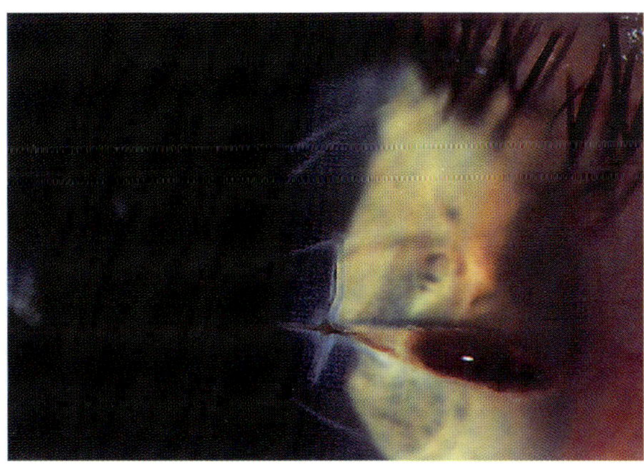

Fig. 15.92 Close-up of the same eye. Note that the chamber is formed. Vision was 20/60, uncorrected before repair.

were found to have opened, and the anterior chamber remained full and deep with no evidence of leakage or secondary glaucoma.

On the other hand, a female patient 1½ years after RK, was thrown through the windshield of an automobile during an accident, sustaining severe head trauma. The cornea of one eye was found to have ruptured along the 12 to 6 o'clock meridian in the incisions, and the ocular contents herniated anteriorly (Figure 15.90). Several of the other incisions were said to have been split as well. The eye was not lost, but vision was reduced to "count fingers." A similar case involved a male approximately 1 year after RK. Again, the eye was not lost, but vision was impaired.

Recently, a case of a rupture following a blow from an elbow was reported; the eye was saved. The latest incident involved a case of the author's in which a macroperforation had occurred during a reoperation that required suturing. Approximately 3 months after suture removal, the patient was struck in the face by an automobile "half-axle" while repairing his car. The axle fell some 12 in. and struck the eye directly. In this instance, the previously sutured (but currently unsutured) wound opened, and the chamber collapsed. The patient sought consultation after 3 days only because of persistent irritation and mild tearing (Figures 15.91 and 15.92). The unaided visual acuity was 20/60, corrected to 20/20, on the initial visit. Resuturing of the wound with repositioning of the iris was accomplished with minimal trauma. The anterior chamber was clear and full by the next day. The patient retains good unaided vision to this day (20/25) and is correctable to 20/20. No lens complications have occurred in this patient to date—2 years after the trauma.

Forstot and Damiano have reported eight cases of ocular trauma following RK in seven accident-prone patients in their own practice; one patient got hit with a tennis ball—twice. All patients retained the same visual acuity after the trauma that they had before the trauma. Only two of the eight cases received a direct injury, which opened one incision in each case, resulting in flat chambers. Both were 16-incision cases, and one incision opened at the site of a microperforation. In one of the other cases, the laceration was oblique to the RK incisions [61].

Spivack reported a case in which a woman had received severe facial trauma consequent to a plane crash in which the globes remained intact [63]. That these corneas may be vulnerable for some time is shown by the case reported by McDermott and colleagues. A woman suffered corneal rupture after trauma in an eye that had had RK 10 years previously [57].

Ocular injury accounts for a considerable number of accident cases each year. Visual loss occurs in an appalling number of these. It is obvious that RK does not necessarily predispose a patient to such a sad fate, however. Still, in both rupture cases described by Forstot, each occurred in eyes that had had 16 incisions. Is this evidence that

16-incision eyes are more vulnerable than those with fewer incisions? Possibly, but both of these oases were in eyes injured within 1 year of the original surgery—one of them at 2 weeks. It is possible that while the shear strength of an eye that has had 16 incisions is less than one with 8 or fewer incisions, it is also true that such eyes tend to be easily distorted, thus possibly absorbing the shock of trauma through this distortion. The author treated a police officer who suffered a kick in the face and in whom a radial incision split open; this was an 8-incision case, and the trauma occurred 13 years after the surgery. An iris prolapse sealed the wound, which saved the eye, but the patient required cataract removal a year later.

At least one rupture has been reported following blunt trauma after HK [64]. Approximately 6 months after HK, the patient's left eye collided with a fist. Both nasal and temporal transverse incisions opened. It was noted that incisions at the apices were joined (some overlapped). The patient never regained useful vision in the damaged eye.

Critics of RK have pointed to the work of Larson showing that eyes do not regain normal tensile strength even after 3 months and are prone to rupture along the incisions [65]. This study, while interesting, used rabbit eyes, and each eye was subjected to repeated trauma until rupture occurred. Rabbits do not have a Bowman's layer in any event, which adds considerably to the integrity of the human cornea. Thus all we can conclude from this study is that rabbit eyes undergoing RK should not be exposed to repeated blunt trauma. Luttrull's study, on the other hand, is more significant [66]. The safety of deep corneal incisions in RK was evaluated in a porcine model. All eyes were subjected to standard blunt trauma. Control eyes ruptured at the equatorial sclera. Eyes with radial incisions cut through approximately 70% of corneal thickness also ruptured at the equator. When incisions of this depth (70%) were extended across the limbus rather than stopping at the corneal-scleral junction, all ruptures occurred at the limbal portion of the incisions—which further reinforces our decision not to carry the incisions across the limbus. Eyes cut 95% to 100% of corneal thickness tended to rupture at the incisions, as would be expected. However, this tendency in pig eyes does not explain the oblique lacerations in Forstot's cases, nor does it explain Figure 15.93, which shows an RK eye that received severe blunt trauma in which the resulting laceration crosses the RK incisions—none of which opened.

Patients in whom transverse incisions cross radials may be more vulnerable to such injury nonetheless. Karr and colleagues reported persistent wound gape in a patient with just such an incisional pattern [67]. This patient's case was complicated by a sterile keratitis. Girard described a patient in whom the radials reopened 6 months postoperatively when a circumferential incision was made in an effort to correct postoperative astigmatism [68].

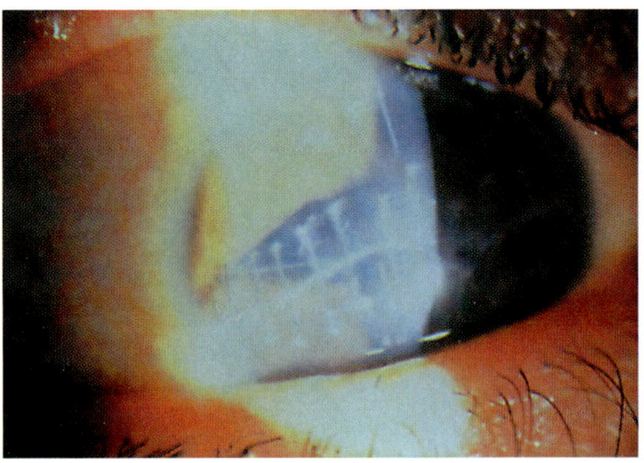

Fig. 15.93 Blunt trauma (auto accident) corneal laceration crossing an RK incision obliquely. (Courtesy of Villasenor.)

All this means is that RK eyes may be vulnerable to trauma, and patients should be so cautioned. Still in question is how to explain the author's patient who, 1 month after bilateral RK surgery, completed a free ocean descent with scuba equipment to a depth of 435 ft. Despite the enormous pressures to which he was subjected during the dive and the hours spent in the decompression chamber, he experienced only mild, transient blurring of vision upon surfacing. No evidence of ocular injury was found.

Hyphema (not associated with external trauma)

One case is known to have developed a small hyphema after RK. This is believed to have been caused by one of the incisions perforating at the limbus. The blood cleared spontaneously within 24 hours, and no sequelae have been reported [69].

Cataract formation

A small number of cases of cataract formation have been reported to date. Five followed perforation into the anterior chamber (Figures 15.94 through 15.96). Four of these showed frank evidence of direct lens injury [26,70]. It is presumed that the fifth lens also was injured, but no injury site could be unequivocally identified [71]. It is difficult to postulate how entry into the anterior chamber of the blade tip alone without trauma to the lens could produce a cataract in the immediate postoperative period. Unless withdrawal of the blade is instantaneous in the event of a microperforation, the chamber can deflate sufficiently to allow contact of the blade tip with the lens capsule. That this can occur without notice of the physician and in the absence of evident lens trauma is borne out by the case of Nozik. In this instance, phakoanaphylaxis occurred in a female patient some considerable

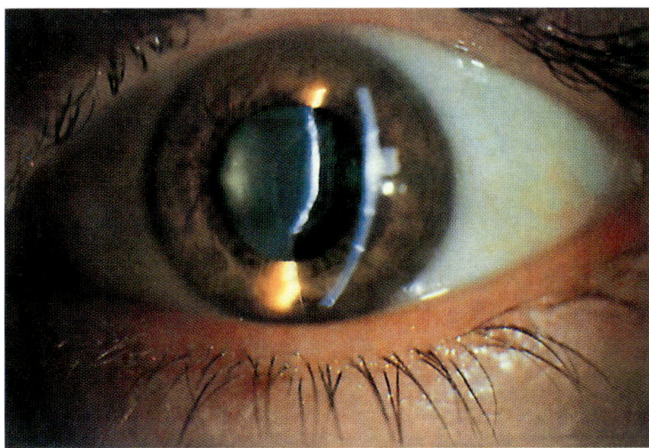

Fig. 15.94 Cataract following surgical trauma during RK. (Courtesy of B. Hewitt.)

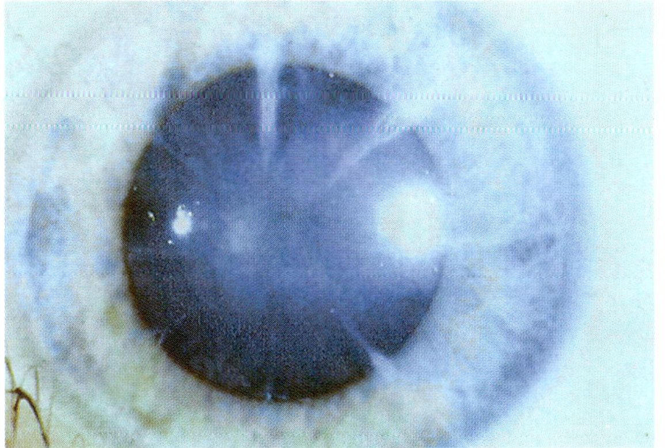

Fig. 15.95 Cataract developing in an eye following presumed intrasurgical lens trauma. (Courtesy of J.I. Barraquer.)

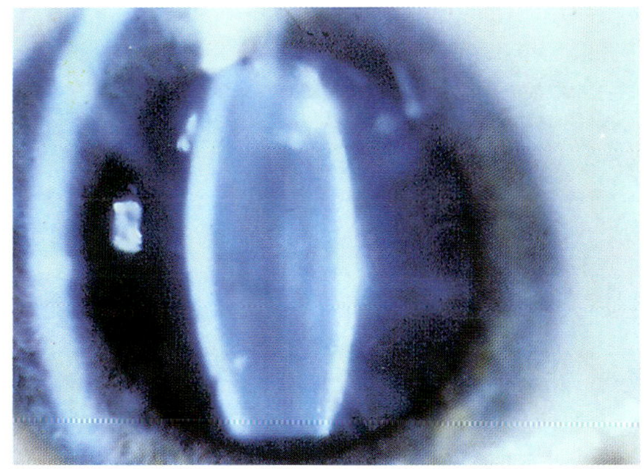

Fig. 15.96 Slit-lamp view of the same eye. (Courtesy of J.I. Barraquer.)

time after a 16-incision RK was performed. The surgeon acknowledged that a microperforation had occurred but that the chamber had not flattened in any way (Figures 15.97 and 15.98). Care in blade setting, reduced blade speed, avoidance of manipulation of the incision when

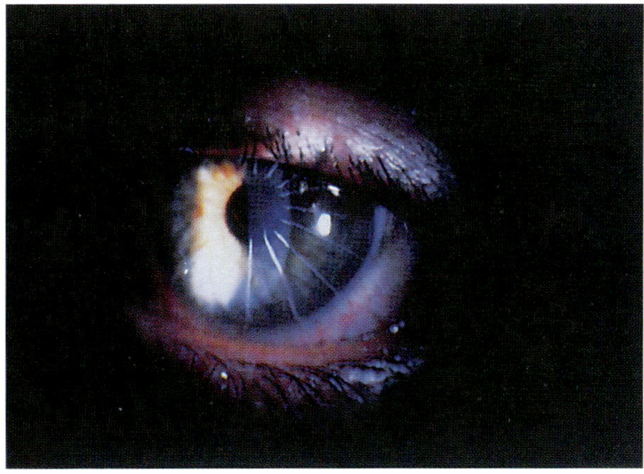

Fig. 15.97 Sixteen-incision RK case 3 months postsurgery. (Courtesy of R. Nozik.)

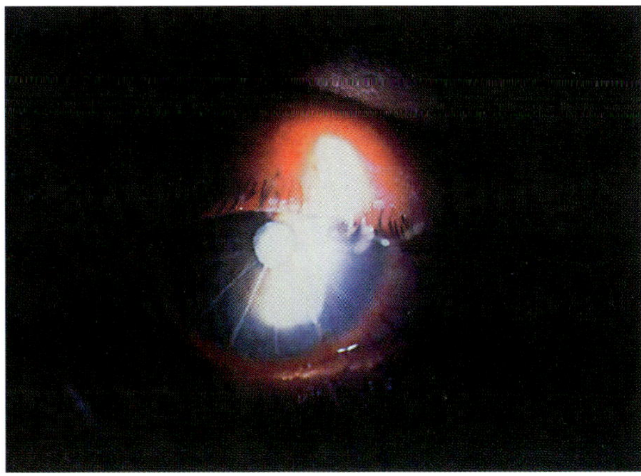

Fig. 15.98 The same eye shortly after having developed phakoanaphylaxis and cataract formation—6 months postsurgery. (Courtesy of R. Nozik.)

the chamber is shallow (free-hand deepening), and an undilated pupil should prevent the occurrence of this major complication.

Two cases of steroid-induced cataract formation have been reported. In each case the surgeon was attempting to enhance the effect of the surgery by inducing an IOP rise with topical steroids [47]. It has not been shown that increasing the IOP above normal has any permanent effect on the outcome of the surgery; nonetheless, some surgeons persist in this attempt. Because of the serious side effects reported with long-term topical steroid usage, this method of "treating" undercorrection is not recommended. Additionally, the steroid itself may interfere with the healing process and negate any possible gain. Our experience with the use of steroids at 8 weeks in which the correction was consequently reduced leads us to believe that the hazards of the long-term use of steroids far outweigh its possible benefits. Furthermore, it does not seem logical to induce a disease (glaucoma) in order to cure another (myopia).

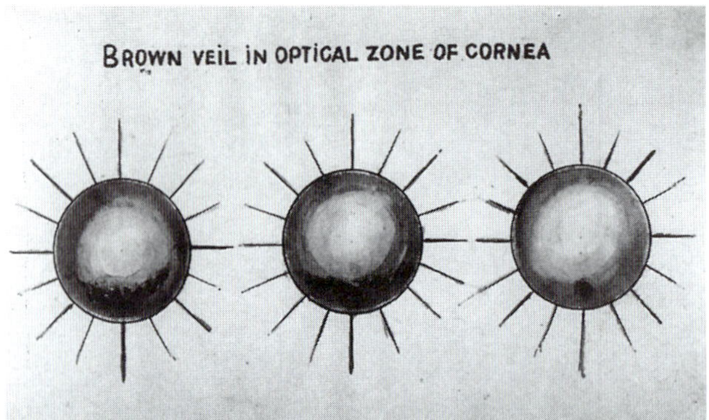

Fig. 15.99 Hudson–Stähli iron lines.

Iron (Hudson-Stähli) lines

These areas of small brownish pigment deposits are sometimes seen in the inferior aspect of the OZ and are due to pooling of tears admixed with various electrolytes—especially iron [50,72–74] (Figure 15.99). They are less often seen with well-irrigated incisions and do not appear to degrade vision. They do not progress but may be quite large. Such lines have been seen after other forms of refractive surgery as well [75,76].

Retinal detachment

A number of cases of this complication have been reported to date. In one case, the patient had been placed on a strong miotic (phospholine iodide) postoperatively in an attempt to ameliorate an overcorrection [47,77–85]. Strong miotics, particularly phospholine iodide, have been implicated in numerous instances of retinal detachment in myopic patients, and their use in these cases is decried [78,80,86–89].

Optical atrophy

The use of retrobulbar anesthesia in this surgery has led, tragically, to acute optical atrophy in a number of cases [90]. In each instance, irretrievable visual loss has occurred. In at least three of these cases, penetration of the globe has been demonstrated [91] (Figure 15.100). The myopic eye, being long and thin, is much more vulnerable to this hazard than the older, shorter cataractous eye (Figure 15.101). The indiscriminant use of this type of anesthesia has never been advocated in this surgery for the reason that it is fraught with known hazards and inappropriate to the situation. The fact that thousands of patients have had this surgery performed under topical anesthesia alone and under all sorts of differing conditions strengthens this viewpoint.

The author recognizes that there may be those occasions where the use of local, injectable anesthesia may be appropriate. In these rare instances, the surgeon is advised to use peribulbar anesthesia, which has been put forward as an effective and less hazardous alternative to retrobulbar injection. The author would agree with this point of view, but it is this author's strong recommendation that injectable anesthetics be avoided in these cases. In the unlikely event that such anesthesia must be used, the patient should look down toward the needle, thus swinging the posterior pole away from the tip instead of toward it—which would be the case if the patient is instructed to look up as usual (Figures 15.102 and 15.103).

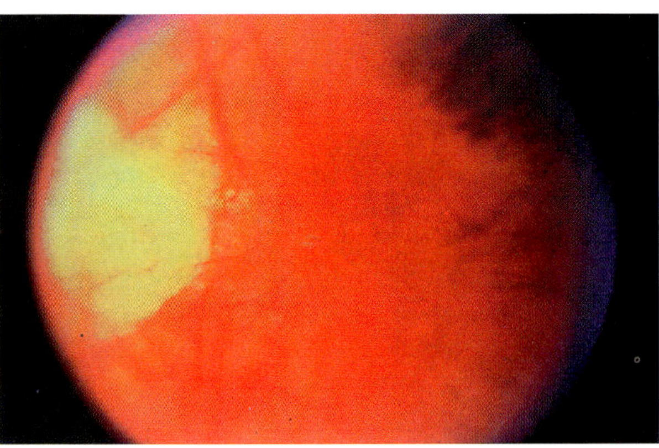

Fig. 15.100 Penetration of the globe with a retrobulbar needle. This case had a cataract as well from direct lens trauma during surgery.

Lamellar refractive surgery

The complications of this surgery are those which can be expected of any nonpenetrating surgical procedure on the cornea. Infection is usually rare, typically confined to the corneal stroma, and generally localized. It responds well to topical antibiotics but in some cases may require subtenon injection. Severe intraocular infections have been reported, with rare cases of endophthalmitis leading to visual loss having occurred. Induced astigmatism is by far the most common complication with this surgery, and it occurs in about 4% of the cases, tending to group in the higher myopia ranges. The following is applicable to LASIK and intracorneal implants as well. Specific problems with these modalities are detailed in their respective sections.

Intraoperative problems and complications

Reference mark incorrectly placed

The reference mark may be placed either too central or too peripheral. In either case, when the corneal disk is resected, the entire mark may end up in the periphery or on the disk. When measuring the diameter of the keratectomy with the applanator, it may be seen clearly if the location of the mark is incorrect—if it is, it must be corrected.

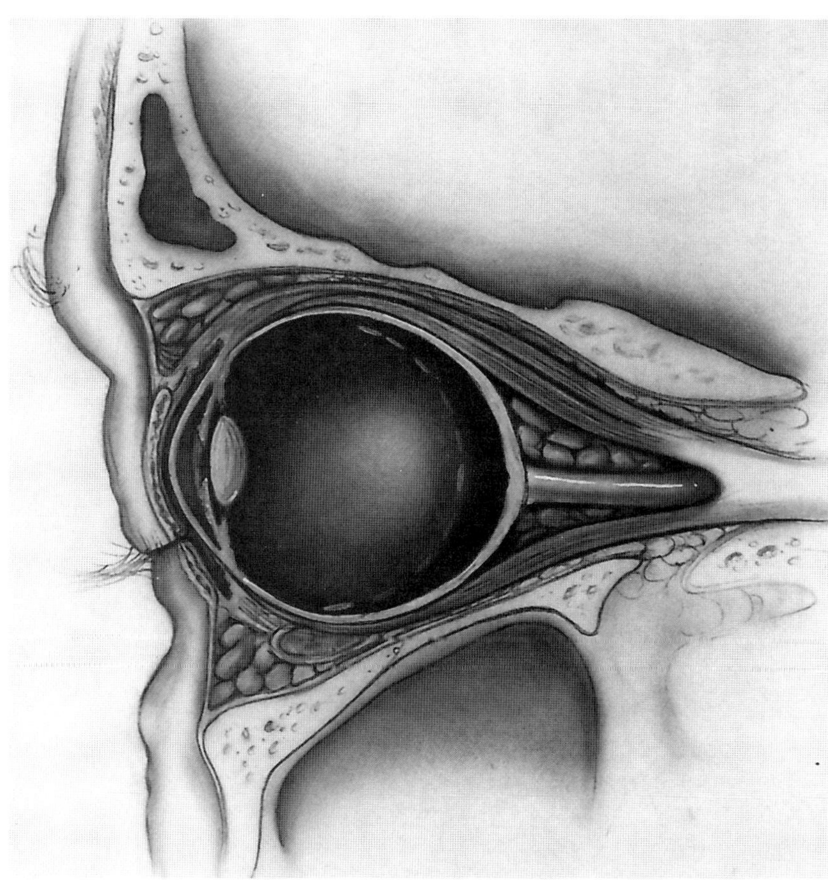

Fig. 15.101 Myopic versus emmetropic eye within the orbit.

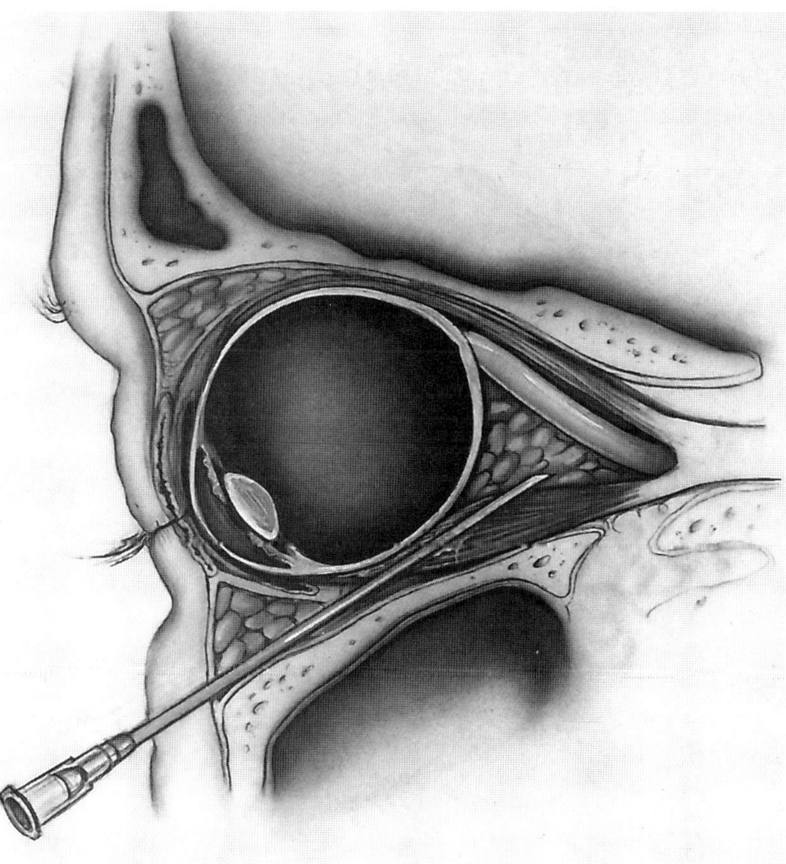

Fig. 15.102 If the patient looks down, the vulnerable posterior pole swings away from the needle tip.

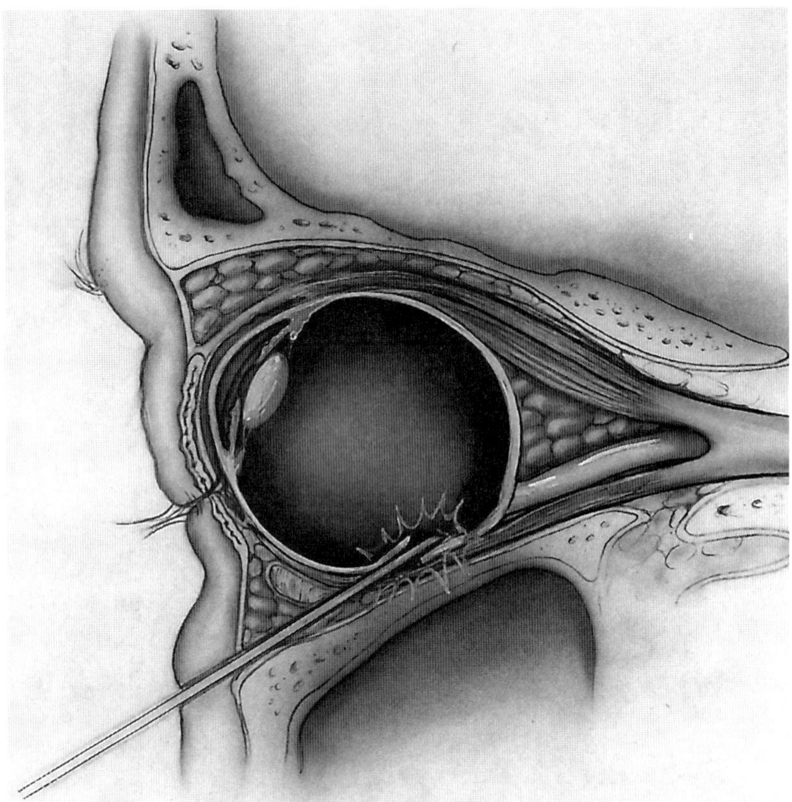

Fig. 15.103 If the patient looks up, the posterior part of the eye swings into the needle tip.

Prophylaxis At the beginning of the surgery, use a caliper set to the diameter of the section to make sure the mark straddles the edge. Use of a 4.0-mm. RK marker will work as well. Simply scribe the line from the edge of the OZ to the limbus. Be certain to make the mark as shown in Figure 15.104.

Treatment (disk upside down) Remove disk, and clean it and resuture it in place correctly. Rarely, the lenticule may be irreparably damaged by collagenase secreted by the corneal epithelium and will have to be replaced by donor tissue. This is rarely a problem in LASIK unless the hinge tears. In this case, a Woods lamp may help because the epithelium is naturally fluorescent, whereas stroma is not.

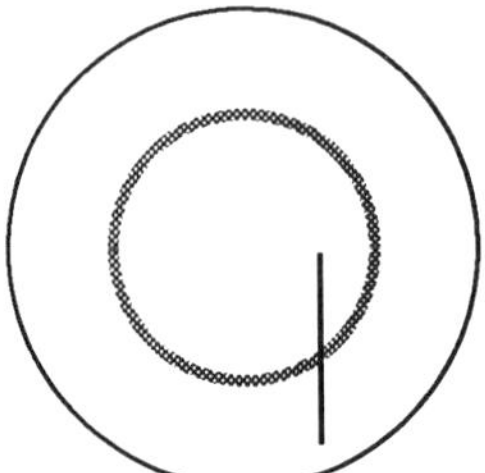

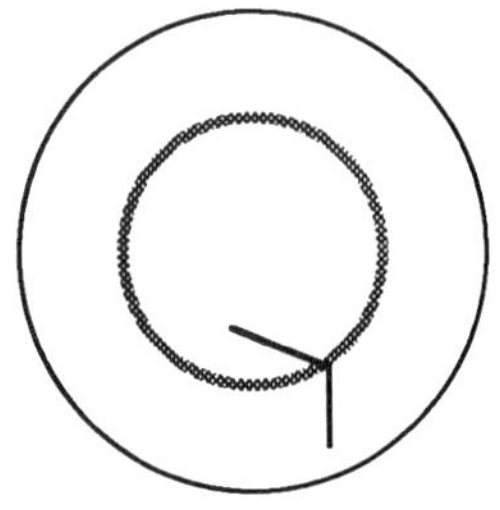

Fig. 15.104 Mismatched reference marks. The tissue has been replaced with the epithelial side down.

Retrobulbar injection

Hematoma

The retrobulbar (or peribulbar) injection may cause a retrobulbar hematoma, which, if small, will not hinder continuation of the surgery because it is not necessary to open the eye. However, a large hematoma may produce difficulty with opening the lids and can interfere with placement of the ring and/or obtaining sufficient suction.

Prophylaxis Use blunt needles for injection, and inject a small quantity of fluid as the needle is introduced.

Anterior infiltration

If the injection is not placed within the muscle cone, it may infiltrate toward the subtenons or subconjunctival space. This will cause perilimbal swelling that will prevent correct adaptation of the fixation ring to the globe. In this case, performing several small incisions 5 or 6 mm from the limbus to evacuate the fluid may be tried, or a peritomy may be done to place the ring directly over the sclera. Surgery may have to be postponed.

Prophylaxis Inject only when certain the muscle cone has been entered.

Perforation of the globe

This complication is vision threatening and a real danger. The myopic globe is not only longer but also thinner. Consequently, it is much easier to penetrate with a retrobulbar needle than is that of a normal (see Figure 15.101).

Prophylaxis When administering the retrobulbar, use a shorter, more flexible needle and have the patient look down (see Figure 15.102). It helps to blunt the needle slightly by rubbing the tip across a sterile towel.

Pneumatic fixation ring

Insufficient lid clearance

If the interpalpebral opening is insufficient to place the pneumatic fixation ring owing to its shape or to proptosis due to retrobulbar injection, a small lateral canthotomy may be performed. Remember to suture it at the end of the surgery. In children, use the smaller-diameter rings.

Difficulty with fixation

The scleral radius differs from that of the ring. If the scleral radius is larger than the radius of the ring, the latter makes contact only by its peripheral edge, and the central edge does not contact the limbus (Figure 15.105). If the scleral radius is smaller than that of the ring, the reverse case exists (Figure 15.106). Fortunately, this occurs very rarely.

Prophylaxis Ensure that the rings at hand are the correct size for the patient. Remember that the rings for children are 110 mm in diameter, whereas those for adults are 125 mm in diameter.

Lax or edematous conjunctiva blocking the suction aperture

In some cases, the conjunctiva may be so lax as to become aspirated into the ring suction aperture, thereby preventing full suction from occurring (Figure 15.107). In this case, the first step is to reorient the ring to move the hole. If, despite this, the same thing happens, a small peritomy must be performed, leaving the conjunctiva of the upper area outside the pneumatic ring and the bare sclera directly in front of the hole. Too large a peritomy may cause a tendency for the ring to decentrate. If small enough, this peritomy will not cause this problem nor require suturing. The keratectomy must not be attempted unless the fixation provided by the ring is perfect.

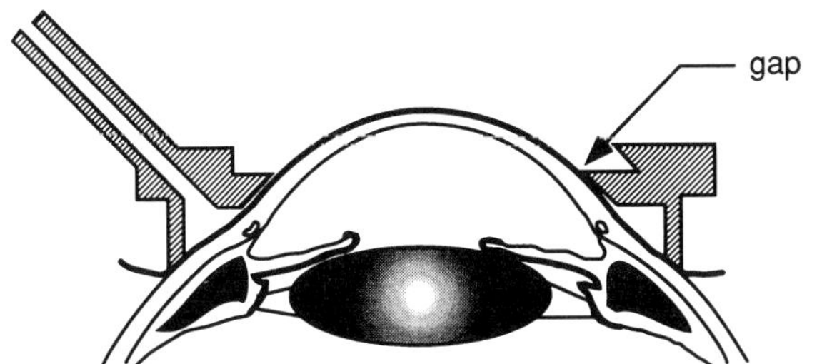

Fig. 15.105 Ring too big for eye.

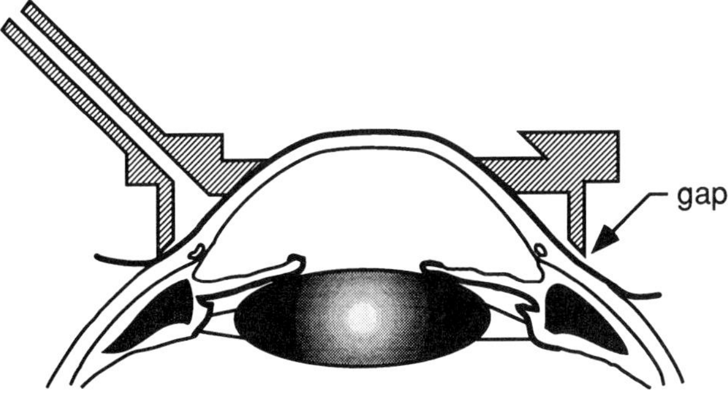

Fig. 15.106 Ring too small for eye.

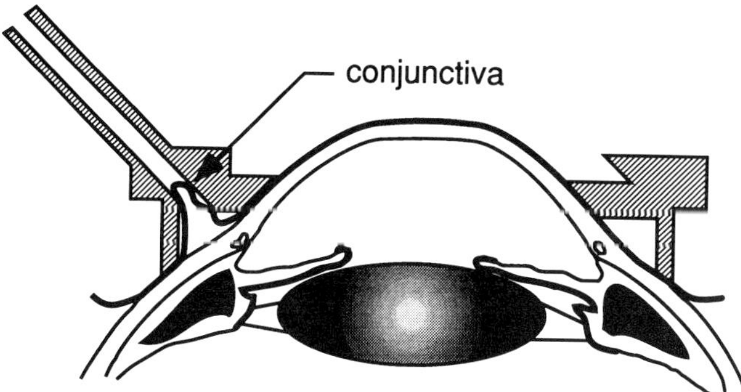

Fig. 15.107 Aspirated conjunctiva.

Insufficient pump suction on startup

This is something that will occur on check-out of the instrument preoperatively. This will occur if there is partial blockage of the vacuum path or if there is a leak in the system.

Prophylaxis Ensure proper functioning of the vacuum system before the surgery starts.

Difficulty with centration

In some globes with a somewhat irregular sclera, the cornea tends to be out of center in relation to the ring aperture (Figure 15.108). A small decentration of 0.50 mm toward the superotemporal side is desirable in myopia and to the inferonasal side in hyperopia. If the decentration is greater than this, the conjunctiva should be disinserted near the limbus on the side where the conjunctiva is showing mostly (Figure 15.109).

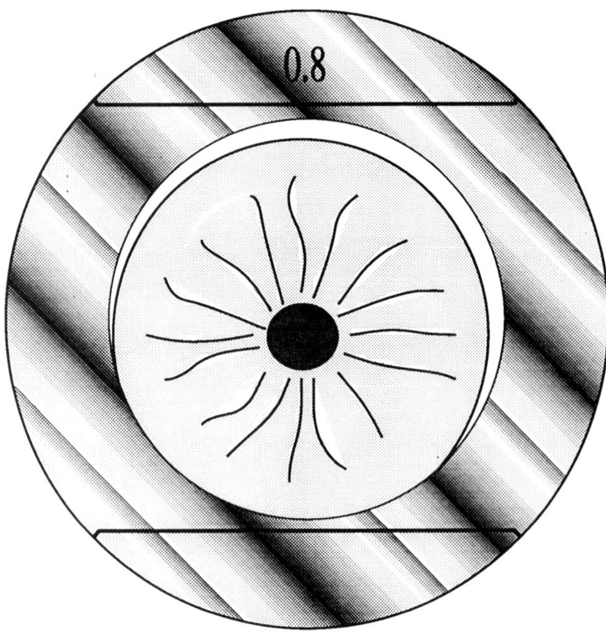

Fig. 15.108 Decentration of ring.

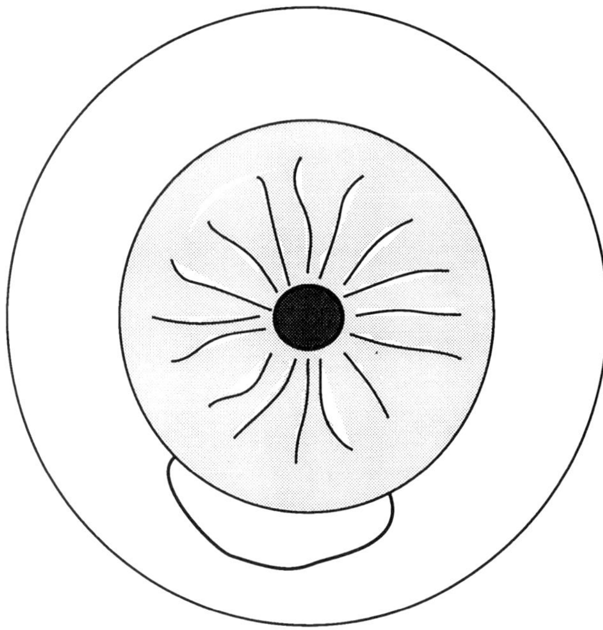

Fig. 15.109 Peritomy for decentration. The peritomy must be on the opposite side of the decentration.

Section with the microkeratome

Obstacles to movement

Lid speculum problems Care must be taken to prevent the blades of the lid speculum from extending into the path of the microkeratome. If the microkeratome strikes the speculum during its translation across the cornea, an irregularity in the section will result. Generally, an assistant can move the blades out of the way with forceps. If this cannot be done, it is better to remove the fixation ring and the lid speculum and use lid sutures—4-0 silk is adequate for this purpose. Be careful to place the sutures in the skin and away from the lid margin vascular arcade. Sometimes a problem will arise if the retrobulbar injection has been excessive or the speculum is too small. Beware of using a Guyton-Park type of speculum with lockable blades. This device has been implicated in postoperative ptosis secondary to levator aponeurosis dehiscence [92].

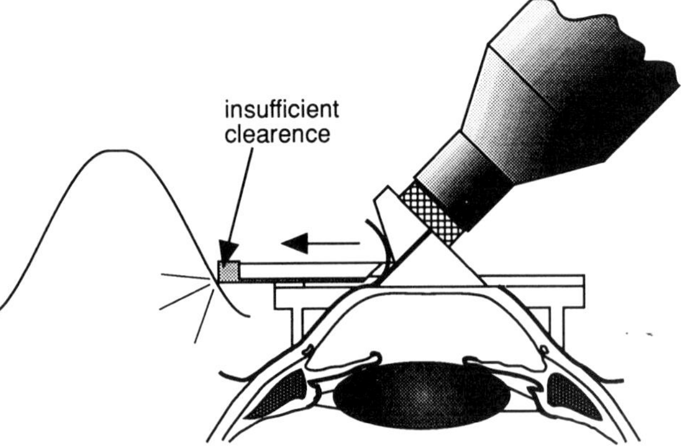

Fig. 15.110 The keratome may strike the nose, preventing complete resection of the disk.

Nose gets in the way In cases of large noses, the head of the microkeratome may hit the nose before completing the pass (Figure 15.110). This can be prevented by taking measurements over the ring with the microkeratome off. If there is insufficient space, the globe can be abducted with the ring handle. It is recommended that prior to moving the keratome across the eye the eye be adducted (rotated outward) slightly with the suction ring handle (Figure 15.111).

Disk of size other than selected

Smaller disk The cornea was wet, and liquid meniscus falsified the reading, making it appear larger.

Prophylaxis Dry the cornea before applanating. Check the blades for proper dimensions. The latter cause is very unlikely today because all blades are examined and measured at the factory.

Larger disk Inadequate seating of the applanator to the surface of the fixation ring.

Prophylaxis Ensure that applanator seats against the ring surface.

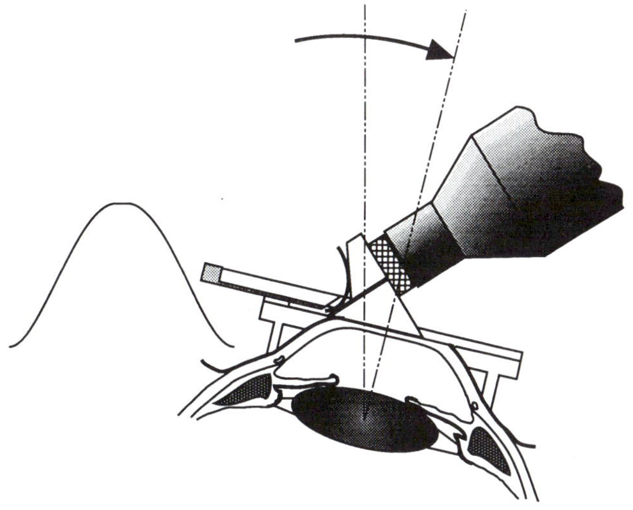

Fig. 15.111 Rotating the eye temporally will provide more clearance for the keratome.

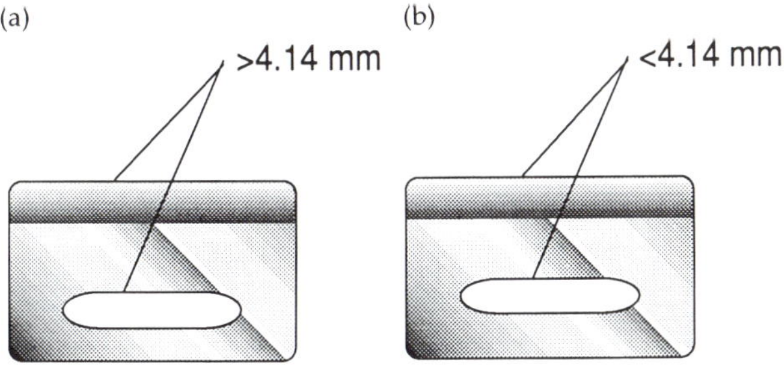

Fig. 15.112 (a) Blade too big; (b) blade too small.

Thicker disk

1 Higher IOP
2 Wider blade (Figure 15.112a)
3 Large-diameter disk

Thinner disk

1 Low IOP
2 Narrower blade (Figure 15.112b)
3 Smaller-diameter disk

Incomplete section

If the section with the microkeratome is incomplete but the corneal disk is attached by only a small bridge of tissue, it may be sectioned with a small sharp spatula or knife. If the microkeratome stops halfway or two-thirds of the way through the resection, the surgery must be postponed.

Prophylaxis Observe the disk as it exits the microkeratome. As soon as it stops emerging, the section is complete. Take care to retain pressure on both the motor and vacuum foot switches during the keratectomy.

Sectioning of the disk halfway or in the final third This may occur for two reasons:

1 From having withdrawn the microkeratome from the eye too soon—with the motor running
2 From detachment of the fixation ring during the section

Prophylaxis If the vacuum breaks for any reason, stop the keratome motor immediately. Ensure that fixation is adequate prior to starting, and do not pull up strongly on the vacuum ring. Stop the motor in any case before removing it from the ring.

Entering the anterior chamber

This can occur from a number of causes. The most obvious is setting the plate incorrectly or an error in pachymetry. Too-slow translation during the keratectomy or stopping with the motor running also can cause it. The most common cause in fixed-plate microkeratomes is operating the microkeratome without a plate (Figures 15.113 and 15.114).

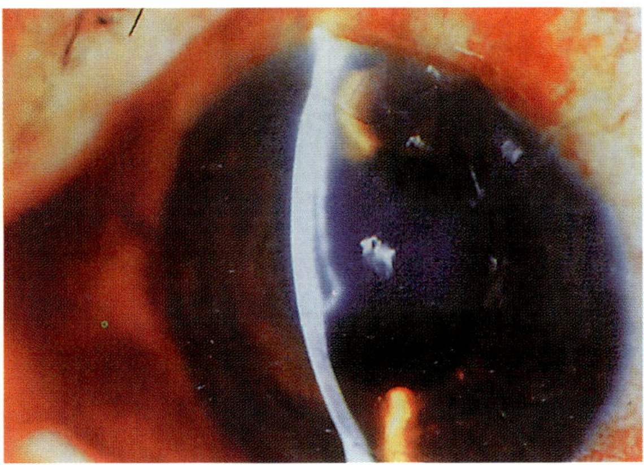

Fig. 15.113 Entry into the anterior chamber during keratectomy. (Courtesy of J.I. Barraquer.)

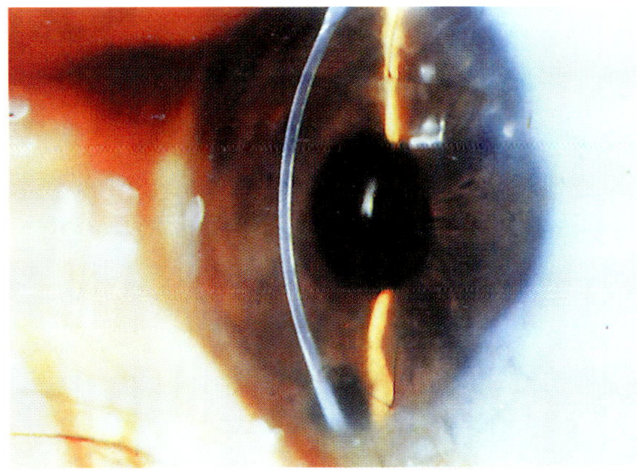

Fig. 15.114 The same eye at 1 month. (Courtesy of J.I. Barraquer.)

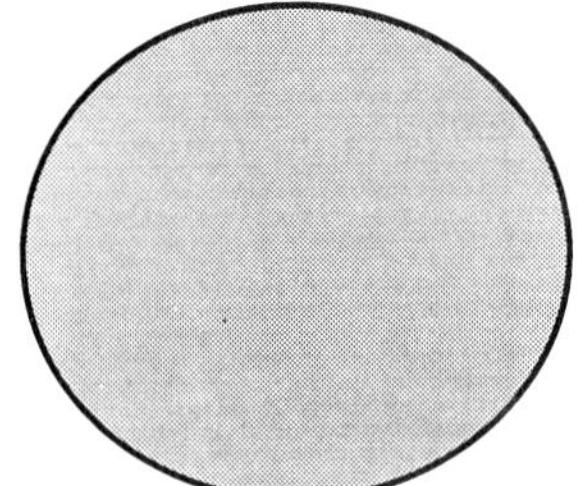

Fig. 15.115 Oval disk.

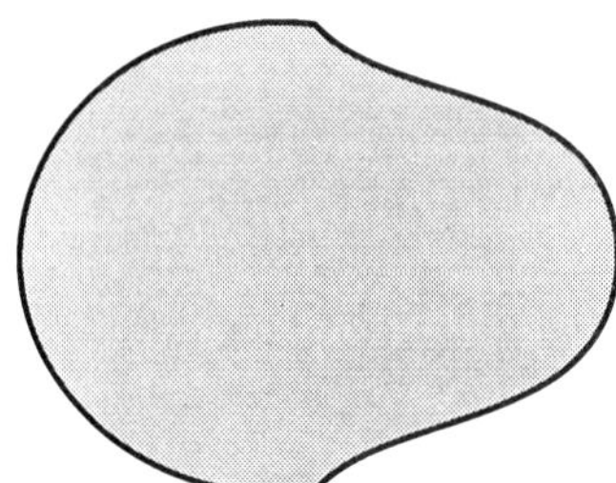

Fig. 15.116 Piriform disk.

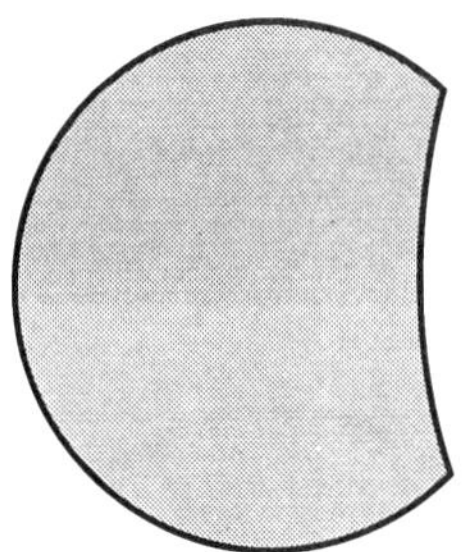

Fig. 15.117 D or kidney-shaped disk.

Irregularity in the corneal disk

Irregularity in shape The shape of the disk may be defective because it is to a greater or lesser extent oval (Figure 15.115), piriform (Figure 15.116), or kidney-shaped (Figure 15.117).

These accidents may be due to

1 An irregularly shaped cornea
2 An irregularity in the limbus (pterygium, etc.)
3 Variation in IOP during the resection
4 Defective fit of the microkeratome into the ring guides
5 Faster translation of the microkeratome at the end of the resection than at the beginning

Prophylaxis
1 Preoperative examination of the corneal surface and limbus
2 Keeping the ring in a constant position—not pushing down
3 Uniform microkeratome motion

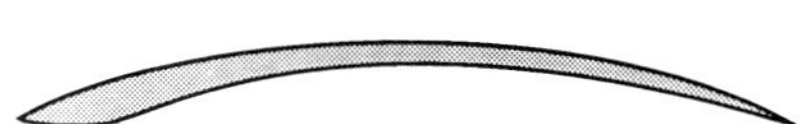

Fig. 15.118 Irregular section thickness.

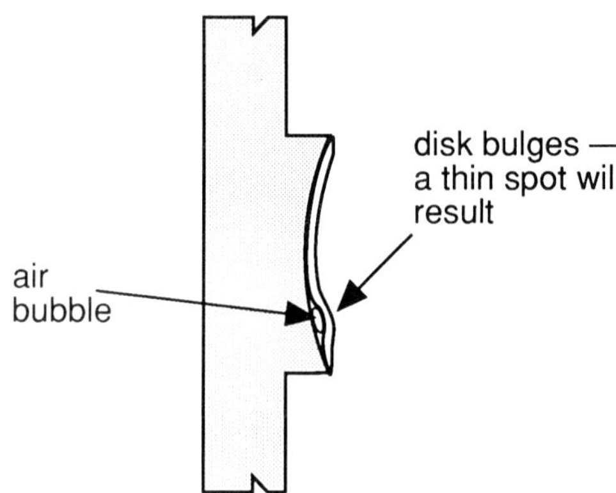

Fig. 15.119 Air under the tissue during lathing can produce an eccentric thin spot and postoperative irregular astigmatism.

Irregularity in thickness This can occur as a result of insufficient or variable IOP during the resection (Figure 15.118). Also, if the microkeratome is moved too rapidly during the keratectomy, the tissue will be thinner. Occasionally, this will occur because of use of a dull blade. If the corneal surface is highly irregular, the resection bed also will be irregular. If a parallel-sided disk of sufficient thickness is sutured into the bed, it is possible for a smooth external surface to result. However, the center of myopic lenticules is thin and is likely to reshape itself to the bed. In this case, irregular astigmatism may result. When lathing, make sure that no air remains between the disk and the Delrin base (Figure 15.119).

Prophylaxis
1 Check the blade edge.
2 Do prekeratectomy tonometry.
3 Keep the ring stable (see above).
4 Keep the motion of the microkeratome uniform (see above).

Irregularity in the section The section looks like a Ruffles potato chip (Figure 15.120).

Prophylaxis Slow and uniform movement of the microkeratome. In case of a small defect, the operation can continue. Otherwise, the best solution is to replace the disk, suturing it into place and postponing the surgery.

Foreign bodies in the section interface

Interface inclusions—everything from dust to lint—can find its way between the tissues—and usually will (Figure 15.121). Working without gloves, using lint-free drapes,

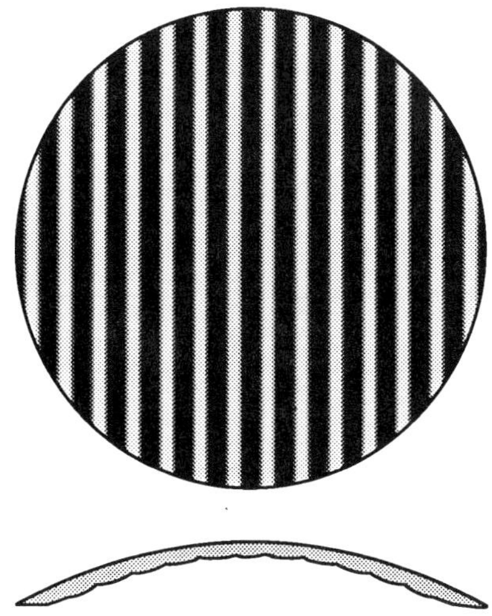

Fig. 15.120 "Ruffled" section.

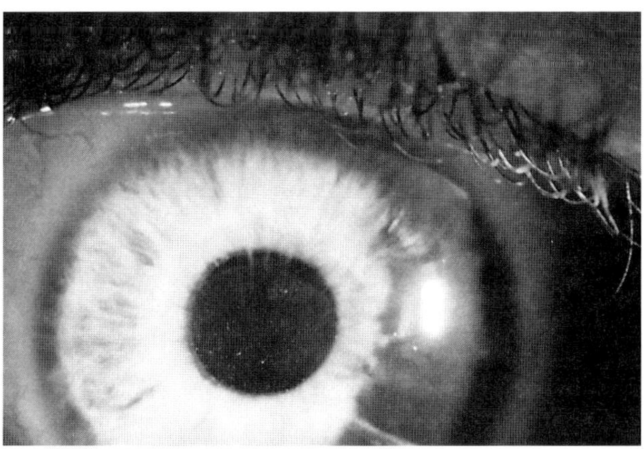

Fig. 15.121 Metallic particles and dust in the interface.

and having a laminar airflow unit in the operating room can minimize this problem. The most common source of such substances is from the air (lint, hair, talcum, dust) or from small chips off the blade caused by its striking the lid speculum (see discussion on minimizing interface particulates in the LASIK section, below).

Prophylaxis Use a laminar flow filter and avoid striking any metallic surfaces. Examine both the bed and the disk under the microscope with oblique lighting. Carefully scrub both surfaces with a sable brush, and pick away pieces not dislodged by the scrubbing or irrigation. Do not lay the disk on the eye to clean it. This is sure to sow epithelial cells into the interface.

Suture difficulties

When suturing the disk, the needle used must be very sharp to minimize trauma to the disk edges. Make sure that you expose the needle tip before passing it through the keratectomy edge.

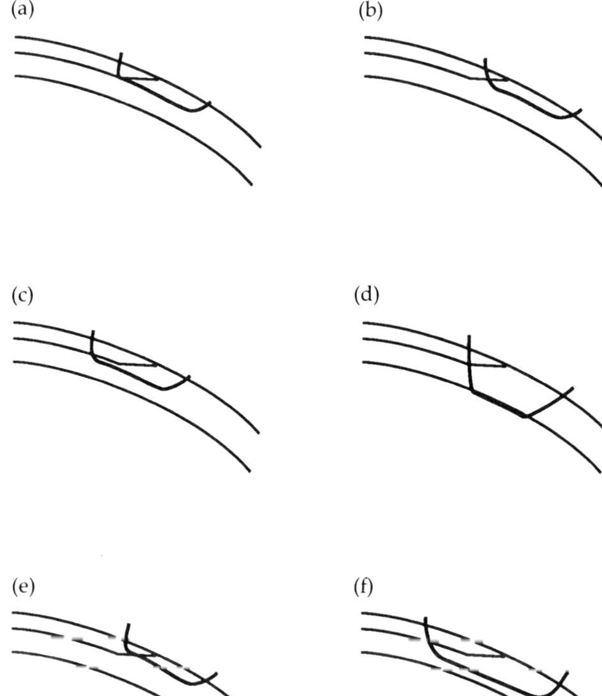

Fig. 15.122 Suturing mistakes. (a) Correct suture placement; (b) too close to lenticule edge; (c) too central and includes the resection bed; (d) too deep, enters the anterior chamber; (e) too superficial; (f) too deep and too broad.

Edge tearing

The bites must be placed at least 1.0 mm from the edge of the disk (Figure 15.122). If they are placed more peripherally, the tissue can be torn easily. Torn edges provide easy access to the interface for the epithelium (see Chapter 10).

Perforating or superficial suture

If a suture penetrates into the anterior chamber, it should be replaced, although the use of 10-0 nylon makes this less imperative. When the suture is superficial, there is a risk of the tissue tearing, which will result in a loose running suture and displaced disk. In addition, torn tissue impedes re-epithelialization and promotes epithelial invasion of the interface. Use of ⅜-in. curved needles will assist placing the bites correctly—do not use the fish-hook configuration. The author uses 10-0 black nylon on an Alcon A-3 needle.

Suture breakage

If the suture breaks after the ends have been cut, prior to burying (or during) the knot, loosen the suture sufficiently so as to provide length for tying onto an additional suture. Tie the knot with a 2-1-1 throw, and pull the knot into the corneal side (Figure 15.123). Replace the suture bite (it

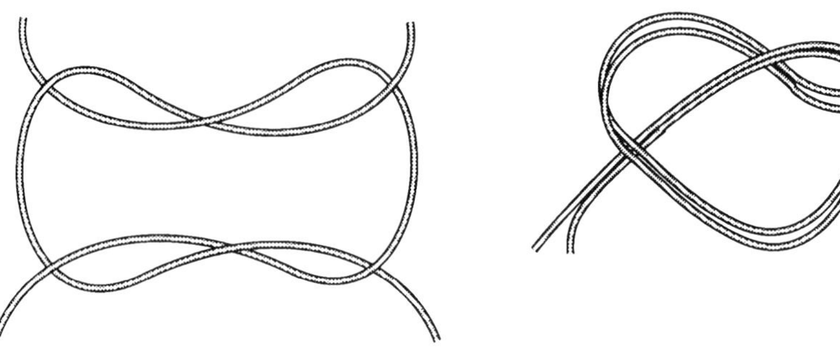

Fig. 15.123 Recommended knots to be used with broken sutures.

should pass through the original hole easily), and try to tie it to the other end so that the new knot can be pulled into the cornea as well. Suture breakage before finishing usually occurs at the needle—the solution is obvious, if not pleasant.

Sowing epithelial cells

This can occur during cleaning (as explained earlier) but also can happen during suturing. If the needle is blunt or rough, it can drag cells into the interface. Likewise, sutures placed too close to the edge of the disk could cause tearing or gaping, allowing epithelium to "sneak" in under the disk. Transfer of cells can occur from handling with the Colibri forceps as well. This can be minimized by not handling the disk with forceps once the first cardinal suture is in place. Keep all instruments scrupulously clean during the procedure.

Irregular coaptation or edge gap

In lamellar refractive surgery, the edges of the disk must not be allowed to extend beyond the edge of the resection (Figure 15.124). This can occur if the disk is too large for the bed—something that can happen in homoplastic cases—and also if care is not taken to center the tissue before completing the knotting. The epithelium will dive under the edge rather than climb over it. It is better that

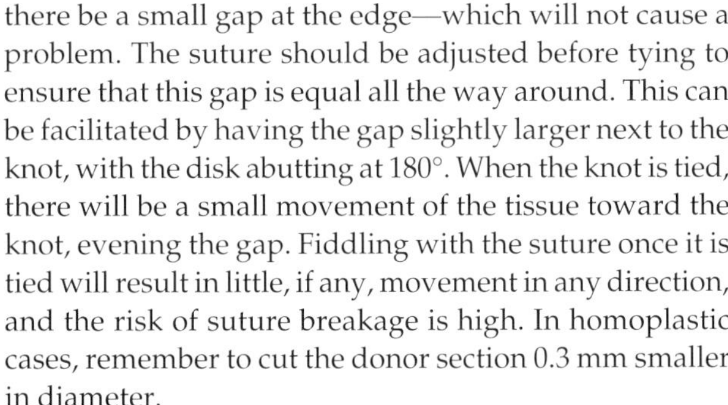

there be a small gap at the edge—which will not cause a problem. The suture should be adjusted before tying to ensure that this gap is equal all the way around. This can be facilitated by having the gap slightly larger next to the knot, with the disk abutting at 180°. When the knot is tied, there will be a small movement of the tissue toward the knot, evening the gap. Fiddling with the suture once it is tied will result in little, if any, movement in any direction, and the risk of suture breakage is high. In homoplastic cases, remember to cut the donor section 0.3 mm smaller in diameter.

Loose suture

Apart from providing a bad coaptation, a loose running suture will produce discomfort for the patient by accumulating mucus in the loose suture limbs and may interfere with epithelialization as well as possibly promote neovascularization. To prevent this from happening, before knotting, it will help to "snug up" the suture with a 2-1 knot so that it will hold for the final throw. Avoid using the usual 3-2-2 throw, which results in a large knot that is difficult (if not impossible) to pull into the needle hole. If after knotting the suture it is seen to be loose, it may be tightened by placing a radial stitch in the periphery of the cornea, taking in one of the loops (limbs) of the running suture and tightening it until the running suture takes up the proper tension. More than one of these can be done (Figure 15.125).

Excessively tight suture

If the running suture is too tight, the edges of the disk can overlap the peripheral epithelium, and the coaptation will

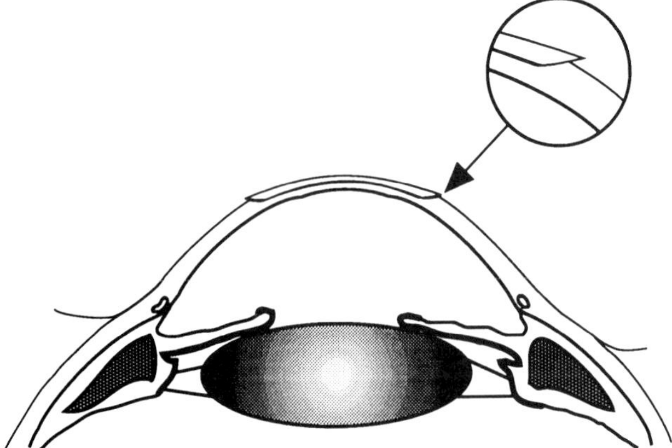

Fig. 15.124 Avoid the lenticule overriding the resection edge.

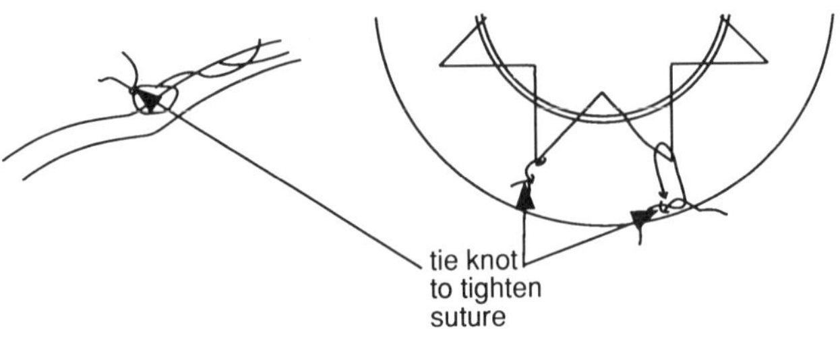

Fig. 15.125 Dealing with a loose suture.

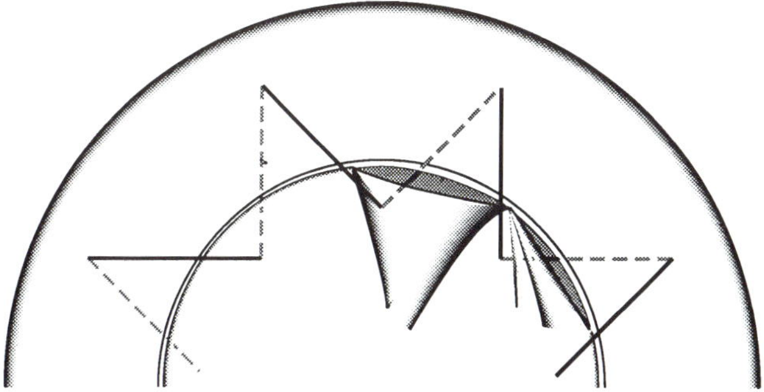

Fig. 15.126 Tight sutures produce edge-gaping.

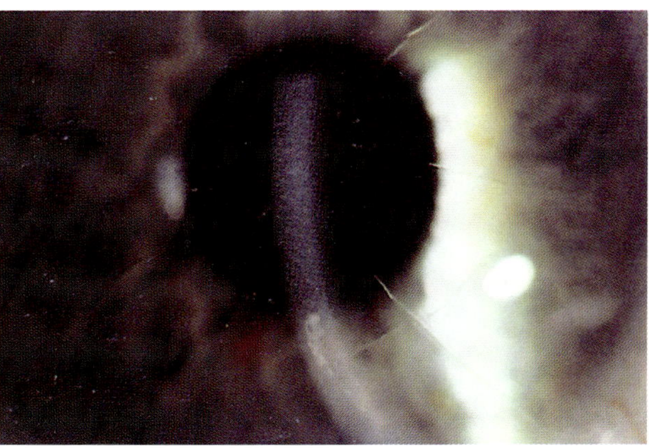

Fig. 15.127 Epithelial implantation—at lenticule edge.

be irregular and scalloped (Figure 15.126). Sublenticular epithelialization can occur under these circumstances, as well as astigmatism from the furrowing.

Postoperative complications

The postoperative complications are generally those of any operation on the cornea of the eye such as keratitis, ulcer, etc. Those peculiar to these procedures are induced or residual astigmatism, irregular astigmatism, sublenticular epithelialization, disk slough, residual refractive error, infection, and interface foreign bodies interfering with vision.

Astigmatism

Irregular astigmatism has been reported with this surgery and occurs as a result of a severely torn disk or decentration of the resection. It also can occur in keratomileusis with a disk whose thickness is not uniform. This may not always be apparent by examination at the time of surgery. The incidence of induced astigmatism is approximately 11% after keratomileusis in situ (KMIS or automated lamellar keratoplasty), which is about twice that of classic or freeze-lathing keratomileusis. In HLK, induced astigmatism is approximately 4%, indicating that decentration of the second pass is the operative factor in the increased astigmatism seen in KMIS. Approximately 50% of the complications associated with laser in situ keratomileusis (LASIK) are due to irregular astigmatism.

If it occurs, it is best handled by attempting to "regularize" the astigmatism through the application of relaxing incisions after some months of healing. Removal and replacement of the disk are not the solution because the repeat section also may be irregular due to irregular applanation. This is unlikely to occur in HLK because nothing is removed. Irregular astigmatism may occur in KMIS if the diameter of the second pass is less than 4.5 mm. You are advised to avoid secondary sections less than 4.5 mm—it is suggested that 5.0 mm be the minimum.

Residual or induced regular astigmatism is treated by allowing 3 to 4 months to elapse or until the keratometry readings stabilize. Relaxing incisions appropriate to the degree of astigmatism are then made (see Chapter 9). The same is true for residual myopia in the case of KMIS. Relaxing incisions have been used successfully in conjunction with MKM for some time.

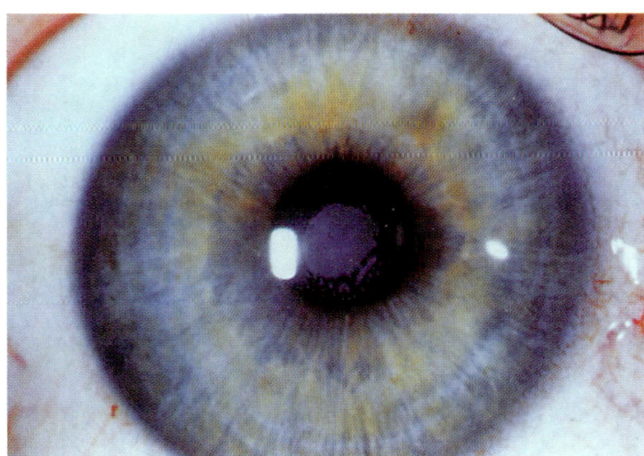

Fig. 15.128 Epithelial ingrowth—central. (Courtesy of J.I. Barraquer.)

Epithelial ingrowth

Epithelialization of the interface is a serious complication in lamellar refractive surgery because it is progressive and usually results in loss of vision. In classic keratomileusis, it is the leading cause of lenticular loss. Rarely, epithelial cells will stop proliferating if they have been sown into the interface, but if they migrate in from the edge—usually they do not stop growing (Figures 15.127 through 15.132). Epithelial ingrowth is often accompanied by serous elevation and clouding of the disk (Figure 15.133).

In these cases, the disk must be totally removed from the resection bed and the epithelial cell mass carefully peeled away and removed from both surfaces. This is best accomplished by placing a single "hinge" of interrupted

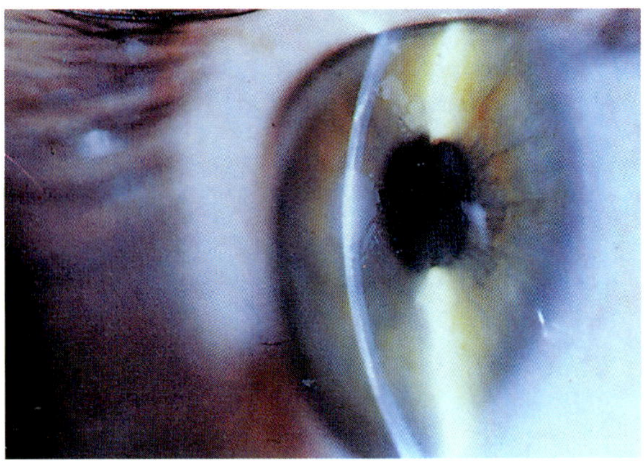

Fig. 15.129 Epithelial ingrowth—central. Slit-lamp view. (Courtesy of J.I. Barraquer.)

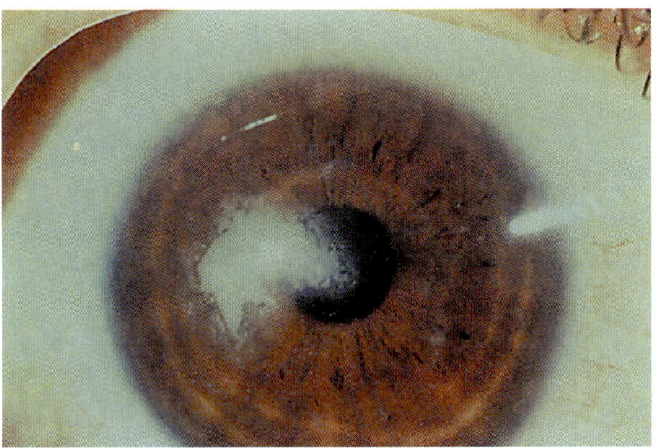

Fig. 15.130 Epithelial ingrowth—peripheral. (Courtesy of J.I. Barraquer.)

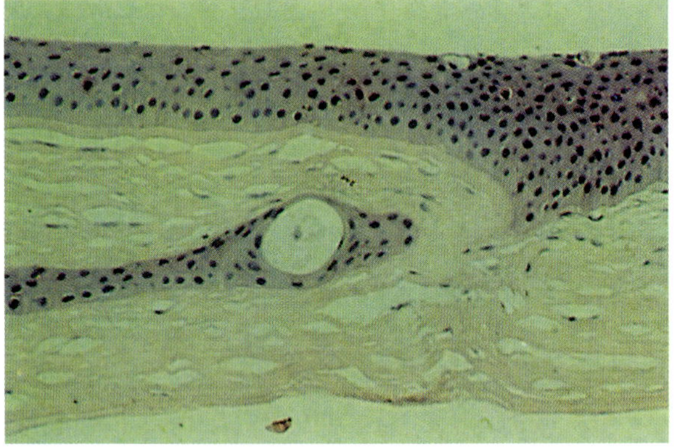

Fig. 15.131 Epithelial ingrowth—peripheral. Histologic section. (Courtesy of J.I. Barraquer.)

10-0 nylon before removing the running suture. The epithelium must be completely removed from the coapted edge before lifting the edge of the disk. A small amount of 10% cocaine on a microsponge will loosen and destroy some of the cells.

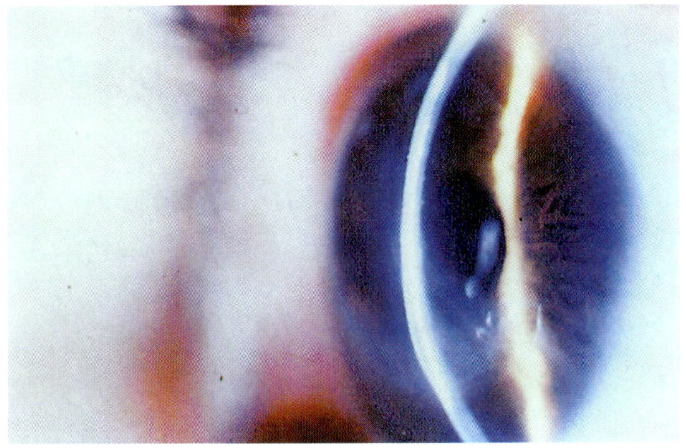

Fig. 15.132 Typical reaction to active epithelium in the interface. (Courtesy of J.I. Barraquer.)

The running suture is removed and the lenticule carefully freed from the interface. Use a gentle lifting movement with a flat, blunt iris spatula such as the Katena Jaffe spatula (Figure 15.134). As the disk is lifted, the underlying ingrown epithelium probably will come up with it (Figure 15.135). At this juncture, the disk must be lifted carefully so as to leave the epithelial "sheet" intact—if possible. Hinge the disk over onto its top surface—Bowman's layer down. Using a dry or lightly moistened microsponge (not a Weck-Cel), remove the epithelium from the resection bed. Do this by making repeated one-way passes with the sponge, using a clean, new sponge each time. Repeat the process with the stromal side of the lenticule.

After the mechanical scrubbing is done, gently brush both surfaces with a red sable brush while irrigating with copious quantities of BSS (Jorge Krumeich suggests distilled water). Once clean, the disk can be replaced and resutured, taking care not to duplicate the circumstances that caused the problem in the first place (Figure 15.136).

Lenticular necrosis and sloughing

Only two cases of disk decompensation with necrosis not due to trauma have been observed in classic keratomileusis; the cause is still unknown but believed to be due to contamination of the lenticule by Cidex during the surgery in one case and diabetic glycemic crisis in the other (Figure 15.137). In the former case, two subsequent lenticules failed due to poor coaptation. The problem was finally solved with a modified form of epikeratophakia. Most sloughing or displacement will occur due to direct trauma or through suture breakage (Figure 15.138). Occasionally, a suture is sufficiently loose to allow the lid blink to tear the lenticule loose from the bed. Lathing without cryopreservative or prolonged freezing also can lead to lenticular failure (Figures 15.139 and 15.140). In these

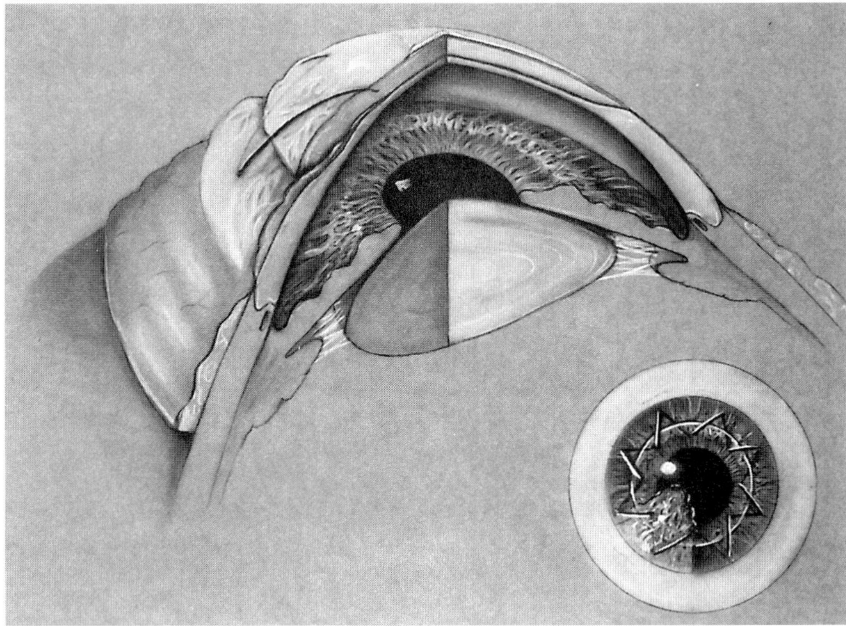

Fig. 15.133 Epithelial ingrowth.

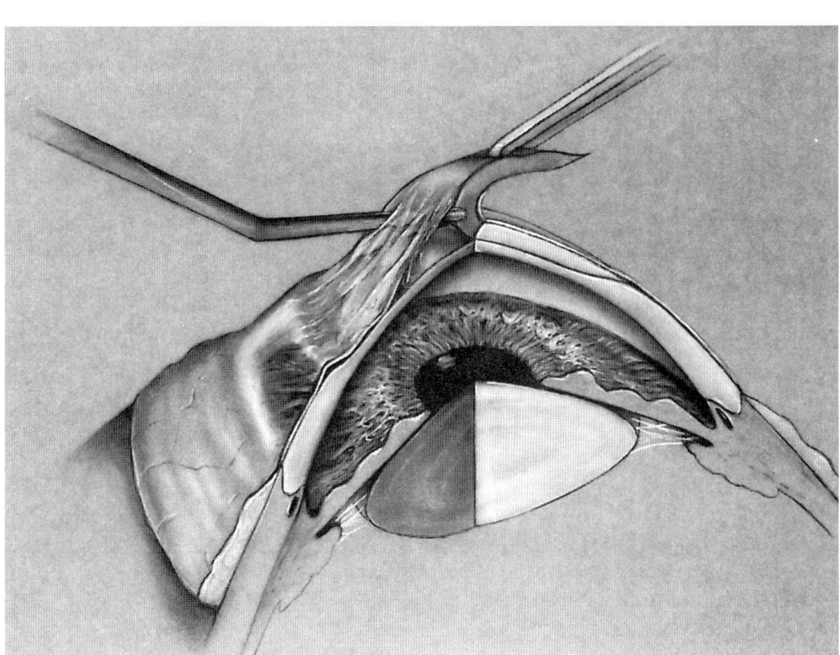

Fig. 15.134 Elevate lenticule and epithelial sheet, using spatula to separate the epithelial sheet.

cases, a replacement with donor tissue must be done as soon as possible.

Interface foreign bodies

Interface foreign bodies result from particulate matter entering the interface during surgery. These are most frequently lint and dust particles but sometimes may be talc and, rarely, metallic pieces caused by "spalling." Particles not interfering with vision are best left alone. Their damage is to the surgeon's pride alone—who, if he or she is doing this surgery, should possess sufficient ego to cope with it. However, if these particles interfere with vision because of glare or obstruction, they must be removed. It may be necessary, in some cases, to separate and lift the disk from the bed over the foreign body. Begin at one edge by first removing the epithelium in the area with a cotton-tipped applicator moistened with 10% cocaine. This will swell and loosen the epithelial layer without damaging the lenticule—avoid alcohol. Gently

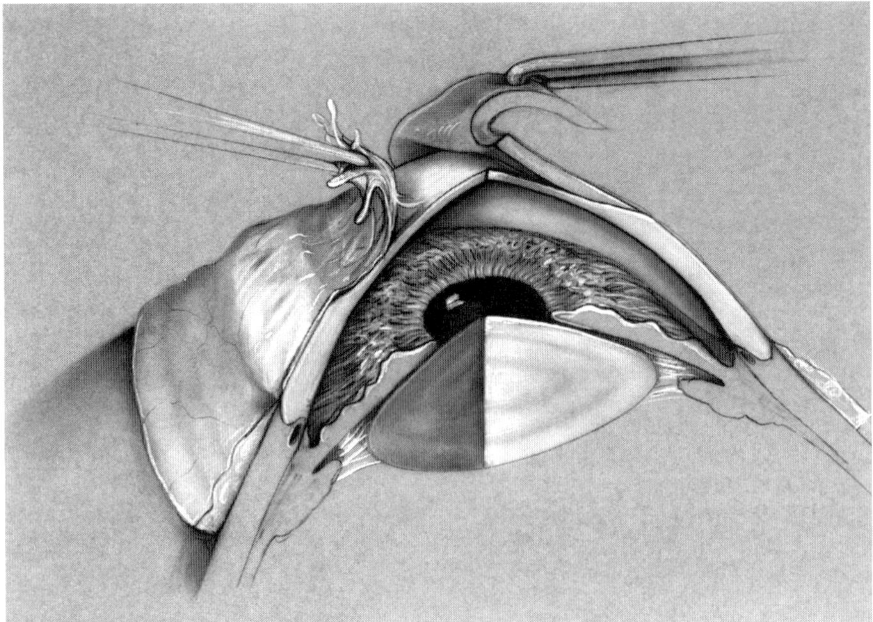

Fig. 15.135 Peel epithelium away from disk bed and lenticule.

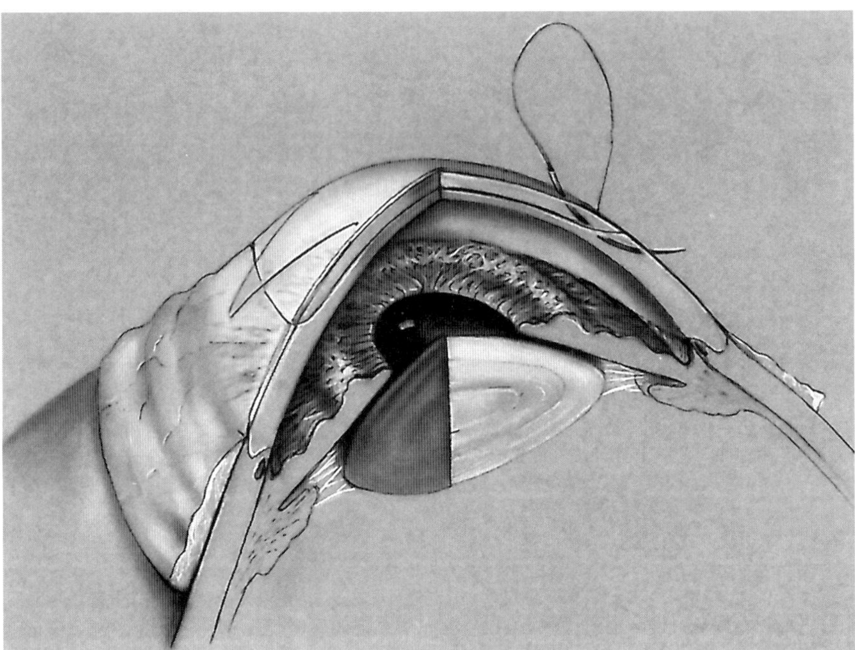

Fig. 15.136 Resutured lenticule.

elevate the edge of the disk with a fine spatula and tease the disk away from the bed until the foreign body can be reached (Figure 15.141). Avoid handling the tissue edge with forceps of any kind to prevent tearing or fraying. If the disk tends to bend excessively, it will have to be freed up still more. Rarely will it be necessary to remove it completely. Remove the offending material with a smooth, fine-tipped forceps. If the area of elevation is not extensive, no resuturing will be required, but generally, resuturing is recommended. Patch overnight after administering antibiotic/steroids and possibly a cycloplegic/mydriatic.

Infection

Fortunately, infection is usually very rare in these cases and manifests—when it occurs—as a clouding within the interface. This can mimic an ingrowth of epithelium and

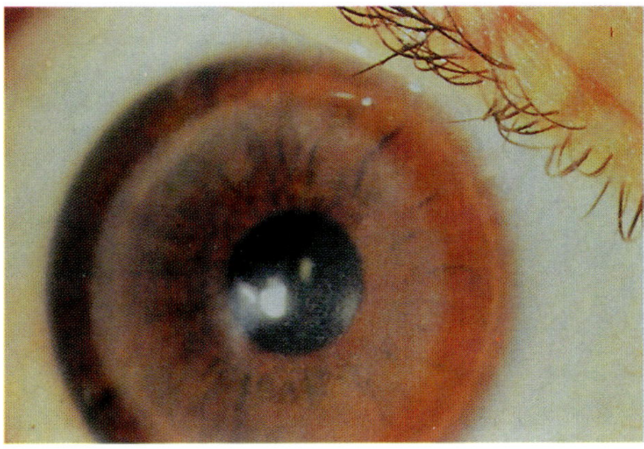

Fig. 15.137 Asceptic necrosis of MKM lenticule. (Courtesy of J.I. Barraquer.)

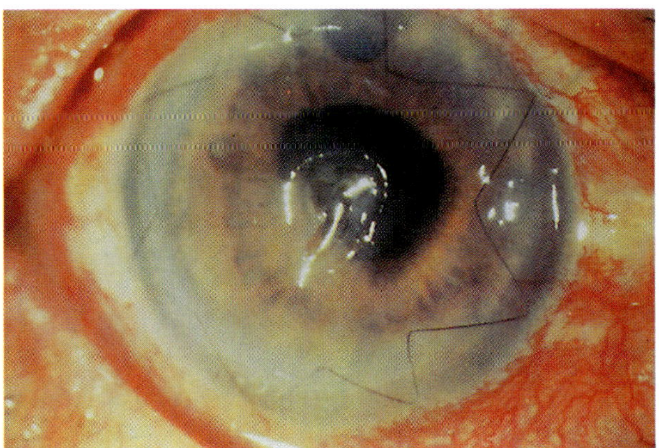

Fig. 15.138 Central necrosis of MKM lenticule following corneal abrasion. (Courtesy of J.I. Barraquer.)

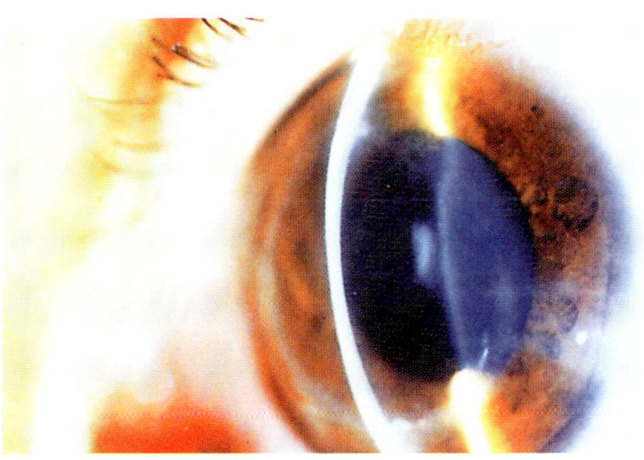

Fig. 15.139 Lenticular clouding following lathing without use of cryopreservative. (Courtesy of J.I. Barraquer.)

could prove to be a diagnostic dilemma (Figures 15.142 through 15.145). Such an infection is unlikely to be present, however, within the first few days—if the recommended postoperative injection of subtenon gentamicin has been administered. If infection is suspected, vigorous treatment with broad-spectrum topical antibiotic/steroid drops must be instituted immediately.

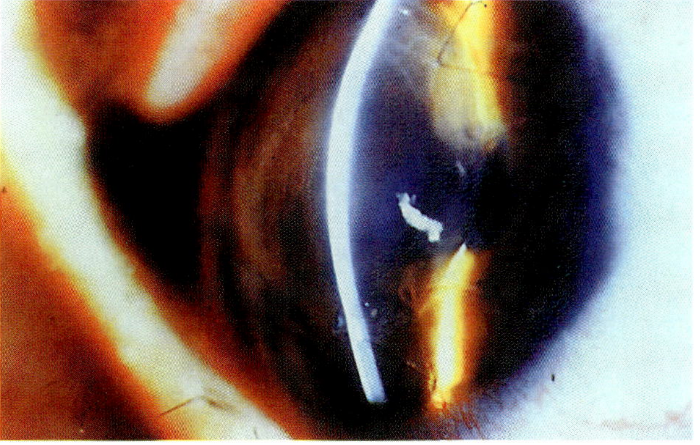

Fig. 15.140 Prolonged freezing (8 min in this case) can lead to prolonged lenticular edema and possible loss of the tissue. (Courtesy of J.I. Barraquer.)

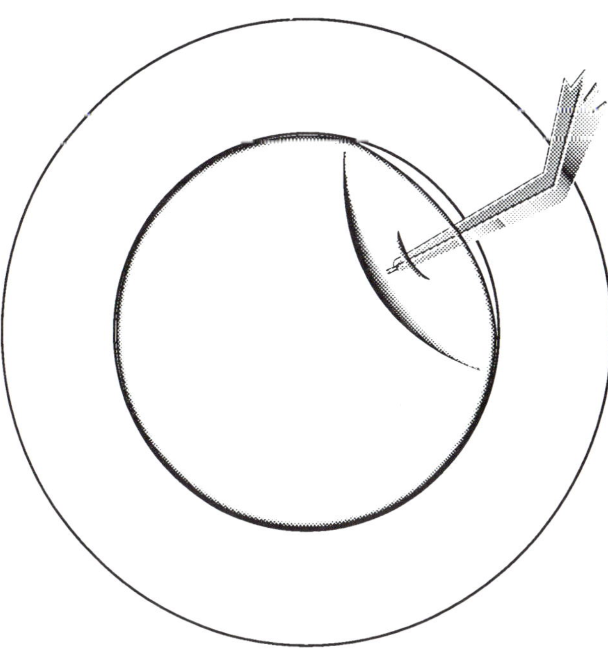

Fig. 15.141 Elevate the edge of the lenticule near the foreign body to be removed.

Over- or undercorrection

The nature of surgery on living tissue is such that accurate prediction of the outcome is not entirely possible. Therefore, the occurrence of over- and undercorrections of the myopia or hyperopia is inevitable.

Undercorrections

In *keratomileusis*, if the residual myopia is less than 5 D and greater than 1 D, RK incisions may be employed to complete the reduction of the correction toward plano. In

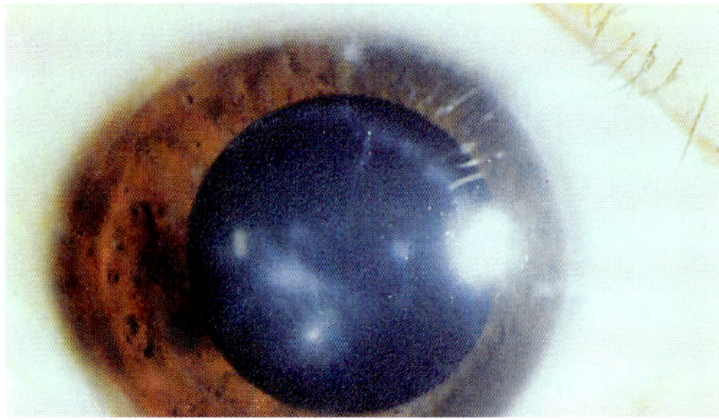

Fig. 15.142 Infection involving lenticule. In the early stages it may be difficult to distinguish from epithelium in the interface. (Courtesy of J.I. Barraquer.)

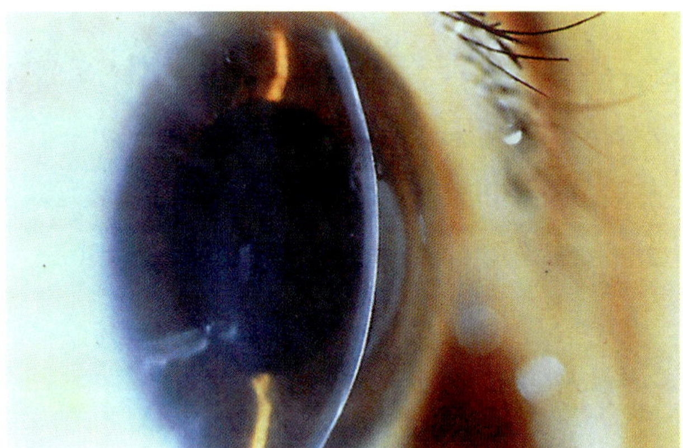

Fig. 15.143 Slit-lamp view of the same eye. (Courtesy of J.I. Barraquer.)

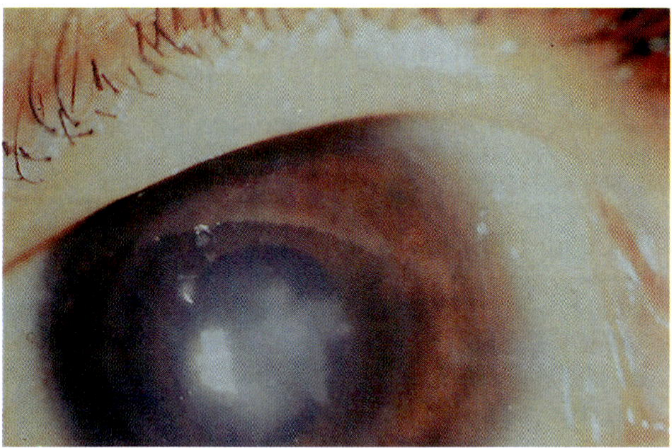

Fig. 15.144 Interface bacterial growth occurring after early contact lens use. (Courtesy of J.I. Barraquer.)

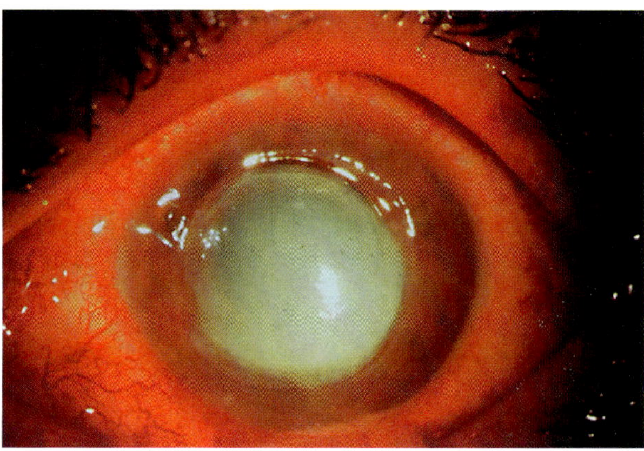

Fig. 15.145 Complete loss of epilenticule following infection. (Courtesy of J.I. Barraquer.)

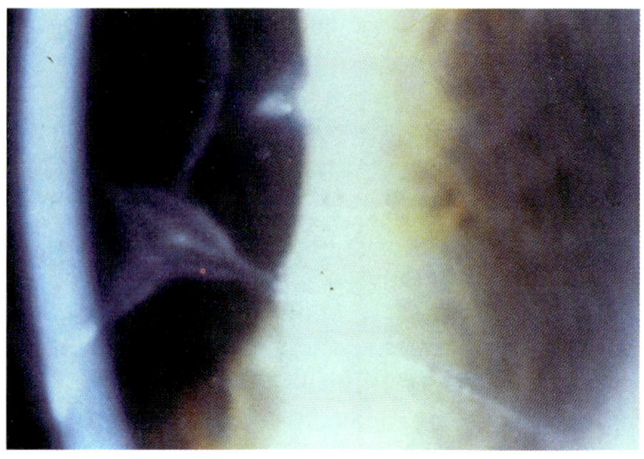

Fig. 15.146 Tissue "melting" at the intersection of RK incisions and lenticular edge. (Courtesy of J.I. Barraquer.)

these cases it is best to wait for at least 4 months to ensure stabilization of the residual refractive error. *"When in doubt—wait it out."* When using the calculations, input the original preoperative K-readings (remember that your postoperative K-readings are meaningless). Use the sharpest blade in your armamentarium—preferably a new, double-edged one. However, be advised that incisions through the edge of the lenticule can result in a tissue response similar to that seen when T-cuts join radials (Figure 15.146).

In *hyperopic lamellar keratotomy* (HLK), the solution here really depends on the degree of residual hyperopia. If it is not very great, the best solution is to do nothing—surgically. If greater than 2 D, it is best to wait for at least 6 months and repeat the section at a deeper setting. Be careful when selecting the depth, however. If the section is too deep, myopia of the progressive, possibly never-ending variety can occur. Additionally, the new resection must be larger in diameter—by at least 0.5 mm—than the first one; do not attempt to make the new section inside the first one.

In *epikeratophakia,* if the residual hyperopia is of sufficient magnitude, removal and replacement with an appropriately powered fresh epilenticule are in order.

Overcorrections

In *keratomileusis,* these are much more difficult to deal with than undercorrections. If the degree of induced hyperopia is creating difficulties for the patient and spectacles or contact lenses are not an option, it may seem desirable to perform HLK. In these cases, at least 6 months must be allowed to elapse to ensure that adequate adhesion of the lenticule to the underlying cornea has occurred. Typically, the disk diameter in HLK is much smaller than that in keratomileusis, and the resulting annulus remaining of the original resection may opacify or part company with the parent cornea. Most overcorrections are of a low order, however; therefore, a more viable alternative would be application of a low-power hyperopic epikeratophakia lenticule. This choice is more likely to effect a reduction of the hyperopia and has the advantages that it will overlay and extend beyond the edges of the first resection. Additionally, it is replaceable in the event of difficulty. This latter alternative may not be viable for individual surgeons with no access to either a lathe or source of an appropriate lenticule; therefore, it would be prudent to plan for undercorrection in subsequent patients. Considering the improved communication and transportation facilities currently available, the enterprising surgeon will no doubt be able to come up with a solution to this dilemma of obtaining epilenticules in such an event.

In *hyperopic lamellar keratotomy* (HLK), it may seem obvious that this problem is easily corrected with RK. *Beware!* This complication is frequently due to sections that are too deep. Here, the myopia is likely to be progressive. Sufficient time must be allowed to elapse to make sure that progression has stopped—a minimum of 9 months. If it does stop, then RK may be able to reduce the myopia to acceptable levels. If the myopia continues to progress, however, the alternative is myopic epikeratophakia—preferably of the wet variety using an MKM-type meniscus or lenticule. Avoid a PKP unless the induced keratoconus is associated with severe irregular astigmatism. Even in these cases, an epikeratoplasty can save the day.

In *epikeratophakia,* as in undercorrections, the choice is removal and replacement of the lenticule.

Summary

While some of these problems may seem formidable, they do not occur with frequency. For example, epithelial ingrowth occurs in about 3% of cases. Overcorrection is even rarer in HLK or keratomileusis. You must be aware that these problems are discussed because they have occurred to someone—they are *not* theoretical! Therefore, you must be prepared to face them some time in your career as a refractive surgeon. This is why the author has stated that this branch of surgery is not a sometime thing! You are either going to devote yourself wholly to it or you are better advised to look elsewhere for "entertainment." This surgery can be a most fulfilling and rewarding challenge. Please give it the attention and respect that it and your patients deserve.

Laser in-situ keratomileusis (LASIK)

LASIK is the new darling of the laser crowd and has caught on well around the world. It is a good procedure, but it requires thinking. Greater care needs be taken with lamellar surgery—which this most assuredly is, the principles of which are laid out in Chapter 10—than with relaxing incisions.

LASIK came about in the late 1980s because some thought that an operation like photorefractive keratectomy (PRK), in destroying Bowman's membrane, would affect corneal innervation and healing [93]. As with any procedure, LASIK has its propensity for complications. These most commonly include difficulties making the corneal flap and not with the laser ablation itself. When one performs the partial keratectomy, a suction ring is used to hold the eye and bring the cornea up so that a planar stromal flap is made. If one has low or loss of suction, as the microkeratome passes across the eye, a free flap will result. Newer microkeratome units have safety features to shut down if vacuum is lost. If the microkeratome jams or power is lost, an incomplete corneal flap will be created. Laser treatment should be aborted and the flap replaced, to be recut several weeks to 3 months later. Newer microkeratome units have battery backups to prevent stoppage from power failures.

Although there appear to be fewer complications with LASIK than with other refractive procedures, the complications that can occur usually are much more severe. Irregular astigmatism, epithelial ingrowth, displaced flaps, stromal melts, and poorly cut flaps can be very hard to manage. Fortunately, most such complications are treatable without loss of best-corrected acuity, but patients always should be informed of the potential beforehand. Patients need to be informed that many times a second operation or enhancement is required, and they need to be told what the typical frequency is—in your hands. If they are told in advance of this, most accept it very well. However, since some of the complications that occur can be serious and difficult to correct, the best treatment is prevention. This can be done, in part, by obtaining the best possible training for yourself and your surgical staff and by meticulously paying attention to the details of laser calibration, setup, and performance of the surgery (see also Chapter 10).

The most common side effect encountered by LASIK patients is residual refractive error. This may be a result of the nomogram the practitioner is using. Nomograms usually require individual input, and manufacturers are reluctant to give out nomograms directly. Basically, nomograms are developed by individual surgeons based on their individual techniques with their individual results, and surgeons vary tremendously in their techniques. Thus you would only expect the nomogram to be helpful to you if the surgeon who developed it for the company during clinical trials performs the surgery with a technique that is similar to your own. To find a more closely suited nomogram, visit a surgeon who has experience with the laser you are using, with an eye toward how his or her technique varies from your own. He or she then may recommend obtaining a copy of the individualized nomogram and cautiously trying it. If, after doing a few of your own patients, you see that you are getting an undercorrection of an extra 5% or so, you will cut back accordingly—then you essentially have your nomogram.

A suction break or a decentered or uneven resection of the corneal flap can induce irregular astigmatism, as well as improper replacement of the flap or a decentered ablation. A bad or damaged blade also can create irregular astigmatism. Scanning lasers coupled with real-time topography are becoming the instruments of choice for correcting these problems.

Epithelial ingrowth occurs as a result of the microkeratome blade implanting rests of cells as it cuts across the cornea (see Figure 15.133). Epithelium also can grow beneath a loosely adherent flap or into the interface through epithelial plugs when operating over old RK incisions. Generally, epithelium should not be removed unless it is causing irregular astigmatism or undercorrection or blocks the visual axis. A sheet of epithelium that covers both sides of the corneal flap can cause it to melt.

Epithelium is not a mole nor any other burrowing creature. It will not insinuate itself between cap and stromal bed unless it is either placed there or a gap exists. If there is enough of it, it will obey the first law of life—to grow and to thrive. This is why it is so important to make sure that the cap is replaced smoothly and on a reasonably dry bed so as to ensure adherence all around.

The *first rule* is: *"If it ain't broke, don't fix it."* Isolated islands of epithelium in the midperiphery are best left alone. These usually do not get larger and eventually will go away, leaving, at worse, a small area of haze and a damaged ego. Larger patches, particularly if near an edge, can be very troubling and often are associated with edge melting or worse. I have seen a case in which the intrusion extended across the entire resection bed beneath the cap within 24 hours; epithelium can be bodacious if given a chance.

The *second rule* is: *"Don't use anti-inflammatories and assume that they will limit epithelial growth by themselves."* What they will do instead is ensure a corneal melt, interface inflammation, or worse.

The *third rule* is: *"Don't try to irrigate it out."* The mechanics of epithelial removal have been detailed in the section on classic keratomileusis above; however, a few points need to be reemphasized. Irrigation as a primary removal method is typically useless; the cap must be lifted sufficiently to unroof the implanted material. The usual advice is to tease up an edge and then, holding the cap with forceps, strip the cap away from the resection bed. *Don't do it!* I've got as much, if not more, experience with lamellar surgery as anyone, and I'm saying that this isn't the way—unless you want to tear the cap (flap), hinge, or both. The best way, IMHO (in my humble opinion), is to delineate the edge of the cap with a blunt, flat spatula, thereby stripping away the epithelium covering the gap. Then tease an edge up, preferably at 180° to the inclusion, and gently slide the blunt, flat, rounded-edge spatula between the lamellae until it appears at the opposite edge. Then sweep the spatula toward the inclusion and out, hence freeing the cap. I typically then fold the flap back with the spatula and remove the inclusion—open sky. Irrigate and then gently brush both the cap and the bed with a sable brush—not a Murocel sponge—and then replace the cap, smoothing it from the initial insertion toward the former inclusion site.

Do not lift the cap with forceps if you can avoid it. This tissue is very thin and easy to tear. If you must use a forceps, avoid those with teeth and employ those with Pearse-Hoskins-type tips with great care. My favorite is a Harms-Tubingen curved tying forceps. Of course, the tissue will slip away if trying to grasp with just the tip of the instrument; you have to grasp across the flap, thereby limiting the chance for tears. And gently does it. The argument against using a spatula is that it is likely to implant epithelial cells. Not! Because you're going to irrigate afterward—not before. I have never had a case wherein I reimplanted epithelium in this manner. I have seen cases, however, where this happened when the surgeon attempted to introduce a tunnel for irrigation. *The flap must be lifted over the inclusion.* 'Nuff said.

Minimizing interface particulates The Chayet sponge (Visitec) is made of the same material as the Murocel sponge. It is an oval with a 10-mm round cut-out in the center and a small tail trailing off one side. The sponge is placed after the microkeratome dissection but before the flap is reflected and acts as a 360° barrier around the limbus. This prevents any cul-de-sac material from moving centrally; it also absorbs any debris that is irrigated from the center outward. Because it is larger nasally and temporally than it is superiorly and inferiorly, it covers the nasal conjunctiva nicely. When the nasally hinged flap is reflected, the sponge protects the flap from falling into the cul-de-sac, ultimately preventing any cul-de-sac material from entering the stromal interface. Once the flap is repositioned, with the Chayet drain still in place, irrigate under the flap copiously with a Moria irrigator or similar. Any material irrigated out of the interface is absorbed by the sponge.

An *aspirating lid speculum,* such as the American Surgical Instruments product, is very important in maintaining a clean interface. Some surgeons use it in lieu of the sponge; some use both. My advice is that while I use both these aids, my most important tool in the LASIK room is a laminar flow filter by Oto-Med, of Lake Havasu, Arizona. This inexpensive device hangs on the wall, and if it is run at full speed about 15 minutes before performing your first surgery (and leaving it at low speed throughout the session), the incidence of interface particulates will be reduced to a minimum. It can produce a CRC (Clean Room Condition) rating of 15 within 25 minutes; this is equivalent to that within an integrated-circuit assembly room.

Maintaining a clean, hydrated flap to reduce striae Steinert employs a disposable Banaji sponge (Visitec) to the flap's stromal side while it is reflected. This is an 8-mm disk cut at one side to match the hinge location. He saturates it with ofloxacin to provide antibiotic as well as moisture. It is placed on the stromal side to prevent dehydration and contamination. After ablation, the disk is removed, and the flap is reflected into position. The result is a reasonably hydrated flap instead of one that has developed fixed folds. In addition, the peripheral margin is closer to the original cut if the flap has not shrunk from dehydration. Ordinarily, you should expect no more than a 0.2-mm shrinkage of the flap (see also Chapter 10).

Flap displacements Corneal flaps can be displaced several different ways. They can be moved out of position or wrinkled. A number of people know exactly when their flaps slipped—usually 1 to 2 hours after surgery. This corresponds to about the time they removed their shields and pried their eyes open or started to blink. Examination of such patients generally will reveal folds that radiate from the upper edge or striae. If the wrinkled or displaced area includes the visual axis, irregular astigmatism can be present. The longer wrinkles are present in the flap, the more difficult they are to treat. The flap must be lifted and replaced after gently massaging the wrinkles out. This encourages many practitioners to employ disposable contacts after surgery. Some feel that this may delay recovery of best vision, but the alternative is a torn or lost cap.

The 9.5-mm flap Hansatome may reduce the incidence of flap displacement. Large flaps seem to adhere better in patients who do not have excessive limbal vascularization. Many practitioners have had no displacements, and when tested during surgery, 9.5-mm flaps seem to adhere much better than the 8.4- or 8.5-mm flaps. This and a superior hinge might be helpful in preventing flap displacement.

Extremely thin corneal flaps and those so thin as to have a central hole (doughnut flaps) should be replaced, having the patient wait up to 3 months before recutting the flap and performing the laser ablation. Extremely thin flaps that include little more than central epithelium have a greater tendency to scar and develop haze postoperatively if not replaced and recut deeper at a later date. Incomplete flaps, flaps that bisect the visual axis, and free flaps that do not leave enough area for laser ablation also should be replaced and recut deeper at a later date.

Dry eyes

A troubling link between refractive surgical procedures such as laser in situ keratomileusis (LASIK) and dry eyes is beginning to emerge and is taking some patients and practitioners by unwelcome surprise [94]. One dissatisfied patient even went so far as to recount her experience in a *Time* magazine article entitled, "The Laser Fix." The journalist featured in the article claimed that following LASIK, she found herself suddenly besieged by extremely dry eyes. Her surgeon advised the woman to apply drops every 15 minutes, which seems a trifle impractical for a journalist, and it did not solve the problem in any event. This case is by no means an isolated incident—there appears to be an emerging dry-eye syndrome that affects many LASIK patients. While no one knows for certain what is causing the rash of complaints, many LASIK surgeons have offered theories about it and how to best manage the condition.

So what's up? It is probably no coincidence that sands of the Sahara syndrome was first described in LASIK patients. It would not surprise the author to find that the two are connected in some way. Be that as it may, for the time being, the occurrence of dry eyes following LASIK is on the rise, and the best treatment is to avoid it happening, if at all possible.

Many dry-eye patients are contact lens wearers who can no longer tolerate lenses due to dryness and who, as a result, may self-select for LASIK. Another group of self-selecting patients may be women in or approaching middle age, who are affected by hormonal factors, such as the dipping estrogen levels that accompany menopause; the incidence of keratitis sicca is higher in this group [95]. A lot of patients are older by the time they can afford surgery. The average myope seeking surgery is typically 40 years of age and the average hyperope is 50.

While dissatisfied contact lens wearers and those with autoimmune diseases, hormonal declines, and other associated causes suffer post-LASIK dry eyes, the crucial link may lie in the nerves of the central cornea, which are cut during the procedure. An 8.5-mm LASIK flap severs the fibers that innervate about 60% of the corneal surface. Initially, this affects the reflex of corneal sensation, which has a bearing on the level of tear secretion [96–98]. In the later stages, however, there is a whole unexplored area of patients who get an abnormal sensation after LASIK. There may be a supersensitivity—an abnormal return to sensation of the cornea in some patients. In short, the nerves grow back, in some cases, with abnormal parameters.

Other factors may cloud the issue [99]. The incidence of dry eyes in the general population also may be on the

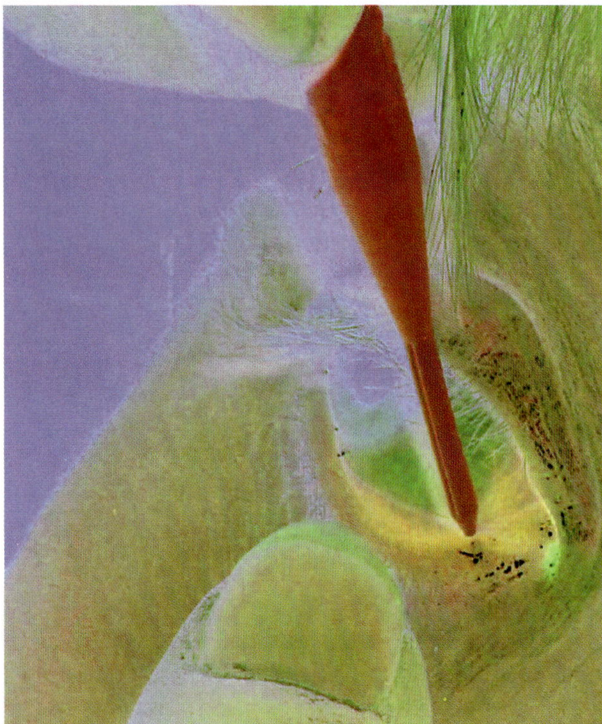

Fig 15.147 Punctal occlusion will solve most dry-eye problems associated with LASIK.

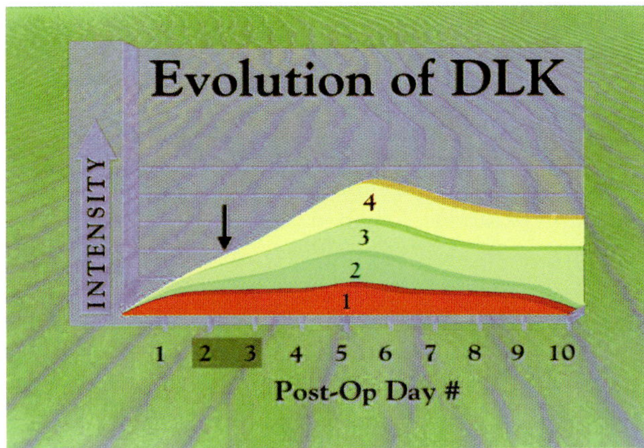

Fig 15.148 Sands of the Sahara or diffuse interlamellar keratitis (DLK) showing evolution of pathology. (Slide courtesy Eric J. Linebarger, M.D., used with permission.)

rise. This could be the result of environmental factors [100,101], as well as subtle side effects of medications such as antidepressants, whose use is increasing in the middle-aged and older people [102]. Our population as a whole is also aging.

Pinpointing the borderline patient

Many post-LASIK dry-eye patients are those who have gone undiagnosed before the procedure or who are borderline cases pushed over the edge afterward. Such a patient's eyes may be aggravated by post-LASIK steroid treatment, which is known to dry the cornea. Many of these patients may be borderline dry-eye cases and opt for LASIK surgery because they can no longer wear contact lenses comfortably. If a dry-eye diagnosis is made, treating the patient aggressively from the start—even if it means punctal occlusion—is probably the best course (Figure 15.147).

The most common reason patients choose LASIK surgery is contact lens intolerance related to dry eye. Other common dry-eye causes include hormonal factors, systemic medications, Meibomian gland dysfunction, and chronic ocular allergy in contact lens wearers. The microkeratome damages or destroys the cilia that hold the mucous layer of the tear film as it goes across. The liberal use of nonpreservative artificial tears following the procedure is recommended for these patients, who often have decreased tear breakup times. Preserved artificial tears, when they are used frequently, can slow visual rehabilitation and result in variable acuity [103]. In severe cases, cyclosporine applied topically [104] has been shown to be effective, as has autologous serum [105].

It is important to aggressively treat associated blepharitis and meibomianitis with good lid hygiene and erythromycin ointment—doxycycline 100 mg every day. Counseling patients before surgery that it may take 4 to 6 months to get better will relieve some anxiety associated with this problem, but the fact remains that many will not recover normal tear function completely.

It would not surprise me to find a connection between the high incidence of dry eyes and the following problem, which also enjoys a certain notoriety in LASIK patients.

Sands of the Sahara

Another problem after LASIK is interface inflammation [106]. In recent years, with the increased volumes of LASIK procedures being performed, a mysterious postoperative condition known as *diffuse lamellar keratitis* (DLK) has been reported. Bobby Maddox, who termed it "sands of the Sahara" because of the swirling desertlike appearance of the stroma, first described this in 1996 (Figure 15.148). Grainy small infiltrates appear at the periphery of the flap shortly after the LASIK procedure and migrate toward the center of the ablation. It is a nonspecific inflammatory insult to the cornea and can be precipitated by a host of variables. There is an influx of polymorphonucleocytes (neutrophils) into the interface, and these neutrophils produce proteolytic enzymes that may end up digesting or "melting" the cornea. These instances can vary in intensity from minimal blurring to a rare corneal melt.

Theories abound regarding the cause of SOS/DLK. Several etiologies have been proposed, with no definite identifying cause. Speculation seems to point toward contamination of the corneal interface during surgery [107].

Implicated sources include oil, epithelial defects, silicates, metallic fragments, Betadine, and bacterial endotoxins [108]. Prevention is suggested by keeping the interface as clean as possible and employing strict aseptic technique in the laser suite. Some believe the cause to be the lubricant from the microkeratome motor head, and others, the microkeratome blades. Some feel it is due to secretions from the Meibomian glands, lid debris, and necrotic cells, and still others believe it is from the heat of the laser. Others feel that it is due to using warm as opposed to chilled balanced saline solution. Sands of the Sahara is not an infectious entity—it is sterile. There have been no positive cultures associated with it, and it resolves without antibiotics. It does not invade other tissue layers, other than secondary or spillover effects, like collagenase liberation and melts. It often appears within 8 hours of LASIK surgery. This condition is believed to be as common as 1 in 50 cases in its mild form, but in 1 in 5000 cases can be so severe as to cause stromal melting and permanent scarring.

Typically, patients present 1 to 3 days after surgery, sometimes reporting sudden increased pain, but usually with photophobia, redness and/or tearing, and an infiltrate with the following characteristics:

1 It is confined to the interface without extension into the anterior or posterior stroma.

2 The multiple foci are diffusely distributed in several possible patterns but are more concentrated around surgical debris.

3 There is little or no anterior-chamber reaction and no associated epithelial defect.

4 The conjunctiva is relatively noninflamed, with little or no ciliary flush.

5 Although uncommon, it is possible to observe discrete areas of stromal loss several weeks later.

It may seem more than passingly strange that the so-called sands of the Sahara problem only showed up when LASIK came along and only after its popularity soared. It does not seem strange to me, however, not after observing many neophytes (and sad to say "oldtimers") at work with LASIK and the results of their endeavors. I am appalled at what I have seen both within the operating theater and without. However, I am not surprised. I predicted that the incidence of RK complications would skyrocket once it became "okay to do it"; now we see the same phenomenon with LASIK.

When I studied keratomileusis with Nordan and later with Barraquer and Ruiz, part of what we learned (aside from the critical importance of centration of the fixation ring) was cleanliness of the interface. Using a sable brush and copious quantities of normal saline, we scrubbed the corneal bed to a fare-thee-well. We were less diligent with the lenticule only because the underside had been lathed and with that lathing, debris was removed. Besides, we stored the completely removed cap in a covered receptacle and treated it to some brush strokes before returning it to the patient's eye. Interface debris was a rarity, and when it existed at all, it was mostly observed in the periphery of the resection bed. Not so today. Today we see debris scattered throughout the interface, and today we see sands of the Sahara. But why?

Someone wrote that they believed that the SOS phenomenon was related to chemical debris left on the surface of the microkeratome blade. This may be true. Sometimes manufacturers get sloppy. Witness the "dry pack" debacle in the formative years of intraocular lens (IOL) implantation when "mysterious" occurrences of postimplant uveitis surfaced and finally were traced to remnants of silver-based polishing compound remaining on the IOL surface. Many of us used the same IOLs without experiencing uveitis for the simple reason that we adhered to a quaint notion that anything put into an eye should be clean. Consequently, we continued to treat the "dry pack" IOLs as if they were "wet pack" (soaking in sodium hydroxide) and soaked them first in bicarbonate solution and then in balanced salt (or in my case—and my residents/fellows if they knew what was good for them—Eagles Tissue Culture Medium No. 1), finally irrigating them off before implantation.

Blade manufacturing has not changed all that much over the years, from what I've seen. The possibility of residuals on the surface of a blade is as real today as it was back in the days of MKM. So what is the difference? The answer is cleanliness. Cleanliness and a dust/lint-free atmosphere. Of the two, cleanliness is the most important, because the process of cleaning generally takes care of most airborne particles. There is one salient feature of LASIK that is the nexus of the problem, however, and that is the need for speed. Or perhaps the *perceived* need for speed, since I do not see this need. There are two things that make LASIK popular aside from the fact that it pays well, and these are 1) with the automated keratome and the excimer laser, the procedure is perceived as a no-brainer, and 2) it is fast. It also weakens the cornea to a much lesser degree, which is—of course—a major plus. However, this has always been true of lamellar surgery; LASIK did not make it true. Today—as in cataract surgery's halcyon days—the hallmark of the "successful" eye surgeon is how many cases he or she can push through his or her operating theater (rather like pork through a goose). And implant surgery is also a no-brainer. All that is required is a modicum of manual dexterity and the wit to discern that the lens has indeed become opaque. Rocket science it isn't. Fyodorov said in the early days of RK—and I agree—that a good cataract surgeon does not necessarily make a good refractive surgeon because refractive surgery requires attention to minute details—microns counted. The ranks of LASIK practitioners are replete with cataract surgeons today bringing with them some bad habits, chief among them the need for speed.

In the beginning, LASIK was not all that popular, the chief reason being that it was necessary to make a keratome section on the cornea. This aspect was seen as fraught with peril and the most important and dangerous part of the procedure. And this perception was correct—the microkeratome sectioning was the most important part of the procedure, and it still is. But the making of the section—as difficult as it may have been—was only part of the story. It is that remaining part that seems to have become lost.

When I took up keratomileusis—first lathing and then in situ—I was introduced to the *first principles of lamellar microkeratome corneal surgery*. Chief among these was that absolute centration of the section be accomplished and maintained. This required careful observation of the relationship of the ring opening with the premarked visual axis and the maintenance of this relationship while the ring fastened itself onto the eye through the vacuum applied. The next was that the section must be of uniform thickness. This was hard to achieve with a manual translation of the cutter across the corneal surface, but it *was* achievable. The third of these was that the resection bed must be smooth. This latter was a factor of the uniformity of the translation and the speed of the blade oscillation, as well as the blade sharpness. The fourth principle was that of absolute cleanliness of the interface. To this end, not only was the resection bed cleaned thoroughly after the sectioning, but the blade also was wiped clean, and an absolute minimum of lubrication was used on the motor spindle and none anywhere else aside from normal saline prior to its use. Some of us went a step further and employed laminar flow filters in our refractive surgical theaters to minimize particulates. Attention to minutiae? Perhaps, but with portable laminar flow filters available for around $1200, I am at a loss to explain their absence from most laser rooms, not to mention the lack of attention to sterility.

The problem of the microkeratome sectioning was "solved" by introduction of the self-propelled gear-driven microkeratome, which, while it moved at the same speed across the cornea each time, tended to "hobble" or dip. This resulted in a tendency of the resection bed to become ribbed or rugous. To be sure, a certain amount of this also occurred with the manual-driven devices, but it seems to be more pronounced with this device. Such ditches tend to collect debris, even though they may not have contributed overmuch to visual degradation.

Then too, there was the "problem" of the cap. Since it had been cut free, it must be reattached to the eye from whence it came. This meant employing the eight-bite Barraquer nontorquing suture technique, which is not easy; it certainly takes time to do it right. Consequently, early cases resulted in quite a number of incidences of irregular astigmatism caused by wrinkled or displaced caps, quite apart from those caused by decentration simply because insufficient pains were taken in suturing. Then someone got the bright idea of not suturing at all. Properly treated, the cap could be made to adhere to the bed without benefit of sutures, which—of course—reduced the chance for irregular astigmatism to a great degree. However, to get the cap to stick down, the bed had to be dry, and the only way to achieve this was to reduce the amount of irrigation applied to the lenticule and the bed, hence violating a *first principle*—that of cleanliness, since many made only minor gestures of irrigation. In fact, some actually taught that irrigation/cleaning of the resection bed was totally unnecessary! Needless to say, "dusty" interfaces were the order of the day; in point of fact, this is still seen today.

This is true because the use of the hinge exposes the resected cap to airborne detritus while it is exposed during the laser ablation, and a dry bed is still important to promote adherence of the cap. Thus painstaking cleaning of the resection bed is not performed. I have yet to witness anyone wiping off a blade prior to use either, and I have seen too many technicians spray microkeratomes with silicone spray such as used to protect surgical instruments. It is enough to make a Klingon weep! But it can't just be the blade alone, nor the number of cases being done—after all, no such cases were seen with cryo-MKM or ALK. It probably has to do with the laser acting on some introduced foreign substance, but no source has been proven yet. However, surgeons do agree that cleanliness seems to be a key to prevention.

Treatment

Early diagnosis and treatment with an aggressive topical steroid and perhaps antibiotic drops are critical for the management of this complication, which has been tentatively classified by Hatsis into four progressive grades depending on the signs and symptoms at presentation (Figures 15.148 and 15.149).

With prompt initiation of aggressive topical steroid treatment every half to 1 hour and antibiotics four or five times a day, there should be a complete resolution without sequelae. Even with prompt, correct treatment, however, some vision loss can occur and has been reported. If the DLK is mild (i.e., details can be seen underneath the white cells, and the patient's visual acuity is 20/25 or better), treat aggressively with steroids without lifting the flap to culture and irrigate. Because the progression can be rapid and serious, keep an eye on these patients, seeing them daily for several days. Although it is not completely clear, I believe that the interface cellular infiltration, left on its own, may become a tissue-destroying lesion and cause irregular astigmatism and loss of best spectacle-corrected visual acuity over time.

If the infiltrate is significant (i.e., obscuring details of the iris rim or forming waves of localized inflammation), lift the flap, take a culture, and then copiously irrigate the bed before replacing the flap (Figure 15.150). Treat these

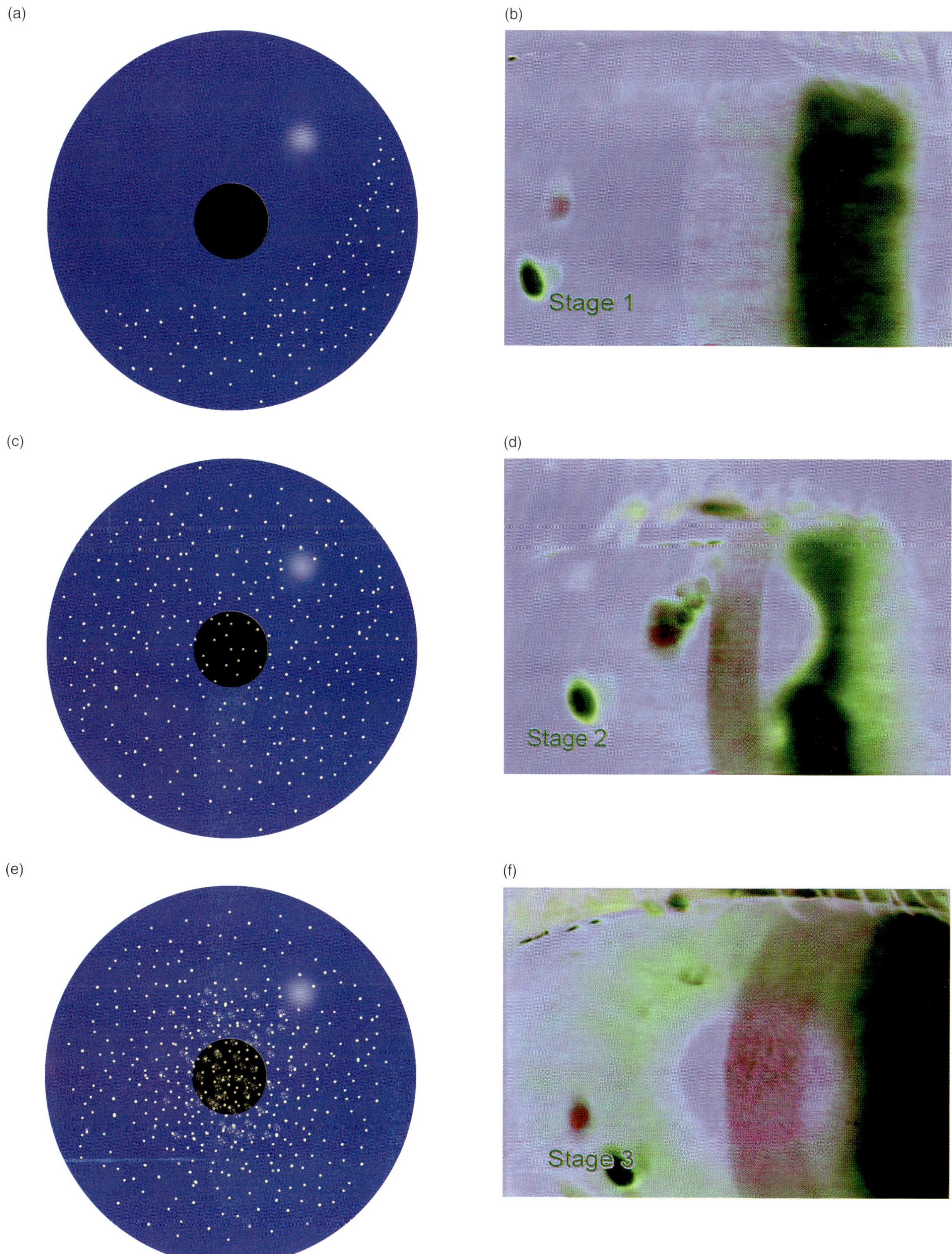

Figure 15.149 The stages of diffuse lamellar keratitis (sands of the Sahara) (a) Stage 1 – localized in inferior corneal. (b) Stage 1 – slit-lamp photo of Stage 1. (c) Stage 2 – diffuse. (d) Stage 2 – slit-lamp photo. (e) Stage 3 – diffuse with central aggregations. (f) Stage 3 – slit-lamp photo. Patient's vision may become impaired; increased glare, etc. (g) Stage 4 – typical sand of the Sahara pattern. (h) Stage 4 – slit-lamp photo. This stage may require surgical intervention (see Figure 15–150). (Figures courtesy Eric J. Linebarger, M.D., used with permission.)

(g)

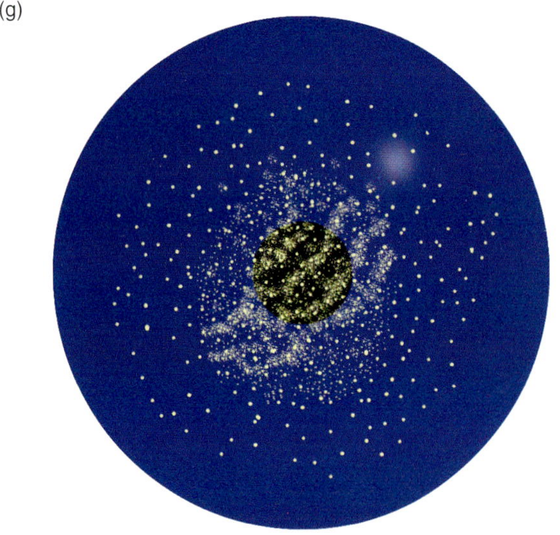

(h)

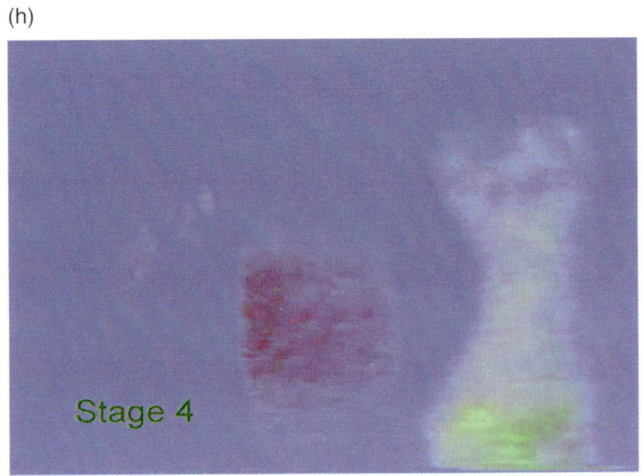

Figure 15.149 (*Continued*)

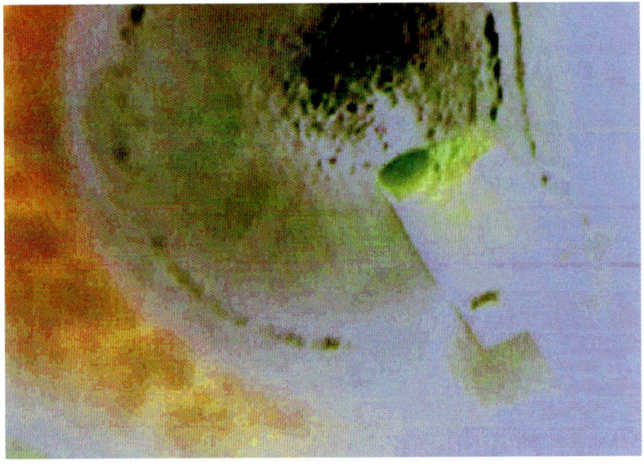

Fig 15.150 Sands of the Sahara or diffuse interlamellar keratitis, Grade 3. In severe cases the flap must be lifted and the underlying stroma irrigated and wiped clean. (Slide courtesy Alexander Hatsis, M.D., used with permission.)

patients aggressively with topical 1% prenisolone or fluoromethalone as frequently as every hour, with a quick taper once the inflammation resolves.

It is also very important to identify potentially infectious infiltrates and treat them. In such a situation, management will include dissection of the corneal flap, culture, debridement, and intensive topical antibiotics, if necessary. If infection is suspected, institute an antibiotic (such as ofloxacin) every hour while the patient is awake until the culture results are obtained. If the cultures are negative, back off quickly on the antibiotic and reduce the corticosteroid to every few hours. The steroid should be tapered over a period of several weeks as the leukocytes in the bed disappear. If there are any doubts about the clinical presentation of the syndrome, it is better to treat more aggressively than wait for possible stromal melt and permanent irregular astigmatism.

As in most clinical situations, prevention is the best treatment. Precautions include preoperatively treating and controlling any Meibomian gland dysfunction or lid disease; completely cleaning and sterilizing the microkeratome blade holder, blade cavity, and suction ring, but not the motor; storing the microkeratome motor or turbine upside down; using talc-free gloves; using proper technique for cleaning the stromal interface and a new multipore-protected cannula for each case; using a new blade for each case; and advising patients with previous atopic or autoimmune skin or mucosal reactions about the potential problems. And, of course, instituting laminar flow filtration in the laser space.

Anti-inflammatory drugs in PRK and LASIK

Although pain is considerably less of a problem following LASIK than PRK, LASIK patients can be very light-sensitive in the early postoperative period, and nonsteroidal anti-inflammatory drugs (NSAIDs) provide effective relief from photophobia [109]. Corticosteroids can provide relief as well, but probably less effectively than NSAIDs. This is understandable because there are differences between the mechanisms of action of steroids and NSAIDs (Figure 15.151).

The sequence of biochemical events that leads from a corneal insult to an inflammatory reaction has a number of steps and proceeds along two pathways: the cyclooxygenase pathway and the leukotriene pathway. NSAIDs and corticosteroids block these pathways in different places and therefore have different degrees of effectiveness in blocking specific aspects of the inflammatory reaction.

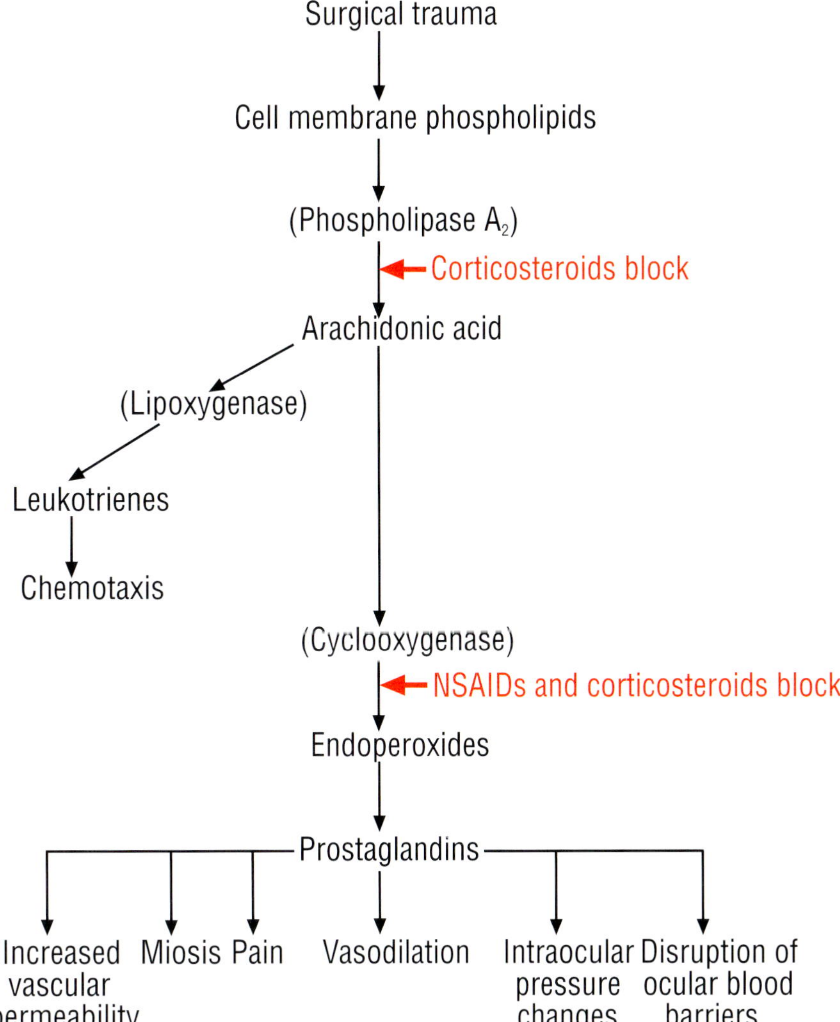

Fig 15.151 Prostaglandin and leukotriene synthesis resulting from surgical trauma (adapted from Flach, AJ., Cyclo-oxygenase inhibitors in ophthalmology. Surv Ophthalmol 1992; 36(4): p. 259–84).

The cascade of events

When there is an injury to the cornea, from, for example, the creation of a LASIK flap or laser ablation, cell membranes are disrupted. The injured membranes release phospholipids, which are first transformed to arachidonic acid via phospholipase A_2 (inhibited by corticosteroids). Cyclooxygenase then mediates the transformation of arachidonic acid to prostaglandin precursors [110].

NSAIDs, both diclofenac and ketorolac, are very effective at blocking cyclooxygenase (both constitutive COX 1 and inducible COX-2). Thus NSAIDs prevent, or significantly diminish, the transformation of arachidonic acid to prostaglandins. Corticosteroids, which inhibit constitutive COX-1 but not inducible COX-2, also block this pathway, but less effectively. In the other arm of the inflammatory reaction, arachidonic acid is transformed in the presence of lipoxygenase to leukotrienes, chemotactic agents that attract white blood cells to the affected area.

Since NSAIDs block the breakdown of arachidonic acid to prostaglandins, the use of an NSAID alone risks creating a buildup of arachidonic acid. This accumulation of arachidonic acid may shift the equilibrium toward the leukotriene pathway and result in the attraction of leukocytes to the wound. Concomitant use of a corticosteroid will inhibit phospholipase A_2 and thus limit arachidonic acid buildup. This explains why some PRK patients (who received NSAIDs but no corticosteroids) presented with sterile infiltrates following their procedure.

Rationale

One's first thought may be to use a corticosteroid, since this would block, at least partially, both the production of arachidonic acid and the cyclooxygenase-mediated transformation of arachidonic acid to prostaglandins. Unfortunately, if you do not use an NSAID, the patient can experience significant light sensitivity and pain following the procedure.

It would be attractive to use only an anti-inflammatory in LASIK. This, however, creates problems of its own.

(a)

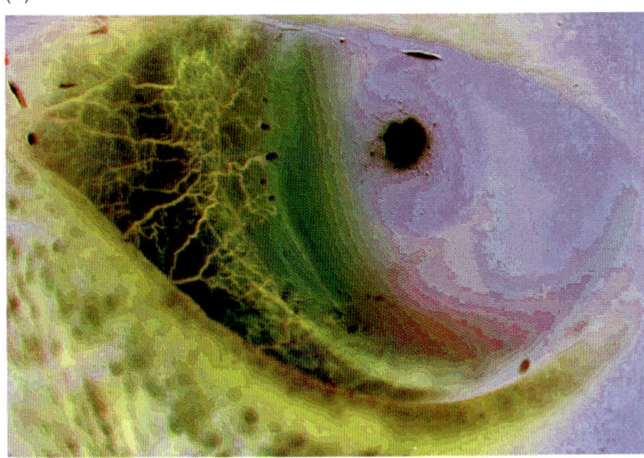

(b)

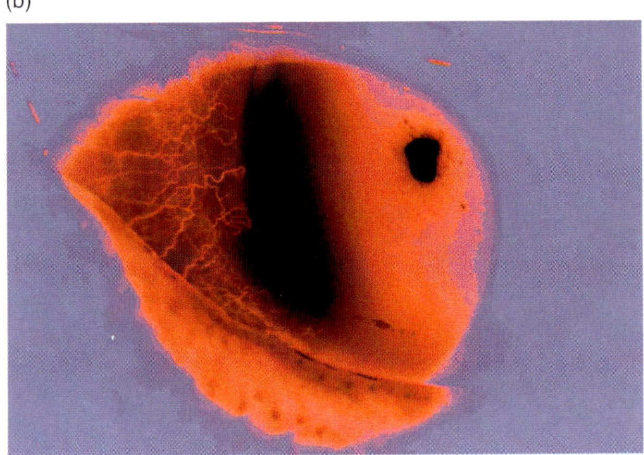

Fig 15.152 (a) Cataract incision melting following administration of an NSAID postsurgery. (b) Same flowing fluorescein showing that wound is not leaking. (Slides courtesy James Gills, M.D.)

If the only postoperative anti-inflammatory used is an NSAID, the buildup of arachidonic acid and the potential shift in the equilibrium toward the leukotriene pathway increase the risk of conditions such as DLK (sands of the Sahara; see above). Because corticosteroids block the transformation of cell membrane phospholipids to arachidonic acid, they reduce the production of leukotrienes, and fewer leukocytes are attracted to the wound. As a result, LASIK patients should receive both an NSAID and a steroid.

The trouble with NSAIDs

Developing a responsible approach to NSAIDs

The late NSAID controversy has brought to light lessons for all of us involved in patient care. We have learned—again, regrettably—that seemingly benign pharmaceutical agents can, in fact, do harm. We have learned again that physicians often prescribe drugs in an off-label manner, and we have learned again that physicians tend to underreport adverse reactions. Perhaps of greater significance, we have learned (also again) that the laws governing the dispensing of generic drugs may allow patients to receive agents other than those prescribed by physicians, and we have relearned that the U.S. Food and Drug Administration (FDA) may not be as vigilant as generally believed.

NSAID safety

In the wake of concerns about postoperative corneal complications associated with the use of topical NSAIDs after cataract or refractive surgery, a product was recalled, and the American Society of Cataract and Refractive Surgery initiated a comprehensive study. The study, already underway, is designed to pinpoint the cause of the complications.

To review, Alcon's generic subsidiary, Falcon, released a product, Diclofenac Sodium Ophthalmic Solution (DSOS) as a generic equivalent of Voltaren (diclofenac sodium, CIBA Vision). As a result of competitive pricing and the fact that generics may be legally substituted for brand-name products in many HMO plans in many states, the product enjoyed widespread use. Within a few months, however, physicians observed a number of patients with corneal melting problems following cataract surgery.

In July of 1999, the American Society of Cataract and Refractive Surgery (ASCRS) Cataract Special Interest Group became aware of the problem and surveyed the U.S. membership. Approximately 20% (1000) of the members replied, and of those, roughly 130 indicated that they had noticed corneal healing problems associated with the use of NSAIDs after surgery and in patients with dry eyes, rheumatoid arthritis, and the like.

The survey data suggested that severe corneal epithelial defects and/or melts were associated with the use of Voltaren, Acular (ketorolac tromethamine, Allergan), and Falcon's generic DSOS (Figure 15.152a,b). This information was based on the fact that physicians would prescribe a given agent and presume that the patient was using the medication for which he or she had written the prescription. However, generic DSOS was being freely substituted by many pharmacies and managed-care programs in those states where generic substitution is permissible. The preliminary results of the survey indicated that while DSOS 0.1% (Falcon Pharmaceuticals, Ltd./Alcon Laboratories, Inc.) was observed as causing corneal melts more frequently, corneal melts also were seen with other NSAIDs, including Acular (ketorolac tromethamine, Allergan) and Voltaren (diclofenac sodium, CIBA Vision). Given the information at hand, ASCRS suggested a moratorium on the use of all NSAIDs after surgery because it was unclear if all agents were casual.

After more information became available, it was apparent that the preponderance of cases were associated

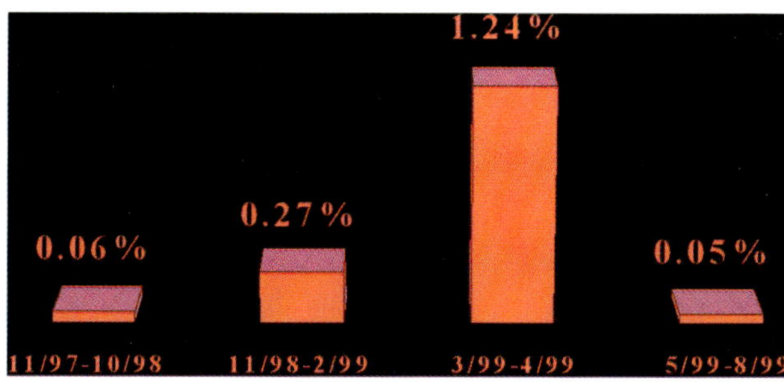

Fig 15.153 Incidence of corneal incision melting following use of generic diclofenac in one clinic. (Courtesy James Gills, M.D.)

with the use of the Falcon DSOS and that 22 of the reported cases would require surgical intervention to treat corneal melting (Figure 15.153). Additionally, the practice patterns of physicians were not in keeping with the package insert provided by the manufacturers. Typically, physicians had prescribed topical NSAIDs prior to surgery, on the day of surgery, and for prolonged postoperative applications. The package insert directions are an aberration when compared with common clinical practice, but the manufacturers suggested that closer adherence to the package insert would result in better outcomes. Accordingly, after 2 weeks, the ASCRS rescinded the moratorium, indicated that most problems were associated with the generic agent, and suggested judicious use and careful follow-up of all patients on topical NSAIDs. Alcon, after initial reticence but acting responsibly, suspended shipment of the generic product and ultimately withdrew it from the marketplace.

Comprehensive study

The ASCRS embarked on a project to study the reported cases with the help of Oliver Schein, professor of ophthalmology at Johns Hopkins University School of Medicine. Schein and colleagues would analyze the data. He estimated that the study would be completed 6 months after all the data were gathered and processed, but as of this writing, no definite conclusions have been drawn.

It became apparent that 1) physicians tend to underreport adverse events, 2) that physicians often prescribe medications in an off-label fashion, 3) that HMOs and certain state laws give generic agents a commercial advantage, 4) that physicians are often unaware of what medications patients actually receive and use, and 5) that NSAIDs, perhaps as a class of drugs, may create a spectrum of corneal problems, particularly when used in patients prone to healing defects (severe dry eye, rheumatoid arthritis, etc.) and when used more aggressively than suggested by the manufacturer.

It is hoped that the study will determine the cause of these occurrences. We may find out that we have to reeducate physicians as to how these drugs should be used properly. For example, if one of the conclusions is that the product is being overused, the industry may have to look at dosages, time intervals, and how the products are labeled and packaged. Ophthalmologists need to be aware of the conditions other physicians are seeing and to closely monitor their use of NSAIDs. If complications arise in connection with topical NSAID use, they should be reported to the manufacturer.

Product recalled

Alcon Laboratories, Inc., and its affiliate, Falcon Pharmaceuticals, Ltd., introduced DSOS in August 1998, distributing and extensively sampling the product primarily to cataract surgeons. In the first year, more than 650,000 units were distributed. According to Alcon, it was unknown at the time that the prevalence of off-label use of NSAIDs was rapidly growing as well. When Alcon realized the predominance of off-label use associated with adverse event reports on DSOS and other NSAIDs, it voluntarily withdrew its product in September 1999.

Two separate well-controlled, double-blind clinical studies comparing DSOS with Voltaren conducted in over 700 patients demonstrated that Falcon diclofenac is safe and effective, according to Stella Robertson, vice president of pharmaceutical products research and development. These studies, in which the NSAIDS were dosed postoperatively four times daily for 14 days beginning the day after surgery, demonstrated no difference between Voltaren and DSOS in the occurrence or severity of adverse events. However, during the investigation of adverse events reported with DSOS, it was found that aggressive off-label use is prevalent not only for DSOS but also for other marketed NSAIDs as well.

In a letter to eye care professionals in August, Alcon emphasized the importance of using topical NSAIDs according to the labeled instructions. The importance of understanding NSAIDs and labeling them accurately has been further emphasized by examining diclofenac labeling in other countries. For instance, in Japan, 40 corneal erosions were noted in postmarketing surveillance of diclofenac. In addition, an October 1999 AAO poster by Ira Udell and associates presented cases of keratitis, ulceration, melt, and perforation in conjunction with all NSAIDs. This poster presented 16 patients (18 eyes) with keratitis, ulcerations, and perforations after initiation of topical NSAIDs (range 4 days to 15 months).

Among these cases, nine patients used DSOS, one used Voltaren (diclofenac sodium, CIBA Vision) and DSOS, one used Voltaren, three used Acular (ketorolac tromethamine, Allergan), one used Acular PF, and one used both Acular and Acular PF. Four patients (six eyes) using Acular developed corneal complications prior to the release of DSOS in August 1998.

Some of these patients had associated systemic or ocular conditions that placed them at risk for these complications. In the study, two patients had known rheumatoid arthritis, one had previously undiagnosed Sjögren's syndrome, and two had rosacea. Other systemic diseases occurring in these patients included diabetes, anemia, and sarcoidosis. Concurrent ocular conditions included glaucoma, uveitis, and ABM dystrophy.

Other members of the class

Not all NSAIDs are the same; industry leaders believe that the differences are apparent after extended study and commercial use. For the purpose of registration, Acular has undergone well-controlled, double-blind studies to minimize any biases in the collection of data. During the course of these studies, including those for postoperative inflammation after cataract surgery, as well as refractive surgery, there were over 1500 patients using ketorolac, and the safety profile was extremely good. In the clinical trials, the primary adverse event was burning and stinging.

Joseph Lambert, medical director of ophthalmology clinical research at Allergan, said that, to date, the company has not documented a single case of corneal melt in a postoperative patient. According to Lambert, only two reports of corneal melt are in the database. Neither was postoperative, and both patients had underlying corneal disease that could explain the corneal melt.

NSAIDS—Origins, efficacy, and potential complications

NSAIDs were developed in ophthalmology primarily because of concerns for the potential complications associated with long-term corticosteroid use—elevation of IOP, potentiation of bacterial infections, and reactivation of herpes. However, the real benefit of NSAIDs is not because of the risk associated with steroids; it is because of their unique properties. NSAIDs, in their inhibition of cyclooxygenase, are much more potent in terms of reducing the amount of prostaglandins present in the eye than are topical steroids.

The first NSAID on the U.S. market was Ocufen (flurbiprofen sodium, Allergan), which was effective for potentiation of intraocular mydriasis but was not particularly effective as an anti-inflammatory. Next was Profenal (suprofen, Alcon), which had properties very similar to Ocufen. However, the market for NSAIDs changed dramatically in 1991, when CIBA Vision introduced its diclofenac product, because Voltaren was the first NSAID that showed real anti-inflammatory properties. The other potent NSAID is Allergan's Acular and its preservative-free formulation, Acular PF. Profenal was removed from the market when the generic diclofenac was removed. At this writing, there are three NSAIDs on the market, Ocufen; Acular (ketorolac tromethamine, Allergan), regular and the preservative-free formulation; and Voltaren.

Indications for NSAIDs

Acular has two indications—temporary relief of itching due to seasonal allergic conjunctivitis and treatment of postoperative inflammation in patients who have undergone cataract extraction.

Voltaren also has two indications—relief of pain after refractive or incisional refractive surgery and the treatment of inflammation 24 hours after cataract surgery, continuing through the first 2 postoperative weeks.

But the most significant usage, particularly associated with cataract surgery, is the belief that it reduces the incidence of cystoid macular edema. Acular is also used in overcorrected myopic LASIK patients to induce regression. This has not been studied formally, but it is common knowledge.

For almost 3 years, I have started NSAIDs prophylactically the day of surgery. I use them four times daily for a month and slowly wean the patients off over several months. This is considerably beyond the scope of what has been the manufacturers' recommended usage. There have been no adverse outcomes other than the rare superficial punctate keratopathy or, perhaps, aggravated dry eye. Mild superficial problems have been recognized by many but never discussed much because of the minor significance, until the recent concentrated problem we have seen.

Whether patients are treated with steroids or NSAIDs, those with rheumatoid arthritis constitute the biggest risk group that I have had the experience of treating. They seem to have a higher likelihood of developing corneal melts than any other treatment group I am familiar with. In any dry-eye patient, if you are going to use a high dosage of NSAID, the eye would be at greater risk for developing an epithelial problem. Anyone wearing a soft contact lens who is also adding an NSAID on top of it belongs in another high-risk group.

Other risk factors are epithelial keratopathy, whether it be bullous keratopathy or anything that will produce a chronic punctate keratopathy (e.g., dry eye), including patients who are chronically treated with NSAIDs and ultimately develop punctate keratopathy as a result of being on the NSAID. Another risk factor, based on anecdotal reports, is peripheral limbal astigmatic relaxing incisions performed at the time of cataract surgery. These may result in an epithelial defect and have the potential to result in a melt.

While it is clear that certain specific NSAIDs may be worse actors than others, the entire class of NSAIDs has some potential to cause serious problems. Even though the incidence of these serious complications may be very low for some of the NSAIDs, it is important to understand that the incidence is not zero. Hence this is a class-of-drugs problem that the prescribing physician must be aware of.

It is not my intention to condemn the entire medley of drugs that fall under the NSAID class but rather to warn of the potential problems that can occur with any of them. Anti-inflammatory drugs continue to play a key role in laser vision correction. In photorefractive keratectomy (PRK), both steroids and NSAIDs are used: NSAIDs to control pain and photophobia and steroids to limit haze and modulate the healing response. The need for anti-inflammatory medication is greatly lessened in LASIK, but NSAIDs remain an important part of the pre- and post-LASIK regimen.

A number of excellent NSAIDs are available that have a definite role in our treatment armamentarium. Use them wisely and recognize that there is some potential for serious side effects.

A conservative approach

NSAIDs have a very modest but real inhibitory effect on epithelial cell migration; therefore, the amount used should be limited. In PRK, NSAIDs are usually only necessary for the first 24 to 48 hours after surgery. If pain control with an NSAID is necessary for longer, look for an underlying problem (e.g., a too-tight contact lens, infection, etc.). Because pain is much less of a factor in LASIK, it is possible to use the NSAID only, and on the day of surgery.

Some believe that corticosteroids inhibit epithelial migration, but there are no conclusive data to support this belief. Other than the preservative effect and the effect of putting another toxic foreign material on the cornea, there is no firm evidence that corticosteroids have any intrinsic inhibitory effect on epithelial migration.

Choosing an NSAID

Both diclofenac and ketorolac cause a very modest delay in epithelial healing. However, with preservative-free ketorolac, there is a statistically significant decrease in inhibition of the epithelial healing. Because of this, I strongly recommend using preservative-free ketorolac for PRK patients. Preservative-free dosing is also very convenient for LASIK patients. Give patients a unit-dose vial or two; this way, you do not have to worry about NSAID abuse because the patient simply does not have enough NSAIDs to abuse.

The bottom line

The recommended anti-inflammatory regimen for LASIK patients includes both an NSAID to control postoperative photophobia and a corticosteroid to reduce the chance of DLK. Preservative-free ketorolac is begun one-half hour before surgery and continued with one drop immediately after surgery. The patient is given a unit-dose vial to use later that day, if needed. Fluorometholone can be used as prophylaxis against DLK.

Kerectasis

It has been said that the hallmark of an intelligent species is that it learns from its mistakes, which is an indictment of *Homo sapiens* in general and *Homo sapiens* var *doctorus ophthalmicorum lasikae* in particular—at least some of them, from what I've seen of their work, because they have not read anything by Barraquer on the subject of keratomileusis. Many are quick to indict hyperopic automated keratotomy (HLK) for its propensity to expose patients' corneas to the possibility of kerectasia on the basis of the deep lamellar cut and the resulting thinned posterior layer. Why is it that this aspect seems to be ignored in LASIK? Some ablations have produced posterior layers that are less than 300 μm thick—sometimes 260 μm or even less [111]. Adding the 135 to 150 μm for the flap gives you a central thickness of 395 to 410 μm or less—which is in the range of central corneal thickness found in most cases of keratoconus. In pocket billiards, the word is *"cut it thin to win"*—this is bad advice in LASIK. Even using a "thick flap" does not solve the problem. Harken again to the example of HLK. If a surgeon follows the rules for LASIK, the risk of having an ectasia is very rare.

Ectasias, which usually develop within the first year or 2 postoperatively, occur in cases where the practitioner has performed LASIK on an inappropriate cornea, such as one that was already too thin [112,113]. In a normal cornea, ectasis results when too large an OZ has been used or a flap is too thick, leaving a part of the cornea too thin, or too high a myopic correction has been attempted.

To improve results on a second eye, one surgeon expanded the OZ from 5 to 5.25 mm. Even with the larger zone and increased tissue removal, the patient was still believed to be 50 μm short of the widely accepted 250-μm posterior layer limit. However, at 9 months, the patient returned with 20/200 vision in this second eye, compared with 20/30 vision in the first. Topography revealed the ectasia, which was the result of a pachymetric miscalculation that had, in fact, left the patient with a 235-μm bed in the eye. This surgeon now does pachymetry in all quadrants and will not knowingly operate on cases involving forme fruste keratoconus (FFK), which involve inferior pachymetries that are much thinner than those seen centrally.

Infection

Finally, the most devastating complication of LASIK most likely would be infection [114,115]. This is extremely rare if proper precautions are taken. Aggressive diagnosis and antibiotic treatment should be instituted at any indication of such possibility.

Today or not today

Simultaneous bilateral LASIK surgery is considered by many refractive surgeons to be within the standard of care [116]. Patients seem to prefer the convenience of having both eyes done on the same day, but the ultimate decision lies with the operating surgeon and his or her hopefully fully informed patient. Others feel differently on the matter. Personally, I am opposed to performing bilateral simultaneous elective eye surgery other than of muscle or lids; there is too much at stake. A little "inconvenience" with respect to time spent or short-lived anisometropia is nothing compared with the "inconvenience" of permanently impaired vision.

Intrastromal corneal implants (ICS)—Intacs

Mechanical complications

The Intacs segments are to be inserted into a lamellar pocket that lies at two-thirds corneal depth. In the early FDA clinical trials, one posterior perforation occurred due to inaccurate initial diamond blade setting. This created a channel deeper than the intended depth, and the metal glide inadvertently entered the anterior chamber during lamellar dissection. The segments were inserted without apparent complication. On postoperative day 1, the perforation was noted, and the segment was retrieved from the anterior chamber without complication. This emphasizes the importance of properly setting the diamond blade before creating the initial superior incision. Similarly, anterior perforations also may occur with the channel dissector intraoperatively. This can happen if the diamond blade was set too shallow or the dissector inserted at a shallow depth.

Another mechanical complication occurs when a properly inserted Intacs segment migrates within the lamellar channel. Segments are most commonly displaced inferiorly. This is believed to result from eye rubbing, which mechanically moves the segments to the base of the channel, although blinking and gravity also may play a role. No adverse refractive effect has been noted with inferiorly displaced segments. However, if the segments are displaced superiorly to lie under the incision, proper healing of the incision is prevented. This often results in the refractive effect of undercorrection, but there is also a risk of infection because the incision may remain open. If the segment remains under the incision site, there is a greater risk of thinning and eventual melting of the overlying stroma. This has been observed in patients even after 9 months from initial implantation. If a segment cannot be repositioned away from the incision, it most likely should be removed. The evolution from a 360° ring to the 150° segments was made to eliminate having the PMMA directly under the incision site and to avoid anterior stromal thinning from keratolysis.

Medical complications

Sterile infiltrates are believed to be an immunologic response to debris or tissue cells introduced during surgery. Such reactions tend to occur at the superior end of the segment in proximity of the entry incision. They tend to be localized within the lamellar channel and anterior to the segment and may be accompanied by a mild iritis. Similar to peripheral sterile infiltrates, those associated with Intacs are not typically light blocking and do not have an epithelial defect. They respond quickly to topical steroids. Managing such infiltrates requires daily surveillance to ensure that the process is not exacerbated by topical steroids, which may indicate an infectious etiology.

Infectious infiltrates may manifest as diffuse, dense lamellar infiltrates with localized stromal edema. Significant anterior-chamber cellular reaction is commonly observed with significant conjunctival injection. Standard culture procedures are warranted to identify the infectious agent. Swabbing the incisional area often helps in identifying the organism. Topical fortified antibiotics and/or fluoroquinolones every hour are recommended as the initial regimen. Explantation of the segment should be considered if the keratitis does not improve with aggressive topical therapy, followed by irrigation with antibiotic throughout the channel. There was one case of this reported in the clinical trials, and it was found to be secondary to *Staphylococcus epidermidis* [117]. It resolved with topical antibiotics.

Optical complications

The complications discussed earlier are unique to intrastromal implant technology. Adverse optical effects are common with other refractive surgical procedures. These include overcorrection, undercorrection, induced astigmatism, halos, and glare.

For over- and undercorrections, the segments can either be exchanged or explanted. With Intacs exchange, a segment of different thickness may be inserted to give the desired refractive effect. The other option is to explant the segments and perform another type of procedure such as LASIK. This second procedure can be performed once refractive stability has been documented, which usually occurs within 2 to 3 months after explantation.

Induced with-the-rule astigmatism has been observed from aggressive wound healing at the superior incision site (Figure 15.154). Astigmatic keratotomy has not proven effective for management of such induced astigmatism. If there is still significant astigmatism at the 6-month visit, the incision can be reincised and either loosely sutured or left unsutured in a patient who shows aggressive healing.

Glare and halos may occur at night as pupils dilate, although it is not a common symptom. In these patients,

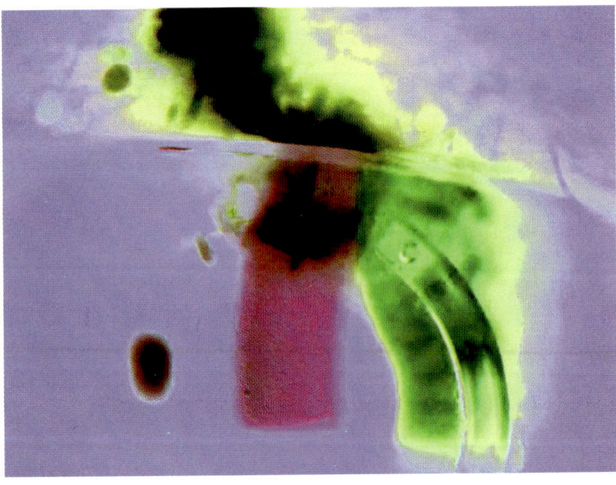

Fig 15.154 Aggressive wound healing following insertion of intracorneal ring segments led to induced with-the-rule astigmatisms. (Slide courtesy Daniel Durrie, M.D.)

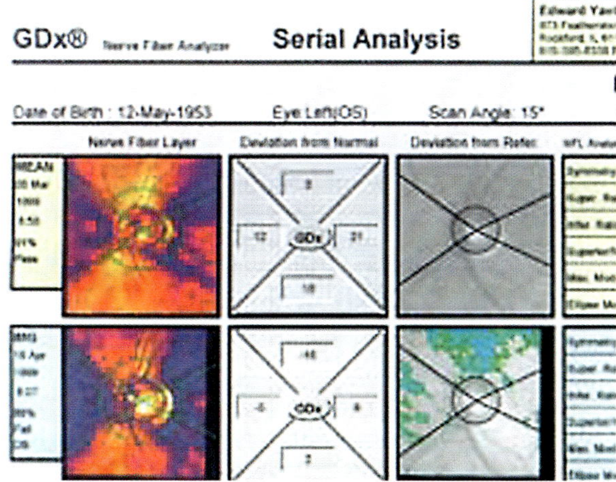

Fig 15.155 Nerve fiber thinning after LASIK. (Courtesy Edward Yavitz, M.D.)

the edge of the segment may be exposed to the entrance pupil and cause spherical aberration, manifested as halos. In some patients, the segment can be slightly repositioned. Glare may occur from light scatter from the lamellar deposits. Glare and halos often improve over time. Rarely, such aberrations may require explantation of the segment for resolution of the symptoms.

Optic nerve damage—Fact or artifact?

Yavitz reported on a series of patients scheduled for the LASIK procedure who were examined with the Laser Diagnostics GDx Nerve Fiber Analyzer both before and after the procedure. In this series he found a short-lived measurable thinning of the fibers of the optic nerve [118] (Figure 15.155). On the other hand, patients pretreated with brimonidine did not show the same changes after LASIK. In no case did any measurable change in either best-corrected visual acuity or visual fields occur.

The author and his colleagues, Guillermo Avalos and John LiVecchi, were unable to duplicate these findings either in normal individuals or in glaucoma patients subjected to the pneumatic trabeculoplasty (PNT) treatment for glaucoma (Figure 15.156). The question of whether or not the LASIK procedure might possibly damage the optic nerve in patients has not been completely answered. Arevalo, in examining almost 30,000 consecutive LASIK cases over a 2-year period, found only 20 vitreoretinal complications, none of which involved the optic nerve [119].

References

1 Bourque LB, Cosand BB, Drews C, *et al.* Reported satisfaction, fluctuation of vision, and glare among patients one year after surgery in the Prospective Evaluation of Radial Keratotomy (PERK) Study. Arch Ophthalmol 1986; 104(3): p. 356–63.

2 Steel D, Jester JV, Salz J, *et al.* Modification of corneal curvature following radial keratotomy in primates. Ophthalmology 1981; 88(8): p. 747–54.

3 Kuster A. Myopieprogression bei Kontaktlinsen und bei Brillentragern in 400 Fallen. [The progression of myopia in wearers of contact lenses and spectacles. 400 cases]. Klin Monatsbl Augenheilkd 1971; 159(2): p. 213–9.

4 Hemenger RP, Tomlinson A, and McDonnell PJ, Explanation for good visual acuity in uncorrected residual hyperopia and presbyopia after radial keratotomy. Invest Ophthalmol Vis Sci 1990; 31(8): p. 1644–6.

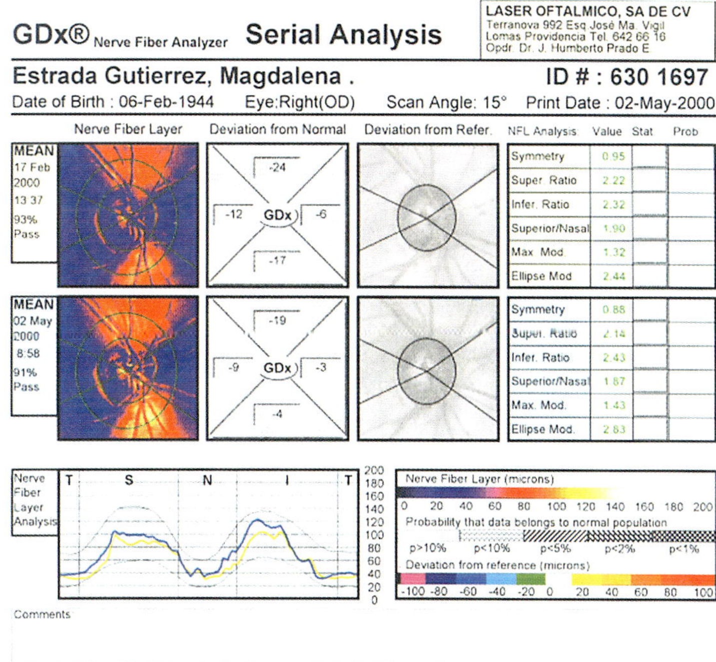

Fig 15.156 Laser Diagnostics examination of a patient with chronic open angle glaucoma before and after being subjected to a 60-second exposure to an IOP of 65 mm Hg from a suction ring used to treat glaucoma. (Courtesy Guillermo Avalos, M.D.)

5 Maguire LJ, and Bourne WM. A multifocal lens effect as a complication of radial keratotomy. Refract Corneal Surg 1989; 5(6): p. 394–9.
6 Bores L. Pseudo–accomodation following radial keratotomy. In: *Quintum Forum*. Instituto Barraquer, Bogota, 1987.
7 Helmholtz HLF. Üeber die Accomodation des Auges. Graefes Arch Ophthalmol 1855; 1(2): p. 1–74.
8 Feldman ST, Frucht-Pery J, Weinreb RN, *et al.* The effect of increased intraocular pressure on visual acuity and corneal curvature after radial keratotomy. Am J Ophthalmol 1989; 108(2): p. 126–9.
9 Wyzinski P, and O'Dell LW. Diurnal cycle of refraction after radial keratotomy Ophthalmology 1987; 94: p. 120–4.
10 Wyzinski P. Daily refractive changes persisting after radial keratotomy. Am J Ophthalmol 1989; 108(2): p. 205–6.
11 Kiely PM, Carney LG, and Smith G. Diurnal variations of corneal topography and thickness. Am J Optom Physiol Opt 1982; 59(12): p. 976–82.
12 Santos VR, Waring GO, Lynn MJ, *et al.* Morning-to-evening change in refraction, corneal curvature, and visual acuity 2 to 4 years after radial keratotomy in the PERK Study [see comments]. Ophthalmology 1988; 95(11): p. 1487–93.
13 Schanzlin DJ, Santos VR, Waring GO, *et al.* Diurnal change in refraction, corneal curvature, visual acuity, and intraocular pressure after radial keratotomy in the PERK Study. Ophthalmology 1986; 93(2): p. 167–75.
14 Deitz MR, Sanders DR, and Marks RG. Radial keratotomy: an overview of the Kansas City study. Ophthalmology 1984; 91(5): p. 467–78.
15 Fyodorov SN. Surgical correction of myopia and astigmatism. In: *Keratorefraction*. LAL Publishing, New York, 1980.
16 Bates WH. *The Bates Method for Better Eyesight without Glasses*. Henry Holt, New York, 1943.
17 Waring GO, Lynn MJ, Strahlman ER, *et al.* Stability of refraction during four years after radial keratotomy in the prospective evaluation of radial keratotomy study [see comments]. Am J Ophthalmol 1991; 111(2): p. 133–44.
18 Sawelson H, and Marks RG. Two-year results of radial keratotomy. Arch Ophthalmol 1985; 103(4): p. 505–10.
19 Kogan L. Personal communication, 1985.
20 Rowsey JJ, and Balyeat HD, Preliminary results and complications of radial keratotomy. Am J Ophthalmol 1982; 93(4): p. 437–55.
21 Salz JJ. Multiple complications following radial keratotomy in an elderly patient: a case report. Ophthalmic Surg 1985; 16(9): p. 579–80.
22 McDonnell PJ, Caroline PJ, and Salz J. Irregular astigmatism after radial and astigmatic keratotomy. Am J Ophthalmol 1989; 107(1): p. 42–6.
23 Salz JJ, Lee T, Jester JV, *et al.* Analysis of incision depth following experimental radial keratotomy. Ophthalmology 1983; 90(6): p. 655–9.
24 O'Donnell FE. Short incision radial keratotomy: A comparative study in rabbits Journal of Refractive Surgery 1987; 3: p. 102–3.
25 Schachar R, Black T, and Huang T. Surgical implications of the theory of radial keratotomy. In: *Radial Keratotomy*, R Schacher, *et al*, Editor. LAL, Dennison, p. 269–82, 1980.
26 Bores LD. Unpublished data, 1991.
27 Bores LD. Radial keratotomy. I. A safe, effective way to correct a handicap. Surv Ophthalmol 1983; 28(2): p. 101–5.
28 Deitz MR, Sanders DR, and Raanan MG. Progressive hyperopia in radial keratotomy. Long-term follow-up of diamond-knife and metal-blade series. Ophthalmology 1986; 93(10): p. 1284–9.
29 Richmond RD. Radial keratotomy as seen through operated eyes: Part I. Journal of Refractive Surgery 1987; 3: p. 22–7.
30 Richmond RD. Radial keratotomy as seen through operated eyes: Part II. Journal of Refractive Surgery 1987; 4: p. 91–5.
31 Deitz M, and Sanders D. Progressive hyperopia with long-term follow-up of radial keratotomy. Arch Ophthalmol 1985; 103(6): p. 782–4.
32 Waring GO, Lynn MJ, Culbertson W, *et al.* Three year results of the Prospective Evaluation of Radial Keratotomy (PERK) study. Indian J Ophthalmol 1990; 38(3): p. 107–13.
33 Lindquist TD, Rubenstein JB, and Lindstrom RL. Correction of hyperopia following radial keratotomy: quantification in human cadaver eyes. Ophthalmic Surg 1987; 18(6): p. 432–7.
34 Rowsey JJ. Personal communication, 1988.
35 Grady FJ. Hexagonal keratotomy for corneal steepening. Ophthalmic Surg 1988; 19(9): p. 622–3.
36 Jensen RP. Experience with hexagonal keratotomy [letter]. J Cataract Refract Surg 1988; 14(5): p. 580–1.
37 Schachar RA. Radial thermokeratoplasty. Int Ophthalmol Clin 1991; 31(1): p. 47–57.
38 Starling JC, and Hoffmann RF. A new surgical technique for the correction of hyperopia after radial keratotomy: An experimental model. J Refract Surg 1986; 2: p. 9–14.
39 Bores LD, Myers W, and Cowden J. Radial keratotomy: an analysis of the American experience. Ann Ophthalmol 1981; 13(8): p. 941–8.
40 Fyodorov SN. Personal communication. Vestn Oftalmol, 1990.
41 Myers W. Personal communications, 1988.
42 Gelender H, Flynn HWJ, and Mandelbaum SH. Bacterial endophthalmitis resulting from radial keratotomy. Am J Ophthalmol 1982; 93(3): p. 323–6.
43 Santos CI. Herpes keratitis after radial keratotomy <original>. Am J Ophthalmol 1982; 93(3): p. 370.
44 Santos CR. Herpetic corneal ulcer following radial keratotomy. Ann Ophthalmol 1983; 15(1): p. 82–5.
45 Fyodorov SN, and Durnev VV. Operation of dosaged dissection of corneal circular ligament in cases of myopia of mild degree. Ann Ophthalmol 1979; 11(12): p. 1885–90.
46 Mandelbaum S, Waring GO, Forster RK, *et al.* Late development of ulcerative keratitis in radial keratotomy scars. Arch Ophthalmol 1986; 104(8): p. 1156–60.
47 O'Day DM, Feman SS, and Elliott JH. Visual impairment following radial keratotomy. A cluster of cases. Ophthalmology 1986; 93(3): p. 319–26.
48 Shivitz IA, and Arrowsmith PN. Delayed keratitis after radial keratotomy. Arch Ophthalmol 1986; 104(8): p. 1153–5.
49 Stern GA, Weitzenkorn D, and Valenti J. Adherence of Pseudomonas aeriginosa to the mouse cornea: epithelial vs stromal adherance. Arch Ophthalmol 1982; 100(12): p. 100.
50 Steinberg EB, Wilson LA, and Waring GO. Stellate iron lines in the corneal epithelium after radial keratotomy. Am J Ophthalmol 1984; 98: p. 416–21.
51 Jester JV, Villasenor RA, and Miyashiro J. Epithelial inclusion cysts following radial keratotomy. Arch Ophthalmol 1983; 101 (4): p. 611–5.
52 Perry L, and Taylor L. Worsening of myopia following a circular keratotomy. Ophthalmic Surg 1982; 13(2): p. 104–7.
53 Smith RS, and Cutro J. Computer analysis of radial keratotomy. CLAO J 1984; 10(3): p. 241–8.
54 Nelson JD, Williams P, Lindstrom RL, *et al.* Map-fingerprint-dot changes in the corneal epithelial basement membrane following radial keratotomy. Ophthalmology 1985; 92(2): p. 199–205.
55 McKnight SJ, Fitz J, and Giangiacomo J. Corneal rupture following radial keratotomy in cats subjected to BB gun injury. Ophthalmic Surg 1988; 19(3): p. 165–7.
56 Pearlstein ES, Agapitos PJ, Cantrill HL, *et al.* Ruptured globe after radial keratotomy. Am J Ophthalmol 1988; 106(6): p. 755–6.

57 McDermott ML, Wilkinson WS, Tukel DB, *et al.* Corneoscleral rupture ten years after radial keratotomy. Am J Ophthalmol 1990; 110(5): p. 575–7.

58 Zhaboedov GD, and Bondareva GS. [Traumatic rupture of the eyeball after radial keratotomy]. Vestn Oftalmol 1990; 106(2): p. 64–5.

59 Bloom HR, Sands J, and Schneider D. Corneal rupture from blunt trauma 22 months after radial keratotomy. Refract Corneal Surg 1990; 6(3): p. 197–9.

60 Binder PS, Waring GO, Arrowsmith PN, *et al.* Histopathology of traumatic corneal rupture after radial keratotomy. Arch Ophthalmol 1988; 106(11): p. 1584–90.

61 Forstot SL, and Damiano RE. Trauma after radial keratotomy. Ophthalmology 1988; 95(6): p. 833–5.

62 John ME, and Schmitt TE. Traumatic hyphema after radial keratotomy. Ann Ophthalmol 1983; 15: p. 930–2.

63 Spivack LE. Case report: radial keratotomy incisions remain intact despite facial trauma from plane crash. J Refract Surg 1987; 3: p. 59–60.

64 McDonnell PJ, Lean JS, and Schanzlin DJ. Globe rupture from blunt trauma after hexagonal keratotomy. Am J Ophthalmol 1987; 103(2): p. 241–2.

65 Larson BC, Kremer FB, Eller AW. *et al.* Quantitated trauma following radial keratotomy in rabbits. Ophthalmology 1983; 90(6): p. 660 7.

66 Luttrull JK, Jester JV, and Smith RE. The effect of radial keratotomy on ocular integrity in an animal model. Arch Ophthalmol 1982; 100(2): p. 319–20.

67 Karr DJ, Grutzmacher RD, and Reeh. Radial keratotomy complicated by sterile keratitis and corneal perforation. Histopathologic case report and review of complications. Ophthalmology 1985; 92(9): p. 1244–8.

68 Girard LJ, Rodriguez J, Nino N, *et al.* Delayed wound healing after radial keratotomy. Am J Ophthalmol 1985; 99(4): p. 485–6.

69 Dodick J. Personal communication, 1984.

70 Gelender H, and Gelber EC. Cataract following radial keratotomy. Arch Ophthalmol 1983; 101(8): p. 1229–31.

71 Baldone JA, and Franklin RM. Cataract following radial keratotomy. Ann Ophthalmol 1983; 15(5): p. 416–8.

72 Steinberg EB, Waring GO, and Wilson LA. Slitlamp microscopic study of corneal wound healing after radial keratotomy in the PERK study. (AMA) Abstracts. Invest Ophthalmol Vis Sci 1985; 26(suppl): p. 203.

73 Waring GO, Steinberg EB, and Wilson LA. Slit-lamp microscopic appearance of corneal wound healing after radial keratotomy. Am J Ophthalmol 1985; 100: p. 218–24.

74 Wharton KR. Corneal stellate iron lines following radial keratotomy. J Am Optom Assoc 1989; 60(5): p. 362–4.

75 Koenig SB, McDonald MB, Yamaguchi T., *et al.* Corneal iron lines after refractive keratoplasty. Arch Ophthalmol 1983; 101(12): p. 1862–5.

76 Grabner G. [New central, epithelial iron deposit following epikeratophakia in high-grade myopia] <original> Eine neue zentrale, epitheliale Eisenablagerung nach Epikeratophakie bei hohergradiger Myopie. Klin Monatsbl Augenheilkd 1987; 190 (5): p. 424–7.

77 Feldman RM, Crapotta JA, Feldman ST, *et al.* Retinal detachment following radial and astigmatic keratotomy. Refract Corneal Surg 1991; 7(3): p. 252–3.

78 Rodriguez A, and Camacho H. Retinal detachment after refractive surgery for myopia. Retina 1992; 12(3 Suppl): p. s46–50.

79 Hofmann RF, Starling JC, and Hovland KR. Retinal Detachment After Radial Keratotomy Surgery. (Case Report) J Refract Surg 1985 1(5) p. 226–30.

80 Weinberger D, Fink-Cohen S, and Axer-Siegel R. Rhegmatogenous retinal detachment operation after radial keratotomy. Acta Ophthalmol Scand 1997; 75(2): p. 214–5.

81 Classe JG. Five liability claims involving the cornea and how they could have been prevented. Optom Clin 1995; 4(3): p. 75–85.

82 Davis DB. 2nd, Radial keratotomy before and after retinal detachment surgery [letter]. J Cataract Refract Surg 1997; 23(1): p. 10–1.

83 Gelisken O, Ozcetin H, and Dogru M. Retinal detachment after radial keratotomy. Bull Soc Belge Ophtalmol 1993; 249: p. 63–5.

84 Grimmett, M.R. and E.J. Holland, Complications of small clear-zone radial keratotomy [see comments]. Ophthalmology 1996; 103(9): p. 1348–56.

85 Panda A, Sharma N, and Kumar A. Ruptured globe 10 years after radial keratotomy. J Refract Surg 1999; 15(1): p. 64–5.

86 Kraushar MF, and Steinberg JA. Miotics and retinal detachment: upgrading the community standard. Surv Ophthalmol 1991; 35(4): p. 311–6.

87 Kraushar MF. Miotics and retinal detachment. Arch Ophthalmol 1991; 109(12): p. 1659.

88 Casanovas J, and Casanovas R. [Dangers of various recent ophthalmologic drugs]. Ann Ocul (Paris) 1969; 202(1): p. 1–22.

89 Rengstorff R, and Royston M. Miotic drugs: a review of ocular, visual, and systemic complications. Am J Optom Physiol Opt 1976; 53(2): p. 70–80.

90 Jindra LF. Blindness following retrobulbar anesthesia for astigmatic keratotomy. Ophthalmic Surg 1989; 20(6): p. 433–5.

91 Schneider ME, Milstein DE, Oyakawa RT, *et al.* Ocular perforation from a retrobulbar injection. Am J Ophthalmol 1988; 106 (1): p. 35–40.

92 Linberg JV, McDonald MB, Safir A, *et al.* Ptosis following radial keratotomy. Performed using a rigid eyelid speculum. Ophthalmology 1986; 93(12): p. 1509–12.

93 Pallikaris IG, Papatzanaki ME, Georgiadis A, *et al.* A comparative study of neural regeneration following corneal wounds induced by an argon fluoride excimer laser and mechanical methods. Lasers Light Ophthalmol 1990; 3: p. 89–95.

94 Hong JW, and Kim HM. The changes of tear break up time after myopic excimer laser photorefractive keratectomy. Korean J Ophthalmol 1997; 11(2): p. 89–93.

95 Caffery BE, Richter D, Simpson T, *et al.* CANDEES. The Canadian Dry Eye Epidemiology Study. Adv Exp Med Biol 1998; 438: p. 805–6.

96 Linna TU, Perez-Santonja JJ, Tervo KM, *et al.* Recovery of Corneal Nerve Morphology Following Laser in situ Keratomileusis. Exp Eye Res 1998; 66(6): p. 755–63.

97 Linna TU, Vesaluoma MH, Perez-Santonja JJ, *et al.* Effect of myopic LASIK on corneal sensitivity and morphology of subbasal nerves. Invest Ophthalmol Vis Sci 2000; 41(2): p. 393–7.

98 Murphy PJ, Corbett MC, O'Brart DP, *et al.* Loss and recovery of corneal sensitivity following photorefractive keratectomy for myopia. J Refract Surg 1999; 15(1): p. 38–45.

99 Whitcher JP, Jr., Gritz DC, and Daniels TE. The dry eye: a diagnostic dilemma. Int Ophthalmol Clin 1998; 38(4): p. 23–37.

100 Citterio A, Sinforiani E, Verri A, *et al.* Neurological symptoms of the sick building syndrome: analysis of a questionnaire. Funct Neurol 1998; 13(3): p. 225–30.

101 Versura P, Profazio V, Cellini M, *et al.* Eye discomfort and air pollution. Ophthalmologica 1999; 213(2): p. 103 9.

102 Crandall DC, and Leopold IH, The influence of systemic drugs on tear constituents. Ophthalmology 1979; 86(1): p. 115–25.

103 Wilson FM. Adverse external ocular effects of topical ophthalmic therapy: an epidemiologic, laboratory, and clinical study. Trans Am Ophthalmol Soc 1983; 81: p. 851–965.

104 Tauber J. A dose-ranging clinical trial to assess the safety and efficacy of cyclosporine ophthalmic emulsion in patients with keratoconjunctivitis sicca. The Cyclosporine Study Group. Adv Exp Med Biol 1998; 438: p. 969–72.

105 Tsubota K, Goto E, Fujita H, *et al.* Treatment of dry eye by autologous serum application in Sjogren's syndrome [see comments]. Br J Ophthalmol 1999; 83(4): p. 390–5.

106 Smith RJ, and Maloney RK. Diffuse lamellar keratitis. A new syndrome in lamellar refractive surgery. Ophthalmology 1998; 105(9): p. 1721–6.

107 Kaufman SC, Maitchouk DY, Chiou AG, *et al.* Interface inflammation after laser in situ keratomileusis. Sands of the Sahara syndrome [see comments]. J Cataract Refract Surg 1998; 24(12): p. 1589–93.

108 Holland SP. Update in cornea and external disease: solving the mystery of "sands of the Sahara" syndrome (diffuse lamellar keratitis). Can J Ophthalmol 1999; 34(4): p. 193–4.

109 Arshinoff S, D'Addario D, Sadler C, *et al.* Use of topical nonsteroidal anti-inflammatory drugs in excimer laser photorefractive keratectomy. J Cataract Refract Surg 1994; 20 Suppl: p. 216–22.

110 Flach AJ. Cyclo-oxygenase inhibitors in ophthalmology. Surv Ophthalmol 1992; 36(4): p. 259–84.

111 Joo CK, and Kim TG, Corneal ectasia detected after laser in situ keratomileusis for correction of less than -12 diopters of myopia. J Cataract Refract Surg 2000; 26(2): p. 292–5.

112 Seiler T, Koufala K, and Richter G. Iatrogenic keratectasia after laser in situ keratomileusis. J Refract Surg 1998; 14(3): p. 312–7.

113 Geggel HS, and Talley AR. Delayed onset keratectasia following laser in situ keratomileusis [see comments]. J Cataract Refract Surg 1999; 25(4): p. 582–6.

114 Mulhern MG, Condon PI, and O'Keefe M. Endophthalmitis after astigmatic myopic laser in situ keratomileusis. J Cataract Refract Surg 1997; 23(6): p. 948–50.

115 Wilson SE. LASIK: management of common complications. Laser in situ keratomileusis. Cornea 1998; 17(5): p. 459–67.

116 Gimbel HV, van Westenbrugge JA, Penno EE, *et al.* Simultaneous bilateral laser in situ keratomileusis: safety and efficacy. Ophthalmology 1999; 106(8): p. 1461–7; discussion 1467–8.

117 Schanzlin DJ, Asbell PA, Burris TE, *et al.* The intrastromal corneal ring segments. Phase II results for the correction of myopia. Ophthalmology 1997; 104(7): p. 1067–78.

118 Yavitz EQ. *Effect of elevated IOP on optic nerve in LASIK cases.* 2000.

119 Arevalo JF, Ramirez E, Suarez, *et al.* Incidence of vitreoretinal pathologic conditions within 24 months after laser in situ keratomileusis. Ophthalmology 2000; 107(2): p. 258–62.

Epilogue—Dealing with the Extremes

Not all refractive errors are "nails"

Everyone is agog over the laser; the term *laser in situ keratomileusis* (LASIK) is used so much it seems as if it were a mantra. However, I fail to understand the tendency of so many surgeons to labor with only one tool in their toolbox. The old saying is *"If you only have a hammer, everything looks like a nail."* Having only one tool at one's disposal is not the mark of a craftsman. Nor is the laser a Swiss army knife.

Low-order myopia

A mere perusal of the literature will reveal in an instant that there are problems associated with the LASIK procedure. Not the least of these is epithelial ingrowth, displacement of the cap, irregular astigmatism, and decentration of the laser ablation, to name but a few (see Chapter 15 for a discussion on these problems and the so-called sands of the Sahara). The Dublin group has shown that decentration is twice as frequent in LASIK compared with PRK, and double the amount of eccentricity is seen after LASIK compared with PRK. Cutting errors and flap problems can occur in about 0.5% to 1% of LASIK cases.

Ask yourself this question: *Why is the occurrence of decentration twice as much for LASIK as PRK?* Now ask: *Why in the name of all that's holy would you have LASIK done on yourself for less than 4 D of myopia?* Although patients tend toward LASIK because it is easier to tolerate and the visual rehabilitation is faster, PRK is clearly safer for corrections up to 4 D, according to Theo Seiler, professor and chairman of the University Eye Clinic, in Dresden, Germany, an early pioneer in PRK. Cutting off the top of the cornea with a microkeratome—never mind that the process is automated—with all its attendant risks is too much surgery for these patients, yet it is being done. Is it because, as Waring recently said, "LASIK is a breeze?" Is it because "LASIK lends itself to bilateral simultaneous surgery?" Color me old-fashioned, but bilateral surgery should not be a criterion for choosing surgical methods. My experience has shown that most patients can tolerate short periods of anisometropia (nonexistent if they can tolerate a disposable soft contact lens) without too much difficulty. This is especially true with low-order myopia. And to do simultaneous bilateral surgery on a myope with greater than −15 D is begging for trouble.

The force behind the upsurge in LASIK is not the patients. It is often said that the patients will demand LASIK, but patients do not do this at all—some want LASIK and some don't, some are confused and decide to sit in the middle, and a high percentage just go for the price, and in my clinic, many lower myopes choose radial keratotomy (RK) when faced with the facts. It is the practitioner who generally decides for the patient in most cases.

As for the practitioners, many have been trained into favoring LASIK over the time-proven RK and PRK techniques. They have taken courses and have spent $5000 or $10,000 and have been told that this is the route that they have to go, that RK and PRK are dead, and that if you are going to be an adult, you have to learn how to do LASIK. You have to have a strong sense of self (read *"big ego"*) to become an eye surgeon in the first place. On a even deeper level, it is a turf issue, with many surgeons concerned about protecting their territory from optometrists, who are not qualified to handle the surgical aspects of LASIK.

Overall, in published studies on acuity, however, PRK seems to be holding its own. In the end, results are essentially the same or, as in one or two studies, PRK is actually slightly superior. The one exception appears to be in cases of high myopia of −12 D and above, in whom LASIK pulls definitively ahead (see below). However, in my view, LASIK should not be performed on eyes with greater than −9 D of myopia.

Although scarring is one of the most important problems after PRK, the incidence of scarring for corrections of up to 4 D is extremely low; above 4 D, however, the incidence and density of post-PRK haze/scarring increase steeply.

Thus, is PRK the answer for low myopia? Perhaps, but RK will do just as well, and the recovery will be faster. The cost to the patient will also be lower. The caveat here is the structural weakening of the cornea with RK. Not a major problem with three to four incisions, but the risk is there. And −1 D? Why would surgery be indicated here at all, especially in a middle-aged patient?

The other end of the string—High myopia

Extreme cases require extreme measures. PRK is definitely not the poster child for myopia greater than −12 D, and LASIK begins to show its seams above −9 D. PRK loses for the reasons that the incidence of postlaser scarring and irregular corneal surfaces is much higher in this group. Aberrations in visual acuity are also much higher here because of the small ablation zone both on a decentration and an edge phenomenon basis. But this is also true for LASIK. Just because the ablation zone is covered by a cap does not change the fact that peripheral light pencils are going to be refracted off the transition zone. Then there is the issue of the thinner central corneas seen in the higher degrees of myopia and the risk of ectasia.

High myopia (−9 D or greater) is a high-order problem and requires a different approach. One size does not fit all in this case. Here I would recommend consideration of either a phakic implant or even a clear lens extraction with implant. In either case, I might opt for a partially corrective intraocular lens (IOL) implanted *after* I first did a LASIK to reduce the overall refractive error—it would depend on just how high the myopia is. I am aware of both the difficulty in determining IOL power after LASIK and the higher incidence of retinal detachments following clear lens extraction in an already high-risk group. Laser photocoagulation of the retina prior to surgery is probably indicated. As I said, this is not an easy problem to solve, and there is no easy, low-risk method to solve it. I do not consider keeping the patient in his or her optical correction low risk, by the by. The field of vision in these patients is very limited, and the minification caused by the high correction also limits best-corrected visual acuity in most cases.

In any event, LASIK is likely to create more problems than it solves in extreme cases.

The operation from hell

(excerpted with permission from Ophthalmology Management)

When HK was first introduced, I refused to do it, and for good reasons—not the least of these was the circular keratotomy (CK) debacle (see Chapter 15), but also because the procedure violated first principles. I predicted that isolating the central cornea in such a way ultimately would result in what can best be described as "flail cornea," a corneal surface that would never stabilize given that it was bereft of any anchors and totally at the mercy of fluctuations in intraocular pressure (IOP), lid movement, and atmospheric pressure. Healing, slow in the best of circumstances, would be even slower, if it ever happened at all, and marsupialization of the incisions was riding high on the list of probable outcomes. Time proved me right, but unfortunately for some five to six of my patients—unlike Laacoön, I was not devoured on the spot by a sea monster sent by the gods.

Nordan raised a cry publicly shortly after we had discussed it. Thus, given all this, why did I stoop to performing HK at all? For several reasons. First among these is a character flaw that sometimes overrides my better judgment or intuition. This flaw sends forth a little voice that constantly whispers, *"You could be wrong, you know."* Some say that this is a good flaw—but not in this case. Add a little hubris into the mix and combine it with the fact that the "crowd" was boarding the train and that several of my friends, fellows who had stuck by me when I introduced what became known as radial keratotomy, were claiming good results. Therefore, I threw caution (and several eyes, as it turned out) to the wind and did some HKs. The upshot was that it took me almost 5 years per eye before I was finally able (with the help of Mother Nature, a modicum of luck, and some surgical skills) to stabilize these corneas to the point that the patients had near-normal vision again. I say *near-normal* because none were ever truly normal again.

So what lessons can be gained from this experience? First and foremost, make sure that you remain a physician. Too many of our colleagues treat patients by rote. Too many treat problems in the same way time and again and with methods adopted from others "with more experience" combined with the phenomenon of enthusiastic presentations by "pioneers" from eye institutes. Too many surgeons equate numbers with skill and just because they have high numbers of surgical cases assume for themselves the mantle of guru when what they really are are machines. Machines that—no doubt—are excellent at what they do, but they are machines nonetheless. And machines do not think. Many of us adopt ideas (which others slavishly follow) as if these had sprung forth from the forehead of Zeus; thereby falling into the trap of believing that we, above all others, have *"the answer."* I cannot count the occasions during the introduction of RK that I was approached by ophthalmologists who were only too willing to share with me "where I had gone wrong with RK" and despite the fact that they had never done a case knew "how to fix it"; of course, they all had degrees in engineering as well.

A true physician follows first principles, that is, basic tenants that apply to the problem at hand and which exist—and have existed—since the dawn of time. What first principle(s) did I violate in this case? I knew about the CK debacle; I knew about the work of Sato and Akiyama with similar incisions; and I knew from my own carefully studied experience that such incisions could be trouble. The first principle I violated was this: *"Is what you are going to do materially different from that which previous physicians have tried and failed?"* The answer was an unqualified no. And yet I did HK. Why? Because I violated another first principle: *"When in doubt—don't!"* The corollary of this is: *"There is no eraser on a knife."* Halstead said it best when he said: *"The only difference between a good surgeon and a bad surgeon is that the good surgeon knows when* not *to cut."* My intuition was screaming at me, and to my everlasting sorrow, I ignored it. See that you are not overwhelmed by the same sort of arrogance. Have the courage of your convictions and most of all—think before you leap!

Index